Textbook of
OPERATIVE DENTISTRY

Textbook of
OPERATIVE DENTISTRY

Second Edition

Editors

Nisha Garg MDS
(Conservative Dentistry and Endodontics)

Reader
Sri Sukhmani Dental College and Hospital
Dera Bassi, Mohali, Punjab, India

Ex-Resident
Postgraduate Institute of Medical Education and Research (PGIMER)
Chandigarh, India

Ex-Resident, Government Dental College
Patiala, Punjab, India

Amit Garg MDS
(Oral and Maxillofacial Surgery)

Consultant
Faridabad, Haryana, India

Ex-Resident, Postgraduate Institute of Medical Sciences
Rohtak, Haryana, India

Foreword

Neelam Mittal

JAYPEE BROTHERS MEDICAL PUBLISHERS (P) LTD

New Delhi • Panama City • London • Dhaka • Kathmandu

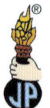
Jaypee Brothers Medical Publishers (P) Ltd.

Headquarters

Jaypee Brothers Medical Publishers (P) Ltd.
4838/24, Ansari Road, Daryaganj
New Delhi 110 002, India
Phone: +91-11-43574357
Fax: +91-11-43574314
Email: **jaypee@jaypeebrothers.com**

Overseas Offices

J.P. Medical Ltd.
83, Victoria Street, London
SW1H 0HW (UK)
Phone: +44-2031708910
Fax: +02-03-0086180
Email: **info@jpmedpub.com**

Jaypee-Highlights Medical Publishers Inc.
City of Knowledge, Bld. 237, Clayton
Panama City, Panama
Phone: +507-301-0496
Fax: +507-301-0499
Email: **cservice@jphmedical.com**

Jaypee Brothers Medical Publishers (P) Ltd.
17/1-B, Babar Road, Block-B
Shaymali, Mohammadpur
Dhaka-1207, Bangladesh
Mobile: +08801912003485
Email: **jaypeedhaka@gmail.com**

Jaypee Brothers Medical Publishers (P) Ltd.
Shorakhute
Kathmandu, Nepal
Phone: +00977-9841528578
Email: **jaypee.nepal@gmail.com**

Website: www.jaypeebrothers.com
Website: www.jaypeedigital.com

© 2013, Jaypee Brothers Medical Publishers

Inquiries for bulk sales may be solicited at: jaypee@jaypeebrothers.com

This book has been published in good faith that the contents provided by the contributors contained herein are original, and is intended for educational purposes only. While every effort is made to ensure accuracy of information, the publisher and the editors specifically disclaim any damage, liability, or loss incurred, directly or indirectly, from the use or application of any of the contents of this work. If not specifically stated, all figures and tables are courtesy of the editors. Where appropriate, the readers should consult with a specialist or contact the manufacturer of the drug or device.

Textbook of Operative Dentistry

First Edition: 2010
Second Edition: **2013**

ISBN 978-93-5025-939-9

Printed at Ajanta Offset & Packaging Ltd., New Delhi

Dedicated to

Prisha and Vedaant

Contributors

Amit Garg MDS
(Oral and Maxillofacial Surgery)
Consultant
Faridabad, Haryana, India

Amita MDS
Reader
(Conservative Dentistry and Endodontics)
BRS Dental College and Hospital
Panchkula, Haryana, India

Anil Chandra MDS
Professor
(Conservative Dentistry and Endodontics)
King George Medical College
Lucknow, Uttar Pradesh, India

Anil Dhingra MDS
Professor and Head
(Conservative Dentistry and Endodontics)
DJ Institute of Dental Sciences and
Research, Modinagar, Ghaziabad
Uttar Pradesh, India

Arundeep Singh MDS
Professor and Head
(Conservative Dentistry and Endodontics)
Manav Rachna Dental College
Faridabad, Haryana, India

Gauri Malik MDS
Senior Lecturer
(Conservative Dentistry and Endodontics)
Gian Sagar Dental College
Patiala, Punjab, India

J William Robbins DDS MA
Clinical Professor
Department of Comprehensive Dentistry
University of Texas Health Science Center
Dental School, At San Antonio
Texas 78258, USA

JS Mann MDS
Associate Professor
(Conservative Dentistry and Endodontics)
Government Dental College
Patiala, Punjab, India

Kanishka Dua MDS
Consultant
(Conservative Dentistry and Endodontics)
Max Healthcare
Pitampura, New Delhi, India

Lekh Santosh MDS
Professor
(Conservative Dentistry and Endodontics)
Oxford Dental College
Bengaluru, Karnataka, India

Manoj Hans MDS
Reader
(Conservative Dentistry and Endodontics)
Vyas Dental College and Hospital
Jodhpur, Rajasthan, India

Martin J Tyas
AM BDS PhD (Birm DDSc (Melb) Graduate
Diploma, Health Science (WAIT) FADM
FICD FRACDS FADI
Professor
Professorial Fellow
Melbourne Dental School
University of Melbourne
720 Anston St
Carlton 3053, Australia

Navjot Singh Khurana MDS
Lecturer
(Conservative Dentistry and Endodontics)
Government Dental College
Patiala, Punjab, India

Niels Oestervemb DDS
322 Dental Sciences
College of Dentistry
Iowa City, IA 52242-1001

Nisha Garg MDS
Reader
(Conservative Dentistry and Endodontics)
Sri Sukhmani Dental College and Hospital
Dera Bassi, Mohali
Punjab, India

Poonam Bogra MDS
Senior Professor
(Conservative Dentistry and Endodontics)
DAV Dental College
Yamuna Nagar, Haryana, India

R Anil Kumar MDS
Professor
(Conservative Dentistry and Endodontics)
Ragas Dental College and Hospital
Chennai, Tamil Nadu, India

RS Kang MDS
Associate Professor
(Conservative Dentistry and Endodontics)
Government Dental College
Patiala, Punjab, India

Rakesh Singla MDS
Reader
(Conservative Dentistry and Endodontics)
Jan Nayak Chaudhary Devi Lal
Dental College
Sirsa, Haryana, India

Régia Luzia Zanata PhD
Operative Dentistry
Bauru School of Dentistry
University of São Paulo
Health Department
University Health Care Centre
(UBAS /Bauru), Alameda Octavio
Pinheiro Brisolla 9-75
Bauru, CEP 17012-901
SP, Brazil

Ruchi Vashisht MDS
Senior Lecturer
(Conservative Dentistry and Endodontics)
National Dental College
Dera Bassi, Mohali
Punjab, India

S Ramachandran MDS
Principal and Professor
(Conservative Dentistry and Endodontics)
Ragas Dental College and Hospital
Chennai, Tamil Nadu, India

Sachin Passi MDS
Professor and Head
(Conservative Dentistry and Endodontics)
Sri Sukhmani Dental College
Dera Bassi, Mohali, Punjab, India

Sarjeev Yadav MDS
Professor and Head
(Conservative Dentistry and Endodontics)
Government Dental College and Hospital
Hyderabad, Andhra Pradesh, India

Suresh K Saini MDS
Reader
Department of Prosthodontics
BRS Dental College and Hospital
Panchkula, Haryana, India

Sandhya Kapoor Punia MDS
Senior Lecturer
(Conservative Dentistry and Endodontics)
Darshan Dental College
Udaipur, Rajasthan, India

Saru Kumar MDS
Senior Lecturer
(Conservative Dentistry and Endodontics)
Himachal Institute of Dental Sciences
Ponta Sahib, Himachal Pradesh, India

Vikas Punia MDS
Senior Lecturer
Department of Prosthodontics
Darshan Dental College
Udaipur, Rajasthan, India

Foreword to the Second Edition

I am delighted to write the foreword of the second edition of *Textbook of Operative Dentistry*. I have gone through the chapters of the book and found that Dr Nisha Garg and Dr Amit Garg have made all efforts to make subject simpler and user friendly for the undergraduate students, clinicians and also a reference for dentists and specialists.

The book is organized right from the basic chapters, i.e. Introduction, structure and physiology of teeth to the management of carious and noncarious lesions by esthetic restorations to precise metallic restorations with a latest trend of minimal intervention dentistry and conscious efforts to practice maximum conservation as per today's need of the patients. We are in the era of nanotechnology and nanodentistry is coming up in a bigger way, which is very well taken care in the book.

As the life expectancy is increasing in the population, the dental problems of these patients are highlighted with the solution and management with special emphasis of geriatric patients.

Nowadays, evidence-based dentistry is in practice and now it is an important aspect of the profession. The textbook concises an elaborated chapter based on this issue.

I am delighted and enlightened to read the book highlighting problems of dental patients in general and operative dentistry in particular. All the chapters of the textbook are described in a simple manner with more diagrammatic illustrations, graphs, charts and photographs. Befitting the quote of great Elbert Einstein, *It is the Supreme Art of the Teacher to Awaken Joy in Creative Expression and Knowledge.*

Professor Neelam Mittal
Dean and Head
Faculty of Dental Sciences
Institute of Medical Sciences
Banaras Hindu University
Varanasi, Uttar Pradesh, India

Foreword to the First Edition

A textbook written with the undergraduate students in mind has seldom come in my hands till I went through the contents of the book in question. I am extremely pleased with the efforts put by authors in penning down the chapters in a systematic and flowing order such that one leads to the other. The commendable expression of the text has been painstakingly selected for the student to understand and grasp the subject of operative dentistry. The flow charts and the apt illustrations add to the understandability of the subject in various chapters. The authors who have already written two well-accepted books have left no stone unturned to include each and every part of the subject. They have tried to drive into the minds of students the basics along with reference to the advancements in the field of operative dentistry. I recognize it as a perfect blend of the age-old accepted concepts with the emerging trends. I would recommend it as a must-read book for one and all in the specific branch of dentistry.

Ravi Kapur
Registrar and Dean (Dental Faculty)
MM University, Mullana
Professor and Head
Department of Conservative Dentistry and Endodontics
MM College of Dental Sciences and Research
Mullana, Ambala, Haryana, India

Preface to the Second Edition

The need for a second edition of this book in less than three years of its publication is good evidence that professionals and students have appreciated the labor of editors and publisher.

In presenting the second edition of the book, we desire to express our appreciation in the kindly manner in which the previous edition was received by the professionals and the dental students. That this book has met the needs and filled the place of operative dentistry is confirmed by its extensive sale and general acceptance by dental professionals of various countries.

The text has been carefully revised and brought up-to-date. Almost all the chapters have been modified. Many new clinical photographs have been added and latest new material has been added.

In order to make the book as comprehensive as possible, several prominent personalities were invited to support, write and modify important chapters.

Dr Anil Chandra, Dr Lekh Santosh and Dr Sachin Passi took "Cutting Instruments", "Cast Metal Restorations", and "Cervical Lesions" respectively and modified these chapters with their clinical expertise. Dr Martin J Tyas made corrections in "Tooth Nomenclature".

Dr J William Robbins modified the chapter "Esthetics in Dentistry", Dr Niels Oestervemb suggested many changes in the "Bonding in Dentistry" and Dr Règia Luzia Zanata modified the chapter "Glass Ionomer Cements" with his suggestions.

We especially thank Dr Poonam Bogra, Dr Sarjeev Yadav, Dr Manoj Hans, Dr Navjot Singh Khurana, Dr Rakesh Singla, Dr Ruchi Vashisht, Dr Arundeep Singh, and Dr Kanishka Dua for contributing in form of photographs.

We are indebted to Dr S Ramachandran and Dr Anil Nair of Ragas Dental College for writing the chapter "Esthetics in Dentistry". We are thankful to Dr Amita, Dr Suresh K Saini and Dr Gauri Malik for writing the chapter "Selection of Restorative Materials".

We would like to especially thank Dr RS Kang, Dr JS Mann, Dr Anil Dhingra, Dr Sandhya Kapoor Punia, Dr Vikas Punia, Dr Rakesh Singla, and Dr Saru Kumar for their critical evaluation of the text and helping us in improvement of the book.

We are really grateful to Dentsply, Coltene Whaledent and GC Fuji for providing high magnification images and videos of products related to conservative dentistry.

It is hoped that all these modifications will be appreciated and render the book still more valuable basis for conservative practice.

We are thankful to Shri Jitendar P Vij (Group Chairman), Mr Ankit Vij (Managing Director), Mr Tarun Duneja (Director-Publishing) and staff of M/s Jaypee Brothers Medical Publishers (P) Ltd, New Delhi, India, for showing personal interest and trying to the level best to bring this book in present form.

Nisha Garg
Amit Garg

Preface to the First Edition

Operative dentistry is one of the oldest branches of dental sciences forming the central part of dentistry as practised in primary care. The clinical practice of operative dentistry is ever evolving as a result of improved understanding of etiology, prevention and management of common dental diseases. The advances and developments within last two decades have drastically changed the scope of this subject.

Since effective practice of operative dentistry requires not only excellent manual skills but also both understanding of disease process and properties of dental materials available for use. The main objective of the book is to provide students with the knowledge required while they are developing necessary clinical skills and attitude in their undergraduate and postgraduate training in operative dentistry. We have tried to cover wide topics like cariology, different techniques and materials available for restorations, recent concepts in management of carious lesions, infection control, minimally intervention dentistry and nanotechnology.

So we can say that after going through this book, the reader should be able to:

- Understand basics of cariology, its prevention and conservative management
- Tell indications and contraindications of different dental materials
- Apply modern pulp protective regimens
- Know the importance of treating the underlying causes of patient's problems, not just the restoration of the damage that has occurred
- Select suitable restorative materials for restoration of teeth
- Know recent advances and techniques like minimally intervention dentistry (MID), nanotechnology, lasers, diagnosis of caries and advances in dental materials.

Nisha Garg
Amit Garg

Contents

Introduction to Operative Dentistry

CHAPTER 1

Chapter Outline

Operative dentistry plays an important role in enhancing dental health and now branched into dental specialities. Today operative dentistry continues to be the most active component of most dental practice. Epidemiologically, demand for operative dentistry will not decrease in the future.

DEFINITION

According to Mosby's dental dictionary, "Operative dentistry deals with the functional and esthetic restoration of the hard tissues of individual teeth".

According to Sturdvent, "Operative dentistry is defined as science and art of dentistry which deals with diagnosis, treatment and prognosis of defects of the teeth which do not require full coverage restorations for correction".

Such corrections and restorations result in the restoration of proper tooth form, function and aesthetics while maintaining the physiological integrity of the teeth in harmonious relationship with the adjacent hard and soft tissues. Such restorations enhance the dental and general health of the patient.

According to Gilmore, "Operative dentistry is a subject which includes diagnosis, prevention and treatment of problems and conditions of natural teeth vital or nonvital so as to preserve natural dentition and restore it to the best state of health, function and aesthetics."

HISTORY

The profession of dentistry was born during the early middle ages. Barbers were doing well for dentistry by removing teeth with dental problems. Till 1900 AD, the term 'Operative dentistry' included all the dental services rendered to the patients, because all the dental treatments were considered to be an operation which was performed in the dental operating room or operatory. As dentistry evolved dental surgeons began filling teeth with core metals. In 1871, GV Black gave the philosophy of "extension for prevention", for cavity preparation design. Dr GV Black (1898) is known as the "Father of operative dentistry". He provided scientific basis to dentistry because his writings developed the foundation of the profession and made the field of operative dentistry organized and scientific. The scientific foundation for operative dentistry was further expanded by Black's son, Arthur Black.

In early part of 1900s, progress in dental sciences and technologies was slow. Many advances were made during the 1970s in materials and equipment. By this time, it was also proved that dental plaque was the causative agent for caries. In the 1990s, oral health science started moving toward an evidence-based approach for treatment of decayed teeth. The recent concept of treatment of dental caries comes under minimally invasive dentistry. In December 1999, the World Congress of Minimally

Prehistoric era	5000 BC	A Sumerian text describes "tooth worms" as the cause of dental decay.
	500-300 BC	Hippocrates and Aristotle, wrote about dentistry, including the eruption pattern of teeth, treating decayed teeth.
	166-201 AD	The Etruscans practiced dental prosthetics using gold crowns and fixed bridgework.
	700	A medical text in China mentioned the use of "silver paste," a type of amalgam.
Pre 1700	1530	Artzney Buchlein, wrote the first book solely on dentistry. It was written for barbers and surgeons who used to treat the mouth, it covered topics like oral hygiene, tooth extraction, drilling teeth and placement of gold fillings.
	1563	Batholomew Eusttachius published the first book on dental anatomy, 'Libellus de dentibus'.
	1683	Antony van Leeuwenhoek identified oral bacteria using a microscope.
	1685	Charles Allen, wrote first dental book in English 'The operator for the teeth'.
1700-1800	1723	Pierre Fauchard published "Le Chirurgien dentiste". He is credited as Father of Modern Dentistry because his book was the first to give a comprehensive system for the practice of dentistry.
	1746	Claude Mouton described a gold crown and post for root canal treated tooth.
	1764	James Rae gave first lectures on the teeth at the Royal College of Surgeons, Edinburgh.
	1771	John Hunter published "The natural history of human teeth" giving a scientific basis to dental anatomy.
	1780	William Addis manufactured the first modern toothbrush.
	1790	John Greenwood constructed the first known dental foot engine by modifying his mother's foot treadle spinning wheel to rotate a drill.
1800-1900	1832	James Snell invented the first reclining dental chair.
	1830s-1890s	The 'Amalgam War' conflict and controversy generated over the use of amalgam as filling material.
	1855	Robert Arthur introduced the cohesive gold foil method for inserting gold into a preparation with minimal pressure.
	1864	Sanford C. Barnum, developed the rubber dam.
	1871	James Beall Morrison invented foot engine.
	1890	WD Miller formulated his "chemicoparasitic" theory of caries in "Microorganisms of the human mouth"
	1895	Lilian Murray became the first woman to become a dentist in Britain.
	1896	GV Black established the principles of cavity preparation.
1900-2000	1900	Federation Dentaire Internationale (FDI) was founded.
	1903	Charles Land introduced the porcelain jacket crown.
	1907	William Taggart invented a "lost wax" casting machine.
	1930-1943	Frederick S. McKay, a Colorado dentist showed brown stains on teeth because of high levels of naturally occurring fluoride in drinking water.
	1937	Alvin Strock develoed Vitallium dental screw implant.
	1950s	The first fluoride toothpastes were marketed.
	1949	Oskar Hagger developed the first system of bonding acrylic resin to dentin.
	1955	Michael Buonocore described the acid etch technique
	1957	John Borden introduced a high-speed air-driven contra-angle handpiece running up to 300,000 rpm.
	1960s	Lasers were developed.
	1962	Rafael Bowen developed Bis-GMA.
	1989	The first commercial home tooth bleaching product was made available.
	1990s	New advances in esthetic dentistry including tooth-colored restorative materials, bleaching materials, veneers and implants.

Invasive Dentistry (MID) was formed. Initially MI dentistry focused on minimal removal of diseased tooth structure but later it evolved for preventive measures to control disease.

Current minimally intervention philosophy follows three concepts of disease treatment:

1. Identify—identify and assess risk factors early.
2. Prevent—prevent disease by eliminating risk factors.
3. Restore—restore the health of the oral environment.

INDICATIONS OF OPERATIVE DENTISTRY PROCEDURES

Indications for operative procedures are divided into the following main sections:

Caries

Dental caries is an infectious microbiological disease of the teeth which results in localized dissolution and destruction of the calcified tissue, caused by the action of microorganisms and fermentable carbohydrates.

Based on anatomy of the surface involved dental caries can be of following types:

- Pit and fissures carious lesions (**Fig. 1.1**)
- Smooth surface carious lesions (**Fig. 1.2**)
- Root caries (**Fig. 1.3**).

Noncarious Loss of the Tooth Structure due to Attrition, Abrasion, Abfraction and Erosion

Attrition

Mechanical wear between opposing teeth commonly due to excessive masticatory forces (**Fig. 1.4**).

Abrasion

Loss of tooth material by mechanical means other than by opposing teeth (**Fig. 1.5**).

Erosion

Loss of dental hard tissue as a result of a chemical process not involving bacteria.

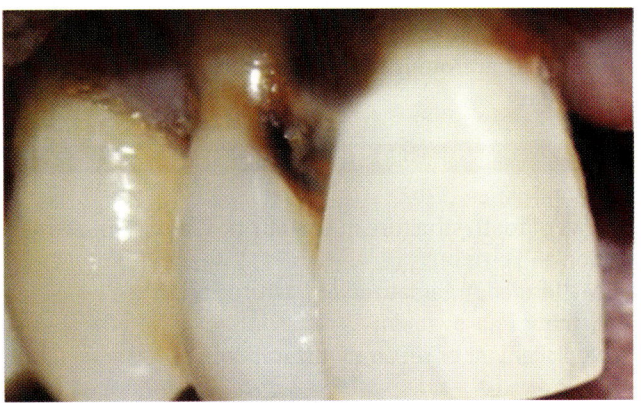

Figure 1.3: Root caries

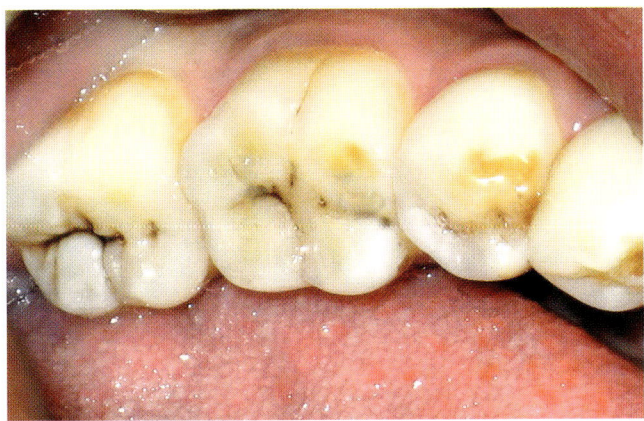

Figure 1.1: Pit and fissure caries

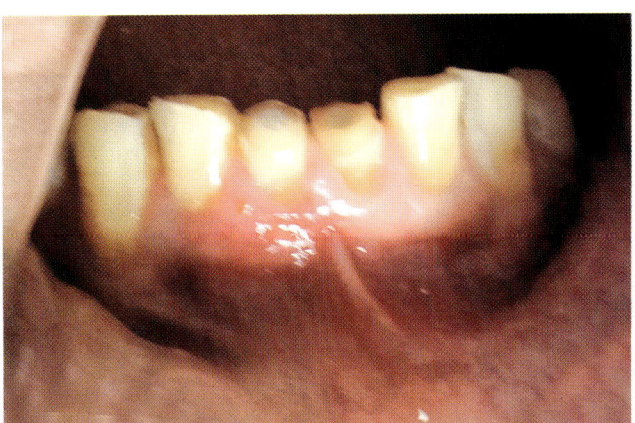

Figure 1.4: Attrition of teeth

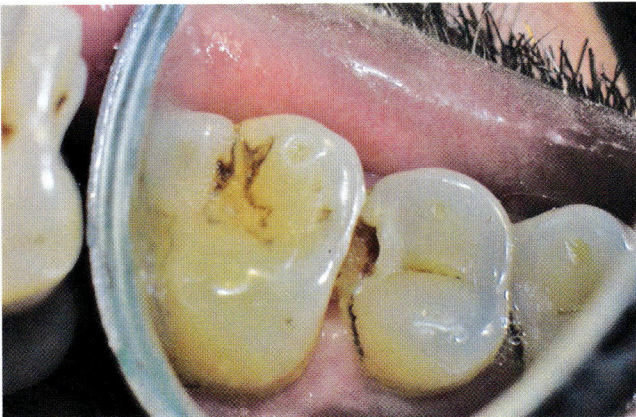

Figure 1.2: Smooth surface caries

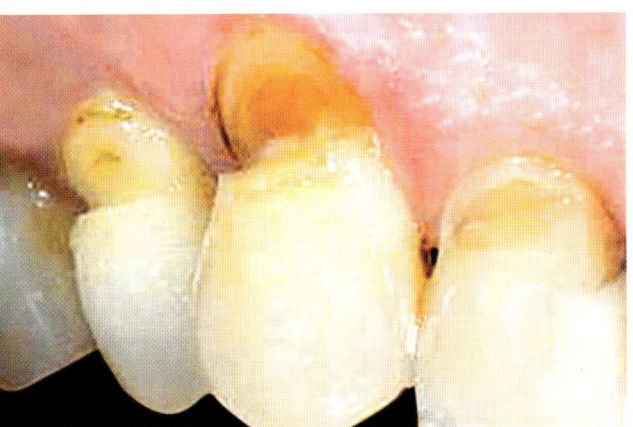

Figure 1.5: Abrasion of teeth

Malformed, Traumatized, or Fractured Teeth (Fig. 1.6)

Traumatic injuries may involve the hard dental tissues and the pulp which require restoration.

Sometimes teeth do not develop normally and there are number of defects in histology or shape which occur during development and become apparent on eruption. These teeth are often unattractive or prone to excessive tooth wear.

Indications of operative dentistry
➡ Dental caries
➡ Loss of tooth structure due to attrition, abrasion, abfraction and erosion
➡ Malformed, traumatized or fractured teeth
➡ Esthetic improvement
➡ Replacement or repair of restoration.

Esthetic Improvement (Figs 1.7 and 1.8)

Discolored teeth because of staining or other reasons look unesthetic and require restoration.

Replacement or Repair of Restoration

Repair or replacement of previous defective restoration is indicated for operative treatment (**Fig. 1.9**).

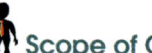

Scope of Operative Dentistry

Scope of operative dentistry includes the following:
- To know the condition of the affected tooth and other teeth.
- To examine not only the affected tooth but also the oral and systemic health of the patient.
- To diagnose the dental problem and the interaction of problem area with other tissues.
- Provide optimal treatment plan to restore the tooth to return to health and function and increase the overall well being of the patient.
- Thorough knowledge of dental materials which can be used to restore the affected areas.
- To understand the biological basis and function of the various tooth tissues.

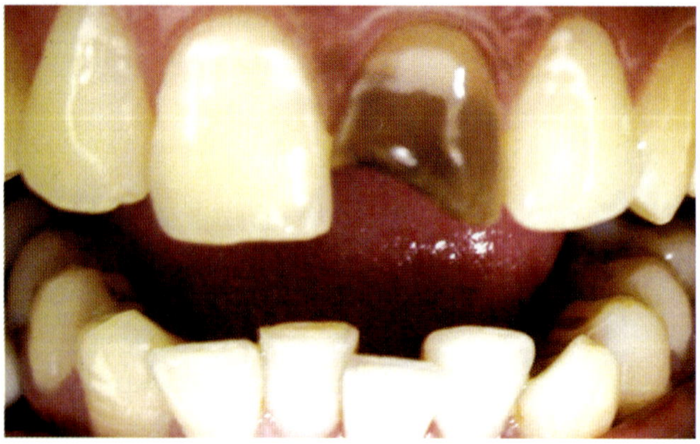

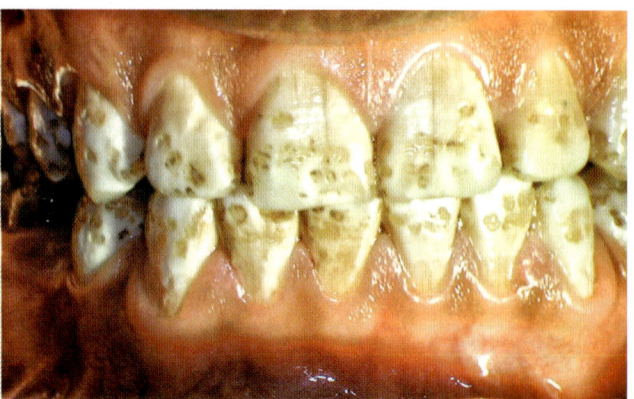

Figure 1.6: Fractured and discolored tooth

Figure 1.8: Discolored teeth needing esthetic treatment

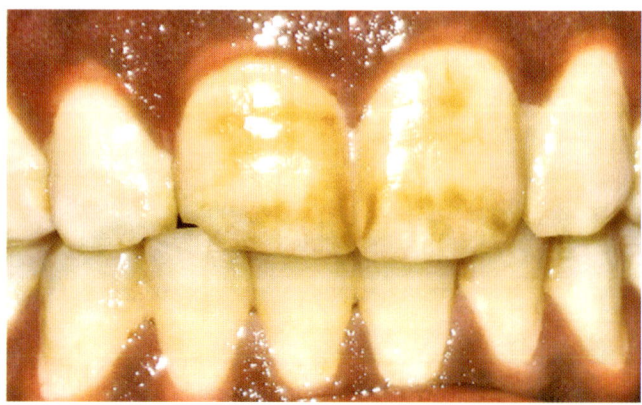

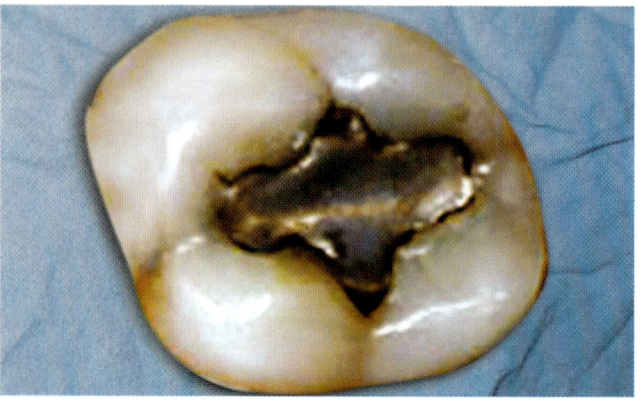

Figure 1.7: Discolored teeth requiring esthetic improvement

Figure 1.9: Defective amalagam restoration requiring replacement

- To maintain the pulp vitality and prevent occurrence of pulpal pathology.
- To have knowledge of dental anatomy and histology.
- To understand the effect of the operative procedures on the treatment of other disciplines.
- An understanding and appreciation for infection control to safeguard both patient and the dentist against disease transmission.

PURPOSE OF OPERATIVE DENTISTRY

Purpose of operative dentistry basically is:

Diagnosis

Proper diagnosis is vital for treatment planning. It is the determination of nature of disease, injury or other defect by examination, test and investigation.

Prevention

To prevent any recurrence of the causative disease and their defects, it includes the procedures done for prevention before the manifestation of any sign and symptom of disease.

Interception

Preventing further loss of tooth structure by stabilizing an active disease process. It includes the procedures undertaken after signs and symptoms of disease have appeared, in order to prevent the disease from developing into a more serious or full extent. Here teeth are restored to their normal health, form and function.

Purpose of operative dentistry
➡ Diagnosis
➡ Prevention
➡ Interception
➡ Preservation
➡ Restoration
➡ Maintenance.

Preservation

Preservation of the vitality and periodontal support of remaining tooth structure. Preservation of optimum health of teeth and soft tissue of oral preparation is obtained by preventive and interceptive procedures.

Restoration

Includes restoring form, function, phonetics and aesthetics.

Maintenance

After restoration is done, it must be maintained for providing service for longer duration.

 Recent Advances in Restorative Dentistry

Concept of tooth preparation has been remained the same as given by GV Black for many decades. That is extension for prevention for treatment of dental caries. Later on, scope of operative dentistry widened to involve all lesions affecting the hard tooth tissues, i.e. caries, fracture, attrition, erosion, abrasion and developmental and acquired defects. The modern concept of operative dentistry is based on conservation and prevention of diseases. Many advancements have been made in the area of operative dentistry so as to meet its goals in better ways.

Basically advances in operative dentistry has occurred in following areas:
- Advances in diagnosis
  - Advances in visual method
    - i. Ultrasonic illumination
    - ii. Ultrasonic imaging
    - iii. Fiberoptic transillumination (FOTI)
    - iv. Digital imaging fiberoptic transillumination (DIFOTI)
    - v. Caries detecting dyes
  - Recent advances in radiographic techniques
    - i. Digital imaging
    - ii. Computerized image analysis
    - iii. Tuned aperture computerized tomography (TACT)
    - iv. Magnetic resonance microimaging (MRMI).
  - Electrical conductance measurement
  - Lasers
    - i. Qualitative laser fluorescence
    - ii. Diagnodent (quantitative laser fluorescence)
    - iii. Optical coherence tomography
    - iv. Computerized occlusal analysis
- Recent advances in treatment planning
  - Minimal intervention dentistry
  - Ozone therapy.
- Recent advances in tooth preparation
  - Use of air abrasion technique
  - Chemomechanical caries removal
  - Use of lasers in tooth preparation
  - Use of ultrasonics in tooth preparation
  - Management of smear layer.
- Recent advances in restorative materials
  - Modification in silver amalgam:
    - i. Mercury free alloys

    ii. Gallium-based silver alloy

    iii. Bonded amalgam restorations

  – Advances in other restorations:

    i. Packable composites

    ii. Flowable composites

    iii. Modifications in glass ionomers cements

    iv. Compomers

    v. Giomers

    vi. Ormocers

    vii. Ceromers

    viii. Tooth colored inlays.

- Recent advances in techniques and equipment
  - Incremental packing and C-factor concept in composites
  - Soft start polymerization
  - High intensity QTH polymerization.
- Recent advance in handpieces and rotary instruments like
  - Fiberoptic handpiece
  - Smart prep burs
  - CVD burs
  - Fissurite system.

Key Points

- According to Mosby's dental dictionary, "Operative dentistry deals with the functional and esthetic restoration of the hard tissues of individual teeth".
- According to Sturdvent, "Operative dentistry is defined as science and art of dentistry which deals with diagnosis, treatment and prognosis of defects of the teeth which do not require full coverage restorations for correction".
- In 1871, GV Black gave the philosophy of "extension for prevention", for cavity preparation design.
- Dr GV Black is known as the "Father of operative dentistry". The scientific foundation for operative dentistry was further expanded by Black's son, Arthur Black.

Want to Know More

- First dental chair was manufactured by SS white dental company, it was called "Harris"
- First hydraulic dental chair was manufactured in 1877, it was called Wilkinson dental chair.

REVIEW QUESTIONS

1. Define operative dentistry. What is scope of operative dentistry?
2. Write short notes on:
   a. Scope and purpose of operative dentistry.
   b. Recent advances in operative dentistry.

BIBLIOGRAPHY

1. American Dental Association, Health Policy Resources Center: Future of Dentistry, Chicago, 2001, American Dental Association. 2001;88-113.
2. Berkey DB, et al. The old-old dental patient: the challenge of clinical decision-making. J Am Dent Assoc. 1996;127:321-32.
3. Berry J. The demographics of dentistry. J Am Dent Assoc. 1996;127:1327-30.
4. Brown LJ, et al. Dental caries, restoration and tooth conditions in US adults, 1988-1991. J Am Dent Assoc. 1996; 127:1315-25.
5. Brown LJ, Lazar V. Dentist work force and educational pipeline. J Am Dent Assoc. 1998;129:1700-7.
6. Brown LJ, Lazar V. Dentists and their practices. J Am Dent Assoc. 1998;129:1692-9.
7. Christensen GT. Intracoronal and extracoronal tooth restorations. J Am Dent Assoc. 1999;130:557-60.
8. Giangrego E. Dentistry and the older adult. J Am Dent Assoc. 1987;114:299-307.
9. Grainger DA. What are you, operative dentistry, and why are they saying all of those nasty things about you? Amer Aced Gold Foil Oper J. 1972;15:67.
10. Hicks J, et al. Root-surface caries formation: effect of *in vitro* APF treatment. J Am Dent Assoc. 1998;129:449-53.
11. Hume WR. Restorative dentistry: current status and future directions. J Dent Educ. 1998;62:781-90.
12. Kidd EA, et al. Secondary caries. Int Dent J. 1992;42:127-38.
13. Mueller CD, et al. Access to dental care in the United States. J Am Dent Assoc. 1998;129:429-37.
14. Ortiz RM, Kuri MD. Women in Dentistry. J History of Dentistry. 2001;49:1.
15. Resine S, Litt M. Social and psychological theories and their use for dental practice. Int Dent J. 1993;43:279-87.
16. Suitti OW. Origins of Argentinean Dentistry and Development of Teaching. J History of Dentistry. 2001;49:2.

Tooth Nomenclature

CHAPTER
2

Dental anatomy or anatomy of teeth is the branch of anatomy which deals with the study of human teeth structures. It includes development, appearance and classification of teeth. Dental anatomy is also a taxonomical science; it is concerned with the naming of teeth and the structures of which they are made.

For convenience human dentition is divided into four quadrants viz; upper (maxillary) right, upper (maxillary) left, lower (mandibular) right and lower (mandibular) left (**Fig. 2.1**). Right and left here relate to patient's right and left side.

Why it is important to know anatomy of teeth?

It is important to understand anatomy of teeth because of following reasons:

➡ For maintenance of supporting tissues in a healthy state
➡ For restoration of a damaged tooth to its original form
➡ For optimal function of teeth.

TYPES OF HUMAN TEETH (FIG. 2.2)

Depending upon their form and function human teeth can be divided into following types:

Incisors (Fig. 2.3)

- The square-shaped teeth located in front of the mouth, with four in the upper jaw and four in the lower jaw, are called incisors
- Incisors are important teeth for phonetics and esthetics
- They help in cutting and shearing the food.

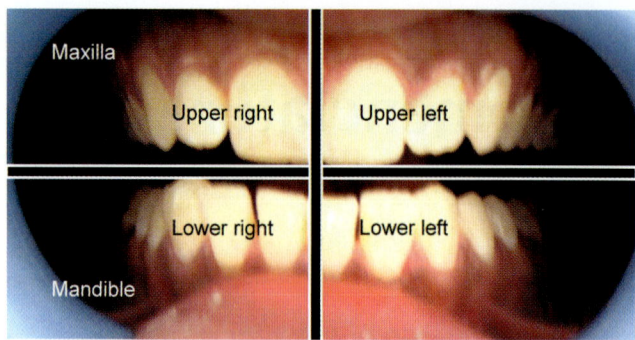

Figure 2.1: Division of whole dentition into four quadrants, i.e. upper right, upper left, lower right and lower left. Right and left relate to patient's right and left

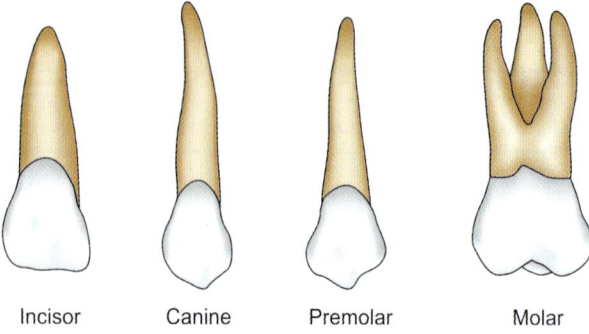

Figure 2.2: Maxillary central and lateral incisors

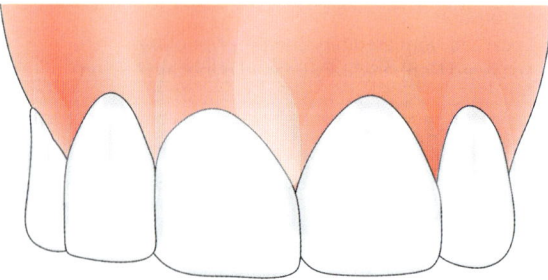

Figure 2.3: Maxillary canine showing sharp tip and long root

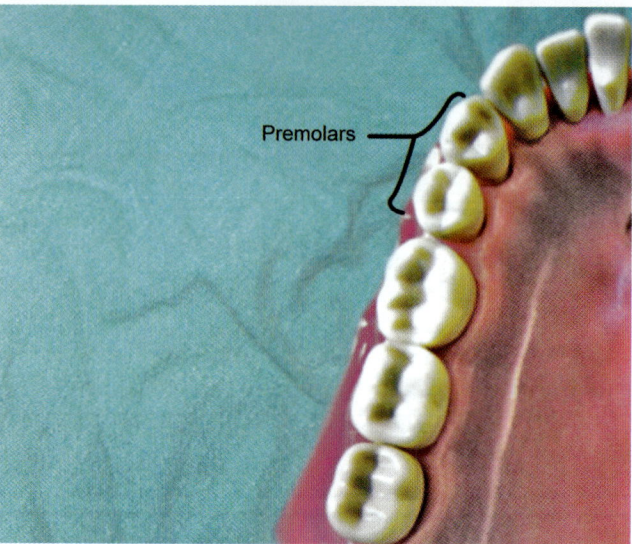

Figure 2.4: Premolars

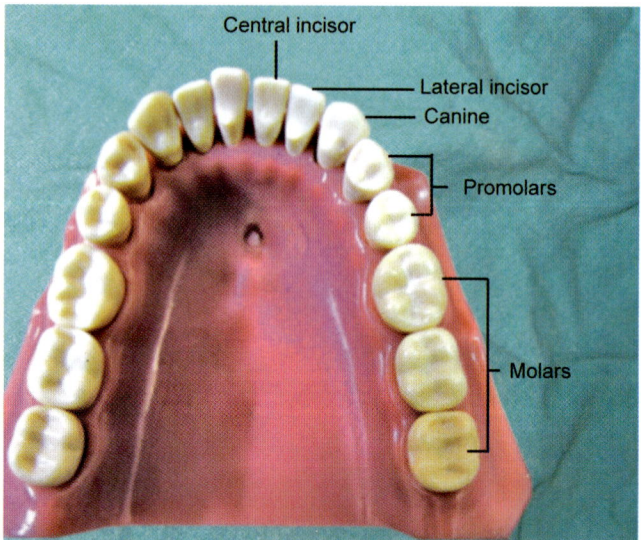

Figure 2.5: Molars

Canines (cuspids)

- The sharp teeth located near the corner of the mouth.
- Because of their anatomy and long root, they are strong teeth. They help in tearing and cutting of food.

Premolars (bicuspids) (Fig. 2.4)

- They are similar to canine in tearing the food, and similar to molar in grinding the food. So, they serve dual role in function.

- They are present in permanent dentition only, not in primary dentition.
- There are a total of eight premolars, four premolars are present in upper and lower arch, two on each side of the canine.
- Facially they resemble canines and lingually as molars.

Molars (Fig. 2.5)

- Distal to premolars are the molars.
- There are six molars in each arch (three in each side), therefore a total of 12.

- They have multi-cusped which help in crushing and grinding the food.
- Also help in maintenance of vertical height of the face.

SETS OF TEETH

There are two sets of teeth that develop in a person's mouth (**Fig. 2.6**). The first set of teeth is termed the "milk", "baby," "deciduous" or "primary" teeth. The total number of teeth in this set are twenty. Primary teeth erupt at between 6 months and 2 years of age. Most children develop all their primary teeth at the age of three years.

The second set of teeth, i.e. the permanent teeth, erupt at the age of six years. There are 32 permanent teeth in an adult mouth. The teeth are present in two jaws (arches), i.e. an upper and a lower arch each, being the upper and lower jaws respectively. Normally, 16 teeth are found in each complete arch.

TOOTH NOTATION SYSTEMS

There are different tooth notations for identifying specific tooth. The three most commons systems are the "FDI World Dental Federation" notation, the "Universal" system and the "Zsigmondy-Palmer" system. The FDI system is used worldwide and the universal is used predominantly in the USA.

Most commonly used tooth notation systems
➡ Zsigmondy-Palmer system
➡ Universal (National) system (American Dental Association system)
➡ FDI system (FDI World Dental Federation).

Zsigmondy-Palmer System (Fig. 2.7)

It was originally termed as "Zsigmondy system" after the Austrian dentist Adolf Zsigmondy who developed the idea in 1861, using a "Zsigmondy cross" to record quadrants of tooth positions.

Adult teeth were numbered 1 to 8 and the primary teethas Roman numerals I, II, III, IV, V, starting at the midline. Palmer changed this to A, B, C, D, E. This makes it less confusing and less prone to errors in interpretation.

The Zsigmondy Palmer notation consists of a symbol (⌐⌐ ⌐⌐) designating in which quadrant the tooth is found and a number indicating the position from the midline. Permanent teeth are indicated by the numerals 1 to 8, and primary teeth by the letters A to E.

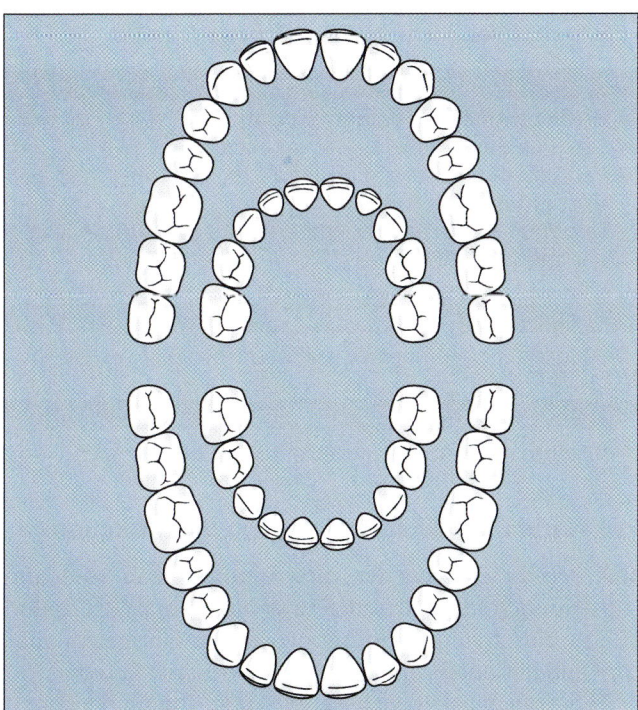

Figure 2.6: Two sets of teeth. The outer ring represents the permanent teeth. The inner ring represents the deciduous teeth

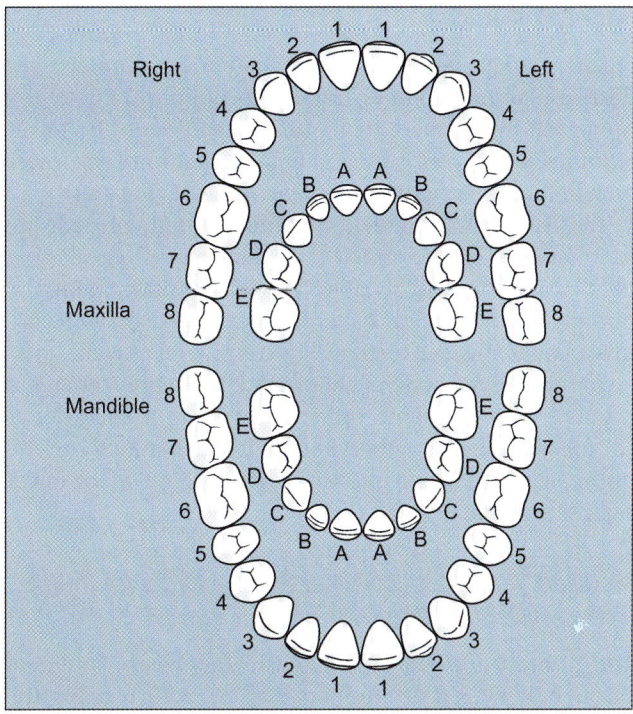

Figure 2.7: Presentation of Zsigmondy-Palmer notation of both deciduous and permanent dentitions

Universal (National) System

This system was introduced by the American Dental Association in 1968. This system is most popular in the United States. The universal numbering system uses a unique letter or number for each tooth.

The Universal or National System is represented as following:

Permanent Teeth

For permanent teeth, tooth 1 is the patient's upper right third molar and follows around the upper arch to the upper left third molar, tooth 16, descending to the lower left third molar, tooth 17, and following around the lower arch to the lower right third molar, tooth 32 (**Fig. 2.8**).

In this system, the teeth that are normally present are numbered. If a third molar ("wisdom tooth") is missing, the first number will be 2 instead of 1, acknowledging the missing tooth. If teeth have been extracted or teeth are missing, the missing teeth will be numbered as well.

In the original system, children's 20 primary teeth were numbered in the same order, except that a small letter "d" followed each number, thus a child's first tooth on the upper right side would be 1d and the last tooth on the lower right side would be 20d.

Modified Version of Universal System Order for the Primary Dentition (Fig. 2.8)

The primary teeth are by English upper case letters A through T instead of numbers 1 to 20, with A being the patient's upper right second primary molar and T being the lower right second primary molar, for example:

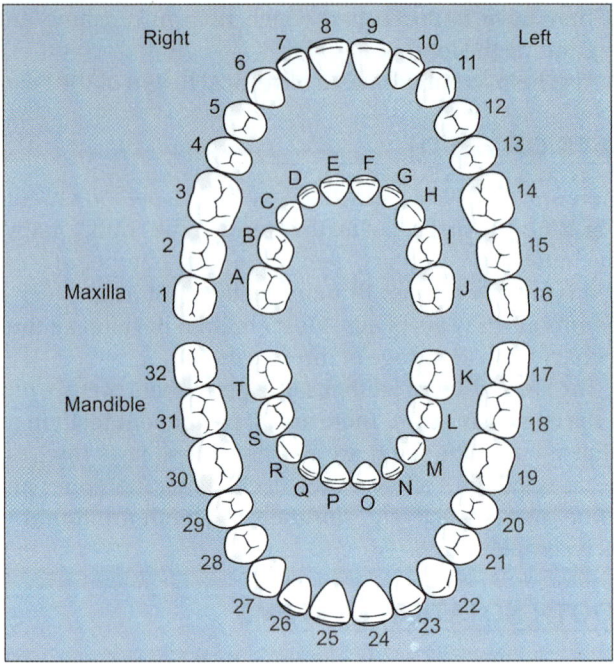

Figure 2.8: Presentation of modified version of universal system of tooth nomenclature for both deciduous and permanent teeth

B   is maxillary right deciduous first molar
P   is mandibular right deciduous central incisor
5   is maxillary right permanent first premolar.

FDI World Dental Federation (Two-digit Notation)

This two-digit system was first introduced in 1971 and subsequently adopted by the American Dental Association (1996). This system is commonly used in European countries and in Canada and is gaining popularity in India.

This system is known as a 'two-digit' system because it uses two digits; the first number represents a tooth's quadrant, and the second number represents the number of the tooth from the midline of the face. Both digits should be pronounced separately in communication. For example, the lower left permanent second molar is '37'; however, it is not said as 'thirty-seven', but rather 'three seven'. It should not be preceded by the 'hash' mark (#), which is often used as shorthand for 'number'.

Permanent Teeth (Fig. 2.9)

In the FDI notation, '1' is a central incisor, '2' is a lateral incisor, '3' is a canine, '4' and '5' 1st and 2nd premolars respectively and '6', '7' and '8' are the 1st, 2nd and 3rd molars respectively. The quadrants are designated 1 to 4, such that '1' is upper right, '2' is upper left, '3' is lower left and '4' is lower right, with the resulting tooth identification a two-digit combination of the quadrant and tooth, e.g. the upper right canine is '13' (one three) and the upper left canine is '23' (two three) (**Figs 2.10 and 2.11**).

Deciduous Teeth

In the deciduous dentition the numbering is correspondingly similar except that the quadrants are designated 5, 6, 7 and 8. Teeth are numbered from number 1 to 5, 1 being central incisor and 5 is second molar.

Features

- Introduced in 1971
- Also known as two-digit notation
- In two digit system, first number represents tooth's quadrant while second number is the number of tooth from midline
- Permanent upper right central incisor is designated as 11
- Deciduous upper right central incisor is designated as 51.

Advantages

- Simple to understand
- Simple to teach
- Simple to pronounce
- No confusion
- Each tooth has specific number
- Easy to record on computers
- Easy for charting.

Disadvantage

May be confused with universal tooth numbering system.

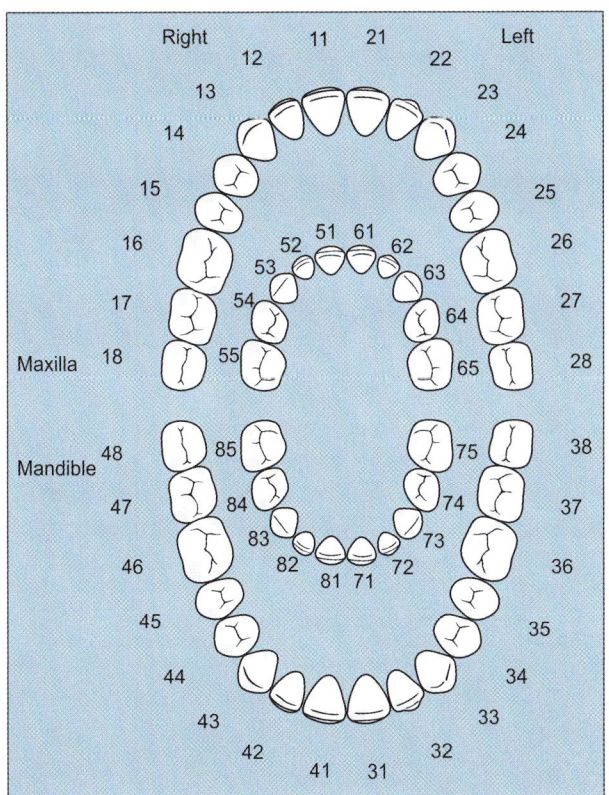

Figure 2.9: Presentation of FDI system of tooth nomenclature for permanent and primary teeth

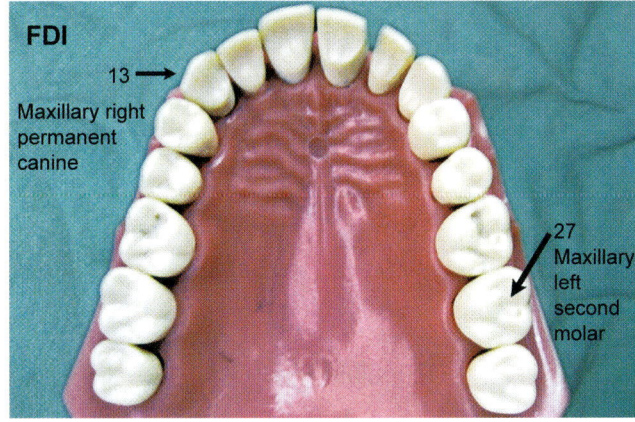

Figure 2.10: FDI notation of maxillary right canine and left second molar

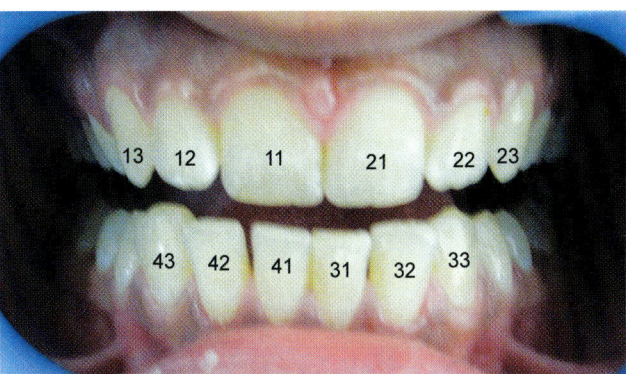

Figure 2.11: FDI system for permanent teeth

Comparison of Tooth Notation Systems

As a result, any given tooth has three different ways to identify it, depending on which notation system is used (**Fig. 2.12**). The permanent left maxillary central incisor is identified by the number "9" in the Universal system, whereas in the FDI system, the same tooth is identified by the 11 number "21". The Palmer system uses the number and symbol, L1, to identify this tooth. Further confusion

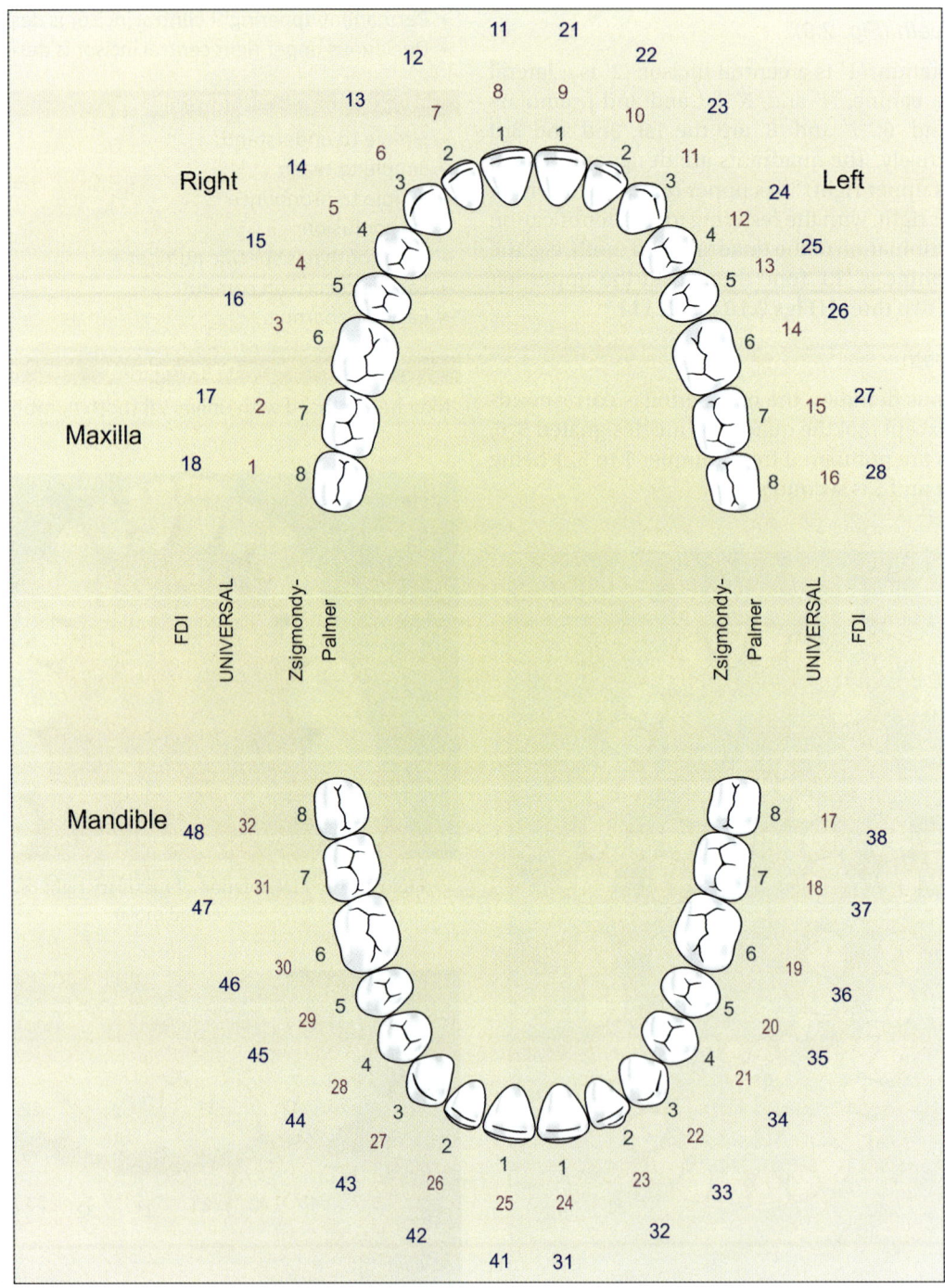

Figure 2.12: All nomenclature (all systems). First row describes—Zsigmondy-Palmer; Second row describes—Universal; Third row describes—FDI

Permanent Teeth

Zsigmondy-Palmer Notation															
8	7	6	5	4	3	2	1	1	2	3	4	5	6	7	8
8	7	6	5	4	3	2	1	1	2	3	4	5	6	7	8

Universal Numbering System															
			Upper right							Upper left					
1	2	3	4	5	6	7	8	9	10	11	12	13	14	15	16
32	31	30	29	28	27	26	25	24	23	22	21	20	19	18	17
			Lower right							Lower left					

FDI Two-digit Notation															
18	17	16	15	14	13	12	11	21	22	23	24	25	26	27	28
48	47	46	45	44	43	42	41	31	32	33	34	35	36	37	38

Deciduous Teeth

Palmer Notation															
			E	D	C	B	A	A	B	C	D	E			
			E	D	C	B	A	A	B	C	D	E			

Universal Numbering System															
			Upper right							Upper left					
			A	B	C	D	E	F	G	H	I	J			
			T	S	R	Q	P	O	N	M	L	K			
			Lower right							Lower left					

FDI Two-digit Notation															
			55	54	53	52	51	61	62	63	64	65			
			85	84	83	82	81	71	72	73	74	75			

may result if a number is given to a tooth without assuming a common notation method. Since the number, "21", may signify the permanent left mandibular first premolar in the Universal system or the permanent left maxillary central incisor in the FDI system, the notation being used must be clearly specified in order to prevent confusion.

NOMENCLATURE OF TOOTH SURFACES

The clinical crown of each tooth is divided into surfaces that are designated according to their related anatomic structures and landmarks (**Fig. 2.13**).

Buccal Surface

Tooth surface facing the check.

Labial Surface

Tooth surface facing the lip.

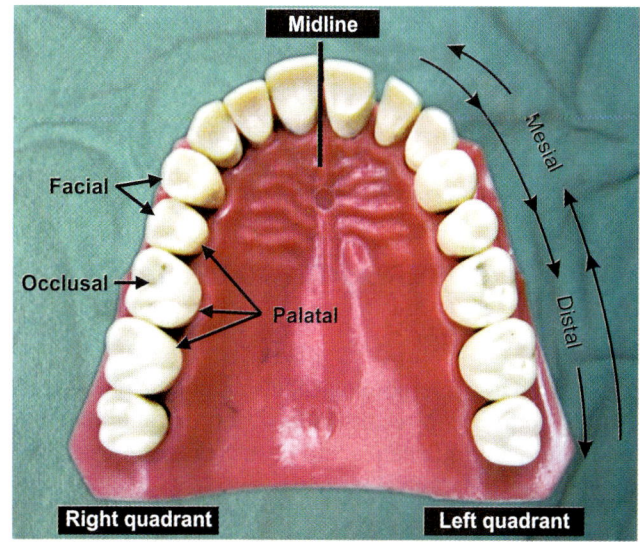

Figure 2.13: Diagrammatic representation of different surfaces of teeth

Facial Surface

Labial and buccal surface collectively form the facial surface.

Mesial Surface

Tooth surface towards the anterior midline.

Distal Surface

Tooth surface away from the anterior midline.

Lingual Surface

Tooth surface towards the tongue.

Occlusal Surface

Masticating surface of posterior teeth (in molars and premolars).

Incisal Surface

Functioning/cutting edge of anterior tooth of incisors and canines (cuspids).

Gingival Surface

Tooth surface near to the gingiva.

Cervical Surface

Tooth surface near the cervix or neck of the tooth.

Anatomic Crown

It is part of tooth that is covered with enamel (**Fig. 2.14**).

Clinical Crown

It is part of tooth that is visible in oral cavity (**Fig. 2.14**). In case of gingival recession, the clinical crown is longer than anatomical crown (**Fig. 2.15**).

NOMENCLATURE RELATED TO DENTAL CARIES

Dental Caries

It is defined as a microbiological disease of the hard structure of teeth, which results in localized demineralization of the inorganic substance and destruction of the organic substance of the tooth (**Fig. 2.16**).

Primary Caries

Denotes lesions on unrestored surfaces.

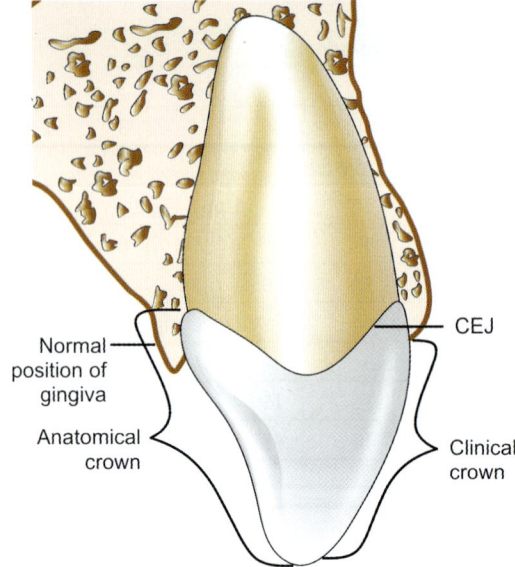

Figure 2.14: Anatomical crown and clinical crown

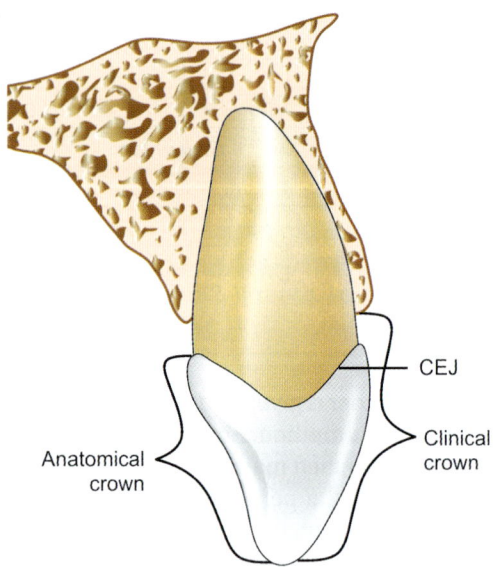

Figure 2.15: When there is gingival recession, clinical crown is longer than anatomical crown

Secondary (Recurrent) Caries

Lesions developing adjacent or beneath existing restorations are referred to as 'secondary' or 'recurrent' caries (**Fig. 2.17**).

Residual Caries

Demineralized tissue left in place before a restoration is placed. It can occur as a result of the clinician's neglect or intentionally.

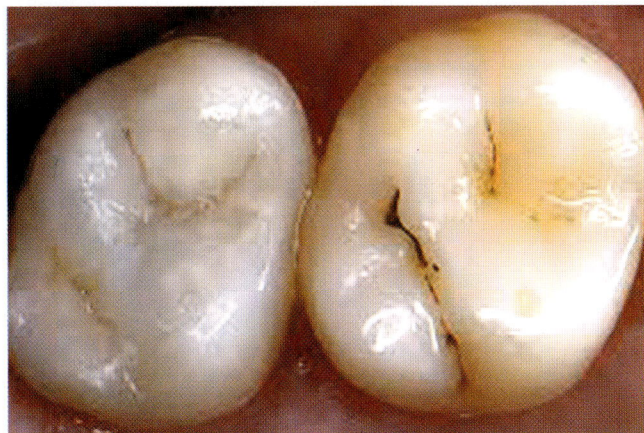

Figure 2.16: Dental caries

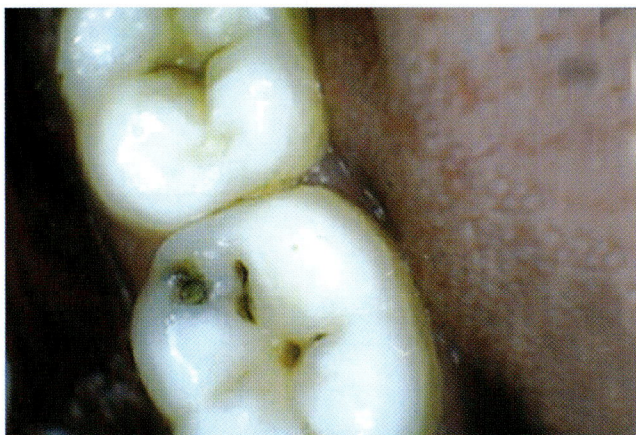

Figure 2.18: Pit and fissure caries

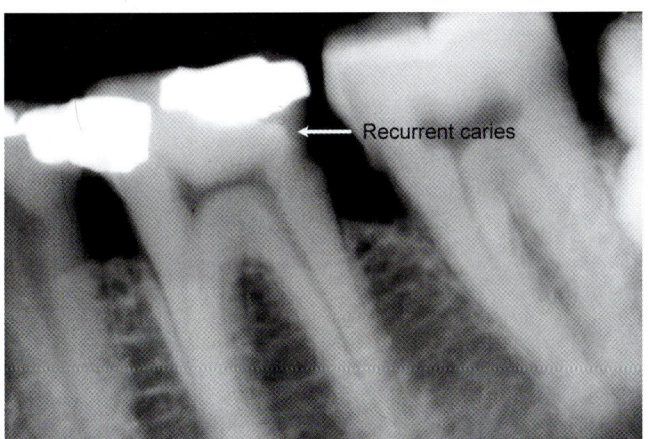

Figure 2.17: Radiograph showing recurrent caries

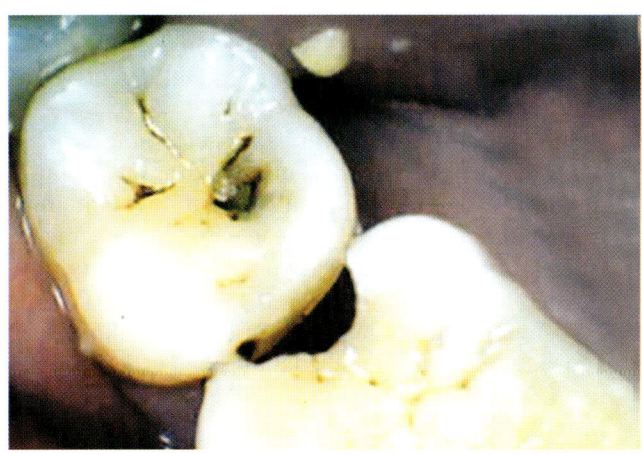

Figure 2.19: Smooth surface caries

Active Carious Lesion

A lesion which is progressing is described as an active carious lesion.

Inactive/Arrested Carious Lesion

A lesion that has formed and then not progressed is referred to as an 'arrested' or 'inactive' carious lesion. Arrested carious lesions are often characterized by a large open cavities which no longer retain food and become self-cleansing.

Pit and Fissure Caries

Pit and fissure caries describes caries which occurs on occlusal surface of posterior teeth, buccal and lingual surfaces of molars and on lingual surfaces of maxillary incisors (**Fig. 2.18**).

Smooth Surface Caries

Smooth surface caries occurs on the gingival third of buccal and lingual surfaces and on approximal surfaces (**Fig. 2.19**).

Root Caries (Fig. 2.20)

Root caries occur on exposed root cementum and dentin, usually following gingival recession:

Acute Dental Caries

Acute caries travels towards the pulp at a very fast speed.

Rampant Caries

The name given to multiple active carious lesions occurring in the same patient, frequently involving surfaces of teeth that are usually caries-free. Rampant caries can be of following three types:

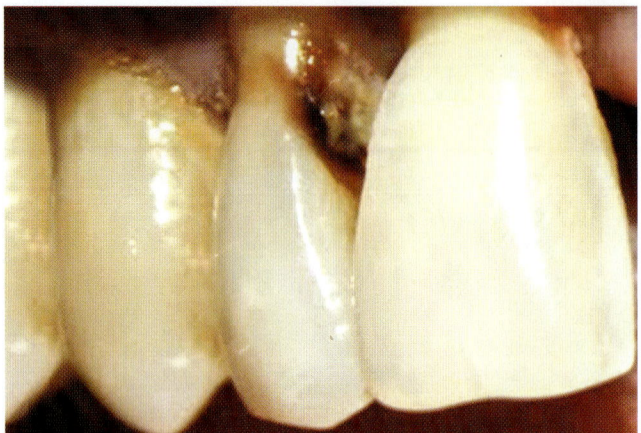

Figure 2.20: Root caries

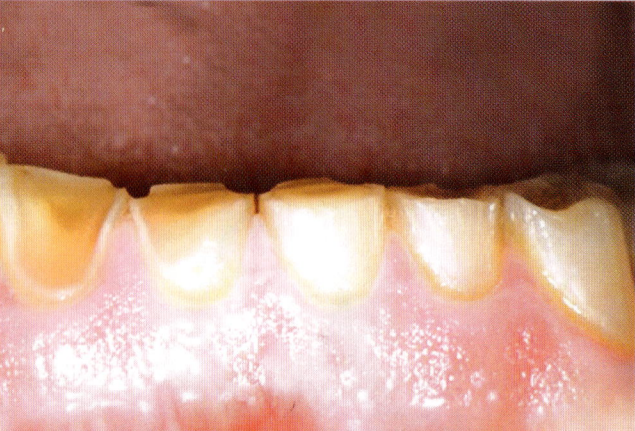

Figure 2.21: Attrition of teeth

- Early childhood caries is a term used to describe dental caries presenting in the primary dentition of young children
- Bottle caries or nursing caries is seen in the primary dentition of infants and young children as a consequence of sucking on a bottle or dummy containing cariogenic liquids. The clinical pattern is characteristic, with the four maxillary deciduous incisors most severely affected.
- Xerostomia induced rampant caries is commonly seen after radiotherapy of malignant lesions of the jaws, as the salivary glands may be damaged by the radiation resulting in reduced salivary flow.

Chronic Dental Caries

Chronic caries progresses very slowly towards the pulp. Such lesions appear dark in color and hard in consistency.

NOMENCLATURE RELATED TO NONCARIOUS DEFECTS OF TEETH

Attrition (Fig. 2.21)

It is defined as a physiological, continuous, process resulting in loss of tooth structure from direct frictional forces between contacting teeth. It occurs both on occlusal and approximal surfaces. Attrition is accelerated by parafunctional mandibular movements, especially bruxism.

Abrasion

It refers to the loss of tooth substance induced by mechanical wear other than that of mastication. Abrasion results in saucer-shaped or wedge-shaped indentations with a smooth, shiny surface (**Fig. 2.22**).

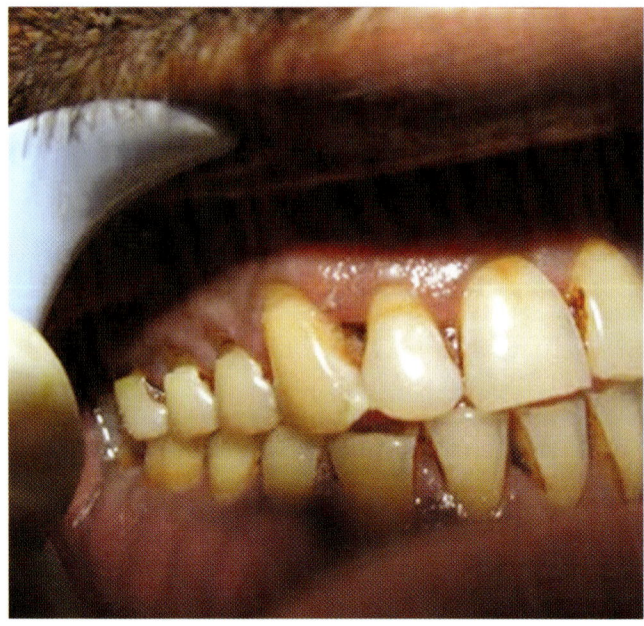

Figure 2.22: Abrasion of teeth

Erosion

It can be defined as a loss of tooth substance by a chemical process that does not involve known bacterial action. The eroded area appears smooth, hard and polished.

Abfraction

Abfractions are the microfractures which appear in the enamel and possibly the dentine caused by flexion of the cervical area of the tooth under heavy loads.

Abfraction lesions usually appear as wedge-shaped defects with sharp line angles.

Resorption

'Resorption' is defined as "a condition associated with either a physiologic or a pathologic process resulting in the loss of dentin, cementum or bone."

If resorption occurs, it is often because of some pathological process, although deciduous tooth roots undergo physiological resorption in order to be shed.

Localized Nonhereditary Enamel Hypoplasia

Refers to the localized defects in the crown of the portion tooth caused by to injury to ameloblasts during the enamel matrix formation stage. These lesions may appear as isolated pits or widespread linear defects, depressions or loss of a part of the enamel. Injury to ameloblasts may be caused by:

- Traumatic intrusion of deciduous teeth
- Fluorosis
- Exanthematous diseases
- Deficiency of vitamins A, C or D
- Hypocalcemia.

Localized Nonhereditary Enamel Hypocalcification

Refers to localized defects in the crown of a tooth due to injury to the ameloblasts during the mineralization stage. In these defects, the enamel is normal in structure but its mineralization is defective. The color of lesion varies from chalky to yellow, brown, dark brown or grayish.

 Key Points

- Dental anatomy or anatomy of teeth is the branch of anatomy which deals with the study of human teeth structures.
- For convenience human dentition is divided into four quadrants viz; upper (maxillary) right, upper (maxillary) left, lower (mandibular) right and lower (mandibular) left.
- The three most commons systems are the FDI World Dental Federation notation, Universal numbering system and Zsigmondy-Palmer notation method.
- The FDI system is used worldwide and the universal is used widely in the USA.
- Zsigmondy-Palmer system was originally termed as "Zsigmondy system" after the Austrian dentist Adolf Zsigmondy who developed the idea in 1861. Adult teeth were numbered 1 to 8 and the primary dentition as Roman numerals I, II, III, IV, V from the midline. Palmer changed this to A, B, C, D, E. This makes it less confusing and less prone to errors in interpretation.
- Universal system was given by American Dental Association in 1968. The universal numbering system uses a unique letter or number for each tooth.
- For permanent teeth, 1 is the patient's upper right third molar and follows around the upper arch to the upper left third molar 16, descending to the lower left third molar 17 and follows around the lower arch to the lower right third molar (32). For the primary dentition, letters A through T are used instead of number 1 to 20.
- FDI, was first introduced in 1971 which later on, was adopted by ADA (1996). This system is known as two digit system because it uses a two-digit numbering system in which the first number represents a tooth's quadrant and the second number represents the number of the tooth from the midline of the face. Both digits should be pronounced separately while communication. For example, the lower left permanent second molar is 37; however, it is not said thirty-seven, but rather three seven.

QUESTIONS

1. What are different nomenclature of teeth. Explain FDI nomenclature in detail.
2. Write short notes on:
   a. Zsigmondy-Palmer system.
   b. Universal system.
   c. FDI system.
   d. Two digit notation.
3. What are different nomenclatures of teeth? Discuss the advantages and disadvantages of FDI system.

BIBLIOGRAPHY

1. Ash Major M, Stanley J Nelson. Wheeler's Dental Anatomy, Physiology, and Occlusion. 8th ed. 2003.p.198.
2. Blinkhorn AS, Choi CLK, Paget HE. An investigation into the use of the FDI tooth notation system by dental schools in the UK Eur J Dent Educ. 1998;2:39.
3. Ten Cate AR, Oral Histology. Development, Structure, and Function, 5th ed. Saint Louis: Mosby-Year Book, 1998.p.95.
4. Ten Cate AR, Oral Histology. Development, Structure, and Function, 5th ed. Saint Louis: Mosby-Year Book, 1998.pp.86 and 102.

3
CHAPTER

Structure of Teeth

Chapter Outline

Good knowledge of dental anatomy, histology, physiology and occlusion is the foundation stone of operative dentistry. In other words, thorough knowledge of morphology, dental anatomy, histology, is essential to get optimal results of operative dentistry. Though the dental tissues are passive, the occurrence of caries can only be understood when the structure of the teeth is understood.

The teeth consist of enamel, dentin, pulp and cementum (**Fig. 3.1**).

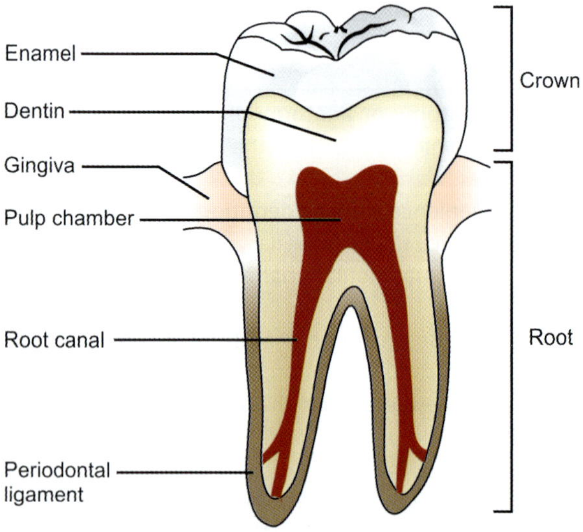

Figure 3.1: Enamel, dentin, pulp and supporting structures

ENAMEL

Tooth enamel is the hardest and most highly mineralized substance of the body which covers the crown of the tooth. It is the normally visible dental tissue of a tooth which is mainly responsible for color, esthetics, texture and translucency of the tooth. One of the main goal in operative dentistry is preservation of enamel. So today's dentistry mainly revolves around simulating natural enamel in its color, esthetics, contours and translucency by replacing with synthetic restorative materials.

Although enamel can serve lifelong, but it is more susceptible to caries, attrition (physical forces) and fracture due to its structural make up, i.e. mineralized crystalline structure and rigidity. One of the interesting features of enamel is that it cannot repair itself. So, loss in enamel surface can be compensated only by restorative treatment.

Composition

It is highly mineralized structure which mainly contains inorganic contents in the form of crystalline structure. Main inorganic content in the enamel is hydroxyapatite. In addition to inorganic content, it also contains a small portion of organic matrix along with small amount of water which is present in intercrystalline spaces.

Composition
→ Inorganic content (by volume)
♦ Hydroxyapatite—90 to 92 percent
♦ Other minerals and trace elements—3 to 5 percent
→ Organic content (by volume)
♦ Proteins and lipids—1 to 2 percent
♦ Water—4 percent.

Structure

Enamel is mainly composed of millions of enamel rods or prisms as well as sheaths and a cementing inter-rod substance. Each rod has a head and tail. The head is directed occlusally and the tail is directed cervically. The rod is formed of number of hydroxyapatite crystals which vary in size, shape and number. Each rod formed of about 300 unit crystal length and 40 units wide and 20 unit thick in three-dimensional hexagon. In transverse sections, enamel rods appear as hexagonal and occasionally round or oval. Rods may also resemble fish scales.

The diameter of rods increases from dentino-enamel junction towards the outer surface of enamel in a ratio of 1:2.

The rods or the prisms run in an alternating coarse of clockwise and anticlockwise direction (twisting course). Initially there is wavy coarse in one-third of enamel thickness adjacent to DEJ, then the coarse becomes more straight in the remaining thickness.

Enamel rods are arranged in such planes so as to resist the maximum masticatory forces. Rods are oriented at prependicular to the dentinoenamel junction. Towards the incisal edge these become increasingly oblique and are almost vertical at the cusp tips. In the cervical region, there is difference in the direction of the enamel rods of deciduous and permanent teeth (**Fig. 3.2**).

Clinical Significance

The cervical enamel rods of deciduous teeth are inclined incisally or occlusally, while in permanent teeth they are inclined apically clinical significance of derections of rods.

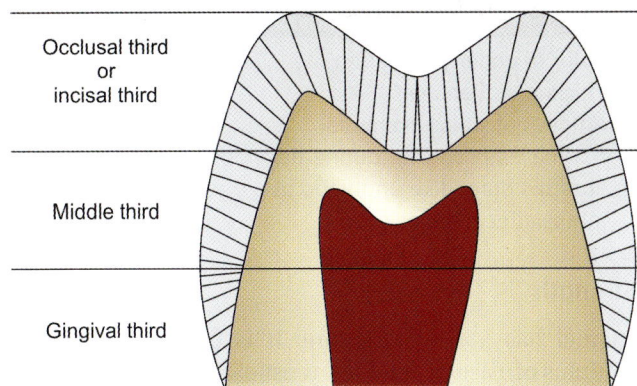

Figure 3.2: Direction of enamel rods in deciduous and permanent teeth

This change in direction of enamel rods should be kept in mind during tooth preparation so as to avoid unsupported enamel rods.

Structure
→ Composed of millions of rods or prisms
→ Diameter of enamel rod increases from dentin enamel junction towards outer surface of enamel in 1:2
→ Enamel rods lie perpendicular to dentino-enamel junction
→ In cervical region, direction of enamel rod is incisally/occlusally in deciduous while in permanent, it is apically.

Thickness

The thickness of enamel varies in different areas of the same tooth and from one type of tooth to another type of tooth. The average thickness of enamel at the incisal edges of incisors is 2 mm; at the cusp of premolar and molar it ranges from 2.3 to 3.0 mm. Thickness of enamel decreases gradually from cusps or incisal edges to cemento-enamel junction.

Thickness of enamel	
Tooth type	*Thickness*
→ Anterior tooth (incisal edges)	2.0 mm
→ Premolar tooth (cusp)	2.3 to 2.5 mm
→ Molar tooth (cusp)	2.5 to 3.0 mm

Color

The color of enamel is usually gray and translucent in nature. Color of tooth mainly depends upon three factors:
1. Color of underlying dentin
2. Thickness of enamel
3. Amount of stains in enamel. The translucency of enamel is directly related to degree of mineralization and homogenicity. Anomalies occurring during developmental and mineralization stage, antibiotic usage and excess fluoride intake affect the color of tooth.

Color of enamel is affected by

➡ Color of underlying dentin
➡ Thickness of enamel
➡ Amount of stains in enamel
➡ Anomalies occurring during developmental and mineralization stage like antibiotic usage and excess fluoride intake affects the color.

Strength

Enamel has a rigid structure. It is brittle, has a high modulus of elasticity and low tensile strength. The specific gravity of enamel is 2.8. Hardness of enamel is different in different areas of the external surface of a tooth. The hardness also decreases from outer surface of the enamel to its inner surface. Also the density of enamel increases from dentino-enamel junction to the outer surface. When compared, dentin has high compressive strength than the enamel.

Significance

Because of high compressive strength of dentin than enamel, the dentin acts as a cushion for enamel when masticatory forces are applied on it. For this reason, during tooth preparation, for maximal strength of underlying remaining tooth structure all enamel rods should be supported by healthy dentin base.

Structure present in enamel

➡ Gnarled enamel
➡ Bands of Hunter-Schreger
➡ Enamel tufts
➡ Enamel lamellae
➡ Enamel spindles
➡ Striae of Retzius
➡ Prismless layer
➡ Dentino-enamel junction
➡ Occlusal pits and fissures.

Structure Present in Enamel (Fig. 3.3)

Gnarled Enamel

There are group of irregular enamel that is more resistant to cleavage called Gnarled enamel present mostly in cervical, incisal and occlusal portion. This consists of bundles of enamel rods which interwine in an irregular manner with other group of rods, finally taking a twisted and irregular path towards the tooth surface.

Significance: This part of enamel is resistant to cutting while tooth preparation.

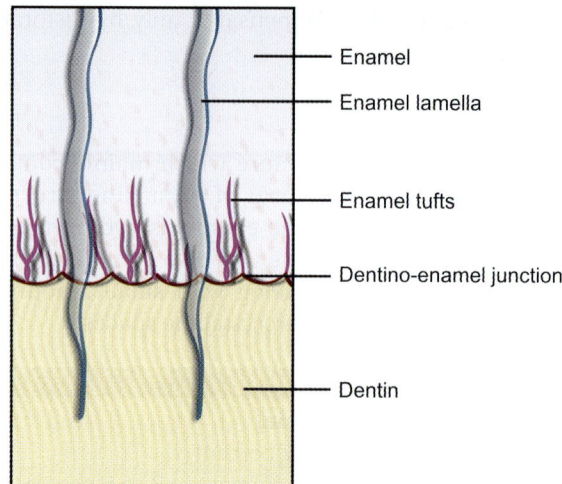

Figure 3.3: Different structures present in enamel

Bands of Hunter-Schreger

Hunter-Schreger bands usually occur because of alteration of light reflection (optical phenomenon) due to changes in rod direction. This results in alternating light and dark zones under the microscope. It is best seen in longitudinal ground sections seen under reflected light. They are mainly found in the inner surface of tooth. H-S bands are composed of different contents of organic material and varied permeability.

Significance: They are considered to resist and disperse the strong forces.

Enamel Tufts

Enamel tufts are ribbon-like structures which run from dentin to enamel. They are named so because they resemble tufts of grass. They contain greater concentration of enamel proteins.

Significance: Enamel tufts are hypomineralized structure in the enamel, thus play role in spread of dental infection.

Enamel Lamellae

These are leaf like defects present in enamel and may extend to DEJ. They contains organic substances. Lamellae are commonly found at the base of occlusal pits and fissures. Bodecker in 1906 was the first to describe these developmental defects of enamel which he named 'lamellae'.

These are caused by 'imperfect calcification of enamel tissue'.

Pincus suggested that if developing cusps fail to coalesce when forming a fissure, a gap in the enamel occurs. Such a gap may vary in size from a crack or lamella.

Three types of lamellae are commonly seen:
1. Type A composed of 'poorly calcified rod segments'
2. Type B composed of degenerated cells
3. Type C arising after eruption where the crack is filled with mucoproteins from the oral preparation

Type A lamellae is confined to enamel while types B and C may extend into dentin.

Significance

Various studies have shown that lamellae might be the site of entry of caries.

Ten Cate stated that tufts and lamellae are of no significance and do not appear to be sites of increased vulnerability to caries attack.

A lamella at the base of an occlusal fissure provides an appropriate pathway for bacteria and initiate caries.

Enamel Spindles

Odontoblastic processes sometimes cross DEJ and their ends are thickened, called enamel spindles

Significance: Spindles serve as pain receptors, that is why, when we cut in the enamel patient complains of pain.

Striae of Retzius

They appear as brownish bands in the ground sections and illustrate the incremental pattern of enamel. These represent the rest periods of ameloblast during enamel formation, therefore also called as growth circles. When these circles are incomplete at the enamel surface, they result in alternating grooves called imbrications lines of pickerills, the elevations in between are called Perikymata. Perikymata are shallow furrows where the striae of Retzius end. These are continuous around the tooth and parallel to the CEJ.

Striae of Retzius are stripes that appear on enamel when viewed microscopically in cross-section. Formed from changes in diameter of 'Tomes' processes, these stripes demonstrate the growth of enamel, similar to the annual rings on a tree.

Prismless Layer

There is structureless layer of enamel near the cervical line and to a lesser extent on the cusp tip which is more mineralized.

Dentino-enamel Junction

Dentino-enamel junction is pitted/scalloped in which crests are toward enamel and shallow depressions are in dentin. This helps in better interlocking between enamel and dentin. This is a hypermineralized zone and is about 30 microns thick.

Significance: Shape and nature of the dentino-enamel junction prevents tearing of enamel during functions.

Occlusal Pits and Fissures

Pits and fissures are formed by faulty coalescence of developmental lobes of premolars and molars (**Fig. 3.4**). These are commonly seen on occlusal surfaces of premolars and molars. These are formed at the junction of the developmental lobes of the enamel organs. Grooves are developed by smooth coalescence of developmental lobes.

Significance:
• Thickness of enamel at the base of pit and fissure is less.
• Pits and fissures are the areas of food and bacteria impaction which make them caries prone (**Fig. 3.5**).

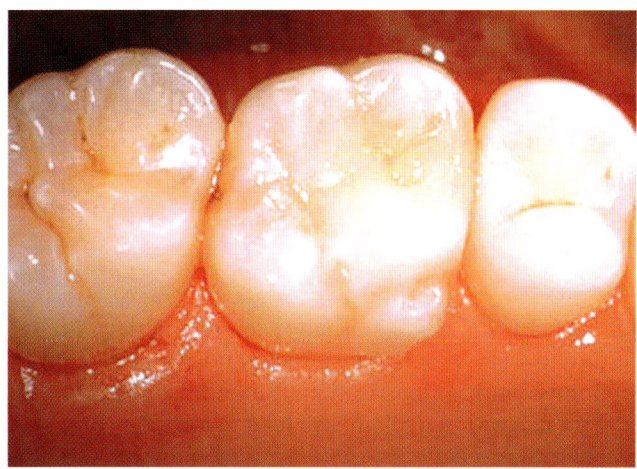

Figure 3.4: Pits and fissures of premolars and molars

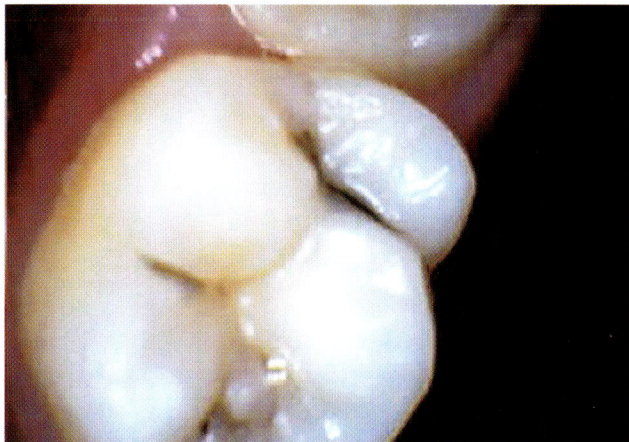

Figure 3.5: Deep pits and fissures making areas favorable for food impaction

- V-shaped grooves provide escapement of food when cusps of teeth of opposite arch occlude during mastication.

Functions of Enamel

- It is hardest structure of tooth which supports masticatory forces
- It is mainly responsible for color, esthetics, surface texture and translucency of the tooth
- It also supports the underlying dentin and pulp.

Functions of enamel
➡ Hardest structure of tooth supporting the masticatory forces
➡ Responsible for color and esthetics
➡ Responsible for surface texture and translucency of tooth
➡ Supports underlying dentin and pulp.

Clinical Significance of Enamel

- *Color*: Color of the enamel varies because of following factors:
  - Age
  - Ingestion of tetracycline during the formative stages
  - Ingestion of fluoride
  - Extrinsic stains
  - Developmental defects of tooth.
- *Attrition*: The change usually seen in enamel with age due to wear of occlusal surfaces and proximal contact points during mastication. Sometimes bruxism or contacts with porcelain also lead to attrition (**Fig. 3.6**). So, in these patients, try to avoid placing the margins of restoration in occlusal contact area or place a restorative material that wears at a same rate as enamel.
- *Acid etching*: Acid etching is used in fissure sealants and bonding of restorative material to enamel. Acid etching has been considered as accepted procedure for improving the bonding between resin and enamel. Acid etching causes preferential dissolution of enamel surface and helps in increasing the bonding between resin and enamel.
- *Permeability*: Enamel has been considered to be permeable to some ions and molecules. Hypomineralized areas present in the enamel are more permeable than mineralized area. So, these hypomineralized areas are more sensitive to dental caries.
- Defective surfaces like hypoplastic areas, pits and fissures are at more risk for dental caries
- Cracks present on the enamel surface sometimes lead to pulpal death and fracture of tooth.
- To avoid fracture of tooth and restoration, enamel walls should be supported by underlying dentin. Also the preparation walls should be made parallel to direction of enamel rods since enamel rod boundaries are natural cleavage lines through which fracture can occur.
- *Remineralization*: Remineralization is only because of enamel's permeability to fluoride, calcium and phosphate (available from saliva or other sources).

DENTIN

Dentin, the most voluminous mineralized connective tissue of the tooth, forms the hard tissue portion of the dentin-pulp complex, whereas the dental pulp is the living, soft connective tissue that retains the vitality of dentin. Enamel covers the dentin in crown portion while cementum covers the dentin in root portion. Dentin contains closely packed dentinal tubules in which the dentinal fluid and the cytoplasmic processes of the odontoblasts, are located. Hence, dentin and bone are considered as vital tissues because both contain living protoplasm. Dentin is type of specialized connective tissue which is mesodermal in origin, formed from dental papilla.

The unity of dentin-pulp is responsible for dentin formation and protection of the tooth.

Composition

Dentin contains 70 percent inorganic hydroxyapatite crystals and the rest is organic substance and water making it more resilient than enamel.

The organic components consist primarily of collagen type 1.

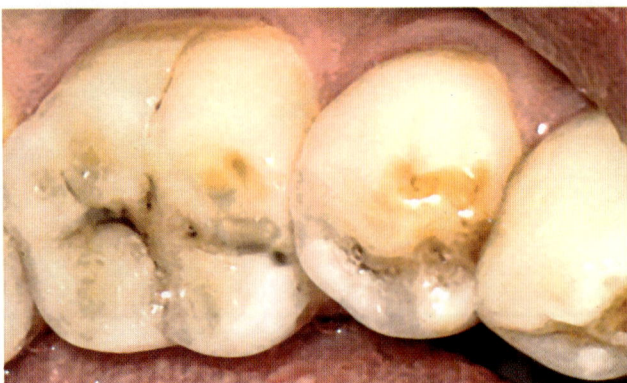

Figure 3.6: Attrition of teeth

Composition (by weight)	
➡ Inorganic material	70 percent
➡ Organic material	20 percent
➡ Water	10 percent

Color

The color of dentin is slightly darker than enamel and is generally light yellowish in young individuals while it becomes darker with age. On constant exposure to oral fluids and other irritants, the color becomes light brown or black (**Fig. 3.7**).

Thickness

Dentin thickness is usually more on the cuspal heights and incisal edges and less in the cervical areas of tooth. It is around 3 to 3.5 mm on the coronal surface. With advancing age and various irritants, the thickness of secondary and tertiary dentin increases.

Hardness

The hardness of dentin is one-fifth that of enamel. Hardness is not the same in all its thickness. Its hardness at the DEJ is 3 times more than that near the pulp so it is important to keep the depth of preparation near the DEJ. Hardness of dentin also increases with advancing age due to mineralization. Compressive hardness is about 266 MPa. The modulus of elasticity is about 1.67×106 Psi. As the modulus of elasticity of dentin is low, so it indicates dentin is flexible in nature. The flexibility of dentin provides support or cushion to the brittle enamel. The tensile strength of dentin is 40 to 60 MPa. It is approximatcly onc-half of that of enamel.

Hardness of dentin
➟ 1/5th of enamel
➟ Compressive hardness is 266 Mpa
➟ Tensile strength—40 to 60 Mpa
➟ Hardness increases with age.

Structure of dentin
➟ Dentinal tubules
➟ Predentin
➟ Peritubular dentin
➟ Intertubular dentin
➟ Primary dentin
◆ Mantle
◆ Circumpulpal
➟ Secondary dentin
➟ Reparative dentin
➟ Sclerotic dentin.

Dentinal Tubules (Table 3.1)

- The dentinal tubules follow a gentle 'S' shaped curve in the tooth crown and are straighter in the incisal edges, cusps and root areas
- The ends of the tubules are perpendicular to dentino-enamel and dentino-cemental junctions (**Fig. 3.8**)
- The dentinal tubules have lateral branches throughout the dentin, which are termed as canaliculi or microtubules
- Each dentinal tubule is lined with a layer of peritubular dentin, which is much more mineralized than the surrounding intertubular dentin
- Number of dentinal tubules increase from 15,000-20,000/mm² at DEJ to 45,000-65,000/mm² toward the pulp

Table 3.1: Dentinal tubules

	Pulp	DEJ
Diameter	2-3 μm	0.5-0.9 μm
Numbers	45,000-65,000/mm²	15,000-20,000/mm²

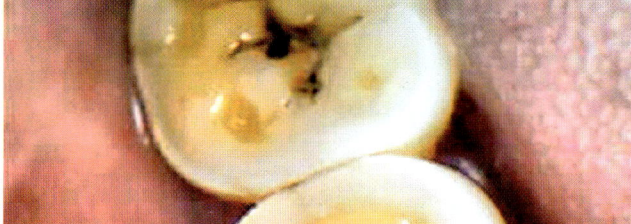

Figure 3.7: Dark colored dentin because of irritants

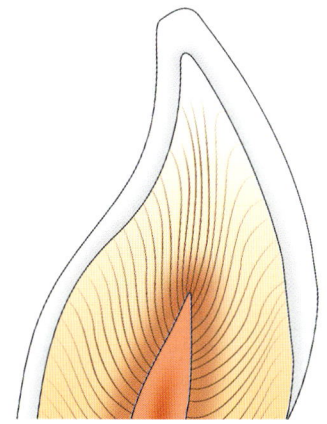

Figure 3.8: Course of dentinal tubules

- Dentinal tubules may extend from the odontoblastic layer to the dentino-enamel junction and give high permeability to the dentin. In addition to an odontoblast process, the tubule contains dentinal fluid, a complex mixture of proteins such as albumin, transferrin, tenascin and proteoglycans.

Predentin

- The predentin is 10 to 30 μm unmineralized zone between the mineralized dentin and odontoblasts.
- This layer of dentin, lie very close to the pulp tissue which is just next to cell bodies of odotoblasts. It is first formed dentin and is not mineralized.

Peritubular Dentin (Fig. 3.9)

This dentinal layer usually lines the dentinal tubules and is more mineralized than intertubular dentin and predentin.

Intertubular Dentin (Fig. 3.9)

- This dentin is present between the tubules which is less mineralized than peritubular dentin
- Intertubular dentin determines the elasticity of the dental matrix.

Primary Dentin

This type of dentin is formed before root completion, gives initial shape of the tooth. It continues to grow till 3 years after tooth eruption.

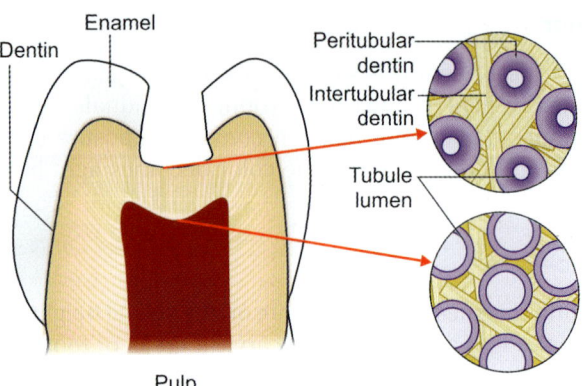

Figure 3.9: Pattern of intertubular and peritubular dentin

- **Mantle dentin**: At the outermost layer of the primary dentin, just under the enamel, a narrow zone called mantle dentin exists. It is formed as a result of initial mineralization reaction by newly differentiated odonto blasts. In other words, it is first formed dentin in the crown underlying the dentino-enamel junction.
- **Circumpulpal dentin**: It forms the remaining primary dentin and is more mineralized than mantle dentin. This dentin outlines the pulp chamber and therefore it may be referred to as circumpulpal dentin. It is formed before root completion.

Secondary Dentin

- Secondary dentin is formed after completion of root formation

Difference between Enamel and Dentin

	Enamel	Dentin
Color	Whitish blue or white gray	Yellowish white or slightly darker than enamel
Sound	Sharp, high pitched sound on moving fine explorer tip	Dull or low pitched sound on moving fine explorer tip
Hardness	Hardest structure of the tooth	Softer than enamel
Reflectance	More shiny surface and reflective to light than dentin	Dull and reflects less light than enamel

Difference between Primary, Secondary and Reparative/Tertiary Dentin

	Primary	Secondary	Tertiary
Definition	Dentin formed before root completion	Formed after root completion	Formed as a response to any external stimuli such as dental caries, attrition and trauma
Type of cells	Usually formed by primary odontoblasts	Formed by primary odontoblasts	Secondary odontoblasts or undifferentiated mesenchymal cells of pulps
Location	Found in all areas of dentin	It is not uniform, mainly present over roof and floor of pulp chamber	Localized to only area of external stimulus
Orientation of tubules	Regular	Irregular	Atubular
Rate of formation	Rapid	Slow	Rapid between 1.5 and 3.5 μm/day depending on the stimuli
Permeability	More	Less	Least

- In this, the direction of tubules is more asymmetrical and complicated as compared to primary dentin. Secondary dentin forms at a slower rate than primary dentin.

Reparative Dentin/Tertiary Dentin

- Tertiary dentin;s frequently formed in response to external stimuli such as dental caries, attrition and trauma
- If the injury is severe and causes odontoblast cell death, odontoblast like cells synthesize specific reparative dentin just beneath the site of injury to protect pulp tissue
- The secondary odontoblasts which produce reparative dentin are developed from undifferentiating mesenchymal cells of pulp
- Unlike physiological dentin, reparative dentin is irregular, with cellular inclusions
- The tubular pattern of the reparative dentin ranges from a irregular to an atubular nature
- Reparative dentin matrix matric is less permeable, this prevents the diffusion of noxious agents from the tubules.

Sclerotic Dentin

- It occurs due to aging or chronic and mild irritation (such as slowly advancing caries) which causes a change in the composition of the primary dentin
- In sclerotic dentin, peritubular dentin becomes wider due to deposition of calcified materials, which progress from enamel to pulp
- This area becomes harder, denser, less sensitive and more protective of pulp against irritations.

Types of Sclerotic Dentin

Physiologic sclerotic dentin: Sclerotic dentin occurs due to aging.

Reactive sclerotic dentin: Reactive sclerotic dentin occurs due to irritants.

Eburnated dentin: It is type of reactive sclerotic dentin which is formed due to destruction by slow caries process or mild chronic irritation and results in hard, darkened cleanable surface on outward portion of reactive dentin.

Dead Tracts

- This type of dentin usually results due to moderate type of stimuli such as moderate rate caries or attrition
- In this case, both affected and associated odontoblasts die, resulting in empty dental tubules which appear black when ground sections of dentin are viewed under transmitted light. These are called dead tracts due to appearance of black under transmitted light.

Functions of dentin
➡ Provide strength to the tooth
➡ Offers protection of pulp
➡ Provides flexibility to the tooth
➡ Affects the color of enamel
➡ Defensive in action (initiating pulpal defence mechanism).

Clinical Considerations of Dentin

- As dentin is known to provide strength and rigidity to the tooth, care should be taken during tooth preparation
- Tooth preparations should be done under constant air water spray to avoid build up of heat formation which, in further, damages dental pulp
- Dentinal tubules are composed of odontoblastic processes and dentinal fluid. The dehydration of dentin by air blasts causes outward fluid movement and stimulates the mechanoreceptor of the odontoblast, resulting in dentinal sensitivity (**Fig. 3.10**)
- Dentin should always be protected by liners, bases or dentin bonding agents
- When tooth is cut, considerable quantities of cutting debris made up of small particles of mineralized collagen matrix are formed. This forms a layer on enamel of dentin called smear layer for bonding of restorative materials to tooth structure, this smear layer has to be removed or modified. This can be done by etching or conditioning.

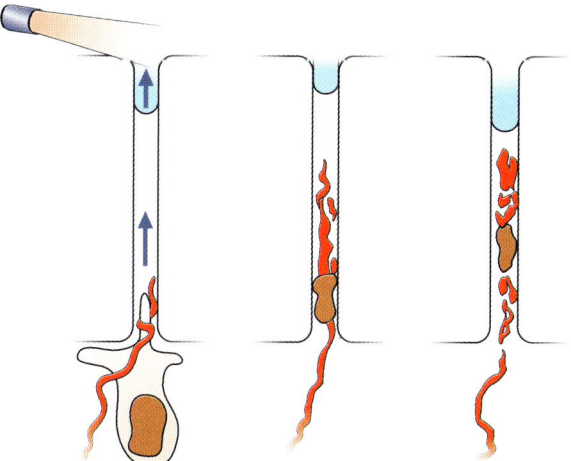

Figure 3.10: Fluid movement in dentinal tubules resulting in dentin hypersensitivity

- Etching of dentin causes removal of smear layer and etching of intertubular and peritubular dentin for micromechanical bonding.
- Restoration should be well adapted to the preparation walls so as to prevent microleakage and thus damage to underlying dentin/pulp.

DENTAL PULP

The dental pulp is soft tissue of mesenchymal origin located in the center of the tooth. It consists of specialized cells, odontoblasts arranged peripherally in direct contact with dentin matrix. This close relationship between odontoblasts and dentin is known as 'Pulp – dentin complex'. The pulp is connective tissue system composed of cells, ground substances, fibers, interstitial fluid, odontoblasts, fibroblasts and other cellular components. Pulp is actually a microcirculatory system consists of arterioles and venules as the largest vascular component. Due to lack of true collateral circulation, pulp is dependent upon few arterioles entering through the foramen. Due to presence of the specialized cells, i.e. odontoblasts as well as other cells which can differentiate into hard tissue secreting cells. The pulp retains its ability to form dentin throughout the life. This enables the vital pulp to partially compensate for loss of enamel or dentin occurring with age.

Histology of Dental Pulp

Basically the pulp is divided into the central and the peripheral region. The central region of both coronal and radicular pulp contains nerves and blood vessels.

The peripheral region contains the following zones (**Fig. 3.11**):
- Odontoblastic layer
- Cell free zone of Weil
- Cell rich zone.

Odontoblastic Layer

Odontoblasts consist of cell bodies and their cytoplasmic processes. The odontoblastic cell bodies form the odontoblastic zone whereas the odontoblastic processes are located within predentin matrix. Capillaries, nerve fibers and dendritic cells may be found around the odontoblasts in this zone.

Cell Free Zone of Weil

Central to odontoblasts is subodontoblastic layer, termed as cell free zone of Weil. It contains plexuses of capillaries and fibers ramification of small nerve.

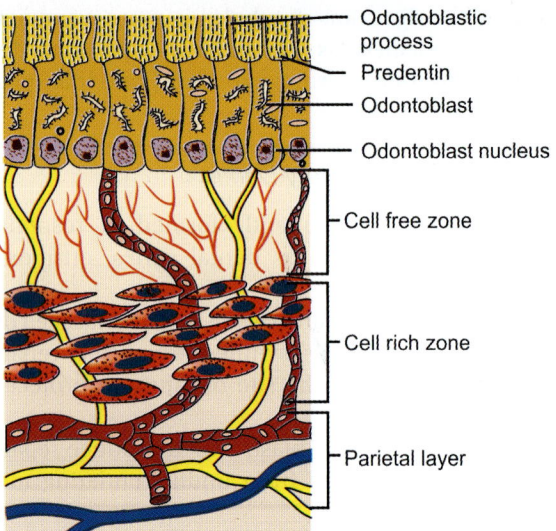

Figure 3.11: Different zones of dental pulp

Cell Rich Zone

This zone lies next to subodontoblastic layer. It contains fibroblasts, undifferentiated cells which maintain number of odontoblasts by proliferation and differentiation.

Contents of pulp		
➡ Cells		
◆ Odontoblasts		
◆ Fibroblasts		
◆ Undifferentiated mesenchymal cells		
◆ Defense cells	Macrophages	
	Plasma cells	
	Mast cells	
➡ Matrix		
◆ Collagen fibers	Types I and II	
◆ Ground Substance	Glycosaminoglycans	
	Glycoproteins	
	Water	
◆ Blood vessels	Arterioles, venules, capillaries	
◆ Lymphatics	Draining to submandibular, submental and deep cervical nodes	
◆ Nerves	Subodontoblastic plexus of Rashkow sensory afferent from Vth nerve and superior cervical ganglion	

Structural or Cellular Elements

Odontoblasts

- They are first type of cells encountered as pulp is approached from dentin.

- The number of odontoblasts range from 59,000 to 76,000/mm^2 in coronal dentin with lesser number in root dentin.
- In the crown of the fully developed tooth, the cell bodies of odontoblasts are columnar and measure approximately 500 μm in height, whereas in the midportion of the pulp, they are more cuboid and in apical part, more flattened.
- Ultrastructure of the odontoblast shows (**Fig. 3.12**) large nucleus which may contain up to 4 nucleoli. Nucleus is situated at basal end. Golgibodies is located centrally. Mitochondria, rough endoplasmic reticulum (RER), ribosome are also distributed throughout the cell body.
- Odontoblasts synthesize mainly type I collagen, proteoglycans. They also secrete sialoproteins, alkaline phosphatase, phosphophoryn (phosphoprotein involved in extracellular mineralizations).
- Irritated odontoblast secretes collagen, amorphous material and large crystals into tubule lumen which result in dentin permeability to irritating substance.

Fibroblasts

- The cells found in greatest numbers in the pulp are fibroblasts.
- These are particularly numerous in the coronal portion of the pulp, where they form the cell-rich zone.
- These are spindle shaped cells which secrete extracellular components like collagen and ground substance (**Fig. 3.13**).
- They also eliminate excess collagen by action of lysosomal enzymes.

Undifferentiated Mesenchymal Cells

Undifferentiated mesenchymal cells are descendants of undifferentiated cells of dental papilla which can dedifferentiate and then redifferentiate into many cells types.

Defence Cells (Fig. 3.14)

- *Histiocytes and macrophages*: They originate from undifferentiated mesenchymal cells or monocytes. They appear as large oval or spindle shaped cells which are involved in the elimination of dead cells, debris, bacteria and foreign bodies, etc.
- *Polymorphonuclear leukocytes*: Most common form of leukocyte is neutrophil, though it is not present in healthy pulp. They are major cell type in micro abscesses formation and are effective at destroying and phagocytising bacteria and dead cells.
- *Lymphocytes*: In normal pulps, mainly T-lymphocytes are found. They are associated with injury and resultant immune response.
- *Mast cells*: On stimulation, degranulation of mast cells release histamine which causes vasodilatation, increased vessel permeability and thus allowing fluids and leukocytes to escape.

Extracellular Components

The extracellular components include fibers and the ground substance of pulp:

Fibers

The fibers are principally type I and type III collagen. Collagen is synthesized and secreted by odontoblasts and fibroblasts.

Ground Substance

It is a structureless mass with gel like consistency forming bulk of pulp.

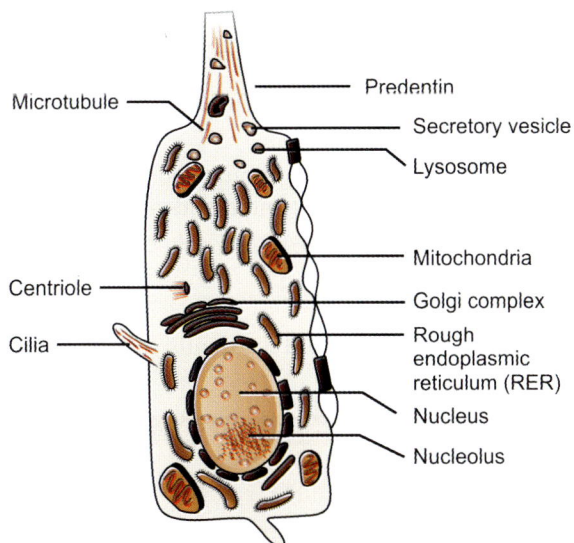

Figure 3.12: Odontoblasts

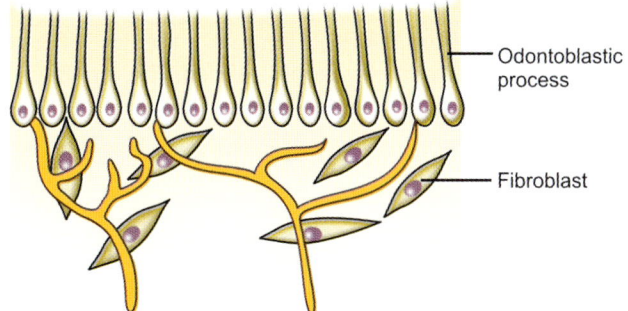

Figure 3.13: Histology of pulp showing fibroblasts

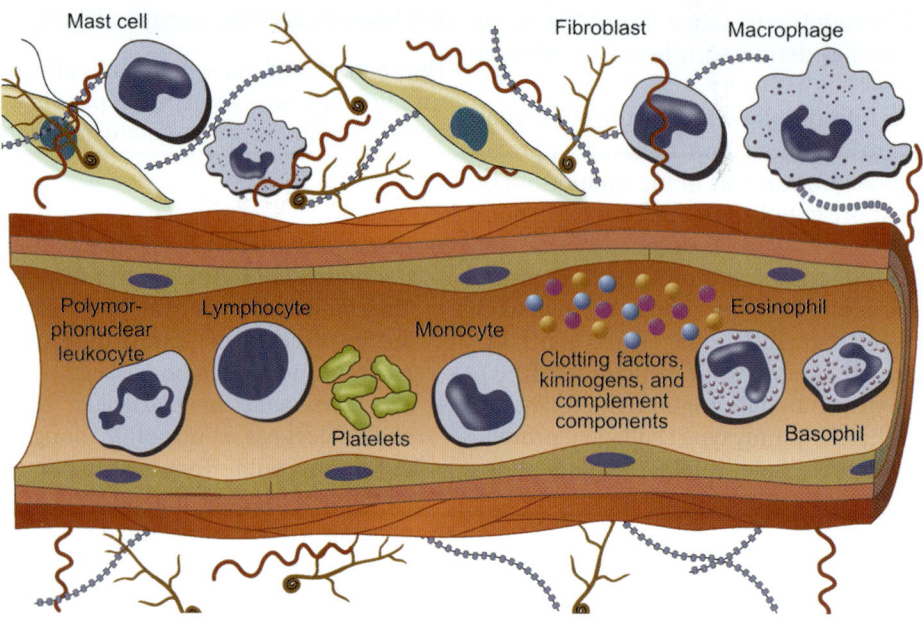

Figure 3.14: Cells taking part in defence of pulp

Components of ground substance are:
- Glycosaminoglycans
- Glycoproteins
- Water.

Functions of ground substance:
- Forms the bulk of the pulp.
- Supports the cells.
- Acts as medium for transport of nutrients from the vasculature to the cells and of metabolites from the cells to the vasculature.

Anatomy of Dental Pulp

Pulp lies in the center of tooth and shapes itself to miniature form of tooth. This space is called pulp cavity which is divided into pulp chamber and root canal (**Fig. 3.15**).

Pulp Chamber

It reflects the external form of enamel at the time of eruption, but anatomy is less sharply defined. The roof of pulp chamber consists of dentin covering the pulp chamber occlusally.

Root Canal

It is that portion of pulp preparation which extends from canal orifice to the apical foramen. The shape of root canal varies with size, shape, number of the roots in different teeth.

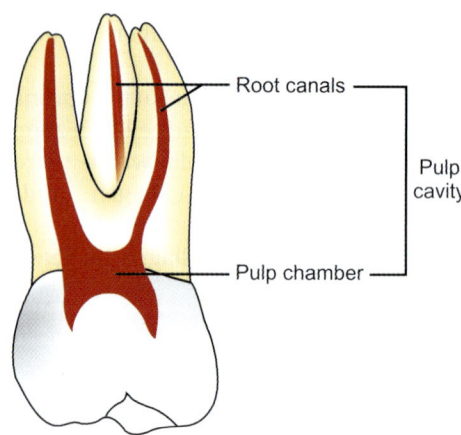

Figure 3.15: Pulp cavity

The apical foramen is an aperture at or near the apex of a root through which nerves and blood vessels of the pulp enter or leave the pulp cavity.

Functions of Pulp

The pulp lives for dentin and the dentin lives by the grace of the pulp.

Basic functions of pulp
➡ Formation of dentin
➡ Nutrition of dentin
➡ Innervation of tooth
➡ Defense of tooth.

Formation of Dentin

It is primary function of pulp both in sequence and importance. Odontoblasts are differentiated from the dental papilla adjacent to the basement membrane of enamel organ which later deposits dentin. Pulp primarily helps in:

- Synthesis and secretion of organic matrix
- Initial transport of inorganic components to newly formed matrix
- Creates an environment favorable for matrix mineralization.

Nutrition of Dentin

Nutrients exchange across capillaries into the pulp interstitial fluid, which in turn travels into the dentin through the network of tubules created by the odontoblasts to contain their processes.

Innervation of Tooth

Through the nervous system, pulp transmits sensations mediated through enamel or dentin to the higher nerve centers. Pulp transmits pain, also senses temperature and touch.

Defense of Tooth

Odontoblasts form dentin in response to injury particularly when original dentin thickness has been compromised as in caries, attrition, trauma or restorative procedure.

Age Changes in Pulp

Pulp like other connective tissues, undergoes changes with time. Pulp can show changes in appearance (morphogenic) and in function (physiologic).

Morphologic Changes

- Continued deposition of intratubular dentin-reduction in tubule diameter
- Reduction in pulp volume due to increase in secondary dentin deposition (**Fig. 3.16**)
- Presence of dystrophic calcification and pulp stones (**Fig. 3.17**)
- Decrease in sensitivity
- Reduction in number of blood vessels.

Physiologic Changes

- Decrease in dentin permeability provides protected environment for pulp-reduced effect of irritants
- Possibility of reduced ability of pulp to react to irritants and repair itself.

PERIRADICULAR TISSUE

Periradicular tissue consists of cementum, periodontal ligament and alveolar bone (**Fig. 3.18**).

Cementum

Cementum can be defined as hard, avascular connective tissue that covers the roots of the teeth. It is light yellow in color and can be differentiated from enamel by its lack of luster and darker hue. It is very permeable to dyes and chemical agents, from the pulp canal and the external root surface.

Cementum consists of approximately 45 to 50 percent inorganic matter and 50 to 55 percent organic matter and water by weight. It is softer than dentin. Sharpey's fibers,

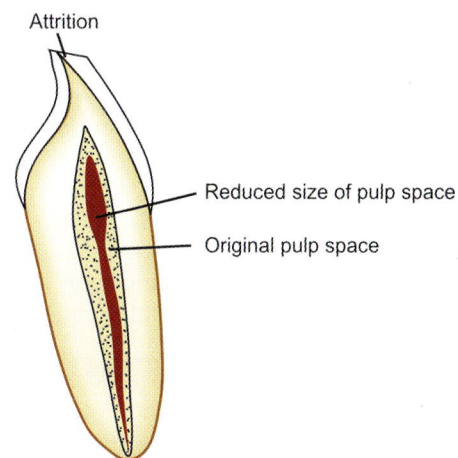

Figure 3.16: Reduced volume of pulp cavity because of secondary dentin deposition

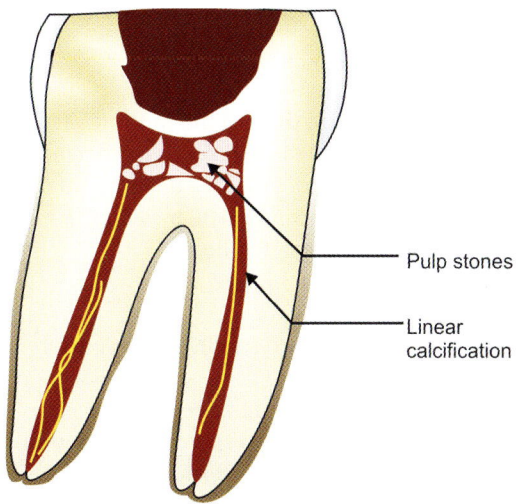

Figure 3.17: Pulp stones

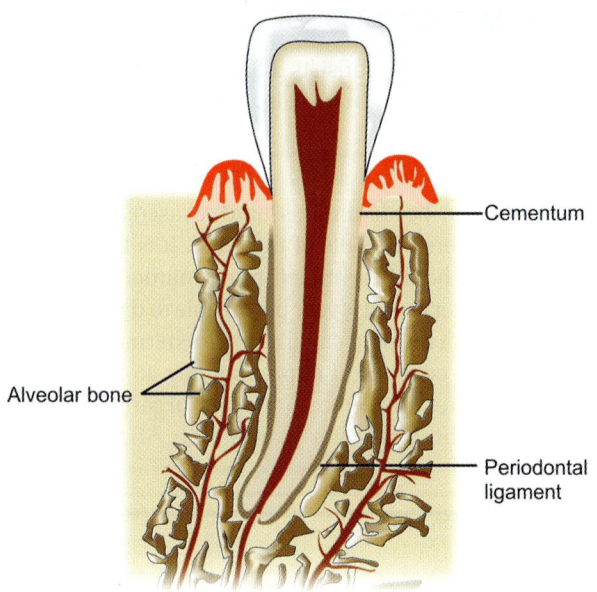

Figure 3.18: Cementum periodontal ligament and alveolar bone

which are embedded in cementum and bone, are the principal collagenous fibers of periodontal ligament.

Composition
➡ Inorganic content—45 to 50 percent (by wt.)
➡ Organic matter—50 to 55 percent (by wt.)
➡ Water.

Types

There are two main types of root cementum:
1. **Acellular (Primary)**
2. **Cellular (Secondary)**

- Acellular cementum:
  - Covers the cervical third of the root.
  - Formed before the tooth reaches the occlusal plane.
  - As the name indicates, it does not contain cells.
  - Thickness is in the range of 30 to 230 µm.
  - Abundance of sharpey's fibers.
  - Main function is anchorage.
- Cellular cementum:
  - Formed after the tooth reaches the occlusal plane.
  - It contains cells.
  - Less calcified than acellular cementum.
  - Sharpey's fibers are present in lesser number as compared to acellular cementum.
  - Mainly found in apical third and interradicular.
  - Main function is adaptation.

Periodontal Ligament

Periodontal ligament is a unique structure as it forms a link between the alveolar bone and the cementum. It is continuous with the connective tissue of the gingiva and communicates with the marrow spaces through vascular channels in the bone. Periodontal ligament houses the fibers, cells and other structural elements like blood vessels and nerves.

Components of periodontal ligament
➡ Periodontal fibers
➡ Cells
➡ Blood vessels
➡ Nerves.

Periodontal Fibers (Fig. 3.19)

The most important component of periodontal ligament is principal fibers. These fibers are composed mainly of collagen type I while reticular fibers are collagen type III. The principal fibers are present in six arrangements.

Horizontal group: These fibers are arranged horizontally emerging from the alveolar bone and attached to the root cementum.

Alveolar crest group: These fibers arise from the alveolar crest in fan-like manner and attach to the root cementum. These fibers prevent the extrusion of the tooth.

Oblique fibers: These fibers make the largest group in the periodontal ligament. They extend from cementum to bone obliquely. They bear the occlusal forces and transmit them to alveolar bone.

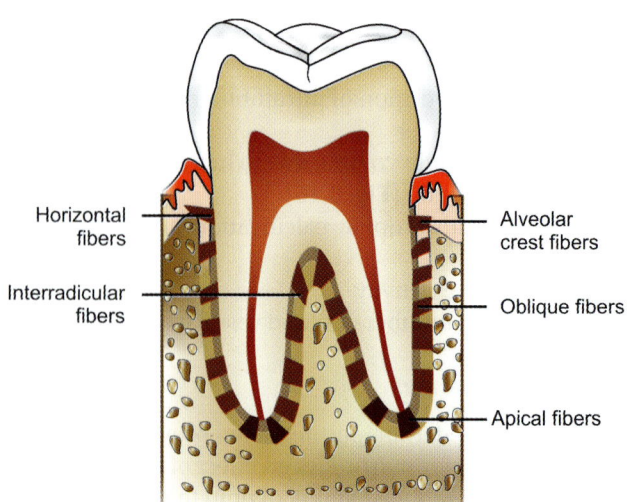

Figure 3.19: Periodontal ligament fibers

Transeptal fibers: These fibers run from the cementum of one tooth to the cementum of another tooth crossing over the alveolar crest.

Apical fibers: These fibers are present around the root apex.

Interradicular fibers: Present in furcation areas of multi-rooted teeth.

Apart from the principal fibers, oxytalan and elastic fibers are also present.

Cells

The cells present in periodontal ligament are:
- Fibroblast
- Macrophages
- Mast cells
- Neutrophil
- Lymphocytes
- Plasma cells
- Epithelial cells rests of Mallassez.

Nerve Fibers

The nerve fibers present in periodontal ligament, is either of myelinated or nonmyelinated type.

Blood Vessels

The periodontal ligament receives blood supply from the gingival, alveolar and apical vessels.

Functions
- It supports the tooth and is suspended in alveolar socket.
- This tissue has very rich blood supply. So, it supplies nutrients to adjoining structures such as cementum, bone and gingiva by way of blood vessels.
- It also provides lymphatic drainage.
- These fibers perform the function of protection absorbing the occlusal forces and transmitting to the underlying alveolar bone.
- The cells of PDL help in formation of surrounding structures such as alveolar bone and cementum.
- The resorptive function is also accomplished with the cells like osteoclasts, cementoclasts and fibroblasts provided by periodontal ligament.

Functions of periodontal ligament
➡ Supportive
➡ Nutritive
➡ Provides lymphatic drainage
➡ Protective
➡ Formative
➡ Resorptive function is accomplished with cells like osteoclasts and cementoclasts.

Alveolar Bone

Bone is specialized connective tissue which comprises of inorganic phases that is very well designed for its role as load bearing structure of the body.

Cells and Intercellular Matrix

- *Cells present in bone are*:
  - Osteocytes
  - Osteoblasts
  - Osteoclasts.
- *Intercellular matrix*: Bone consists of two-third inorganic matter and one-third organic matter. Inorganic matter is composed mainly of minerals calcium and phosphate along with hydroxyapatite, carbonate, citrate, etc. while organic matrix is composed mainly of collagen type I (90%).

Bone consists of two plates of compact bone separated by spongy bone in between. In some area, there is no spongy bone. The spaces between trabeculae of spongy bone are filled with marrow which consists of hemopoitic tissue in early life and fatty tissue latter in life. Bone is a dynamic tissue continuously forming and resorbing in response to functional needs. Both local as well as hormonal factors play an important role in metabolism of bone. In healthy conditions, the crest of alveolar bone lies approximately 2 to 3 mm apical to the cemento-enamel junction but it comes to lie more apically in periodontal diseases. In periapical diseases, it gets resorbed easily.

🔑 Key Points

- Tooth enamel is the hardest and most highly mineralized substance of the body which covers the crown of the tooth.
- Enamel is mainly composed of millions of enamel rods or prisms, sheaths and a cementing inter rod substance. Each rod has a head and tail. The head is directed occlusally and the tail is directed cervically.
- Rods are oriented at prependicular to the dentino-enamel junction. Towards the incisal edge, they become increasingly oblique and are almost vertical at the cusp tips. In the cervical area, in deciduous teeth, rods are inclined incisally or occlusally, while in permanent teeth they are inclined apically.

- The average thickness of enamel at the incisal edges of incisors is 2 mm, at the cusp of premolar and molar from 2.3 to 3.0 mm. Thickness of enamel decreases gradually from cusps or incisal edges to cemento-enamel junction.
- Color of tooth mainly depends upon three factors, color of underlying dentin, thickness of enamel and stains in enamel.
- The translucency of enamel is directly related to degree of mineralization and homogenicity.
- Enamel is brittle, has a high modulus of elasticity and low tensile strength. The specific gravity of enamel is 2.8.
- The color of dentin is slightly darker than enamel and is generally light yellowish in young individuals while it becomes darker with age.
- The dentinal tubules follow a gentle 'S'-shaped curve in the tooth crown and are straighter in the incisal edges, cusps and root areas. The ends of the tubules are perpendicular to dentino-enamel and dentino-cemental junctions.
- Reparative dentin is irregular, with cellular inclusions, and the tubular pattern of the reparative dentin ranges from a irregular to an atubular nature. Reparative dentin matrix has decreased permeability, therefore helping in prevention of diffusion of noxious agents from the tubules.
- Sclerotic dentin occurs due to aging or chronic and mild irritation. Here peritubular dentin becomes wider due to deposition of calcified materials. This area becomes harder, denser, less sensitive and more protective of pulp against irritations.
- In dead tracts, both affected and associated odontoblasts die, resulting in empty dental tubules which appear black when ground sections of dentin are viewed under transmitted light.
- Pulp lies in the center of tooth and shapes itself to miniature form of tooth. This space is called pulp cavity which is divided into pulp chamber and root canal.
- Pulp chamber reflects the external form of enamel at the time of eruption, but anatomy is less sharply defined. The roof of pulp chamber consists of dentin covering the pulp chamber occlusally.
- Root canal is that portion of pulp preparation which extends from canal orifice to the apical foramen. The shape of root canal varies with size, shape, number of the roots in different teeth.

- The apical foramen is an aperture at or near the apex of a root through which nerves and blood vessels of the pulp enter or leave the pulp cavity.
- Periradicular tissue consists of cementum, periodontal ligament and alveolar bone.
- Cementum can be defined as hard, avascular connective tissue that covers the roots of the teeth. It is light yellow in color and can be differentiated from enamel by its lack of luster and darker hue.
- Periodontal ligament forms a link between the alveolar bone and the cementum. It is continuous with the connective tissue of the gingiva and communicates with the marrow spaces through vascular channels in the bone. Periodontal ligament houses the fibers, cells and other structural elements like blood vessels and nerves.

QUESTIONS

1. Describe the composition and structure of enamel in brief. Also discuss the clinical significance of enamel.
2. Write short notes on:
   a. Difference between primary, secondary and tertiary dentin.
   b. Functions of pulp.
   c. Difference between acellular and cellular cementum.
   d. Functions of periodontal ligament.

BIBLIOGRAPHY

1. Brännström M, Aström A. The hydrodynamics of the dentine: its possible relationship to dentinal pain. Int Dent J. 1972;22:219.
2. Butler WT, Ritchie H. The nature and functional significance of dentin extracellular matrix proteins. Int J Den Biol. 1995;39:169.
3. Sasaki T, Garant PR. Structure and organization of odontoblasts. Anat Rec. 1995;245:235.
4. Silverstone LM, et al. Variation in the pattern of acid etching of human dental enamel examined by scanning electron microscopy. Caries Res. 1975;9:373.
5. Warshawsky H, Nanci A. Stereo electron microscopy of enamel crystallites. J Dent Res. 1982;61:1504.
6. Weber DF, Glick PL. Correlative microscopy of enamel prism orientation. Am J Anat. 1975;144:407.
7. Yoshida S, Ohshima H. Distribution and organization of peripheral capillaries in dental pulp and their relationship to odontoblasts. Anat Rec. 1996;245:313.

CHAPTER

4

Physiology of Tooth Form

As we have already discussed that there are different types of teeth (incisors, canines, premolars and molars) which have specific form to perform their functions. In general, teeth perform different functions viz; mastication, esthetics, speech and protection. To perform all these functions to the optimal level, teeth should have normal form and proper alignment (**Fig. 4.1**). Form and alignment of anterior as well as posterior teeth helps in articulation of sounds which has an important effect on phonetics.

For esthetics, anterior teeth also need to have proper form and alignment. Similarly proper form and alignment of teeth help in maintenance of teeth in dental arches along with the development and the protection of the periodontium which support them. Therefore, we should always make an effort to have a dental restoration that would comply with normal form and alignment for periodontal physiology and health.

FUNCTIONS OF TEETH

Functions of teeth
➡ Mastication
➡ Speech
➡ Esthetics
➡ Protection.

Mastication

Teeth play an important part during mastication of food. Every class of teeth serves different functions in the arch. For example:

- Incisors — Cutting and shearing
- Canines — Tearing
- Premolars and molars — Grinding

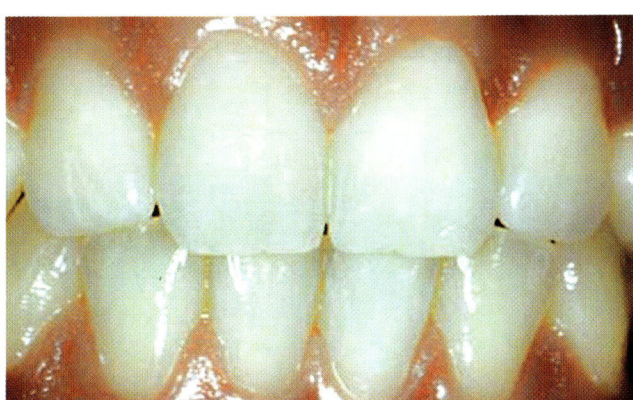

Figure 4.1: Maxillary and mandibular arches showing teeth in proper alignment

Speech

Teeth are important in pronunciation of certain sounds and thus play vital role during speech.

Esthetics

The form, alignment and contour of anterior teeth has been considered to play important role in maintaining esthetics of face.

Protection of Supporting Tissues

Teeth also help in protection of certain supporting tissues such as gingiva, periodontium and alveolar bone.

PHYSIOLOGY OF TOOTH FORM

Before going into detailed description of this topic, we should have an idea about normal periodontium.

Gingiva

Gingiva covers the cervical portion of the crown (**Fig. 4.2**). Anatomically gingiva is divided into three parts:
- Marginal or unattached gingiva
- Attached gingiva
- Gingival sulcus or crevice.

Marginal/Unattached Gingiva

It is border of gingiva encircling the tooth in collar like fashion. It can be differentiated from attached gingiva by free gingival groove.

Attached Gingiva

It is continuous with marginal gingiva. It is usually firm, resilient and tightly bound to underlying periosteum of alveolar bone. The width of attached gingiva vary in different areas of the oral cavity. It is greatest in the incisor region (3.5–4.5 mm in maxilla, 3.3–3.9 mm in mandible) and narrower in posterior segments.

Gingival Sulcus/Crevice

Gingival sulcus is the sulcus present between the free gingiva and tooth. It is lined with sulcular epithelium which is not keratinized. It extends from free gingival margin to functional epithelium. The average depth of gingival sulci is about 1.8 mm.

The health of periodontal tissue is one of the important aspect in restorative dentistry. It is important to note that margins of restorations should be placed supragingivally to preserve the gingival health.

PRESERVATION OF THE PERIODONTIUM

Periodontal health should be optimal before placement of dental restoration. Adequate time should be given after scaling and root planning. Surface gingival appearance and health depends on adequate supragingival plaque control.

Desirable characteristics of gingival health prior to restorative procedure are:
- There should be thin gingival margin closely adapted to enamel
- Color of gingival tissue should be uniform pale pink
- Gingival tissue should be firm and dense
- There should be no bleeding on probing.

Long-term success of restoration and preservation of periodontium depends upon following factors:

Contour

A prominent contour present on the crowns of teeth (on mesial, distal, buccal and lingual surfaces) is of great importance as it protects the gingival tissue against bruising and trauma caused from food. It also prevents the food being packed into gingival sulcus (**Fig. 4.3**).

All protective contours are most functional when the teeth are in proper alignment. The buccal and lingual

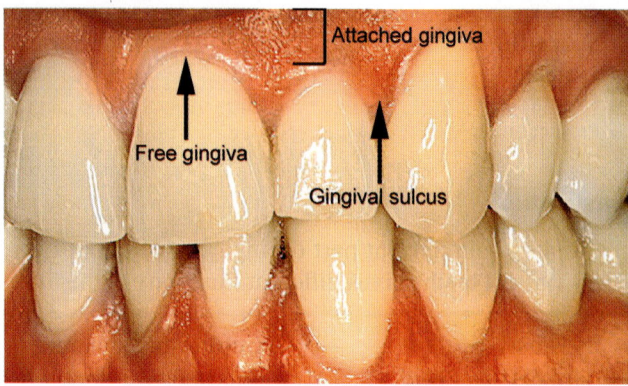

Figure 4.2: Normal gingiva

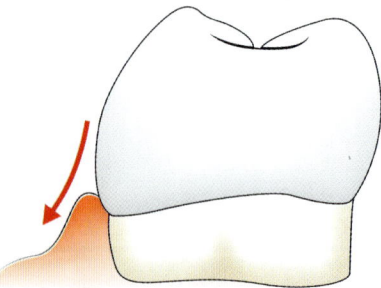

Figure 4.3: Normal contour of a tooth helping in stimulation of gingiva

surfaces of teeth possess some degree of convexity (**Fig. 4.4**) . This convexity is generally located at :

- Cervical third of facial surfaces (all teeth)
- Cervical third of lingual surfaces (anterior teeth)
- Middle third of lingual surfaces (posterior teeth).

Significance of contours

The type of curvature determines the direction in which the food would be passed either in buccal vestibular area or lingual area (**Fig. 4.5**). The two clinical conditions, usually seen in practice are:

➡ *Over-contouring*: This type of contouring is considered more health hazard to periodontal tissues than under contouring as it enhances the supragingival and subgingival plaque accumulation at the overcontoured crowns (**Fig. 4.6**). These are commonly seen in interproximal restorations, cast restorations and pontics.

➡ *Under-contouring (Fig. 4.7)*: It means too little contouring. Consequences of under-contouring are food impaction and trauma to attachment apparatus.

Height of Epithelial Attachment

The epithelial attachment seals the soft tissue to the tooth. This is unique system which is capable of adjusting normal physiologic changes but vulnerable to physical/pathological injury. The teeth may be injured by careless probing during examination, improper sealing and in tooth preparation techniques.

The height of normal gingival tissue, mesially and distally on approximating teeth is directly dependent on the heights of the epithelial attachment on these teeth. Normal attachment of tissue follows the curvature of cementoenamel junction if teeth are in normal alignment and in contact (**Fig. 4.8**).

The extent of curvature usually depends upon two main factors:

1. Location of contact area above the crown cervix

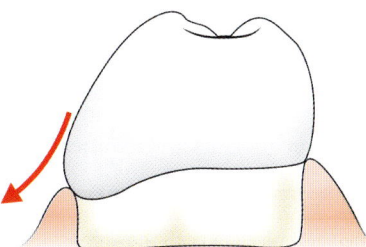

Figure 4.6: Overcontoured surface deflecting the food away from gingiva resulting in its understimulation

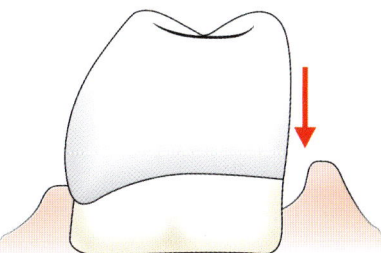

Figure 4.7: Undercontoured tooth results in food impaction and irritation to gingiva

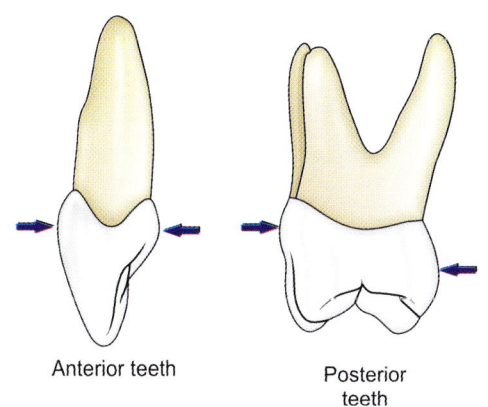

Anterior teeth   Posterior teeth

Figure 4.4: Height of contour

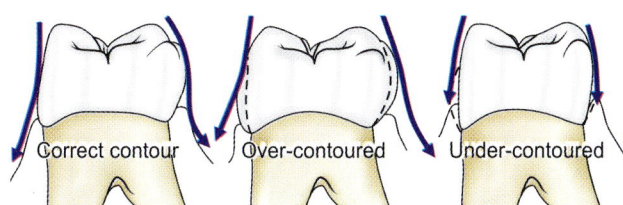

Correct contour   Over-contoured   Under-contoured

Figure 4.5: Type of curvature determines the direction in which food is deflected, i.e. buccal or lingual area

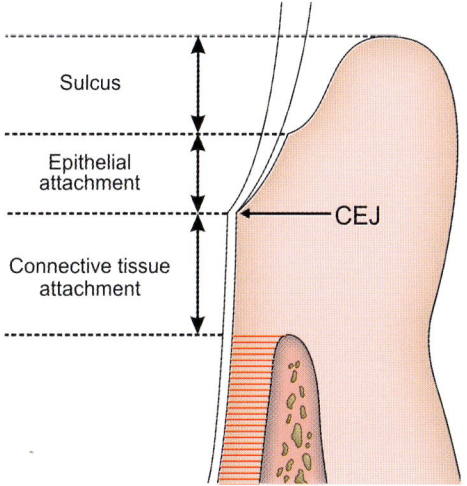

Figure 4.8: Height of epithelial attachment

2. Diameter of crown faciolingually or buccolingually.

Usually crowns of anterior teeth show greatest curvature while premolars and molars have rather uniform but slight curvatures.

Significance of epithelial attachment
To avoid possibility of injuring the mesial and distal periodontal attachment during tooth preparation, height of attachment must be ascertained by careful probing and by the continuous observation of landmarks during the operation.

Marginal Ridges

Marginal ridges are defined as rounded borders of enamel which form the mesial and distal margins of occlusal surfaces of premolars and molars and mesial and distal margins of lingual surfaces of the incisors and canines (**Fig. 4.9**).

Significance of marginal ridges
➡ Help in balancing of teeth in both the arches
➡ Improve the efficiency of mastication
➡ Prevent food impaction in interproximal areas.

During restoration, marginal ridges should be restored in two planes, i.e. buccolingually and cervico-occlusally and also restore adjacent marginal ridges at the same height. One should always try to the level best to avoid common faults in restoration of marginal ridges (**Fig. 4.10**).

Embrasures

When two teeth are in contact with each other, their curvatures adjacent to contact areas form spillway spaces called embrasures (**Fig. 4.11**). In other words, embrasures can be defined as V-shaped spaces that originate at proximal contact areas between adjacent teeth and are named for the direction towards which they radiate. These are:

- *Labial/buccal and lingual embrasures:* These are spaces that widen out from the area of contact labially or buccally and lingually (**Fig. 4.12**).
- *Incisal/occlusal embrasures:* These are spaces that widen out from area of contact incisally/occlusally (**Figs 4.11 and 4.13**).

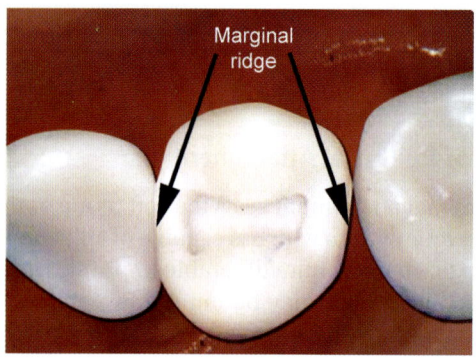

Figure 4.9: Marginal ridges

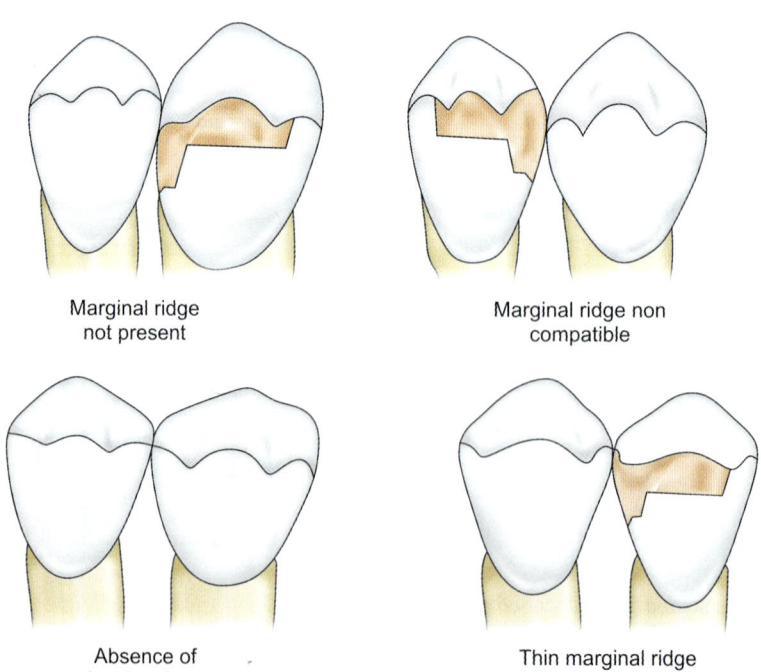

Marginal ridge not present

Marginal ridge non compatible

Absence of occlusal embrasure

Thin marginal ridge

Figure 4.10: Common faults in the restoration of marginal ridge

- *Gingival embrasure:* These are the spaces that widen out from the area of contact gingivally (**Fig. 4.14**).

Functions of Embrasure

- Provides a spillway for food during mastication
- Prevents food for being forced through contact area.

Significance of embrasure

The correct relationships of embrasures, marginal ridges, contours, grooves of adjacent and opposing teeth provide for escape of food from the occlusal surfaces during mastication (**Fig. 4.15**).

→ In case embrasure size is decreased/absent, then additional forces are created in teeth and supporting structures during mastication (**Fig. 4.16**).

→ If embrasure size is enlarged, they provide little protection to supporting structures as food is being forced into interproximal space by opposing cusp.

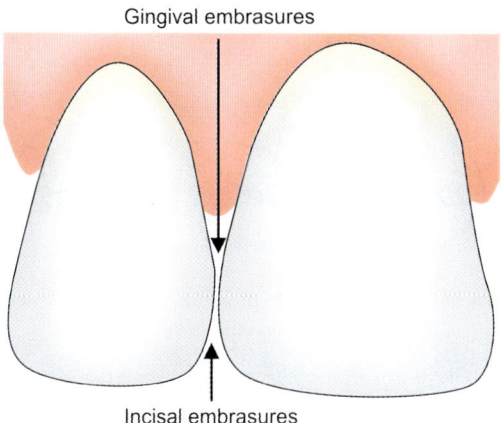

Gingival embrasures

Incisal embrasures

Figure 4.11: Embrasures/Spillway spaces

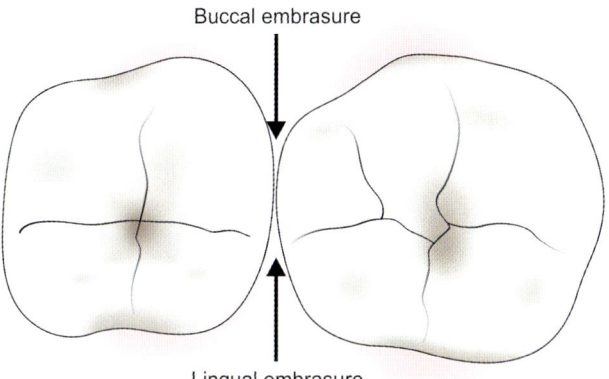

Buccal embrasure

Lingual embrasure

Figure 4.12: Buccal and lingual embrasure

Interproximal Spaces (Fig. 4.17)

Interproximal space is triangular shaped area that is usually filled by gingival tissue. In this triangular area, the base is formed by alveolar process, the sides are proximal

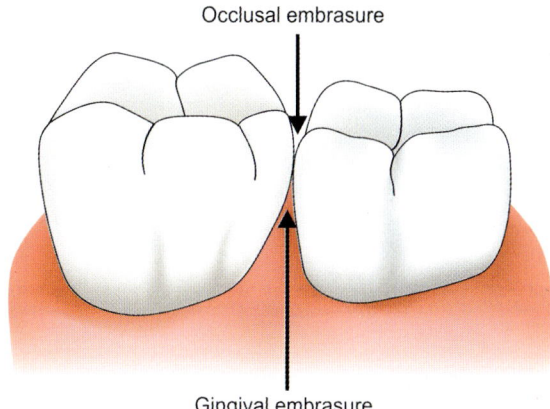

Occlusal embrasure

Gingival embrasure

Figure 4.13: Occlusal embrasure

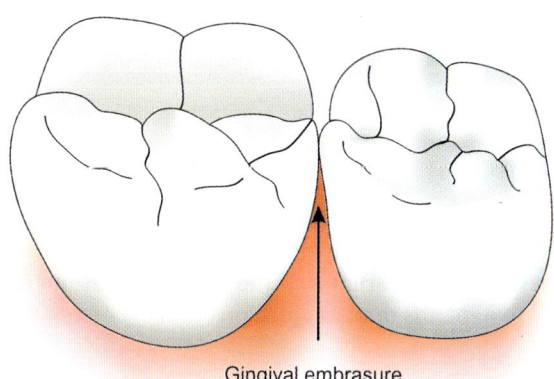

Gingival embrasure

Figure 4.14: Gingival embrasure

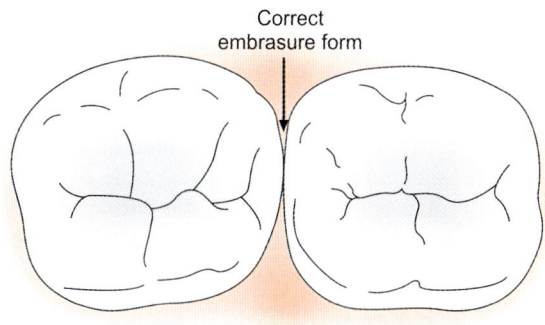

Correct embrasure form

Figure 4.15: Correct embrasure resulting in stimulation of supporting tissues

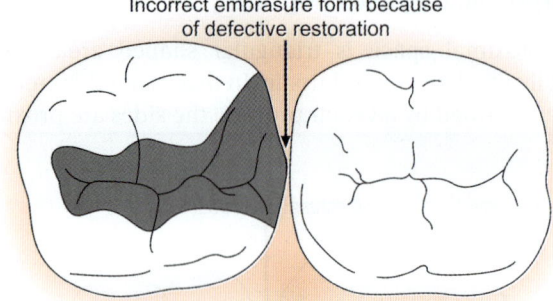

Figure 4.16: Improper contour of restoration resulting in improper embrasure form

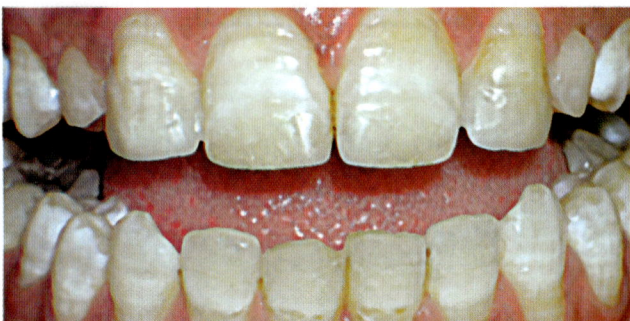

Figure 4.17: Interproximal space is triangular shaped area filled by gingival tissue

1. Labial/buccal aspect.
2. Incisal/occlusal aspect.

Labial/buccal aspect: It shows the relative position of contact area cervicoincisally or cervico-occlusally (**Fig. 4.21**).

Incisal/occlusal aspect (Fig. 4.22): It shows the relative position of contact area labiolingually or buccolingually.

Importance of proper contact relation:

➡ Stabilize the dental arches by combined anchorage effect of all the teeth.
➡ Serves to keep food away from packing between the teeth.
➡ Protect interdental papillae.

Improper proximal contact area (Fig. 4.23) can result in:

➡ Food impaction
➡ Periodontal disease
➡ Carious lesions
➡ Mobility of teeth.

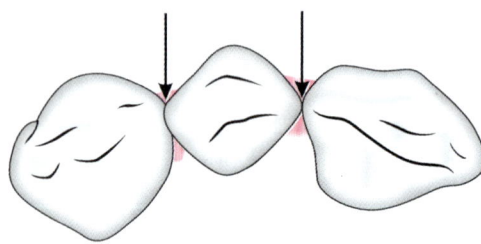

Figure 4.18: In anterior teeth, proximal contact area is located at incisal third and is centered faciolingually

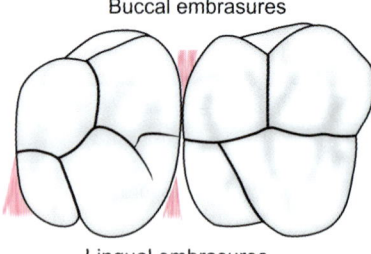

Figure 4.19: In posterior teeth, contact area is placed more in buccal 1/3rd

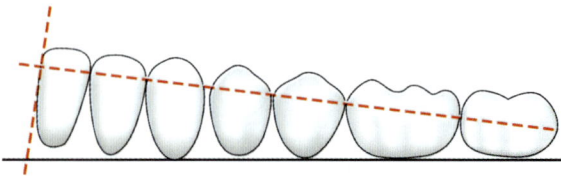

Figure 4.20: Mesial contact area of a tooth is more occlusally placed than the distal contact area

surfaces of contacting teeth and apex is area of contact. This area usually varies with the form of teeth in contact and also depends upon relative position of contact areas.

Proximal Contact Areas

The periodontal importance of proximal contact areas was first observed by Hirschfeld long ago. Each tooth in the arch has two contacting members adjoining it, one on mesial side and other on distal side. Except third molar, positive contact relation should take mesially and distally of one tooth with another in each arch.

Proximal contact area denotes area of proximal height of contour of the mesial or distal surface of a tooth that contacts its adjacent tooth in the same arch. In maxillary and mandibular central incisors, the proximal contact area is located in incisal third (**Fig. 4.18**). Proceeding posteriorly from the incisor region through all remaining teeth, proximal contact area lies near the junction of incisal and middle third or in middle third (**Figs 4.19 and 4.20**).

Proximal contact areas must be observed from two different aspects:

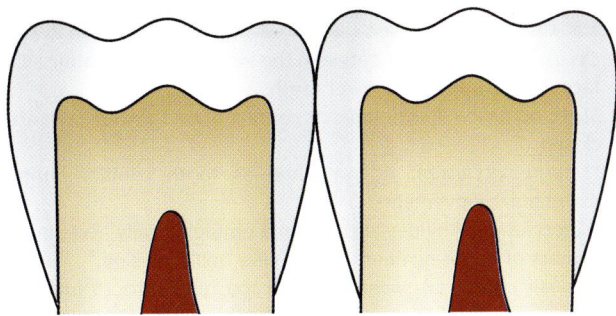

Figure 4.21: Cervicoocclusal contour

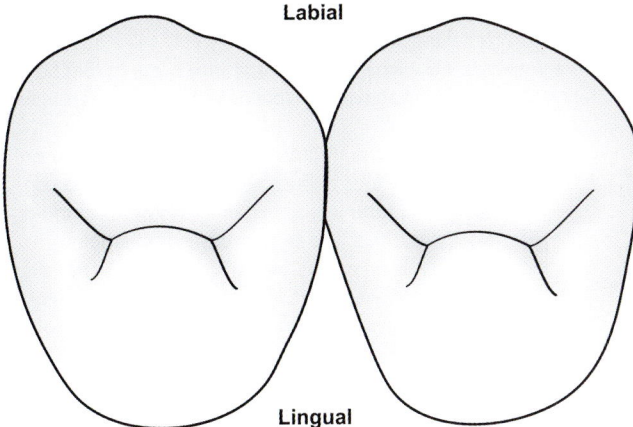

Figure 4.22: Labiolingual contour

Trauma From Occlusion (TFO)

Periodontal tissue injury caused by repeated occlusal forces that exceeds the physiological limits of tissue tolerance is called trauma from occlusion (TFO).

The periodontium tries to accommodate the forces exerted on the crown of tooth. The adaptive capacity of periodontium may vary from one person to another and may be different in different tooth at same time.

Types of Trauma from Occlusion

Types of trauma from occlusion based on etiology:
- *Primary trauma from occlusion*: Usually results when occlusion is primary etiological factor, for example:
  - Insertion of new restoration placed above the line of occlusion
  - Movement or extrusion of teeth into spaces created by unreplaced missing tooth.
- *Secondary trauma from occlusion*: Usually results when excessive force is applied on a tooth with bone loss and inadequate alveolar bone support.

Type of trauma from occlusion based on chronicity:
- *Acute*: Usually results from abrupt change in occlusal biting such as on hard object or placement of new restoration high above the occlusal line
- *Chronic*: Usually results from gradual change in occlusion such as attrition, extrusion of teeth, parafunctional habits such as bruxism.

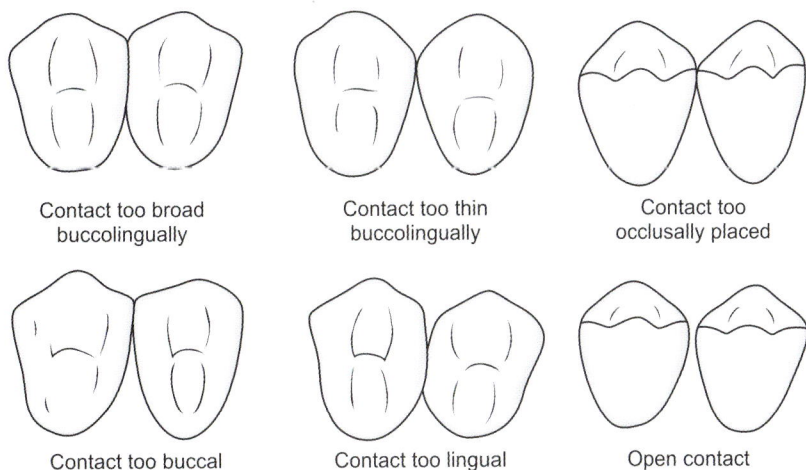

Contact too broad buccolingually

Contact too thin buccolingually

Contact too occlusally placed

Contact too buccal

Contact too lingual

Open contact

Figure 4.23: Common faults in restoration of contact area

Clinical Findings

- Tooth mobility
- Fremitus (Palpable vibration of the roots of the teeth that close into contact)
- Sensitivity of teeth to pressure/percussion
- Pathologic migration of teeth
- Open contacts leading to food impaction
- Occlusal wear leading to attrition
- Temporomandibular joint symptoms
- Muscle spasm.

Radiographic Findings of TFO

- Root resorption in some cases
- Widening of periodontal ligament
- Vertical bone loss
- Thickening of lamina dura.

Diagnosis of premature contacts

- Study casts
- Palpation of suspected tooth
- Radiographs
- Articulating paper markings
- Modelling wax impression
- Visual examination.

Management of TFO

In order to correct adverse effects of occlusion, occlusal adjustment is mandatory to achieve the satisfactory result.

Occlusal adjustment can be done by grooving, spheroiding and pointing.

Grooving: Means restoring the depth of developmental grooves which has become shallow due to attrition.

Spheroiding: Means to reduce premature contacts and restoring original contour of the tooth.

Pointing: Means to restore cusp point contours.

Occlusal adjustment is done to improve the masticatory efficiency, speech problems, and to provide comfort to temporomandibular problems. It also helps in establishment and maintenance of stable and functional occlusion.

OCCLUSION AND OPERATIVE DENTISTRY

The term "occlusion" means the contact relationship of opposing teeth in function or parafunction.

An ideal occlusion is defined as the most dynamic position, arrangement and relationship of one tooth with other tooth, of one arch with opposite arch with the base of skull so as to perform optimal functions of mastication, phonetics and esthetics maintaining the integrity and longevity of individual tooth and the stomatognathic system.

Definitions

- *Occlusion*: Any contact between the incising or masticating surfaces of the upper and lower teeth.
- *Static occlusion*: It is defined as contact of teeth when jaws are closed.
- *Dynamic occlusion*: It is defined as tooth contact during mandibular movements.
- *Malocclusion*: Any deviation from a physiologically acceptable contact of opposing dentition is called "malocclusion."
- *Occlusal contact*: Any contacting or touching of tooth surfaces is called occlusal contact. Unmodified, contact should involve a normal, nonpathologic touching of tooth surfaces. Harmful occlusal contacts can occur in following forms:
  - *Parafunctional (nonfunctional) contacts*: Normal tooth contacts that have been subjected to excessive use through bruxism, clenching, etc. (**Fig. 4.24**).
  - *Interferences*: Abnormal contacts that may occur in functional or parafunctional activity. Following occlusal interferences are usually present:
    - i. *Occlusal prematurity*: It is an occlusal contact that interrupts the harmonious closure of the teeth along the centric relation arc. It can result in damage to periodontium, masticatory muscles, and temporomandibular joint.
    - ii. *Occlusal interference*: It is an occlusal contact that disrupts the smooth excursive movements of teeth against each other. Presence of occlusal interference can result in disclusion of the anterior guidance.
    - iii. *Working side interference*: It is an interference present between posterior teeth on the side of the dental arches to which the mandible is moving laterally in excursion. It usually occurs when stamp cusp moves against a shear cusp.
    - iv. *Nonworking side interference*: It is an interference which occurs between posterior teeth on the side of the dental arches away from which the mandible is moving laterally in excursion. It occurs when stamp cusp moves against stamp cusp.
    - v. *Protrusive interference*: An interference between posterior teeth on either side of the dental arches caused by a protrusive movement of the mandible is called protrusive interference.
- *Hyperfunction*: An abnormal amount of a normal or parafunctional activity is called hyperfunction.
- *Bruxism*: It is parafunctional grinding of teeth which generally takes place during sleep and patient is not aware of the condition.
- *Bruxomania*: It is the condition which occurs during the day time and patient is conscious about it.
- *Clenching*: The exertion of force in a static tooth-to-tooth relationship is called clenching.
- *Centric occlusion*: In centric occlusion, there is maximum intercuspation of upper and lower teeth when jaws are closed. It is in harmony with the neuromuscular mechanism.
- *Centric relation*: This is maxilla to mandible relationship in which the condyles are in most retruded position in the glenoid fossa, regardless of any tooth to tooth relationship. Here the condyles are in the most superior position they can attain in the glenoid fossa. If a healthy joint is correctly positioned and aligned in centric relation, it can resist maximum loading in function with no sign of tension or tenderness.

➡ *Maximum intercuspation*: It is the maximum occlusal contact or intercuspation irrespective of condylar position (**Fig. 4.25**). This type of contact may or may not occur on the path of the centric relation closure.

Angle's Classification for Interarch Relationship

It describes the position of mesiobuccal cusp of maxillary first molar in relation to mandibular first molar. This can be of following types:

Class I (Neutrocclusion)

It is normal anteroposterior relationships of the jaws, as indicated by correct intercuspation of maxillary and mandibular molars. Here the mesiobuccal cusp of maxillary first molar falls on the mesiobuccal groove of mandibular first molar (**Fig. 4.26**). It can be associated with possible crowding and rotation of teeth elsewhere. In the absence of first molars, the cuspids may be used for reference.

Class II (Distocclusion)

Here the mandibular dental arch is posterior to the maxillary arch in one or both lateral segments. In this the mesiobuccal cusp of maxillary first molar is located in the buccal embrasure between mandibular first molar and second premolar. It is of the following types:

- ***Division 1:*** Unilaterally or bilaterally distal retrusion with narrow maxillary arch and protruding maxillary incisors (**Fig. 4.27**).
- ***Division 2:*** Unilaterally or bilaterally distal retrusion with normal or square-shaped maxillary arch, retruded maxillary central incisors, labially malposed maxillary lateral incisors, and an excessive vertical overlap (**Fig. 4.28**).

Class III (Mesiocclusion)

In this malocclusion, the mandibular arch is anterior to the maxillary arch in one or both lateral segments. Here the mesiobuccal cusp of maxillary first molar fits into distobuccal groove of mandibular first molar. In this type, mandibular incisors are usually in anterior reverse occlusion (**Fig. 4.29**).

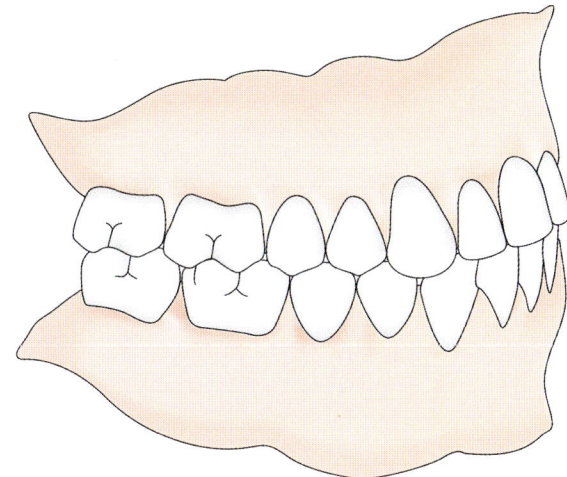

Figure 4.26: Angle's class I occlusion

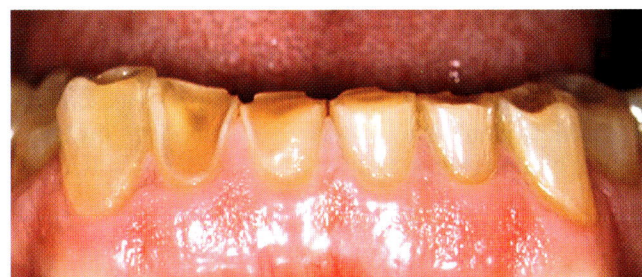

Figure 4.24: Attrition of teeth resulting from excessive occlusal forces

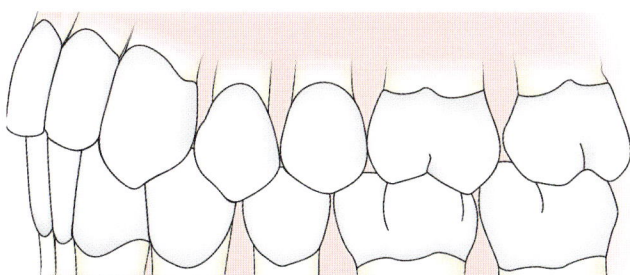

Figure 4.25: Upper and lower teeth during maximum intercuspation

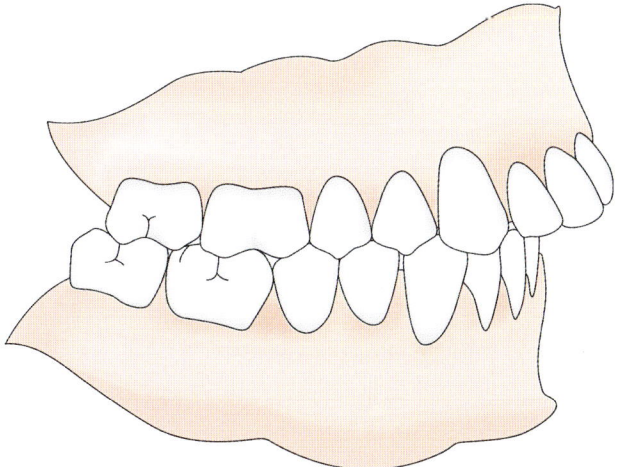

Figure 4.27: Angle's class II div. I malocclusion

Occlusal Schemes

Mutually Protected Occlusion/Anterior Protected Occlusion/Posterior Disclusion

It is an occlusal arrangement in which the posterior teeth contact in maximum intercuspation but not in lateral or protrusive movements. Here the anterior teeth protect posteriors teeth during eccentric contacts. The posterior teeth protect the anterior teeth in maximum intercuspation. Canines are the only teeth contacting in lateral movement and the incisors the only teeth contacting in protrusive movement in this type of occlusion (**Fig. 4.30**).

Unilaterally Balanced Occlusion/Group Function Articulation

In this type of occlusion during lateral excursions, the posterior teeth on the working side contact as a group simultaneously with contact on the anterior guidance. The effect of this is to distribute lateral forces to multiple teeth rather than a single cuspid or other anterior guiding teeth. Group function occlusion is useful when anterior teeth are weak or nonfunctional.

Bilaterally Balanced Occlusion

This type of occlusion is seen in dentures where there is group contact between posterior teeth simultaneously with contact on the anterior guidance in both working and balancing excursions. This type of occlusion provides stability for dentures in excursive movement.

Various Mandibular Movements During Function

Interocclusal Records

A record of the positional relation of the teeth or jaws to each other is referred to as interocclusal record.

Freeway Space or Interocclusal Space

It is the difference between the physiologic rest position and the vertical dimension of occlusion. It is measured when the mandible is in rest position. In different patients it varies. Position of the head is also responsible for the variation in the measurement.

Physiologic rest position: It is the position attained by the mandible when the head is in an upright position, the muscles are in equilibrium in tonic contraction, and the condyles are in a neutral unstrained position. It is not a reproducible position.

Envelope of motion: The three dimensional space circumscribed by mandibular border movements forms the envelope of motion (**Fig. 4.31**).

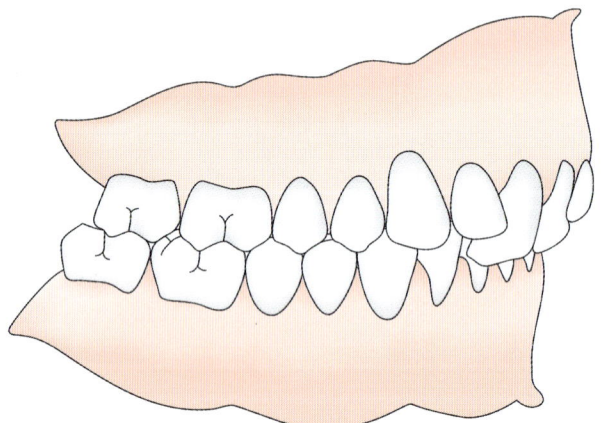

Figure 4.28: Angle's class II div. II malocclusion

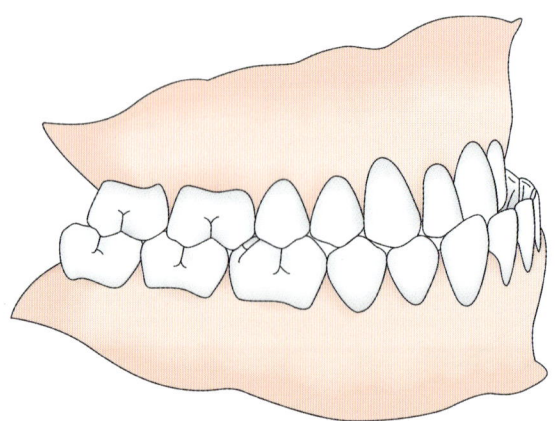

Figure 4.29: Angle's class III malocclusion

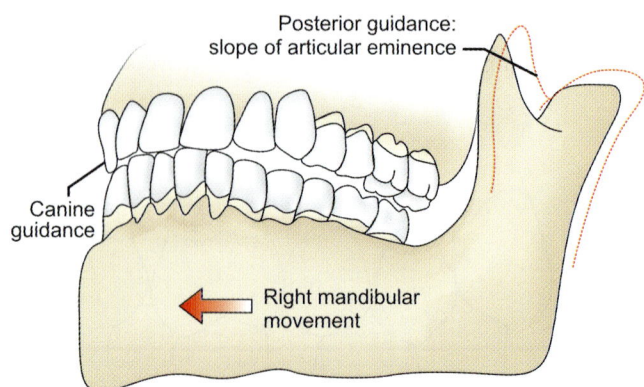

Figure 4.30: Canine guided occlusion showing that canines are only teeth contacting during lateral movement

Envelope of function: The three dimensional space contained within the envelope of motion that defines mandibular movement during masticatory function, phonation forms the envelope of function.

Anterior guidance: It is the anterior determinant of mandibular movement. Anterior guidance in the natural dentition can be defined as the dynamic relationship of the mandibular anterior teeth against the maxillary anterior teeth through all ranges of function.

Condylar guidance: It determines the pathway of the condyles in the temporomandibular joints. It is influenced by shape of the articulating surfaces, the ligaments and muscles. Condylar guidance is the posterior determinant of mandibular movement. It allows a range of motion limited only by the bones, ligaments, and muscles.

Axis of condylar rotation: It is the conceptual axis through the mandibular condyles around which the mandible rotates. An actual mandibular movement may involve rotation about all three axis combined with translation. These are:
- *Vertical:* A vertical axis through one "rotating" condyle imposes an "orbiting" function upon the other condyle.

Since the orbiting condyle must descend the eminence, there can be no pure rotation about a vertical axis.
- *Horizontal:* This axis passes through both condyles and is the axis of opening and the centric relation axis.
- *Sagittal:* This axis passes horizontally through the rotating condyle in an anteroposterior direction. It takes place because of the downward component of movement by the orbiting condyle.

Hinge axis: An imaginary line between the mandibular condyles around which the mandible can rotate without translatory movement is the hinge axis. In other words, the hinge axis is a stationary line drawn between the condyles when they are in the centric relation position.

Hinge movement: Opening or closing movement of the mandible on the hinge axis forms the hinge movement (**Fig. 4.32**).

Translation: Translation is the motion of a rigid body in which a straight line passing through any two of its particles always remain parallel to its initial position (**Fig. 4.33**).

Christensen's phenomenon: Phenomenon of creation of a space between the posterior teeth bilaterally during protrusion or on the balancing side during lateral excursions is called as Christensen's phenomenon.

Excursion: Any mandibular movement produced by movement of the condyles away from their most retruded position is excursion. It is associated with transitory movement of one or both condyles. The pattern of tooth contact in excursions defines the occlusal scheme.

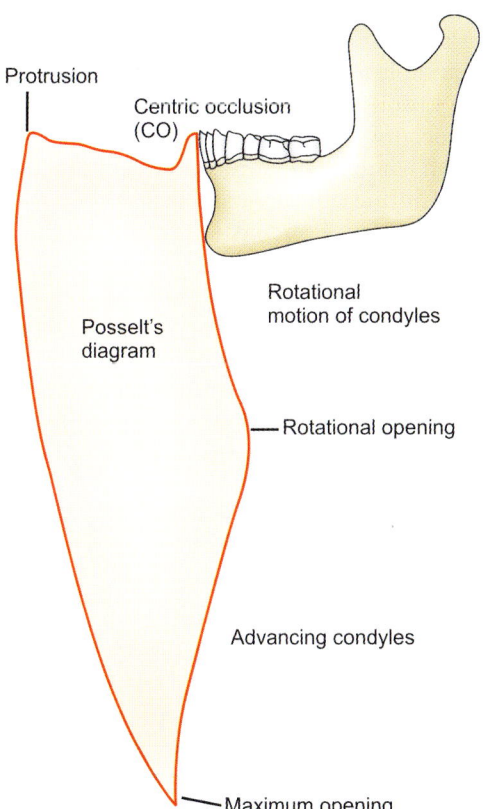

Figure 4.31: Envelope of motion showing mandibular motion

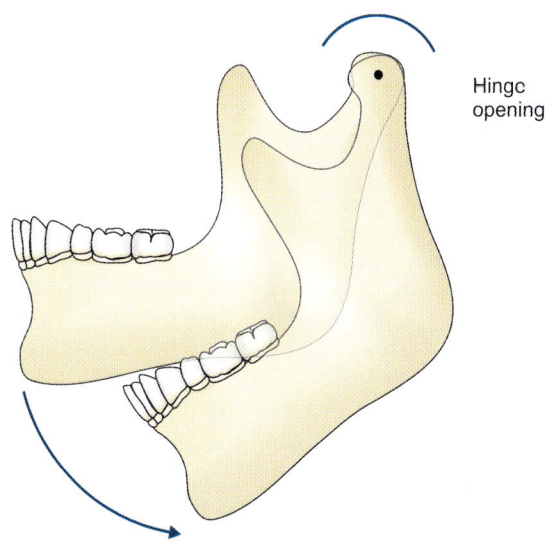

Figure 4.32: Hinge movement

- *Lateral excursion (**Fig. 4.34**):*
  - *Working side:* The lateral segment of a dentition toward which the mandible is moved is working side. In lateral excursions, it is the side of rotating condyle.
  - *Nonworking side:* The side opposite the working side is called nonworking side.

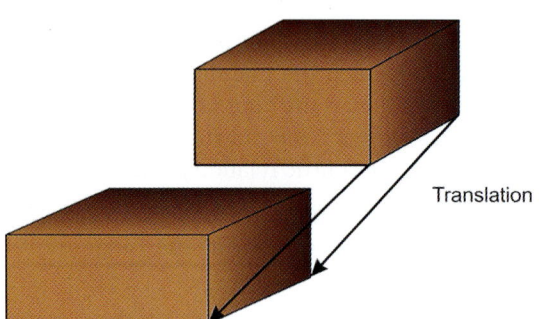

Figure 4.33: Translation motion

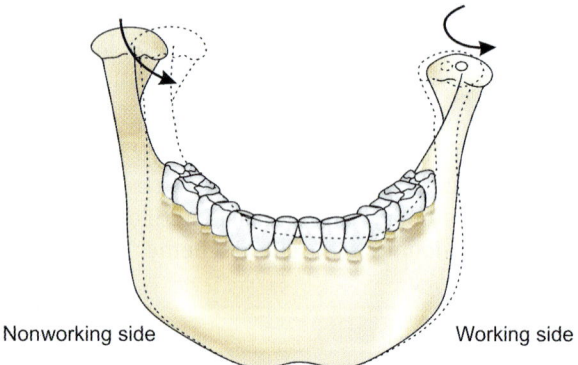

Figure 4.34: Lateral movement of mandible showing working and nonworking side

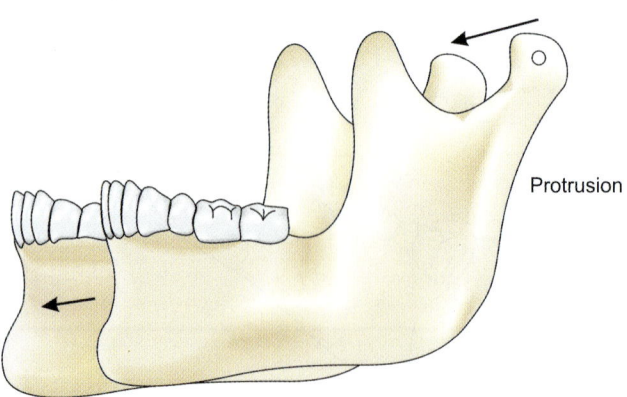

Figure 4.35: Mandible in protrusion

- *Protrusion:* A position of the mandible anterior to centric relation is protrusion (**Fig. 4.35**).
- *Lateral protrusion:* It is the protrusive movement of the mandible in which there is a lateral component.

Features of an Ideal Occlusion

Many concepts have been given to explain the ideal occlusion. Ideal occlusion is not observed in any person because there is wide variation in size of the jaws and arrangement of teeth within the jaws. Since masticatory system has high adaptability, it can show wide range of differences in jaw size and tooth alignment. But despite of great adaptability, any change in tooth contacts often brought about by operative procedures can result in patient discomfort, and minor discrepancies in vertical dimension can produce pain in temporomandibular joint, which may require further correction.

Since restored occlusal surface has important effects on the number and location of occlusal contacts. The occlusion should be restored in both dynamic and static conditions. Therefore, the clinician must understand the precise details of occlusion.

An ideal occlusion has following characteristic features:

- When the teeth come in contact in centric relation and in centric occlusion, then there should be firm and stable jaw relationship.
- The mandible should freely move forward.
- During various excursions, gliding of occlusal contacts should occur smoothly.
- No tooth should get any thrust either buccally or lingually during centric closure.
- Occlusal guidance should always be on the working side.
- Soft tissue should be free of any kind of strain or trauma.
- The center of the disk of the TMJ should bear even pressure on both the sides when the jaws are closed in centric relation and the teeth are in centric occlusion.
- There should be no restriction of the gliding between the centric relation and centric occlusion.

Factors of Occlusion Affecting Operative Dentistry

Important features of posterior cusps:

- Cusps are blunt, rounded or pointed projections of crowns of the teeth which are separated by distinct developmental grooves (**Fig. 4.36**).
- Cusps have four cusp ridges or slopes and the name of cusp ridge is derived from the direction of incline of cusp. For example, lingual cusp ridge is the ridge, which occurs on lingual surface of cusp.

- There are inner ridges of cusps which are wider at base and narrower when they reach at cusp tip, and are termed as triangular ridges (named so because the slopes of each side of ridge are inclined to resemble two sides of a triangle). Triangular ridges are named according to the cusps to which they belong.

Supporting Cusp/Stamp Cusp or Centric Holding Cusp (Fig. 4.37)

A centric holding cusp is that which ideally occludes along the line of the central grooves of opposing teeth. Normally, these are the lingual cusps on the maxillary and buccal on the mandibular teeth.

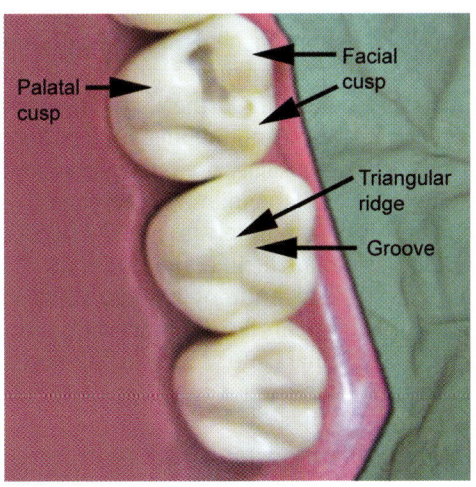

Figure 4.36: Molar showing cusps and grooves

Five common characteristic features of supporting cusps are:

1. Contact the opposing tooth in centric occlusion
2. Lie nearer to the faciolingual center of the tooth in comparison to nonsupporting cusps
3. Support the vertical dimension of the face
4. Outer incline has the potential for contact
5. Have broader, more rounded cusp ridges.

Significance of nonsupporting cusps
➡ During mastication, the maximum forces and longest duration of contact occur at centric occlusion. Since they also prevent drifting and passive eruption of the teeth, they are also known as centric holding cusps.
➡ During restorations of teeth, the supporting cusps should not contact the opposing tooth, because it can cause lateral deflection of tooth.

Nonsupporting Cusp/Noncentric Cusp/Gliding Cusps (Fig. 4.38)

These cusps overlap the opposing tooth without contacting the tooth. They are usually present on buccal cusps of maxillary teeth and lingual cusps of mandibular teeth.

Significance nonsupporting
Nonsupporting cusps keep soft tissue such as tongue and cheek away from teeth and prevent self-injury to these soft tissues during chewing.

Alignment of Teeth and Dental Arches

In both mandible and maxilla, the cusps are aligned in a parabolic curve. The maxillary cusps overlap the

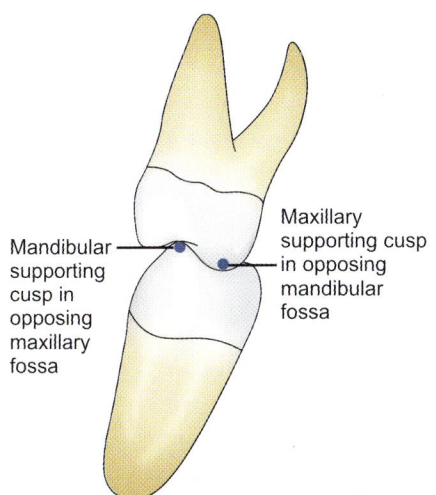

Figure 4.37: Maxillary and mandibular supporting cusps

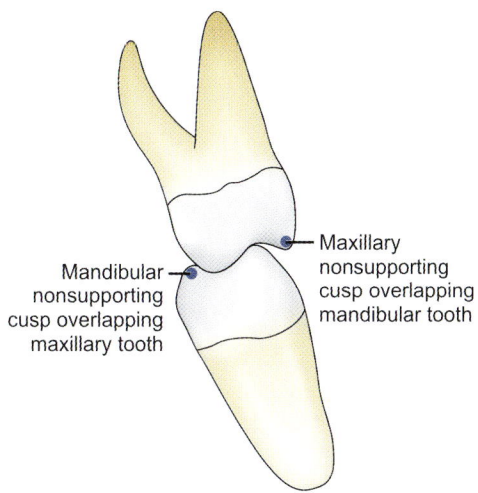

Figure 4.38: Maxillary and mandibular nonsupporting cusps

mandibular cusps during maximum intercuspation because maxillary arch is frequently wider and larger than mandibular arch. To evaluate the arch form, two imaginary curved lines are drawn over the teeth. The alignments of functioning cusps or fossae are also identified by these curved lines. Facial occlusion line is drawn on the left side of arches, this is an imaginary line which connects the mandibular facial cusps (**Fig. 4.39**). This line coincides with an imaginary line connecting the maxillary central fossae. In the similar way, on the right side, maxillary palatal occlusion line and mandibular central fossae line coincides (**Fig. 4.40**).

When the mandibular arches are in complete contact with maxillary arches, mandibular facial occlusion line coincides with maxillary central fossae and the maxillary palatal occlusion line coincides with mandibular central fossae line.

Interarch Tooth Relationships

The interarch relationship of an individual tooth can be of following two types:
1. Surface contact
2. Cusp and fossa apposition.

- **Surface contact:** It occurs in incisor teeth in which the incisal edges of mandibular incisors contact palatal surfaces of maxillary incisors during function. This type of contact results in overjet (horizontal overlap) and overbite (vertical overlap) (**Fig. 4.41**).

  Any variation in size of maxilla and mandible can result in variations in incisor relationships. These can be openbite, deepbite or crossbite (**Figs 4.42A to C**).

- **Cusp and fossa apposition (Figs 4.43A and B):** In a normal occlusion, the mesiolingual cusp of maxillary first molar falls in central fossa of mandibular first molar. This relationship helps in mastication and acts as a stabilizer in alignment of teeth. The distolingual cusps of maxillary molars lie in the distal triangular fossae and marginal ridge of mandibular molars. Similarly the palatal cusps of maxillary premolars lie in contact with triangular fossae of mandibular premolars.

  In the similar manner, the mesiobuccal cusps of mandibular molars lie in contact with distal fossa, or marginal ridge surrounding it and distobuccal cusps of mandibular molars lie in contact with central fossae of maxillary molars. But these cusp fossa relationships can be changed in cases of posterior crossbite.

Curve of Spee (Anteroposterior Curve)

It is drawn to show anatomic curvature of the occlusal alignment of teeth starting at the tip of the lower canine and

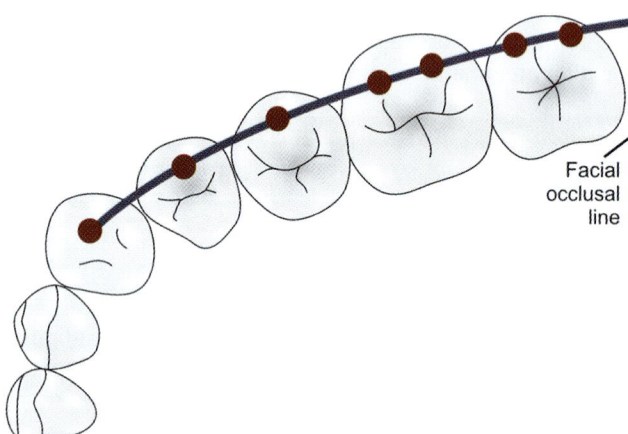

Figure 4.39: Facial occlusal line connects facial cusps of mandibular teeth. Markings show the supporting cusps

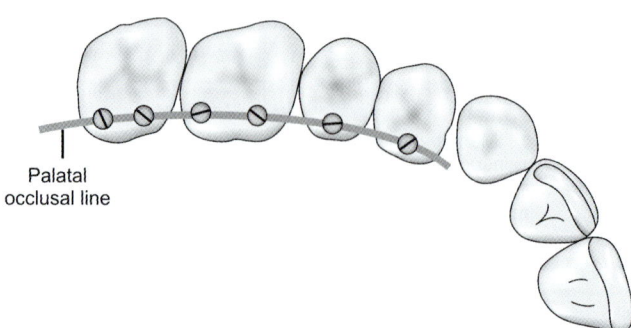

Figure 4.40: Occlusal line on maxillary palatal cusps. Markings show the supporting cusps

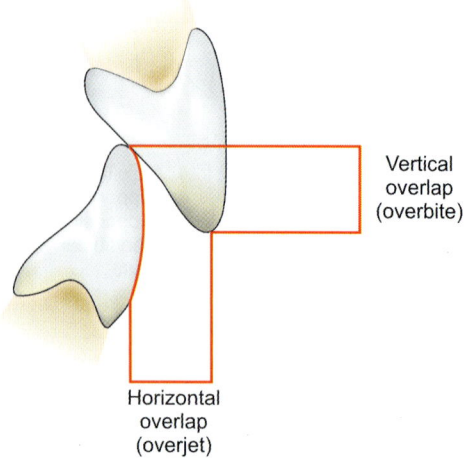

Figure 4.41: Overjet and overbite

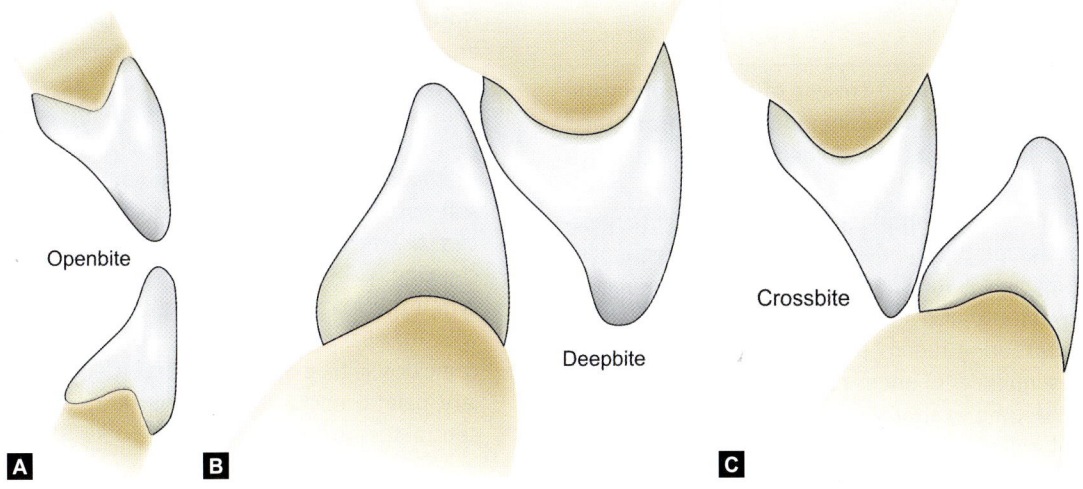

Figures 4.42A to C: Different incisor relationships

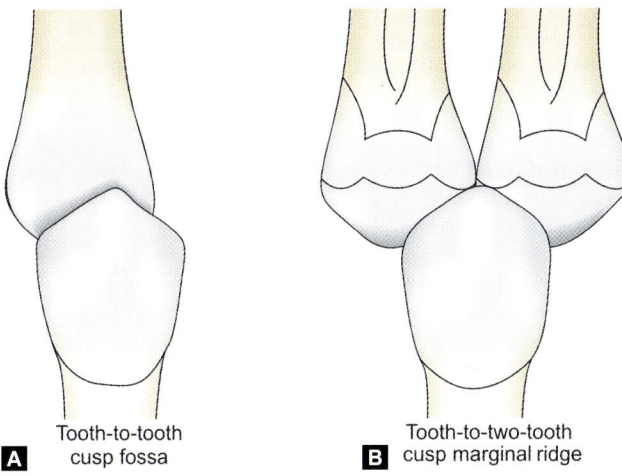

Figures 4.43A and B: Different tooth-to-tooth relationships: (A) Cusp fossa relation; (B) Cusp marginal ridge

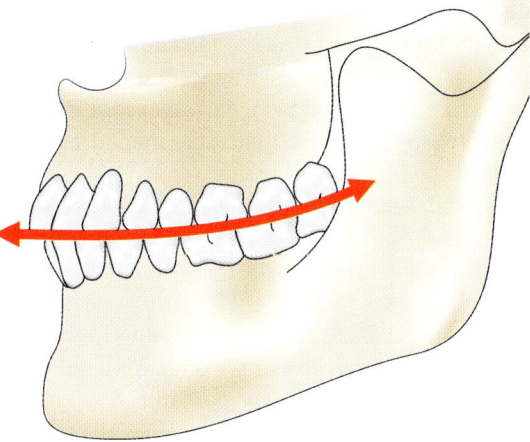

Figure 4.44: Curve of Spee

following the buccal cusps of posterior teeth continuing to the anterior border of the ramus (**Fig. 4.44**).

Curve of Wilson

This is the concave plane which contacts the buccal and lingual cusps of the mandibular molars (**Fig. 4.45**).

So we can say that understanding the concept of occlusion and applying it in operative dentistry can prevent failures which occur in restorations.

The restoration whether for single tooth for or multiple teeth should be in harmony with TMJ, supporting tissues and the neuromuscular system.

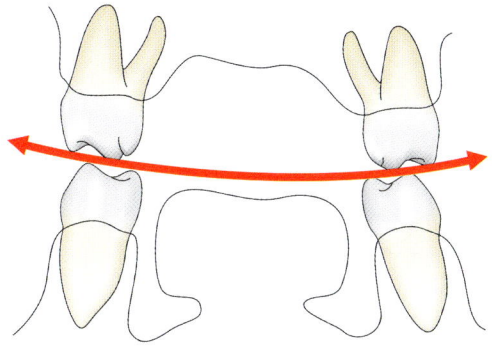

Figure 4.45: Curve of Wilson

Key Points

- Contours present on the crowns of teeth protect the gingival tissue against bruising and trauma from food and they also prevent the food being packed into gingival sulcus.
- Overcontouring is considered more harmful to periodontal tissues than under contouring as it enhances the supragingival and subgingival plaque accumulation at the overcontoured crowns.
- Under-contouring means too little contouring. Important consequences of under-contouring are food impaction and trauma to attachment apparatus.
- Marginal ridges are defined as rounded borders of enamel which form the mesial and distal margins of occlusal surfaces of premolars and molars and mesial and distal margins of lingual surfaces of the incisors and canines.
- Embrasures are defined as V-shaped spaces that originate at proximal contact areas between adjacent teeth and are named for the direction towards which they radiate. They provide a spillway for food during mastication and prevent food being forced in contact area.
- Interproximal space is triangular shaped area that is usually filled by gingival tissue.
- Periodontal tissue injury caused by repeated occlusal forces that exceeds the physiological limits of tissue tolerance is called trauma from occlusion (TFO).
- Grooving means to restore the depth of developmental grooves which has become shallow due to attrition.
- Spheroiding means to reduce premature contacts and restoring original contour of the tooth.
- Occlusal adjustment is done to improve the masticatory efficiency, speech problems, and to provide comfort to temporomandibular problems. It also helps in establishment and maintenance of stable and functional occlusion.
- An ideal occlusion is defined as the most dynamic position, arrangement and relationship of one tooth with other tooth, of one arch with opposite arch with the base of skull so as to perform optimal functions of mastication, phonetics and esthetics maintaining the integrity and longevity of individual tooth and the stomatognathic system.
- Bruxism is parafunctional grinding of teeth which generally takes place during sleep and patient is not aware of the condition.
- bruxomania is the condition which occurs during the day time and patient is conscious about it.
- A centric holding cusp is that which ideally occludes along the line of the central grooves of opposing teeth.

Normally, these are the lingual cusps of the maxillary and buccal cusps of the mandibular teeth.
- Nonsupporting cusps/noncentric cusps/gliding cusps overlap the opposing tooth without contacting the teeth. These are present on buccal cusps of maxillary teeth and lingual cusps of mandibular teeth. They keep soft tissue such as tongue and cheek away from tooth and prevent self-injury to these soft tissues during chewing.
- When the mandibular arches are in complete contact with maxillary arches, mandibular facial occlusion line coincides with maxillary central fossae and the maxillary palatal occlusion line coincides with mandibular central fossae line.

QUESTIONS

1. Explain in detail the physiology of tooth form.
2. What are different factors affecting oclusion in operative dentistry?
3. Write short note on importance of contacts and contours.

BIBLIOGRAPHY

1. Angle EH. Classification of malocclusion, Dent Cosmos. 1899;41:248-64,350-7.
2. Celenza FV, Nasedkin JN. Occlusion: the state of the art, Chicago, 1978, Quintessence.
3. Gibbs CH, et al. Functional movements of the mandible. J Prosthet Dent. 1971;26:601-10.
4. Lund JP. Mastication and its control by the brain stem. Crit Rev Oral Biol Med. 1991;2:33-64.
5. Lundeen HC, et al. An evaluation of mandibular border movements: their character and significance. J Prosthet Dent. 1978;40:442-52.
6. Lundeen TF, Mendosa MA. Comparison of two methods for measurement of immediate Bennett shift. J Prosthet Dent. 1984;51:243-5.
7. Celenza, FV. The centric position—Replacement and character. JPD. 1973;30:591.
8. Christensen, GJ. Now is the time to observe and treat dental occlusion. JADA. 2001;132:100.
9. Danveniza M. Full occlusal protection- theory and practice of occlusal therapy. Aust Dent J. 2001;46:70.
10. Lee WC, Eakle WS. Possible role of tensile stress in the etiology of cervical erosive lesions of teeth. JPD. 1984; 52:374.
11. Small BW. Location of incisal edge position for esthetic restorative dentistry. Gen Dent. 2000;48:396.
12. Small BW. The importance of contact and embrasures and their effect on periodontium. Gen Dent. 2000;48:239.

5 CHAPTER

Dental Caries

Chapter Outline

Dental caries is a process that may take place on any tooth surface especially when there is continuous deposition of dental plaque. Plaque is an example of a biofilm, which means it is not a disorganized collection of bacteria but a group of metabolically active microorganisms attached to a surface. This group works together, having a collective physiology. The organisms are organized into a three-dimensional structure enclosed in a matrix of extra-cellular material derived from the cells themselves and their environment.

Many of the bacteria are capable of fermenting a dietary carbohydrate substrate and produce acid, resulting in plaque pH to fall below 5 within 1-3 minutes. Repeated falls in pH may result in demineralization of the tooth surface. Though, the acid produced by bacteria is neutralized by saliva resulting in increase in the pH. This causes regain of lost minerals, called remineralization. When the collective results of the demineralization and remineralization processes results in a net loss of mineral, a carious lesion occurs that can be seen. Thus we can say that the

carious process is an ubiquitous, natural process. Since caries activity is highly variable, so the course of individual lesion is not always predictable. Progression of carious lesions is characterized by a series of exacerbations and remissions, because the pH at the tooth surface varies with changes in plaque metabolism.

Definition
➡ Dental caries is defined as a microbiological disease of the hard structure of teeth, which results in localized demineralization of the inorganic portion and destruction of the organic substances of the tooth.
➡ Cariology is a science which deals with the study of etiology, histopathology, epidemiology, diagnosis, prevention and treatment of dental caries.

SITES OF DENTAL CARIES (FIGS 5.1A TO D)

As we know that plaque is the essential forerunner of caries and therefore the sites on the tooth surface which

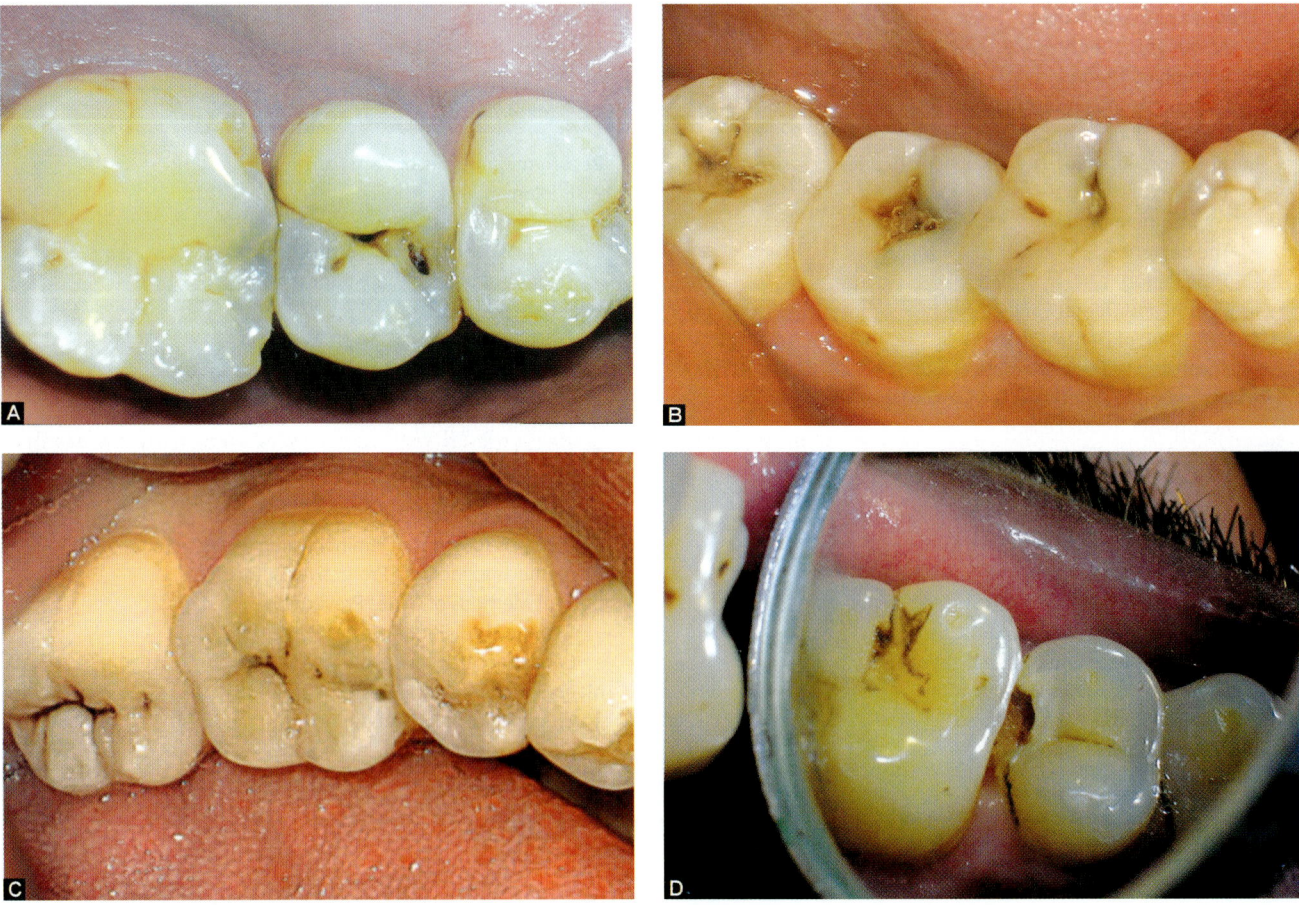

Figures 5.1A to D: Most common sites of caries development

encourage plaque retention and stagnation are particularly prone to progression of lesions. These sites are:

- Pits and fissures on occlusal surfaces of molars and premolars
- Buccal pits of molars
- Palatal pits of maxillary incisors
- Enamel of the cervical margin of the tooth just coronal to the gingival margin
- Proximal enamel smooth surfaces apical to the contact point
- In teeth with gingival recession occurring because of periodontal disease
- The margins of restorations predominantly which are deficient or overhanging
- Tooth surfaces adjacent to dentures and bridges.

EPIDEMIOLOGY OF DENTAL CARIES

Epidemiology is the study of health and disease state in populations rather than individuals. In this, the epidemiologist defines the frequency and severity of health problems in relation to factors such as age, sex, geography, race, economic status, nutrition and diet.

Measuring Caries Activity

Epidemiologists measure both the prevalence and the incidence of caries.

Prevalence

Prevalence is the proportion of a population affected by a disease at a particular time.

Incidence

Incidence measures the rate at which a disease progresses.

To measure incidence, two examinations are required one at the beginning and one at the end of a given time period. The incidence of the condition is the increase or decrease in the number of new cases occurring in a population within that time period.

In dental caries, the measurements of disease is done by applying DMF index in permanent teeth and def for the primary dentition.

D = decayed, M = missing, F = filled tooth; DMF may be used as DMFT which means D = decayed, M = missing, F = filled, T = number of teeth or DMFS which means D = decayed, M = missing, F = filled, S = Surfaces of teeth. In def, d is decayed, e is extracted and f is filled.

Disadvantages of DMF/def Index:

- In young children missing deciduous teeth may have been lost as a result of natural exfoliation so they must be differentiated from teeth lost due to caries.

- Permanent teeth are lost for reasons other than caries, such as trauma, extraction for orthodontic purposes and periodontal disease. Thus missing teeth may be skipped from the index.

DENTAL PLAQUE/BIOFILM

Dental plaque is an adherent deposit of bacteria and their products, which forms on all tooth surfaces.

Biofilm is defined as a microbiologically derived community, characterized by cells which are irreversibly attached to substrate or interface or with each other, embedded in matrix of extracellular polymeric substances that they have produced and exhibit an altered phenotype with respect to growth rate and gene transcription.

Features of Biofilm

Microorganisms in biofilm show distinct character to survive under difficult environmental conditions. This distinct and unique feature of microorganism is due to following characteristic features of biofilm:

- *Protection of bacteria in biofilm*: Many bacteria can produce polysaccharides which cover the communities of biofilm and create favorable conditions for functioning. This protects the bacteria from number of environmental factors such as ultraviolet radiation, metal and toxins.
- *Trapping nutrients in biofilm*: Microorganisms present in biofilm have tendency to degrade large nutrient molecules that could not be effectively degraded by single microorganisms.
- *Providing favorable conditions for different bacterial species in biofilm*: A biofilm displays organized internal compartments for distribution of nutrients, pH, oxygen and metabolic products as well as bacterial species. This would create a different microniche that can favor the growth of diverse bacterial species with in a biofilm.
- *Exchange of genetic material between different species of bacteria in a biofilm*: This features helps in evolution of new microbial communities with different trails.

According to Coldwell, a biofilm should meet the following criteria
➡ Homeostasis
➡ Autopoiesis
➡ Synergy
➡ Communality.

A biofilm should have following characteristics:

- Resist environmental changes
- Should have ability to self-reorganize.
- Should be more effective in association with each other rather than alone.

Components of Biofilm

Inorganic Components

Calcium, phosphorus and fluoride are more in biofilm than in saliva.

Organic Components

- **Carbohydrates**: These are produced by bacterias. Commonly present carbohydrates are glucans, fructans and glucans.
- **Proteins**: Proteins are derived from saliva (in supragingival part) and gingival sulcus fluid (in subgingival part).
- **Lipids**: They include endotoxins from Gram-negative bacterias.

Development of Biofilm

Bacteria can form biofilms on different surfaces ranging from hard to soft tissue. It can form in three basic steps:

1. *Formation of pellicle (Fig. 5.2)*: Pellicle is an acellular, proteinaceous film, derived from saliva formed on tooth surface. In this stage, different bacteria reversibly or irreversibly attach to tooth surface resulting in formation of enamel pellicle which acts as foundation for multilayered biofilm.
2. *Colonization of bacteria (Fig. 5.3)*: In this stage, bacteria which attach in preliminary stage, start dividing and form microcolonies. This bacterial composition further grow into more mature complex flora in three stage scenario. The stages are as follows:
   - *1st stage*: Gram-positive cocci. For example, streptococcal species.
   - *2nd stage*: Fusobacterium species.
   - *3rd stage*: Gram-negative organisms.
3. *Maturation of biofilm (Fig. 5.4)*: In two weeks, the plaque becomes more mature. As the biofilm matures, vibrios and spirochetes start growing into this.

There is site-to-site differences in its composition. That is why caries progress in some sites but not others in the same mouth.

Pathogenic Properties of Cariogenic Bacteria and Pathogenesis of Dental Caries

Cariogenic bacterias have some characteristics which make them special:

- *Acidogenic nature*: This means bacterias should be able to transport sugars and convert them to acid.
- *Aciduric nature*: Bacterias should be able to thrive at low pH.
  - Bacterias should be able to produce extracellular and intracellular polysaccharides which contribute to the plaque matrix. These intracellular polysaccharides can be used for energy production and converted to acid when sugars are not available (**Fig. 5.5**).

Hypothesis Concerning Relation Between Plaque and Caries

- The specific plaque hypothesis says that only a few organisms out of the diverse collection in the plaque flora are actively involved in the disease. Preventive measures against these bacteria can control occurrence of the disease.
- The nonspecific plaque hypothesis believes that the carious process is caused by the overall activity of the total plaque microflora. Accordingly all plaque should be removed by mechanical plaque control.

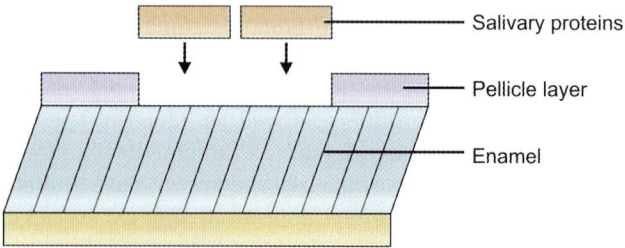

Figure 5.2: Formation of pellicle—1st stage

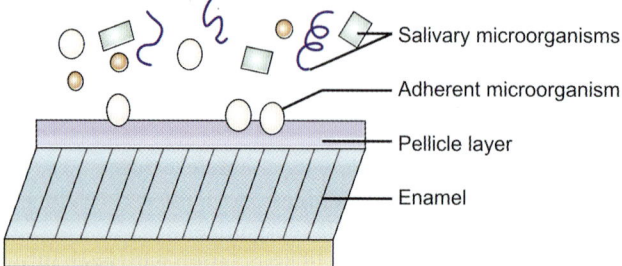

Figure 5.3: Colonization of bacteria—2nd stage of biofilm formation

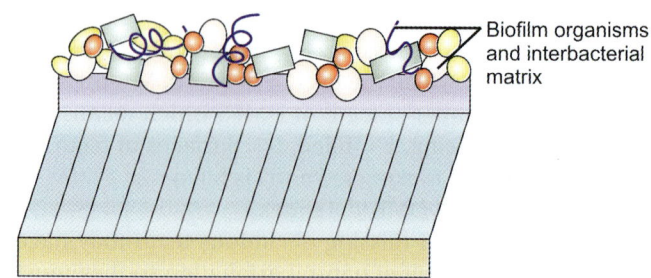

Figure 5.4: Maturation of biofilm—3rd stage

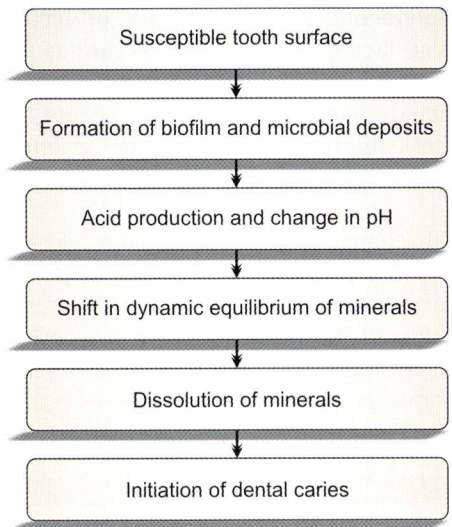

Figure 5.5: Pathogenesis of dental caries

- The ecological plaque hypothesis says that the organisms associated with disease may be present at sound sites. Demineralization results if there is shift in the balance of these resident microflora by a change in the local environment. Frequent sugar intake encourages the growth of acidogenic and aciduric species, thus predisposing to caries. According to this hypothesis, both mechanical cleaning and restriction of sugar intake are important in controlling caries progression.

THEORIES OF DENTAL CARIES

As we know, dental caries is a multifactorial disease of tooth which has been explained by many theories. Though there is no universally accepted theory of the etiology of dental caries, but following three theories are considered in etiology of dental caries:
1. Acidogenic theory
2. Proteolytic theory
3. Proteolysis-chelation theory.

Acidogenic Theory

- WD Miller was the first known investigator of dental caries. He published his results in 1882.
- This theory is most accepted.
- Miller said "Dental decay is a chemicoparasitic process consisting of two stages, the decalcification of enamel, which results in its total destruction, as a preliminary stage; followed by dissolution of the softened residue of the enamel and dentin.
- In the first stage there is destruction which is done by the acid attack where as the dissolution of the residue

(2nd stage) is carried out by the proteolytic action of the bacterias.
- This whole process is supported by the presence of carbohydrates, microorganisms and dental plaque.
- All the preventive steps have been based on this theory.

Role of Dental Plaque

Dental plaque also known as microbial plaque is important for beginning of caries because it provides the environment for bacteria to form acid, which causes demineralization of hard tissue of teeth.

Role of Carbohydrates

Carbohydrates exert cariogenic effect which depends upon the following factors:
- Frequency of intake
- Chemical composition, for example, monosaccharides and disaccharides are more carious than polysaccharides
- Physical form like solid, sticky jelly like or liquid
- Time of contact of carbohydrate with the tooth
- Presence of other food components like presence of high fat or proteins makes carbohydrate less cariogenic.

Role of Microorganisms

Though many microorganisms are involved in the etiology of dental caries but most commonly associated are streptococci mutans. On coronal surface initiation of caries is caused by *Streptococcus mutans* and on root surface mainly by *Actinomyces viscosus*. Presence of high *Lactobacillus acidophilus* count in saliva designates the occurrence of active carious lesion.

Role of Acids

For initiation of dental caries, presence of acids (lactic acid, butyric acid) on the tooth surface is necessary.

Proteolytic Theory

- Heider, Bodecker (1878) and Abbott (1879) thrown considerable light to this theory
- According to this theory, organic portion of the tooth plays an important role in the development of dental caries
- It has been recognized that enamel contains 0.56 percent of organic matter out of which 0.18 percent is keratin and 0.17 percent is a soluble protein
- Enamel structure which are made of the organic material such as enamel lamelle and enamel rods prove to be the pathways for the advancing microorganisms
- Microorganisms invade the enamel lamelle and the acid produced by the bacterias causes damage to the organic pathways.

Proteolysis-Chelation Theory

This theory was put forward by Schatz and his coworkers.

Chelation

- It is a process in which there is complexing of the metal ions to form complex substance through coordinate covalent bond which results in poorly dissociated/or weakly ionized compound. Example of chelation reaction is hemoglobin in which 4 pyrrole nuclei are linked to iron by a similar bond.
- Chelation is independent of the pH of the medium.
- Bacterial attack on the surface of the enamel is initiated by keratinolytic microorganisms. This causes the breakdown of the protein chiefly keratin. This results in the formation of soluble chelates which decalcify enamel even at neutral pH.
- Enamel contains mucopolysaccharides, lipids and citrate which are susceptible to bacterial attack and act as chelators.

Reduced incidence of caries because of fluoridation has been explained by this theory. According to this, due to formation of fluoroapatite, strength of linkage between organic and inorganic phases of enamel is increased which helps in reducing their destruction.

"Caries Balance Concept" (Proposed by Featherstone) (Fig. 5.6)

According to the caries balance theory, caries does not result from a single factor; rather, it is the outcome of the complex interaction of pathologic and protective factors. Pathological factors involved in a carious lesion are bacteria, poor dietary habits, and xerostomia. Protective factors include saliva, antimicrobial agents (chlorhexidine, xylitol), fluoride, pit and fissure sealants and an effective diet.

A balance between pathologic and protective factors dynamically changes throughout the day, even in healthy individuals. Any change in balance of these factors can result in carious lesion. So these risk factors must be evaluated from time to time because the effect of each factor can change over time. For example, if a person is healthy today and develops xerostomia, he can develop severe decay months later.

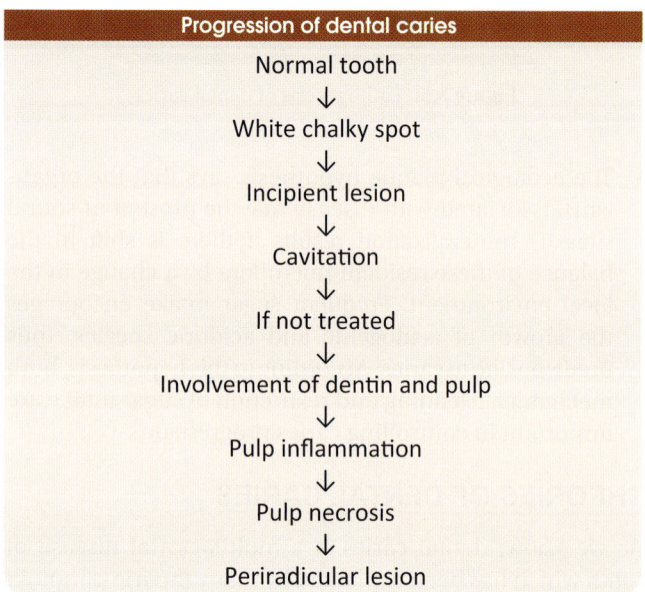

Progression of dental caries
Normal tooth
↓
White chalky spot
↓
Incipient lesion
↓
Cavitation
↓
If not treated
↓
Involvement of dentin and pulp
↓
Pulp inflammation
↓
Pulp necrosis
↓
Periradicular lesion

LOCAL FACTORS AFFECTING THE INCIDENCE OF CARIES (FIG. 5.7)

Dental caries is an ecological disease in which the diet, the host and the microbial flora interact in a way which increases demineralization of the tooth structure with resultant caries formation.

Some races have higher incidence of dental caries, for example, white American and English people. Some races (e.g. Indians and black Americans) due to hereditary patterns have lower incidence of dental caries. There are some local factors which can easily alter the manifestation of caries activity based on heredity pattern.

In 1960s, Keyes showed that there are three prerequisite factors for the development of dental caries, known as Keyes's triad (**Fig. 5.8**). These factors are plaque, tooth and the diet. Later on many studies were conducted which

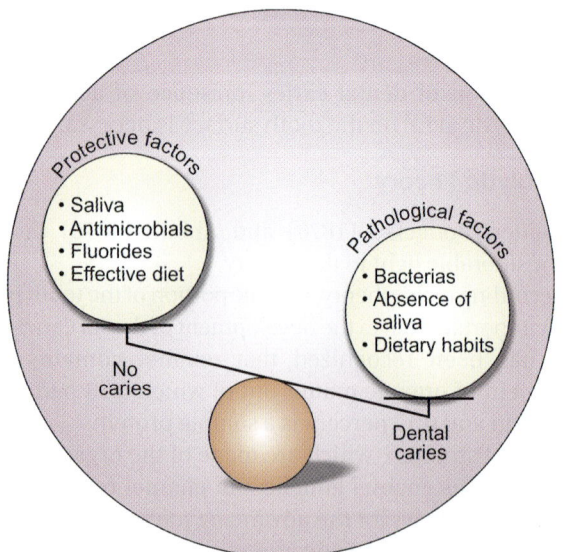

Figure 5.6: Caries balance concept. If pathological factors overweight then caries progress

extended Keyes model with many other factors affecting the interplay between these primary factors.

The difference in occurrence of dental caries in different individuals of same age, sex, race and geographic area, diet, and similar living conditions is because of various factors that manipulate the etiology of caries (**Fig. 5.9**):

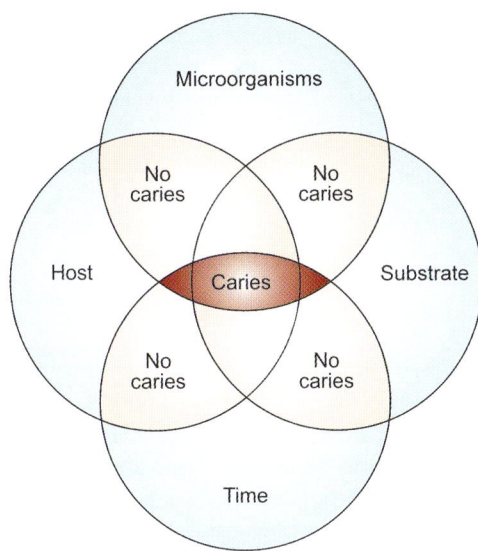

Figure 5.7: Local factors affecting incidence of dental caries

- Tooth (Host)
  - Variation in morphology
  - Composition
  - Position.
- Substrate (Environmental factors)
  - Saliva
    - i. Composition
    - ii. Quantity
    - iii. pH
    - iv. Viscosity
    - v. Antibacterial factors.
  - Diet
    - i. Physical factors
    - ii. Local factors
      - a. Carbohydrate content: Presence of refined cariogenic carbohydrate particles on the tooth surface
      - b. Vitamin content
      - c. Fluoride content.
      - d. Fat content
- Microorganisms: Most commonly seen microorganisms associated with caries are *Streptococcus mutans* and *Lactobacillus*.
- Time period.

The Host

Structure of enamel can be changed by a various factors. Lack of enamel maturation or the presence of developmental

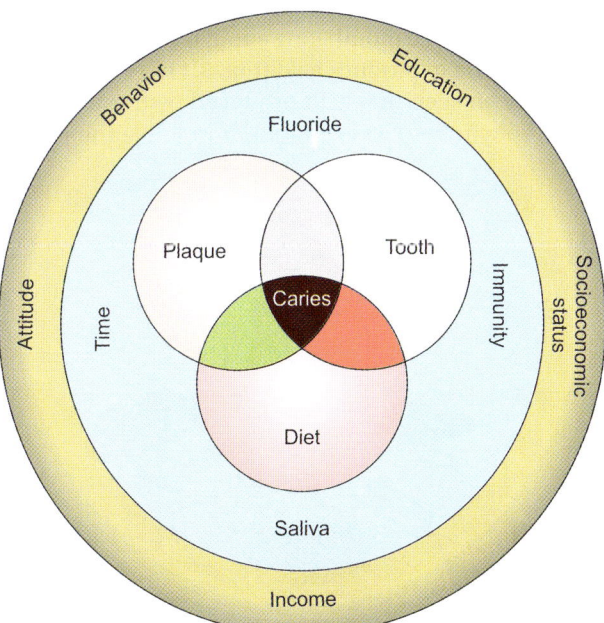

Figure 5.8: Factors affecting caries. Here plaque, tooth and diet are shown as three main prerequisites for caries development (Keyes's triad). Other factors modify the interplay between these factors

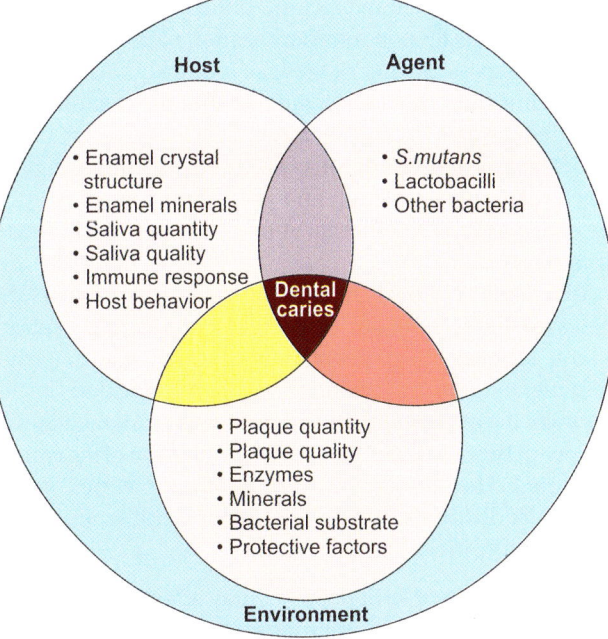

Figure 5.9: Variations in host, agent and environmental factors affect incidence of caries

defects in enamel may result in increase the caries risk. These defects increase plaque retention, increase bacterial colonization, and in some cases, the loss of enamel make it more susceptible to tooth demineralization.

Physical characteristics of teeth like deep and narrow occlusal fissures, deep buccal or lingual pits and enamel hypoplasia, etc. affect the initiation of dental caries. Also it is the shape, size and order of the teeth which affects the cleaning effects of saliva.

There is no difference in the chemical composition of carious and sound enamel in contents of calcium, phosphorus, magnesium and carbon, but there is difference in their fluoride content. It is lesser in carious enamel and dentin as compared to a sound tooth. In carious enamel and dentin it is 139 ppm and 223 ppm, whereas in sound enamel and dentin it is 410 ppm and 873 ppm, respectively.

Tooth position also affects the initiation of dental caries. If a tooth is out of position, rotated or in any abnormal position, it becomes difficult to clean, and hence retains more food and debris.

Environment of the Tooth: Saliva and Diet

Saliva

Saliva is the body's natural protective mechanism against decay. It contains salivary proteins which get deposited onto the tooth surface which help the enamel against acid dissolution. This protective layer is referred to as the pellicle. Salivary proteins also act as antibacterial agents.

Since saliva is rich in calcium, phosphate and fluoride, these materials help in remineralization of the enamel.

Saliva acts as cleaner of teeth as it quickly washes away food debris from the mouth and to buffer the organic acids that are produced by the bacteria.

Under normal conditions, the tooth is continually in touch with saliva. Calcium and phosphate ions present in the saliva help in remineralization of the very early stages of carious lesion.

When salivary flow is reduced or absent, there occurs the increased food retention. Since salivary buffering capacity is lost, an acid environment is encouraged which further promotes the growth of aciduric bacteria. These aciduric bacterias savor the acid conditions and metabolize carbohydrates in the low-pH environment. This results in initiation of the caries.

Though the susceptibility of tooth for caries varies among individuals, following factors influencing the susceptibility include:

- **Composition of saliva**: Saliva may affect caries rate by influencing bacteria, immune status, plaque formation.
- Saliva has a very important role in the balance between demineralization and remineralization. Dental enamel

is susceptible to acid dissolution during the process of demineralization. This demineralization process is counterbalanced by the repair process known as remineralization. The balance between demineralization and remineralization of the enamel determines whether caries occurs.

Functions of saliva	Components of saliva
Antimicrobial action	Lysozyme, lactoperoxides, mucins, cystins, immunoglobulins, IgA
Maintaining mucosa integrity	Water, mucins, electrolytes
Lubrication	Mucin, glycoproteins, water
Cleansing	Water
Buffer capacity and remineralization	Bicarbonate, phosphate, calcium, fluorides

Diet (Fig. 5.10)

Physical nature of diet: In the earlier times, the primitive man used to eat rough and raw unrefined foods which had self-cleansing capacity. But in present times, soft refined foods are eaten which stick stubbornly to the teeth and are not removed easily due to lack of roughage. This is the reason for higher incidence of dental caries now-a-days than the past.

Nature of carbohydrate content of the diet: To cause demineralization of dental enamel, it is essential for fermentable carbohydrates and plaque to be present on the tooth surface for a minimum length of time. These need to be retained in the mouth long enough to be metabolized by oral bacteria to produce acid (**Fig. 5.11**).

It has been seen that acid produced by these fermentable carbohydrates cause a rapid drop in plaque pH to a

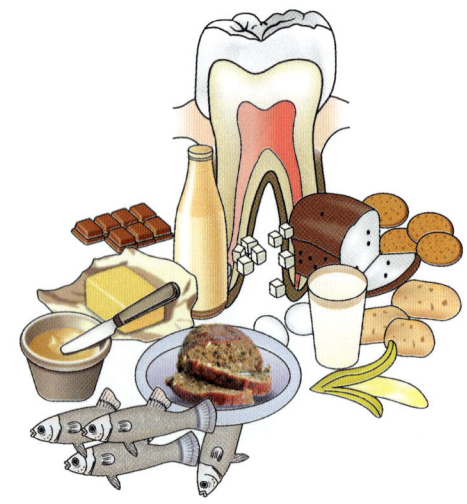

Figure 5.10: Physical nature of diet affects the incidence of dental caries

level which results in demineralization of the tooth structure. But since acids produced in plaque diffuse out of the plaque combined with buffering capacity of saliva exerting a neutralizing effect, this acidic nature of plaque remains for sometime only, and with in 30 to 60 minutes, plaque returns to its normal pH. However, repeated and frequent consumption of sugar will keep plaque pH depressed which results in demineralization of the teeth.

Stephan has shown the relationship between change in plaque pH over a period of time following a glucose rinse in form of a graph. This graph is called a 'Stephan curve' (Stephan and Miller, 1943) (**Fig. 5.12**). The drop in pH is the result of fermentation of carbohydrates by plaque bacteria. The gradual return of the pH occurs because of buffers present in plaque and saliva. This drop in pH can demineralize tooth structure depending on the absolute pH decrease, as well as the length of time that the pH is below the "critical pH" level. ***The critical pH value for demineralization usually ranges between 5.2 and 5.5***.

Since both plaque and saliva are saturated with calcium and phosphate ions, the pH returns rises rapidly from the 5.3 resulting in remineralization. This remineralization process takes more time in an acid environment. Caries is unusual in those parts of the oral cavity near the areas where the teeth are constantly bathed with the buffers and concentrated calcium ions of saliva like lower incisors.

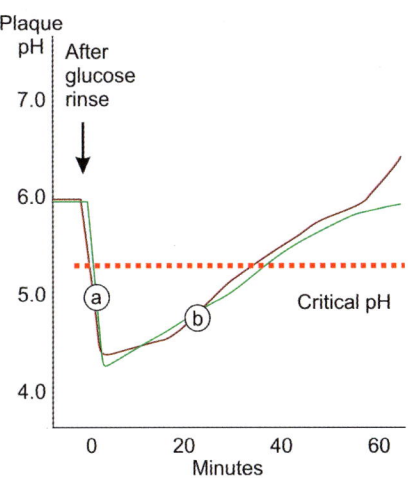

Figure 5.12: Stephan curve graph showing plaque pH before and after glucose rinse. (a) pH decreases because of acids produced by bacteria; (b) pH increases, due to buffering of plaque and saliva

Caries occurs when the process of remineralization is slower than the process of demineralization and there is a net loss of mineral into the environment. It can be prevented by restricting the intake of dietary sugars, and removing plaque.

Tooth remineralization can take place if the pH of the environment adjacent to the tooth is high due to
➡ Lesser number of cariogenic bacteria
➡ Availability of fluoride
➡ Lack of substrate for bacterial metabolism
➡ Elevated secretion rate of saliva
➡ Strong buffering capacity of saliva
➡ Presence of inorganic ions in saliva
➡ Quick washing of retained food.

Researches have shown reduced caries activity with sugar alcohols (viz; sorbitol, mannitol, and xylitol) sweeteners. These are not metabolized by bacteria and are metabolized at a slower rate.

Extensive studies have shown that foodstuff or drink containing fermentable carbohydrate are likely to cause significant acid production, followed by demineralization of the enamel, but all carbohydrates are not equally cariogenic. Complex carbohydrates such as starch are relatively harmless because they are not completely digested in the mouth, but low molecular weight carbohydrates diffuse readily into plaque and are metabolized quickly by the bacteria. The production of extracellular polysaccharides from sucrose is faster than glucose, fructose, or lactose. Accordingly, sucrose is the most cariogenic sugar, although the other sugars are also harmful.

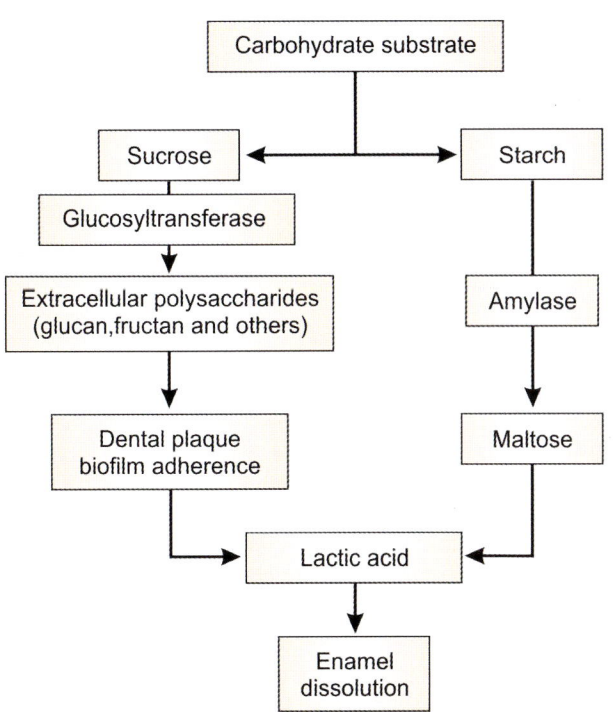

Figure 5.11: How presence of carbohydrate substrate initiates dental caries

Moreover, *Streptococcus mutans* make use of sucrose to produce the extracellular polysaccharide glucan. Glucan polymers help the *Streptococcus mutans* to adhere firmly to teeth and inhibit diffusion properties of plaque.

Frequency of carbohydrate intake: It is widely documented that it is not quantity but the frequency of carbohydrate intake which affects the occurrence of dental caries. In a person with normal salivary function, after intake of fermentable carbohydrate foods or drinks, the acidic pH lasts 30 to 60 minutes. Greater time between acid attacks allows greater time for the repair process (remineralization) to occur.

Recently researches have been done to establish the dynamic interactions between frequency of eating/drinking and oral hygiene and the use of fluoride. Nowadays the commonly given advice to patient that 'three meals a day' is safe for teeth, and 'frequent snacking is undesirable', is no longer recommended because:

- Though there is increase in frequency of eating and drinking, fluoride especially in dentifrices has compensated and overridden the effect of increased snacking.
- Studies have shown that occurrence of caries depends on alternating periods of demineralization and remineralization. Appropriate use of fluoride has been seen to 'neutralize' the effect of frequent snacking.

Vitamin content of the diet: As we know vitamin are essential components of daily diet. Deficiency of some vitamins increases the incidence of dental caries.

Vitamin A: Deficiency or excess are not related to dental caries.

Vitamin D: Vitamin D helps in normal development of teeth. Enamel hypoplasia can result due to vitamin D deficiency. It can result in early attack of caries. It has been seen that supplement of vitamin D in children helps in the formation of healthy teeth and thus helps in reduction in the dental caries.

Vitamin K: Deficiency does not affect the dental caries incidence.

Vitamin B Complex: Its deficiency may exert a caries protective Influence on the tooth. Several types of vitamin B are important growth factors for the oral acidogenic flora which serve as component of the coenzymes involved in glycolysis. Vitamin B_6 acts as an anticaries agent because it promotes the growth of noncariogenic organisms.

Vitamin C: Directly vitamin C does not help in protection of tooth against dental caries, but it is required for the normal health of the gingiva.

Some minerals other than calcium and phosphorus which are seen to affect the incidence of dental caries are Vanadium and selenium. It has been seen that when concentration of vanadium in drinking water is increased, it results in decrease in the incidence of dental caries. Whereas increase in the incidence of dental caries is seen in those areas where high concentration of selenium is present in drinking water.

The Bacteria

Dental caries do not occur if the oral cavity is free of bacteria. Of the many types of bacteria in the mouth, the most caries active appear to be *Streptococcus mutans*, *Lactobacillus* spp., *Veillonella* spp. and *Actinomyces* spp. These bacteria can be transferred from mother to child and are present at varying levels in all human mouths.

Among these streptococci *mutans* are most commonly seen microorganism associated with the dental caries. They are considered main causative factors for caries because of their ability to adhere to tooth surfaces, produce abundant amounts of acid, and survive and continue metabolism at low pH conditions. Colonization with *Streptococcus mutans* at an early age is an important factor for early caries initiation.

However, most researchers have shown that other organisms present in the oral cavity are also capable of plaque formation and acid production from fermentable carbohydrates.

Time Period

The time period during which all above three direct factors, i.e. tooth, microorganisms and substrate are acting jointly should be adequate to produce acidic pH which is critical for dissolution of enamel to produce a carious lesion. Time required for acid production from the fermentation of the carbohydrates by bacteria and for demineralization of tooth, is allowed by poor oral hygiene and not cleaning teeth immediately after eating.

IRRADIATION AND DENTAL CARIES

Rapid development of rampant dental caries is one of most commonly seen expression of irradiation injury in patients undergoing radiation therapy.

According to Frank and Baden, three types of dental defects are observed as a result of irradiation:

1. The first type is a characteristic caries like lesion completely encircling the neck of the tooth.
2. The second type of lesion begins with brown to black discoloration of the crown. In this type, occlusal and incisal surfaces of teeth wear away.
3. The third type of lesion begins as a spot depression which spreads from incisal or occlusal edges on labial or buccal and lingual surfaces. Later on the enamel is

smashed and coronal dentin becomes partially disintegrated leaving an irregular discolored root stump projecting over the gingiva.

Irradiation results in increase in the incidence of caries because of:

- Xerostomia, one of the main complication of radiation therapy.
- Increase in viscosity and decrease in pH of saliva after irradiation.
- Increased migration of neutrophils into the oral cavity and increased excretion of lysosomal enzymes into the oral environment.

CLASSIFICATION OF DENTAL CARIES

Carious lesions can be classified in different ways.

According to Their Anatomical Site

- *Pit and fissure caries (Fig. 5.13)*: Pit and fissure caries occur on occlusal surface of posterior teeth and buccal and lingual surfaces of molars and on lingual surface of maxillary incisors.
- *Smooth surface caries (Fig. 5.14)*: Smooth surface caries occurs on gingival third of buccal and lingual surfaces and on proximal surfaces.
- *Root caries (Fig. 5.15)*: When the lesion starts at the exposed root cementum and dentin, it is termed as root caries.

According to Whether It is a New Lesion or Recurrent Carious Lesion

- *Primary caries*: It denotes lesions on unrestored surfaces (**Fig. 5.16**).

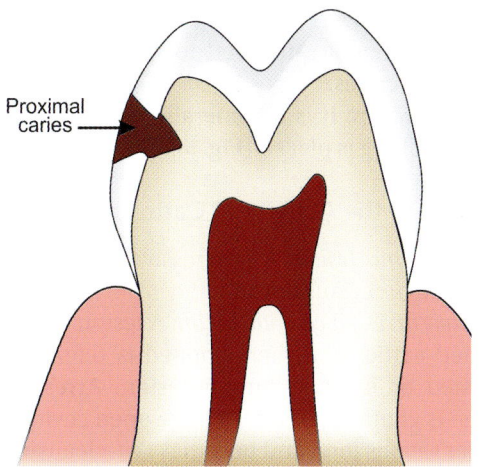

Figure 5.14: Smooth surface caries

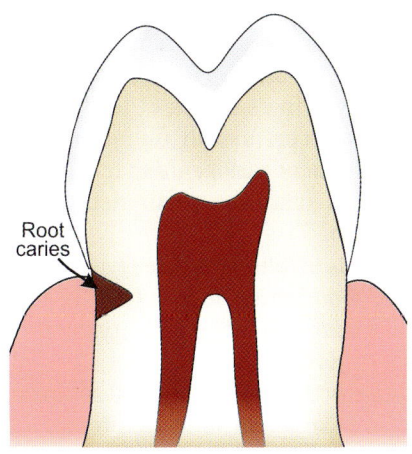

Figure 5.15: Root caries

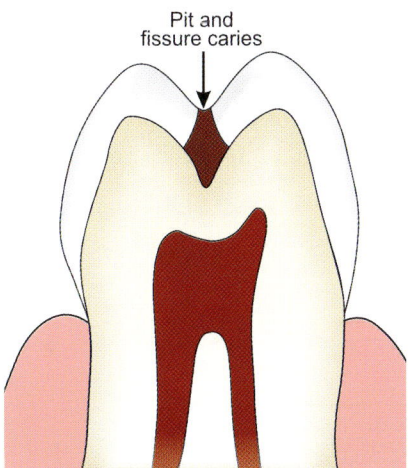

Figure 5.13: Pit and fissure caries

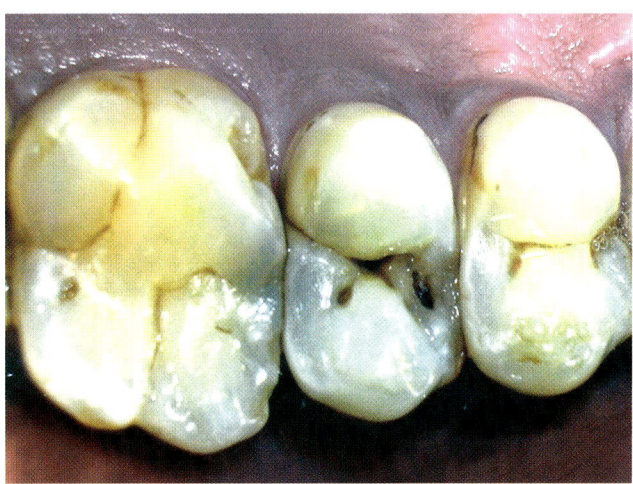

Figure 5.16: Primary caries

- *Recurrent caries (Fig. 5.17)*: Lesions developing adjacent to fillings are referred to as either recurrent or secondary caries.
- *Residual caries*: It is demineralized tissue left in place before a filling is placed (**Fig. 5.18**).

According to the Activity of Carious Lesion

- *Active carious lesion*: A progressive lesion is described as an active carious lesion.
- *Inactive/arrested carious lesion*: A lesion that may have formed earlier and then stopped is referred to as an arrested or inactive carious lesion. Arrested carious lesion is characterized by a large open cavity which no longer retains food and becomes self-cleansing.

According to Speed of Caries Progression

- *Acute dental caries*: Acute caries travels towards the pulp at a very fast speed.
- *Rampant caries*: It is the name given to multiple active carious lesions occurring in the same patient, frequently involving surfaces of teeth that are usually caries free. It occurs usually due to poor oral hygiene and taking frequent cariogenic snacks and sweet drinks between meals. It is also seen in mouths where there is hyposalivation.

Rampant caries is of following three types:
1. *Early childhood caries*: It is a term used to describe dental caries present in the primary dentition of young children.
2. *Bottle caries or nursing caries*: These are names used to describe a particular form of rampant caries in the primary dentition of infants and young children. The clinical pattern is characteristic, with the four maxillary deciduous incisors most severely affected.

3. *Xerostomia induced rampant caries (radiation rampant caries)*: These are commonly observed that after radiotherapy of malignant areas of or near the salivary glands. Because of radiotherapy salivary flow is very much reduced. This results in rampant caries even in those teeth which were free from caries before radiotherapy.
   - *Chronic dental caries*: Chronic caries travel very slowly towards the pulp. They appear dark in color and hard in consistency.

Based on Treatment and Restoration Design

- *Class I*: Pit and fissure caries occur in the occlusal surfaces of premolars and molars, the occlusal two-third of buccal and lingual surface of molars, lingual surface of incisors (**Fig. 5.19**).
- *Class II*: Caries in the proximal surface of premolars and molars (**Fig. 5.20**) .
- *Class III*: Caries in the proximal surface of anterior (incisors and canine) teeth and not involving the incisal angles (**Fig. 5.21**)
- *Class IV*: Caries in the proximal surface of anterior teeth also involving the incisal angle (**Fig. 5.22**).
- *Class V*: Caries on gingival third of facial and lingual or palatal surfaces of all teeth (**Fig. 5.23**).

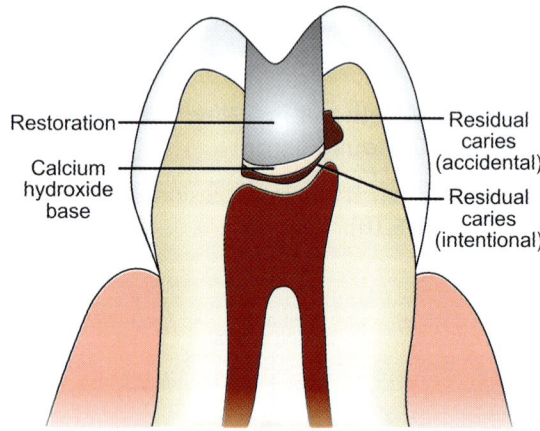

Figure 5.18: Residual caries

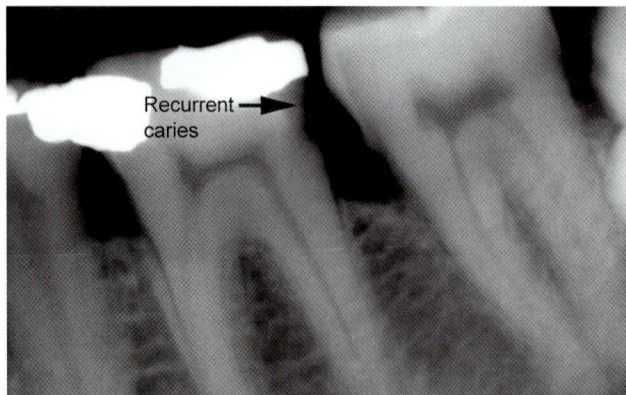

Figure 5.17: Radiograph showing recurrent caries adjacent to proximal restoration

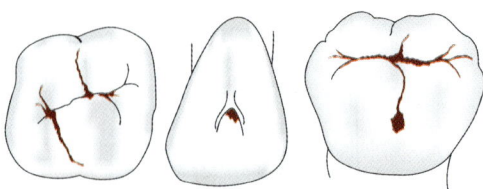

Figure 5.19: Class I caries present on occlusal surface of posterior teeth, occlusal two-third of buccal and lingual surface of molars and lingual surface of incisors

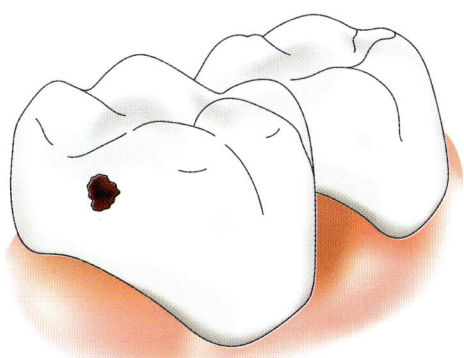

Figure 5.20: Class II caries on proximal surface of molars and premolars

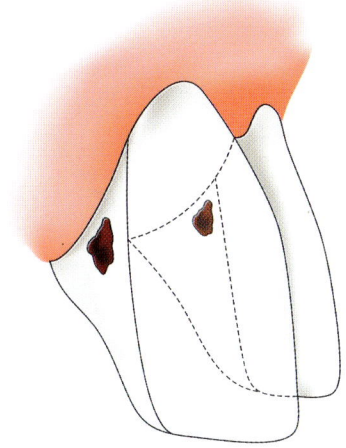

Figure 5.21: Class III caries on proximal surfaces of anterior teeth not involving incisal edge

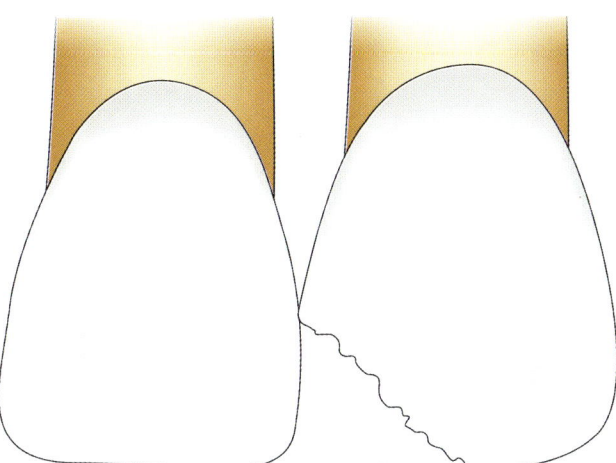

Figure 5.22: Class IV caries on proximal surfaces of anterior teeth involving incisal angle

- *Class VI*: Caries on incisal edges of anterior and cusp tips of posterior teeth without involving any other surface (**Fig. 5.24**).

Visual Classification (Occlusal Surfaces)

0 No or slight changes in enamel translucency after prolonged air drying.
1 Opacity hardly visible on the wet surface but distinctly visible after air drying.

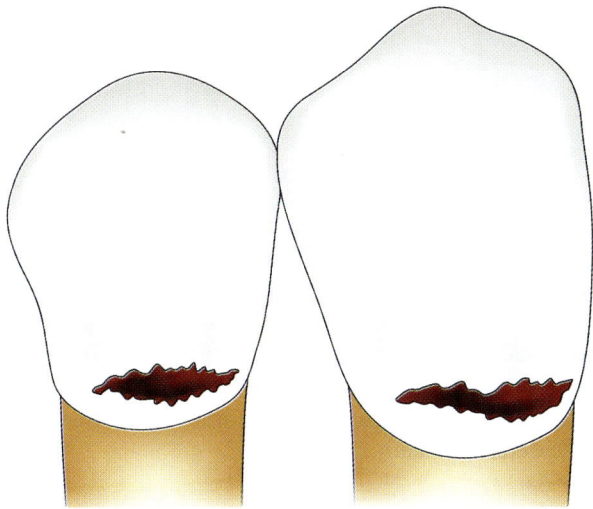

Figure 5.23: Class V caries on gingival third of facial or lingual surfaces of all teeth

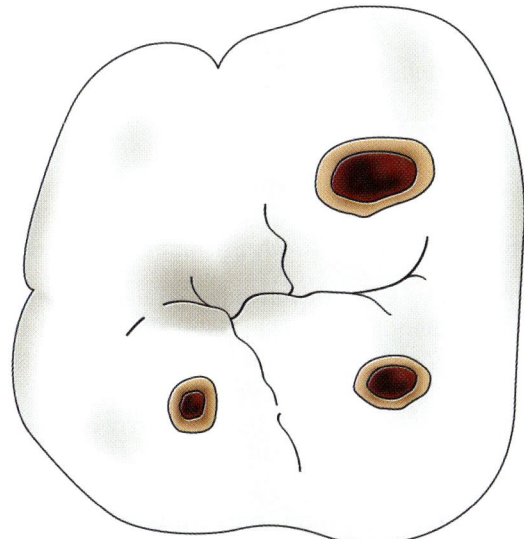

Figure 5.24: Class VI caries on incisal edges of anterior teeth and cusp tips of posterior teeth

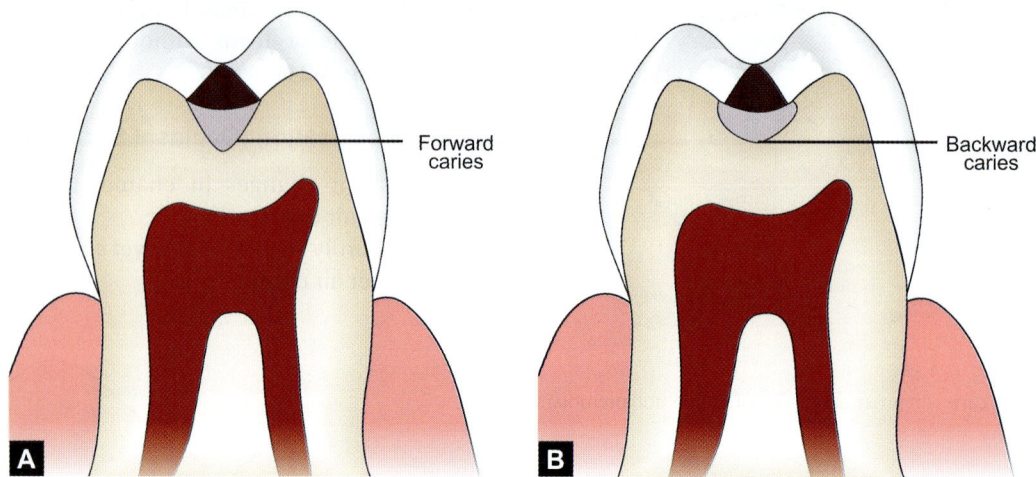

Figures 5.25A and B: (A) Forward caries; (B) Backward caries

2 Opacity (white or yellow) distinctly visible without air drying.
3 Localized enamel breakdown in opaque or discolored enamel and/or grayish discoloration from underlying enamel.
4 Cavitation in opaque or discolored enamel exposing the dentin beneath.

Based on Pathway of Caries Spread (Figs 5.25A and B)

Forward Caries

When the caries cone in enamel is larger or of same size as present in dentin, it is called as forward caries.

Backward Caries

When spread of caries along dentinoenamel junction exceeds the adjacent caries in enamel, it is called backward caries (here caries extend from DEJ to enamel).

Based on Number of Tooth Surfaces Involved

- *Simple caries*: Caries involving only one tooth surface is termed as simple caries (**Fig. 5.26**).
- *Compound caries (Fig. 5.27)*: If two surfaces are involved it is termed as compound caries.
- *Complex caries (Fig. 5.28)*: If more than two surfaces are involved it is called as complex caries.

Classification According to the Severity

- *Incipient caries (Fig. 5.29)*: It involves less than half the thickness of enamel

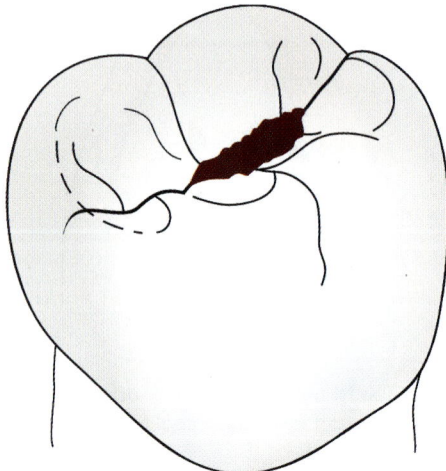

Figure 5.26: Simple caries

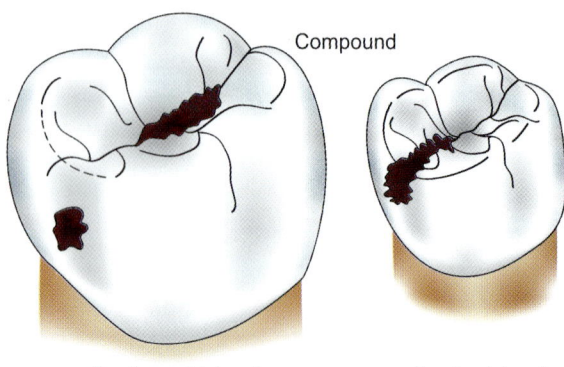

Figure 5.27: Compound caries

- *Moderate caries (Fig. 5.30)*: It involves more than half the thickness of enamel, but does not involve dentinoenamel junction.
- *Advanced caries (Fig. 5.31)*: It involves the dentinoenamel junction and less than half distance to pulp cavity.
- *Severe caries (Fig. 5.32)*: It involves more than half distance to pulp cavity.

WHO System of Caries Classification

This classification is based on shape and depth of carious lesion which can be scored on a four point scale:

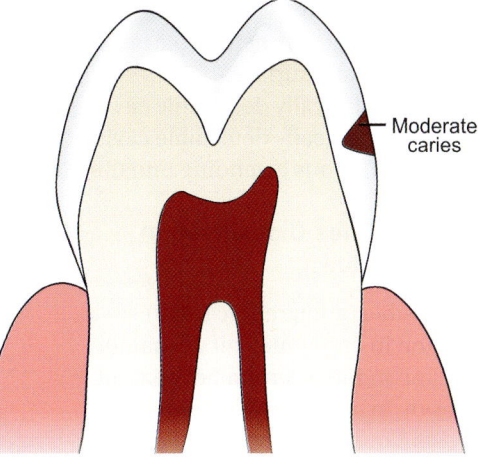

Figure 5.30: Moderate caries

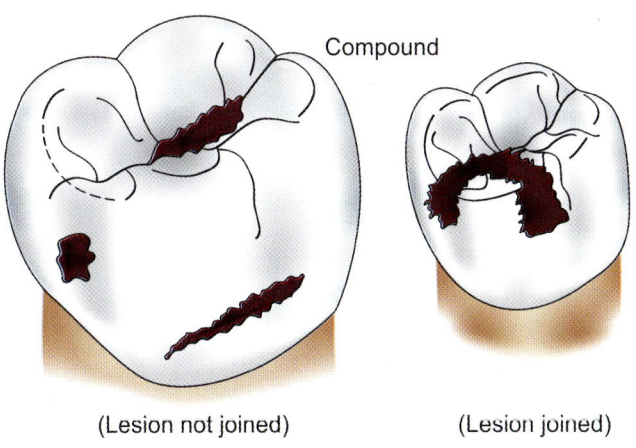

Figure 5.28: Complex caries

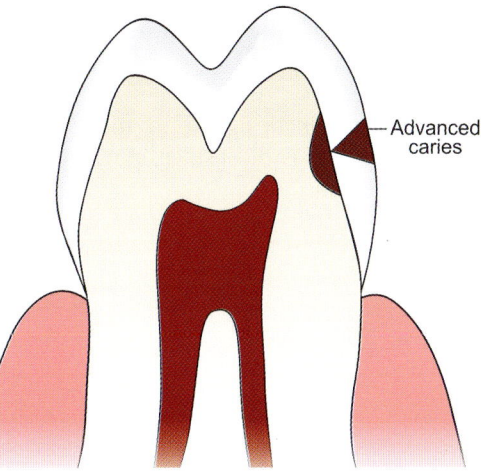

Figure 5.31: Advanced caries

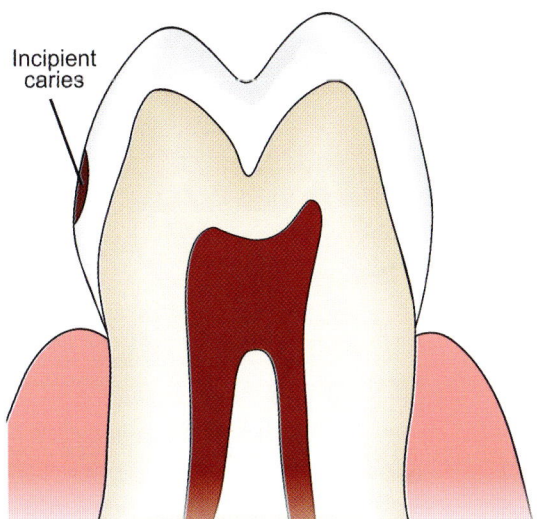

Figure 5.29: Incipient caries

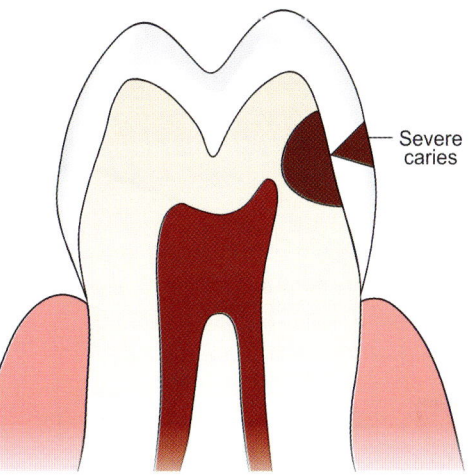

Figure 5.32: Severe caries

Scale points	Features
1. D1	Clinically detectable enamel lesions with intact surfaces
2. D2	Clinically detectable cavities in enamel
3. D3	Clinically detectable cavities in dentin
4. D4	Lesions extending into the pulp.

Radiographic Caries Classification (See Figs. 5.53A to E)

E0 – No visible radiographic lesion
E1 – Lesion in outer one half of enamel
E2 – Lesion in inner one half of enamel
D1 – Lesion in outer third of dentin
D2 – Lesion in middle third of dentin
D3 – Lesion in inner third of dentin.

Graham Mount's Classification

This classification system is based on two simple parameters:
1. Location of carious lesion
2. Size of carious lesion.

Here, the system is designed to recognize carious lesions beginning at the earliest stage, in which remineralization is the indicated:

Cavity site	Size 1 (Minimal)	Size 2 (Moderate)	Size 3 (Enlarged)	Size 4 (Extensive)
Site 1 Pit and fissure	1.1	1.2	1.3	1.4
Site 2 Contact area	2.1	2.2	2.3	2.4
Site 3 Cervical region	3.1	3.2	3.3	3.4

Comparison between enamel hypoplasia and white spot

Characteristic features	Enamel hypoplasia	Caries/ white spot
Surface	Hard	Softer than enamel
On drying the surface	Opaque in appearance	Opaque in appearance
On wetting the surface	Opaque in appearance	Translucent in appearance

HISTOPATHOLOGY OF DENTAL CARIES

Enamel Caries (Fig. 5.33)

Caries of enamel initiates by deposition of dental plaque on tooth surface. We will discus the carious process of the enamel according to its location on tooth surface, i.e. smooth surface caries, and pit and fissure caries.

Smooth Surface Caries (Figs 5.34A to D)

- Smooth surface caries occurs on gingival third of buccal and lingual surfaces and on proximal surfaces below the contact point (**Fig. 5.35**).
- The earliest manifestation of incipient caries (early caries) of enamel is usually seen beneath dental plaque as areas of decalcification (white spots). As caries progresses it appears bluish-white in color.
- The first change seen histologically is the loss of interprismatic/interrod substance of enamel with increased prominence of the rods.
- There is also accentuation of the incremental lines of Retzius.
- This is followed by the loss of mucopolysaccharides in the organic substance.

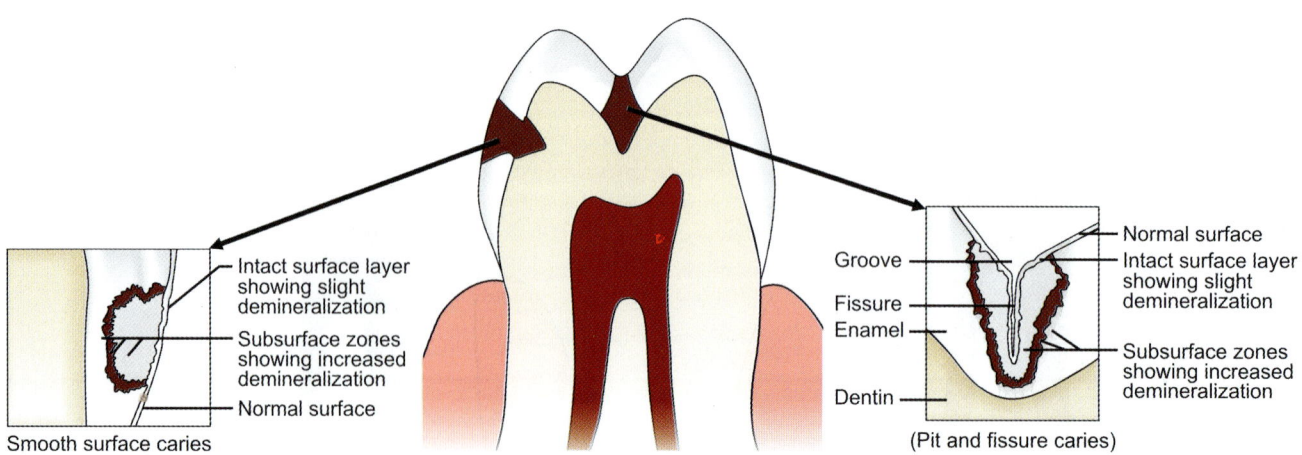

Figure 5.33: Magnified schematic presentation of smooth surface caries (Pit and fissure caries)

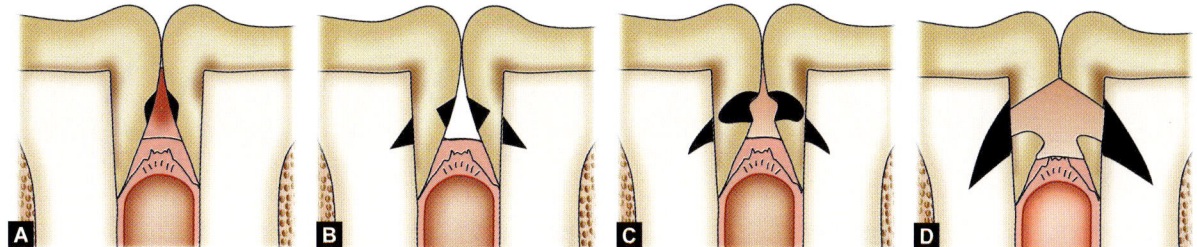

Figures 5.34A to D: Progression of smooth surface caries: (A) Initial lesion on proximal surface, it can be remineralized by salivary fluoride; (B) Demineralization of dentin, but intact enamel; (C) Cavitation of enamel; (D) Advanced caries with Frank cavitation of enamel and dentin followed by progression towards pulp

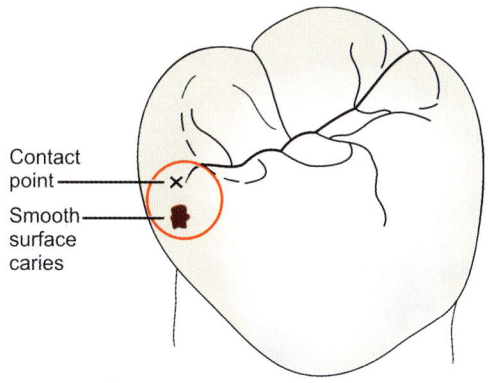

Figure 5.35: The most common site of occurrence of smooth surface caries below the contact point

- As it goes deeper, the caries forms a triangular pattern or cone shaped lesion with the apex towards DEJ and base towards the tooth surface.
- Finally there is loss of enamel structure, which gets roughened due to demineralization, and disintegration of enamel prisms.

Pit and Fissure Caries (Figs 5.36A to D)

- The shape of pits and fissures contributes to their high susceptibility to caries because of entrapment of bacteria and food debris in them.
- Initially caries of pits and fissures appears brown or black in color and with a fine explorer, a 'catch' is felt. Enamel at the margins of these the pits and fissures appears opaque bluish-white.
- Caries begin beneath plaque resulting in decalcification of enamel.
- Enamel in the bottom of pit or fissure is very thin, so early dentin involvement frequently occurs.
- Here the caries follows the direction of the enamel rods.
- It is triangular in shape with the apex facing the surface of tooth and the base towards the DEJ.
- When reaches DEJ, greater number of dentinal tubules are involved.

- It produces greater cavitation than the smooth surface caries and there is more undermining of enamel.
- When undermined enamel fractures, it causes exposure of cavitation and caries.

Zones in Enamel Caries

Different zones are seen before complete disintegration of enamel. Early enamel lesion seen under polarized light reveals four distinct zones of mineralization (**Fig. 5.37**). These zones begin from the dentinal side of the lesion.

- *Zone 1*: Translucent zone
  - Represent the advancing front of the lesion
  - Ten times more porous than sound enamel
  - Not always present.
- *Zone 2*: Dark zone
  - It lies adjacent and superficial to the translucent zone
  - Usually present and thus referred as positive zone
  - Called dark zone because it does not transmit polarized light
  - Formed due to demineralization.
- *Zone 3*: Body of the lesion
  - Largest portion of the incipient caries
  - Found between the surface and the dark zone
  - It is the area of greatest demineralization making it more porous.
- *Zone 4:* Surface zone
  - This zone is not or least affected by caries
  - Greater resistance probably due to greater degree of mineralization and greater fluoride concentration
  - It is less than 5 percent porous
  - Its radiopacity is comparable to adjacent enamel.

Dentinal Caries

Although caries of enamel is clearly a dynamic process, it is not a vital process because it does not defend itself from trauma. But since pulp and dentin are vital tissues, they are capable of defending. Relationship between pulp and

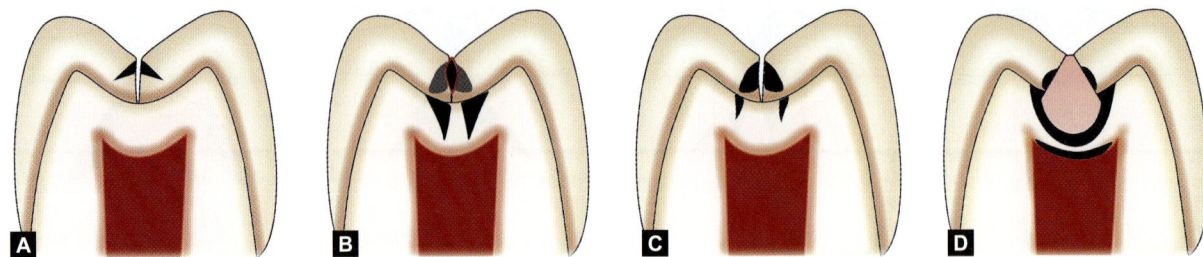

Figures 5.36A to D: Progression of pit and fissure caries: (A) Initial caries start at the lateral walls of fissure and spread laterally as it progresses to DEJ; (B) Appearance of discoloration and opacification of enamel close to the fissure; (C) Opacification is similar to stage B, slight cavitation of enamel which is difficult to detect because of surface remineralization; (D) Frank cavitation of dentin and enamel

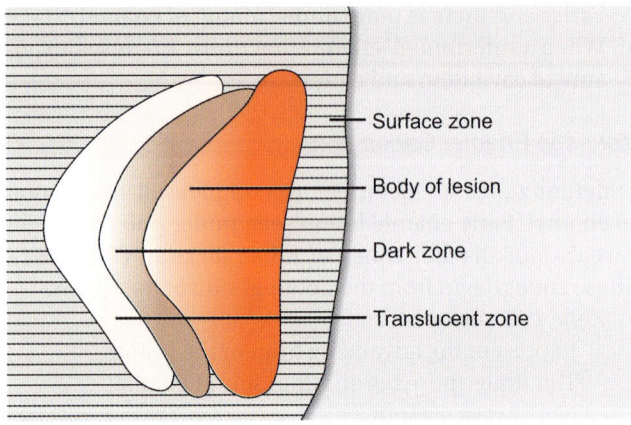

Figure 5.37: Zones in caries of enamel

dentin is termed as pulp-dentin complex, it acts as a structural and functional biological unit.

When enamel caries reaches the dentinoenamel junction it spreads rapidly laterally because it is least resistant to caries.

Dentinal caries appear brown because of color produced by
➡ Pigment producing microorganisms
➡ Chemical reaction which occurs when proteins break down in presence of sugar
➡ Exogenous stains.

The caries process in dentin involves the demineralization of the inorganic component and breakdown of the organic component of collagen fibers. The caries process in dentin is twice as fast in enamel because dentin provides much less resistance to acid attack. When caries attacks the dentin, the following changes occur in dentin:

Early Dentinal Changes (Fig. 5.38)

- Initial penetration of the dentin by caries causes an alteration in dentin, known as dentinal sclerosis.

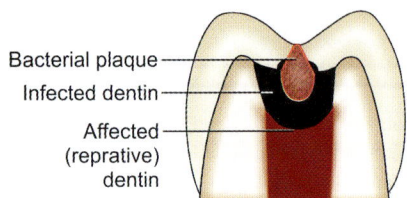

Figure 5.38: Dentinal changes because of caries

- In this reaction there occurs the calcification of dentinal tubules which seals off from further penetration by microorganisms.
- More prominent in slow chronic caries.
- When dentinal tubules are completely occluded by the mineral precipitate, section of the tooth gives a transparent appearance in transmitted light, this dentin is termed as transparent dentin.
- In transparent dentin, intertubular dentin is demineralized and lumen is filled by calcified materials, which provides softness and transparency to the dentin compared to sound dentin.
- In the earliest stages, when only few tubules are involved, microorganisms may be found penetrating the tubules, called *Pioneer Bacteria*.
- In early caries, fatty degeneration of Tome's fibers and deposition of fat globules in these processes act as predisposing factor for sclerosis of the tubules.
- This initial decalcification involves the walls allowing them to distend as the tubules are packed with microorganisms. Each tubule is seen to be packed with pure forms of bacteria, e.g. one tubule packed with coccal forms the other tubule with bacilli.
- As the microorganisms proceed further they are distanced from the carbohydrates substrate that was needed for the initiation of the caries. Thus the high protein content of dentin must favor the growth of the microorganisms. Therefore, proteolytic organisms might appear to predominate in the deeper caries of

dentin while acidophilic forms are more prominent in early caries.

Advanced Dentinal Changes

- In advanced lesion, decalcification of the wall of the individual tubules takes place, resulting in confluence of the dentinal tubules.
- Sometimes the sheath of Neumann shows swelling and thickening at irregular intervals in the course of dentinal tubules.
- The diameter of dentinal tubules increases because of packing of microorganisms.
- There occurs the formation of tiny *liquefaction foci*, described by Miller. They are formed by the focal coalescing and breakdown of dentinal tubules. These are ovoid areas of destruction parallel to the course of the tubules which are filled with necrotic debris and increase in size by expanding. This expansion produces compression and distortion of adjacent dentinal tubules, leading to course of dentinal tubules being bent around the *liquefaction focus.*
- The destruction of dentin by decalcification and then proteolysis occurs in numerous focal areas. It results in a necrotic mass of dentin with a leathery consistency.
- Clefts occur in the carious dentin that extends at right angles to the dentinal tubules. These account for the peeling off of dentin in layers while excavating.
- Shape of the lesion is triangular with the apex towards the pulp and the base towards the enamel.

Zones of Dentinal Caries (Fig. 5.39)

Five zones have been described in dentinal caries. These zones are clearly distinguished in chronic caries than in acute caries. These zones begin from the pulpal side:

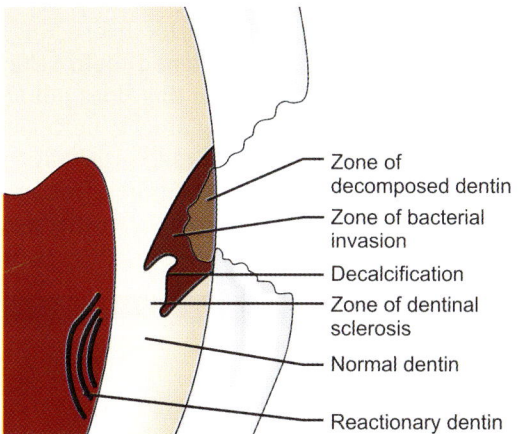

Figure 5.39: Zones of dentinal caries

- *Zone 1*: Normal dentin
  - Zone of fatty degeneration of Tome's fibers
  - Formed by degeneration of the odontoblastic process
  - Otherwise dentin is normal and produces sharp pain on stimulation.
- *Zone 2*: Zone of dentinal sclerosis
  - Intertubular dentin is demineralized
  - Dentinal sclerosis, i.e. deposition of calcium salts in dentinal tubules takes place
  - Damage to the odontoblastic zone process is apparent
  - There are no bacteria in this zone. Hence, this zone is capable of remineralization.
- *Zone 3*: Zone of decalcification of dentin
  - Further demineralization of intertubular dentin lead to softer dentin.
- *Zone 4*: Zone of bacterial invasion
  - Widening and distortion of the dentinal tubules which are filled with bacteria
  - Dentin is not self-repairable, because of less mineral content and irreversibly denatured collagen
  - This zone should be removed during tooth preparation.
- *Zone 5*: Zone of decomposed dentin due to acids and enzymes
  - Outermost zone
  - Consists of decomposed dentin filled with bacteria
  - It must be removed during tooth preparation.

Difference between infected and affected dentin

Affected dentin	Infected dentin
• Soft, demineralized dentin invaded with bacteria	• Demineralized dentin but not invaded by bacteria
• Soft leathery tissue which can be flaked easily	• Does not flake easily though soft in nature
• Irreversible denaturation of collagen	• Uninterrupted collagen cross-linking
• Cannot be remineralized	• Can be remineralized
• Caries detecting dyes can stain	• Does not stain

DIAGNOSIS OF DENTAL CARIES

As we know dental caries is an infectious disease, but there are many terms which describe the symptoms of the disease, for example, cavitation, white or brown spot, affected or infected dentin, etc. (**Fig. 5.40**). In order to conserve tooth structure and perform minimally invasive dentistry, carious lesions must be detected at the earliest possible time. By doing so, caries progress can be arrested, thus avoiding a more invasive operative intervention.

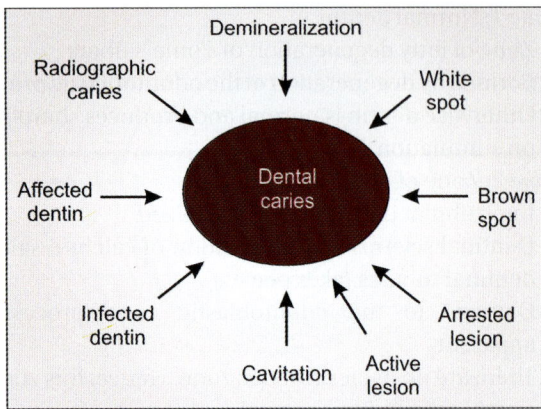

Figure 5.40: Synonyms of dental caries

Accurate diagnosis of the noncavitated lesion is extremely valuable because an increased prevalence of difficult to diagnose caries can be an indication of high caries activity, a circumstance that must be treated with a more aggressive preventive program.

The assessment of accuracy of any method of caries detection must be accomplished through clinical and basic science research.

The accuracy of any diagnostic test or evaluation is typically measured according to its sensitivity and specificity.

Sensitivity and specificity: They refer to the capability of a test to diagnose disease correctly when disease is actually present and to rule out the disease when it is absent.

The essential anatomic-pathophysiologic problem is that the carious lesion occurs within a small, highly mineralized structure following penetration through the structure's surface in a manner which may be difficult to detect using current methods. Additionally, carious lesions occur in a variety of anatomic locations, often adjacent to existing restorations, and have unique aspects of configuration and rate of spread. These differences make it unlikely that any one diagnostic modality will have adequate sensitivity and specificity of detection for all sites.

The application of multiple diagnostic tests to the individual patient increases the overall efficacy of caries diagnosis. Existing diagnostic modalities require stronger validation, and new modalities with appropriate sensitivities and specificities for different caries sites, caries severities, and degrees of caries activity are needed.

Various methods for diagnosis of dental caries

- Visual-tactile method
  - Conventional methods
    - i. Tactile examination
    - ii. Visual examination.

- Advances in visual method
  - i. Illumination
    - a. Ultrasonic illumination
    - b. Ultrasonic imaging
    - c. Fiberoptic transillumination (FOTI)
    - d. Wavelength dependent FOTI
    - e. Digital imaging FOTI (DIFOTI).
  - ii. Dyes
  - iii. Endoscopy filtered fluorescence (EFF) method.
- Radiographic methods
  - Conventional methods
    - i. Intraoral periapical X-rays (IOPA)
    - ii. Bitewing radiographs
    - iii. Panorex radiography
    - iv. Xeroradiography.
  - Recent advances in radiographic techniques
    - i. Digital imaging
    - ii. Computerized image analysis
    - iii. Substraction radiography
    - iv. Tuned aperture computerized tomography (TACT)
    - v. Magnetic resonance microimaging (MRMI).
- Electrical conductance measurement
- Lasers
  - Argon laser
  - Diode lasers
  - Qualitative laser fluorescence
  - Diagnodent (Quantitative laser fluorescence)
  - Optical coherence tomography
  - Polarization sensitive optical coherence tomography (PSOCT)
  - Dye enhanced laser fluorescence.

Visual-Tactile Method of Diagnosis

This method is most commonly used method for tooth examination. This method involves the use of mirror, explorer and light for detecting caries.

Conventional Methods

Tactile examination: In this method explorer has been used for the tactile examination of the tooth for a long time. The explorer is used to detect softened tooth structure. Since demineralization is a process that does not always involve sufficient softening of the enamel to be detectable by an explorer. When an explorer sticks, it's usually a good indication that there is decay beneath; however, when it does not stick, it does not necessarily mean that decay is not present.

Types of explores

- Right angle probe
- Shepherds Crook
- Backaction probe
- Cowhorn with curved end
- Sharp curved probe.

In Volume 1 of GV Black's text "Operative Dentistry" published in 1924, it was stated that "a sharp explorer should be used with some pressure and if a very slight pull is required to remove it, the pit should be marked for restoration even if there are no signs of decay."

Simon (1956) explained the use of a mirror and an explorer to distinguish change around a previously placed restoration.

Disadvantages

- Sturdevant said cavitation at the base of a pit or fissure can be detected tactilely as softness, but mechanical binding of an explorer in the pits or fissures may be due to noncarious causes, like shape of the fissure, sharpness of the explorer, or the force of application (**Fig. 5.41**).
- Sharp edge of explorer may fracture the demineralized enamel, if left alone, such lesion could have remineralized and reverted back to normal.
- Use of a sharp explorer tip within a pit and fissure can cavitate the enamel and actually create an opening through which cariogenic bacteria can penetrate.
- The cariogenic bacteria on the tip of the probe can be seeded into other pits and fissures so that an uninfected tooth can be infected.
- Interproximal caries account for more than 40 percent of caries in adults. The dental explorer is not an effective tool for interproximal caries detection.
- For pit and fissure caries, the explorer is incapable of determining the presence of most occlusal caries.
- Use of an explorer has a low sensitivity and low specificity. This means an explorer used for diagnosis of caries may give false positives.

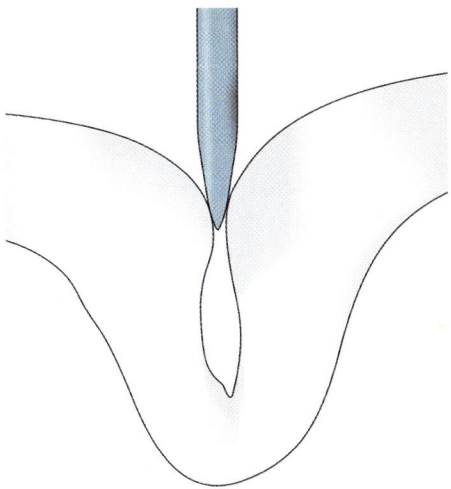

Figure 5.41: An explorer can stick to a healthy deep fissure giving false positive result

Visual examination

Use of visual examination only, is known as the *European method*, while use of sharp or blunt probe in visual tactile system is popularly known as the *American system* for diagnosis of dental caries.

Visual examination for diagnosing dental caries is a very popular method. It is based on the criteria such as cavitation, surface roughness, opacification and discoloration of clean and dried teeth under adequate light source.

Advantage
Preferred over probing because of harmful effects of probing.

Disadvantages
→ Visual examination by a skilled clinician, in some cases, can be successful, but oftentimes, a large percentage of the occurrence of decay is too small to generate a distinctive visual signature for proper detection of caries even in advanced stages.
→ Discoloration of the pits and fissures which is found in normal healthy teeth, can be mistaken for the presence of caries.
→ Caries in enamel are white, opaque, because of its color and opacity. Even when demineralization is detected in the pits and fissures, it is difficult to assess the level of caries penetration.

Advances in Visual Method

Illumination

Ultraviolet illumination: Ultraviolet light increases optical contrast between carious area and the surrounding healthy tissue. The natural fluorescence of enamel as seen under UV light is decreased in areas of less mineral content such as carious lesion, artificial demineralization and developmental defects. The carious lesion appears as a dark spot against a fluorescent background.

Advantages
→ More sensitive method as compared to the visual tactile methods
→ More reliable results.

Disadvantages
→ Difficult to differentiate developmental defects and caries
→ It is not a quantitative method.

Ultrasonic imaging: Ultrasonic imaging was introduced for detecting the early carious lesions on the smooth surfaces. The demineralization of enamel is assessed by ultrasound pulse echotechnique. It has been seen that there is a definite relation between the mineral content of the lesion and the relative echo amplitude changes.

The ultrasonic probe is used which sends longitudinal waves to the surface of the tooth and also serves the function of receiving the waves:

- Initial white spot lesions, which extend only up to enamel, produce no or weak surface echoes
- The sites with visible cavitation produce echoes with substantially higher amplitude.

Advantage
More sensitive than visual tactile method.

Disadvantage
It is not a quantitative method.

Fiberoptic transillumination (FOTI): Transillumination takes advantage of the opacity of a demineralized tooth structure over more translucent healthy structures. The decalcified area will not let light pass through as much as it does in a healthy area, generating a shadow corresponding to decay. In other words, a carious lesion has a lowered index of light transmission in an area of caries and appears as a darkened shadow that follows the spread of decay through the dentin. Illumination is delivered by means of fiberoptics from the light source to the tooth surface using a fiberoptic handpiece. The light propagates from the fiber illumination across tooth tissue to nonilluminated surface resulting in image formation used for diagnosis.

Advantages
➡ Noninvasive method
➡ Useful in patients with posterior crowding
➡ No radiation hazards
➡ Comfortable to patients
➡ Lesions which cannot be diagnosed radiographically can be diagnosed by this method.

Disadvantages
➡ Not possible in all anatomic locations
➡ Considerable intra and interobserver variation
➡ No permanent records

Wavelength dependent FOTI: The distance light propagates through tooth material from the light source to the detector is called "effective decatic optical thickness" and is dependent on the wavelength of light. In case of small lesions, the effective *decatic* optical thickness increases linearly with mineral loss.

Advantages
➡ Quantitative information about lesion depth
➡ No radiation hazards.

Digital imaging fiberoptic transillumination (DIFOTI): The DIFOTI unit was developed as advanced diagnostic tool for early detection of caries without using ionizing radiation. The light from the DIFOTI probe is positioned on the tooth to be assessed, then the tooth is illuminated and the resultant images are captured by a digital electronic charged coupled device camera (CCD) and sent to a computer where these are analyzed using proprietary algorithms. The illumination and imaging conditions are controlled and repeatable. The DIFOTI appears to have the potential to both detect early carious lesions and assess their progression.

These digitally processed images helped in reducing the intra and interobserver variations.

Advantages
➡ Noninvasive
➡ DIFOTI provides clear signal of different types of frank caries
➡ Instant image projection
➡ Shows surface changes associated with early demineralization as early as two weeks
➡ DIFOTI images can indicate the presence of incipient and recurring caries even when radiological images failed to show their presence.

Disadvantages
➡ Not able to measure the depth of the carious lesions
➡ Cannot differentiate dental caries and stained deep fissures.

Dye penetration method

Dyes can visualize a subject from its routine background or if several objects have similar appearance, coloring by a dye helps in their identification. The observation of the coloring can be qualitative or quantitative. In caries diagnosis, qualitative examination is sufficient; observation of colored dye signifies presence of caries.

Dyes should fulfill the following criteria
➡ Should be absolutely safe for intraoral use
➡ Should be specific and stain only the tissues, it is intended to stain
➡ Should be easily removed and not lead to permanent staining.

Dyes for detection of carious enamel: As early as 1940, Gomori used silvernitrate to stain carious lesions. Fluorescein dye has been used in the detection of carious lesions by use of ultraviolet illumination (Hefferren, 1971).

Procion has been used to stain enamel lesions, but the staining is irreversible because the dye reacts with nitrogen and hydroxyl groups of enamel and acts as a fixative.

Calcein makes a complex with calcium and remains bound to the lesion.

Fluorescent dye like Zyglo ZL-22 which is made visible by ultraviolet illumination has been used *in vitro*, but it is not used *in vivo*.

Use of dyes for diagnosing early enamel lesions has not been fully established as yet. If possible, it will allow lesions to be visualized at an early stage and thus allow remineralization procedures to be carried out early in the treatment plan.

Dyes for carious dentin detection: In carious dentin, two layers of decalcification can be identified:

One layer which is soft and cannot be remineralized and a second layer, which is hard with intermediate calcification and can be remineralized. It is now clearly established that these dyes donot stain bacteria but instead stain the organic matrix of less mineralized dentin. This make them less specific because dyes donot stain bacteria nor delineate the bacterial front but stain collagen associated with less mineralized organic matrix.

Use of *basic fuschin in propylene glycol* for the diagnosis and treatment of carious dentin has been given by Fusayama, 1980. The dye was found to be carcinogenic. To overcome this disadvantage, methylene blue was used, but methylene blue is slightly toxic.

Disadvantages
➡ Dyes are carcinogenic/toxic
➡ Dye staining and bacterial penetration are independent phenomena, this limits the usefulness of these dyes.
➡ Dyes donot discriminate between healthy and diseased tooth structures, i.e. these are not caries specific, their routine use may lead to over treatment.

Endoscopic filtered fluorescence method (EFF): Endoscope technique is based on observing the fluorescence that occurs when tooth is illuminated with blue light (wavelength range 400-500 nm). Difference is seen in the fluorescence of sound enamel and carious enamel. When this fluoresced tooth is viewed through a specific broadband gelatin filter, white spot lesions appear darker than enamel.

Videoscopy is the procedure in which camera is attached with this. Light endoscopy is the technique in which white light source can be connected to an endoscope by a fiber-optic cable so that the teeth can be viewed without a filter.

Advantages
➡ It offers a magnified image
➡ Clinically feasible

Disadvantages
➡ Necessitate thorough drying and isolation of teeth
➡ Time consuming
➡ Expensive.

Radiographic Method of Diagnosis

Radiographs play an important role in diagnosis of the dental diseases. Dental radiographs provide useful information for diagnosing carious lesions. Although radiographs may show caries which are not visible clinically, the minimal depth of a detectable lesion on a radiograph is about 500 μm.

The interpretation of radiographs should be done in a systematic manner. The clinician should be familiar with normal radiographic landmarks.

Normal radiographic landmarks (Fig. 5.42)
➡ *Enamel*: It is the most radiopaque structure
➡ *Dentin*: Slightly darker than enamel
➡ *Cementum*: Similar to dentin in appearance
➡ *Periodontal ligament*: Appears as a narrow radiolucent line around the root surface
➡ *Lamina dura*: It is a radiopaque line representing the tooth socket
➡ *Pulp cavity*: Pulp chamber and canals are seen as radiolucent lines within the tooth.

Caries of Different Surfaces of Teeth

Caries of occlusal surfaces:
- Combined use of visual examination and radiographic examination enhances diagnostic sensitivity for occlusal caries.
- By the time caries is evident on radiograph, dentin is usually affected.
- X-ray diagnosis of pits and fissures decay is difficult in earlier stages of the carious process because the decalcified, radiolucent tooth structure is small in percentage compared to the healthy surrounding tooth structure.
- Since the evolution of enamel decay is slower and smaller than dentin decay, occlusal detection is often only possible when the decay is more advanced in the dentin and where it has created a greater damage to the tooth integrity (**Fig. 5.43**).
- Once in dentin, the classical radiographic appearance of a broad based thin radiolucent zone in the dentin with little or no change apparent in the enamel is seen.

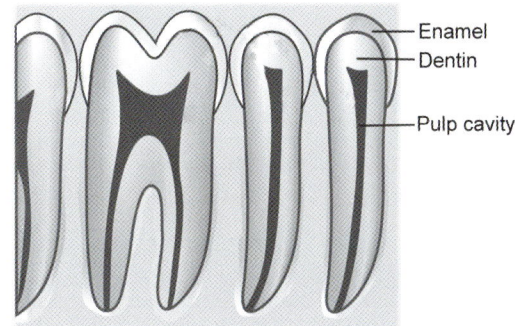

Figure 5.42: Normal radiographic landmarks

- In advanced occlusal caries in dentin, there is a band of increased opacity between the carious lesion and the pulp chamber. The white band represents the calcification within the primary dentin, which will not be evident in buccal caries.

Caries of proximal surfaces:
- Small lesions are difficult to detect radiographically.
- A considerable loss of mineral content is necessary before it becomes evident on a radiograph.
- Lesions confined to enamel may not be evident radiographically until approximately 30 to 40 percent demineralization has occurred (**Fig. 5.44**).
- Radiolucent demineralized enamel is more easily detectable in interproximal areas.
- Because of tooth convexity interproximally and the buccolingual trajectory of the X-ray radiations, the percentage of radiolucent tooth structure decayed over a healthy radiopaque is larger in the interproximal area for a same volume of pit and fissure carious structure. Still, X-rays lack sensitivity in the interproximal region because of the variability in tooth morphology, internal structure and positioning.
- The shape of early lesion in the enamel is a triangle with its broad base at the tooth surface. Once the lesion crosses the DEJ and invades into the dentin, it appears as another triangle with base at DEJ and apex towards the pulp chamber. Collectively, these may appear as two triangles with their bases facing towards the external surface.
- Bitewing radiographs are preferably utilized to detect interproximal caries.

Caries of buccal and lingual surfaces:
- Difficult to differentiate between buccal and lingual caries on a radiograph.
- Appear as well defined radiolucency surrounded by a uniform, noncarious region of enamel.
- More than one radiographs are needed to diagnose because the buccal or lingual lesion may be superimposed on the DEJ and suggest occlusal caries.

Root surface caries:
- It should be detected clinically as radiographs are not needed for diagnosis.
- Drawbacks in the radiographic detection of root lesion are:
  - The surface may appear to be carious as a result of "cervical burnout phenomenon".
  - Diffuse radiolucent areas with ill defined borders may be radiographically evident on the mesial or distal aspects of teeth in the cervical regions between the cervical edge of the enamel and the crest of the alveolar bone.

Cervical burnout is an apparent radiolucency found just below the CE junction on the root due to anatomical variation or a gap between the enamel and bone covering the root (anteriorly) mimicking root caries.

Posterior cervical burnout (Fig. 5.45): It appears because the invagination of the proximal root surfaces allow more X-rays to pass through this area, resulting in a more radiolucent appearance on the radiograph. When radiograph is taken at different angle, these pass through more tooth structure and the radiolucency disappears.

Anterior cervical burnout (Fig. 5.46): The space between the enamel and the bone overlying the tooth appears more radiolucent than either the enamel or the bone-tooth combination.

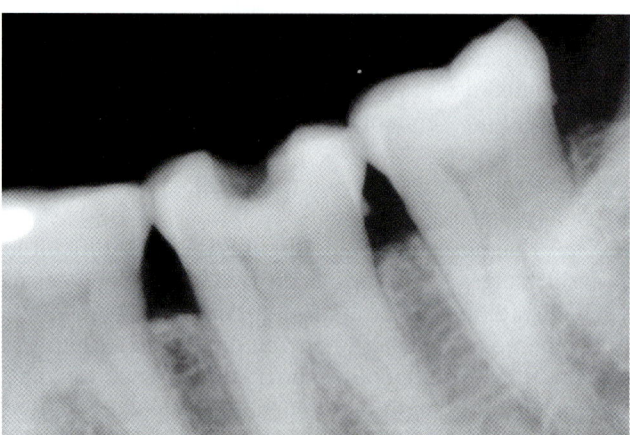

Figure 5.43: Radiograph showing occlusal caries

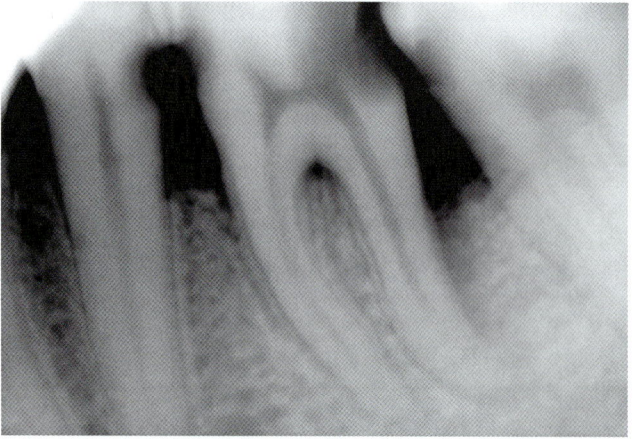

Figure 5.44: Radiograph showing proximal caries of premolar and molar

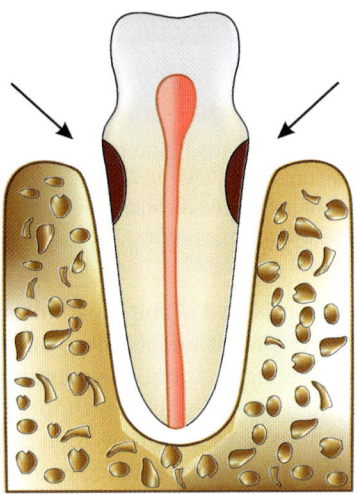

Figure 5.45: Posterior cervical burnout

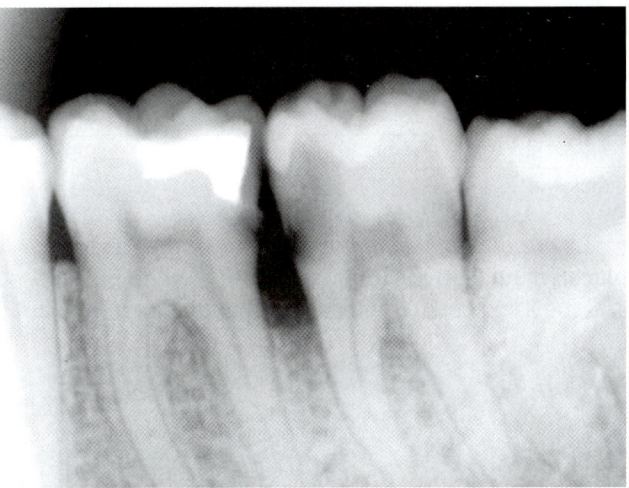

Figure 5.47: Radiograph showing secondary caries

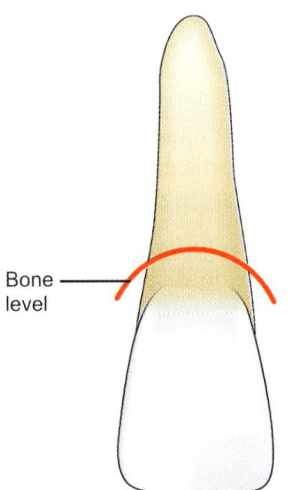

Figure 5.46: Anterior cervical burnout

Secondary Caries (Fig. 5.47)
- Diagnosis mainly depends on the clinical examination.
- Radiographs may not be helpful until the lesion is at an advanced stage.
- Lesion next to a restoration may be obscured by the radiopaque image of the restoration.
- Recurrent caries at cervical margins are best observed in bitewing films, since the central ray is directed along the plane of the cervical areas.

Types of Radiographic Method Used

- Conventional
  - Intraoral periapical radiography
  - Bitewing radiographs
  - Occlusal and panoramic radiograph (rarely used)
  - Xeroradiography.
- Recent advances in radiographic techniques
  - Digital imaging
  - Computerized image analysis
  - Substraction radiography
  - Tuned aperture computed tomography (TACT)
  - Magnetic resonance microimaging (MRMI).

Conventional Methods of Radiography

Intraoral Periapical Radiography

These radiographs can show the pathologic conditions in relation to the supporting bone, the periodontal membrane, the roots and the crowns of the teeth.

A properly placed film permits the visualization of approximately three teeth and at least 3 to 4 mm beyond the apex.

Intraoral periapical (IOPA) radiographs are available in three sizes:
1. Size 0 (For children)—22 mm × 35 mm
2. Size 1 (For adult-anterior teeth)—24 mm × 40 mm
3. Size 2 (Standard size)—31 mm × 41 mm.

There are two types of techniques for exposing teeth viz; *bisecting angle technique* and *paralleling technique*.

In *bisecting angle technique* (**Fig. 5.48**) the X-ray beam is directed perpendicular to an imaginary plane which bisects the angle formed by recording plane of X-ray film and the long axis of the tooth. This technique can be performed without the use of film holders, it is quick and comfortable for the patient. But it also has certain disadvantages like incidences of cone cutting, image distortion, superimposition of anatomical structures and difficulty to reproduce the periapical films.

Various angulations used

Tooth	Maxilla	Mandible
Incisors	+40°	–15°
Canine	+45°	–20°
Premolar	+30°	–10°
Molar	+20°	–5°

In *paralleling technique* (**Fig. 5.49**), the X-ray film is placed parallel to the long axis of the tooth to be exposed and the X-ray beam is directed perpendicular to the film.

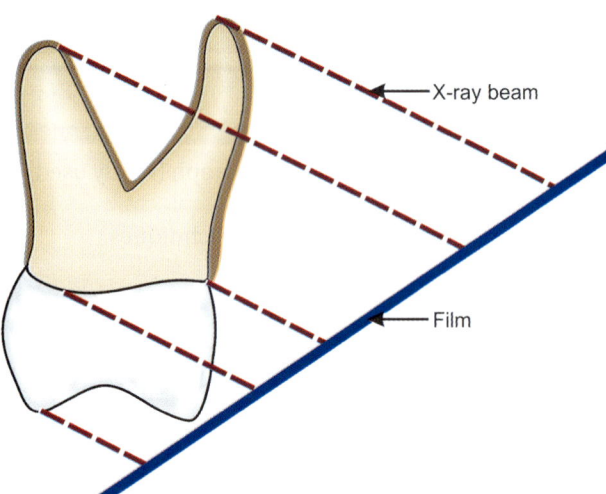

Figure 5.48: Bisecting angle technique

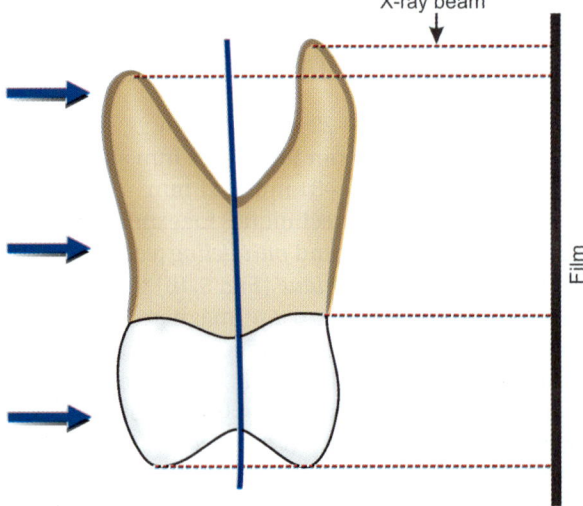

Figure 5.49: Paralleling technique

Advantages of paralleling technique
- Better accuracy of image
- Reduced dose of radiation
- Reproducibility
- Better images of bone margins, interproximal regions and maxillary molar region
- Disadvantages of paralleling technique are difficult to use in patients with shallow vault gag reflex
- When rubber dam is in place.

Cone angulation is one of the most important aspects of radiography because it affects the quality of image. It is seen that paralleling technique is superior to bisecting angle technique especially in reproduction of apical anatomy of the tooth. As the angle increases away from parallel, the quality of image decreases. This happens because with increase in angle, the tissue that the X-rays must pass through includes greater percentage of bone mass thus anatomy becomes less predictable. To limit this problem, Walton gave a *modified paralleling technique* in which central beam is oriented perpendicular to radiographic film but not to teeth. Modified paralleling technique is also beneficial for some special situations in which paralleling technique is not feasible, for example, shallow palatal vault, maxillary tori, extremely long roots, uncooperative and gagging patient.

Cone image shift technique: The proper application of this technique helps in distinguishing the objects which have been superimposed, differentiating the different types of tooth defects. The main concept of technique is that as the vertical or horizontal angulations of X-ray tube head changes, the object buccal or closest to the tube head moves to opposite side of radiograph when compared to lingual object (**Fig. 5.50**). In other words, we can say that the cone image shift technique separates and identifies the facial and lingual structures.

As the cone position moves from parallel either towards horizontal or vertical, the object on the film shifts away from the direction of cone, i.e. in the direction of central beam. In other words, when two objects and the film are in fixed position and the tube head is moved, images of both objects move in opposite direction. The resultant radiograph shows lingual object that moved in the same direction as the cone and the buccal object moved in opposite direction. This is also known as "SLOB" rule (same lingual opposite buccal).

Synonyms of cone image shift technique
- BOR (Buccal object rule)
- SLOB (Same lingual opposite buccal)
- BOMM (Buccal object moves most)
- Clark's rule
- Walton's projection.

Bitewing Radiographs (Fig.5.51)

It is reliable methods for estimation of the proximal tooth surfaces before they are detected clinically, because these areas usually are not readily assessed visually or tactilely.

These are specially important to detect incipient lesions at the contact points. In bitewing films we can also notice height of alveolar crest, cervical margins of the restoration, lamina dura and pulp cavity.

Different sizes of bitewing X-ray films are
➡ Size 0 (for children)—22 mm × 35 mm
➡ Size 1 for adult (anterior teeth)—24 mm × 40 mm
➡ Size 2 for adult (posterior teeth)—31 mm × 41 mm
➡ Size 3 (for all posterior teeth of one side in one film)—27 mm × 54 mm.

Occlusal and Panoramic Radiographs (Fig. 5.52)

These are mainly used for detecting lesions of the oral cavity, for educating the public and for having a broader view of the oral cavity. Most common size of occlusal X-ray film is 57 mm × 76 mm.

Since this technique uses intensifying screen which may obstruct finer details, so these are not indicated for diagnosis of incipient carious lesions.

Advantages
➡ Relatively low patient radiation dose
➡ Provides information about the size of the lesion
➡ Can tell whether the lesion is present lingually or facially
➡ Broad anatomic region covered
➡ Convenience, ease and speed of performance
➡ Useful in patients with limited mouth opening.

Disadvantages
➡ Lack of fine anatomic detail
➡ Geometric distortion
➡ Overlapping
➡ Cost factor
➡ Occlusal technique does not determine the angulation of a tooth in that particular arch.

Xeroradiography

It is new method for recording images without film. In this technique the image is recorded on an aluminum plate coated with selenium particles.

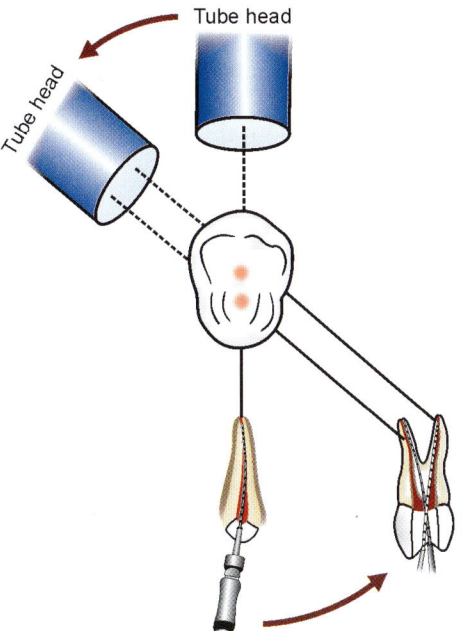

Figure 5.50: Cone image shift technique

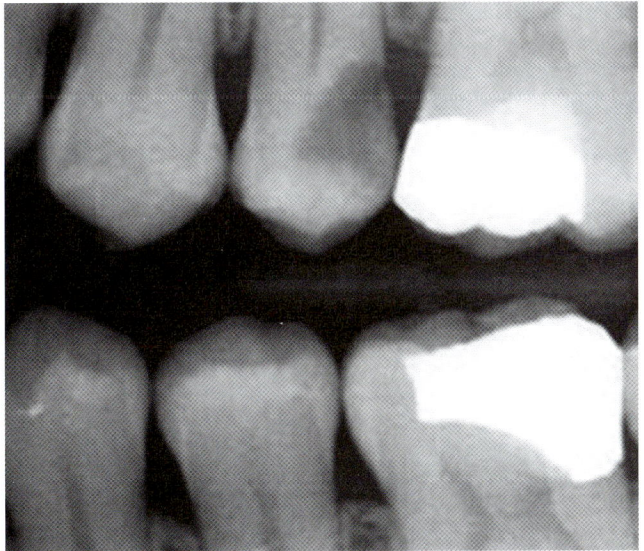

Figure 5.51: Bite wing radiograph

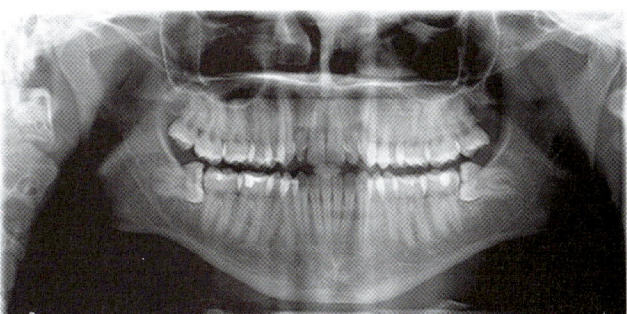

Figure 5.52: OPG

The plate is removed from the cassette and subjected to relaxation which removes old images, then these are electrostatically charged and inserted into the cassette. Radiations are projected on film which cause selective discharge of the particles. This forms the latent image and is converted to a positive image by a process called 'development' in the processor unit.

Advantages of xeroradiography

- This technique offers 'edge enhancement' and good detail ('Edge enhancement' means differentiating areas of different densities especially at the edges)
- The ability to have both positive and negative prints together
- It is two times more sensitive than conventional D-speed films.

Disadvantages of xeroradiography

- Since saliva may act as a medium for flow of current, the electric charge over the film may cause discomfort to the patient.
- Exposure time varies according to thickness of the plate.
- The process of development cannot be delayed beyond 15 minute.

Classification of Caries as seen on Radiograph (Figs 5.53A to E)

E0 – No visible radiographic lesion
E1 – Lesion in outer one-half of enamel
E2 – Lesion in inner one-half of enamel
D1 – Lesion in outer third of dentin
D2 – Lesion in middle third of dentin
D3 – Lesion in inner third of dentin.

Recent Advances in Radiographic Techniques

Digital Radiography

Digital imaging uses the standard radiology technique in which film is used to record the image and then final image is subjected to digital processing to produce the final result.

The backlot film image is converted to a digital signal by a scanning device, such as videocamera. First the image is divided into a grid or matrix of uniformly sized pixels, each of which is assigned a gray scale value based on its optical diversity. This value is stored in computer.

Once the image is in computer, a number of operations can be performed on computer program used.

One of the most useful operations is a comparison of images called digital substraction. The computers can compare two images. Some use for this type includes determination of progression of disease over time and evaluation of treatment outcomes for periodontal and endodontic therapy.

For digital substraction, this is standardization of the process used to make the images as well as adjustments of the film density and contrast.

Another use is in detection of lesion on radiographs. This is where an endodontist can use this application for diagnosis. The computers can detect lesion with pattern recognition and boundary determination. Sometimes, density changes on radiographs are so subtle that human eye has trouble identifying them, but machines are able to discriminate at density level beyond what human eye can see.

Advantages

- The amount of information available from these radiographs is greater than from radiographs that have not been digitalized.
- The storage of radiographs and quality of image is better.
- Photographs of radiographs can be produced.

Disadvantages

The radiation dose to the patient is the same as that used during radiographs. However, depending on the task required, less dense radiographs requiring low doses, could be used because computer can differentiate between areas of low contrast better than the human eye.

E1	E2	D1	D2	D3
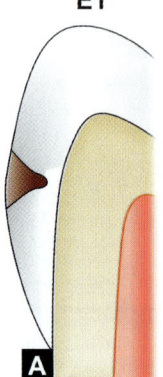	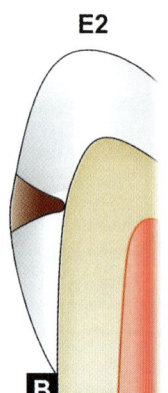	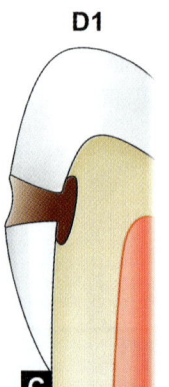	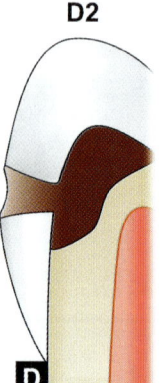	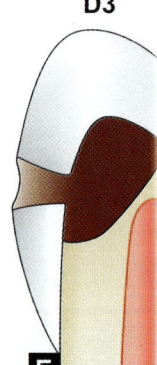
A	B	C	D	E

Figures 5.53A to E: Classification of caries when seen on radiograph

Digital dental radiology: Images in digital form can be readily manipulated, stored and retrieved on computer. Furthermore, technology makes the transmission of images practicable. The general principles of digital imaging are:
- The chemically produced radiograph is represented by data that is acquired in a parallel and continuous fashion known as analogue.
- Computers use binary (0 or 1) language, where information is usually handled in 8 character words called bytes.
- If each character can be either 0 or 1. This result in 28 possible combination (words) that is 256 words. Thus digital dental images are limited to 256 shades of gray.
- Digital images are made-up of pixels (picture elements), each allocated a shade of gray.
- The spatial resolution of a digital system is heavily dependent upon the number of pixels available per millimeter of image.

Methods of digital dental radiology
➡ One uses charged couple devices
➡ Other uses photostimulable phosphor imaging plates.

Both methods can be used in dental surgery with conventional personal computers.

Digital imaging systems require an electronic sensor or detector, an analog to digital converter, a computer, and a monitor or printer for image of the components of imaging system. It instructs the X-ray generator when to begin and end the exposure, controls the digitizer, constructs the image by mathematical algorithm, determines the method of image display, and provides for storage and transmission of acquired data.

The most common sensor is the CCD, the other being phosphor images.

When a conventional X-ray unit is used to project the X-ray beam on to the sensor, an electronic charge is created, an analog output signal is generated and the digital converter converts the analog output signal from CCD to a numeric representation that is recognizable by the computer.

The radiographic image then appears on the monitor and can be manipulated electronically to alter contrast, resolution, orientation and even size.

The CCD system: The CCD is a solid state detector composed of array of X-ray or light sensitive phosphores on a pure silicon chip. These phosphore convert incoming X-rays to a wavelength that matches the peak response of silicon.

RVG: RVG is composed of three major parts. The radio part consists of a conventional X-ray unit, a precise timer for short exposure times and a tiny sensor to record the image. The sensor has a small (17 × 24 mm) receptor screen which transmits information via fiberoptic bundle to a miniature CCD. The sensor is protected from X-ray degradation by a fiberoptic shield and can be cold sterilized for infection control. Disposable latex sheaths are used to cover the sensor when it is in use (**Fig. 5.54**).

Because the sensor does not need to be removed from mouth after each exposure, the time to take multiple images is greatly reduced.

The 'visio' portion of the system receives and stores incoming signals during exposure and converts them point by point into one of 256 discrete gray levels. It consists of a video-monitor and display processing unit (**Fig. 5.55**). As the image is transmitted to the processing unit, it is digitalized and memorized by the computer. The unit magnifies the image four times for immediate display on video-monitor and has additional capability of producing colored images (**Figs 5.56 and 5.57**). It can also display multiple images simultaneously, including a full mouth series on one screen. A zoom feature is also available to enlarge a portion of image up to face-screen size.

The 'graphy' part of RVG unit consists of digital storage apparatus. That can be connected to various print out or mass storage devices for immediate or later viewing.

Advantages of RVG
➡ Low radiation dose
➡ Darkroom is not required as instant image is viewed
➡ Image distortion from bent radiographic film is eliminated
➡ The quality of the image is consistent
➡ Greater exposure latitude

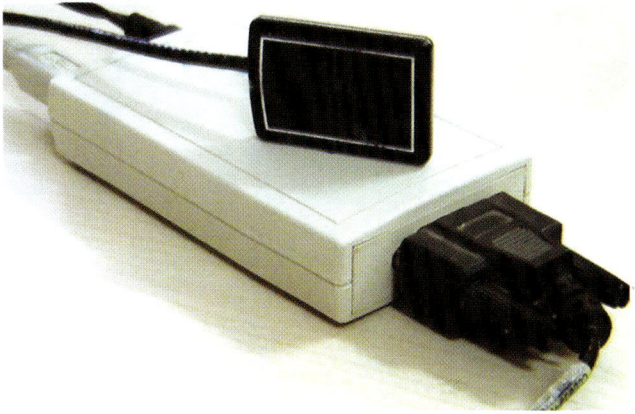

Figure 5.54: Sensor and CCD system

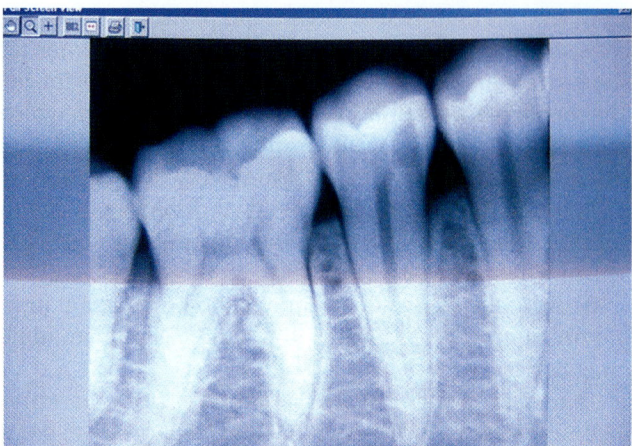

Figure 5.55: Video monitor displaying images

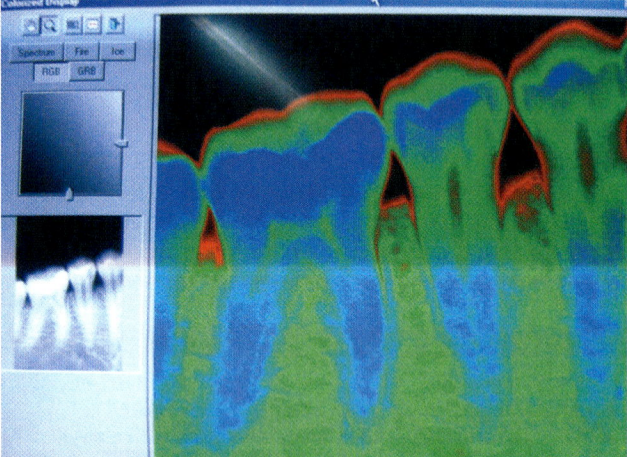

Figure 5.56: Colored images produced in RVG

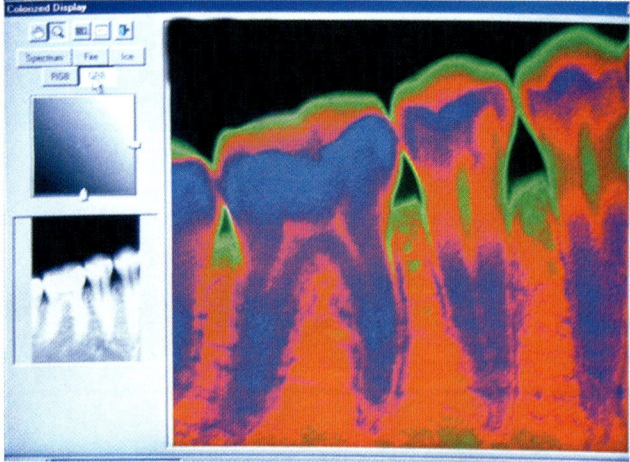

Figure 5.57: Different color contrasts can be produced in RVG

- Elimination of hazards of film development
- Diagnostic capability is increased through digital enhancement and enlargement of specific areas for closer examination
- Contrast and resolution can be altered, and images can be viewed in black and white color
- Images are displayed instantly
- Full mouth radiographs can be made within seconds
- Storages and archiving of patient information
- Transfer of images between institutions (teleradiology)
- Infection control and toxic waste disposal problems associated with radiology are eliminated.

Disadvantages of RVG

- Expensive
- The life expectancy of CCD is not fixed
- Solid state sensors when used for bitewing examination are small as compared to size-2 film
- Large disk space required to store images
- Bulky sensor with cable attachment, which can make placement in mouth difficult
- Soft tissue imaging is not very nice.

Phosphor imaging system: Imaging using a photostimulable phosphor can also be called as an indirect digital imaging technique. The image is captured on a phosphor plate as analogue information and is converted into a digital format when the plate is processed.

Two sizes of phosphor plates, similar in size to conventional intraoral film packets are provided. They have to be placed in plastic light-tight bags, before being used in the mouth. They are then positioned in the same manner as film packets, using holders, incorporating beam-aiming devices, and are exposed using conventional dental X-ray equipment. The dose is highly reduced. The image is displayed and manipulated. A hard copy can be obtained if necessary.

Advantages

- Low radiation dose (90% reduction)
- Almost instant image (20-30 seconds)
- Wide exposure latitude (almost impossible to burn out information)
- Same size receptor as films
- X-ray source can be remote from PC
- Image manipulation facilities.

Disadvantages

- Cost
- Storage of images (same as with CCD systems)
- Slight inconvenience of plastic bags.

Recent studies have shown that accuracy of caries diagnosis was as high or better with a digital storage phosphor system as with conventional film in the permanent dentition.

Computerized Image Analysis

Development of computer has made it possible to use automated procedures which are able to overcome the shortcomings of human eye. Softwares have been developed for automated interpretation of digital radiographs in order to standardize image assessment.

Advantages
➡ Automated analysis may provide sensitive and objective observation of smaller lesions which otherwise are not perceptible to naked eye
➡ It is possible to monitor the progression of the lesion
➡ Quantification of smaller lesions is possible.

Disadvantages
➡ There is always a need for standardization of exposure geometry
➡ Sensitivity is higher but specificity is less
➡ Time consuming and less economical.

Substraction Radiography

In this technique, to increase the noticeable changes in radiographs, the structured noise is reduced. The structured noises are the images which obstruct the routine examination of radiographs are not of diagnostic value.

Substraction images can be achieved from photographic, electronic and digital method.

Digital substraction radiographs can be used for:
- Demonstration of approximal carious lesions.
- Estimation of alveolar bone height.
- Detecting little mineral loss of bone.
- Detecting artificially produced recurrent caries.
- Detecting progress of remineralization and demineralization pattern of dental caries.

Tuned Aperture Computed Tomography (TACT): TACT is a tomosynthetic technique which conquers the shortcomings of conventional radiography. With this technique a three-dimensional image can be formed by generating a series of cross-sectional images of an object and then combining them.

Advantages
➡ More accurate than radiographic films
➡ Does not require much new equipment as it can be added to basic digital imaging systems.

Magnetic Resonance Microimaging (MRMI)

For diseases of the mineralized dental tissues the detection of changes, particularly early changes, is of considerable importance. However, such changes are below the limit of detection of clinical MRI instrumentation. Hence, magnetic resonance microimaging was developed by which is a refinement of the whole body.

The two main differences between whole body MRI and MRMI are:
- MRI uses a magnetic field in the range of 1.0 to 1.5 tesla (T), while MRMI uses greater field strength, i.e. 7T.
- The MRMI has a considerably smaller bore, i.e. = 2.5 than the whole body imager.

Advantages
➡ MRMI is noninvasive and nondestructive
➡ It's use allows a specimen to be reimaged after further exposure to a clinically relevant environment
➡ Teeth examined with MRMI do not suffer the sectioning artifacts that can occur during conventional histologic examination
➡ MRMI produces high resolution, three-dimensional images of internal and external tooth morphologies
➡ MRMI will provide information not available through other methods of investigation on the site, extent and structure of carious lesions.

Disadvantages
➡ Very expensive
➡ Still in initial developmental stages.

Electrical Resistance Measurement

Sound tooth enamel is a good electrical insulator due to its high inorganic content. Caries results in increased porosity. Saliva fills the pores and forms conductive pathways for electrical current. The electrical conductivity is hence directly proportional to the amount of demineralization that has occurred. Electrical resistance refers to measuring the electrical conductivity through these pores.

Vanguard Electronic Caries Detector

It has been designed to measure the electrical conductivity of the tooth. The electrical conductivity is expressed numerically on a scale from 0 to 9, indicating a change from sound tooth to an increased degree of demineralization.

Advantages
➡ Very effective in detecting early pit and fissure caries
➡ It can also monitor the progress of caries.

Disadvantages
➡ Can only recognize demineralization and not caries specifically
➡ Presence of enamel cracks may lead to false positive diagnosis
➡ A sharp metal explorer is utilized which is pressed into the fissure causing traumatic defects
➡ Separate measurements are required for different sites making full mouth examination quite time consuming
➡ Area of diagnosis is confined to the dimensions of the probe.

Lasers

Different types of lasers used for the diagnosis of caries are

➠ Argon laser
➠ Diode laser
➠ Qualitative laser fluorescence
➠ Diagnodent quantitative laser fluorescence
➠ Optical coherence tomography
➠ Dye enhanced laser fluorescence.

Argon Laser

When the Argon laser light illuminates the tooth; the diseased carious area appears of dark orange-red color and is easily discernible from the surrounding healthy structures.

Diode Laser

A visible red diode with a wavelength of 655 nm and 1MW of power is used. This red energy excites fluorescence reflected back into a detector in the unit, which analyses and quantifies the degree of caries.

Qualitative Laser Fluorescence

This technique uses argon laser (488 nm) with a filtered blue light source. This technique depends upon the ability of enamel to autofluorescence under certain conditions.

It has been suggested that fluorescence of tooth structure is due to the presence of chromophores within the enamel. Sound and carious enamel have differences in fluorescence due to the loss of chromophores when there are caries, some of the mineral content of enamel is lost and replaced by water, which results in an increase in light scattering and consequently the less fluorescence (**Fig. 5.58**).

A reduction in the fluorescence of demineralized enamel, helps in detection of caries.

In this technique, blue light is used to irradiate the surface of the tooth and the resultant fluorescent image is captured in a computer. The lesion appears dark against the bright fluoresced background of the sound enamel. It causes the carious lesion to appear as a different color. QLF shows demineralization or incipient lesions as a dark spot. Caries and plaque appear red in color, indicating a bacterial presence. The images can be stored, measured and quantified in terms of shape of an area.

For the patient, the differences in color can be motivational since the invasion of bacteria is understandable. In conjunction with the operative microscope, some consider laser fluorescence to be the most consistent method for diagnosing pit and fissure caries.

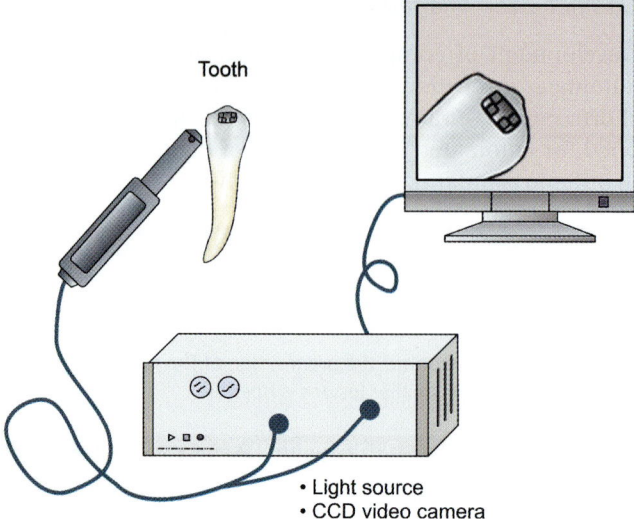

Tooth

- Light source
- CCD video camera

Figure 5.58: QLF principle

Advantages

➠ Helps in detecting incipient caries
➠ Detect early caries adjacent to orthodontic brackets and restorations
➠ Can detect failing fissure sealants
➠ Can monitor enamel erosion
➠ Convenient and fast.

Disadvantages

➠ It provides moderate sensitivity and specificity
➠ High cost
➠ Not able to differentiate caries, calculus or hypoplasia.

Diagnodent

Based on principle of fluorescence. It uses a diode laser light source and a fiber optic cable that transmits light to a hand held probe. Light is absorbed induces infrared fluorescence by organic and inorganic materials. Emitted fluorescence is collected at probe tip, processed and presented on display as an integer between 0 and 99. (**Fig. 5.59**).

Technique: Before using the diagnodent, the unit must be calibrated with the selected tip and a patient-specific baseline must be established. Switch on the diagnodent, set the diagnodent so that the readout confirms the correct position of the unit to the tip selected.

The numeric readout on the device (00-99) indicates the amount of fluorescence.

Place the tip on the area to be evaluated. Use a rocking motion with the tip. Note and record the peak value. Based upon *in vivo* studies, the following correlations can be made.

Value 0 to 14 : No caries
Value 15 to 20 : Histological caries within enamel
Value 21 to 99 : Histological dentinal caries

The restorative suggestion from the above data is as follows:

For 0 to 14 : No treatment other than preventive
For 15 to 20 : Pit and fissure sealants
For 21 to 30 : Risk
For > 30 : Operative treatment.

Advantages of diagnodent

- Good reproducibility
- For detection of nonpreparation occlusal carious lesions, diagnodent is considered as superior to other aids in terms of both correlation with histopathology and specificity/sensitivity
- Because of its good reproducibility, it can be used to monitor caries regression or progression.

Disadvantages of diagnodent

- Increased likelihood of false positive diagnosis
- Sensitive to the presence of stains
- Any changes in the physical structure of enamel like hypoplasia may give false readings
- It cannot detect secondary caries.

Optical Coherence Tomography (OCT)

It utilizes broad band-width light sources and advanced fiberoptics to achieve images. Similar to ultrasound, OCT uses reflections of near infrared light with considerable penetration into tissue and no known detrimental biological effect. This is helpful to determine not only the presence of decay but also the depth of caries progression.

Advantages OCT

- High probing depth in scattering media
- High depth and transverse resolution
- Contact free
- Noninvasive operation
- Microstructural tissue detail is revealed
- More sensitive method for detection of recurrent caries
- Also it shows extent and severity of the carious lesion.

Disadvantage OCT

Loss of penetration depth occurs in OCT images, thus it is difficult to use it in early decay.

Polarization Sensitive Optical Coherence Tomography (PSOCT)

PSOCT is a nondestructive imaging system that can utilize near infrared light to produce depth resolved images of dental enamel and has the potential to monitor early enamel occlusal caries. PSOCT overcomes the limitation of depth loss of OCT and can be used to quantify lesion severity in topographically challenging areas such as occlusal pits and fissures.

Dye Enhanced Laser Fluorescence (DELF)

With the addition of a fluorescent dye, QLF can be used to detect early demineralization in dentin.

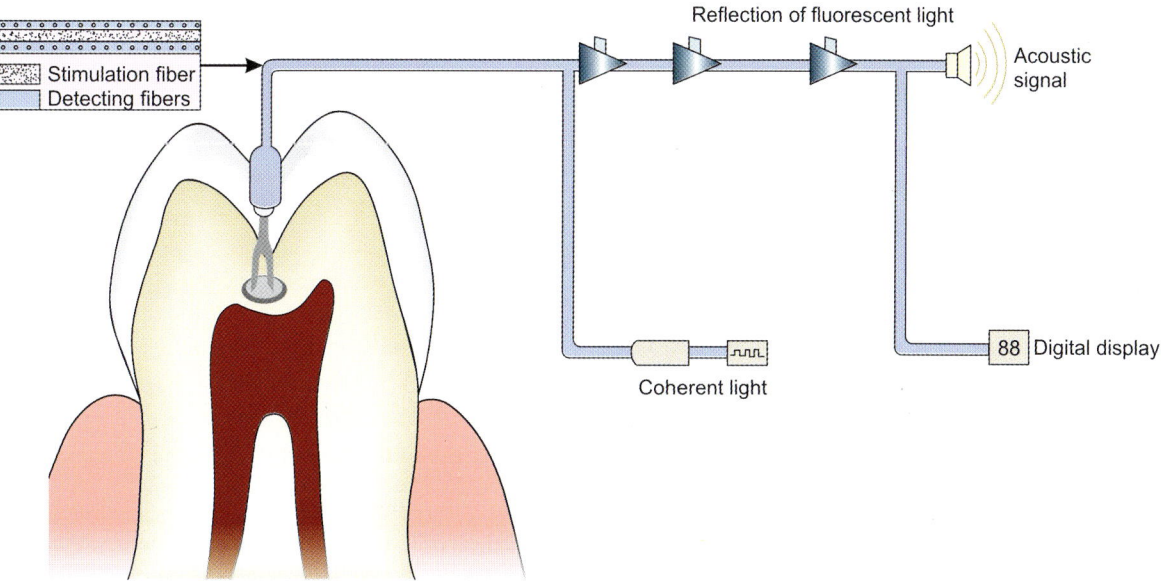

Figure 5.59: Principle of diagnodent

DELF approach is based on the hypothesis that if a fluorescent dye penetrates an early carious lesion, current laser fluorescence method for detection and qualification of early mineral loss could be enhanced. One of the dyes used is Pyromethane 556.

Advantages

→ In the absence of plaque, DELF is a better diagnostic tool than LF in detection of demineralization in artificial tissues.
→ It is seen that optical measurement of dye uptake may be a useful technique to detect approximal subsurface caries.

Zandona AGF et al (1998) concluded that DELF was a better diagnostic tool than LF for detection of demineralization in artificial fissures.

 Want to Know More

Other devices for detecting caries

Ultrasonics
Use of sound waves for detection. Sonic velocity and specific acoustic impedance can be determined for dentin and enamel as well as for soft tissue and bone. *Velocity of sound on enamel surfaces (V_s) = 3,143,121m/s.* All sites with visible cavitation and dentinal radiolucencies produce echoes with higher amplitude.

Intraoral camera
It is indispensable diagnostic and magnification tool. The camera moves around inside the mouth and generate video examination of mouth and also helps in patient education.
Magnification
Loupes and microscope tremendously increase visibility thus improving diagnosis and treatment.
Digora
It is an indirect digital radiography that uses phosphor luminescence flexible filmlike radiation sensor placed intraorally and exposed to X-ray. A laser sensor reads exposed plates offline and reveals a digital image data.

ARRESTED CARIES

Arrested carious lesion is a lesion that may have formed earlier and then stopped. It usually presents as a large open cavity which no longer retains food and becomes self-cleansing.

Arrested carious lesions are most commonly seen on lingual and labial aspects of teeth and less commonly interproximally. On the proximal surface, it appears as brown-stained area just below contact point of retained tooth. Here, the caries process is arrested because proximal surface becomes self-cleansing due to extraction of

adjacent teeth. In arrested caries, superficially softened and decalcified dentin is gradually burnished away due to mastication until it takes on a brown, stained, polished appearance which is hard. This type of dentin is referred as eburnated dentin.

Stages of Development of Arrested Caries

The development of arrested caries occurs in the following stages (**Figs 5.60A to C**).

First Stage

- The acids produced by bacteria dissolve the minerals of the surrounding intertubular dentin
- The tubule fluid becomes saturated with calcium magnesium and phosphate ions
- If less acid is produced then the second stage can occur.

Second Stage

Large crystals of tricalcium phosphate are formed by precipitation of saturated crystals.

Third Stage

- The odontoblast process secretes collagen into the dentin tubule

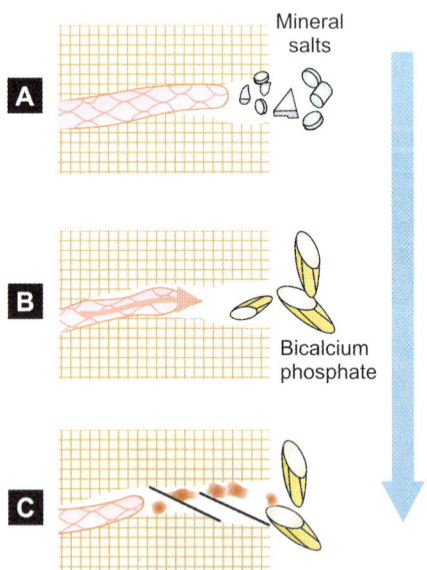

Figures 5.60A to C: Steps of development of arrested caries: (A) High concentration of mineral salts deposited in dentinal tubules; (B) With reduced acid production, pH rises resulting in deposition of salts in crystals of tricalcium phosphate to block the tubule; (C) Blockage of dentinal tubules because of further deposition of crystals and calcium salts

- Hydroxyapatite crystals accumulate and block the tubule
- The growth of crystals takes place in the intertubular dentin.

RECURRENT CARIES/SECONDARY CARIES

Secondary or recurrent caries can be defined as contact caries, which refers to caries on the tooth surface which is in contact with the restoration. Similar to the primary caries, the enamel or root surface adjacent to the restorative material may possess an inactive arrested lesion, an active incipient lesion, or a frankly cavitated lesion. With enamel surfaces, recurrent caries may be seen as a white spot, or a brown spot lesion. The enamel lesion color varies depending upon the adjacent restorative material. When the cavosurface is involved and undermined by caries, the adjacent enamel surface takes on a brown to gray to blue hue.

Since, secondary caries may be present at surface enamel surrounding the restoration or extend below it along the margins (**Fig. 5.61**). Therefore, these are also referred as caries adjacent to restorations and sealants (CARS).

Though restorations are placed to restore a damaged tooth to its form, functions and esthetics but none of the restorations can last for ever. Most of the restorations are replaced because of the clinical diagnosis of recurrent caries which is thought to be within a range of 45 to 55 percent. The recurrent caries are seen more often in resin-based composite restorations than the amalgam restorations.

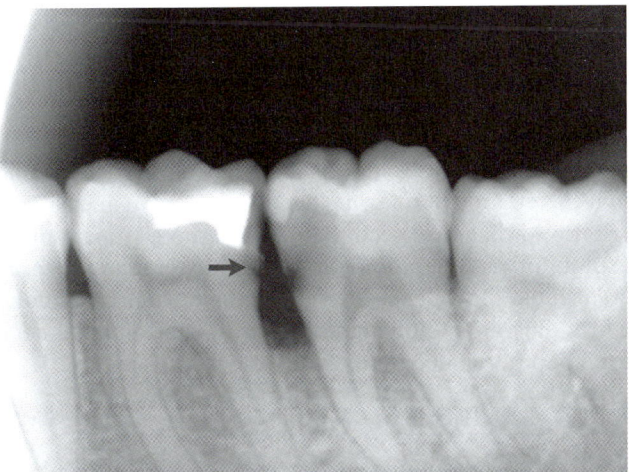

Figure 5.61: Secondary caries in first molar

Etiology

- The main causative factor for recurrent caries is marginal leakage around the restorations
- Factors which predispose to recurrent caries are ditching or fracture of the restoration at the edges
- Fracture of the marginal tooth structure, microleakage.
- Presence of overhangs
- Rough surface of the restoration along with poor oral hygiene
- An improper tooth preparation
- Unpolished enamel surfaces.

Microbiology

Studies have shown not much significant differences in the microflora in primary and recurrent caries. Secondary caries are caused by the action of acids produced by bacteria.

In the outer surface lesion, acid production is predisposed by bacterias present on the tooth surface.

Most common microorganisms with recurrent caries are
➡ *Streptococcus mutans*
➡ Lactobacilli
➡ Actinomyces viscosus.

In wall lesion, acid production is predisposed by the penetration of bacteria along the tooth–restoration interface. This depends upon type and amount of plaque present on tooth surface.

Clinical Diagnosis of Recurrent Caries

The diagnosis of secondary caries depends upon visual inspection, tactile sensation with judicious explorer usage, and radiographic interpretation.

Secondary caries has been described as occurring in two ways: An "outer lesion" and a "wall lesion" (**Fig. 5.62**).

The chemical and histological processes involved in "outer lesions" are the same as primary caries and it has been suggested that it occurs as the result of a new, primary, attack on the surface of the tooth adjacent to the restoration. The 'wall lesion' is the lesion which is present on the preparation walls. It occurs because of microleakage of oral fluids, percolation of hydrogen ions and lytic enzymes from plaque, and bacterial colonization along the cavosurface wall. Thus, these lesions only occur secondary to the presence of a restoration.

- Usually both wall lesion and outer surface lesion occur.
- If there is only outer lesion is present but not the wall lesion, it can be due to closure of the interface between the preparation wall and the restoration because of corrosion products.

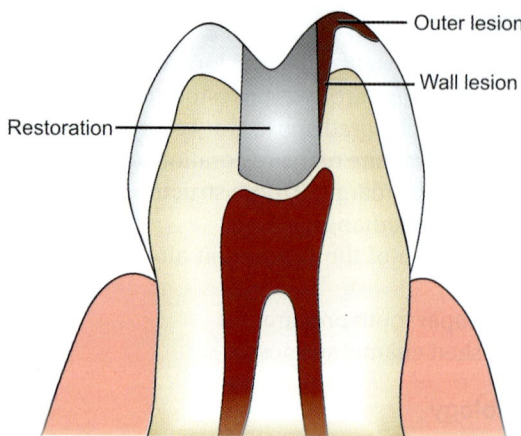

Figure 5.62: Outer and wall lesion of secondary caries

- If only wall lesion is present, it can be due to the resistance of the occlusal enamel to demineralization.

Some of features which make the diagnosis of secondary caries difficult are:

- Difficulties in the differentiation among restoration margin discrepancies (marginal integrity, discoloration of the tooth at restoration margin).
- Sharp probing can be misleading as a probe may become impacted in a margin discrepancy that is not in fact carious.
- Discoloration at the restoration margin is difficult to evaluate, as it can be due to the other causes like discoloration found next to amalgam or slowly progressing lesions.

Recurrent caries at proximal or gingival locations in restorations can be diagnosed by radiography provided that X-rays are projected at an optimal angle in relation to the lesion. Recent advances in diagnostic methods like digital imaging, digital substraction radiography and computer based digital systems which provide image enhancement and Tuned aperture computer tomography (TACT) which presents three-dimensional images, may help in diagnosis of secondary caries. Studies have shown that recurrent caries are mostly seen on the gingival margins of all types of Class II and Class V restorations, and less commonly on Class I restorations or on the occlusal part of Class II restorations.

Factors predisposing occurrence of recurrent caries on the gingival surface are:

- Gingival area is prone to contamination during the restoration by gingival fluid and saliva leaking between the matrix and the cavosurface margin. Insufficiency in the adaptation of the restorative materials may cause empty space that may lead to secondary caries.

- Polymerization shrinkage of resin-based materials at the gingival margins tends to pull the material away from the gingival part of the tooth preparation.
- Bonding to dentin and cementum is less effective at the gingival cavosurface margin than is bonding to enamel.
- Besides, it is more difficult for patients to keep plaque-free gingival area of the restoration, which further leads tooth decay.
- Also the gingival margins of Class II restorations are difficult to examine.

Difficulties in diagnosis of secondary caries is due to
➡ Small size of the initial lesion
➡ Color change is, dusty white to brownish, difficult to interpret in amalgam restorations
➡ It is difficult to examine wall lesion clinically unless there is adequate demineralization which is seen through the overlying enamel
➡ Stains at the margins of tooth-colored restorations are difficult to differentiate from recurrent caries
➡ Catch formed while probing tooth restoration interface may not be carious, though it appears to be
➡ Two-dimensional radiographic picture
➡ Radiopacity of restoration obstruct the lesion
➡ The burnout at the cervical margin may make the interpretation difficult.

Classification by Espelid and Tveit (1991)
➡ S-1: Initial carious lesion characterized by discoloration only
➡ S-2: Lesions characterized by softness in enamel
➡ S-3: Lesions with cavitation on the root surfaces.

Treatment of Secondary Caries

An accurate diagnosis of recurrent caries is mandatory before instigating any treatment because it could be just a discoloration but not a carious lesion **Flow chart 5.1**.

If recurrent caries is a marginal defect rather than a carious lesion, it is doubtful that fluoride or fluoride releasing materials will reduce the frequency of recurrent caries.

One should consider reburnishing and repairing the defects at restoration margins rather than going for replacement of restoration.

Secondary carious lesions are all localized defects that may be repaired or reburnished. Even if after using clinical criteria to diagnose secondary caries there is any doubt, exploratory preparations into the restorative material adjacent to the defects determines their extent and allows a firm diagnosis to be made. This will determine the need for repair or replacement of the restoration.

ROOT CARIES (FIG. 5.63)

Root caries as defined by Hazen, is a soft, progressive lesion that is found anywhere on the root surface that has

Flow chart 5.1: Diagnosis and management of secondary/recurrent caries

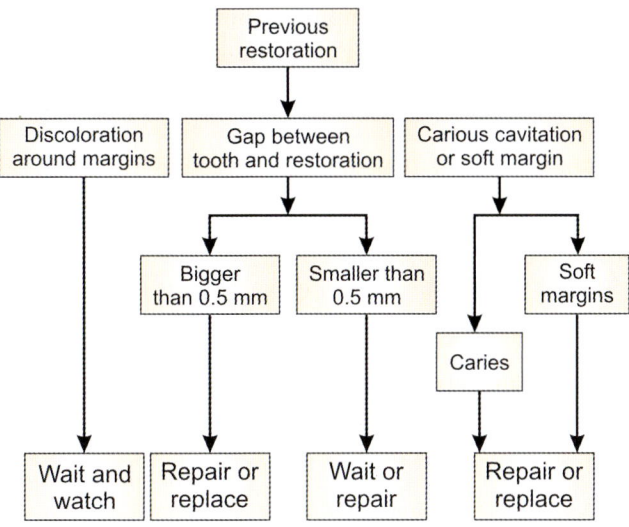

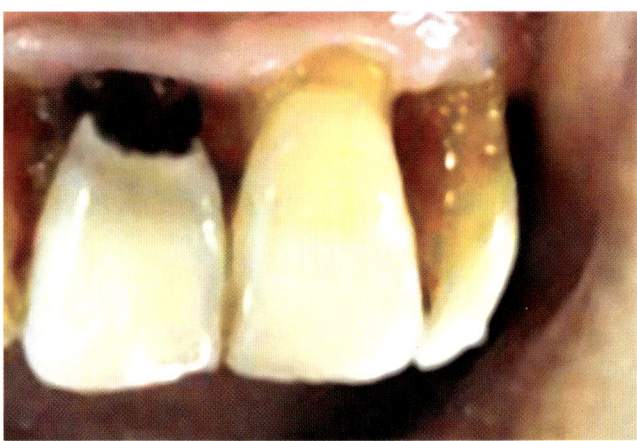

Figure 5.63: Cervical caries

Features of root caries

→ Root surface caries are initiated when there is periodontal attachment loss exposing the root surface to the oral environment
→ Root caries is a soft, irregular, progressive lesion occurring at or apical to the CEJ
→ An area where root caries has taken place may appear as round or oval in shape which then may spread radially and join other areas of root caries
→ These areas appear as white or discolored having irregular outline, with or without a cavity at an exposed root surface
→ Root caries are more common in males than females
→ Most commonly they are seen in mandibular molars, followed by premolars, canines and incisors. This order is reversed in the maxilla.

Etiology of the Root Caries

The microflora responsible for root caries consists of *Streptococcus mutans*, *Lactobacillus* and *Actinobacillus*. Micro-organisms metabolize sugars into organic acids, these acids then pass through the root structure and start the process of demineralization. This process takes place at the pH of 6.4 (5.5 for demineralization of enamel). The rate of demineralization of root occur at higher pH and is much faster than that of enamel because the root has much less mineral content (55%) than that of enamel (99%).

Intraoral factors

→ Xerostomia
→ Low salivary buffer capacity
→ Poor oral hygiene
→ Periodontal disease and periodontal surgery
→ Gingival recession
→ Frequency of carbohydrate intake
→ Unrestored and restored coronal and root caries
→ Overdenture abutments and removable partial dentures
→ Malocclusion
→ Abfraction lesions
→ Tipped teeth which make areas of teeth inaccessible for cleaning.

Extraoral factors

→ Advanced age
→ Medications that decrease the salivary flow
→ Lower educational and socioeconomic levels
→ Antipsychotics, sedatives, barbiturates, and antihistamines
→ Diabetes, autoimmune disorders (e.g. Sjögren's syndrome)
→ Radiation therapy
→ Gender—males are affected more than females
→ Physical disability where patients have limited manual dexterity for cleaning of teeth
→ Limited exposure to fluoridated water
→ Consumption of alcohol or narcotics.

Diagnosis

• Clinical examination is best carried out with an explorer. Tooth surface should be cleaned before

lost its connective tissue attachment and is exposed to the environment.

Root caries occurs at or apical to the cementoenamel junction (CEJ). Generally root caries lesions have been described as having a distinct outline and presenting with a discolored appearance in relation to the surrounding noncarious root.

Most common reason for their occurrence is gingival recession, though other causes can also be present. With advanced age, there is more gingival recession, which leaves the root surface exposed to the oral environment and leads to an increase in the root caries rate. Root caries can occur in the areas of abrasion, erosion, and abfraction, or as primary root caries and recurrent decay.

examination since plaque covering the lesion can lead to misdiagnosis.

- Accurate radiographs can also help in diagnosis but they should be free from overlapping or burnout.
- Special dyes can be useful for detecting root caries, these dyes stain the infected dentin and thus allow the clinician to detect caries.

Differential diagnosis of root caries			
	Active root caries	Arrested root caries	Extrinsic stain on root surface
Color	Light brown	Dark brown to black	Dark in color
Surface texture	Soft, leathery, and elastic in nature	Hard and can-not be com-pressed	Hard and rough texture

Prevention

- Proper preventive measures of plaque removal, diet modification, and the use of topical fluoride should be advocated.
- Preventive measures like educating patients, assisting them to avoid high sugar-containing meals and maintaining a proper toothbrushing technique should be practiced.
- Special attention should be given to root caries-prone patients who are wearing dental prostheses. This can be done by proper management of soft tissues during fixed prosthesis procedures and avoiding the placement of restoration margins apical to the surrounding tissue to avoid plaque accumulation.
- In patients with low salivary flow, xylitol-containing chewing gum which stimulates salivary flow and decreases plaque formation has shown to decrease the caries.

Treatment of Root Caries

- Treatment plan for root caries depends on the following factors:
  - Clinical examination
  - Size of the lesion
  - Type, extent, and site of the lesion
  - Esthetic requirements
  - Physical and mental condition of the patient.
- Root caries lesions are difficult to restore because of their location, which is usually subgingival. For proper restoration, sufficient access and isolation are needed.
- To begin with, root surface is cleaned with pumice to remove the plaque.
- Then the excavation of carious tooth tissue is done and restoration walls are prepared. The margins and retention design depends on the restorative material

used. For example, when a tooth is to be restored with amalgam, retention grooves are required occlusally and gingivally. For composites, beveling of the coronal margins of the preparation is required.

Restorative Materials Used for Treatment of Root Caries

Different restorative materials are used for the treatment of root caries, all having different characteristics. One should chose the restorative material according to the location, accessibility, margins and oral hygiene.

Direct filling gold was material of choice because of its ability to adapt the preparation walls with good marginal adaptation. But since isolation of these areas is difficult, the use of direct filling gold is decreased.

Dental amalgam is easy to manipulate, can be used in areas which are difficult to isolate and has self-sealing property.

Traditional glass-ionomer cements have the desirable properties of being biocompatible, achieving a chemical bond to tooth structure and releasing fluoride over extended periods of time. But they have poor aesthetics and excessive wear with time.

Resin-modified glass ionomers are biocompatible, *bond to tooth*, have thermal expansion and contraction characteristics that match tooth structure, and fluoride releasing feature. They are aesthetic and less brittle than the traditional glass ionomers.

Resin composites are highly aesthetic materials, and bond to enamel and dentin but do not have any anticariogenic effect. Hybrid composites possess improved strength and improved aesthetics compared with traditional resin composites. Microfilled composites are recommended for root surface restorations as they have lower elastic modulus than hybrid composites. This is an advantageous property, since the teeth flex during mastication and a flexible material will be a better choice to restore the root surface. Diagnosis and management of root caries are shown in **Flow chart 5.2**.

CARIES RISK ASSESSMENT

The main objective of caries risk assessment in dentistry is to deliver preventive and restorative care specific to an individual patient. Many factors may affect the caries susceptibility of different individuals. For example, low birth weight children are more prone to caries because it is associated with enamel hypoplasia and other enamel defects. Other caries risk indicators are sociodemographic factors, such as education and income of parents, systemic and topical fluoride exposure, toothbrushing behavior, bottle use and dietary habits.

Caries risk assessment of a person can also be done by caries activity tests. Assessment of a caries risk at

Flow chart 5.2: Diagnosis and management of root caries

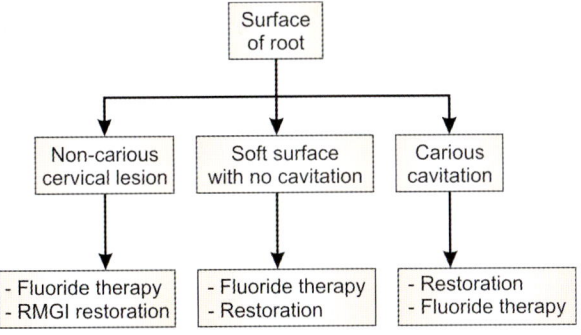

RMGI: Resin modified glass ionomer

screening or initiation of therapy, allows better appraisal of caries activity and refinement of the treatment planning. For example, children at high risk of caries require intense prevention to primarily prevent caries initiation and secondarily to arrest caries progression.

A patient is said to be at high caries risk if there is

- One new lesion on smooth surface during past one year
- New carious lesion on root surface
- Patient on medication which causes hyposalivation
- Systemic disorder
- Past dental history with multiple restorations
- Exposure to sugary snacks for more than three times a day
- Senility
- Following factors are commonly seen in patients with high-risk caries:
- Status of oral hygiene
  - Poor oral hygiene
  - Nonfluoridated toothpaste
  - Low frequency of tooth cleaning
  - Orthodontic treatment
  - Partial dentures
- Dental history
  - History of multiple restorations
  - Frequent replacement of restorations
- Medical factors
  - Medications causing xerostomia
  - Gastric reflux
  - Sugar containing medications
  - Sjögren's syndrome
- Behavioral factors
  - Bottle feeding at night
  - Eating disorders
  - Frequent intake of snacks
  - More sugary foods
  - Nonfluoridated toothpaste
- Socioeconomic factors
  - Low education status
  - Poverty
  - No fluoride supplement.

Caries Activity Tests

Cries activity in a patient can be determined by doing caries activity tests.

Caries activity tests help in the following ways:
- In determining the need for caries control measures
- To determine the optimal time for restoration
- In determining the results of preventive measures.

Unstimulated Salivary Flow Test

In this, resting saliva from submandibular gland is measured. Patient is asked to sit upright in chairs to drool into a collection cup for 5 minutes.
- More than 0.25   –   Normal
- 0.1 to 0.25   –   Low
- Less than 0.1   –   Very low

It can also be done by visually assessing the saliva production from the minor salivary glands on the lower labial mucosa. For this revert, the lower lip, block with labial mucosa with a piece of tissue and observe the time taken for droplets of saliva to form.
- Less than 30 sec.   –   High
- 30 to 60 sec.   –   Normal
- More than 60 sec.   –   Low

Saliva Viscosity Test

For this test, visually inspect the viscosity of resting saliva. If it is frothy or bubbly, it indicates low water content in saliva because of low saliva production.

Resting pH of Unstimulated Saliva (Fig. 5.64)

To measure pH of resting saliva, drop the saliva on pH paper strip, and note the value.

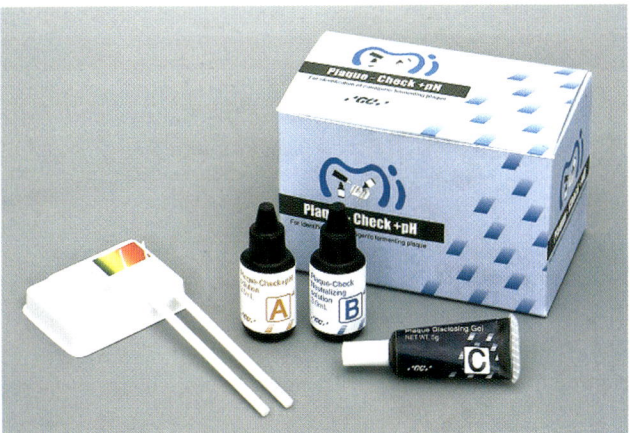

Figure 5.64: Commercially available kit to check plaque pH

- Healthy resting pH = 6.8 to 7.8
- Moderately acidic resting pH = 6.0 to 6.6
- Acidic resting pH = 5.0 to 5.8

Salivary Buffering Capacity Test

For this test, add stimulated saliva to a test strip. Acids present in test strip dissolve and there occurs decrease in the pH. If saliva can buffer, the pH will rise and the indicator will show final pH.

S Mutans, Lactobacillus Test

In this test, *S mutans* count is estimated. For this, rotate the *spatula* on the patient's tongue and incubate it in a special culture medium. After this, compare the results with the manufacturer's chart to estimate the *S mutans* count.

PREVENTION OF DENTAL CARIES

Method of dental caries control can be classified into two main types (**Fig. 5.65**):

Methods to reduce demineralizing factors
➡ Dietary measures ➡ Methods to improve oral hygiene ➡ Chemical measures.

Methods to increase protective factors

➡ Methods to improve flow, quantity and quality of saliva
➡ Chemicals altering the tooth surface or tooth structure:
  ♦ Fluorides
  ♦ Iodides
  ♦ Zinc chloride
  ♦ Silver nitrate
  ♦ Bisbiguanides
➡ Application of remineralizing agents
➡ Use of pit and fissure sealants.

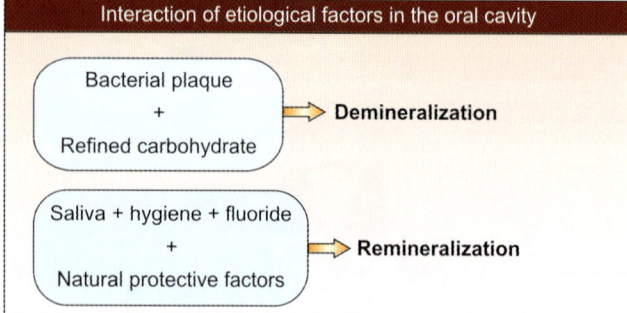

Figure 5.65: Factors promoting demineralization and remineralization of the tooth surface

Methods to Reduce Demineralizing Factors

Dietary Measures

Diet has been considered one of the main step in influencing the dental caries. Different nutritional substitutes are:
- Sugar substitutes
  - Xylitol
  - Sorbitol

Xylitol is a five-carbon sugar alcohol derived primarily from forest and agricultural materials with the taste almost identical to that of table sugar. Though the dental benefits of xylitol first were recognized in Finland in 1970, the first chewing gum was introduced in Finland in 1975. Currently, xylitol is available in many forms like chewing gums, chewable tablets, lozenges, toothpastes, mouthwashes. It is nonfermentable, noncariogenic sugar and has anticaries effects. Though it is yet not clear whether xylitol is actually lethal to bacteria or if bacteria are washed from the mouth by saliva.

Anticariogenic effects of xylitol
➡ Xylitol reduces plaque formation ➡ It reduces bacterial adherence ➡ It inhibits enamel demineralization ➡ It has a direct inhibitory effect on *S mutans* ➡ Increases salivary flow ➡ It is nonfermentable ➡ It increases concentration of amino acids which neutralize the plaque acidity.

Because of Xylitol's anticaries effects, it is recommended for pregnant mothers. Studies have shown that mothers using xylitol gum during the first-two years of their child's age show much lower caries in the children later.
- *Fibrous food*: One should avoid excessive intake of sugary and sticky foods such as cakes, biscuits, jams and sweets. Intake of raw fruits and vegetables helps in increasing the salivary flow, thereby removal of food debris from the oral cavity. Intake of raw vegetables, fruits and grains increases caries protective mechanism because these foods contain natural phosphates, phytates and nondigestable fibers, moreover they do not stick to teeth.
- *Low caloric sweeteners*: In this, several sweetener such as aspartame, saccharin and cyclamate considered to have some role.
- *Fats*: Fats form a protective barrier on enamel or carbohydrate surface so that it is less available for bacteria. They also speed up the clearance of carbohydrate from oral cavity, thus decreasing cariogenic potential.

- *Cheese*: Cheese is considered as responsible for:
  - Increasing the salivary flow
  - Increasing the pH
  - Promoting the clearance of sugar.

  All these factors help in reducing the incidence of caries.
- Trace elements.

Effect	Mineral
Cariostatic	Fluoride (F), Phosphate (Po_4)
Mild cariostatic	Fe, Li, Cu, B, Mo, V, Sr, Au
Doubtful	Co, Zn, Br, I
Caries inert	Al, Ni, Ba, Pd
Caries promoting	Mg, Cd, Pb, Si

Methods to Improve Oral Hygiene (Fig. 5.66)

Measures for preventing dental caries include the following:
- Dental prophylaxis
- Toothbrushing
- Interdental cleaning.

Dental prophylaxis: In dental prophylaxis, polishing of roughened tooth surfaces and replacement of faulty restorations is done so as to decrease the formation of dental plaque, therefore, resulting in less incidence of caries.

Toothbrushing: Nowadays, toothbrushing and other mechanical cleaning procedures are considered to be the most reliable means of controlling plaque and provide clean tooth surface. But variations exist in design of toothbrush, brushing techniques, frequency of brushing and brushing time.

Ideally a toothbrush should have the following features (**Fig. 5.67**):

- A handle size according to user's age and handiness
- A head size according to the person's mouth
- Nylon bristles not larger than 0.009 inches in diameter
- Soft bristles as approved by international industry standards (ISO).

Many toothbrushing techniques have been described and being promoted as being effective. Bass technique is most recommended as it emphasizes sulcular placement of bristles while in periodontal cases, sulcular technique with vibratory motion is preferred (**Figs 5.68A to C**).

Technique	Category
Bass technique	Normal patient
Sulcular technique with vibratory motion	Periodontally involved cases

Interdental cleaning (Fig. 5.69): It is well known that toothbrush can clean only the buccal, lingual and occlusal tooth surfaces but proximal and interdental areas are

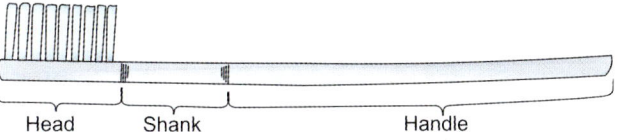

Figure 5.67: Parts of a toothbrush

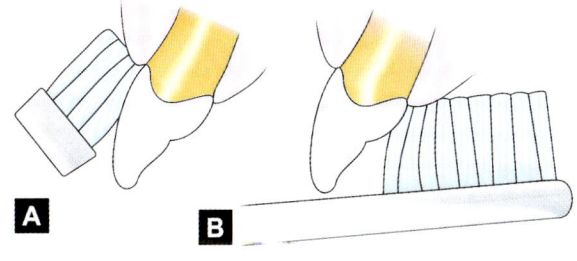

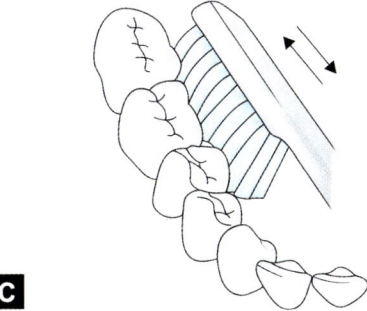

Figures 5.68A to C: Sulcular brushing: (A) Keep the bristles in gingival sulcus at 45° to long axis of tooth; (B) Brushing on palatal surface; (C) Brushing on posterior teeth

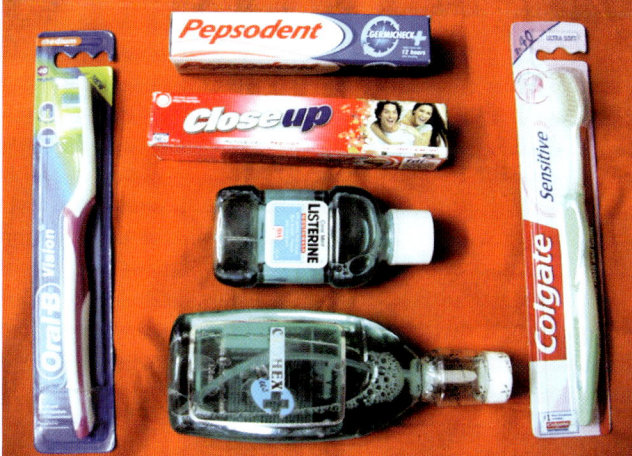

Figure 5.66: Materials used for maintaining oral hygiene

not cleaned. Interdental cleaning devices include following devices (**Figs 5.70A and B**):

- *Dental floss and tape*: Used in persons with normal proximal contact between their teeth
- *Woodsticks and interdental brushes*: They are indicated in patients with wide interdental spaces because of gingival recession and/or loss of periodontal attachment (**Figs 5.71A and B**).
- Other mechanical devices.

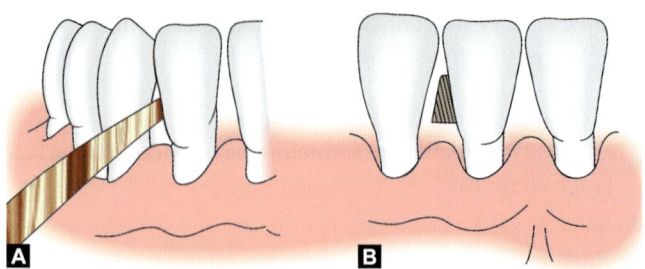

Figures 5.71A and B: Use of wood stick as interdental cleaner

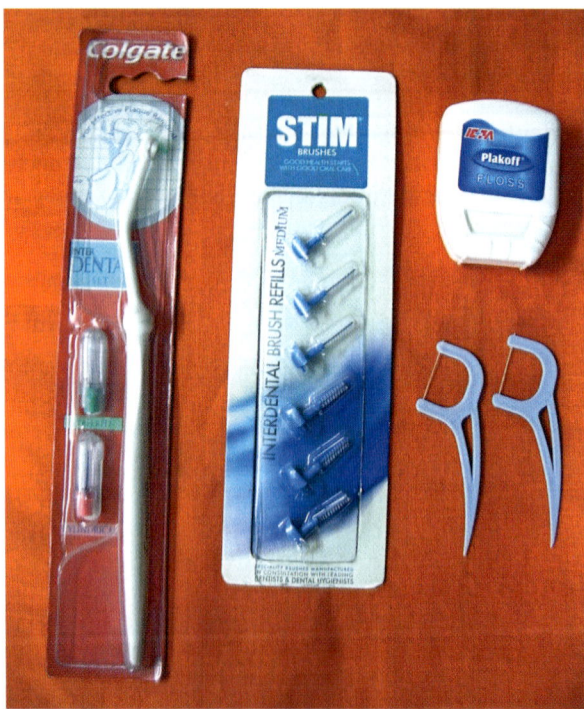

Figure 5.69: Interdental cleaning aids

Chemical Measures

- Substances interfering with carbohydrate degradation through enzymatic alterations:
  - Vitamin K
  - Sarcocide
- Substances interfering with bacterial growth and metabolism
  - Chlorhexidine
  - Iodine
  - Urea and ammonium compounds
  - Nitrofurans
  - Glutaraldehyde.

Properties of ideal chemotherapeutic agent
➡ It should be bacteriocidal in nature
➡ It should be safe for intraoral use
➡ It should have an acceptable taste
➡ It should possesses a degree of specificity to affect the cariogenic organisms
➡ It should be able to penetrate dense microbial plaque
➡ It should retain in oral environment for sufficient period of time.

- Substances interfering with carbohydrate degradation through enzymatic alterations
  - *Vitamin K*: Vitamin K, synthetically made, has been found to prevent acid formation, when added in incubated mixtures of glucose and saliva.
  - Sarcocide.
- Substances interfering with bacterial growth and metabolism
  - *Chlorhexidine*: Chlorhexidine has highly positive charge, which is responsible for reducing the number of *Streptococcus mutans* (**Fig. 5.72**).

Patients are advised to do 0.12 percent chlorhexidine gluconate oral rinse for one minute twice a day for seven days. Nowadays alcohol free 0.12 percent chlorhexidine has been introduced, which has advantages of chlorhexidine gluconate oral rinse without the drying effects of alcohol.

Chlorhexidine treatment is generally followed by topical fluoride like mouthrinse, a fluoride containing dentifrice,

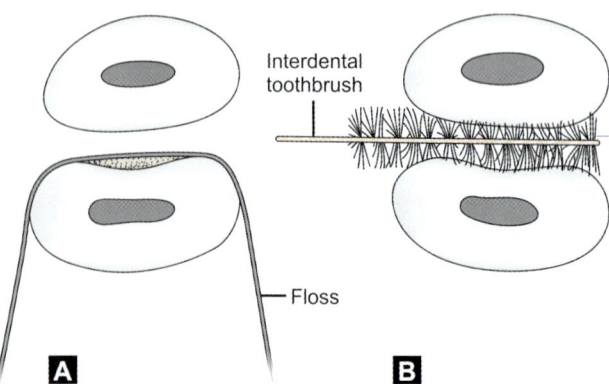

Figures 5.70A and B: (A) Flossing; (B) Use of interdental brush

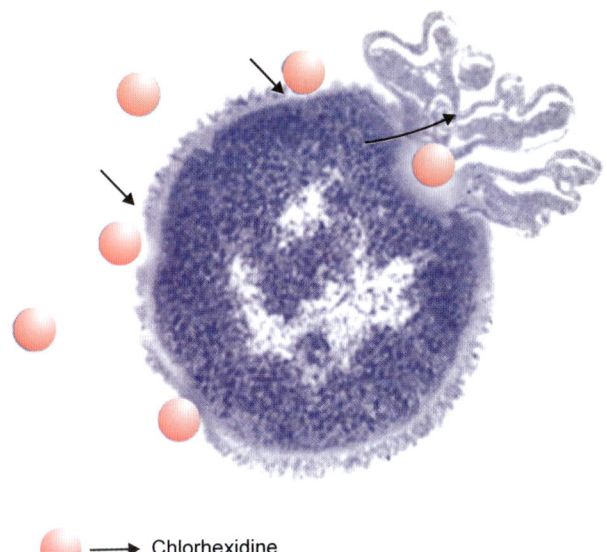

Figure 5.72: Mechanism of action of chlorhexidine

and xylitol gum. Simultaneous use of positively charged chlorhexidine and negatively charged fluoride or iodine therapy is not suggested because they will bind making the results less effective.

- *Iodine*: As we know that iodine is a strong antimicrobial that kills on contact. Application of iodine is done only at office, it is not suggested for patient for home use.
- *Urea and ammonium compounds*: Urea on degradation releases ammonia, neutralizes the acids and interferes with bacterial growth.
- *Nitrofurans*: These compounds are believed to have both bacteriostatic and bacteriocidal action on gram-positive and gram-negative organisms.
- *Glutaraldehyde*: It has been shown that a two minutes daily application of glutaraldehyde reduces mineral loss in dentin caries. The mechanism of action is thought to be:
  – Collagen fixation
  – Reduced diffusion of ions out of the carious lesion
  – Antibacterial action of glutaraldehyde.

Methods to Increase Protective Factors

Methods to Improve Flow, Quantity and Quality of Saliva

In patients with hyposalivation, baking soda may help to neutralize acids. The mouth rinse is prepared by mixing two teaspoons of baking soda in eight oz of water. This solution is used for mouthrinsing after eating.

Chemicals Altering the Tooth Surface or Structure

Fluorides: To increase the resistance of tooth structure to demineralization, small amounts of fluoride should be added. So, fluoride is considered as important component in caries prevention. Fluoride, is important part of natural diet for humans. It is usually required in very small quantity.

The good source of fluoride in human diet includes
- Potatoes
- Bananas
- Tea leaves
- Rock salt
- Salmon and sardines.

Fluoride ions increase the resistance of the hydroxyapatite in enamel and dentin to dissolution by plaque acids. The maximum benefit from fluoride is accomplished when there is a constant low level available for remineralization. The dentin requires higher levels of fluorides for remineralization (100 ppm) than enamel (5 ppm).

Fluoride reacts with enamel and dentin and produce different effects
⇒ Formation of fluoroapatite (less soluble than hydroxyapatite) (**Fig. 5.73**)
⇒ Inhibits demineralization
⇒ Induces remineralization
⇒ Inhibits bacterial metabolism
⇒ Inhibits plaque formation
⇒ Reduces "Wettability of surfaces of tooth".

One should select the fluoride product that the patient will most likely to use as recommended. If there is doubt about patient compliance, the clinician should opt for fluoride varnish which is applied professionally every six months.

Goals of fluoride administration
⇒ Do not harm the patient
⇒ Prevent decay on intact dental surfaces
⇒ Arrest active decay
⇒ Remineralize decalcified tooth surfaces.

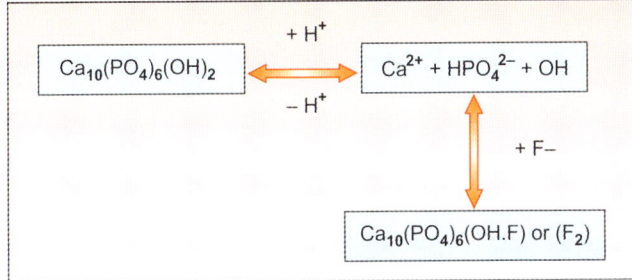

Figure 5.73: Conversion of hydroxyapatite to fluoroapatite

Clinical fluoride products:
- Professional topical fluorides
  - 2.72 percent APF gel
  - 2 percent sodium floride gel
- Fluoride varnishes
  - Duraflor
  - Florprotector
- Fluoride varnishes
- Mouthrinses
- Dentifrices
- Supplements in the form of fluoride tablets and drops
- Fluoridated salt
- *Professional topical fluorides*: Commonly used products under professional applications are
  - *2.72 percent acidulated phosphate fluoride (APF) gel*: It has 3.5 pH and contains 12,300 ppm fluoride. It is made from sodium fluoride and 0.1M phosphoric acid.
  - *2 percent sodium fluoride gel*: It contains 9200 ppm fluoride. It is preferred in composite restorations because APF etches glass filler particles of the composites.
    Methods of use:
    i. Before using first determine total fluoride exposure of the patient.
    ii. Administer 0,1,2,3,4 times a year as indicated by caries risk level.
    iii. Isolate the teeth and apply gel for 4 minutes.
    iv. Advise patient to avoid rinsing, drinking or eating for 30 min after application.
- *Fluoride varnish*: Duraflor is commonly used fluoride varnish which contains 5 percent NaF.
- Flor protector contains 0.7 percent silane fluoride and is used as a cavity varnish. Although the caries benefits are similar to topical fluoride gels, less total fluoride is released into the oral cavity during treatment when compared to fluoride gels.
- *Mouthrinses*: A mouthrinse may contain active ingredients like chlorhexidine gluconate, essential oils, triclosan, and sodium dodecyl sulphate. Daily rinsing with 0.05 percent NaF (226 ppm F) use of 0.2 percent NaF (900 ppm F) once every two weeks has shown to effective.
- Because of chances of fluoride ingestion, mouthrinsing is not recommended for children under six years of age.
- *Dentifrices*: Dentifrices are considered principle means of delivering topical fluoride.

Most fluoride dentifrices contain an active fluoride compound, water, abrasive system, surfactants, binding agents, humectants, sweetening agents, coloring, and preservatives.

Different sources of fluoride used in dentifrices are stannous fluoride (SnF_2), sodium monofluorophosphate (Na_2PO_3F) (MFP) and sodium fluoride (NaF). All dentifrices are formulated to contain either 1000 or 1100 ppm fluoride by and large in the form of NaF and MFP.

Factors affecting anticariogenicity of a dentifrice are
- *Frequency of dentifrice use*: Brushing twice per day is more effective than once per day.
- *Duration of brushing*.
- *Rinsing after brushing*: Rinsing after toothbrushing and salivary flow rate during and after fluoride application influence the rate of fluoride clearance.
- *The time of day that dentifrice is used*: When compared to daytime application, bedtime use of fluoride dentifrice results in retention of fluoride because of decreased salivary flow during sleep.
- *Concentration of fluoride in dentifrice* : Higher the fluoride concentration, the greater is the fluoride diffusion towards the tooth surface.
- *Fluoride supplements*: Fluoride tablets can be suggested for individuals with high caries risk and in patients for general use when other fluoride sources are not available. While prescribing the fluoride supplements, the dosage must take into account and it should be scheduled according to patient need.
- *Fluoridated salt*: Intake of fluoridated salt is an alternative where the water fluoridation is not feasible. Concentration of fluoride in salt should depend on salt intake and the availability of fluoride from other sources.

Silver nitrate: Silver is thought to be responsible for plugging the enamel either by organic invasion or inorganic invasion pathways. This combines with soluble inorganic portion of enamel to form a less soluble combination.

Zinc chloride: Zinc chloride is considered to have some role in prevention of caries.

Application of Remineralizing Agents

Recently the trend for treatment of dental caries follows the "improved diagnosis of early noncavitated lesions and prevention and arrest these lesions." Many studies support the remineralization of early noncavitated lesions.

Ideally, remineralizing agents are required to rapidly precipitate on partially demineralized tooth structure and transform into a more stable, less acid-soluble apatite than the hard tissue replaced.

Since a remineralizing material works in the presence of saliva, if the mineral phase which is formed is soluble in saliva or acids, it will be rapidly lost and its benefits are not achieved. For the optimal remineralization of the tooth surface, the agent must also be able to diffuse into the pellicle covered enamel surface and into the subsurface lesion area and should be hydrolyzed by enzymes present in the plaque or under acidic pH of plaque.

Since it is almost impossible to diffuse calcium and phosphate ions into the deeper layers of the decay, most of the remineralization is restricted to the surface of a decay. Usually during remineralization, calcium gets adsorbed on the surface layer of the decay and precipitate in the pores, this blocks its further entry to the deeper layers.

Remineralizing approaches: Remineralizing agents are available in various forms like dentifrices, mouthwashes, chewing gums, lozenges, and foods and beverages. Various approaches have been employed to enhance the remineralization of teeth. These are

- Combining remineralizing agents with fluoride (to increase anticariogenicity of fluorides).
- Combining remineralizing agents with a lower dosage of fluoride to decrease the possibility of dental fluorosis without losing effectiveness.
- The use of remineralizing materials as independent agents since even a small amount of fluoride can reverse early carious lesions by remineralization by precipitation of calcium phosphates, and the formation of fluorhydroxyapatite in the tooth tissues.

Commonly used agents are calcium glycerophosphate and calcium lactate, dicalcium phosphate dihydrate (DCPD), and calcium carbonate. Recently, casein phosphopeptide (CPP), amorphous calcium-phosphate (ACP) complexes have also been considered as agents for remineralization. Because of high solubility and ability to rapidly hydrolyze to form apatite, Amorphous calcium phosphate agents (ACPs) come under good source for tooth remineralization.

Mechanism of action CPP-ACP

- CPP stabilize calcium phosphate in solution and increases the level of calcium phosphate. Thus CPP-ACP nanocomplexes act as a reservoir of calcium and phosphate ions so as to have supersaturation state with respect to tooth enamel and buffer plaque pH
- Provide ions for tooth remineralization
- CPP-ACP inhibit caries by concentrating ACP in dental plaque, preventing demineralization and increasing remineralization.

Pit and Fissure Sealant

"A pit and fissure sealant is a material that is placed in the pits and fissures of teeth in order to prevent or arrest the development of dental caries".

For better effects, sealants should be placed as soon as possible because of more susceptibility of caries during the posteruption period.

Indications and contraindications for pit and fissure sealants

Indications	Contraindications
• Children and young adults with high risk for caries	• Children and young adults having low risk for caries
• Teeth showing signs of incipient caries	• Teeth with easily cleanable fossa and grooves
• In adult patients with potentially susceptible area like deep fissures	• Stained occlusal pits and fissures • Cases in which isolation of tooth is difficult
• Young permanent teeth having deep retentive pits and fissures	• Teeth showing resistance to caries 3-4 years after

Advantages of pit and fissure sealants

- Seal pits and fissures mechanically making them resistant to food impaction
- Make pits and fissures self-cleansable
- Halt incipient carious lesion.

Types of pit and fissure sealants

Resins: Resin sealants are bonded to enamel by acidetch technique. These make a tight seal with enamel which checks the leakage of nutrients to the microflora in the deeper parts of the fissure.

Compomers: Since the amount of fluoride release is lesser than conventional GIC, their properties should be expected comparable to the resins.

Glass Ionomer Cement (GIC): One of the main advantages of GIC is their ability to bond chemically to dentin and enamel along with active fluoride release into the surround enamel.

Since the resins are most durable, so they should be preferred, but glass ionomer cements should be used in cases where moisture control is difficult, e.g. young permanent teeth.

Technique of resin sealants (**Figs 5.74A to E**)

- *Surface cleaning*: Before application of pit and fissure sealant, there is a need for removal of most organic substance in order to obtain sufficient bonding. But care should be taken to avoid removal of sound tooth tissue by the use of instruments.
- *Isolation*: Isolation is the most critical aspect of sealant application because if enamel porosity created by the etching procedure gets contaminated, the formation of resin tags in the enamel is blocked or reduced resulting in poor retention of resin. Salivary contamination during resin application greatly decreases the bond strength of sealant.

Best way for optimal moisture control is use of the rubber dam, but in young and newly erupted teeth

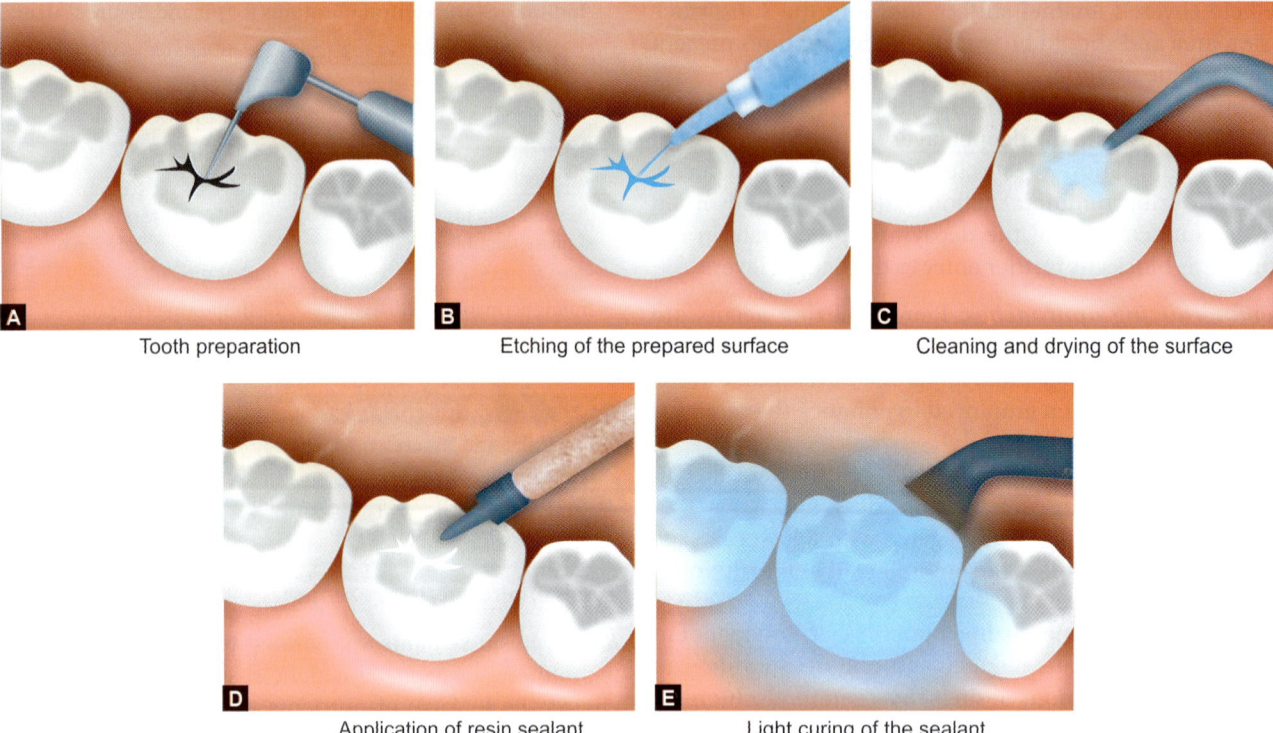

Figures 5.74A to E: Technique of placement of resin sealant

rubber dam is not practical since it requires use of local analgesia for placement of the clamp.

- *Etchants and conditioners*: Etching is done to produce an uncontaminated, dry, frosted surface. Commonly used etchant is orthophosphoric acid (between 30 and 50%).
- *Washing and drying*: The tooth is washed with air and water for about 30 seconds and then dried with compressed air for 15 seconds to give a chalky, frosted appearance.

Patient and tooth selection
- In children with medical, physical or intellectual impairment
- In children with signs of acute caries activity
- Children and young people with no signs of caries activity but having potentially susceptible areas like deep fissures.

Clinical and radiographical examination of restored surfaces should be done on regular basis. If there is any defective sealant, it should be reapplied to maintain the marginal integrity of tooth.

CURRENT METHODS OF CARIES PREVENTION

Genetic Modalities in Caries Prevention

In an attempt to produce the strains of *S mutans* which can not cause caries, various researches were conducted at genetic level to control caries. The genes for enzyme glycosyl transferase were decoded, resulting new strains of *S mutans* which lacked the capability to produce lactic acid responsible for caries.

Genetically Modified Foods

The research have been carried out so to produce genetically modified foods in an attempt to prevent tooth decay. They can be given to patients with 'high caries risk' as 'probiotics'. These modified fruits and vegetables are being developed by incorporating antagonist peptides to work against glycosyl transferase.

Genetically Modified Organisms

S mutans causes tooth decay by converting sugar into lactic acid which causes dissolution of tooth tissue, with the help of enzyme lactodehydrogenase. A new strain of *S mutans* has been created which lacks lactodehydrogenase gene, thus unable to produce lactic acid.

Lactobacillus zeae: Researches have been conducted to find a good bacteria called lactobacillus zeae. These are genetically modified bacteria which produce antibodies so as to attach to surface of *S mutans* resulting in their death.

Probiotic approach: In this approach, *S mutans* strain is modified to increase the production of enzyme urease. This urease converts urea into ammonia which helps in remineralization of enamel.

Caries Vaccine

Even though scientific advancements have led to a decrease in the prevalence of tooth decay, dental caries is still a highly prevalent disease. Fluoridation of water has been one of the major reasons for decrease in prevalence of the disease but the effect is far from adequate. Scientists have been trying to develop a vaccine for dental caries for more than three decades now.

Vaccine is an immunological substance designed to produce specific protection against a given disease. It stimulates production of protective antibody and other immune mechanism.

Although many trials have been carried out on experimental animals in the laboratories, no such vaccine is commercially available till date. *Streptococcus mutans* has for long been identified as the major etiological agent of human dental caries. The main thrust of the scientists has been on immunizing experimental animals with antigens derived from the main causative organisms of dental caries, viz, *S mutans* and *S sobrinus*.

Rationale of caries vaccine

- Rationale for caries vaccine is that immunization with *S mutans* should induce an immune response so as to prevent organisms from colonizing the tooth surface and thus prevent *carious* decay.
- General public should be well exposed to vaccine.
- Vaccine should be given before eruption of deciduous teeth so as to achieve maximum benefits.

Problems in development of caries vaccine

- Since complete etiology of caries is not known, 100 percent effectiveness of vaccine is not possible.
- Due to variation in number of etiological microorganisms, infective dose also varies.
- Even with same level and type of *S mutans*, variation in severity of disease occur due to other factors.
- Cross reactivity of *S mutans* cell antigens is seen with heart muscles.

- Lack of immunological competence can result in lack of response to *S mutans*
- There is nonavailability of human models to study immunological response.

Three routes have been tried to achieve caries immunity in animal studies

- Systemic immunization
- Mucosal immunization
- Passive immunization.

Systemic immunization: This type of immunization has been successfully used in many caries immunization trials in apes. Antibody level especially IgG has been found to be increased in saliva after subcutaneous immunization with *S mutans*.

In this route, mostly the injections of *S mutans* were given in salvary glands so as to increase salivary IgA antibody levels. But this route has drawback that function of salivary gland gets disturbed by repeated injections.

Mucosal route: To cover drawback of above route, mucosal immunization is tried by oral route. When the ingested antigens come in contact with gut, associated lymphoid tissue induce SIgA response at distant mucosal surfaces. Antigens stimulate lymphoblasts which move into lamina propria of mucosal tissue including the salivary glands. On setting the local clonal growth of cells, maturation into IgA antibody producing plasma cells is induced a result of local stimulus by an antigen. This is "common mucosal immune system" which is generated by ingestion of whole cells of *S mutans* encapsulated with gelatin matter.

Passive route: Here systemic immunization of cow is done, with vaccine from whole *S mutan* cells generated IgG. This results in formation of antibodies in both serum and milk which is passed on further. Many studies have been tried to form the yolk with antibodies from eggs of the chicken immunized with *S mutans*.

Appropriate Animal Models for Testing Caries Vaccine

Rodents are animals of choice for conducting studies being economical and easy to maintain. Though they can be made available in large experimental groups, it should be noted that their morphology of teeth, bacterial colonization and composition of saliva completely different from human beings.

Monkeys have morphology and pattern of development of dentition, immune response and microbiology similar to humans, they are considered as more appropriate than rodents in spite of their high cost of maintenance, small size of experimental groups and long-term experiments.

The thought of caries vaccine came after the discovery of mucosal immune system in 1965.

It was assumed that it might be possible to hinder the process of tooth decay by stimulating salivary antibodies to antigens. Initially, these antigens were whole cells of *S mutans*. Currently, the primary virulent factors/antigens of *S mutans* and *S robrinus* are considered. These are:

- Adhesion antigen I/II
- Glucosyl transferases
- Glucan binding proteins.

The duration of immunity achieved is a major factor in determining the success of caries vaccine as caries can occur throughout life and immunological memory has been seen to be particularly short with passive immunization. Many questions regarding the effectiveness of caries vaccine remain unanswered. Some of these are

- Would booster doses be required and would they be effective?
- Would immunizing lactating mothers help in developing immunity in children?
- Can animal trials be considered conclusive and would the results be the same in human beings?
- What would be the potential side effects?
- Cost factor.

Some of the other acute infectious diseases are totally eliminated by immunization but the etiopathogenesis of dental caries is unique so some special considerations need to be given.

All these issues need to be successfully addressed an effective caries vaccine can be commercially available to reduce the burden of this highly prevalent disease of the human race.

MANAGEMENT OF DENTAL CARIES

The restoration of a decayed tooth involves the use of a drill, low or high speed for preparation cutting. But now- a-days other procedures have also been used for removal of caries like air abrasion, chemomechanical caries removal, atraumatic restorative therapy (ART) and latest with lasers.

Chemochemical Caries Removal

Chemochemical caries removal (CMCR) involves the selective removal of carious dentin. The reagent is prepared by mixing solutions of amino acids and sodium hydrochlorite.

Mechanism of Action of Chemochemical Caries Removal Method

Dentin consists of 70 percent mineral, 10 percent water and 20 percent organic matrix. Organic matrix consists of 18 percent is collagen and 2 percent noncollagenous compounds including chondroitin sulphate, other proteoglycans and phosphophoryns.

Collagen contains proline and amino acid content, glycine. The polypeptide chains are coiled into triple helices, called tropocollagen units, which orientated side by side to form a fibril. In dentin, the fibrils are in the form of a dense meshwork which becomes mineralized.

When caries occurs, acids produced by bacteria results in a decrease in pH and thus demineralization of enamel and dentin. When the inorganic gets matrix demineralized, the organic matrix becomes susceptible to enzymatic degradation, by bacterial proteases and hydrolases.

With respect to collagen degradation, two layers are formed

- Inner layer which is partially demineralized and can be remineralized and in which the collagen fibrils are still intact.
- Outer layer where the collagen fibrils are partially degraded and cannot be remineralized.

Goldman and Kronman in 1970 were studying the effect of sodium hypochlorite on the removal of carious material from dentin. Since it is a harmful for use on healthy tissue, so it was mixed with Sorensen's buffer (mix of glycine, sodium chloride and sodium hydroxide). This caused chlorination of glycine to form N-monochloroglycine NMG.

In the later studies they found that this was more efficient if glycine was replaced by amino butyric acid, resulting in the product, N-monochloroaminobutyric acid (NMAB).

The mechanism of action of NMG and NMAB on collagen though unclear but it is assumed that they involve chlorination of the partially degraded collagen in the carious lesion and the conversion of hydroxyproline to pyrrole-2-carboxylic acid. This causes disruption of the collagen fibrils which become more friable and can then be removed.

Reagents commonly available in market are Caridex and Carisolv.

Caridex consists of two solutions viz. Solution I containing sodium hypochlorite and Solution II containing glycine, aminobutyric acid, sodium chloride and sodium hydroxide.

The two solutions are mixed immediately before use. The solution is applied to the carious lesion by means of applicator. Application is done until the sound dentin comes.

Advantages of caridex

➡ No need for local anesthesia
➡ Suited for treatment of anxious and pediatric patients
➡ Indicated in medically compromised patients
➡ Conservation of sound tooth structure
➡ Reduced risk of pulp exposure.

Disadvantages of caridex

➡ Instruments may still be needed for the removal of caries or material
➡ It leaves a surface with many overhangs and undercuts
➡ Large volumes of solution are needed
➡ Procedure is slow
➡ It is ineffective in the removal of hard eburnated parts of the lesion
➡ Unpleasant taste.

In 1998, carisolve was introduced. It is available in two syringes, one containing the sodium hypochlorite and other a pink viscous gel consisting of lysine, leucine and glutamic acid, amino acids, together with carboxymethyl-cellulose to make it viscous and erythrocin to make it readily visible in use.

The contents of the two syringes are mixed together immediately before use. The gel is applied to the carious lesion with hand instruments and after 30 seconds, carious dentin can be gently removed. Another application may be required until no more carious dentin remains.

Advantages of carisolve

➡ Volume required is less
➡ Does not require heating or a delivery system
➡ Since it involves gel not liquid, it is much easier to use than caridex
➡ Better contact with the carious lesion.

Disadvantage of carisolve

Use of rotary instruments may still be required for some cavities.

Ozone Treatment of Dental Caries

At the decay interface inside the tooth preparation, there are three types of dental tissues: soft (decayed dentin and enamel), leathery (infected dentin), and hard (healthy tissue). Very soft tissues must be removed from the cavity. The leathery tissues if are given the proper ionic compartment, can remineralize and harden. Hard tissues are generally healthy and should be left intact. The introduction of aerotherapeutic ozone therapy to completely eliminate bacteria at and below the preparation surface enhances the success of treatment. Ozone is a proven antimicrobial agent that a 10 seconds application eliminates more than 99 percent of the microorganisms found in dental biofilm.

Ozone occurs naturally when molecular oxygen (O_2) is photodissociated into activated ions (O^-) which further combines with other oxygen molecules (O_2) to form transient radical anions (O_3). Ozone ultimately decomposes to a hydroxyl radical which is a powerful oxidant. It oxidizes biomolecules like cysteine, methionine, and histidine resulting in cell death. Just 20 to 40 second exposure of ozone kills all oral microbes and their protective biofilm environment. Because of this change in microenvironment, the remineralization of enamel and dentin can be accomplished. It has been shown that when GIC is placed in direct contact with the demineralized tooth surface, it acts as an brilliant source of ions for tooth remineralization.

Technique of Using Ozone Therapy

Carious lesion is diagnosed visually, tactilely and/or radiographically. Entry through the enamel is made with airotor. Disposable sterile cup on the ozone is used to form a seal around the prepared tooth.

Once the seal is obvious, ozone is delivered, and refreshed 300 times per second, for 40 seconds. Healozone remineralizing solution which contains xylitol, fluoride, calcium, phosphate and zinc, is applied to the demineralized tooth surface. Tooth is restored with glass ionomer cement. Carving and finishing of glass ionomer cement is done. Over it, after confirming remineralization, place composite restoration.

Caries Removal Using Air Abrasion

Here kinetic energy is used to remove carious lesion. In this method, a powerful fine stream of aluminum oxide particles is targeted against the surface to be removed. The abrasive particles hit the tooth with high velocity and remove small amounts of tooth structure. Air abrasion technique is not indicated in patients with dust allergy, asthma, advanced periodontal disease, fresh extraction and recent placement of orthodontic appliances.

Lasers

Lasers have shown to remove caries selectively while leaving the sound enamel and dentin. They can be used without application of local anesthetics. Commonly used lasers for caries removal are Erbium:yttrium-aluminum garnet lasers and erbium, chromium:yttrium-scandium-gallium-garnet lasers. These lasers can remove soft caries, as well as hard tissue. Added advantages of lasers include little noise, no smell and vibrations.

Key Points

- Dental caries is defined as a microbiological disease of the hard structure of teeth, which results in localized demineralization of the inorganic portion and destruction of the organic substances of the tooth.
- Biofilm is defined as a microbiologically derived community, characterized by cells which are irreversibly attached to substrate or interface or with each other, embedded in matrix of extracellular polymeric substances that they have produced and exhibit an altered phenotype with respect to growth rate and gene transcription.
- Cariogenic bacterias should be of acidogenic (able to transport sugars and convert them to acid) and aciduric nature (able to thrive at low pH).
- Dental plaque also known as microbial plaque is important for beginning of caries because it provides the environment for bacteria to form acid, which causes demineralization of hard tissue of teeth.
- Carbohydrates exert cariogenic effect which depends upon frequency of intake, chemical composition, physical form and time of contact of carbohydrate with the tooth.
- On coronal surface initiation of caries is caused by *Streptococcus mutans* and on root surface mainly by *Actinomyces viscosus*.
- Presence of high *Lactobacillus acidophilus* count in saliva designates the occurrence of active carious lesion.
- According to the caries balance concept, caries does not result from a single factor; rather, it is the outcome of the complex interaction of pathologic (bacteria, poor dietary habits, and xerostomia) and protective factors (saliva, antimicrobial agents, fluorides, pit and fissure sealants and an effective diet).
- The physical characteristics of teeth like deep and narrow occlusal fissures, deep buccal or lingual pits and enamel hypoplasia, etc. affect the initiation of dental caries.
- In carious enamel and dentin, fluoride content is 139 ppm and 223 ppm, whereas in sound enamel and dentin it is 410 ppm and 873 ppm, respectively.

- Under normal conditions, the tooth is continually in touch with saliva. Calcium and phosphate ions present in the saliva help in remineralization of the very early stages of carious lesion.
- When salivary flow is reduced, salivary buffering capacity is lost, an acid environment is encouraged which further promotes the growth of aciduric bacteria.
- To cause demineralization of dental enamel, it is essential for fermentable carbohydrates and plaque to be present on the tooth surface for a minimum length of time. These need to be retained in the mouth long enough to be metabolized by oral bacteria to produce acid.
- Stephan showed the relationship between change in plaque pH over a period of time following a glucose rinse in form of a graph. This graph is called a 'Stephan curve' (Stephan and Miller, 1943).
- The critical pH value for demineralization usually ranges between 5.2 and 5.5.
- Dental caries does not occur if the oral cavity is free of bacteria.
- Smooth surface caries occurs on gingival third of buccal and lingual surfaces and on proximal surfaces below the contact point.
- The earliest manifestation of incipient caries of enamel is seen beneath dental plaque as areas of decalcification (white spots). As caries progresses it appears bluish-white in color.
- Although caries of enamel is clearly a dynamic process, it is not a vital process because it does not defend itself from trauma. But since pulp and dentin are vital tissues, they are capable of defending.
- Use of visual examination only, is known as the European method, while use of sharp or blunt probe in visual tactile system is popularly known as the American system for diagnosis of dental caries.
- Transillumination takes advantage of the opacity of a demineralized tooth structure over more translucent healthy structures. The decalcified area will not let the light pass through as much as it does in a healthy area, generating a shadow corresponding to decay.
- Lesion confined to enamel may not be evident radiographically until approximately 30 to 40 percent demineralization has occurred. X-rays are currently the gold standard in interproximal caries assessment. Caries of buccal and lingual surfaces are difficult to differentiate on a radiograph. They appear as well defined radiolucency surrounded by a uniform, noncarious region of enamel.

- Cervical burnout is an apparent radiolucency found just below the CE junction on the root due to anatomical variation (concave root formation posteriorly) or a gap between the enamel and bone covering the root (anteriorly) mimicking root caries. Posteriorly, this radiolucency disappears when radiograph is taken at different angle.
- Cone image shift technique is based on the concept that as the vertical or horizontal angulations of X-ray tube head changes, the object buccal or closest to the tube head moves to opposite side of radiograph when compared to lingual object.
- Digital imaging systems employs an electronic sensor or detector, an analog to digital converter, a computer, and a monitor or printer for image of the components of imaging system. It instructs the X-ray generator when to begin and end the exposure, controls the digitizer, constructs the image by mathematical algorithm, determines the method of image display, and provides for storage and transmission of acquired data.
- RVG comprises of three main parts, the radio part consists of a conventional X-ray unit, a precise timer for short exposure times and a tiny sensor to record the image. The 'visio' portion of the system receives and stores incoming signals during exposure and converts them point by point into one of 256 discrete gray levels. As the image is transmitted to the processing unit, it is digitalized and memorized by the computer.
- The 'graphy' part of RVG unit consists of digital storage apparatus. That can be connected to various printout or mass storage devices for immediate or later viewing.
- In phosphor imaging system, the image is captured on a phosphor plate as analog information and is converted into a digital format when the plate is processed.
- Diagnodent is a device that emits a red laser light which is absorbed by tooth. The tooth then fluoresces under this light and is captured by a probe that sends the light back to a photocell which provides both an analog scale of reflectance and fluorescence combined with an acoustic signal, the sound volume of which can be adjusted.
- Arrested carious lesion is a lesion that may have formed earlier and then stopped. It usually presents as a large open cavity which no longer retains food and becomes self-cleansing. Here superficial softened and decalcified dentin is gradually burnished away by mastication until it takes on a brown stained, polished appearance which is hard. This type of dentin is referred as "eburnation dentin".

- Secondary or recurrent caries can be defined as contact caries, which refers to caries on the adjacent tooth surface in contact with the restoration.
- Since secondary caries may be present at surface enamel surrounding the restoration or extend below it along the margins. Therefore, these are also referred as caries adjacent to restorations and sealants (CARS).
- Root caries as defined by Hazen, is a soft, progressive lesion that is found anywhere on the root surface that has lost its connective tissue attachment and is exposed to the environment.
- The rate of demineralization of root occurs at higher pH and is much faster than that of enamel because the root has much less mineral content (55%) than that of enamel (99%).
- In 1960s, Keyes has showed that there are three prerequisite factors for the development of dental caries, known as Keyes's triad. These factors are plaque, tooth and the diet. Later on many studies were conducted which extended Keyes model with many other factors affecting the interplay between these primary factors.
- Xylitol is nonfermentable, noncariogenic sugar and has anticaries effects. Xylitol reduces plaque formation, bacterial adherence and inhibits enamel demineralization.
- Fluoride ions increase the resistance of the hydroxyapatite in enamel and dentin to dissolution by plaque acids.
- The dentin requires higher levels of fluorides for remineralization (100 ppm) than enamel (5 ppm).
- Commonly used remineralizing agents are calcium glycerophosphate and calcium lactate, dicalcium phosphate dihydrate (DCPD), calcium carbonate, and Casein phosphopeptide (CPP), amorphous calcium phosphate (ACP) complexes.
- CPP stabilize calcium phosphate in solution and increases the level of calcium phosphate. Thus CPP-ACP nanocomplexes act as a reservoir of calcium and phosphate ions so as to have supersaturation state with respect to tooth enamel and buffer plaque pH.
- A pit and fissure sealant is a material that is placed in the pits and fissures of teeth in order to prevent or arrest the development of dental caries.
- *Lactobacillus zeae* are genetically modified bacteria which produce antibodies so as to attach to surface of *S mutans* resulting in their death.
- Rationale for caries vaccine is that immunization with *S mutans* should induce an immune response so as to prevent organisms from colonizing the tooth surface and thus prevent carious decay.

- Chemochemical caries removal (CMCR) involves the selective removal of carious dentin. The reagent is prepared by mixing solutions of amino acids and sodium hydrochlorite. Reagents commonly available in market are Caridex and Carisolv.
- Lasers have shown to remove caries selectively while leaving the sound enamel and dentin. They can be used without application of local anaesthetics. Commonly used lasers for caries removal are Erbium:yttrium-aluminum garnet lasers and erbium, chromium:yttrium-scandium-gallium-garnet lasers.

QUESTIONS

1. Write short notes on:
   a. Caries vaccine
   b. Chemomechanical caries removal
   c. Caries activity tests
2. Define dental caries. What are different theories of dental caries?
3. Explain in detail Keye's triad of dental caries.
4. Classify dental caries. What is histopathology of enamel caries?
5. How will you diagnose dental caries. Explain diagnosis.
6. Explain in detail prevention of dental caries.
7. Write short notes on:
   a. Infected and affected dentin
   b. Diagnosis of initial carious lesion
   c. Role of saliva in prevention of dental caries.
8. Write in short about the current methods of caries prevention.
9. Write short notes on:
   a. Caries vaccine
   b. Chemomechanical caries removal (CMCR)
   c. Caries activity tests
   d. Advantages and disadvantages of caridex.
   e. Advantages and disadvantages of carisolve.
   f. Ozone treatment of dental caries.

BIBLIOGRAPHY

1. Anusavice KJ. Management of dental caries as a chronic infectious disease. J Dent Educ. 1998;62:791-802.
2. Backer DO. Posteruptive changes in dental enamel. J Dent Res. 1966;45:503.
3. Bader JD, Brown JP. Dilemmas in caries diagnosis. J Am Dent Assoc. 1993;123:48-50.
4. Bader JD, Shugars DA. A systematic review of the performance of a laser fluorescence device for detecting caries. J Am Dent Assoc. 2004;135:1413-26.
5. Bandlish LK. Attrition and plaque defence mechanism of teeth. The Probe. 1981;23:67.
6. Bassi G, Chawla S, Patel M. The Nd YAG laser in caries removal. BDJ: 1994;177:248.
7. Baum LJ. Dentinal pulp conditions in relation to caries lesions. Int Dent J. 1970;20:309-37.
8. Beltrán-Aguilar ED, et al. Fluoride varnishes—a review of their clinical use, cariostatic mechanism, efficacy, and safety. J Am Dent Assoc. 2000;131:589-96.
9. Brannström M, Lind PO. Pulpal response to early dentinal caries. J Dent Res. 1965;44:1045-50.
10. Brown JP, Lazar V. The economic state of dentistry, an overview. J Am Dent Assoc. 1998;129:1682-91.
11. Brown LJ. Indicators for caries management from the patient history. J Dent Educ. 1997;61:855-60.
12. Caldwell RC. Physical properties of foods and their caries producing potentials. JDR. 1970;49:1293.
13. Edgar WM. Saliva and dental health: clinical implications of saliva: report of a consensus meeting. Br Dent J. 1990;169:96-8.
14. Elederton RJ, Mjor IA. Changing scenes in cariology and operative dentistry. Int Dent J. 1992;42:165.
15. Elederton RJ. The prevalence of failure of restorations: A literature review. J Dent. 1976;4:207.
16. Fitzgerald J, Adams D, Davis E. A microbiological study of recurrent dentinal caries. Caries Res. 1994;28:409.
17. Frank RM, Voegel JC. Ultrastructure of the human odontoblast process and its mineralization during dental caries. Caries Res. 1980;19:367-80.
18. Fusayama T. Two layers of carious dentin: diagnosis and treatment. Oper Dent. 1979;42:63.
19. Houte JV. Bacterial specificity in the etiology of dental caries. Int Dent J. 1980;30:305.
20. Hudson P. Conservative treatment of the Class I lesion-a new paradigm for dentistry. J Am Dent Assoc. 2004; 135:760-3.
21. Kantor ML, et al. Efficacy of dental radiographic practices: opinions or image receptors, examination selection, and patient selection. J Am Dent Assoc. 1989;119:259-68.
22. Kidd EAM. The histopathology of enamel caries in young and old permanent teeth. BDJ. 1983;155:196.
23. Leverett JB, et al. Cost effectiveness of sealants as an alternative to conventional restorations. J Dent Res. 1978; 1143:130.
24. Mjor IA. Frequency of secondary caries at various anatomical locations. Oper Dent. 1985;10:88.
25. Mjor IA. Glass ionomer cement restoration and secondary caries: a preliminary report Quint Int. 1996;27:171.
26. Mjor IA. The location of clinically diagnosed secondary caries. Quint Int. 1998;29:313.
27. Newman HN, Morgan WJ. opographical relationship between plaque and approximal caries. Car Res. 1980;14:428.
28. Parfitt GJ. The speed of development of the carious cavity. BDJ. 1956;100:204.
29. Ripa LW. Occlusal sealants: rationale and review of clinical trials. Int Dent J. 1980;30:127.

30. Sarnat H, Massler M. Microstructure of active and arrested dentinal caries. JDR. 1965;44(6):1389.

31. Simosen RJ. Cost-effectiveness of pit-and-fissure sealants at 10 years. Quintessence Int. 1989;20:75-82.

32. Stephan RM. Intra-oral hydrogen-ion concentration associated with dental caries activity. J Dent Res. 1944;23:257.

33. Straffon LH, Dennison JB. Clinical evaluation comparing sealant and amalgam after 7 years: final report. J Am Dent Assoc. 1988;117:71-755.

34. Tanzer JM. Xylitol chewing gum and dental caries. Int Dent J 45 (suppl 1): 1996.pp.65-76.

35. Trahan L. Xylitol: A review of its action on mutans streptococci and dental plaque-its clinical significance. Int Dent J 45 (suppl 1): 1995.pp.77-92.

36. Yamada T, et al. The extent of the odontoblastic process in normal and carious human dentin. Dent Res. 1983;62:798.

6 CHAPTER

Cutting Instruments

Chapter Outline

INTRODUCTION

A wide range of specific instruments hand/rotary are required for preparation and cutting of tooth, and for other operative procedures. Rotary instruments help in gross cutting and final refining of the preparation whereas hand instruments are used for examination, producing minor details of the tooth preparation and for insertion, compaction and finishing of the restoration. One must be able to use both hand and rotary instruments judiciously so as to perform the operative procedures accurately. In this chapter we will discuss different types of instruments and instrumentation techniques used in operative dentistry.

In Lilian Lindsay's English translation of 1946, it has been shown that most preparation was carried out by hand instruments. Fauchard advocated the use of the manually operated bow drill, an unwieldy device widely used in the early 18th century and adapted by dentists from the workshops of jewellers, silversmiths and ivory turners. George Greenwood, modified spinning wheel for use as footoperated dental engine in 1790. The first commercially manufactured footpowered engine was patented by Morrison in 1871.

Black described hand instruments such as chisels, hatchets, hoes, excavators and margin trimmers—terms which might have been taken from wood working and gardening.

Metals Used for Manufacturing Cutting Instruments

Carbon steel or stainless steel are most commonly used for manufacturing of cutting instruments.

The Carbon Steel

Carbon steel alloy contains 0.5 to 1.5 percent carbon in iron. Instruments made from carbon steel are known for their hardness and sharpness. But disadvantages with these instruments are their susceptibility to corrosion and fracture. They are of two types:
1. *Soft steel*: It contains < 0.5% carbon
2. *Hard steel*: It contains 0.5 to 1.5% carbon

Stainless Steel

Stainless steel alloy contains 72 to 85 percent iron, 15 to 25 percent chromium and 1 to 2 percent carbon. Instruments made from stainless steel remain shiny bright because of deposition of chromium oxide layer on the surface of the metal which reduces the tendency to tarnish and corrosion. Problem with stainless steel instruments is that they tend to lose their sharpness with repeated use, so they need to be sharpened again and again.

Heat Treatment of Materials

For gaining maximum benefits from instruments made from carbon or stainless steel, they are subjected to two heat treatments—hardening and tempering heat treatment.
- *Hardening heat treatment*: In this, instrument is heated to 815°C in oxygen free environment and then quenched in a solution of oil. By hardening treatment, the alloy becomes brittle.
- *Tempering heat treatment*: In this, instrument is heated at 176°C and then quenched in solutions of oil, acid or mercury. Tempering heat treatment is done to relieve the strains and increase the toughness of alloy.

CLASSIFICATION OF HAND CUTTING INSTRUMENTS

Classification Given by GV Black

This classification is based according to use of the instrument.
- Cutting instruments
  - Hand
    i. Hatchets
    ii. Chisels
    iii. Hoes
    iv. Excavators
    v. Others
  - Rotary
    i. Burs
    ii. Stones
    iii. Others
- Condensing instruments
  Pluggers
  - Hand
  - Mechanical
- Plastic instruments
  - Plastic filling instrument
  - Cement carriers
  - Carvers
  - Burnishers
  - Spatulas
- Finishing and polishing instruments
  - Hand
    i. Orangewood sticks
    ii. Polishing points
    iii. Finishing strips
  - Rotary
    i. Finishing brushes
    ii. Mounted brushes
    iii. Mounted stones
    iv. Rubber cups
- Isolation instruments
  - Rubber dam frame clamps, forceps and punch
  - Saliva ejector
  - Cotton roll holder
  - Evacuating tips and equipment
- Miscellaneous instruments
  - Mouth mirrors
  - Explorers
  - Probes

- Scissors
- Pliers
- Others

Classification Given by Marzouck

This classification is based upon different procedures performed by different instruments.

- Exploring instruments
  - Tweezers/cotton pliers
  - *Retractors*: Mouth mirror, blunt bladed restoring instruments, plastic instruments, tongue depressors
  - *Probes/Explorers*: Straight, right angled, arch explorer, interproximal explorer.
  - Separators
  - Instruments for tooth structure removal
  - Hand cutting instruments
    - i. *Excavators*: Hatchet, hoes, spoon, discoid, cleoid, angle formers.
    - ii. *Chisels*: Straight, monoangle, biangle and triple angle.
    - iii. *Special forms of chisel*: Enamel hatchets, gingival marginal trimmers, Wedelstaedt chisel, offset hatchets, triangular chisel and hoe chisel.
  - *Rotary cutting and abrasive instruments*
    - i. Handpieces
    - ii. Burs
    - iii. Ultrasonic instruments
- Restoring instruments
  - *Mixing instruments*: Stainless steel or plastic spatulas
  - Plastic instruments
  - *Condensing instruments*: Rounded, triangular, diamond, or parallelogram condensers.
  - *Burnishing instruments*: Ball/egg/conical-shaped burnishers
  - *Carvers*: Hollenback's discoid and cleoid, diamond shaped carvers
  - *Files*: Hatchet/parallelogram-shaped
  - *Knives*: Bard parker knife and Stein's knife
- *Finishing and polishing instruments*: Burs, stones, brushes, rubber (wheel, cups or cones), cloth or felt

Nomenclature for the Instruments
Dr GV Black has given a way to describe instruments for their easier identification similar to biological classification.
→ *Order*: Function or purpose of the instrument, e.g. excavator, condenser
→ *Suborder*: Position, mode or manner of use, e.g. push, pull
→ *Class*: Design or form of the working end, e.g. hatchet, spoon excavator
→ Subclass: Shape of the shank, e.g. binangle, contra-angle.

These names are combined to give a complete description of the instrument. Naming of an instrument generally moves from 4 to 1. Sometimes, the suborder is omitted due to variable and nonspecific use of the instrument. For example, the instrument will be named according to the classification as biangle enamel hatchet or biangle spoon excavator.

PARTS OF HAND CUTTING INSTRUMENTS

Though there is great variation among hand cutting instruments, they have certain design features in common.

Each hand instrument is composed of three parts (Figs 6.1A and B)
→ Handle or shaft
→ Shank
→ Blade or nib.

Handle or Shaft

The handle is used to hold the instrument. The handle can be small, medium or large, smooth or serrated for better grasping and developing pressure (**Figs 6.2A to C**). Earlier, instruments had handles of quite large diameter that were to be grasped in the palm of the hand.

Now-a-days, instrument handles are smaller in diameter for ease of their use. On the handle, there are two numbers; one is the instrument formula, which describes the dimensions and angulation of the instrument, the other number is the manufacturer's number which is used for ordering purposes.

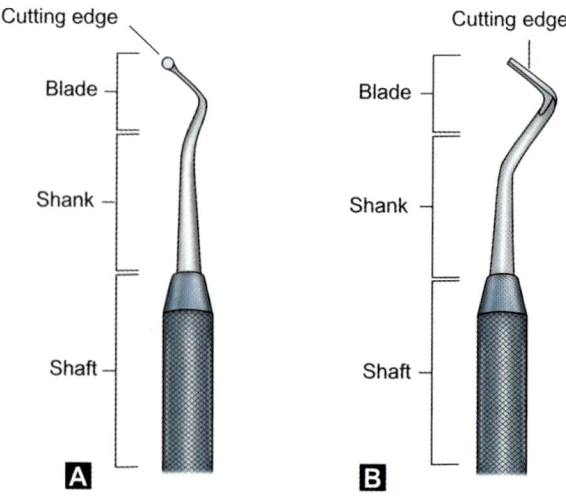

Figures 6.1A and B: Parts of a hand instrument

Shank

Shank connects the handle to the blade. It tapers from the handle down to the blade and is normally smooth, round or tapered. The shank may be straight or angled.

Classification base on number of shank angles (Figs 6.3A to E)
➡ *Straight*: Shank having no angle
➡ *Monoangle*: Shank having one angle
➡ *Binangle*: Shank having two angles
➡ *Tripleangle*: Shank having three angles
➡ *Quadrangle*: Shank having four angles

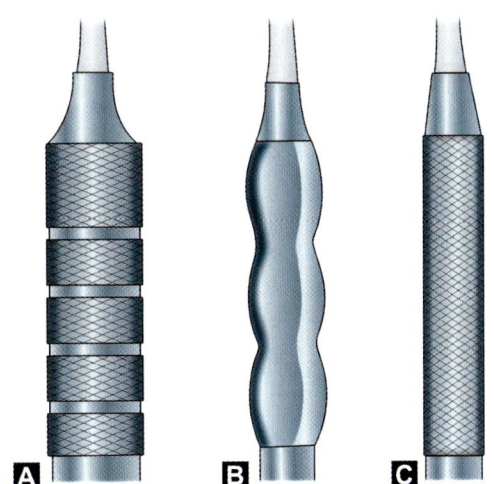

A **B** **C**

Figures 6.2A to C: Different designs of instrument handle for better grasping

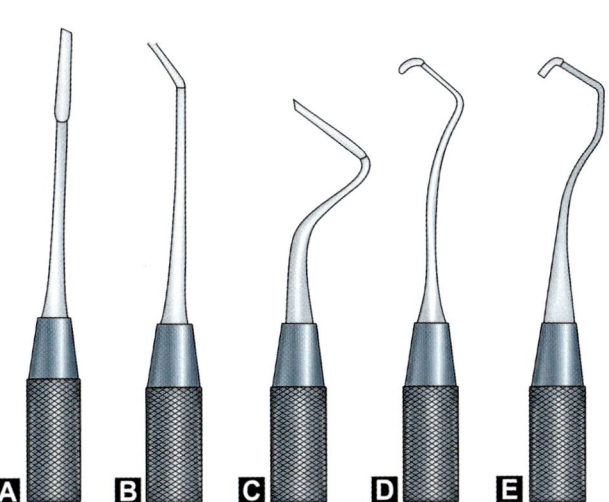

A **B** **C** **D** **E**

Figures 6.3A to E: Instruments with different shank angles

The angulation of instrument is provided for access and stability. Closer the working point to the long axis of the handle, better will be the control on it. For better control, the working point should preferably be within 3 mm of the center of the long axis of the handle (**Figs 6.4A and B**).

Advantages of contrangling of instrument
➡ Better access and stability
➡ Better balance
➡ Clear view.

Blade or Nib

The blade is the last section. It is the working part of the instrument. It is connected to the handle by the shank. For non-cutting instruments, the working part is termed the nib and is used to place, adapt and condense the materials in the prepared tooth. Depending on the materials being used, the surface of the nib may be plain or serrated. To cleave and smoothen the enamel and dentin, the working point of the instrument is beveled to create the cutting edge. If instrument has blade on both the ends of the handle, it is known as 'double-ended' instrument. In such cases, one end is for the left side and other for the right.

In some instruments, there are three bevels. Two are on the side and one is at the end. The edge on the end is called the primary cutting edge and the edges on the sides are called the secondary cutting edges.

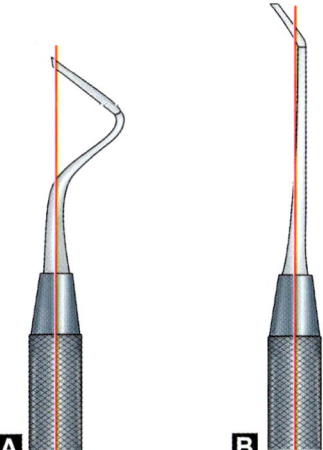

A **B**

Figures 6.4A and B: Balancing of instrument (A) Working end of instrument lies within 2-3 mm to long axis of handle, this provides balancing; (B) Working end is away from long axis of handle, this is not balanced

Instrument Formula

GV Black established an instrument formula for describing dimensions of blade, nib or head of instrument and angles present in shank of the instrument (**Fig. 6.5**). The formula is usually printed on the handle consisting of a code of three or four numbers separated by spaces.

The first number of the formula indicates width of the blade or primary cutting edge in tenths of a millimeter (**Fig. 6.6**).

The second number represents the angle formed by the primary cutting edge and long axis of the instrument handle in clockwise centigrade. The instrument is positioned in such a way that the number always exceeds 50 and is measured in clockwise centigrades. If the cutting edge is at right angle to the length of the blade, then this number is omitted.

The third number (second number in three number code) represents the length of the blade in millimeters, that is, from the shank to the cutting edge (**Fig. 6.7**).

The fourth number (third number in three number code) represents the angle which the blade forms with the long axis of the handle or the plane of the instrument in clockwise centigrade. To calculate the measurement of the angle, place the instrument on the center of the circle and move it until the blade lines up with one line on the ruler. This measurement represents the angulation of the blade from the long axis of the handle. To keep balance during working, tip of blade is brought in the line of the long axis of the handle.

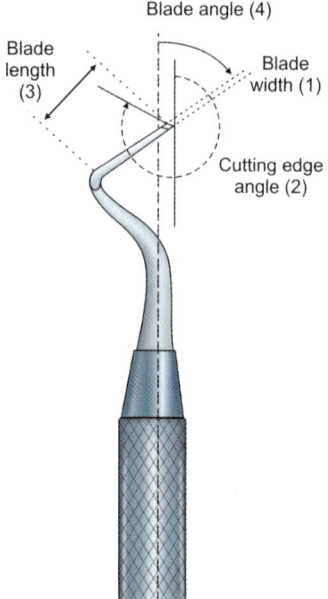

Figure 6.5: Instrument formula

Example of three number formula
➤ An instrument having instrument formula of 15-8-14 (**Figs 6.8A and B**) indicates following: ♦ 15 represents the width of the blade in tenths of a mm, i.e. 1.5 mm ♦ 8 represents the length of the blade in millimeters, i.e. 8 mm ♦ 14 represents the blade angle in centigrades.

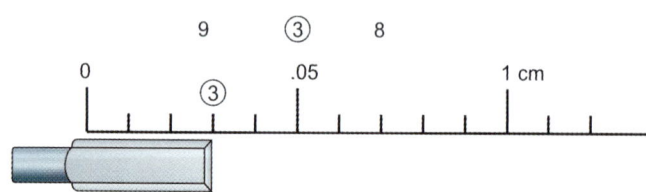

Length of blade

Figure 6.7: Third number indicates length of blade in millimeters

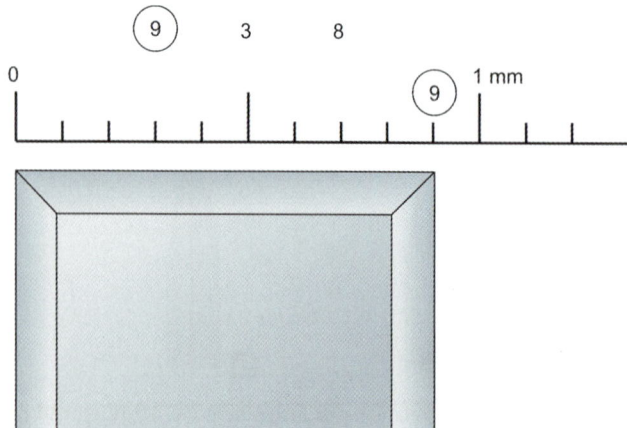

Figure 6.6: First digit of formula indicates width of blade in 1/10th of a millimeter

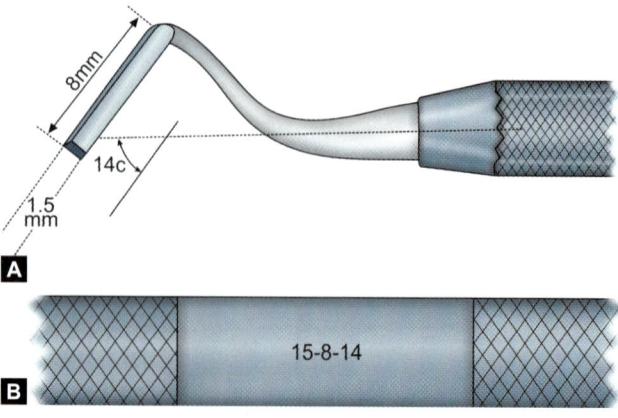

Figures 6.8A and B: Three number formula

→ Instrument with formula 15-95-8-12 (**Figs 6.9A and B**) represents the following:
  - 15 represents width of the blade in tenths of a millimeter, i.e. 1.5 mm
  - 95 represents the cutting edge angle in centigrades
  - 8 represents length of the blade, i.e. 8 mm
  - 12 represents blade angle in centigrades
  - 5 no. formula on handle.

Want to Know More

Manufacturer's number: This number is found on the handle of the instrument. This number is used when ordering the instrument and indicates the instrument's placement in a set of instruments.

Examples of three number formula instruments are chisels, hatchets and hoes.

Examples of four number formula instruments are angle formers and gingival marginal trimmers.

DIFFERENT INSTRUMENT DESIGNS

Bevels in Cutting Instruments

Single Bevel Instruments

Most of the instruments have single bevel that forms the primary cutting edge. These are called single beveled instruments. These can be right or left bevel and mesial or distal bevel instruments (**Figs 6.10A and B**).

Right and left bevel instruments: Single-beveled direct cutting instruments such as enamel hatchets are made in pairs having bevels on opposite sides of the blade. These are named as right and left bevel instruments.

During use, move the instrument from right to left in right beveled instrument and from left to right in left bevel instrument.

Identification of bevel: Hold the instrument in such a way that the primary cutting edge faces downwards and pointing away from operator. If bevel is on the right side of the blade, the instrument is right sided and if bevel is on the left side of the blade the instrument is left sided.

Mesial and distal bevel instrument: If we observe the inside of the blade curvature and the primary bevel is not visible then the instrument has a distal bevel and if the primary bevel can be seen from the similar view point the instrument has a mesial or reverse bevel.

Bibeveled Instrument (Fig. 6.10B)

If two additional cutting edges extend from the primary cutting edges, then the instrument with secondary cutting edges is called bibeveled instrument.

Triple-beveled Instrument

If three additional cutting edges extend from the primary cutting edge, then the instrument is called triple-beveled instrument.

Circumferential Bevel

Here instrument blade is beveled at all its peripheries for example spoon excavator.

Direct and Lateral Cutting Instruments

Direct cutting instruments are those in which force is applied the same plane as that of blade and handle. They

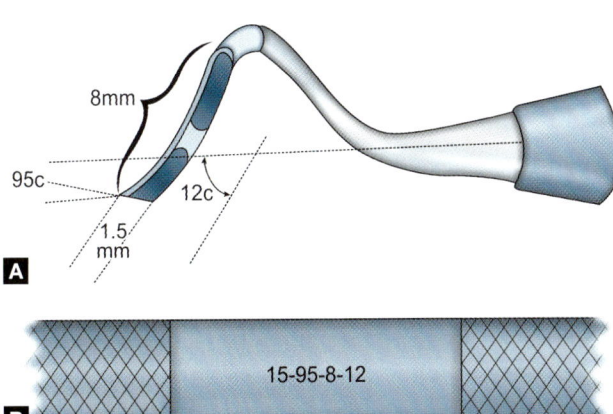

8mm

95c

12c

1.5 mm

A

15-95-8-12

B

Figures 6.9A and B: Four number formula

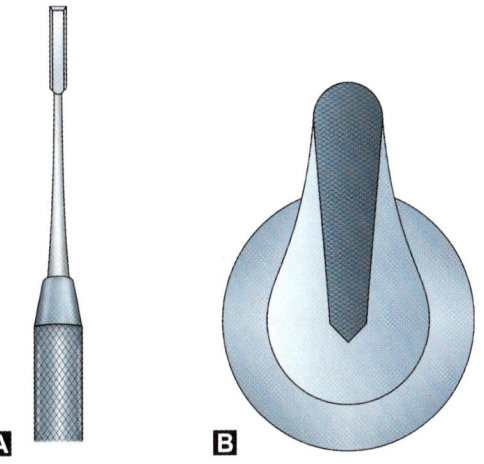

A   **B**

Figures 6.10A and B: Different bevels of an instrument: (A) Straight chisel with single bevel; (B) Bibeveled instrument

are called as single planed instrument. They can be used for both direct and lateral cutting.

Lateral cutting instruments are those in which force is applied at their right angle to the plane of the blade and the handle. They have curved blade, and also called double plane instrument. They can be used lateral cutting only.

Single and Double Ended Instruments

In single ended instruments, working end is present on one side only. In double ended instruments, working end is present on both sides of the instrument. They are used to give mesial and distal or right and left form of the instrument in the same handle.

Instrument motions
➡ *Pulling*: Here, instrument is moved towards operator's hand
➡ *Scraping*: Here, instrument is moved side to side or back and forth on the tooth surface
➡ *Pushing*: Here, instrument is moved away from operator's hand
➡ *Cutting*: Here, instrument is moved parallel to the long axis of handle

EXPLORING INSTRUMENTS

Mouth Mirrors

Mouth mirrors are used as supplement to improve access to instrumentation (**Figs 6.11A and B**).

Types of Mirror Faces (Fig. 6.12)

- *Front surface reflecting mirror:* Here the coating is pressent on front surface of the mirror to prevent image distortion

- *Rear surface reflecting mirror:* It is most commonly used mirror. In this, coating is present on back side of the mirror
- *Plane or flat surface:* It provides clear image without distortion
- *Concave surface:* It is used to provide different degrees of magnification, but it causes image distortion
- *One sided*: Image on one side
- *Two sided*: Image on either side (Advantage—retraction with indirect vision simultaneously).

Uses of Mouth Mirror

- *Direct vision:* Retraction is done with mirror to enhance visibility in specific area. Illumination allows the dentist to use mirror as a spotlight to reflect light from dental light on to a specific area of oral cavity. For example, use in maxillary left palatal aspect
- *Indirect illumination:* In this, mirror is placed in oral cavity that can not be seen directly without compromising dentist's position. For example, use in maxillary right palatal area and for palatal surfaces of anterior teeth (**Fig. 6.13**)
- *Transillumination:* Mirror is placed behind the teeth and direction of light perpendicular to long axis of teeth
- *Retraction:* Retraction of soft tissue such as tongue and cheeks to aid in better visualization of the operating field (**Figs 6.14A and B**).

Uses of mouth mirror
➡ Direct vision
➡ Indirect illumination
➡ Retraction
➡ Transillumination.

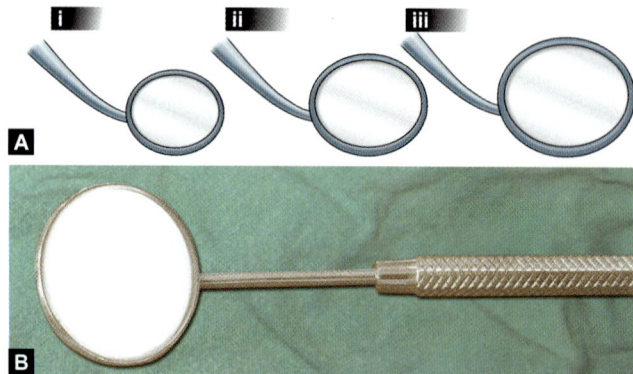

Figures 6.11A and B: Photograph showing mouth mirror. Different sizes of mouth mirrors

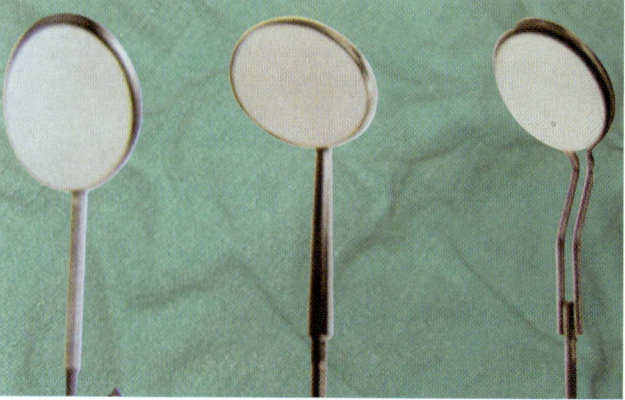

Figure 6.12: Different types of mirror faces

Explorer

Explorer is commonly used as a diagnostic aid in evaluating condition of teeth especially pits and fissures (**Fig. 6.15**).

Parts

- Handle of explorer is straight which could be plain or serrated
- Shank of explorer is curved with one/more angle
- Working tip of explorer is pointed.

Types of Explorer (Figs 6.16A to C)

- *Straight explorer:* It is bent perpendicular to the handle. This is used for examining occlusal surfaces of teeth.
- *Shepherd's Hook or curved explore or arch explorer:* It has semilunar shaped working tip perpendicular to the handle. This is used for examining occlusal surfaces.

- *Interproximal explorer/Briault explorer/Back action probe:* This explorer has two more angles in the shank with working tip-pointed towards the handle.

Uses of interproximal explorer
➡ Examination of interproximal caries
➡ For assessing marginal fit of the restoration.

Cow horn/pigtail explorer: It has smaller arch than curved explorer.

Tweezers

These have angled tip and are available in different sizes (**Figs 6.17A and B**). They are used to place and remove cotton rolls and other small materials.

Probes

Though they almost look like straight explorers but they have blunt end which is marked with graduations (**Fig. 6.18**).

Uses of probes
➡ Mainly used for measuring pocket depth
➡ To determine dimensions of tooth preparation

Types

- William's probe
- PCP 12 probe
- PSR (periodontal screening and recording probe).

These probes differ in:
- Diameter
- Position of markings
- Type of marking (painted/notched).

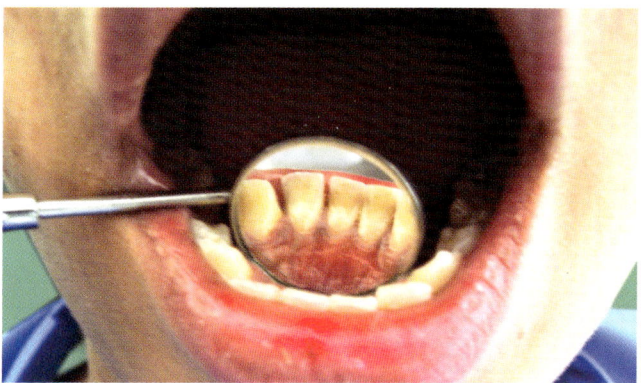

Figure 6.13: Mirror used for indirect vision of lingual surfaces of mandibular anterior teeth

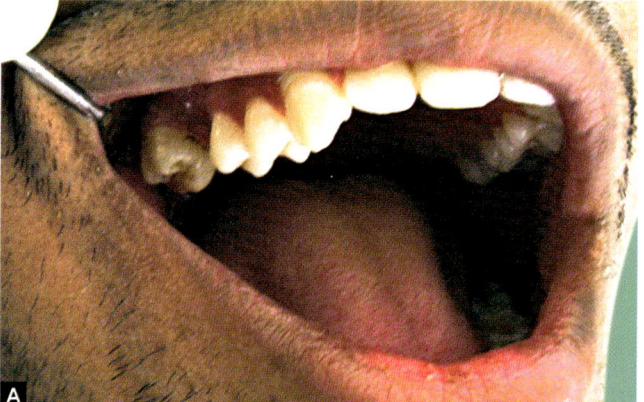

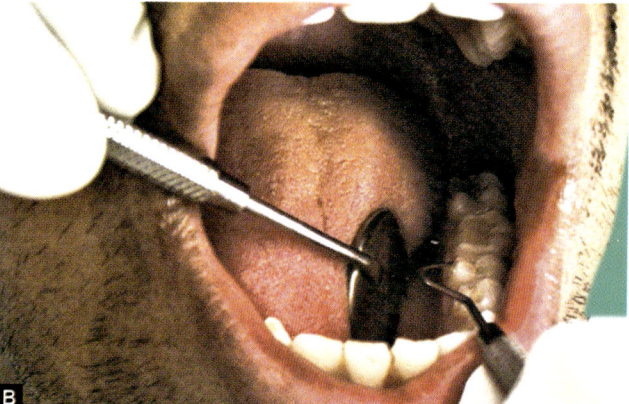

Figures 6.14A and B: (A) Mirror helps in retraction of cheek; (B) Tongue can be retracted using mirror

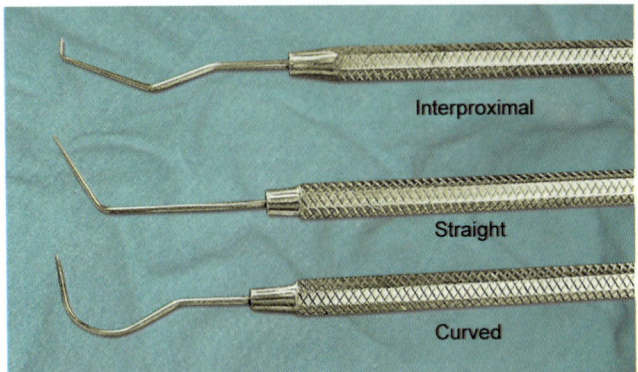

Figure 6.15: Different types of explorers

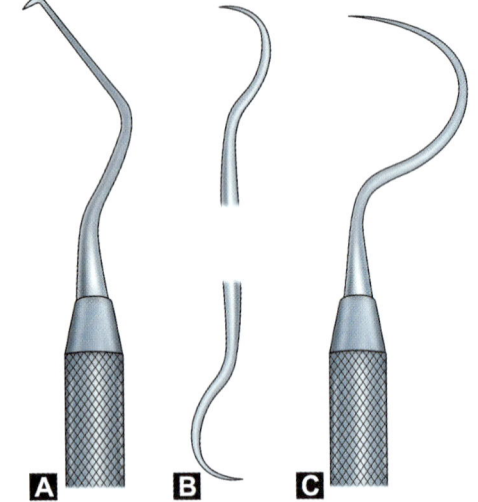

Figures 6.16A to C: Diagrammatic representation of explorers

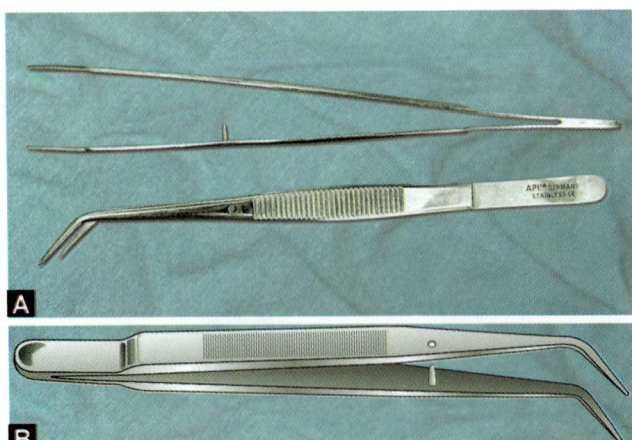

Figures 6.17A and B: (A) Tweezers; (B) Diagrammatic representation of tweezer

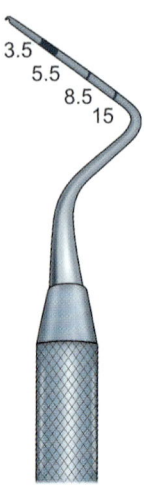

Figure 6.18: Periodontal probe

HAND CUTTING INSTRUMENTS

Instrument families
Chisels
➡ Chisels
◆ Straight chisel
◆ Monoangle chisel
◆ Binangle chisel
◆ Wedelstaedt chisel.
➡ Enamel hatchet
➡ Gingival marginal trimmer.
Excavators
➡ Hatchet
➡ Hoe
➡ Angle former
➡ Spoon excavator.
Others
➡ Knives
➡ Files
➡ Discoid-cleoid.

Chisels

Chisels are used for cleaving, planing and lateral scraping. In other words, they are used to split tooth enamel, to smooth preparation walls and to sharpen the preparations. Chisels are used with a push motion.

Straight Chisel

In straight chisel

- The cutting edge of the chisel makes a 90° angle to the plane of the instrument

- It is used with straight thrust force, push motion.
- It is used for gingival restoration of the anterior teeth (**Fig. 6.19**).

Angled Chisel

In angled chisel
- The primary cutting edge is in a plane perpendicular to the long axis of the shaft and may have either a mesial or distal bevel. Distal bevelled chisel is also called as reverse bevelled or contra-bevelled.
- They are used with a push or pull motion for anterior proximal restorations, smoothening proximal walls and gingival walls for full coverage restorations (**Figs 6.20A and B**).
- Two most common types used are the Wedelstedt and binangle chisels.
- The Wedelstedts chisel is almost similar to straight chisel except for slight vertical curvature in its shank (**Fig. 6.21**). It can be mesially or distally bevelled. It is mainly used on anterior teeth.
- The binangle chisel has two different angles—one at the working end and other at the shank. This design permits access to tooth structures which is not be possible with straight chisels. It is mesially or distally bevelled. It is used to cleave the undermined enamel.

Hatchet
- Any instrument where the cutting edge is parallel or close to parallel to the plane of the instrument is called a hatchet
- Basically, a hatchet is the similar to an axe except that it is much smaller (**Figs 6.22A and B**)
- Hatchet is a paired instrument in which blades makes 45 to 90° angle to the shank
- In paired right and left hatchets, blades are beveled on opposite sides to form their cutting edges (**Figs 6.23A and B**)
- Some hatchets have single cutting ends and some have cutting edges on both ends of the handle
- Hatchets are used for cleaving enamel and planing the dentinal walls so as to have sharp outline of the preparation
- Some hatchets are bibeveled, i.e. blade has two bevels with cutting edge in the center. These bibeveled binangle hatchets are used in a chopping motion to refine line and point angles.

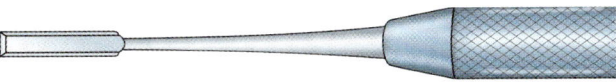

Figure 6.19: Chisel

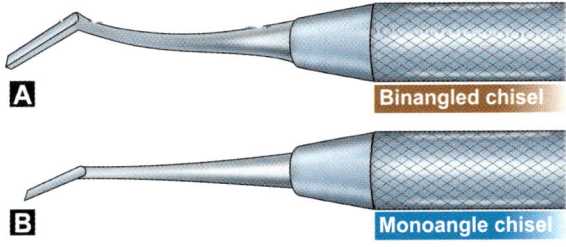

A

Binangled chisel

B

Monoangle chisel

Figures 6.20A and B: Angled chisels (A) Binangled; (B) Monoangle chisel

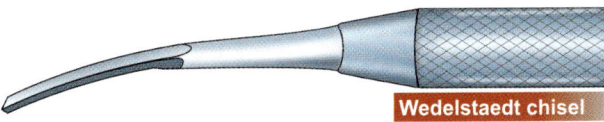

Wedelstaedt chisel

Figure 6.21: Wedelstaedt chisel

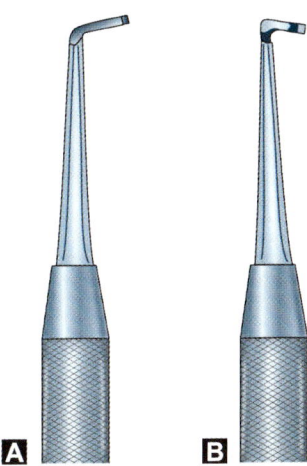

A   B

Figures 6.22A and B: Hatchet

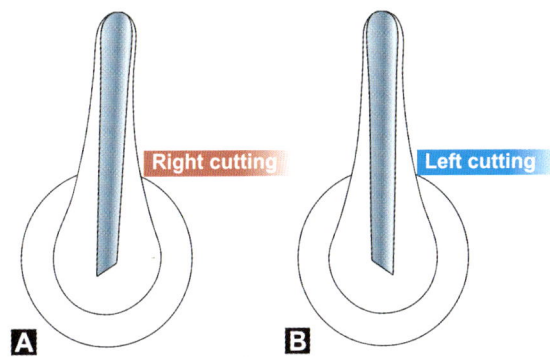

Right cutting   Left cutting

A   B

Figures 6.23A and B: Right and left cutting hatchets

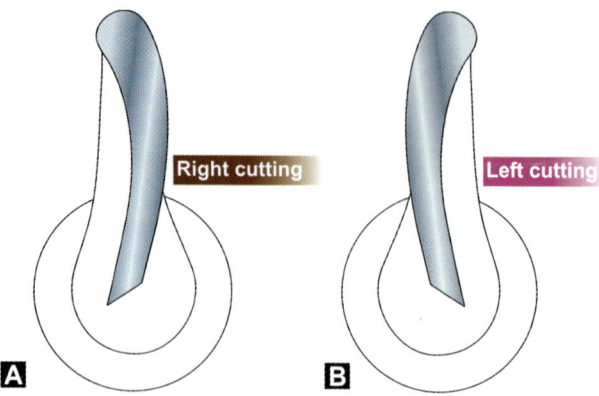

Figures 6.24A and B: (A) Right cutting; (B) Left cutting end of a paired GMT

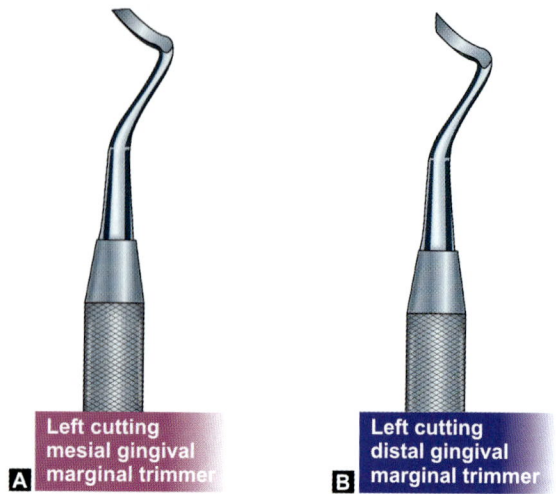

Figures 6.25A and B: Paired gingival marginal trimmer

Gingival Margin Trimmer

- The gingival margin trimmer (GMT) is a modified hatchet which has working ends with opposite curvatures and bevels (**Figs 6.24A and B**)
- The gingival marginal trimmer is available in a set of two double ended styles and is used in pairs, constituting a set of four instruments (**Figs 6.25A and B**)
- Distal gingival margin trimmer is used for the distal surface and the mesial GMT is used for the mesial surface
- If the second number in instrument formula is 75 to 85, it is mesial GMT and if second number is 95 to 100, it is distal GMT
- GMT is used for planing gingival cavosurface margin that is removal of unsupported enamel and to bevel axiopulpal line angle in the class II tooth preparation (**Figs 6.26A and B**).

Main difference between gingival marginal trimmer (GMT) and hatchet
→ GMT has a curved blade, hatchet has straight blade. The curved blade helps in the lateral scraping skill of the GMT
→ The cutting edge of the GMT makes an angle with the plane of the blade whereas cutting edge of the hatchet makes a 90° angle to the plane of the blade.

EXCAVATORS

Ordinary Hatchet

- An ordinary hatchet excavator is a bevelled instrument in which cutting edge of blade is directed in the same plane as that of long axis of the handle.
- Mainly used for preparing and sharpening line angles in anterior teeth.

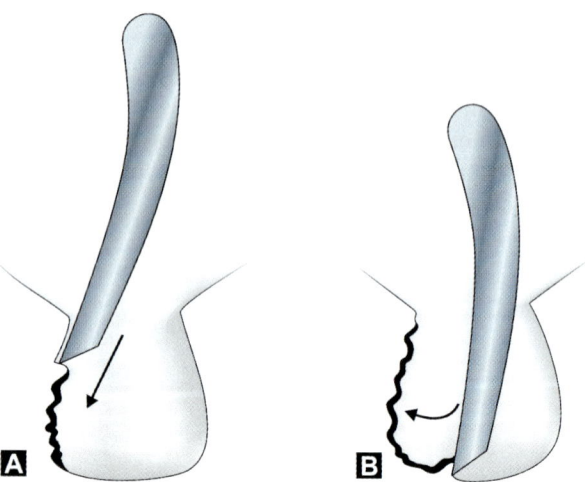

Figures 6.26A and B: Use of GMT in proximal box: (A) GMT in vertical motion to plane facial/lingual wall of proximal box; (B) GMT in horizontal stroke to plane the gingival wall

Hoes

- Dental hoe resembles a miniature garden hoe
- By definition, the hoe is any instrument where the blade makes more than a 12.5° angle with the plane of the instrument (**Figs 6.27A and B**). Usually hoe blades make 45 to 90° angle to the long axis of handle
- Its shank can have one or more angles (**Figs 6.28A and B**)
- Hoe is used with a pulling motion
- Hoe is used to shape and smoothen the floor and form line angles in class III and V restorations.

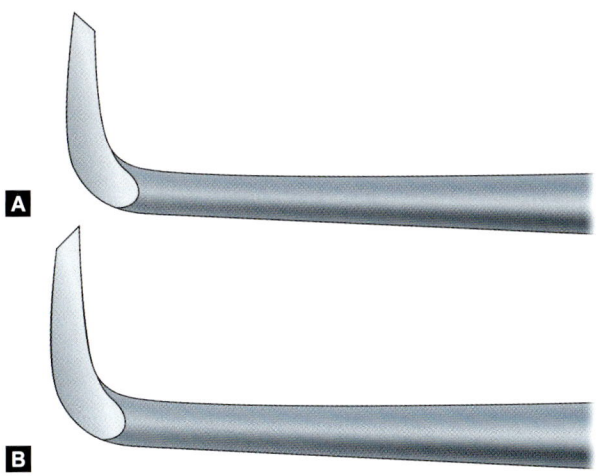

Figures 6.27A and B: Hoe

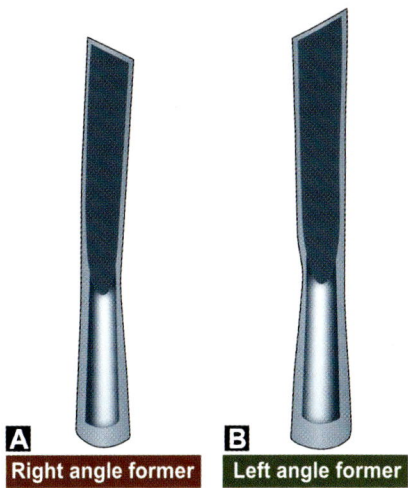

Right angle former **Left angle former**

Figures 6.29A and B: Angle formers

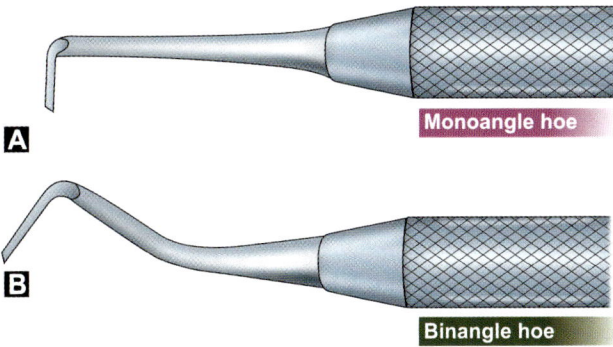

Figures 6.28A and B: Monoangle and binangle hoe

Chisel vs Hoe

By definition, chisel is an instrument where the blade makes up to 12.5° angle with the plane of the instrument, whereas in hoe, the blade is angled more than a 12.5° with the plane of the instrument.

Angle Former (Figs 6.29A and B)

- Angle former is a type of excavator which is monangled with the cutting edge sharpened at an angle to the long axis of the blade
- Angle of cutting edge to blade axis lies between 80 to 85 centigrades
- Blade of angle former is beveled on sides as well as the end, this forms three cutting edges
- It is used with a push or pull motion for accentuating line and point angles, to establish retention form in direct filling gold restoration
- There are two sets of angle formers, mesial and the distal angle former

- Each instrument in the set is a double-ended instrument
- The mesial angle former is used to plane the gingival cavosurface margin in the mesial proximal box. The distal angle former is used to plane the gingival cavosurface margin in the distal proximal box.

Spoon Excavator

- The spoon excavator is a modified hatchet. It is a double-ended instrument with a spoon, claw, or disk-shaped blade (**Figs 6.30A and B**)
- Spoon excavator is used to remove caries and debris in the scooping motion from the carious teeth.

Two main differences between the spoon excavator and hatchet

- The blade of a spoon excavator is curved to emphasize the lateral scraping motion
- The cutting edge of the spoon excavator is rounded.

Knives

They are known as finishing knives, gold knives or amalgam knives. They have thin knife like blade and are used for removing excess material and contouring.

Files

Files are used for trimming excess material especially in the gingival margins.

Cleiod-discoid

- It is modified chisel with different shape of cutting edges (**Figs 6.31A and B**)

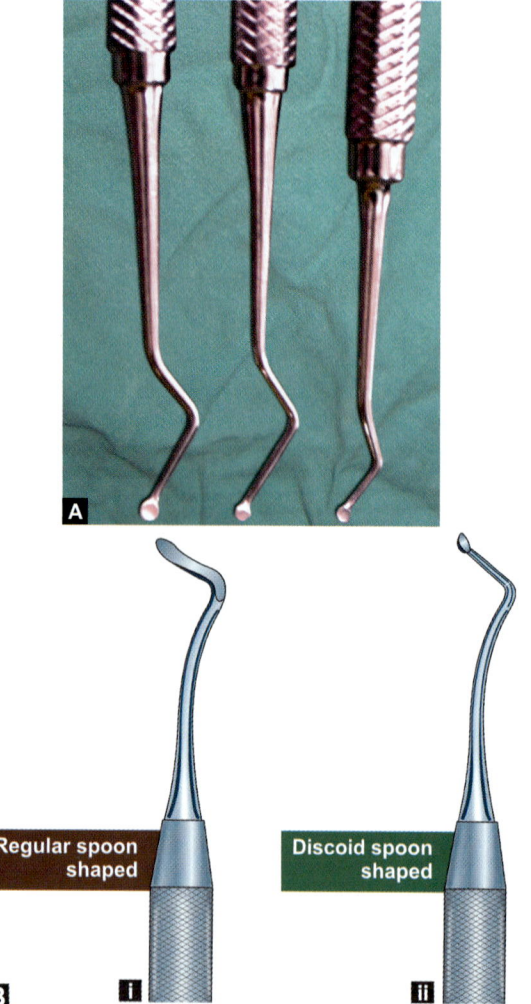

Figures 6.30A and B: Spoon excavators: (i) Regular spoon shaped; (ii) Discoid spoon shaped

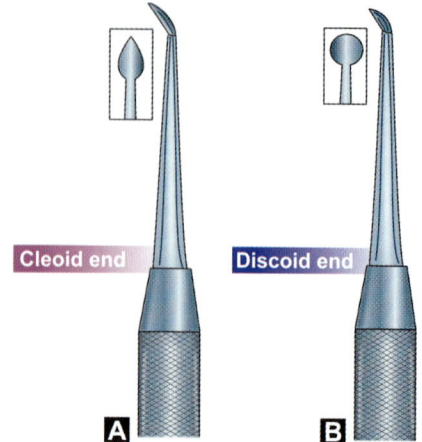

Figures 6.31A and B: Cleoid-discoid

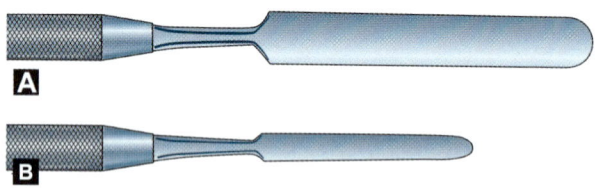

Figures 6.32A and B: Different types of cement spatulas

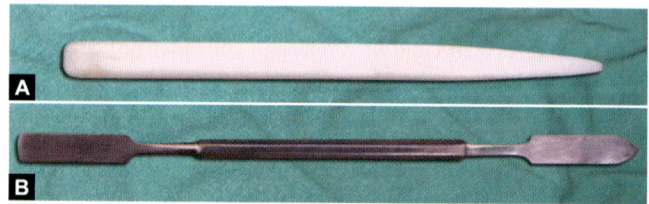

Figures 6.33A and B: Large and small cement spatula

- In cleoid, it is claw-like and in discoid it is disk-like. instead of a sharp edge, the edge is rounded
- These instruments have sharp cutting edges as spoon excavators but blade to shaft relationship is similar to chisels
- They are used for removing caries and carving amalgam or wax patterns.

RESTORATION INSTRUMENTS

Following are the commonly used instruments when temporary or permanent restoration is being done.

Cement Spatulas

- Several types of cement spatulas are available in the market differing in shape and size (**Figs 6.32A and B**)

- On the basis of size, cement spatula can be classified into two types (**Figs 6.33A and B**):
  1. *Large cement spatula*: Mixing of luting cements
  2. *Small cement spatula*: Mixing of liner

Cement spatula also can be classified on the basis of thickness rigid and flexible. Their use depends on viscosity of cement and personal preference.

Plastic Filling Instrument

These instruments have a small metal ball at the working end. They are used to mix, carry and place cements (**Figs 6.34 and 6.35**).

Condensers

Condensers are use to deliver the restoration to the tooth preparation and properly condense it.

- The hammer-like working end of condenser should be large enough to pack the restoration without sinking into it
- Condensers come in single and double-ended designs
- They are available in differently shaped and sized working ends like round, triangular or parallelogram, which may be smooth or serrated

- Condensers can be hand or mechanical in nature (**Figs 6.36 and 6.37**).

Amalgam Carriers

- Amalgam carriers carry the freshly prepared amalgam restorative material to the prepared tooth
- Amalgam carriers have hollow working ends, called barrels, into which the amalgam is packed for transportation (**Figs 6.38 and 6.39**)
- Carriers can be both single and double ended

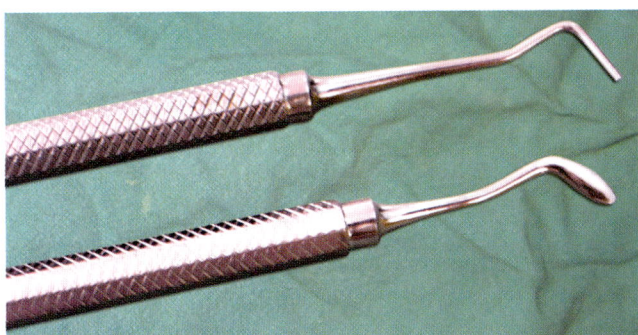

Figure 6.34: Plastic filling instrument

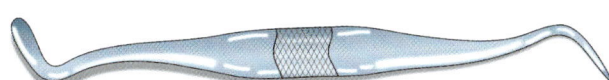

Figure 6.35: Diagrammatic representation of plastic carrier

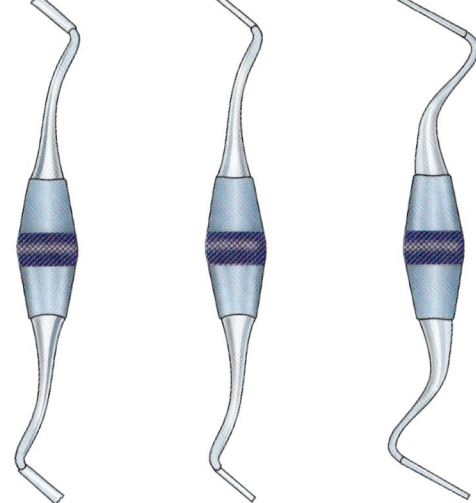

Figure 6.37: Diagrammatic representation of different condensers

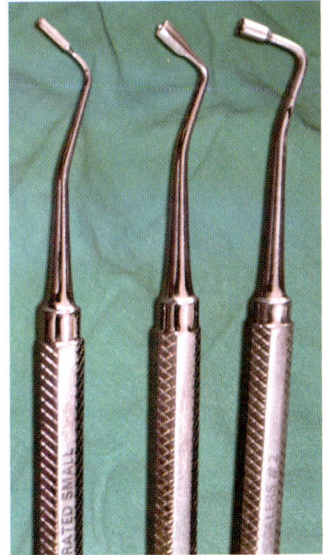

Figure 6.36: Condensers

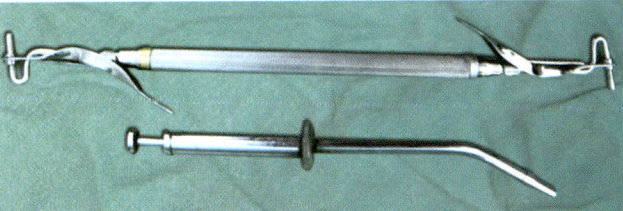

Figure 6.38: Amalgam carriers

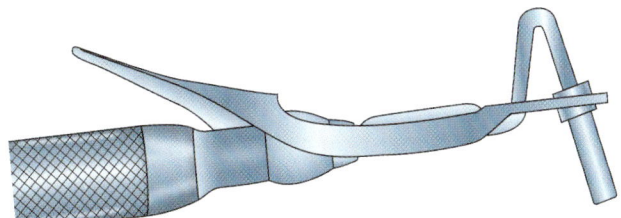

Figure 6.39: Diagrammatic representation of amalgam carrier

- Barrel of amalgam carriers comes in a variety of sizes viz; small, large and jumbo
- Lever of amalgam carrier is located on the top of the carrier. When lever is depressed, the amalgam is expelled into the preparation
- A poorly packed amalgam carrier may result in amalgam fall out before it is ejected into the prepared tooth
- After restoration is completed, any remaining amalgam alloy is expelled out from the carrier into the amalgam well, otherwise carrier will no longer be serviceable if the amalgam is allowed to harden in the carrier.

Carvers (Fig. 6.40)

- Sharp cutting edges present in carvers are used to shape and form tooth anatomy from a restorations
- Carvers come in different shapes and sizes in double ended designs (**Fig. 6.41**)
- Many carvers are designed for carving specific tooth surfaces

- For example, interproximal and hollenback carvers are used for carving proximal surfaces and discoid cleoid and diamond-shaped carvers are used for carving occlusal surfaces (**Fig. 6.42**).

Burnisher (Fig. 6.43)

- Burnishers are the kind of instruments which make the surface shiny by rubbing
- They are used to smoothen and polish the restoration and to remove scratches present on the amalgam surface after its carving
- Burnishers have smooth rounded working ends and come in single and double ended types (see **Figs 6.33A and B**). Different types of burnishers are available but most commonly used are (**Figs 6.44A to C**):
- PKT3—designed by Peter K Thomas
    —Rounded cone-shaped burnisher.
- Beavetail condenser—narrow type of burnisher.
- Ovoid burnisher—comes in various sizes such as 28, 29, 31.

Uses of burnishers
➡ Final condensation of amalgam
➡ Initial shaping of occlusal anatomy of amalgam
➡ Shaping of metal matrix bands
➡ Shaping of occlusal anatomy in posterior resin composite before polymerization of resin
➡ Burnishing margins of cast gold restoration.

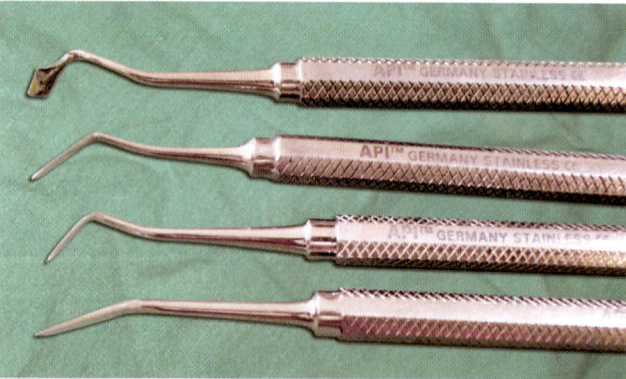

Figure 6.40: Carvers

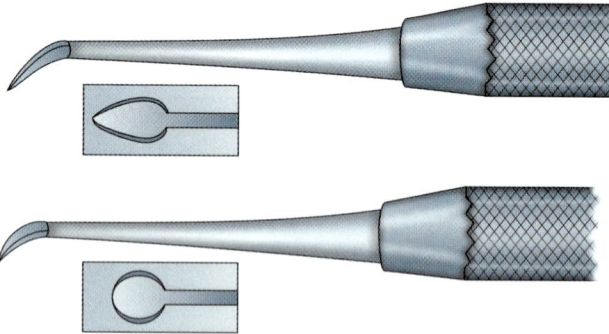

Figure 6.42: Hollenback and discoid cleoid shaped carvers

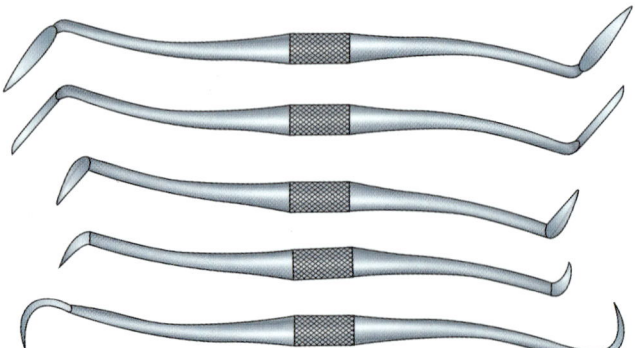

Figure 6.41: Diagrammatic representation of carvers

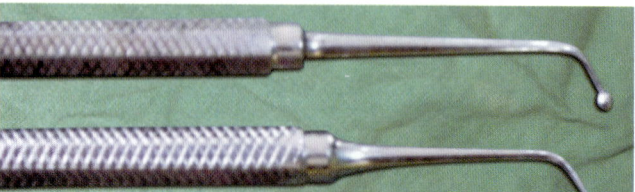

Figure 6.43: Burnishers

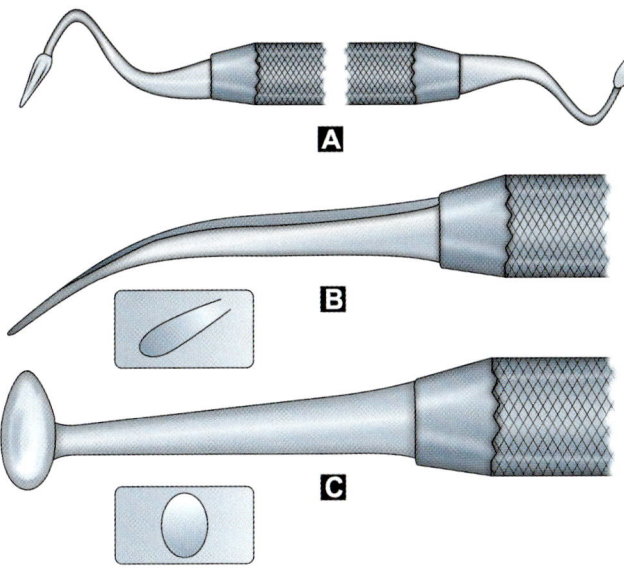

Figures 6.44A to C: Diagrammatic representation of burnishers

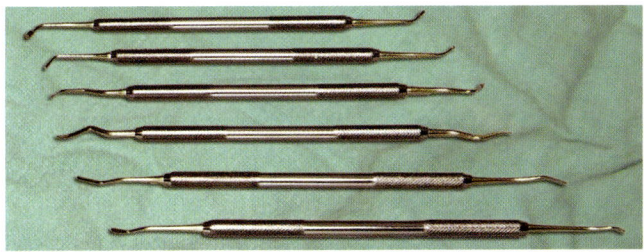

Figure 6.45: Composite resin instruments

Composite Resin Instruments

- For composite resin restorations, a wide range of double ended instruments are used to transport and place resins
- The working ends on these instruments range from small cylinders to angled, paddle like shapes (**Fig. 6.45**)
- Composite resin instruments are made of plastic or titanium coating
- Advantages of using plastic instruments are that they do not discolor or contaminate the composite restoration, and the composite resin material does not stick to the instrument.

INSTRUMENT GRASPS

For accurate and precise control over the instrument certain instrument grasps are suggested which help in increasing efficiency of the operator, offer more flexibility of movements and decrease strain on the operator. In other words, correct instrument grasps are important for achieving success in operative procedures.

The correct grasp is selected according to the instruments being used, position of instrument being used, the operator, the area which is being operated and the specific procedure to be done.

Commonly used instrument grasps in operative dentistry
→ Modified pen grasp
→ Inverted pen grasp
→ Palm and thumb grasp
→ Modified palm and thumb grasp.

Modified Pen Grasp (Fig. 6.46)

This is the most commonly used grasp. The greatest delicacy of touch is provided by this grasp. Normally, a pen is held with the thumb and index finger, with the middle finger placed under the pen. The modified pen grasp is similar to the pen grasp except the operator uses the pad of the middle finger on the handle of the instrument rather than going under the instrument (**Figs 6.47A and B**). The positioning of the fingers in this manner creates a triangle of forces or tripod effect, which enhances the instrument control. It is most commonly used in mandibular teeth. Here palm of the operator faces away from the operator. This position stabilizes the instrument and allows the middle finger to help push the instrument down.

Inverted Pen Grasp

In inverted pen grasp, finger positions are the same as for the modified pen grasp except that hand is rotated so that palm faces towards the operator (**Fig. 6.48**). This grasp is most commonly used for preparing a tooth in the lingual aspect of maxillary anterior and occlusal surface of maxillary posterior teeth (**Fig. 6.49**).

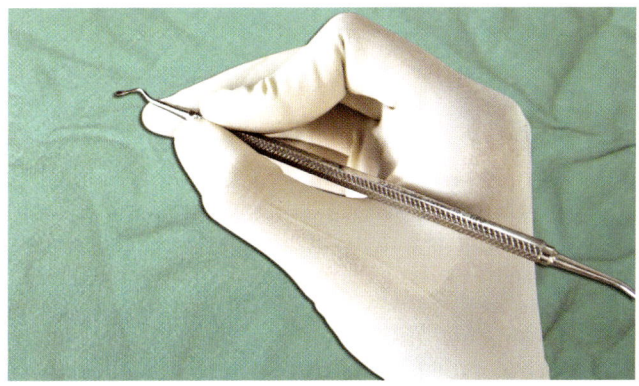

Figure 6.46: Modified pen grasp

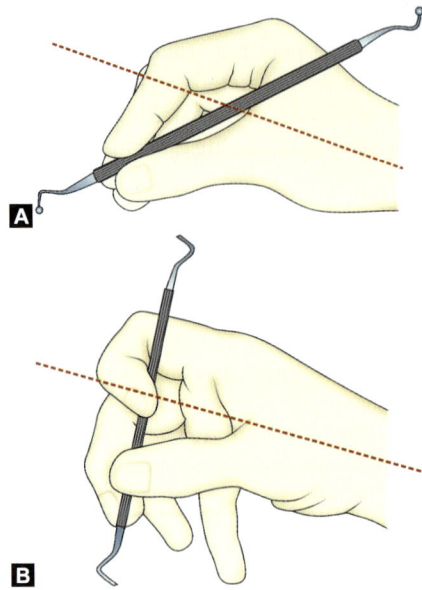

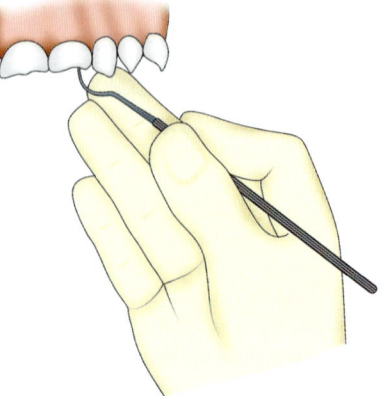

Figure 6.49: Inverted pen grasp is commonly used for preparing lingual aspect of maxillary anterior teeth

Figures 6.47A and B: (A) Pen grasp; (B) Modified pen grasp. There is difference in angle formed by shaft of the instrument and long axis of the forearm

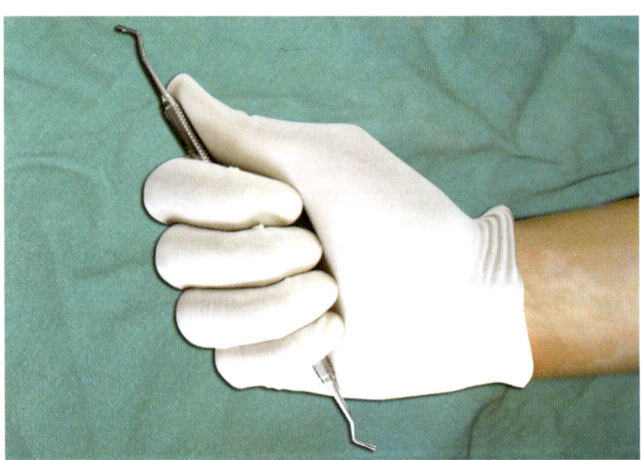

Figure 6.50: Palm and thumb grasp

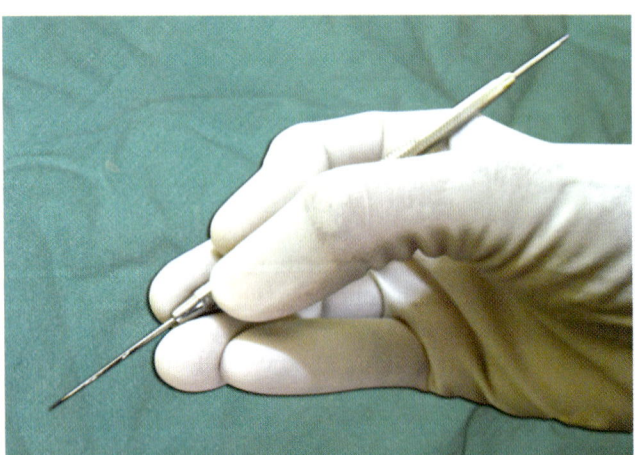

Figure 6.48: Inverted pen grasp

movements and provide rest on a adjacent tooth of the same arch. To achieve the thrust action with the fingers and palm, instrument is forced away from the tip of the thumb which is at the rest position. This grasp has limited use only while operating on maxillary anterior teeth. Since it offers application of heavy force with greater control, it is used for holding a handpiece while cutting incisal retention for a class III preparation in maxillary incisor.

Palm and Thumb Grasp (Fig. 6.50)

This grasp is same as for holding the knife for peeling the skin of an apple. The palm and thumb grasp is commonly used for bulky instruments. In this, instrument is grasped very near to its working end so that thumb can be braced against the teeth so as to provide control during instrument movements. The shaft of the instrument is placed on the palm of the hand and grasped by the four fingers to provide firm control, while the thumb is free to control

Modified Palm and Thumb Grasp (Figs 6.51A and B)

The instrument is held like the palm grasp but the pads of all the four fingers press the handle against the palm and pad and first joint of the thumb. Here tip of the thumb rests on the tooth being prepared or the adjacent tooth.

Modified palm and thumb grasp provides more control to avoid slipping of instrument. This grasp is commonly used in maxillary anterior teeth.

FINGER RESTS

The finger rest helps to stabilize the hand and the instrument by providing a firm rest to the hand during operative procedures. Finger rests may be intraoral or extraoral.

- **Intraoral finger rests**:
  - *Conventional*: In this, the finger rest is just near or adjacent to the working tooth (**Fig. 6.52**)
  - *Cross-arch*: In this, the finger rest is achieved from tooth of the opposite side but of the same arch (**Fig. 6.53**)
  - *Opposite arch*: In this, the finger rest is achieved from tooth of the opposite arch
  - *Finger on finger*: In this, rest is achieved from index finger or thumb of nonoperating hand.
- **Extraoral finger rest**: It is used mostly for maxillary posterior teeth.
  - *Palm up*: Here rest is obtained by resting the back of the middle and fourth finger on the lateral aspect of the mandible on the right side of the face (**Fig. 6.54**)

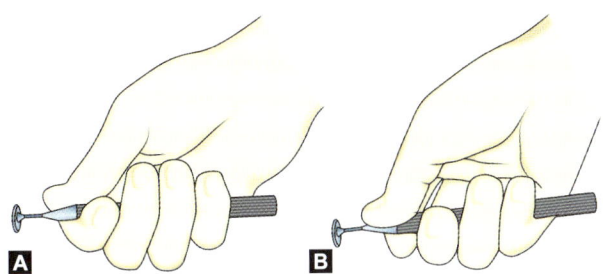

Figures 6.51A and B: (A) True palm grasp; (B) Modified palm grasp. See the difference lies in position of the index finger

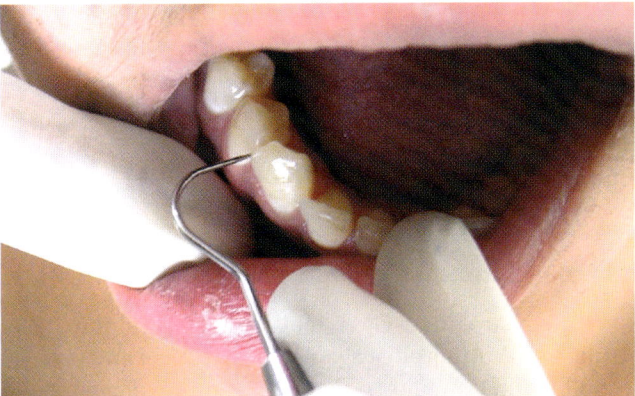

Figure 6.52: Conventional finger rest

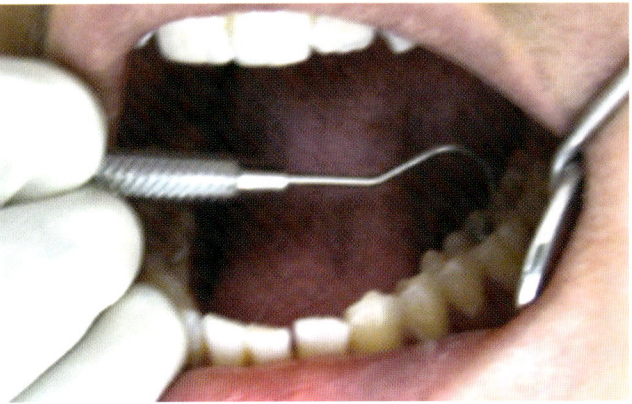

Figure 6.53: Cross-arch finger rest

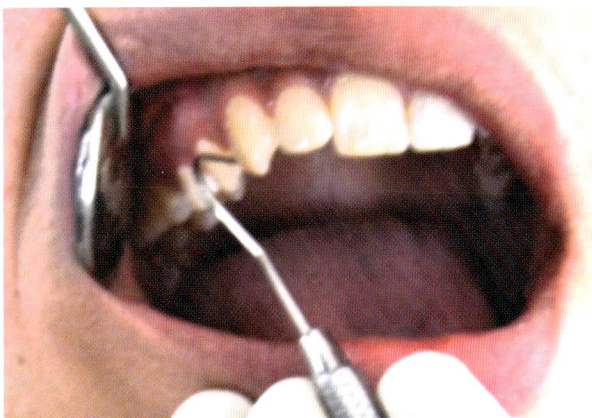

Figure 6.54: Palm up finger rest

- *Palm down*: Here rest is obtained by resting the front surface of the middle and fourth fingers on the lateral aspect of the mandible on the left side of the face (**Fig. 6.55**).

Methods of use of instruments
➡ The instruments are effectively used when they are used from the bevel side to the non-bevel side
➡ Instrument should be held in such a way that allows the cutting edge to remove any unsupported enamel from the preparation walls
➡ Instrument should always be held parallel to the wall being worked upon. Holding an instrument at this angle may increase its cutting but it may also cause damage or fracture of the tooth
➡ For the buccal wall, one side of the instrument is used and on the lingual wall, the other side of the instrument should be used.

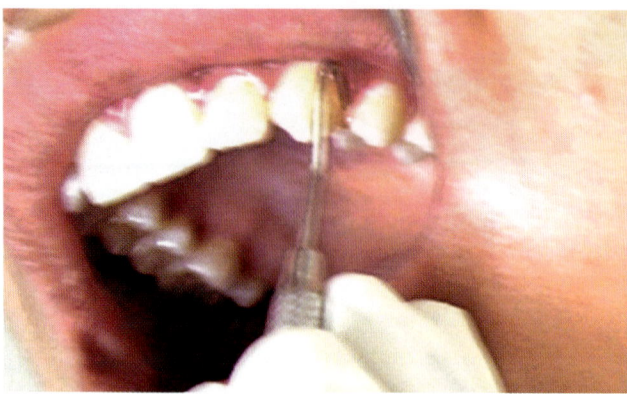

Figure 6.55: Palm down finger rest

SHARPENING OF HAND INSTRUMENTS

Instrument sharpening is a critical component of operative dentistry. It is impossible to carry out procedures with dull instruments. A sharp instrument cuts more precisely and quickly than dull instruments. Therefore to avoid wasting time on using dull instruments, dentists must be thoroughly familiar with principles of sharpening.

Goals of sharpening
➡ To produce a functionally sharp edge
➡ Maintain the contour (shape) of instrument
➡ Maintain the life of instrument.

Advantages of sharp instruments
Use of well sharpened instruments results in:
➡ Improved efficiency
➡ Improved tactile sensations
➡ Less pressure and force
➡ Improved instrument control
➡ Minimized patient discomfort
➡ Less treatment time.

Principles of Sharpening

Some basic principles used during sharpening are:
- Select the appropriate type of stone for type of instrument to be used
- Instrument should be clean and sterile before sharpening
- Establish proper angle between stone and surface of instrument on the basis of design
- Lubricate the stone during sharpening as it reduces the clogging of sharpening stone and heat generated during sharpening
- Stable and firm grip of both instrument and stone is required during sharpening. Maintain the proper angulation throughout sharpening strokes

- Sharpening should be done with light stroke or pressure. Avoid excessive pressure
- When sharpening is completed observe the cutting edge for wire edges. Wire edges should be removed. (Wire edges are unsupported metal fragments that extend beyond the cutting from the lateral side or face of blade)
- Resterilize the sharpened instruments.

Devices Used for Sharpening

- Mechanical
- Mounted stone
- Handhold stones (Unmounted).

Mechanical

It is bench type piece of equipment in which honing disks are mounted. On top disk rotates up to 7,000 rpm. It saves time, e.g. honing machine.

Mounted Stones

In this, stones are mounted on metal mandrel and used with slow speed handpiece. Most common mounted stones are Arkansas and ruby. Various shapes such as cylindrical, conical or disk shaped are available. Mounted stones are not preferred in routine because they:
- Tend to wear down quickly
- Result in generation of frictional heat
- Difficult to control during sharpening.

Unmounted/Handhold Stones

These are commonly used for instrument sharpening. These come in variety of sizes and shapes. Stone can be rectangular with flat, rectangular with grooved surfaces or cylindrical in shape.
- Flat stone is ideal for moving technique
- Cylindrical stone for removing wire edges.

Stone type can come in natural or synthetic form:
- Natural–Arkansas (preferred)
- Synthetic:
  - India stone
  - Ceramic stone
  - Composition stone.

Guidelines for Sharpening Operative Instruments

- When sharpening GMT, chisels, hatchets and hoes, place the cutting edge against the flat stone and push or pull the instrument so that acute cutting angle moved forward (**Fig. 6.56**)

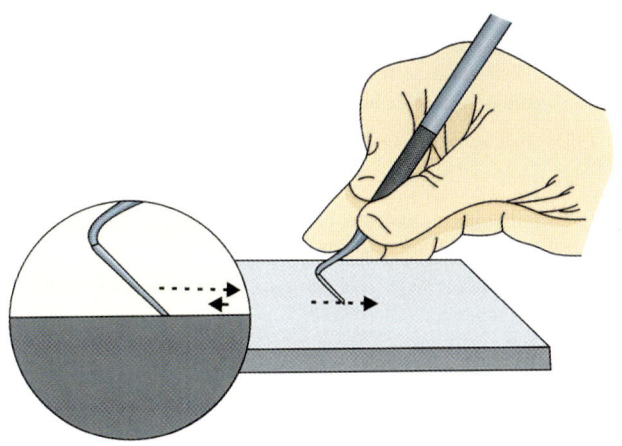

Figure 6.56: Sharpening the bevel end of hoe

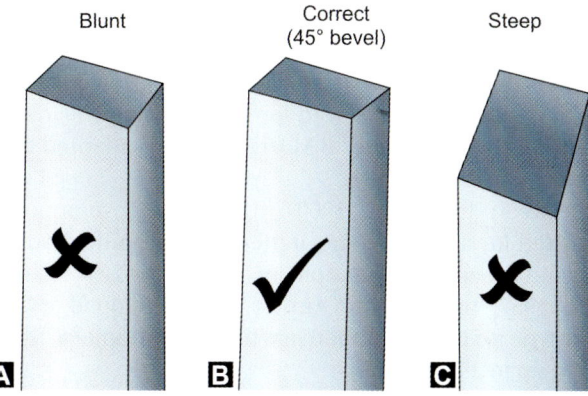

Figures 6.57A to C: Different bevels of sharpened instrument: (A) Blunt bevel—incorrect; (B) Correct bevel with 45°; (C) Steep bevel—incorrect

- Bevel of instrument should make 45° angle with face of blade. So, while sharpening, blade should make a 45° angle with the sharpening surface (**Figs 6.57A to C**)
- While sharpening spoon excavators, cleoid and discoid carvers, rotate the instrument as the blade is moved on the sharpening stone
- Move the instrument with bevel against the stone surface and cutting edge placed perpendicular to the path of movement (**Fig. 6.58**)
- For curved or round cutting edge instrument, handle of edge instrument should be moved in an arc to keep the cutting edge perpendicular to direction of cutting stroke.

Advantages of hand cutting instruments
➡ Self-limited in cutting enamel
➡ They can remove large pieces of undermined enamel quickly
➡ No vibration or heat accompanies the cutting
➡ Efficient means of precise cutting
➡ Create smooth surface on cutting
➡ Long lifespan and can be resharpened.

ROTARY CUTTING INSTRUMENTS

Rotary cutting instruments are those instruments which rotate on an axis to do the work of abrading and cutting on tooth structure.

Types of Rotary Cutting

- *Handpiece*: It is a power device
- *Bur*: It is a cutting tool.

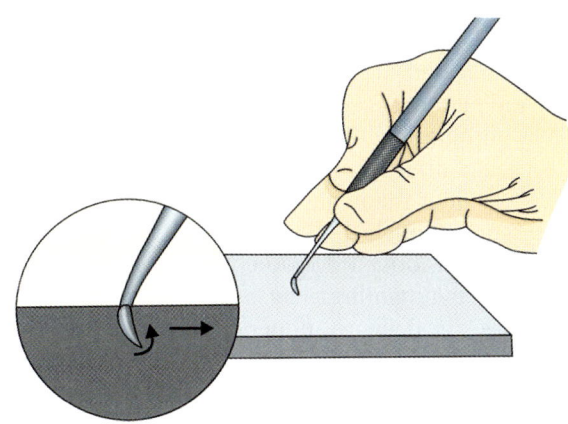

Figure 6.58: Sharpening of cleoid carver is done in such a way that handle is moved in an arc to the rotate the blade as bevel end is pulled on sharpening stone surface

Handpieces

The first rotary instruments were drill or bur heads that were twisted with the fingers for crude cutting of the tooth tissue. Drilling came as the modification (1728) where seat for the drill was provided by a socket fitting against the palm and the ring was adapted to the index or middle finger. In the mid 19th century, the invention and development of both mechanical and pedal powered handpieces occurred in 1864, British dentist George Fellows invented the "clockwork" drill. Here the bur was attached to it by a shaft with a rotating spindle inside. The drill was wound up like a clock, with a key inserted into the back. Drill used to spin for 2 minutes before needing to be rewound.

In 1868, American dentist GF Green developed a pneumatic handpiece powered by pedal operated bellows.

First "dental engine" to provide enough power to spin the bur with sufficient speed for tooth cutting was developed in 1871 by Dr James B Morrison. It was adapted from sewing machine concept.

Between 1950s and 1960s, maximum developments occurred for improvements in design, mechanical operation and speed of the handpieces.

In 1957, the Borden, Airotor was developed as the prototype for today's modern air-turbine handpiece. It had speed up to 250,000 rpm.

Air-turbine systems depend mainly on momentum to produce their power. Since they are powered by the speed of airflow, there is no physical or mechanically connection to the power source. Thus, under load, they tend to slow down. Therefore "touch-and-go" rule should be followed with these air-driven turbines. This means touch the bur to tooth and start cutting by applying pressure. As the bur slows, release pressure until the bur resumes its speed. Because of their ease of use, simple design and patient acceptance air turbine handpieces are still very popular.

Electrically driven handpieces were introduced in the 1970s. They offer many advantages over their air driven predecessors. Though these handpieces are heavier and bigger than air driven handpieces, but they have the advantage of maintaining a constant speed during cutting, which does not decrease under load. Also these handpieces have ability to control the rpm rate.

In general for better efficiency, the diameter and bend of the handpiece should be designed such that it fits optimally between thumb and forefinger and should have balanced center of gravity to make the handpiece feel lighter than its actual weight. Head diameter of handpiece should be smaller in size so as to allow greater visibility and maneuverability.

Development of rotary cutting instruments in dentistry

Year and instrument		Maximum speed (in RPM)
• Ultra low speed		
1728	Finger rotated instruments	300
1871	Foot engine	700
1874	Electric engine motor driven	1000
• Low speed		
1914	Dental unit (Electric motor as a power source)	5000
1942	Diamond cutting instruments	5000

• Medium speed		
1947	High speed electric engines with tungsten carbide burs	12,000
1953	Ball bearings handpieces	25,000
• High speed		
1955	High speed engine with water cooling turbine angle handpiece	50,000
1955	Belt driven water cooling angle handpiece	150,000
• Ultra high speed		
1957	Air turbine angle handpiece with coolant	2,00,000
• Super ultra high speed		
1960	Air turbine angle handpiece with coolant	3,00,000
1961	Air turbine straight handpiece with coolant (Air motor)	25,000
1994	Contemporary air turbine handpiece with coolant	3,00,000 to 4,00,000

Classification of Handpiece

Dental handpiece are classified according to their driving mechanisms.

- *Gear driven handpiece:* Rotary power is transferred by a belt which runs from an electric engine. Power is transferred from the straight handpiece by a shaft and gears inside the angle section. This handpiece is capable of working with wide speed range, though it works best at low speed because of so many moving parts with metal to metal contact.
- *Water driven handpiece:* It was discovered in 1953. It operates at speed up to 100,000 rpm. In this handpiece, a small inner piece transports water under high pressure to rotate the turbine in the handpiece and the larger outer tube returns the water to the reservoir. Advantage of this handpiece is its quiet nature and highest torque.
- *Belt driven handpiece:* Belt driven angle handpiece was made available in 1955. It runs at speed of > 100,000 rpm. This handpieces has excellent performance and great versatility.
- *Air driven handpiece:* This handipiece became available in the later part of 1956. It runs at speed of approximately 300,000 rpm.

Types of Handpiece

- **Contra-angle handpiece:** In this, head of handpiece is first angled away from and then back towards the long axis of the handle. Because of this design, bur head lies close to long axis of the handle of handpiece which improve accessibility, visibility and stability of handpiece while working.

- – *Air-rotor contra-angle handpiece*: It gets power from the compressed air supplied by the compressor. This handpiece has high speed and low torque (**Fig. 6.59**).
- – *Micromotor handpiece*: It gets power from electric micromotor or airmotor. This handpiece has high torque and low speed (**Fig. 6.60**).
- **Straight handpiece**: In straight handpiece, long axis of bur lies in same plane as long axis of handpiece. This handpiece is commonly used in oral surgical and laboratory procedures (**Fig. 6.61**).

Dental Burs

"Bur is a rotary cutting instrument which has bladed cutting head".

Burs are used to remove tooth structure either by chipping it away or by grinding. The earliest burs were handmade. Before 1890s, silicon carbide disks and stones were used to cut enamel since carbon steel burs were not effective in cutting enamel.

William and Schroeder first made diamond dental bur in 1897, modern diamond bur was introduced in 1932 by WH Drendel by bonding diamond points to stainless steel shanks. Diamond burs grind away the tooth. Diamond particles of < 25 µm size are recommended for polishing procedures and > 100 µm are used for cavity preparation.

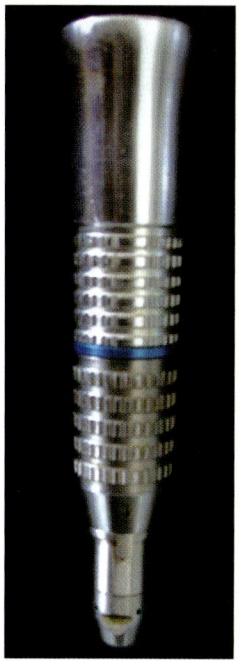

Figure 6.61: Straight handpiece

Diamond particles are attached to bur shank either by sintering or by galvanic metal bond. Degree of bonding and clearance of shavings determine the quantity and effectiveness of bur.

Materials Used for Bur (Fig. 6.62)

- *Stainless steel burs*: These were the first developed burs. Stainless steel burs are designed for slow speed < 5000 rpm. Usually a bur has eight blades with positive rake angle for active cutting of dentin. But this makes steel burs fragile, so they do not have a long life.
  They are used for cutting soft carious dentin and finishing procedures.
- *Tungsten carbide burs*: With the development of high speed handpieces, tungsten carbide burs were designed to withstand heavy stresses and increase shelf life.
  These burs work best beyond 3,00,000. These burs have six blades and negative rake angle to provide better support for cutting edge. Tungsten carbide burs have head of cemented tungsten carbide in the matrix of cobalt or nickel. These burs can cut metal and dentin very well but can produce microcracks in the enamel so weaken the cavosurface margins.
  Diamonds have good cutting efficiency in removing enamel (brittle) while carbide burs cut dentin (elastic material) with maximum efficiency.

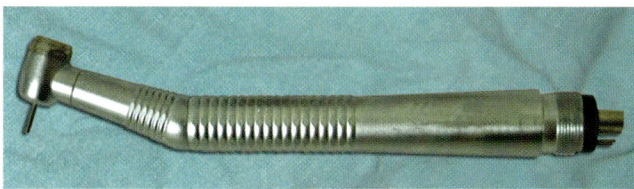

Figure 6.59: Air-rotor contra angle handpiece

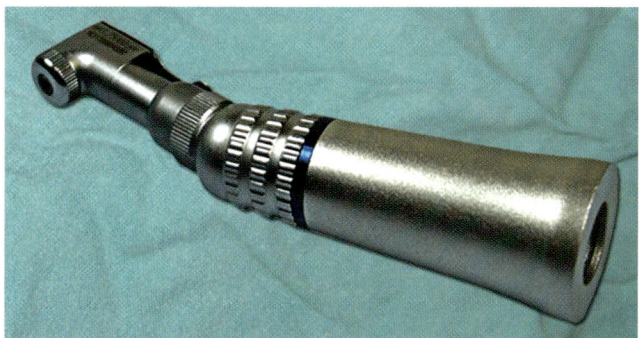

Figure 6.60: Micromotor contra-angle handpiece

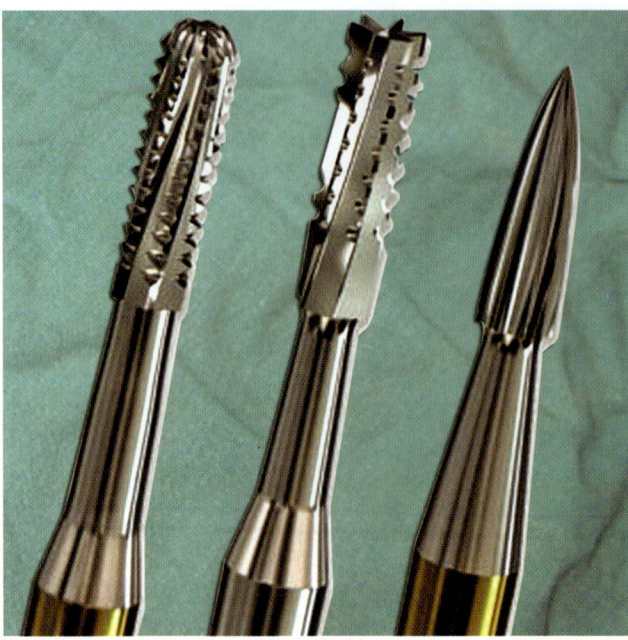

Figure 6.62: Tungsten carbide burs

Classifications of Burs

There are various systems for the classification of burs.
- According to their mode of attachment to the handpiece:
  - Latch type
  - Friction grip type
- According to their composition:
  - Stainless steel burs
  - Tungsten carbide burs
  - A combination of both
- According to their motion:
  - *Right bur:* A right bur is one which cuts when it revolves clockwise.
  - *Left bur:* A left bur is one which cuts when revolving anticlockwise.
- According to the length of their head:
  - Long
  - Short
  - Regular
- According to their use:
  - Cutting burs
  - Finishing burs
  - Polishing burs
- According to their shapes:
  - Round bur
  - Inverted cone
  - Pear-shaped
  - Wheel shaped
  - Tapering fissure
  - Straight fissure
  - End cutting bur

Part of a Bur (Fig. 6.63)

Parts of bur
➡ Shank
➡ Neck
➡ Head.

- **Shank:** The shank is that part of the bur that fits into the handpiece, accepts the rotary movement from the handpiece and controls the alignment and concentricity of the instrument. The three commonly seen instrument shanks are:
  - Straight handpiece shank
  - Latch type handpiece shank
  - Friction grip handpiece shank.
- **Neck:** The neck connects the shank to the hand. Main function of neck is to transmit rotational and translational forces to the head.
- **Head:** It is working part of the instrument. Based upon their head characteristics, the instruments can be bladed or abrasive. These are available in different sizes and shapes.

Different designs of bur shank neck and head.
- **Shank design (Fig. 6.64):** Depending upon mode of attachment to handpiece, shanks of burs can be of following types:
  - Straight handpiece shank
  - Latch type angle handpiece shank
  - Friction grip angle handpiece shank.
    - i. *Straight handpiece shank:* Shank part of straight handpiece is like a cylinder into which bur is held with a metal chuck which has different sizes of shank diameter.

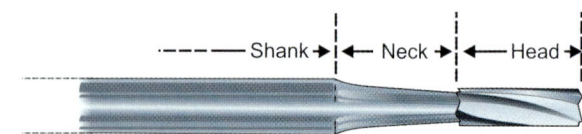

Figure 6.63: Parts of a dental bur

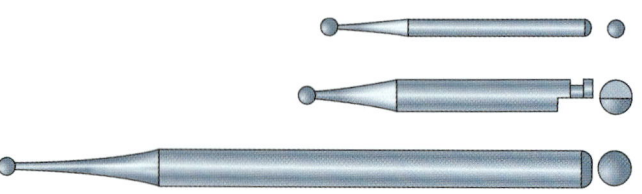

Figure 6.64: Shank design of burs

ii. *Latch type angle handpiece shank*: In this handpiece posterior portion of shank is made flat on one side so that end of bur fits into D-shaped socket at bottom of bur tube. In this, instrument is not retained in handpiece with chuck but with a latch which fits into the grooves made in shank of bur. These instruments are commonly used in contra-angle handpiece for finishing and polishing procedures.

iii. *Friction grip angle handpiece shank*: This was introduced for high speed handpiece. Here the shank is simple cylinder which is held in the handpiece by friction between shank and metal chuck. This design of shank is much smaller than latch type instruments.

- **Design of neck:** Neck connects head and shank. It is tapered from shank to the head. For optical visibility and efficiency of bur, dimensions of neck should be small but at the same time it should not compromise the strength.

- **Design of bur head (Figs 6.65 to 6.67):** The term 'bur shape' refers to the contour or silhouette of the bur head.

  - *Round bur:* Spherical in shape, used for removal of caries, extension of the preparation and for the placement of retentive grooves.
  - *Inverted cone bur:* It has flat base and sides tapered towards shank. It is used for establishing wall angulations and providing undercuts in tooth preparations.

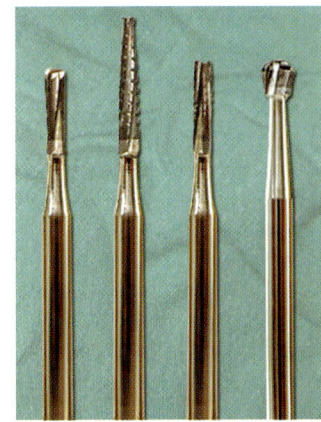

Figure 6.66: Different shapes of cross cut burs

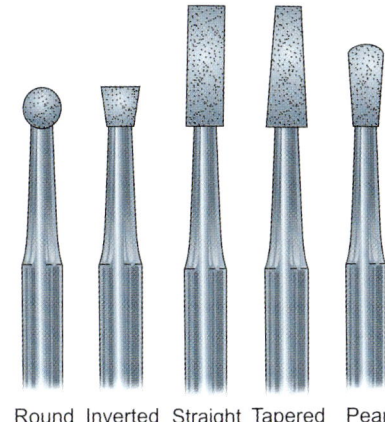

Round Inverted Straight Tapered Pear
cone

Figure 6.67: Different design of bur heads

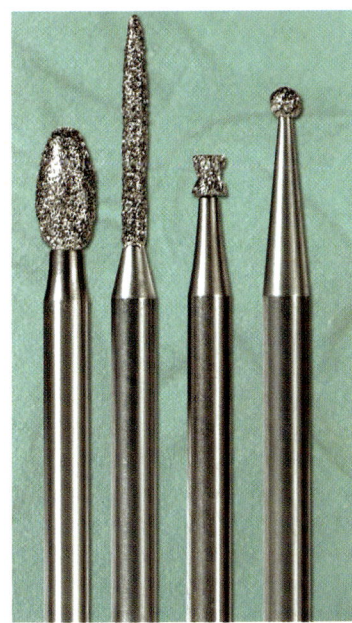

Figure 6.65: Different types of diamond abrasives

- *Pear shaped bur:* Here head is shaped like tapered cone with small end of cone directed towards shank. It is used in class I tooth preparation for gold foil. A long length pear bur is used for tooth preparation for amalgam.
- *Straight fissure bur:* It is parallel sided cylindrical bur of different lengths and is used for amalgam tooth preparations.
- *Tapering fissure bur:* It is tapered sided cylindrical but sides tapering towards tip and is used for inlay and crown preparations.
- *End cutting bur:* It is used for carrying the preparation apically without axial reduction.

Modifications in Bur Design

Because of introduction of handpieces with high speed ranges, many modifications have been made in design of bur. Since cutting efficiency of carbide burs increase with increase in speed, the larger diameter carbide burs have been replaced by small diameter burs.

Head shapes and dimensions of burs

Shape of head	Head diameter (mm)	Number
Round	0.5	¼
	0.6	½
	0.8	1
	1.0	2
	1.2	3
	1.4	4
Straight fissure	0.6	55½
	0.8	56
	1.0	57
	1.2	58
	1.4	59
Tapered fissure	1.0	700
	1.2	701
Inverted cone	0.6	33½
	0.8	34
	1.0	35
	1.2	36
	1.3	37
Straight fissure	0.8	556
Crosscut	1.0	557
	1.2	558
	1.3	559
End cutting	1.0	957
Bur	1.2	958
	1.4	959

Others modifications in bur design are as following:

- *Reduced number of crosscuts:* Since at high speed, crosscuts tends to produce rough surface, newer burs have reduced number of crosscuts.
- *Extended head lengths:* Burs with extended head length have been introduced so as to produce effective cutting with very light pressure.
- *Rounding of sharp tip corners:* Sharp tip corners of burs produce sharp internal angles, resulting in stress concentration. Burs with round tip corners produce rounded internal line angles and thus lower stress in restored tooth.

Bur Size

Bur size represents the diameter of bur head. Different numbers have been assigned to burs which denote bur size and head design. Earlier burs had a numbering system in which burs were grouped by 9 shapes and 11 sizes.

But later because of modifications in bur design this numbering system was modified. For example, after introduction of crosscut burs, 500 numbers was added to the bur equivalent to noncrosscut size and 900 was added for end cutting burs. Thus we can say that no. 58, 558 and no. 958 burs all have same dimensions of the head irrespective of their head design.

Bur Design

Bur head consists of uniformly spaced blades with concave areas in between them. These concave depressed areas are

Speed	Range (RPM)	Commonly used bur (with this speed)	Uses	Advantages	Disadvantages
Low speed	500 to 25,000	Steel burs with or without lubricant	• Polishing, finishing • Drilling holes • For implants • Excavation of caries	Good tactile sense	• Ineffective cutting • Time consuming • Operator fatigue • Produce patient discomfort
High speed	20,000 to 1,20,000	Diamond burs with lubricant	• Tooth preparations • Making small tooth preparations • Refining tooth preparations • Refining occlusions	• Fine tactile sense • Minimum overcutting	• More heat production • Not fit for larger preparations • Preparations can cause operator fatigue
Ultra high speed	2,50,000 to 4,00,000	Tungsten carbide burs with lubricant	• Tooth preparations • Removal of old restorative materials • Crown preparations for fixed prosthesis	• Ease for operator • Faster preparation takes less time • Less fatigue for patient and operator • Quadrant dentistry is possible	• Overcutting is possible • Less tactile sense • Iatrogenic errors are more common

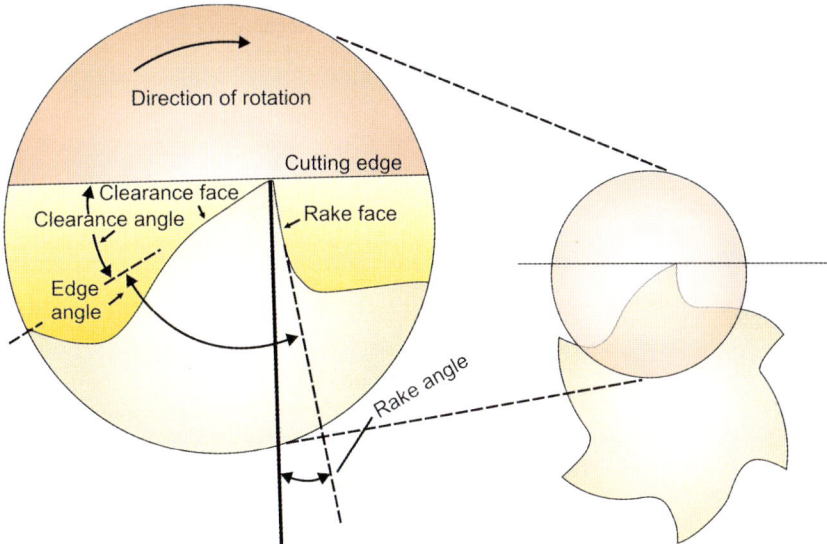

Figure 6.68: Design of bur head

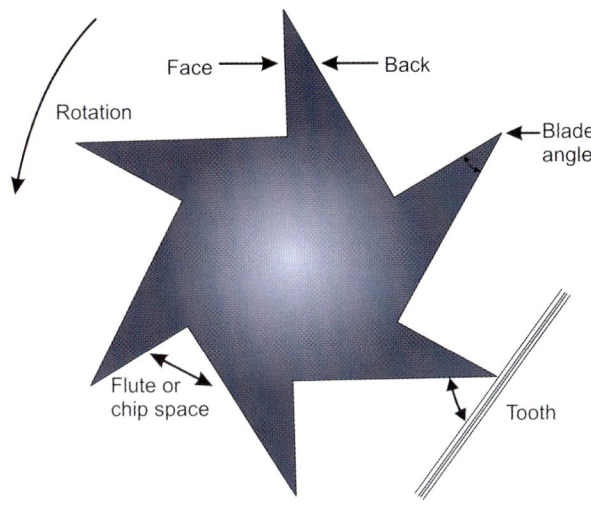

Figure 6.69: Bur blade

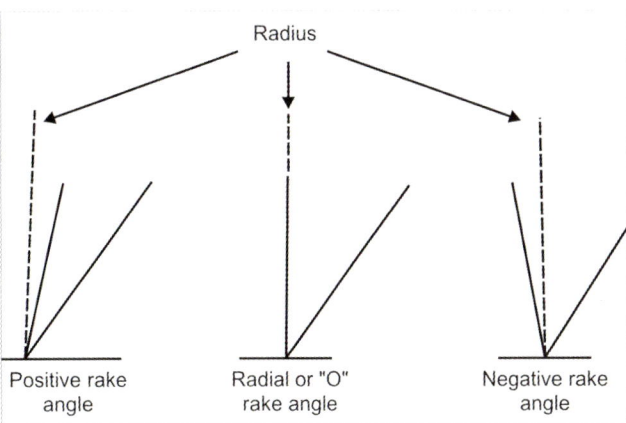

Figure 6.70: Three types of rake angles

called chip or flute spaces. Normally, a bur has 6, 8, or 10 numbers of blades (**Fig. 6.68**).

- **Bur blade (Fig. 6.69):** Blade is a projection on the bur head which forms a cutting edge. Blade has two surfaces:
  - *Blade face/Rake face:* It is the surface of bur blade on the leading edge
  - *Clearance face:* It is the surface of bur blade on the trailing edge.
- **Rake angle:** This is angle between the rake face and the radial line (**Fig. 6.70**).
  - *Positive rake angle:* When rake face trails the radial line

- *Negative rake angle:* When rake face is ahead of radial line
- *Zero rake angle:* When rake face and radial line coincide each other.
- **Radial line:** It is the line connecting center of the bur and the blade.
- **Land:** It is the plane surface immediately following the cutting edge (**Fig. 6.71**).
- **Clearance angle:** This is the angle between the clearance face and the work (**Figs 6.72 and 6.73**).
  Significance: Clearance angle provides a stop to prevent the bur edge from digging into the tooth and provides adequate chip space for clearing debris.
- **Blade angle:** It is the angle between the rake face and the clearance face.

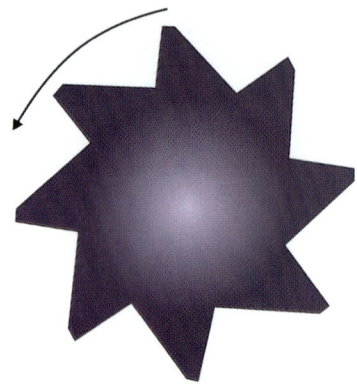

Figure 6.71: Land of bur

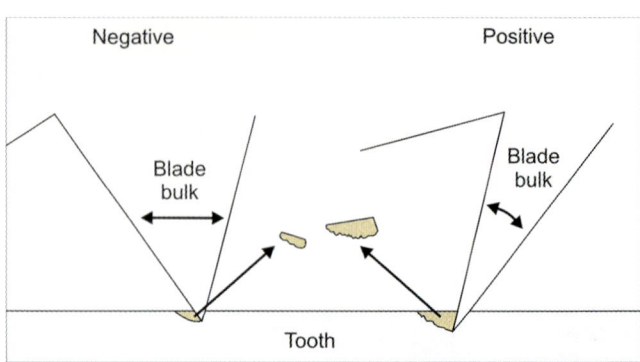

Figure 6.74: Relationship between cutting efficiency and clogging of bur space with change in rake angle

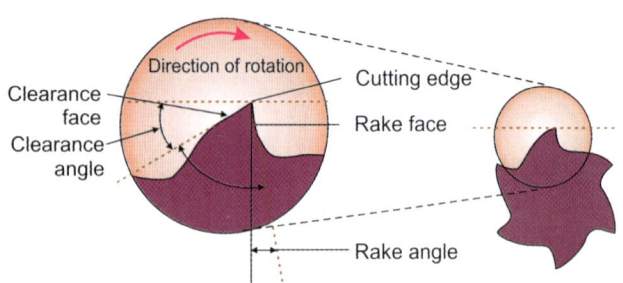

Figure 6.72: Rake angle, clearance angle and edge angle of bur

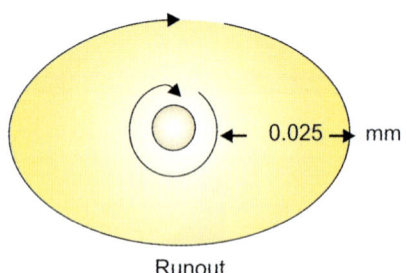

Figure 6.75: Run out

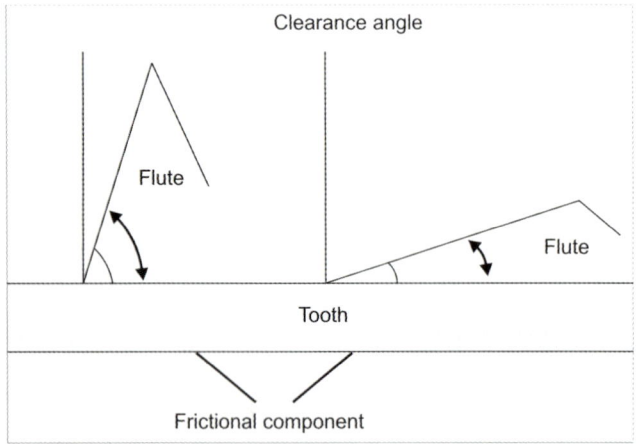

Figure 6.73: Clearance angle provides a stop to present bur edge from digging into the tooth

Significance: Among these, rake angle is one of the most important feature of bur blade design. Negative rake angle increases the life of bur by reducing fracture of cutting edges. Positive rake angle increases the cutting efficiency but since it reduces the bulk of bur blade,

it becomes prone to fracture. Positive rake angle also causes clogging of debris in the chip space (**Fig. 6.74**).

If blade angle is increased, it reinforces the cutting edge and thus reduces their fracture. But clearance angle, blade angle and rake angle cannot be varied independent of each other. For example, increase in blade angle, decreases the clearance angle. Usually, the carbide burs have negative rake angles and 90° of blade angle so as to reduce their chances of fracture. For better clearance of debris, the clearance faces of carbide burs are made curved to provide adequate flute space.

- *Concentricity:* It is a direct measurement of symmetry of the bur head. In other words, concentricity measures whether blades are of equal length or not. It is done when the bur is static.
- *Run out:* It measures the accuracy with which all the tip of blades pass through a single point when bur is moving (**Fig. 6.75**). It measures the maximum displacement of bur head from its center of rotation. In case, there is trembling of bur during rotation, this effect of run out is directly proportional to length of bur shank (**Fig. 6.76**).

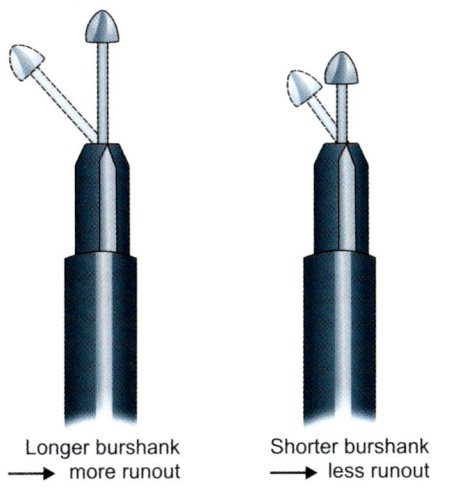

Longer burshank → more runout   Shorter burshank → less runout

Figure 6.76: Relationship between length of bur shank and run out

Run out occurs
→ Bur head is off center on axis of the bur
→ If bur neck is bent
→ If bur is not held straight in handpiece chuck.

Run out causes
→ Increase in vibration during cutting
→ Causes excessive removal of tooth structure.

Definitions related to bur design

• Rake face (Blade face)	Surface of bur blade on leading edge
• Clearance face	Surface of bur blade on trailing edge
• Rake angle	Angle between rake face and the radial line
– Positive rake angle	Rake face trails the radial line.
– Negative rake angle	Rake face ahead of the radial line.
– Zero rake angle	Rake face and radial line coincide each other

Factors Affecting Cutting Efficiency of Bur

Burs remove the tooth tissue at different rates depending upon various factors. It is always desirable to cut a large quantity of tooth in short-time. Following factors affect the cutting efficiency of a bur:

- **Clearance angle, rake angle and blade angle:** Clearance angle reduces the friction between cutting edge and the work. It also prevents the bur from digging excessively into the tooth structure. But an increase in rake angle decreases the blade angle which inturn decreases the bulk of bur blade (**see Fig. 6.74**).

  Positive rake angle increases cutting efficiency of bur, but increase in rake angle causes decrease in bulk

of bur blade and clogging of flute space because of production of larger chips.

- **End cutting or side cutting bur:** According to particular task, choice of bur can be end cutting, side cutting or combination of both. For example, it is preferred to make entry to enamel by end cutting bur, while for making preparation outline, use side cutting bur.
- **Neck diameter of bur:** If neck diameter of bur is large, it may interfere with accessibility and visibility. But if diameter is too short, it will make bur unable to resist the lateral forces.
- **Spiral angle:** Burs with smaller spiral angle have shown better efficiency at high speeds.
- **Linear surface speed:** Within the limit, faster the speed of cutting instrument, faster is the abrasive action and more efficient is the tooth cutting instrument. Bur speed should be increased in limits because with ultrahigh speed, centrifugal force comes into the play.
- **Application of load:** Load is force exerted by operator on tool head. Normally for high speed instruments, load should range between 60 and 120 gm and for low rotational speeds, it should range between 1000 and 1500 gm. Cutting efficiency decreases when load is applied. There is increase in temperature at work face which results in greater wear and tear of handpiece bearings.
- **Concentricity and runout:** The average clinically acceptable runout is 0.023 mm. Increase in runout causes increase in vibrations of the bur and excessive removal of tooth structure.
- **Lubrication:** Lubricant/coolant applied to tooth and bur during cutting increases the cutting efficiency and decreases the rise in temperature during cutting. Absence of coolant can result in increase in surface temperature which may produce deleterious effects on pulp.
- **Heat treatment of bur:** Heat treatment of bur preserves the cutting edges and increases shelf life of the bur.
- **Number of blades:** Usually a bur has 6 to 8 number of blades. Decrease in number of blades reduces the cutting efficiency but causes faster clearance of debris because of larger chip space (**Fig. 6.77**).
- **Visual contact with bur head:** For efficient tooth cutting, it is mandatory to maintain visual contact with bur head while working.
- **Design of flute ends:** There are two types of flute ends (**Figs 6.78A and B**):
  - *Star cut design:* Here the flutes come together in a common point at the axis of bur.
  - *Revelation design:* Here the flutes come together at two junctions near diametrical cutting edge. It has better efficiency in direct cutting.

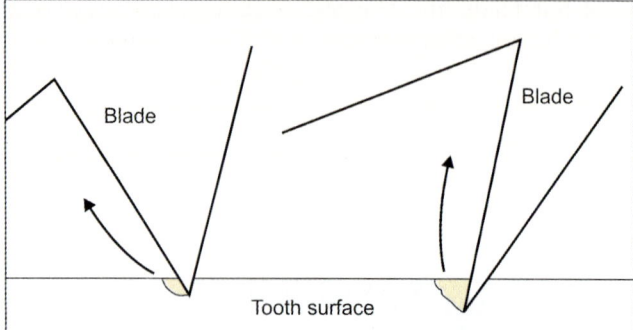

Figure 6.77: As the number of blades reduce, it results in increase in chip size and faster clearance because of larger chip space

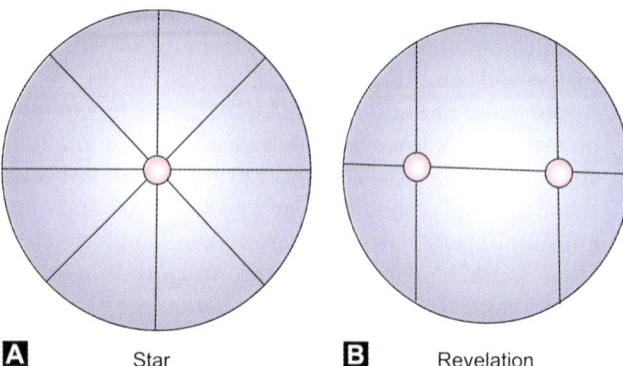

A Star **B** Revelation

Figures 6.78A and B: Flute end designs: (A) Star; (B) Revelation

RECENT ADVANCES IN ROTARY INSTRUMENTS

- Fiberoptic handpiece
- Smart prep burs
- Chemical vapors deposition (CVD) diamond burs
- Fissurotomy burs.

Fiberoptic Handpiece

Now-a-days to avoid shadow or visibility problem associated with external lightening, handpiece with a built in optics has been made available. This fiberoptic delivers a high beam of light to the handpiece head directly on working site.

Smart Prep Burs

Smart prep instrument is also known as polymer bur or smart bur.

This type of instrument is made from polymer that safely and effectively removes decayed dentin without affecting the healthy dentin.

Smart prep bur has property of self-limiting, this means it will not cut the healthy dentin. It cuts dentin only when large amount of force is applied.

Availability
- Sizes 2, 4, 6.
- Used with slow speed handpiece (500–800 rpm).
- Single patient use.

Advantages of smart prep burs
→ Used for deep caries removal in lieu of indirect capping procedure
→ Chances of iatrogenic pulp exposure are less
→ Minimum removal of tooth structure.

Disadvantages of smart prep burs
→ Technique sensitive
→ This instrument leaves large amount of decayed portion unexcavated
→ Expensive
→ Chances of damage of bur are more if it touches the enamel or sound dentin during and after the procedure.

Chemical Vapor Deposition Diamond Burs

In 1996, chemical vapor deposition (CVD) diamond burs attached to an ultrasonic handpiece were introduced to eliminate problems faced with diamond burs.

These diamond burs are obtained by chemical vapor deposition of diamond film over a molybdenum substrate.

These tips are made in a reactor in which mixture of methane and hydrogen gas results in the formation of artificial diamond layer over the molybdenum substrate.

These tips require only slight touch to promote tooth grinding.

If too much pressure and force is applied during cutting, the effects would be:
- Excessive heat generation
- Decrease in cutting efficiency
- Excessive noise production
- Pain
- Fracture of the molybdenum substrate.

Advantages of CVD burs
→ Less noise
→ Greater durability
→ Better access and visibility
→ Better cooling
→ Effective tooth preparation
→ Improved proximal access
→ Reduced risk of metal contamination
→ Preservation of tooth structure and also minimal damage to gingival tissues.

➡ Technique sensitive
➡ Very costly.

Fissurotomy Burs

- New instrument for ultraconservative dental treatment.
- As the name indicates, these are specially designed for pit and fissure lesions.
- Available in three different shapes and sizes:
  - Original fissurotomy
  - Original fissurotomy micro STF
  - Original fissurotomy micro NTF.
- Original fissurotomy and fissurotomy micro NTF has head length of 2.5 mm while fissurotomy micro STF has head length of 1.5 mm
- Fissurotomy micro STF is suitable for deciduous teeth, adult premolars, enameloplasty, etc.
- Fissurotomy bur is mainly indicated for small caries and enlarging the fissure.

Advantages of fissurotomy burs

➡ Minimum heat build up and vibration
➡ Conservation of tooth structure
➡ Increased patient comfort.

Disadvantages of fissurotomy burs

➡ Should be used with suitable restorative materials
➡ Costly.

ABRASIVE INSTRUMENTS

The head of these instruments consists of small angular particles of a hard substance held in a matrix of softer material called as the binder. Different materials used for a binder are ceramic, metal, rubber, shellac, etc.

Abrasive instruments can be divided into:
- Diamond abrasives
- Other abrasives.

Diamond Abrasive Instruments (Fig. 6.79)

They were introduced in 1942. They have greater resistance to abrasion, lower heat generation and longer life to be preferred over tungsten carbide burs. Diamond instruments consist of three parts:
1. A metal blank.
2. *Powdered diamond abrasive*: Abrasive diamond can be natural or synthetic which is crushed to a powder of desired particles.
3. *The bonding agent*: It serves the purpose of holding the abrasive particles together and binding the particles to the metal blank. Most commonly used binding agents for diamond instruments are ceramic and metal.

Classification

- Coarse grit diamonds burs (125–150 µ particle size)
- Medium grit diamond burs (88–125 µ particle size)
- Fine grit diamond burs (60–74 µ particle size)
- Very fine grit diamond burs (38–44 µ particle size).

Abrasive stones are available as mounted and unmounted. The mounted stones have abrading head which is joined to the shank and the attachment part (**Fig. 6.80**). In unmounted stones, the abrading head is supplied separately which can be attached to the mandrel when required.

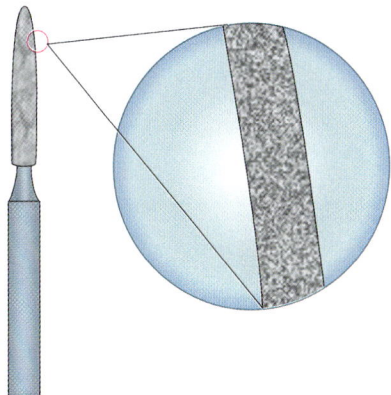

Figure 6.79: Diamond abrasive instrument

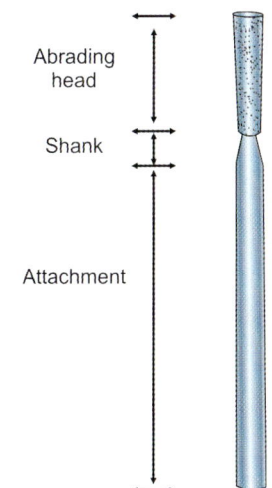

Abrading head

Shank

Attachment

Figure 6.80: Parts of diamond abrasive instrument

Factors Influencing the Abrasive Efficiency and Effectiveness

- *Size of the abrasive particles*: Abrasive nature is directly proportional to size of abrasive particle. Rapid removal of material occurs with coarse grit burs compared to medium or fine grit burs (**Fig. 6.81**).
- *Shape of the abrasive particles*: The abrasive particles with irregular shape show more efficiency because they present a sharp edge (**Fig. 6.82**).
- *Density of the abrasive particles*: Coarse grit burs have a low density compared to fine grit burs.
- *Hardness of the abrasive particle*: The hardness of the abrasive particles should be more than the hardness of the surface on which it is to be used.
- *Clogging of the abrasive surface*: Clogging of the spaces between the particles by grinding debris decreases efficiency.
- *Pressure*: Excessive pressure causes the loss of diamonds, thus, decrease their cutting efficiency.

- *Miscellaneous*: Individual dental techniques, difference in pressure, differences in handpieces, etc. also affect abrasive efficiency of instrument.

Other Abrasive Instruments

They are used for shaping, finishing and polishing restorations in the clinic and in the laboratory. They are of two types:

1. *Moulded abrasive instruments*: These have heads made by moulding mixture of abrasive and matrix around the roughened end to the shank. They are of two types:

    Soft moulded instruments use flexible materials like rubber as matrix while rigid moulded instruments use ceramic as matrix. Soft moulded instruments are used for finishing and polishing procedures while the rigid ones are used for grinding and sharpening procedures.

2. *Coated abrasive instruments*: These are mostly disks which have a thin layer of abrasive cemented to a flexible backing. They are used in the finishing of enamel walls of tooth preparations and restorations. The abrasives used here can be silicon carbide, aluminum oxide, garnet, quartz, pumice, cuttle bone, etc.

Finishing and Polishing Instruments (Fig. 6.83)

Finishing Burs

Finishing burs are usually made of stainless steel or tungsten carbide. Bur should be atleast 12 fluted (**Fig. 6.84**). The main function of finishing bur is to remove excess of restorative material rather than cutting the surface. These

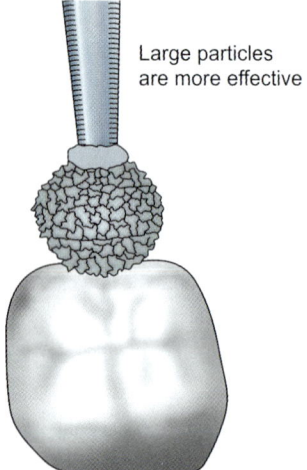

Figure 6.81: Larger particles cause deeper cutting

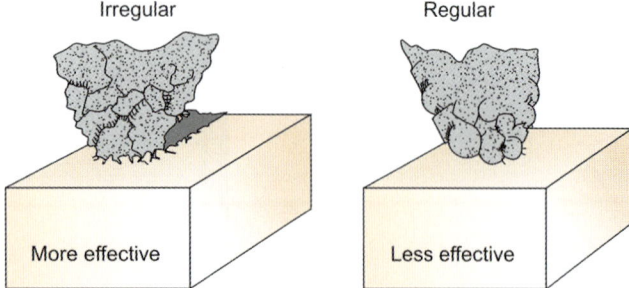

Figure 6.82: Irregular shaped particles have better abrasive efficiency

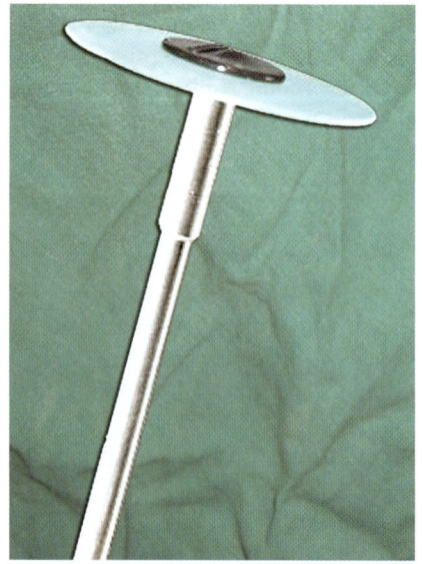

Figure 6.83: Finishing disk

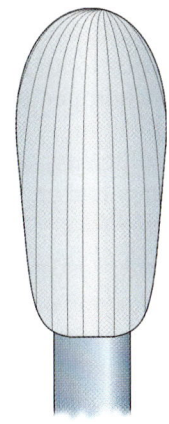

Figure 6.84: Finishing burs

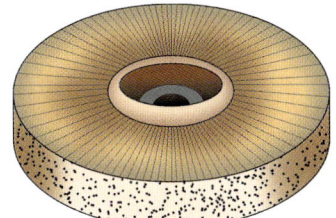

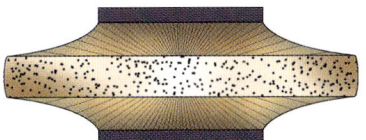

Figure 6.85: Brushes

burs also make the surface smoother. Burs are available in different shapes and sizes, i.e. tapered, inverted cone, rounded and pear-shaped, etc.

Brushes

Several types of shapes, i.e. wheels, cylinders or cones are available, which may be screwed in handpiece either attached to mandrel or having their own attachment (**Fig. 6.85**). These brushes can be used for finishing alone or with abrasive pastes. They are used in polishing cast restorations.

Diamond Instruments and Pastes

They are available in the form of abrasive rotary instruments, metal backed abrasive strips and polishing pastes. These instruments should always be used with light force and copious water spray. These are mainly used on ceramic and composite materials.

Paper-carried Abrasives

These are usually abrasives, i.e. sand, garnet or boron carbide attached to paper disks or strips (**Fig. 6.86**). These are preferably used in back and forth motion polishing (similar to shoe polishing).

Rubber Ended Rotary Tools

These type of instruments are available in variety of shapes, i.e. cups, wheels, etc. (**Fig. 6.87**). These can be attached to handpiece with the help of mandrel or with their own extension. These are used with other abrasive or polishing pastes.

Cloth

Cloth, carried on metal wheel can be used in final stages of polishing with or without polishing medium.

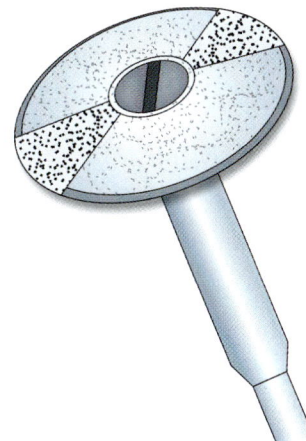

Figure 6.86: Paper disk

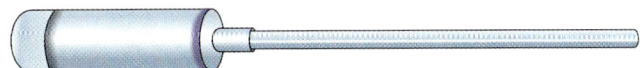

Figure 6.87: Rubber ended rotary tool

Felt

Felt is used for obtaining luster for metallic restorations with polishing agent. It is available in the different shapes such as wheel, cones and cylinders (**Fig. 6.88**).

Advantages of bur cutting
➡ Well-known procedure of tooth cutting
➡ Precision is obtained
➡ Easy to control the cutting
➡ Tactile perception during cutting
➡ Debris can be removed by water and use of suction.

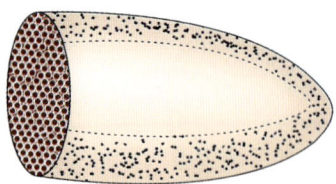 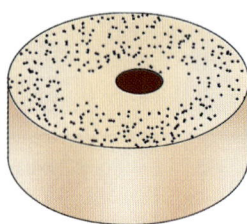

Figure 6.88: Felt

Disadvantages of bur cutting
➡ Pain occurs during cutting
➡ Vibration caused by cutting may crack or fracture tooth structure
➡ Noise production
➡ Constant use and sterilization can cause their breakage
➡ Dull burs produce excessive heat and causes pulpal damage
➡ If operator loses control or the patient moves inadvertently, chances of overcutting.

ULTRASONIC INSTRUMENTS

Ultrasound emerged for caries removal in 1950s. The ultrasonic dental unit consists of an ultrasonic generator and transducer located within the handpiece. The generator transports the energy to the transducer which causes vibrations for removal of tooth. A water cooling system is incorporated into the equipment But the conventional technology for diamond powder aggregation with nickel metallic binders cannot withstand ultrasonic power. Recently an alternative approach using chemical vapor deposition (CVD) resulted in synthetic diamond technology. CVD diamond burs are obtained with high adherence of the diamond on the metal surface with outstanding abrading ability. This technology allows diamond deposition with coalescent granulation in different formats of substrates. When connected to an ultrasonic handpiece, CVD diamond burs show following advantages while tooth preparation:

- Maximizing preservation of tooth structure
- Decreased noise
- Minimal damage to the gingival tissue
- More bur life and better proximal access
- Decreased risk of touching the adjacent tooth
- Minimal patient's risk of metal contamination.

HAZARDS AND PRECAUTIONS WITH ULTRASPEED CUTTING INSTRUMENTS

High speed rotary cutting instruments can result in many hazards, can be avoided or reduced by taking certain precautions. These are as following:

Pulpal Damage

Pulp can be injured during tooth preparation because of mechanical vibration, improper tooth preparation and heat generation during cutting. Dull burs and diamond instruments have poor efficiency and also produce more heat, further resulting in pulpal trauma.

Precautions to Avoid Pulpal Trauma

- Tooth tissue should be done only with adequate finger rests and good visibility of the operating field
- Debris clogging the burs should be cleaned before tooth preparation. Coolant should be used while using rotary instrument to control the heat rise
- For this, air-water spray should be used as it acts as a coolant, moistens the tissues, lubricates and clean the rotary cutting instruments and also cleans the operating site.

Damage to Soft Tissue

Lacerations may occur in the lips, tongue, cheeks and floor of the mouth if proper precautions are not taken.

During cutting procedures, sudden movement by the patient due to gagging, swallowing or coughing can also result in soft tissue injury.

Precautions

- Use good visibility and accessibility to the operative field
- Isolate the operating site preferably by the rubber dam
- Patient should be instructed not to make sudden movement while working
- All the burs and rotary instruments should be perfectly centric. Even a slightly eccentric bur can damage the surrounding dental tissues.

Damage to Ear

When compared to conventional rotary instruments, air turbine handpiece produce high noise level and frequency of vibration (ranges from 75–100 decibels with the frequency more than 2000 cycles per second). But when noise level reaches 85 decibels with frequency ranging more than 5000 cycles per second, it is always preferred to practice protective measures. These are:

- Sound proofing of the room with sound absorbing materials
- Use of ear plugs
- Lubrication of ball bearings so as not to further increase the noise level.

Inhalation Problems

As we know, aerosols and vapors are produced during cutting of tooth structure and restorative materials by rotary instruments. Aerosols are fine dispersions in air consisting of water, cutting debris, microorganisms and restorative materials. While removal of amalgam restoration, mercury vapors are released and while polishing, composite restoration monomers are released. These aerosols can be inadvertently inhaled by the patient or dentist resulting in alveolar (lung) irritation, tissue reactions or may transfer infectious diseases. Their inhalation can be prevented by the use of rubber dam, use of disposable masks and eye wear, etc.

Eye Injuries

When tooth tissue, calculus or any old restorations are removed at high speeds, injury to eyes can occur because of flying particles, microorganisms and other debris. These can be avoided by using protective glasses worn by the patient and the dental personnel. Also plastic shields or protective eyeglasses should be used while using laser equipment or light curing machine.

USE OF LASER

Laser is an acronym for "light amplification by stimulated emission of radiation." Laser produces beams of coherent and very high intensity light. The common principles on which all lasers work is the generation of monochromatic, coherent and collimated radiation by a suitable laser medium in an optical resonator (**Fig. 6.89**).

Common principles of laser
➡ Monochromatic
➡ Coherence
➡ Collimation.

Monochromatic means that the light produced by a particular laser will be of a characteristic wavelength. If the light produced is in the visible spectrum (400–750 nm), it will be seen as a beam of intense color. It is important to have this property to attain high spectral power density of the laser.

Coherence means that the light is all perfectly in phase as they leave the laser. That means that unlike a normal light source, their individual contributions are summated and reinforce each other. In an ordinary light source, much of the energy is lost as out of phase waves cancel each other.

Collimation means that the laser light beam is perfectly parallel when leaving the laser aperture (**Fig. 6.90**). This property is important for good transmission through delivery systems.

Laser systems are capable of modifying hard dental tissues by recrystallization and vaporization. The effects of

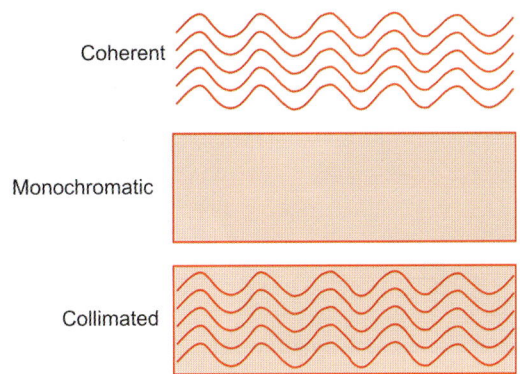

Figure 6.89: Light produced by a laser should be coherent, monochromatic and collimated in nature

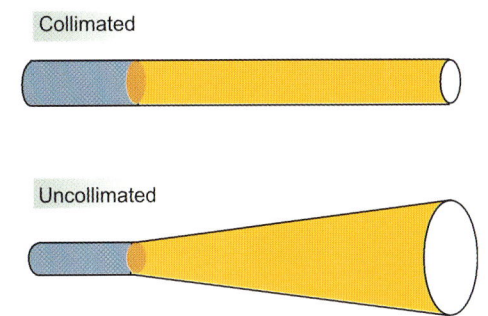

Figure 6.90: Collimation means a laser light beam is perfectly parallel when leaves the laser aperture

laser beam are controlled by its power and the extent of its absorption. Many studies have shown that current laser systems such as Erbium:YAG, Holmium:YAG, Nd:YAG and excimer have the potential to replace the dental drill for a number of uses (**Fig. 6.91**).

Light Absorption and Emission

When light encounters matter, it can be deflected, reflected, scattered or absorbed (**Fig. 6.92**). If a photon is absorbed, its energy is not destroyed, but rather used to increase the energy level of the absorbing atom. The photon then ceases to exist and an electron within the atom jumps to a higher energy level. This atom is thus pumped up to an excited state from the resting ground state. In the excited state, the atom is unstable and will soon spontaneously decay back to the ground state, releasing stored energy in the form of an emitted photon. This process is called spontaneous emission. The spontaneously emitted photon has a longer wavelength and less energy than the absorbed photon. The difference in the energy is usually turned into heat.

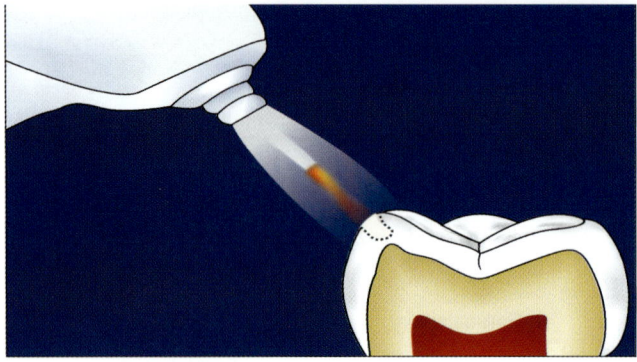

Figure 6.91: Laser used for tooth preparation

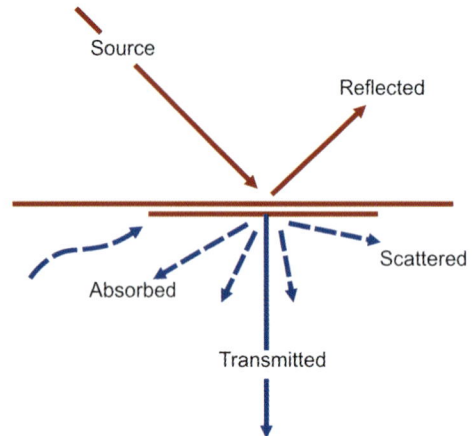

Figure 6.92: When light encounters matter it can be reflected, scattered, transmitted or absorbed

Tissue Effects of Laser Irradiation

The biological interaction of laser photon with tissue occurring along the path of radiation is termed a linear effect and can be categorized broadly into photochemical, photothermal and photomechanical. The ability of the laser photon to produce a biological response after being reflected, deflected, scattered or absorbed is termed non-linear effects.

- Photochemical interaction
  - Biostimulation
  - Photodynamic therapy.
- Photothermal interaction
  - Photoablation
  - Photopyrolysis.
- Photomechanical interaction
  - Photodisruption/photodissociation
  - Photoacoustic interactions.
- Photoelectrical interaction
  - Photoplasmolysis.

Photochemical Effects

The basis of the photochemical effect is the absorption of the laser light without any thermal effect leading to change in the chemical and physical properties of atoms and molecules.

A specific wavelength or photon can be absorbed by a molecular chromophore and convert that molecule to an excited state, thus converting laser energy into stored form of chemical energy. The excited state can subsequently participate in a chemical reaction.

Biostimulation

It is the stimulatory effect of lasers on biochemical and molecular processes that normally occur in the tissues such as healing and repair.

Photothermal Interaction

This class of interaction is the basis for the most types of surgical laser applications. In this interaction, radiant light energy absorbed by tissue substances and molecules become transformed into heat energy which produces the tissue effect. High water content of most oral tissue is responsible for absorption of radiant energy in the target region. This high absorption leads to rapid vaporization of the water component and pyrolysis of the organic matter within the tissue target.

Another important factor, influencing the extent of the thermal damage zone is the relative degree of absorption and scattering of the beam once it enters the tissue. Scattering can directly increase the extent of collateral tissue damage by spatial redistribution of the beam into a larger volume of the surrounding tissue. Much of the scattered beam is transformed into heat energy since it has insufficient power density to cause vaporization.

Thermal effects of laser irradiation range in intensity depending on the level of temperature rise within the target tissue.

Thermal Effects of Laser Irradiation

- Temperature < 60°C
  - Tissue hyperthermia
  - Enzymatic changes
  - Edema.
- Temperature > 60°C
  - Protein denaturation.
- Temperature < 100°C
  - Tissue dehydration
  - Blanching of tissue.
- Temperature > 100°C
  - Superheating
  - Tissue ablation and shrinkage.

Photomechanical and Photoelectrical Interaction

The high energy levels and rapid absorption that occurs during photoablation results in rapid generation of shockwaves that is capable of rupturing intermolecular and atomic bonds. Mechanical disruption or breaking a part of matter is accomplished by conversion of high energy/light energy to vibrational energy.

Photodisruption occurs whenever the photon energy of the incident beam exceeds target tissues.

Laser Effects on Dental Hard Tissues

In the field of mineralized tissues the most thoroughly investigated interactions are photothermal and thermomechanical interactions and the ablative photodecomposition.

The absorption and transmission of laser light in human teeth is mainly dependent on the wavelength of the laser light. The theory that dentinal tubules work as optical fibers transmitting high energy densities to pulpal tissues could explain the unpredictable side effects when lasing dental tissues. The absorption of the laser energy in the superficial tissue layer can alter the optical properties of the affected tissue causing a variation in the intensity of the penetration energy. Therefore laser effects are changing in dependence from the depth of penetration.

Precautions to be Taken While Using Lasers

The surgical lasers currently used in dentistry generally fall in class IV category which is considered the most hazardous group of lasers. The types of hazards that may be encountered within the clinical practice of dentistry may be grouped:

- Ocular injury
- Tissue damage
- Respiratory hazards
- Fire and explosion
- Electrical shock.
- *Ocular hazards*: Injury to the eye can occur either by direct emission from the laser or by reflection from a mirror like surface. Dental instruments have been capable of producing reflections that may result in tissue damage in both operator and patients.
- *Tissue hazards*: Laser induced damage to skin and other nontarget tissue can result from the thermal interaction of the energy with the tissue proteins. Temperature elevations of 21°C above normal body temperature can produce destruction by denaturation of cellular enzymes and structural proteins which interrupt basic metabolic processes.
- *Environmental hazards*: These secondary hazards belong to a group of potential laser hazards referred to as nonbeam hazards. Most surgical lasers used in dentistry are capable of producing smoke, toxic gases and chemicals.

- *Combustion hazards*: Flammable solids, liquids, gases used within the surgical setting can be easily ignited if exposed to the laser beam.
- *Electrical hazards*: Because class IV surgical lasers often use very high currents and high voltage power supplies, there are several associated hazards that may be potentially lethal. Electrical hazards can be in form of electric shock, fire or explosion.

Personal Protective Equipment

Eye protection: Light produced by all class IV lasers by definition presents a potential hazards for ocular damage by either direct viewing or reflection of the beam. Therefore all people must wear adequate eye protection, including the patient.

Control of air borne contamination: Airborne contamination must be controlled by ventilation, evacuation or other method of respiratory protection. Adequate suction should be maintained at all times especially when treating a pathologic condition as it can spread through laser plume.

Procedural controls:

- Highly reflective instruments and those with mirror surfaces should be avoided
- Tooth protection is needed, whenever, the beam is directed at angles other than parallel to the tooth surface
- A No.7 wax spatula can be inserted into the gingival sulcus to serve as an effective shield for the teeth
- If anesthesia is required in place of standard PVC tubes, rubber or silastic tubes should be used. For further protection the tube should be wrapped with an aluminum tape.

Fire and electrical control measures: To avoid an electrical hazard, the operatory must be kept dry. The control panel and its electrical power unit should be protected from any kind of splashing.

 Key Points

- Dr GV Black gave a way to describe instruments for their easier identification in form of order (function), suborder (position of use), class (design of the working end) and subclass (shape).
- The angulation of instrument is provided for access and stability. Closer the working point to the long axis of the handle, better will be the control on it. For better control, the working point should be preferably within 3 mm of the center of the long axis of the handle.
- GV Black established an instrument formula for describing dimensions of blade, nib or head of instrument and angles present in shank of the instrument.

- The first number of the formula indicates width of the blade or primary cutting edge in tenths of a millimeter.
- The second number represents the angle formed by the primary cutting edge and long axis of the instrument handle in clockwise centigrade.
- The third number represents the length of the blade in millimeters, that is, from the shank to the cutting edge.
- The fourth number represents the angle which the blade forms with long axis of the handle or the plane of the instrument in clockwise centigrade.
- Single bevel instruments have single bevel that forms the primary cutting edge. These can be right or left bevel and mesial or distal bevel instruments.
- Bibeveled instrument has two additional cutting edges which extend from the primary cutting edge.
- In triple-bevelled instrument, three additional cutting edges extend from the primary cutting edge.
- Shepherd's Crook or curved explore has semilunar-shaped working tip perpendicular to the handle. This is used for examining occlusal surfaces.
- In straight chisel, the cutting edge of the chisel makes a 90° angle to the plane of the instrument. It is used for gingival restoration of the anterior teeth.
- In angled chisel, the primary cutting edge is in a plane perpendicular to the long axis of the shaft and may have either a mesial or distal bevel. It is used with a push or pull motion for anterior proximal restorations, smoothening proximal walls and gingival walls for full coverage restorations.
- Dental hoe resembles a miniature garden hoe. Basically, hoe is any instrument in which the blade makes more than a 12.5° angle with the plane of the instrument. Hoe is used in pull motion used to smoothen the floor and form line angles in class III and V restorations.
- Angle former is a type of excavator which is monangled with the cutting edge sharpened at an angle to the long axis of the blade. Angle of cutting edge to blade axis lies between 80 to 85 centigrades. It is used with a push or pull motion for accentuating line and point angles, to establish retention form in direct filling gold restoration.
- Cleiod-discoid are modified chisels with claw and disk like cutting edges. These are used for removing caries and carving amalgam or wax patterns.
- Any instrument where the cutting edge is parallel or almost parallel to the plane of the instrument is called a hatchet. Basically, a hatchet is the similar to as an axe except that it is much smaller.
- Spoon excavator is a modified hatchet. It is a double-ended instrument with a spoon, claw, or disk-shaped blade. Spoon excavator is used to remove caries and debris in the scooping motion.

- Gingival margin trimmer (GMT) is a modified hatchet which has working ends with opposite curvatures and bevels. Distal gingival margin trimmer is used for the distal surface and the mesial GMT is used for the mesial surface. If the second number in instrument formula is 75 to 85, it is mesial GMT and if second number is 95 to 100, it is distal GMT. GMT is used for planing of the gingival cavosurface margin and to bevel axiopulpal line angle in the class II tooth preparation.
- Composite resin instruments are made of plastic or titanium coating. These instruments do not stick and discolor the composite restoration.
- First "dental engine" was developed in 1871 by Dr James B Morrison. It was adapted from sewing machine concept.
- "Bur is a rotary cutting instrument which has bladed cutting head".
- William and Schroeder first made diamond dental bur in 1897, modern diamond bur was introduced in 1932 by WH Drendel by bonding diamond points to stainless steel shanks.
- Diamonds have good cutting efficiency in removing enamel (brittle) while carbide burs cut dentin (elastic material) with maximum efficiency.
- Bur head consists of uniformly spaced blades with concave areas in between them. These concave depressed areas are called chip or flute spaces. Normally, a bur has 6, 8, or 10 numbers of blades.
- Rake angle is angle between the rake face and the radial line.
- *Clearance angle:* This is the angle between the clearance face and the work. It provides a stop to prevent the bur edge from digging into the tooth and provides adequate chip space for clearing debris.
- Concentricity is a direct measurement of symmetry of the bur head.
- Run out measures the accuracy with which all the tip of blades pass through a single point when bur is moving. It measures the maximum displacement of bur head from its center of rotation.
- *Number of blades:* Usually a bur has 6 to 8 number of blades. Decrease in number of blades reduces the cutting efficiency but causes faster clearance of debris because of larger chip space.
- Smart prep instrument (polymer bur or smart bur) is made from polymer that safely and effectively remove decayed dentin without affecting the healthy dentin. Smart prep bur has property of self-limiting, this means it will not cut the healthy dentin.
- Chemical vapor deposition (CVD) diamond burs are obtained with high adherence of the diamond on the

metal surface with outstanding abrading ability. This technology allows diamond deposition with coalescent granulation in different formats of substrates. When connected to an ultrasonic handpiece, CVD diamond burs show minimal damage to tooth structure and gingival tissue, minimal noise and decreased risk of touching the adjacent tooth.

- Laser is an acronym for "light amplification by stimulated emission of radiation." Laser produces beams of coherent and very high intensity light.
- The common principles on which all lasers work is the generation of monochromatic, coherent and collimated radiation by a suitable laser medium in an optical resonator.
- Monochromatic means that the light produced by a particular laser will be of a characteristic wavelength. If the light produced is in the visible spectrum (400–750 nm), it will be seen as a beam of intense color.
- Coherence means that the light is all perfectly in phase as they leave the laser. That means that unlike a normal light source, their individual contributions are summated and reinforce each other.
- Collimation means that the laser light beam is perfectly parallel when leaving the laser aperture. This property is important for good transmission through delivery systems.

QUESTIONS

1. Classify hand instruments and its parts.
2. Explain different instrument groups.
3. Classify burs. Explain in detail bur design
4. Enumerate various factors affecting efficiency of bur cutting.
5. Short note:
   a. Instrument formula
   b. GMT (Gingival marginal trimmer)
   c. Sharpening of hand instruments
   d. Hand cutting instruments
   e. Bur design.
6. Write short note on instrument formula for hand cutting instruments.
7. Short notes on:
   a. Use of high speed in dentistry
   b. Abrasives and burs used in operative dentistry.
8. Discuss recent advances in rotary instruments.

BIBLIOGRAPHY

1. Atkinson DR, et al. The effect of an air-powder abrasive system on *in vitro* root surfaces. J Periodontol. 1984;55:13-8.
2. Boyde A. Airpolishing effects on enamel, dentin and cement. Br Dent J. 1984;156:287-91.
3. Chrinstensen GJ. Air abrasion tooth cutting. State of the art. JADA. 1998;129:484.
4. Coluzzi DJ. Fundaments of lasers in dental science. Dent Clin North Am. 2004;48:751-70.
5. Dahlin T. Efficient and high quality cavity preparation. Quint Int. 1982;5:20.
6. Eames WB, et al. Cutting efficiency of diamond stones: effect of technique variables. Oper Dent. 1977;2:156-64.
7. Eames WB, Nale JL. A comparison of cutting efficiency of air-driven fissure burs. J Am Dent Assoc. 1973;86:412.
8. Eames WB, Nale JL. A comparison of cutting efficiency of air-driven fissure burs. J Am Dent Assoc. 1973;86:412-5.
9. Eames WB, Reder BS, Smith GA. Cutting efficiency of diamond stones. Effect of technique variables. Oper Dent. 1977;2:156.
10. Frentzen M, et al. Excimer lasers in dentistry: future possibilities with advanced technology, Quintessence Int. 1992;23:117-33.
11. Grajower R, Zeitchick A, Rajstein J. The grinding efficiency of diamond burs. J Prosth Dent. 1979;42:422.
12. Hartley JL, et al. Cutting characteristics of dental burs as shown by high speed photomicrography. Armed Forces Med J. 1957;8:209.
13. Hartley JL, Hudson DC. Modern rotating instruments: burs and diamond points. Dent Clin North Am. 1958.p.737.
14. Henry EE, Peyton FA. The relationship between design and cutting efficiency of dental burs. J Dent Res. 1954;33:281-92.
15. Henry EE. Influences of design factors on performance of the inverted cone bur. J Dent Res. 1956;35:704-13.
16. Leonard DL, Charlton DG. Performance of high-speed dental handpieces. J Am Dent Assoc. 1999;130:1301-11.
17. Merritt R. Low-energy lasers in dentistry. Br Dent J. 1992;172:90.
18. Morrant GA. Burs and rotary instruments introduction of a new standard numbering system. Br Dent J. 1979;147:97-8.
19. Myers GE. The Air abrasive technique: A report BDJ. 1954;46:241.
20. Myers TD. Lasers in dentistry. J Am Dent Assoc. 1991;122:46-50.
21. Nelson RJ, et al. Hydraulic turbine contra-angle hand-piece. J Am Dent Assoc. 1953;47:324-9.
22. Peyton FA. Effectiveness of water coolants with rotary cutting instruments. J Am Dent Assoc. 1958;56:664-75.
23. Peyton FA. Temperature rise in teeth developed by rotating instruments. J Am Dent Assoc. 1955;50:629-30.
24. Sockwell CL. Dental handpieces and rotary cutting instruments. Dent Clin North Am. 1971;15:219-44.
25. Sockwell CL. Dental handpieces and rotary cutting instruments. Dent Clin North Am. 1971;15:219.
26. Taylor DF, et al. Characteristics of some air turbine handpieces. J Am Dent Assoc. 1962;64:794-805.
27. Westland IN. The energy requirement of the dental cutting process. J Oral Rehabil. 1980;7:51.

Principles of Tooth Preparation

7

CHAPTER

Chapter Outline

INTRODUCTION

Operative dentistry requires essential knowledge of basic tooth preparation, which is important to the dental practitioner. The most important fundamental procedure of operative dentistry is tooth preparation to receive a restoration so that it can fulfill all its requirements. Therefore, it is a must for every operative clinician to be well aware of all the fundamentals of the tooth preparation. A cavity is a defect in the mineralized dental tissues which results from pathological processes like caries, attrition, abrasion and erosion.

The tooth preparation includes all mechanical procedures performed to remove all infected and affected tissues and to give proper design to the remaining hard dental tissues, so that a mechanically and biologically sound restoration can stay in the prepared tooth. Tooth preparation is a surgical procedure that removes the caries till the sound tooth tissue of proper shape is reached which will retain a restorative material that resists masticatory forces, maintains form function and esthetics.

PURPOSE OF TOOTH PREPARATION

Restoration is usually required to repair a diseased, injured or defective tooth structure. The restoration helps in maintaining proper form, function and esthetics.

Preventing and treating caries

➡ Dental caries is one of the most common disease affecting approximately 80 percent of the population in developed countries (**Fig. 7.1**)
➡ The aim of prevention and treatment is to maintain a functioning set of teeth. Interventions can halt and even reverse the development of caries.

Replacing Restorations

Restorations may fail due to a number of 'objective' factors which further depend upon characteristics of the restorative material, operator skill and technique, patients' dental characteristics, and the environment around the tooth.

The decision to replace a restoration is affected by factors such as condition of restoration, health of the tooth, and the criteria used to define failure and patient demand (**Fig. 7.2**).

Treatment of Malformed, Fractured and Traumatized Teeth (Fig.7.3)

Restorations are needed to treat malformed, fractured or traumatized teeth so as to retain them to normal form and function.

Esthetic Improvement (Fig. 7.4)

Teeth which are unesthetic and discolored can be treated by esthetic restorations.

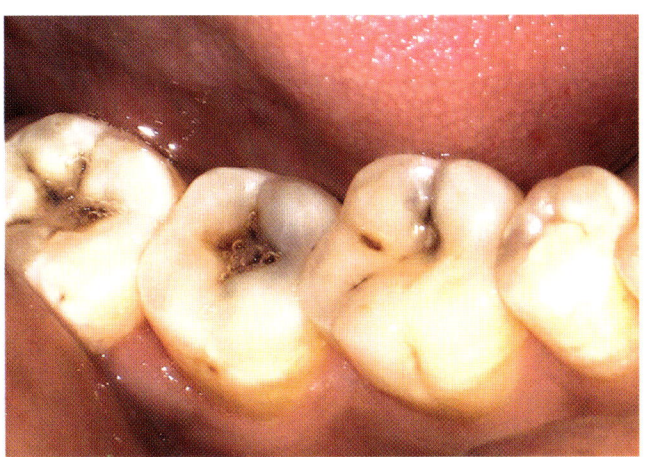

Figure 7.1: Photograph showing carious tooth which needs restoration

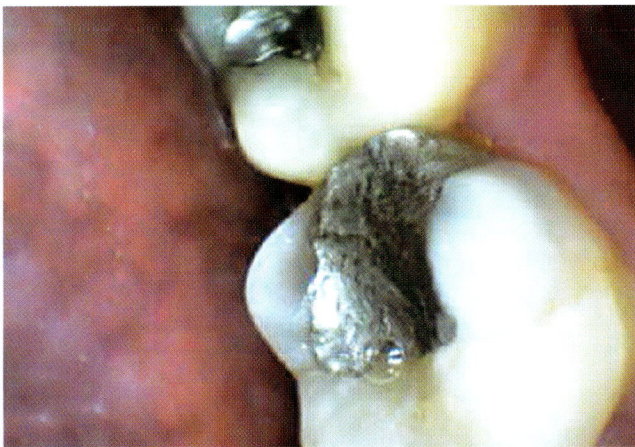

Figure 7.2: Photograph showing an old restoration needing replacement

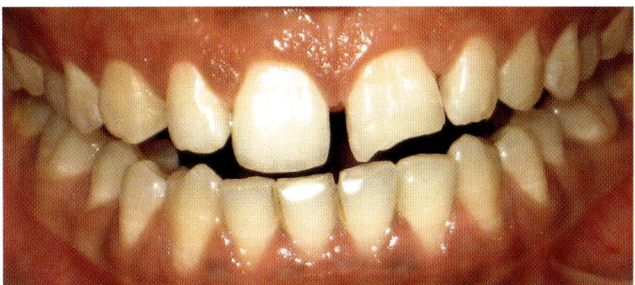

Figure 7.3: Fractured 21 needs restoration

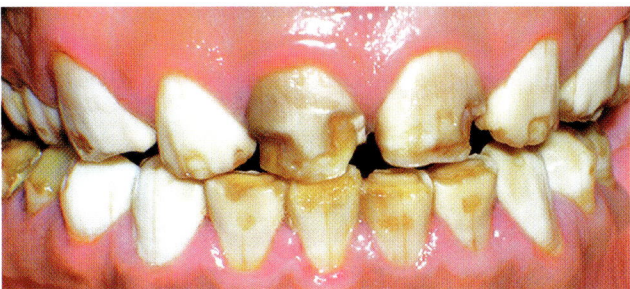

Figure 7.4: Unesthetic teeth require tooth preparation and restoration

Restoration of Tooth Material Loss (Fig. 7.5)

Attrition, abrasion or erosion of teeth can be treated by different restorative materials depending upon the extent and location of the lesion.

TYPES OF RESTORATION (FIGS 7.6A AND B)

Tooth restoration may be classified as intracoronal, when it is placed within a preparation made in the crown of a tooth or extracoronal, when it is placed outside the tooth as in the case of a crown. Intracoronal restoration is placed directly into the tooth preparation while extracoronal restoration uses an indirect technique.

The materials used to restore teeth are: dental amalgam, composite resin, glass ionomer cement, resin-modified glass ionomer cement, compomer and cermet, cast gold and other alloys, and porcelain.

Factors to be considered before restoration of a tooth
Tooth factors
➡ Primary or permanent
➡ Occlusal stresses
➡ Quality of tooth (hypoplasia)
➡ Location of tooth
➡ Type of tooth
➡ Type of tooth preparation.

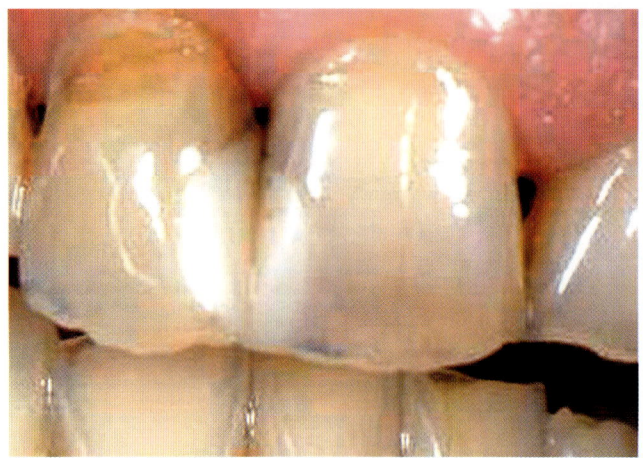

Figure 7.5: Abrasion of tooth requiring restoration

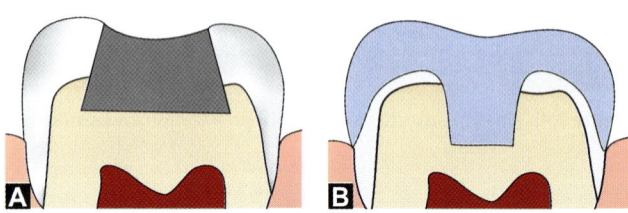

Figures 7.6A and B: (A) Intracoronal amalgam restoration; (B) Extracoronal restoration

General patient factors
- Patient's exposure to fluoride
- Age
- Xerostomia
- Socioeconomic status
- Diet
- Caries status
- General health
- Presence of any parafunctional habit.

Factors related to clinician and the restoration to be used
- Type of restoration
- Physical properties of the restoration
- Whether moisture control can be achieved or not
- Technical expertise.

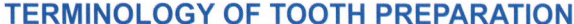

TERMINOLOGY OF TOOTH PREPARATION

Tooth Preparation

It is the mechanical alteration of a defective, injured or diseased tooth in order to best receive a restorative material which will re-establish the healthy state of the tooth including esthetics correction when indicated along with normal form and function (**Fig. 7.7**).

Simple, Compound and Complex Tooth Preparation

Simple Tooth Preparation

A tooth preparation involving only one tooth surface is termed simple preparation (**Fig. 7.8**) for example occlusal preparation.

Compound Tooth Preparation

A tooth preparation involving two surfaces is termed compound tooth preparation (**Fig. 7.9**) for example mesio-occlusal or disto-occlusal preparation.

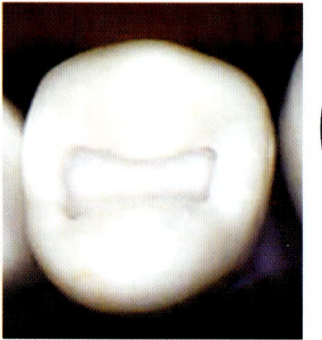

Figure 7.7: Photograph showing tooth preparation on molar

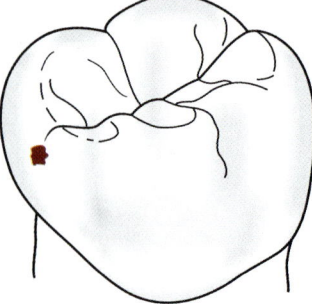

Figure 7.8: Simple tooth preparation involving one tooth surface only

Complex Tooth Preparation

A tooth preparation involving more than two surfaces is called as complex tooth preparation (**Fig. 7.10**) for example MOD preparation.

Tooth Preparation Walls

Internal Wall

It is a wall in the preparation, which is not extended to the external tooth surface (**Fig. 7.11**).

External Wall

An external wall is a wall in the prepared tooth that extends to the external tooth surface (**Fig. 7.12**). External wall takes the name of the tooth surface towards which it is situated.

Pulpal Wall

A pulpal wall is an internal wall that is towards the pulp and covering the pulp (**Fig. 7.13**). It may be both vertical and perpendicular to the long axis of tooth.

Axial Wall

It is an internal wall which is parallel to the long axis of the tooth (**Fig. 7.14**).

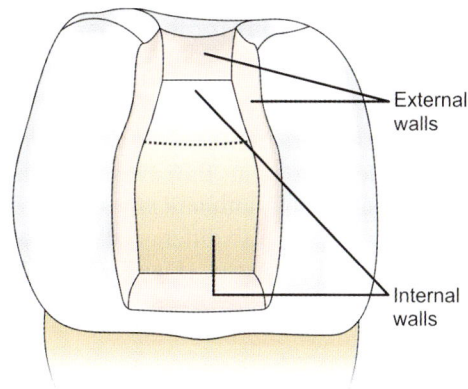

Figure 7.11: Internal and external wall of tooth preparation

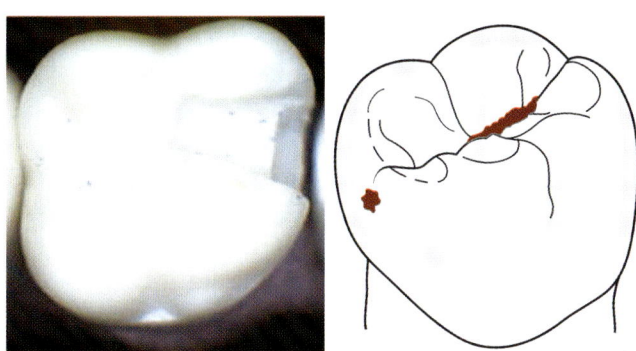

Figure 7.9: Compound tooth preparation involving two surfaces

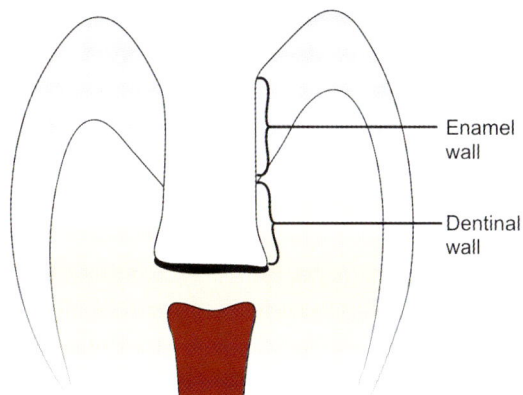

Figure 7.12: External wall of tooth preparation

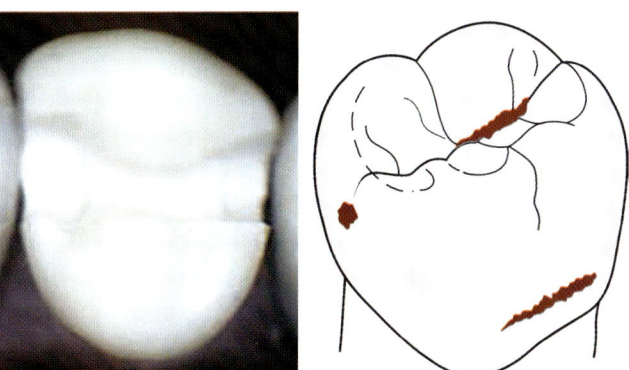

Figure 7.10: Complex tooth preparation involving more than two surfaces

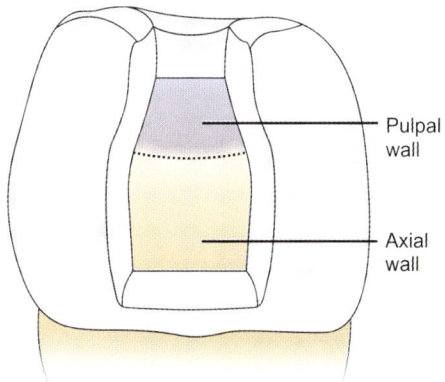

Figure 7.13: Pulpal wall

Floor

Floor is a prepared wall which is usually flat and perpendicular to the occlusal forces directed occlusogingivally, for example, pulpal and gingival walls (**Fig. 7.15**).

Cavosurface Angle Margin/Tooth Preparation Margin

Cavosurface angle is formed by the junction of a prepared tooth surface wall and external surface of the tooth (**Fig. 7.16**). The acute junction is referred to as preparation margin or cavosurface margin. The cavosurface angle may differ with the location of tooth and enamel rod direction of the prepared walls and also differ according to the type of restorative material to be used (**Figs 7.17 and 7.18**).

Line Angle

It is a junction of two surfaces of different orientations along the line and its name is derived from the involved surfaces.

Point Angle

It is a junction of three plane surfaces or three line angles of different orientation and its name is derived from its involved surfaces or line angles.

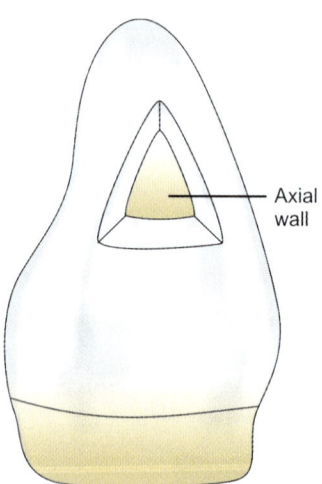

Figure 7.14: Axial wall

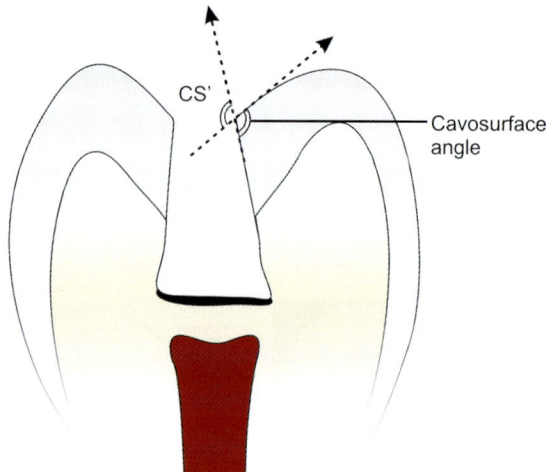

Figure 7.16: Cavosurface angle

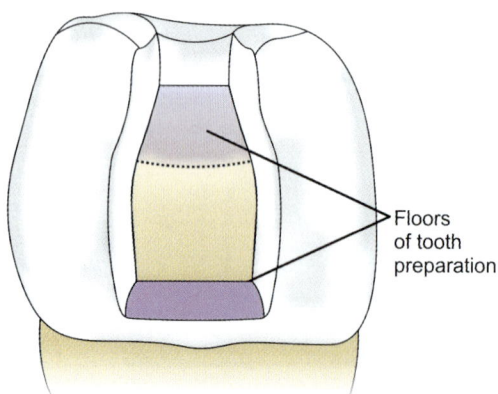

Figure 7.15: Pulpal and gingival floors of a class V tooth preparation

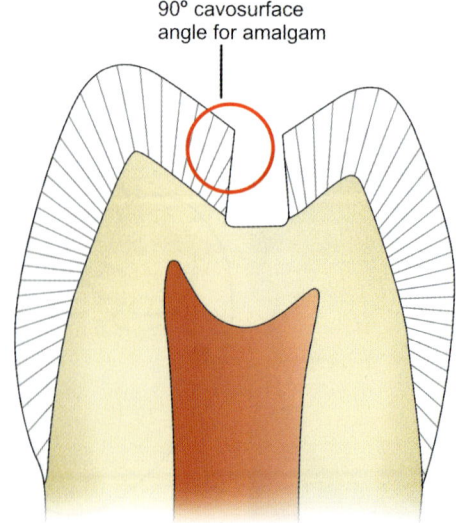

Figure 7.17: Butt joint cavosurface margin for amalgam

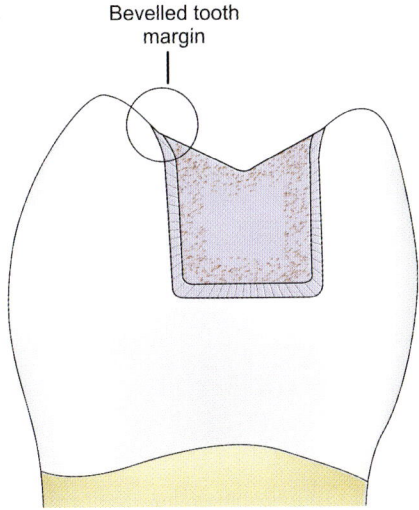

Figure 7.18: Beveled cavosurface margin for cast gold restoration

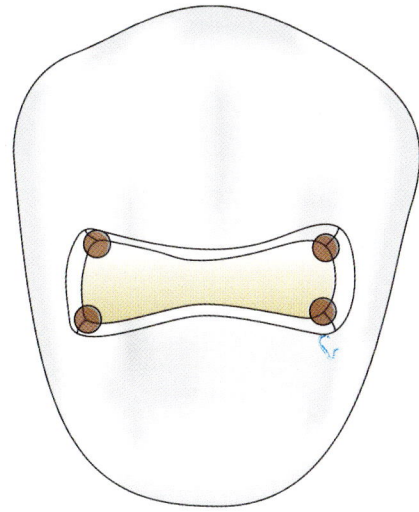

Figure 7.19: Class I tooth preparation showing line angle and point angles

NUMBER OF LINE ANGLES AND POINT ANGLES IN DIFFERENT TOOTH PREPARATION DESIGNS

The line angles and point angles of different tooth preparation designs are as follows:

Number of line angles and point angles in different tooth preparation designs

Type of tooth preparation	Line angles	Point angles
Class I	8	4
Class II	11	6
Class III	6	3
Class IV	11	6
Class V	8	4

Class I Tooth Preparation

For simple class I tooth preparation involving only occlusal surface of molars eight line angles and four point angles are named as follows (**Fig. 7.19**).

Line Angles

- Mesiobuccal line angle
- Mesiolingual line angle
- Distobuccal line angle
- Distolingual line angle
- Faciopulpal line angle
- Linguopulpal line angle
- Mesiopulpal line angle
- Distopulpal line angle.

Point Angles

- Mesiobuccopulpal point angle
- Mesiolinguopulpal point angle
- Distobuccopulpal point angle
- Distolinguopulpal point angle.

Class II Tooth Preparation

For class II preparation (mesio-occlusal or disto-occlusal) 11 line angles and 6 point angles are as follows (**Fig. 7.20**). The following is the nomenclature for mesio-occlusal tooth preparation.

Line Angles

- Distofacial
- Faciopulpal
- Axiofacial
- Faciogingival
- Axiogingival
- Linguogingival
- Axiolingual
- Axiopulpal
- Distolingual
- Distopulpal
- Linguopulpal.

Point Angles

- Distofaciopulpal point angle
- Axiofaciopulpal point angle
- Axiofaciogingival point angle
- Axiolinguogingival point angle

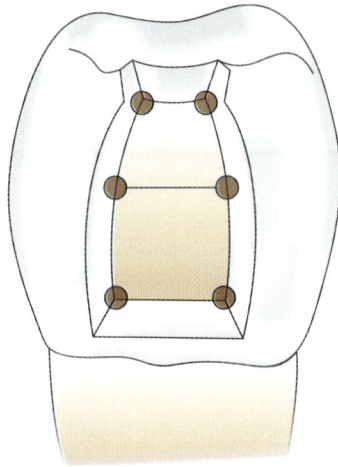

Figure 7.20: Class II tooth preparation showing line and point angles

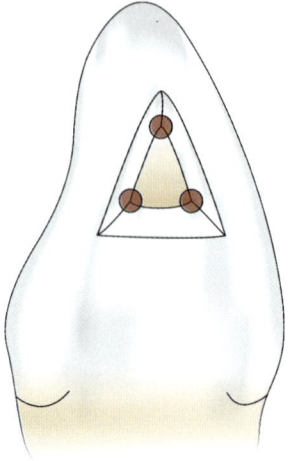

Figure 7.21: Class III preparation showing line and point angles

- Axiolinguopulpal point angle
- Distolinguopulpal point angle.

Class III Tooth Preparation

For class III preparation on anterior teeth 6 line angles and 3 point angles are as follows (**Fig. 7.21**).

Line Angles

- Faciogingival
- Linguogingival
- Axiogingival
- Axiolingual
- Axioincisal
- Axiofacial.

Point Angles

- Axiofaciogingival point angle
- Axiolinguogingival point angle
- Axioincisal point angle.

Class IV Tooth Preparation

For class IV tooth preparation on anterior teeth, 11 line angles and 6 point angles are as follows (**Fig. 7.22**).

Line Angles

- Faciogingival
- Linguogingival
- Mesiofacial
- Mesiolingual
- Mesiopulpal

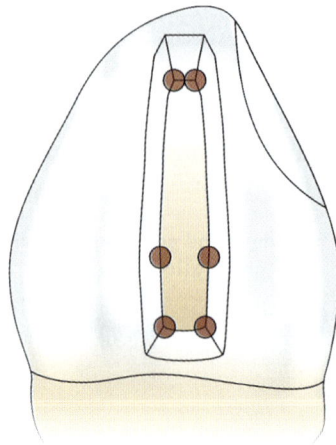

Figure 7.22: Class IV preparation showing line and point angles

- Faciopulpal
- Linguopulpal
- Axiogingival
- Axiolingual
- Axiofacial
- Axiopulpal.

Point Angles

- Axiofaciopulpal point angle
- Axiolinguopulpal point angle
- Axiofaciogingival point angle
- Axiolinguogingival point angle
- Distofaciopulpal point angle
- Distolinguopulpal point angle.

Class V Tooth Preparation

For class V preparation, 8 line angles and 4 point angles are as follows (**Fig. 7.23**).

Line Angles

- Axiogingival
- Axioincisal
- Axiomesial
- Axiodistal
- Mesioincisal
- Mesiogingival
- Distoincisal
- Distogingival.

Point Angles

- Axiodistogingival point angle
- Axiodistoincisal point angle
- Axiomesiogingival point angle
- Axiomesioincisal point angle.

TOOTH PREPARATION

Guidelines of tooth preparation given by black:

Black gave following guidelines for tooth preparation
➡ Providing definite mechanical retention in the preparation
➡ Extension of preparation in adjacent pits and fissures for prevention of recurrent caries
➡ Removal of infected and affected dentin from all surfaces
➡ Removal of even healthy tooth structure to gain access and good visibility

When Black gave classification, following conditions and considerations were prevalent at that time:

- Poor oral hygiene habits
- Poor properties of the existing restorative materials
- The expected longer life of the restoration
- Hard and fibrous food
- Low consumption of refined carbohydrates
- More liking towards gold and silver fillings in teeth
- Prevailing common diagnostic aids such as PMT.

Nowadays because of change in following conditions, design of the tooth preparation has become most conservative
➡ Use of preventive measures like fluoridation of water supply, fluoride toothpaste, topical fluoride applications, proper brushing and flossing, etc.
➡ Understanding of the fact that the remineralization of enamel and affected dentin can take place
➡ Advances in tooth colored, adhesive, fluoride releasing restorative materials
➡ Newer advancements in restorative materials
➡ Improvements in diagnostic aids
➡ Better oral hygiene maintenance
➡ Mechanical retention forms further improve the retention.

Classification of Tooth Preparations

Tooth preparations may be classified according to the location where the carious lesion initiates. Caries often initiate in the developmental pits and fissures of the teeth. These areas are morphologically deeper than the surrounding tooth substance and are thus sites for food impaction and nearly impossible to clean thoroughly, forming ideal conditions for bacterial plaque formation (**Fig. 7.24**).

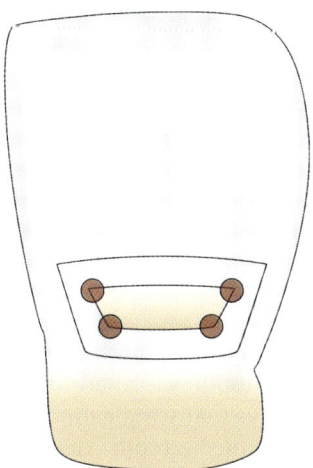

Figure 7.23: Class V preparation showing line and point angles

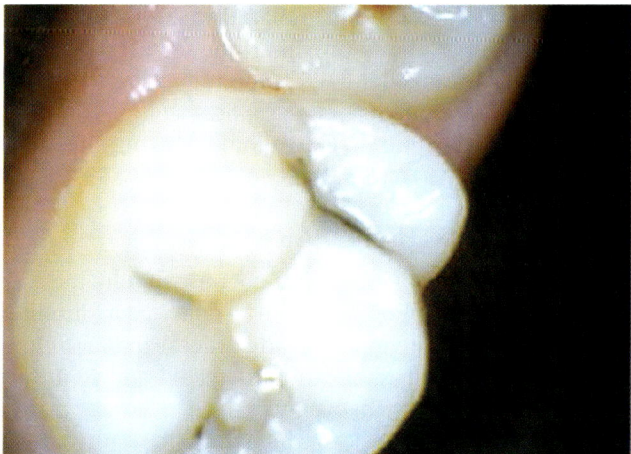

Figure 7.24: Deep pits and fissures are primary areas for food impaction and caries formation

→ Palatal pits of maxillary incisors
→ Palatal grooves and pits of maxillary molars
→ Occlusal surfaces of posterior teeth
→ Facial grooves and pits of mandibular molars
→ Pits occurring in teeth because of irregularities in the enamel formation.

Smooth surface lesions can be found in all teeth on the proximal surfaces, and gingival one-third of the facial and lingual surfaces. GV Black gave a simple classification based on clinical location of the defects, listed as class I, class II, class III, class IV and class V. An additional class VI was later on added by Simon as modification to Black's classification.

Class I is the only pit and fissure preparation whereas rest are smooth surface preparations.

- *Class I*: Pit and fissure preparations occur on the occlusal surfaces of premolars and molars, the occlusal two-third of buccal and lingual surface of molars, lingual surface of incisors and any other abnormal position (**Figs 7.25A and B**).
- *Class II*: Preparations on the proximal surface of premolars and molars are class II (**Figs 7.26A and B**).
- *Class III*: Preparations on the proximal surface of anterior teeth and not involving the incisal angles are class III (**Figs 7.27A and B**).
- *Class IV*: Preparations on the proximal surface of anterior teeth also involving the incisal angle falls under class IV (**Figs 7.28A and B**).
- *Class V*: Preparations on gingival third of facial and lingual or palatal surfaces of all teeth came under Class V (**Figs 7.29A and B**).

Modification of Black's classification was made to provide more specific localization of preparations.

- *Class II*: Preparations on the single or both proximal surface of premolar and molar teeth. When there is involvement of both proximal surfaces, it is called mesio-occlusodistal (MOD) preparation (**Fig. 7.30**).
- *Class VI*: Preparations on incisal edges of anterior and cusp tips of posterior teeth without involving any other surface (**Figs 7.31A and B**) come under Class VI.

STEPS IN TOOTH PREPARATION

Before initiating tooth preparation one should identify presence of caries. There should be an opacity surrounding the pit and fissure indicating demineralization of the enamel. Softened enamel can be detected and removed away with the sharp tip of explorer.

After the clinician decides which tooth to restore, anesthesia is given.

Tooth preparation involves a systemic approach based on the mechanical and physical principles which should

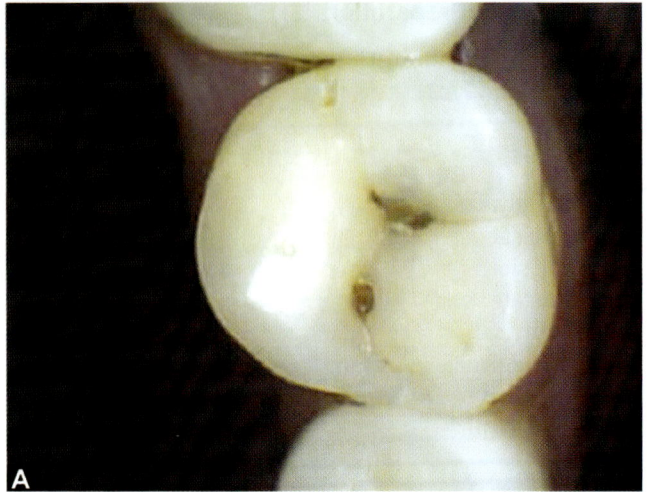
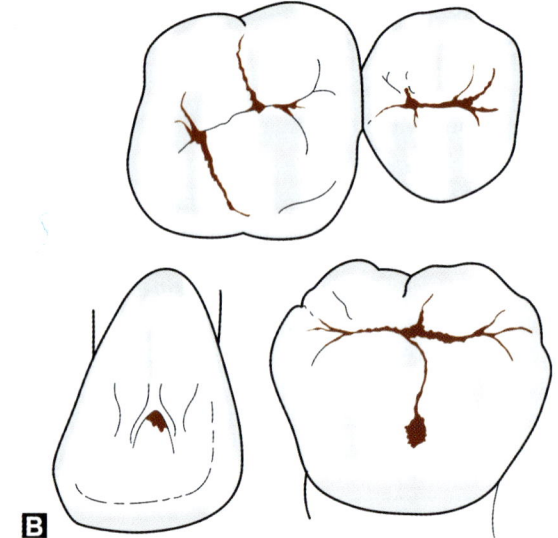

Figures 7.25A and B: (A) Clinical presentation of class I lesion; (B) Diagrammatic presentation of class I lesion

be followed in an orderly sequence. The design of the tooth preparation for either a tooth with initial caries or replacement restoration depends upon location of the caries, the amount and extent of the caries, the amount of lost tooth structure, and the restorative material to be used. But there are some basic principles which should be followed while doing tooth preparation.

Earlier when the affected tooth was prepared because of caries, cutting of tooth was referred to as cavity preparation. But nowadays many indications other than caries lead to preparation of the tooth. Hence, the term cavity preparation has been replaced by tooth preparation.

Tooth preparation is divided into two stages, each consisting of many steps. Though each step should be

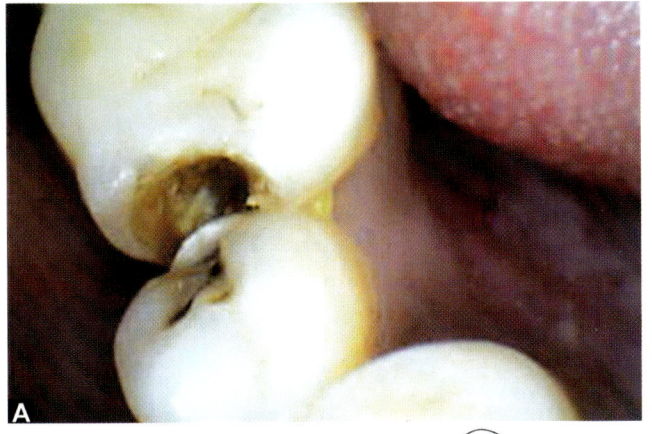

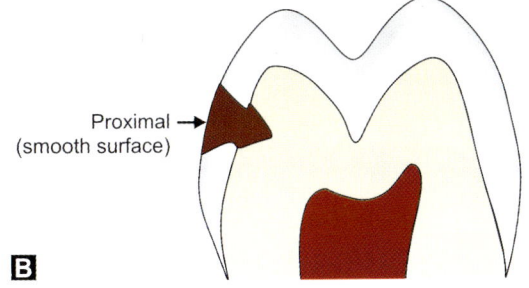

Figures 7.26A and B: (A) Class II lesion; (B) Diagrammatic presentation of Class II lesion

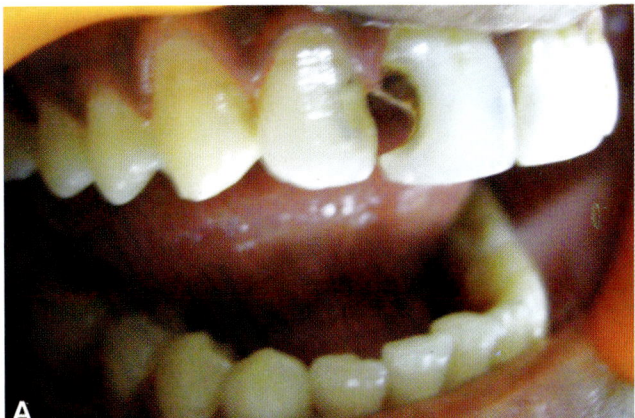

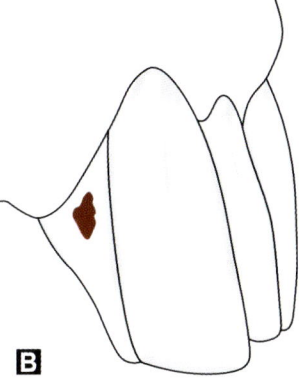

Figures 7.27A and B: (A) Class III lesion; (B) Diagrammatic representation of Class III lesion

done to perfection, but sometimes modifications can be made in steps.

Steps in tooth preparation

→ *Stage I*: Initial tooth preparation steps
  - ♦ Outline form and initial depth
  - ♦ Primary resistance form
  - ♦ Primary retention form
  - ♦ Convenience form.
→ *Stage II*: Final tooth preparation steps
  - ♦ Removal of any remaining enamel pit or fissure, infected dentin and/or old restorative material, if indicated
  - ♦ Pulp protection, if indicated
  - ♦ Secondary resistance and retention form
  - ♦ Procedures for finishing the external walls of the tooth preparation
  - ♦ Final procedures: Cleaning, inspecting and sealing
  - ♦ Under special conditions these sequences are changed.

Initial Tooth Preparation

Outline Form and Initial Depth

The outline form means:
- Placing the preparation margins in the position they will occupy in the final tooth preparation except for finishing enamel walls and margins

- Maintaining the initial depth of 0.2 to 0.8 mm into the dentin.
- Outline form defines the external boundaries of the preparations.

Factors affecting the outline and initial depth form of tooth preparation

→ Extension of carious lesion
→ Proximity of the lesion to other deep structural surface defects
→ Relationship with adjacent and opposing teeth
→ Caries index of the patient
→ Need for esthetics
→ Restorative material to be used.

Before initiating the tooth preparation, outline must be visualized to access the proposed shape of the preparation (**Fig. 7.32**). The outline form includes the external outline form and internal outline form.

The external outline form is established first to extend all margins into sound tooth tissue while maintaining the initial depth of 0.2 to 0.8 mm into the dentin towards

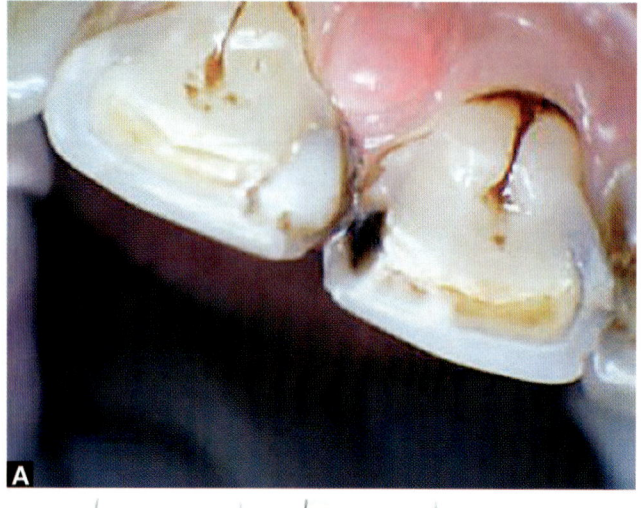

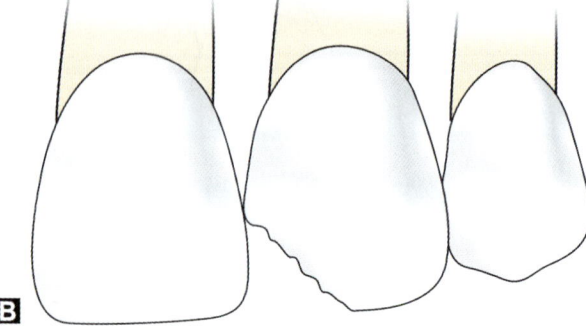

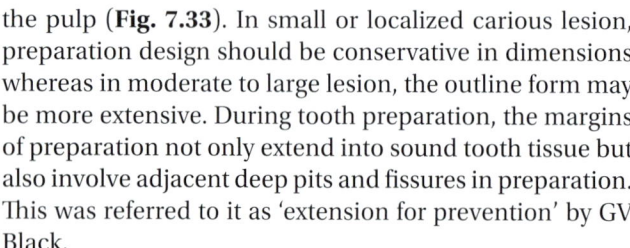

Figures 7.28A and B: (A) Class IV lesion; (B) Diagrammatic representation of Class IV defect

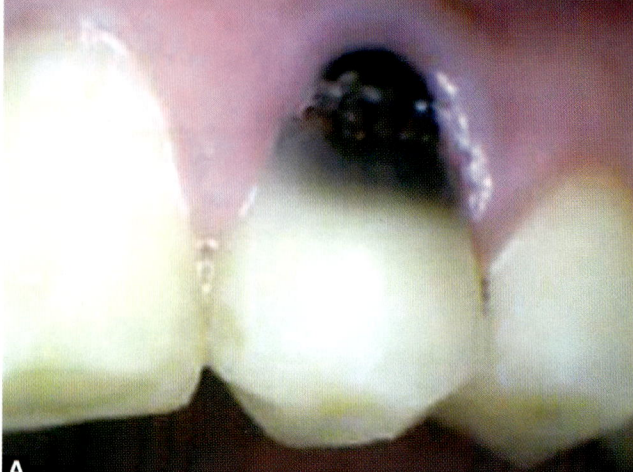

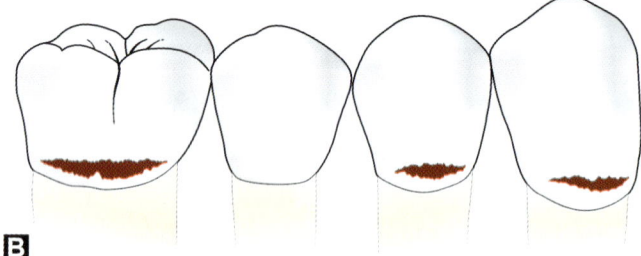

Figures 7.29A and B: (A) Class V lesion; (B) Diagrammatic representation of Class V lesion

the pulp (**Fig. 7.33**). In small or localized carious lesion, preparation design should be conservative in dimensions whereas in moderate to large lesion, the outline form may be more extensive. During tooth preparation, the margins of preparation not only extend into sound tooth tissue but also involve adjacent deep pits and fissures in preparation. This was referred to it as 'extension for prevention' by GV Black.

"Extension for prevention means "placing the margins of preparations at areas that would be cleaned by the excursions of food during chewing". It is done with the objective of preventing the recurrence of caries at the margins of fillings where the recurrence of decay is most commonly seen. His concept also included extending preparations through enamel fissures to allow cavosurface margins to be placed on nonfissured enamel.

For this:

- Margins of the restoration are placed on line angles of the tooth
- Occlusal surface is extended through pits and fissures

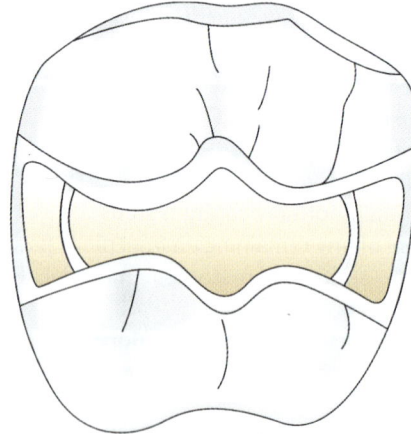

Figure 7.30: MOD preparation

- Proximal line angles extended buccally and lingually through embrasures and cervically below the gingival margin

Advantages

- Prevents recurrence of decay in the tooth surface adjoining restoration
- Results in self-cleaning embrasure areas

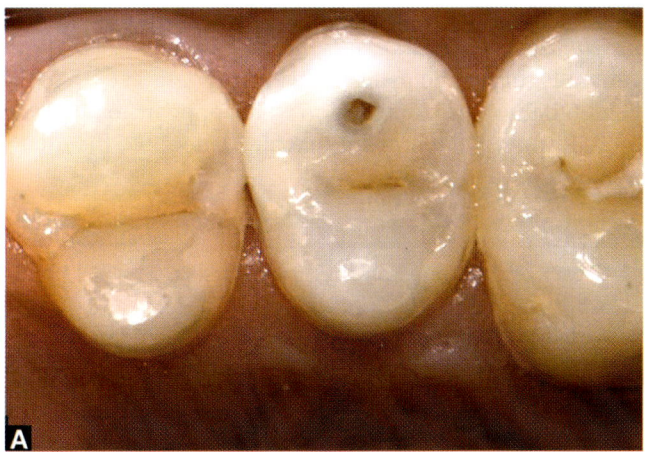

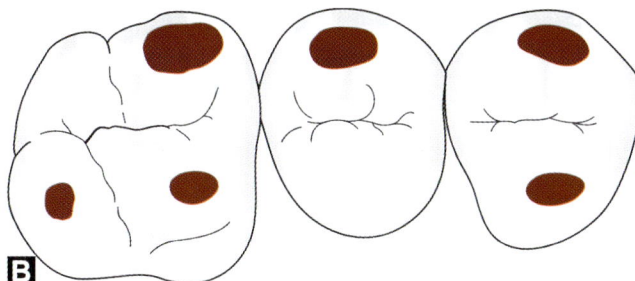

Figures 7.31A and B: (A) Class VI lesion is present on cusp tip; (B) Diagrammatic representation of class VI lesion

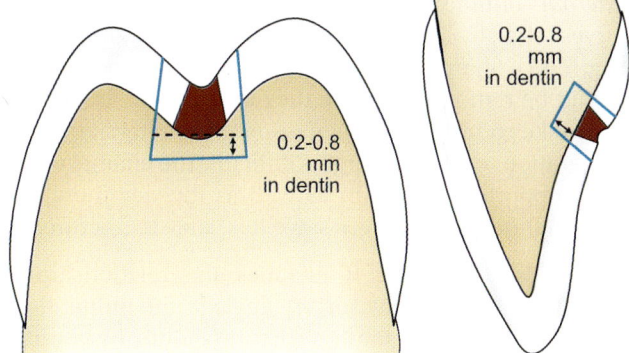

Figure 7.33: Initial depth of preparation should be 0.2 to 0.8 mm into dentin

Following principles are kept in mind while preparing an outline form:

- Removal of all weakened and friable tooth structure
- Removal of all undermined enamel (**Fig. 7.34**)
- Incorporate all faults in preparation
- Place all margins of preparation in a position to afford good finishing of the restoration.

Features for establishing a proper outline form are

- Preserving cuspal strength
- Preserving strength of marginal ridge
- Minimizing the buccolingual extensions
- If distance between two faults is less than 0.5 mm, connect them
- Limiting the depth of preparation 0.2 to 0.8 mm into dentin
- Using enameloplasty wherever indicated

Outline form for pit and fissure lesions:

- Remove all defective portion and extend the preparation margins to healthy tooth structure
- Remove all unsupported enamel rods or weakened enamel margins
- If the thickness of enamel between two preparation sites is less than 0.5 mm, connect them to make one preparation, otherwise prepared as separate tooth preparations
- Avoid ending the preparation margins in high stress areas like cusp eminences
- Extend the preparation margins to include all pits and fissures which cannot be managed by enameloplasty
- Limit the depth of preparation to 0.2 mm into the dentin, though the actual depth of preparation may vary from 1.5 to 2 mm depending on steepness of cuspal slopes and thickness of the enamel
- Extend the outline form to facilitate the convenience for preparation and restoration
- If indicated because of esthetic reasons, make the preparation as conservative as possible.

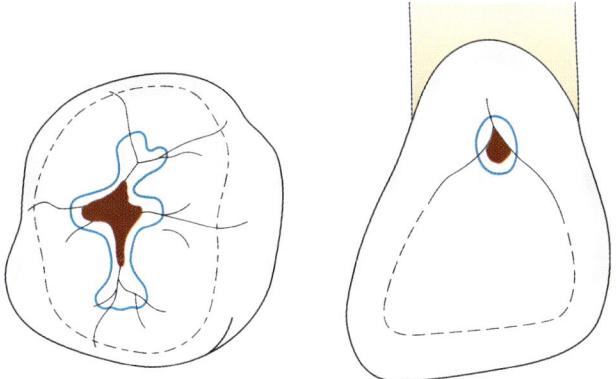

Figure 7.32: Outline form should include all defective pits and fissures

This principle has changed to "Prevention of extension" due to:

- Natural remineralization (via calcium and phosphate from saliva)
- Fluoride-induced remineralization (through water, dentifrices, restorative materials).
- Advancements in instrumentation
- Advancements in restorative materials
- Modifications in tooth preparation designs

External outline form: It should consist of smooth curves, straight lines and rounded line and point angles (**Fig. 7.35**). Sharp and irregular projection of tooth tissue should be removed because they are not only fragile but also make good adaptation of restorative material to tooth preparation walls and margins difficult. The enamel which is unsupported by dentin as well as the demineralized enamel should be removed since it is liable to fracture.

Internal outline form: It includes the relationship of occlusal walls from cavosurface angle to the pulpal floor. Unnecessary loss of tooth structure should be avoided from the inner dimensions of the preparation. Since enamel is brittle and dentin is elastic, one should avoid placing pulpal floor in enamel. The preparation depth should be at least 1.5 to 2.0 mm vertical from the cavosurface margin to the pulpal floor and at least 0.2 to 0.5 mm in dentin so as to provide adequate strength to resist fracture due to masticatory forces (**Fig. 7.36**).

Outline form for smooth surface lesions—Outline form of proximal caries (Class II, III and IV lesions): Class II are generally diagnosed using bitewing radiographs. It should be noted that a proximal lesion which appears to be 2/3 or more toward the dentin has actually penetrated the dentinoenamel junction.

Factors affecting the outline form of proximal preparations
⇒ Extent of the caries on the proximal side (**Figs 7.37 and 7.38**)
⇒ Dimensions of the contact area in the affected tooth
⇒ Contact relationship with adjacent tooth
⇒ Caries index of the patient (**Fig. 7.39**)
⇒ Age of the patient
⇒ Position of gingiva
⇒ Alignment of teeth and masticatory forces likely to fall on restorative material (**Figs 7.40A and B**)
⇒ Esthetic requirement of the patient.

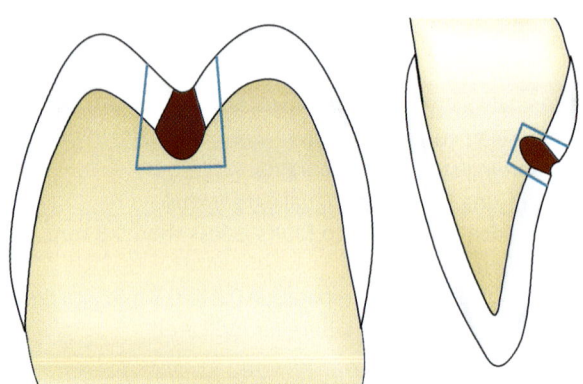

Figure 7.34: Removal of all undermined enamel

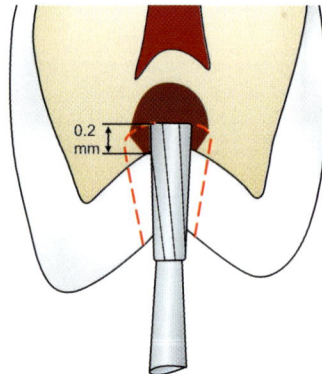

Figure 7.36: Preparation depth should be at least 1.5-2 mm from the cavosurface margin and at least 0.2-0.5 mm into dentin

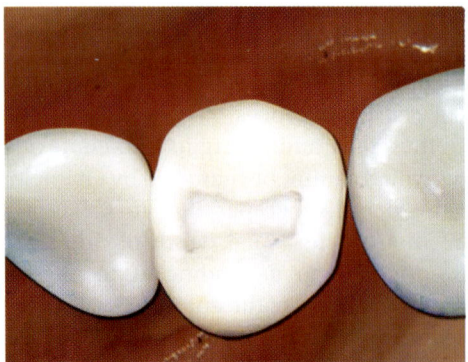

Figure 7.35: Outline form should consist of smooth curves, rounded line and point angles

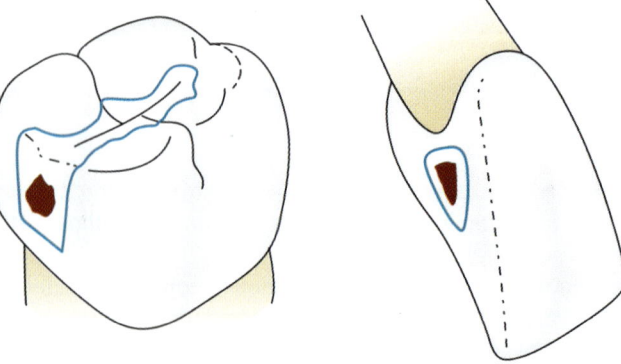

Figure 7.37: Outline form should include all the carious lesion and undermined enamel

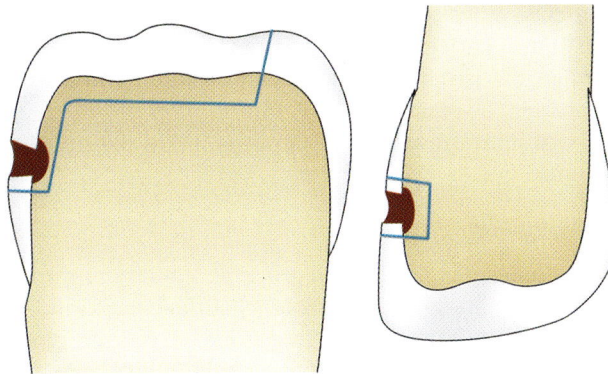

Figure 7.38: Outline form should include all carious lesion

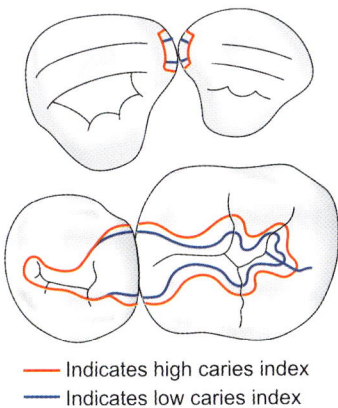

— Indicates high caries index
— Indicates low caries index

Figure 7.39: In a patient with high caries risk it is always preferred to place gingival margin further into the embrasure

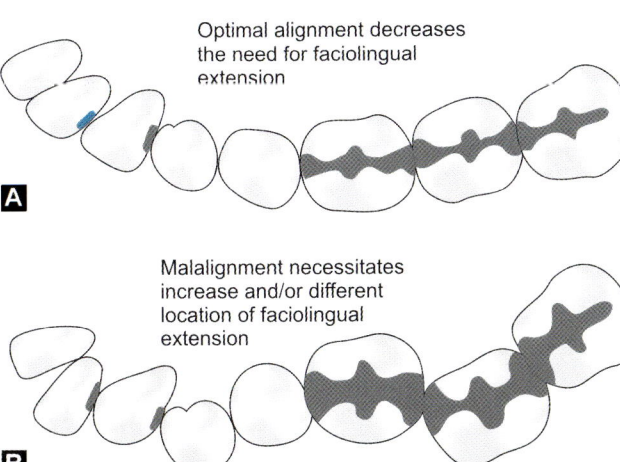

Optimal alignment decreases the need for faciolingual extension

A

Malalignment necessitates increase and/or different location of faciolingual extension

B

Figures 7.40A and B: Proper alignment of teeth requires less faciolingual extensions as compared to malaligned teeth. It also offer better cleanliness of embrasure area

As we saw that Class II tooth preparations varies according to the morphology, anatomy and extent of carious involvement of the individual tooth being restored. Some features are however common to all Class II tooth preparations.

A class II tooth preparation consists of:
- Occlusal segment
- Proximal segment.

Rules for making outline form for proximal preparation:
- Extend the preparation margins until sound tooth structure is reached (**Fig. 7.37**)
- Remove all unsupported enamel rods, extending the margins to allow sufficient access for restoration
- Restrict the depth of axial wall 0.2 to 0.8 mm into dentin (**Fig. 7.41**).
- Axial wall should be parallel to external surface of the tooth (**Fig. 7.42**).

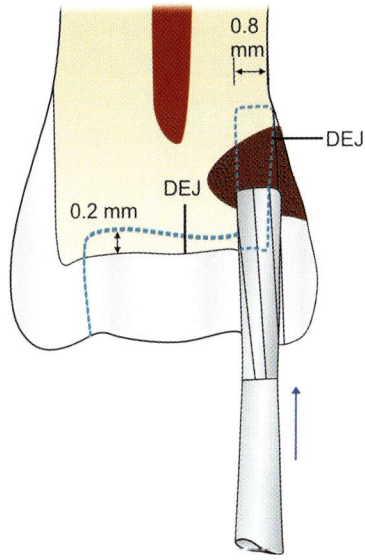

Figure 7.41: Restrict the depth of axial wall 0.2 -0.8 mm into dentin

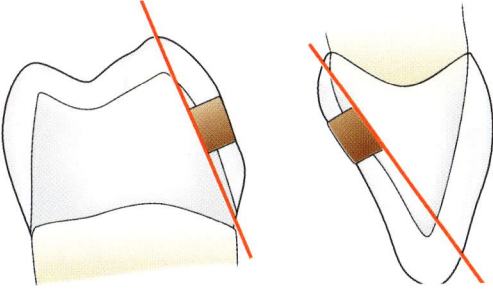

Figure 7.42: Axial wall should be parallel to external surface of tooth

- In class II tooth preparation, place gingival seat apical to the contact but occlusal to gingival margin and have the clearance of 0.5 mm from the adjacent tooth (**Figs 7.43 and 7.44**).
- In class III preparation, position of incisal margins is in the area of contact, especially if esthetic restorative material is used or when incisal embrasure is not large to allow incisal extension out of contact area.

Axial wall should
⇒ Be placed into dentin 0.5-0.8 mm from DEJ.
⇒ Follow curvature of dentinoenamel junction bucco-lingually
⇒ Follow curvature of dentinoenamel junction occlusogingivally

Outline form for class V lesions: Outline form for cervical/root/gingival lesions for buccal and lingual surfaces of class V preparations, is as follows:

- In class V lesions the outline form is governed by the extent of caries. Therefore, extend the cavity mesially, gingivally, distally and occlusally till sound tooth structure may be reached (**Fig. 7.45**).
- The minimum axial wall depth is 0.2 to 0.5 mm into dentin.

Enameloplasty

Enameloplasty is the careful removal of sharp and irregular enamel margins of the enamel surface by 'rounding' or 'saucering' it and converting it into a smooth groove making it self-cleansable, finishable and allowing conservative placement of margins (**Figs 7.46A and B**). Enameloplasty is done when caries is present in the superficial part of the enamel or a fissure in less than one-third thickness of the enamel. The enameloplasty does not extend the outline form, also the use of enameloplasty often confines the preparation to one surface and restoration is not done in the recontoured area.

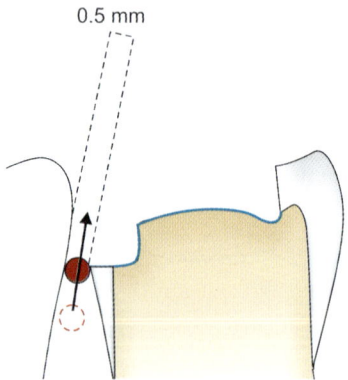

Figure 7.43: In proximal tooth preparation, gingival margin should clear adjacent tooth by 0.5 mm

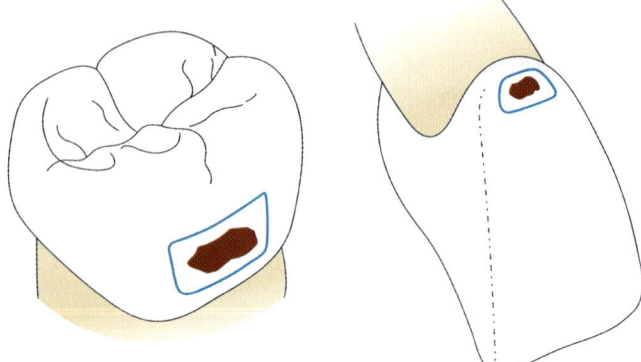

Figure 7.45: Outline form of class V cavity depends upon extent of caries

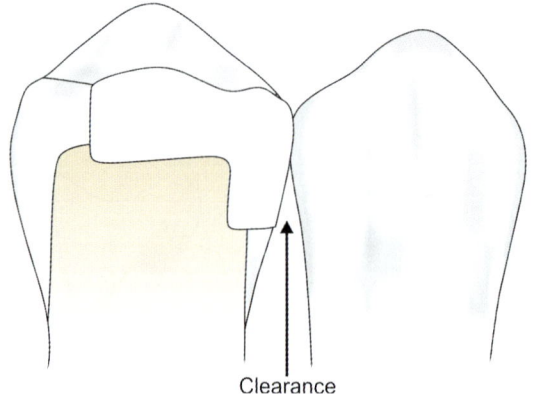

Figure 7.44: 0.5 mm clearance from adjacent tooth

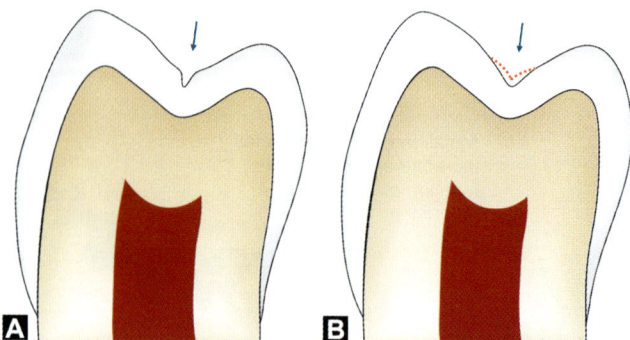

Figures 7.46A and B: Enameloplasty: (A) Tooth with deep pit and fissure; (B) Removal of superficial enamel resulting in rounding of deep pit and fissure caries making it self-cleansable

Primary Resistance Form

Definition: Primary resistance form is that shape and placement of preparation walls to best enables both the tooth and restoration to withstand, without fracture the stresses of masticatory forces delivered principally along the long axis of the tooth.

As we know that masticatory stress pattern is different for each tooth, accordingly, for success of the tooth preparation and restoration, this stress pattern must be recognized.

Factors affecting resistance form
➡ Amount of occlusal stresses
➡ Type of restoration used
➡ Amount of remaining tooth structure.

Features of resistance form
- A box-shaped preparation.
- A flat pulpal and gingival floor, which helps the tooth to resist occlusal masticatory forces without any displacement (**Figs 7.47A and B**).
- Adequate thickness of restorative material depending on its respective compressive and tensile strengths to prevent the fracture of both the remaining tooth structure and restoration. In case of class IV preparations, we check the faciolingual width of anterior teeth, to establish the resistance form.

Type of restoration	*Minimum occlusal thickness*
Cast metal	1–2 mm
Amalgam restorations	1.5 mm
Ceramics	2 mm

- Restrict the extension of external walls to allow strong marginal ridge areas with sufficient dentin support (**Fig. 7.48**)
- Inclusion of weakened tooth structure to avoid fracture under masticatory forces
- Rounding of internal line angle to reduce the stress concentration points in tooth preparation (**Fig. 7.49**)
- Consideration to cusp capping depending upon the amount of remaining tooth structure.

Resistance form also depends upon type of restorative material being used. For example, high copper amalgam requires minimal thickness of 1.5 mm, cast metal requires

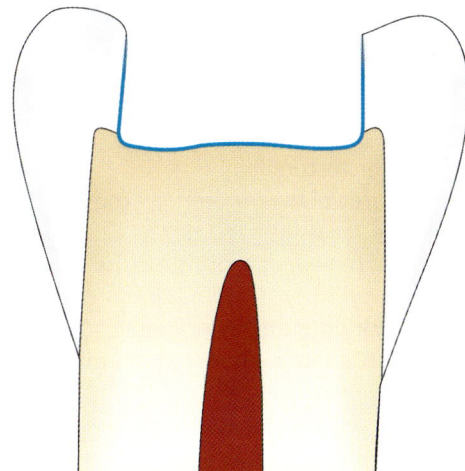

Figure 7.48: Restrict the extensions of external wall so as to have strong marginal ridge area

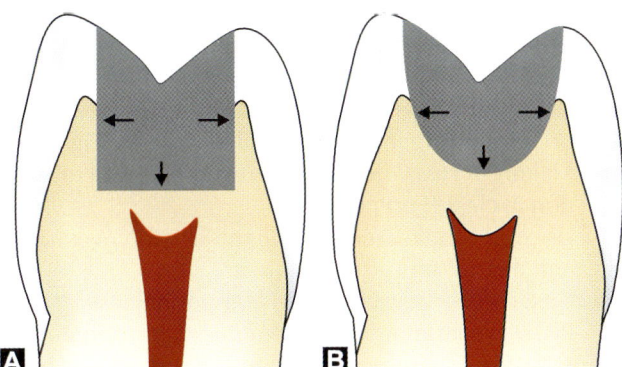

Figures 7.47A and B: (A) Resistance form of tooth provided by flat pulpal and gingival floor; (B) In case of rounded pulpal floor, the rocking motion of restoration results in wedging force which may result in failure of restoration

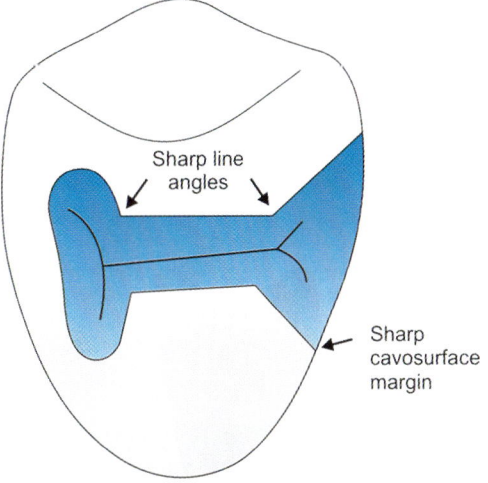

Figure 7.49: Sharp line angle and cavosurface margins can lead to poor resistance form because of concentration of stresses at that point

thickness of 1.0 mm and the porcelain requires a minimum thickness of 2.0 mm to resist fracture. The composite and glass ionomer restorations are more dependent on occlusal wear potential of restorative area and usually require thickness of more than 2.5 mm.

Primary Retention Form

Definition: Primary retention form is that form, shape and configuration of the tooth preparation that resists the displacement or removal of restoration from the preparation under lifting and tipping masticatory forces.

Usually, resistance and retention forms are obtained by providing same features, hence they are sometimes described together. The retention form is affected by the type of the restorative material used.

Factors affecting retention form are
➡ Amount of the masticatory stresses falling on the restoration
➡ Thickness of the restoration
➡ Total surface area of the restoration exposed to the masticatory forces
➡ The amount of remaining tooth structure

Retention form for different restorations:
- *Amalgam:* Retention is increased in amalgam restoration by the following:
  - Providing occlusal convergence (about 2–5%) of the dentinal walls towards the tooth surface (**Fig. 7.50**)
  - Giving slight undercut in dentin near the pulpal wall (**Fig. 7.51**)
  - Conserving the marginal ridges
  - Providing occlusal dovetail (**Fig. 7.52**).

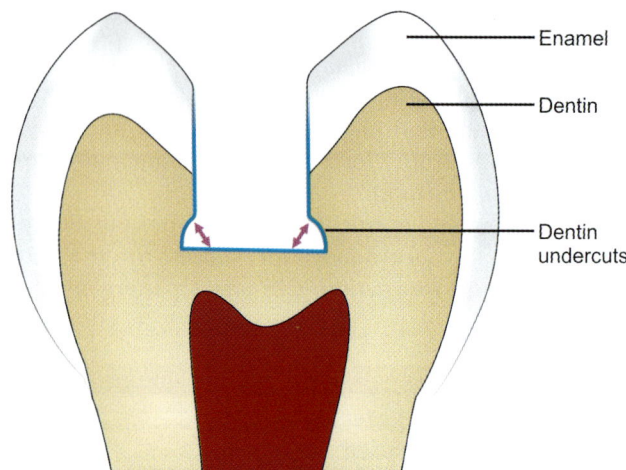

Figure 7.51: Undercut in dentin near the pulpal wall helps in retention of amalgam

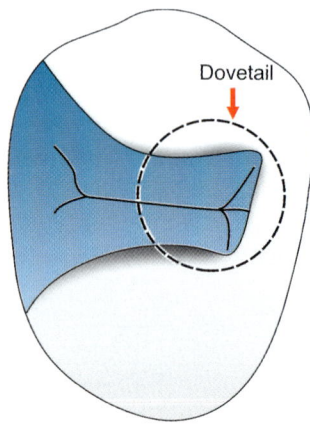

Figure 7.52: Dovetail helps in providing retention

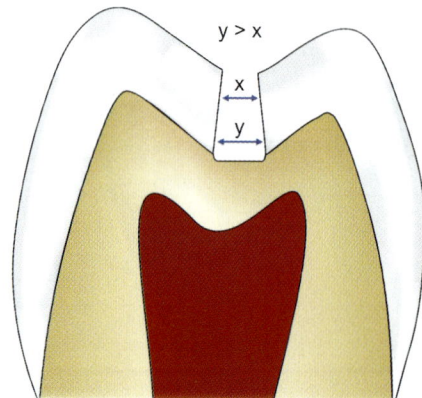

Figure 7.50: Preparation walls should have 2°-5° occlusal convergence for amalgam retention

- *Cast metals:* Retention is increased in cast restorations by the following:
  - Close parallelism of the opposing walls with slight occlusal divergence of two to five degrees (**Fig. 7.53**)
  - Making occlusal dovetail to prevent tilting of restoration in class II preparations
  - Use of secondary retention in the form of coves, skirts and dentin slot
  - Give reverse bevel in class I compound, class II, and MOD preparations to prevent tipping movements
- *Composites:* In composites, retention is increased by:
  - Micromechanical bonding between the etched and primed prepared tooth structure and the composite resin
  - Providing enamel bevels.

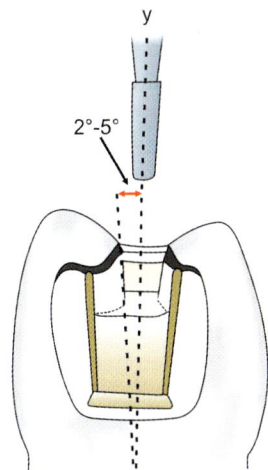

Figure 7.53: Parallelism of opposing walls and slight occlusal divergence provides retention of inlay

- *Direct filling gold:* Elastic compression of dentin and starting point in dentin provide retention in direct gold fillings by proper condensation.

Restoration	Primary retention form
Amalgam class I and II	• Occlusal convergence of external walls (about 2–5%) • Conservation of marginal ridges • Occlusal dovetail
Amalgam class III and IV	• As the external walls diverge outward, retention grooves/coves are the primary retention forms
Cast metals	• Parallel longitudinal walls with slight occlusal divergence of 2–5°. • Occlusal dovetail • Secondary retention in the form of coves, skirts and dentin slot
Composites	• Micromechanical bonding between etched and primed surface with composites • Enamel bevels
Direct filling gold	• Elastic compression of dentin and starting point in dentin provides retention by proper condensation.

Convenience Form

Definition: The convenience form is that form which facilitates and provides adequate visibility, accessibility and ease of operation during preparation and restoration of the tooth.

Features of convenience form

- Sufficient extension of distal, mesial, facial or lingual walls to gain adequate access to the deeper portion of the preparation.
- The cavosurface margin of the preparation should be related to the selected restorative material for the purpose of convenience to marginal adaptation.
- In class II preparations access is made through occlusal surface for convenience form.
- Proximal clearance is provided from the adjoining tooth during class II tooth preparation.
- To make Class II tunnel preparation, for convenience, the proximal caries in posterior teeth is approached through a tunnel initiating from the occlusal surface and ending on carious lesion on the proximal surface without cutting the marginal ridge.
- In tooth preparation for cast gold restorations occlusal divergence is one of the feature of convenience form.

Final Stages of Tooth Preparation

After initial stages of the preparation, the prepared tooth should be carefully examined. For most of the conservative restorations, after initial stages of tooth preparation the tooth is ready for restoration except for some final procedures like varnishing, etching and bonding, etc. For extensive restorations, some of additional steps may be required.

The remaining carious portion should be removed only after the initial tooth preparation has been completed. It provides two advantages:

1. It allows optimal visibility and convenience form for removal of remaining carious lesion.
2. Completion of the initial preparation permits immediate placement of a base and the restoration.

Removal of Any Remaining Enamel Pit or Fissure, Infected Dentin and/or Old Restorative Material, if Indicated

After the establishment of external and internal outline form, if any of the remaining carious tooth structure or defective restorative material is left in tooth, it is to be removed in this stage.

Infected dentin must be removed even if it leads to exposure of pulp which is treated accordingly.

A small isolated carious lesion should be eliminated by a conservative preparation. After the establishment of pulpal and axial wall, if a small amount of carious lesion remains, only this lesion should be removed, leaving concave, rounded area in the wall.

Difference between infected and affected dentin

Infected dentin	Affected dentin
• It is a superficial layer of demineralized dentin	• It is a deeper layer
• Cannot be remineralized	• Can be remineralized
• Lacks sensation	• It is sensitive
• In this, intertubular layer is demineralized with irregularly scattered crystals	• In this, intertubular layer is only partly demineralized
• Collagen fibers are broken down, appear as only indistinct cross bands	• Distinct cross bands are present
• It can be stained with: – 0.2 percent propylene glycol – 10 percent acid red solution – 0.5 percent basic fuschin	• It cannot be stained with any solution.

In the extensive preparations with soft caries, the removal of carious dentin is done early in initial tooth preparation. It is better to remove the extensive caries early in tooth preparation to provide better opportunity to specific needs of retention and resistance form.

Removal of old restorative material is indicated if

➡ It affects aesthetics of new restoration
➡ Has secondary caries beneath (seen on radiograph)
➡ Tooth is symptomatic
➡ It compromises new restoration
➡ Marginal deterioration of old restoration.

Points to remember while removing the remaining carious lesion

➡ Isolate the remaining carious lesion and remove it using the following instruments:
  ◆ Low speed handpiece with the round bur that will fit in the carious lesion used with light force and a wiping motion
  ◆ Spoon excavator that will fit in the carious lesion. Use of a large spoon excavator decreases the chance of a pulpal exposure.
➡ Force for removal of infected dentin should be directed laterally and not towards the center of the carious lesion
➡ Start removal of caries from the lateral borders of the lesion
➡ After removal, confirm it with the explorer applying it laterally. Avoid using excessive force with the explorer as it may cause a pulpal exposure.

Pulp Protection

Pulp protection is a very important step in adapting the preparation for final restoration although actually it is not a step of tooth preparation. When remaining dentin thickness is less, pulpal injury can occur because of heat production, high speed burs with less effective coolants, irritating restorative materials, galvanic currents due to restoration of dissimilar metals, excessive masticatory forces transmitted through restorative materials to the dentin and ingress of microorganisms and their noxious products through microleakage.

Pulp protection is achieved using liners, varnishes and bases depending upon

➡ The amount of remaining dentin thickness
➡ Type of the restorative material used.
  Liners and varnishes are used where preparation depth is shallow and remaining dentin thickness is more than 2 mm. They provide:
➡ Barrier to protect remaining dentin and pulp
➡ Galvanic and thermal insulation.

Bases are the cements used on pulpal and axial walls in thickness of about 0.5 to 2 mm beneath the permanent restorations. They provide thermal, galvanic, chemical and mechanical protection to the pulp. Commonly used restorative materials as base are zinc phosphate cements, glass ionomers, polycarboxylate cements, zinc oxide eugenol, and calcium hydroxide cement.

Secondary Resistance and Retention Forms

This step is needed in complex and compound tooth preparations where added preparation features are used to improve the resistance and retention form of the prepared tooth. These are as follows:

Grooves and coves: Wherever bulk of dentin is present, grooves are prepared without undermining the adjacent enamel (**Fig. 7.54**). Coves are small conical depressions

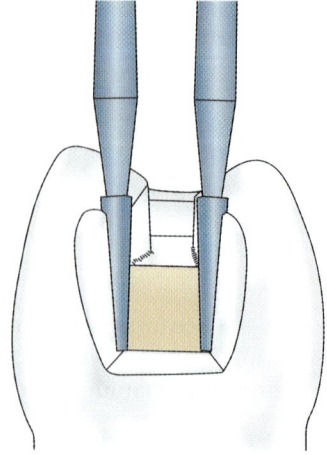

Figure 7.54: Grooves are placed in axiofacial and axiolingual line angles so as to increase retention of the restoration

prepared in healthy dentin to provide additional retention. These are normally prepared in the proximal walls of class II preparations at the axiofacial and axiolingual line angles, thus reducing proximal displacement of the restoration. More than one groove per wall should be avoided as they may weaken the wall. Grooves are especially useful for cast restorations. They are kept parallel to the line of withdrawal of the wax pattern.

Type of tooth preparation	Location of retention grooves
Class II preparation	Proximal wall, at the axiofacial and axiolingual line angles.
Class III preparation	Axiogingival line angle or axiofaciogingival point angle and lingual dovetail
Class V preparation	Axioincisal and axiogingival line angle.

Slots or internal boxes: These are mainly used in amalgam restorations. They are 1.0 to 1.5 mm deep box like grooves prepared in dentin to increase the surface area. These are prepared in occlusal box, buccoaxial, linguoaxial and gingival walls (**Fig. 7.55**). For cast restorations these are prepared by tapered fissure bur to avoid undercuts and for plastic restorative materials like amalgam, these are prepared by inverted cone bur to create slight undercuts in dentin.

Locks (Fig. 7.56): Locks are usually prepared for class II amalgam restorations for increasing resistance and retention form. They are given for wide proximal boxes and for cusp capping cases.

Pins: Different types of pins of various shapes and sizes are used to provide additional retention. They can be used in all types of restorations like amalgam, composite and cast restorations.

Skirts: Skirts are prepared for providing additional retention in cast restorations. They increase the total surface area of the preparation. Skirts can be prepared on one or all four sides of the preparation depending upon the required retention (**Fig. 7.57**). Skirts have shown to improve both resistance and retention form.

Amalgampins: Amalgampins are vertical posts of amalgam anchored in dentin. Dentin chamber is prepared by using inverted cone bur on gingival floor 0.5 mm in dentin with 1 to 2 mm depth and 0.5 to 1 mm width (**Fig. 7.58**). Amalgampins increase the retention and resistance of complete restoration.

Beveled enamel margins: Beveling of the preparation, margins increases the surface area and thus the retention in composite restorations.

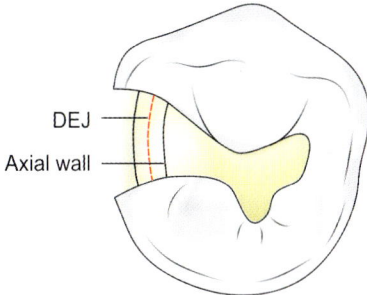

Figure 7.56: Retention locks

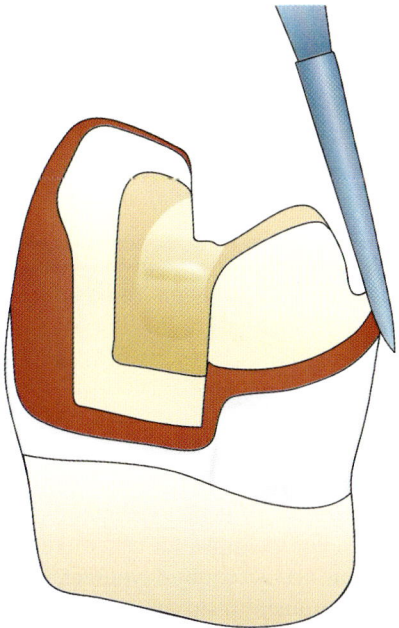

Figure 7.57: Skirt in cast restoration helps in increasing retention

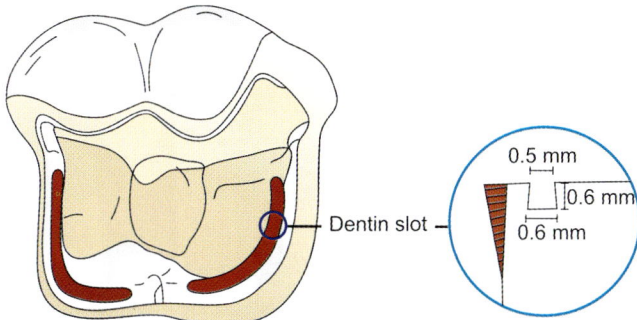

Figure 7.55: Slot

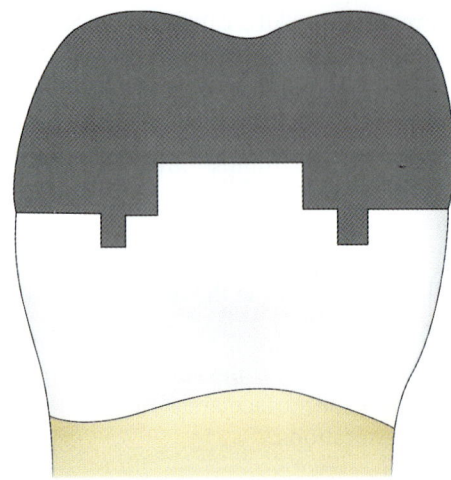

Figure 7.58: Amalgampins increase retention of the restoration

Enamel wall etching: Etching results in microscopic roughness, which increases the surface area and thus helps in enhancing the micromechanical retention.

Dentin conditioning (etching and priming): Etching and priming of the dentin surface done in some restorative materials increases the retention.

Adhesive luting cements: Adhesive luting cements increase the retention of indirect restorations.

Procedures for Finishing the External Walls of the Tooth Preparation

Definition: Finishing of a tooth preparation walls is further development of a specific cavosurface design and degree of smoothness which produces maximum effectiveness of the restorative material being used.

Finishing of the enamel margins should be done irrespective of the restorative material used.

The finishing of the preparation walls results in
➡ Better marginal seal between restoration and tooth structure
➡ Increased strength of both tooth structure and restoration at and near the margins
➡ Strong location of the margins
➡ Increase in degree of smoothness of the margins.

Degree of smoothness of walls: It depends upon type of restoration used. For example, for cast metal restorations, a very smooth surface is required whereas for direct gold, amalgam and composite restorations, slight roughness is needed in the preparation walls.

Location of the margins: During finishing of the preparation walls and margins, one should follow the principles of paralleling the direction of enamel wall. The knowledge of enamel rods is necessary for proper finishing of the preparation margins. At the margins, all the enamel walls should have full length rods supported by dentin (**Figs 7.59A and B**). To remove unsupported enamel rods near gingival margins it should be slightly bevelled. In case of cast gold restorations, a short bevel is given and an ultrashort bevel is given in case of gold foil.

	Butt joint	*Lap/slip joint*
Cavosurface margin	90° at margin	>90° at margin
Nature of prepared walls	Smooth	Roughened
Indications	• Preferred in Amalgam restorations as it produces maximal strength for both tooth and amalgam • Also given in ceramic restorations	• Indicated in cast and composite restorations
Esthetics	• Less esthetic	• More esthetic

Features of finished preparation: The design of cavosurface angle depends on type of restorative material being used. For example, for amalgam restoration, cavosurface angle of 90 degrees affords maximum strength to tooth restoration.

In case of cast metal restoration bevelling of external wall is done to produce stronger enamel margin, as the marginal metal is more easily burnished and adapted.

Final Procedures: Cleaning, Inspecting and Sealing

The final step in tooth preparation is cleansing of the preparation. This includes the removal of debris, drying of the preparation, and final inspection before placing restorative materials.

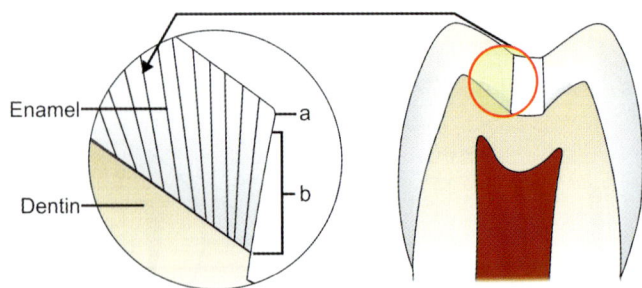

Figures 7.59A and B: At the margins, all the enamel walls should have full length rods supported by dentin

The debridement of the preparation serves the following objectives:

- *Cleaning of preparation walls, floors and margins from enamel and dentin chips resulting during tooth preparation:* Remove all the debris from the preparation, especially on the margins, otherwise deposits left on them consequently dissolve, resulting in microleakage which further can result in secondary caries. Cleaning of preparation can be done by using warm water. Immovable particles of debris can be removed with the help of a small cotton pellet dampened with water or hydrogen peroxide.
- *Drying the tooth preparation before insertion of the restorative materials:* It can be done using air, dry cotton pellets and commercial cleaners. It is important that tooth is not dehydrated by overuse of air or hot air.
- *Sterilization of preparation walls using very mild alcohol free disinfectant:* Use of mild disinfectant in tooth preparation serves the purpose of disinfection.

Noy's structural requirements of finished tooth preparation

- Tooth preparation should rest on sound dentin
- Enamel rods of cavosurface angle should have their inner ends resting on sound dentin
- Outer ends of enamel rods of cavosurface angle should rest on sound dentin with their outer ends to be covered with restorative material.
- Cavosurface angle should be properly trimmed or bevelled so as to prevent harm to tooth structure or restoration.

AIR ABRASION/KINETIC TOOTH PREPARATION

Air abrasion technique involves high energy sandblasting of tooth surface.

It is also called as advanced particle beam technology or microabrasion. This technique was given by Dr Robert Black in 1943. This system is used as an adjunct not as replacement for handpiece. The first air abrasion system was Airdent abrasion unit (SS white company). It was heavy weight (more than 100 pounds) but had small tip to deliver a beam of aluminium oxide particles. Later on many improvements occurred in air abrasion devices like the newer air abrasion devices come in précised designsand have control on flow of abrasive particles with narrow beam.

Technique

Basically in an air abrasion technique, the abrasive particles are emitted in a well defined sharply focused beam to the target.

There are many factors which come into play while evaluating efficiency of air abrasive technology.

- Distance between tip and the tooth.
- *Particle energy:* This is guarded by air pressure.
- *Intensity of beam:* This depends on multiple factors like type of particles, size of nozzle, size of particles, design of nozzle.
- Angle of beam.
- Commonly used particle size is 25 to 30 μ with 60 to 120 pounds per square inch pressure.

Advantages of air abrasion

- Precise and rapid enamel cutting
- Produces less heat and pressure
- Generate less vibrations
- Patient requiring air abrasion do not need local anesthesia
- Less discomfort to patient
- No sound production while tooth preparation.

Disadvantages of air abrasion

- Large and heavy air abrasive units
- Over preparation of tooth can occur
- High cost of the equipment
- Loss of tactile sense
- Can result in soft tissue injury like gingival hemorrhage
- If handled improperly, can damage sound tooth structure
- Inhalation of particles can cause systemic problems.

Uses of Air Abrasion Technology

- *Treatment of pits and fissures:* Using air abrasion technology, deep pits and fissures can be widened and deepened.
- *Diagnosis of pits and fissure caries:* By targeting the particle beam, the discolored portion of tooth can be removed and restored if surface underneath, it is carious. If it is sound, tooth is restored with a sealant.
- It can be used as an adjunct to acid etching.
- Cementation of crown is facilitated by air abrasion technology as sandblasting of internal surface of crown can result in increased adhesion.
- Air abrasion can also be used for removal of debris and repair of defective composite restorations.

So, we have seen the basic steps in a tooth preparation, though specific tooth preparation techniques have been discussed in other chapters. One of the most important thing before carrying tooth preparation is assessment of factors like extent of caries, aesthetics, occlusion, age of patient, operator skill, anatomy of tooth, pulp protection, so as to have a successful long-term restoration which is functionally acceptable with optimal aesthetics and in harmony with occlusion.

Key Points

- Tooth preparation is a mechanical alteration of a defective, injured or diseased tooth in order to best receive a restorative material which will re-establish the healthy state of the tooth including aesthetics correction when indicated along with normal form and function.
- A pulpal wall is an internal wall that is towards the pulp and covering the pulp. It may be both vertical and perpendicular to the long axis of tooth.
- Cavosurface angle is formed by the junction of a prepared tooth surface wall and external surface of the tooth. The acute junction is referred to as preparation margin or cavosurface margin.
- Tooth preparations may be classified according to the location where the carious lesion initiates.
- Smooth surface lesions can be found in all teeth on the proximal surfaces, and gingival one-third of the facial and lingual surfaces.
- Class I is the only pit and fissure preparation whereas rest are smooth surface preparations.
- Class I–Pit and fissure preparations occur on the occlusal surfaces of premolars and molars, the occlusal two-third of buccal and lingual surface of molars, lingual surface of incisors and any other abnormal position.
- Class II preparations occur on the proximal surface of premolars and molars.
- Class III preparations occur on the proximal surface of anterior teeth not involving the incisal angle.
- Class IV preparations occur on the proximal surface of anterior teeth involving the incisal angle.
- Class V preparations are present on gingival third of facial and lingual surfaces of all teeth.
- Class VI (Given by Simon) preparations are present on incisal edges of anterior and cusp tips of posterior teeth without involving any other surface.
- Earlier when the affected tooth was prepared because of caries, cutting of tooth was referred to as cavity preparation. But nowadays many indications other than caries lead to preparation of the tooth. Hence, the term cavity preparation has been replaced by tooth preparation.
- "Extension for prevention (given by Black) means the placing the margins of preparations at areas that would be cleaned by the excursions of food during chewing. It is done with the objective of preventing the recurrence of caries at the margins of fillings where the recurrence of decay is most commonly seen.
- External outline form should consist of smooth curves, straight lines and rounded line and point angles. Sharp and irregular projection of tooth tissue should be removed because they are not only fragile but also make good adaptation of restorative material to tooth preparation walls and margins difficult.
- Internal outline form includes the relationship of occlusal walls from cavosurface angle to the pulpal floor.
- Enameloplasty is the careful removal of sharp and irregular enamel margins of the enamel surface by 'rounding' or 'saucering' it and converting it into a smooth groove making it self-cleansable, finishable and allowing conservative placement of margins.
- Primary resistance form is that shape and placement of preparation walls to best enables both the tooth and restoration to withstand, without fracture the stresses of masticatory forces delivered principally along long axis of the tooth.
- Factors affecting resistance form are amount of occlusal stresses, type of restoration material and amount of remaining tooth structure.
- Primary retention form is that form, shape and configuration of the tooth preparation that resists the displacement or removal of restoration from the preparation under lifting and tipping masticatory forces.
- In amalgam, the retention is achieved by providing occlusal convergence (about 2 to 5%), slight undercut in dentin near the pulpal wall, conserving the marginal ridges and by providing occlusal dovetail.
- In cast metals, the retention is achieved by close parallelism of the opposing walls with slight occlusal divergence, occlusal dovetail, and incorporating secondary retention features.
- In composites, the retention is achieved by enamel bevels and micromechanical bonding between the etched and primed prepared tooth structure and the composite resin.
- The convenience form is that form which facilitates and provides adequate visibility, accessibility and ease of operation during preparation and restoration of the tooth.
- The remaining carious portion should be removed only after the initial tooth preparation has been completed because it allows optimal visibility and convenience form for removal of remaining carious lesion.
- Coves are small conical depressions prepared in healthy dentin to provide additional retention.
- Slots or internal boxes are 1.0 to 1.5 mm deep box like grooves prepared in dentin to increase the surface area. These are prepared in occlusal box, buccoaxial, linguoaxial and gingival walls.
- Skirts are prepared for providing additional retention in cast restorations. They increase the total surface area of the preparation. Skirts can be prepared on one to all

four sides of the preparation depending upon the required retention.

- Amalgampins are vertical posts of amalgam anchored in dentin. Dentin chamber is prepared by using inverted cone bur on gingival floor 0.5 mm in dentin with 1 mm to 2 mm depth and 0.5 to 1mm width.

- Air abrasion technique (advanced particle beam technology or microabrasion) involves high energy sandblasting of tooth surface. Basically in this technique, the abrasion particles are emitted in a well defined sharply focused beam to the target. Commonly used particle size is 25 to 30 µ with 60 to 120 pounds per square inch pressure.

QUESTIONS

1. Define tooth preparation. What are indications of tooth preparation?
2. Write short notes on:
   a. Primary resistance form
   b. Primary retention form
   c. Air abrasion/kinetic tooth preparation
   d. Enameloplasty
   e. Secondary resistance and retention forms
   f. Grooves and coves
   g. Slots or internal boxes
3. Write fundamentals of tooth preparation.

BIBLIOGRAPHY

1. Akimoto N, et al. Biocompatibility of clearfil liner bond 2 and clearfil AP-X systems on nonexposed and exposed primate teeth. Quintessence Int. 1998;29:177-88.
2. Ben-Amar A. Reduction of microleakage around new amalgam restorations. J Am Dent Assoc. 1989;119:725.
3. Boyer DB, Roth L. Fracture resistance of teeth with bonded amalgams. Am J Dent. 1994;7:91-4.
4. Bronner FJ. Mechanical, physiological, and pathological aspects of operative procedures. Dent Cosmos. 1931;73:577.
5. Cantwell KR, et al. Cavity finish with high-speed handpieces. Dent Prog. 1960;1:42.
6. Charbeneau GT, Peyton FA: Some effects of cavity instrumentation on the adaptation of gold castings and amalgam. J Prosthet Dent. 1958;8:514.
7. Frank AL. Protective coronal coverage of the pulpless tooth. J Am Dent Assoc. 1959;59:895.
8. Fusayama T. Two layers of carious dentin: diagnosis and treatment. Oper Dent. 1979;4:63-70.
9. Going RE Massler M. Influence of cavity liners under amalgam restorations on penetration by radioactive isotopes. J Prosthet Dent. 1961;11:298.
10. Going RE. Status report on cement bases, cavity liners varnishes, primers and cleaners. J Am Dent Assoc. 1972;85:654.
11. Hansen EK, Asmussen E. Improved efficacy of dentin-bonding agents. Eur J Oral Sci. 1997;105:434-9.
12. Hosoda H, Fusayama T. A tooth substance saving restorative technique. Int Dent J; 1984.pp.36.
13. Hudson P. Conservative treatment of the class I lesion: a new paradigm for dentistry. J Am Dent Assoc. 2004;135:760-3.
14. Hunt PR. Rational cavity design principals. J Esthe Dent. 1994;6:245.
15. Jokstad A, Mjor IA. Cavity designs for class II amalgam restorations. A literature review and a suggested system for evaluation. Acta Odontol Scand. 1987;45:257.
16. Kanca J III. Replacement of a fractured incisor fragment over pulpal exposure: a long-term case report. Quintessence Int. 1996;27:829-32.
17. Lee WC, Eakle WS. Possible role of tensile stress in the etiology of cervical erosive lesions of teeth. J Prosthet Dent. 1984;52:374-80.
18. Mach Z, et al. The integrity of bonded amalgam restorations: a clinical evaluation after five years. J Am Dent Assoc. 2002;133:460-7.
19. Mahler DB, Terkla LG. Analysis of stress in dental structures. DCNA. 1958;789.
20. Markley MR. Restorations of silver amalgam. J Am Dent Assoc. 1951;43:133.
21. Massler M, Barber TK. Action of amalgam on dentin. J Am Dent Assoc. 1951;43:133.
22. Menegale CM, Swartz ML, Phillips RW. Adaptations of restorative materials as influenced by the roughness of cavity walls. Dent Res. 1960;39:825.
23. Mount GJ, Ngo H. Minimal intervention: Advanced lesions. Quint Int. 2000;31:621.
24. Nelson RJ, et al. Fluid exchange at the margins of dental restorations. J Am Dent Assoc. 1962;44:288.
25. Osborne JW, Summit JB. Extension for prevention. Is it relevant today? Am J Dent. 1998;11:189.
26. Re GJ, Pruitt D, Childers JM, Norling BK. Effect of mandibular molar anatomy on the buccal class I cavity preparation. J Dent Res. 1983;62:997.
27. Ritter AV, Swift EJ. Current restorative concepts of pulp protection. Endod Topics. 2003;5:41-8.
28. Shillinburg HTJr. Conservative preparations for cast restorations. DCNA. 1976;20:259.
29. Simonsen RJ. Preventive resin restoration. Quintessence Int. 1978;9:69-76.

30. Sockwell CL. Dental handpieces and rotary cutting instruments. Dent Clin North Am. 1971;15:219.

31. Sockwell CL. Dental handpieces and rotary cutting instruments. DCNA. 1971;15:219.

32. Street EV. Effects of various instruments on enamel walls. J Am Dent Assoc. 1953;46:274.

33. Swartz ML, et al. Role of cavity varnishes and bases in the penetration of cement constituents through tooth structure. J Prosthet Dent. 1966;16:963.

34. Terkla LG, et al. Analysis of amalgam cavity design. J Prosthet Dent. 1973;29:204.

35. Terklla LG, Mahler DB, Eysden JV. Analysis of amalgam cavity design. JPD. 1973;29:204.

36. Voth ED, et al. Effect of a resin-modified glass ionomer liner on volumetric polymerization shrinkage of various composites. Dent Mater. 1998;14:417-23.

37. Voth ED, et al. Thermal diffusion through amalgam and various lines. J Dent Res. 1966;45:1184.

38. Woolsey GD, Matich JA. The effect of grooves on the resistance form of cast restoration. JADA. 1978;97:978.

39. Zidan O, Abdel-Keriem U. The effect of amalgam bonding on the stiffness of teeth weakened by cavity preparation. Dent Mater. 2003;19:680-5.

Patient Evaluation, Diagnosis and Treatment Planning

8

CHAPTER

Chapter Outline

INTRODUCTION

To provide best treatment and patient satisfaction, thorough clinical history, examination and diagnostic aids are required. Since dental problems are not alike in two patients, thorough examination, evaluation and diagnosis of an individual patient guides the effective treatment plan.

Diagnosis is defined as utilization of scientific knowledge for identifying a diseased process and to differentiate it from other disease process. In other words, literal meaning of diagnosis is determination and judgment of variations from the normal.

It is the procedure of accepting a patient, recognizing that he/she has a problem, determining the cause of problem and developing a treatment plan which would solve the problem. There are various diagnostic tools of diagnosis. Out of all these, art of listening is most important. It also establishes patient-doctor rapport, understanding and trust.

Although diagnostic testing of some common complaints may produce classic results but sometimes tests may produce wrong results, which need to be carefully interpreted by clinician.

PATIENT EVALUATION

The diagnostic process actually consists of four steps:

1. *First step*: Assemble all the available facts gathered from chief complaints, medical and dental history, diagnostic tests and investigations.
2. *Second step*: Analyze and interpret the assembled clues to reach the tentative or provisional diagnosis.
3. *Third step*: Make differential diagnosis of all possible diseases which are consistent with signs, symptoms and test results gathered.
4. *Fourth step*: Select the closest, possible choice.

The importance of making an accurate diagnosis cannot be overlooked. Many a times even after applying all the knowledge, experience and diagnostic tests, a satisfactory explanation for patient's symptoms is not determined. In many cases, nonodontogenic etiology is also seen as a source of chief complaint. To avoid irrelevant information and to prevent errors of omission in clinical tests, the clinician should establish a routine for examination, consisting of chief complaint, past medical and dental history and any other relevant information in the form of case history.

Case History

The purpose of case history is to discover whether patient has any general or local condition that might alter the normal course of treatment. As with all courses of treatment, a comprehensive medical and previous dental history should be recorded. In addition, a description of the patient's symptoms in his or her own words should be noted.

Chief Complaint

The chief complaint of the patient is very important as the overall treatment plan revolves around the chief complaint. It consists of information which promoted patient to visit a clinician. Symptoms are phenomenon or signs of deviation from normal and are indicative of illness. The form of notation should be in patient's own words.

History of Present Illness

Once the patient completes information about his/her chief complaint, a report is made which provides more descriptive analysis about this initial information. It should include signs and symptoms, duration, intensity of pain, relieving and exaggerating factors, etc. Examples of type of the questions which may be asked by the clinician in recording the patient's complaints are as below:

- How long have you had the pain?
- Do you know which tooth it is?
- What initiates pain?
- How would you describe the pain?
  - Quality—Dull, Sharp, throbbing, constant
  - Location—Localized, diffuse, referred, radiating
  - Duration—Seconds, minutes, hours, constant
  - Onset—Stimulation required, intermittent, spontaneous
  - Initiated—Cold, heat, palpation, percussion
  - Relieved—Cold, heat, any medications, sleep

In other words, history of present illness should indicate severity and urgency of the problem.

If a chief complaint is toothache but symptoms are too vague to establish a diagnosis, then analgesics should be prescribed to help the patient in tolerating the pain until the toothache localizes.

A history of pain which persists without exacerbation may indicate problem of nonodontogenic origins. The most common toothache may arise from either pulp or periodontal ligament. Pulpal pain can be sharp piercing if A-delta fibers are stimulated. Dull, boring or throbbing pain occurs if there is stimulation of C-fibers. Pulp vitality tests are usually done to reach the most probable diagnosis. If pain is from periodontal ligament, the tooth will be sensitive to percussion, chewing and palpation. Another hint that pain is of pulpal origin is its intensity. Patient is asked to mark the imaginary ruler with grading ranging from 0 to 10 (**Fig. 8.1**).

0-No pain   10-Most painful

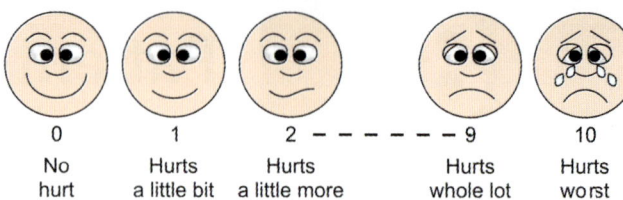

Figure 8.1: Mark the intensity of pain on an imaginary ruler with gradings 0-10

Mild to moderate pain can be of pulpal or periodontal origin but acute pain is commonly a reliable sign that pain is of pulpal origin. Localization of pain also tells origin of pain since pulp does not contain proprioceptive fibers; it is difficult for patient to localize the pain unless it reaches the periodontal ligament.

Past Dental History

This helps to know any previous dental experience, and past restorations.

Medical History

There are no medical conditions which specifically contraindicate operative treatment, but there are several which require special care.

For a proper medical history, importance should be given to the following
➡ Allergies and medications
➡ Communicable diseases
➡ Systemic diseases
➡ Physiological changes associated with aging.

Allergies or Medication

Clinician must be informed about any allergy related to patient. For example, if the patient is allergic to local anesthetic during dental treatment, he/she may go in the state of anaphylactic shock. Allergic reactions may occur in the form of itching, rashes, swellings, gingivitis, ulcers, etc.

The effect of various medicaments should also be evaluated as they can alter the salivary flow, interfere with the metabolism of the other drugs and may cause the pigmentation of oral soft tissues. For example, tricyclic antidepressants make the patient sensitive to epinephrine and use of antiepileptic agents may cause gingival hypertrophy.

Communicable Diseases

Before initiating any treatment, the clinician should check the presence of any communicable disease. The evaluation of communicable diseases should be done cautiously as these can affect the management of the patient and can be transmissible. Since immunocompromised patients are more prone to suffer from various bacterial, fungal and viral infections due to suppression of immune response, they should be evaluated thoroughly. Clinician should seriously assess the condition of a patient because of increasing incidence of AIDS and hepatitis B and C, so that proper measures can be taken.

Systemic Diseases

Patients with valvular defects or heart murmurs are at high risk for development of bacterial endocarditis after surgical and dental procedures, therefore, prophylactic antibiotic coverage should be given to such patients before initiating dental treatment. A screening test should be done to evaluate the status of the diseased person. For this, blood pressure and the patient's pulse should be recorded.

The following types of patients require special examination for systemic diseases.
- Patients with oral lesions due to presence of foci of infection in any other part of the body.
- Patients suffering from systemic complications due to immunocompromised conditions.
- Patients manifesting oral lesions due to reflex neurosis in other parts.
- Patients who manifest systemic disturbances of an inflammatory or infective type which may show oral manifestations.

Scully and **Cawson** have given a checklist of medical conditions which need a special care.

Checklist for medical history (Scully and Cawson)
➡ Anemia
➡ Bleeding disorders
➡ Cardiorespiratory disorders
➡ Drug treatment and allergies
➡ Endocrine disease
➡ Fits and faints
➡ Gastrointestinal disorders
➡ Hospital admissions and attendance
➡ Infections
➡ Jaundice
➡ Kidney disease
➡ Likelihood of pregnancy or pregnant itself.

Physiological Changes Associated with Aging

Physiological changes associated with aging should be examined properly and should not be confused with the pathological changes. Changes in oral cavity occurring due to aging are as follows:

- Attrition, abrasion and wear of proximal surfaces (**Fig. 8.2**)
- Extrinsic staining
- Edematous gingivae
- Diminished salivary flow
- Gingival recession.

Social Status of the Patient

Social status of the patient is evaluated to know his attitudes, expectations, priorities, education, and habits. This helps in planning the line of treatment according to expectations of the patient.

EXAMINATION AND DIAGNOSIS

- *Clinical examination*: It includes both extraoral and intraoral examination
- *Intraoral examination*: It includes the examination of soft and hard tissue.

Clinical Examination

Clinical examination of the patient should be done thoroughly and in proper sequence.

Following sequence is followed during clinical examinations
➡ Inspection
➡ Palpation
➡ Percussion
➡ Auscultation
➡ Exploration.

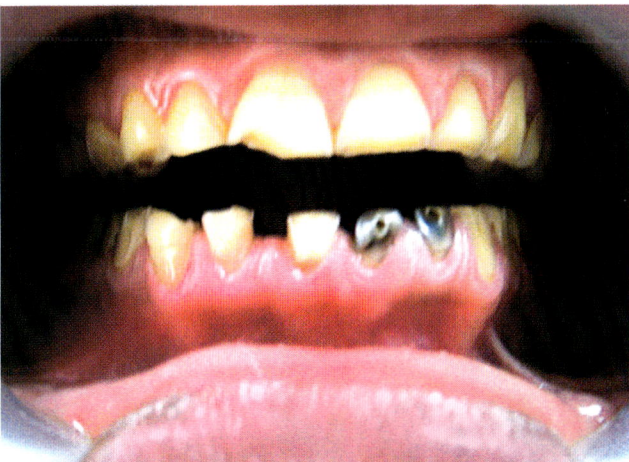

Figure 8.2: Generalized attrition of teeth

Inspection

Extraoral examination begins as soon as patient enters in the clinic and patient should be observed for unusual gait and habits. which may suggest underlying systemic disease, drug or alcohol abuse if any.

Patient should be looked for any facial asymmetry or distention of tissues. Dentist must examine any localized swelling, presence of bruises, abrasions, scars or any other signs of trauma if present. Patient should be looked for size of pupils which may signify systemic disease, premeditation or fear.

Before conducting intraoral examination check the degree of mouth opening. For a normal patient, it should be at least two fingers (**Fig. 8.3**). During intraoral examination, look at the following structures systematically

- The buccal, labial and alveolar mucosa
- The hard and soft palate
- The floor of the mouth and tongue
- The retromolar region
- The posterior pharyngeal wall and facial pillars
- The salivary gland and orifices.

After examining this, *general dental state* should be recorded, which include

- Oral hygiene status
- Amount and quality of restorative work
- Prevalence of caries
- Missing tooth
- Presence of soft or hard swelling
- Periodontal status
- Presence of any sinus tracts
- Discolored teeth
- Tooth wear and facets.

If patient's chief complaint includes symptoms which occur following specific events like chewing and drinking cold liquids, then specific intraoral examination should include tests which reproduce these symptoms. This will help in establishing the proper diagnosis.

Palpation

After extraoral examination of head and neck region, one should go for extraoral palpation by use of fingers. If any localized swelling is present, then look for

- Local rise in temperature
- Tenderness
- Extent of lesion
- Induration
- Fixation to underlying tissues, etc.

Palpation of salivary glands should be done extraorally. Submandibular gland should be differentiated from lymph nodes in the submandibular region by bimanual palpation (**Fig. 8.4**).

Palpation of TMJ can be done by standing in front of the patient and placing the index fingers in the preauricular region. The patient is asked to open the mouth and perform lateral excursion to notice (**Fig. 8.5**).

- Any restricted movement
- Deviation in movement
- Jerky movement
- Clicking
- Locking or crepitus.

Palpation of lymph nodes should be done to note any lymph node enlargement, tenderness, mobility and consistency (**Fig. 8.6**). The lymph nodes frequently palpated are preauricular, submandibular, submental and cervical.

Intraoral palpation is done using digital pressure to check any tenderness in soft tissue overlying suspected tooth (**Fig. 8.7**). Sensitivity may indicate inflammation in periodontal ligament surrounding the affected tooth.

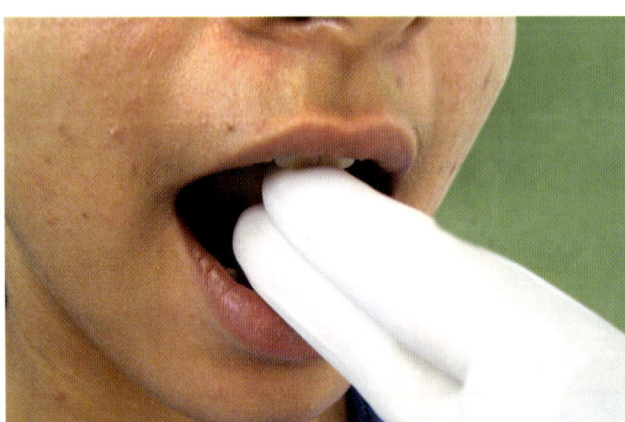

Figure 8.3: Minimum mouth opening should be two fingers for a normal patient

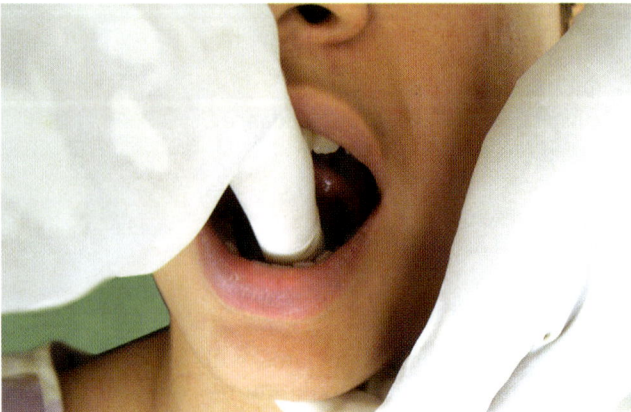

Figure 8.4: Palpation of submandibular salivary glands

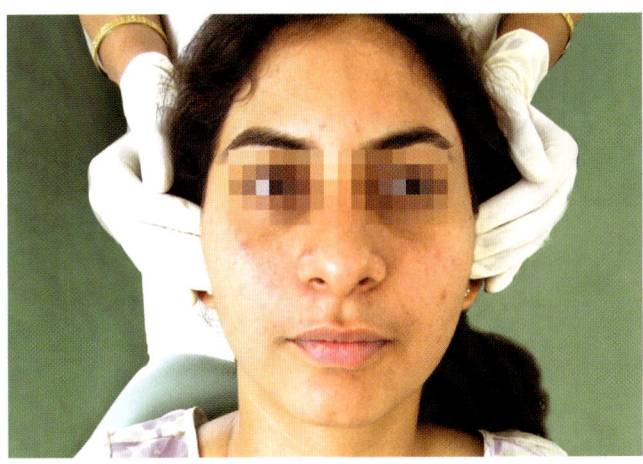

Figure 8.5: Palpation of TMJ

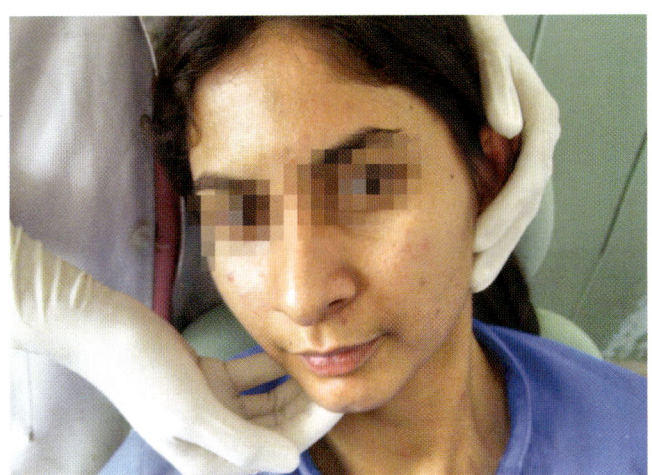

Figure 8.6: Palpation of lymph nodes

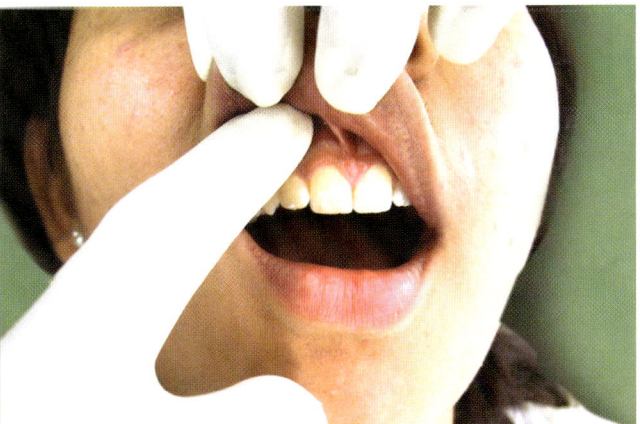

Figure 8.7: Intraoral palpation of suspected tooth is done by using digital pressure of overlying soft tissues

Further palpation can tell any other information about fluctuation or fixation or induration of soft tissue, if any.

Percussion

Percussion gives information about the periodontal status of the tooth.

Percussion of tooth indicates inflammation in periodontal ligament which could be due to trauma, sinusitis and/or PDL disease.

Percussion can be carried out by gentle tapping with gloved finger (**Fig. 8.8**) or blunt handle of mouth mirror (**Fig. 8.9**). Each tooth should be percussed on all the surfaces of tooth until the patient is able to localize the tooth with pain. Degree of response to percussion is directly proportional to degree of inflammation.

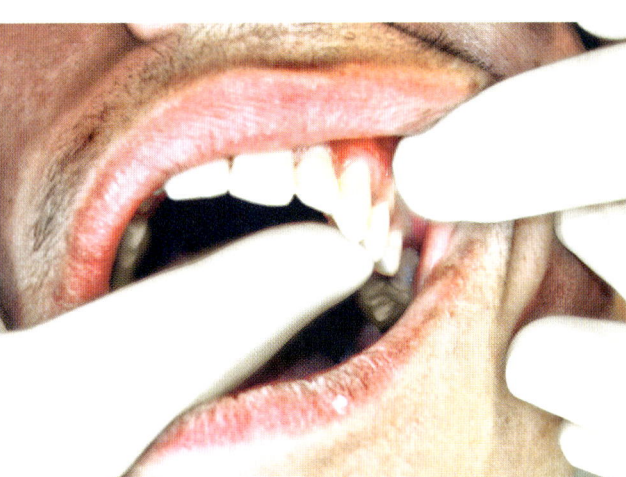

Figure 8.8: Percussion of tooth by tapping with gloved finger

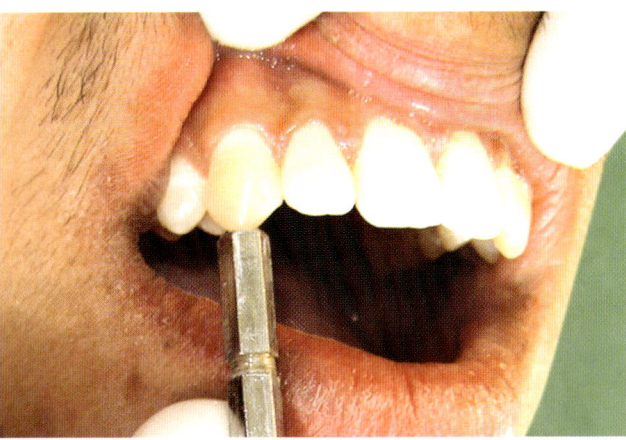

Figure 8.9: Percussion of tooth using blunt end of the instrument

Auscultation

Auscultation is not of much importance, except in some cases. For example, auscultation of TMJ to check the clicking sound.

Exploration

In this, clinical examination of the tooth is done by the use of explorer or probe.

Periodontal Evaluation

Periodontal condition can be assessed by palpation, percussion, mobility of tooth and probing (**Fig. 8.10**). Periodontal examination shows change in color, contour, form, density, level of attachment and bleeding tendency. The depth of gingival sulcus is determined by systemic probing using a periodontal probe. A sulcus depth greater than 3 mm and the sites that bleed upon probing should be recorded in the patient's chart. The presence of pocket may also indicate periodontal disease. If necessary radiographs should be taken at different angulations to assess bone levels.

The presence of plaque, supra- and subgingival calculus should also be checked so that restorations can be contoured accurately to maintain proper periodontal health.

The mobility of a tooth is tested by placing a finger (**Fig. 8.11**) or blunt end of the instrument (**Fig. 8.12**) on either side of the crown and pushing it and assessing any movement with other finger.

Grading of mobility
⇢ Slight (normal)
⇢ Moderate mobility within a range of 1 mm.
⇢ Extensive movement (more than 1 mm) in mesiodistal or lateral direction combined with vertical displacement in alveolus.

Evaluation of Carious Lesions

Dental caries is diagnosed by the following (**Fig. 8.13**).
- Visual changes in tooth surface
- Tactile sensation while using explorer
- Radiography—Definite radiolucency indicating a break in the continuity of enamel is carious enamel (**Fig. 8.14**)
- Transillumination.

A translucency producing a characteristic shadow on the proximal surface indicates presence of caries.

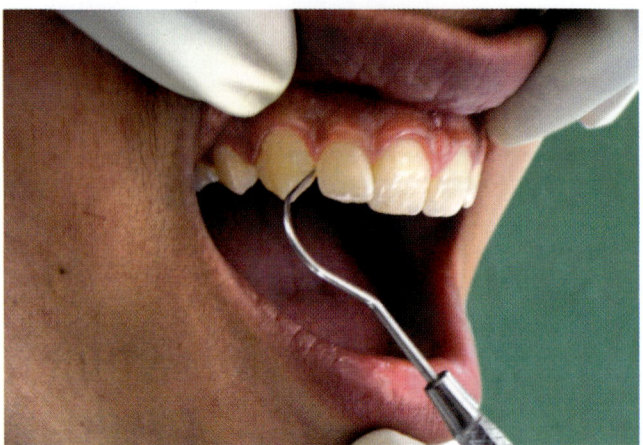

Figure 8.10: Probing of teeth can assess periodontal condition

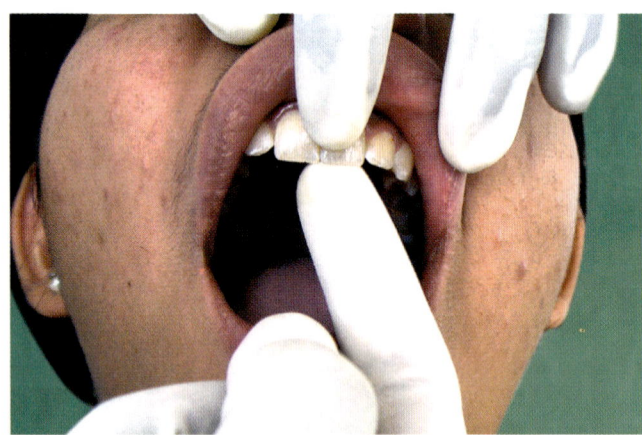

Figure 8.11: To check mobility of tooth using digital pressure

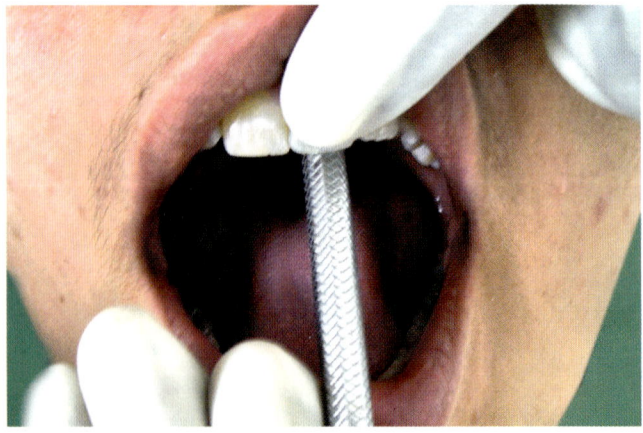

Figure 8.12: Checking mobility of tooth using blunt end of an instrument

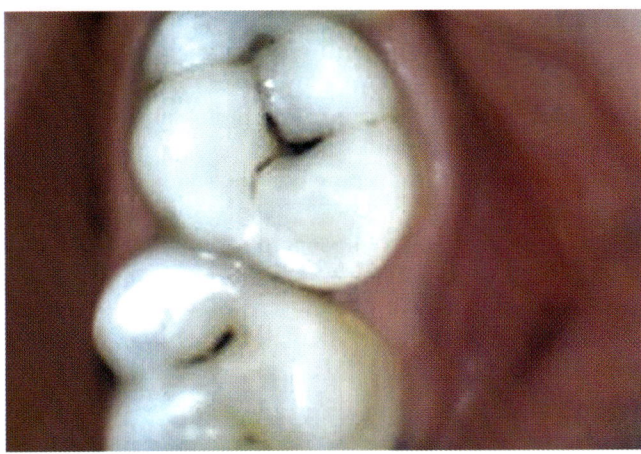

Figure 8.13: Carious teeth

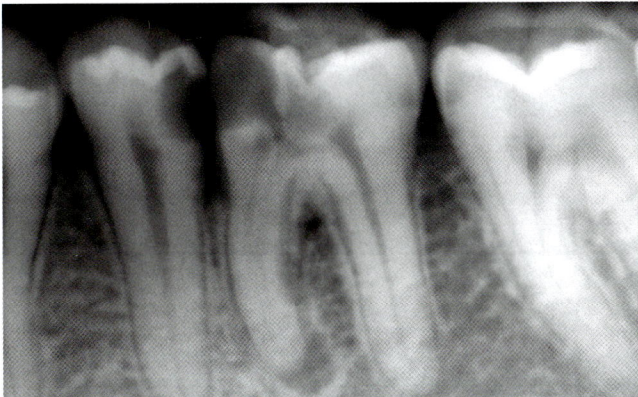

Figure 8.14: Radiograph showing dental caries

Evaluation of Existing Restorations

It should be done to know their life. It can be done by visual examination, tactile and clinical examination using radiographs. On clinical evaluation of restorations, the following conditions may be observed.

- *Proximal overhangs*: Proximal restoration is evaluated by moving the explorer back and forth across it. If the explorer stops at the junction and then moves onto the restoration, an overhang is present. This should be corrected, as it can result in the inflammation of the adjacent soft tissues.
- *Marginal gap or ditching:* It is the deterioration of the restoration-tooth interface on occlusal surfaces as a result of wear or fracture. Shallow ditching, less than 0.5 mm deep usually requires patchwork repair. If ditch is too deep, restoration should be completely replaced.
- *Amalgam blues*: These are the discolored areas seen through the enamel in teeth. The bluish hue results either

from the leaching of corrosion products of amalgam into dentinal tubules or from the color of underlying amalgam as seen through translucent enamel.

- *Voids*: These also occur at the margins of amalgam restorations. If the void is at least 0.3 mm deep and is located in the gingival one-third of the tooth crown, then the restoration should be replaced.
- *Fracture line*: A fracture line that occurs in the isthmus region generally indicates fractured restoration which needs replacement.
- Recurrent caries at the margin of the restoration also indicate repair or replacement of the restoration.

Radiograph

The radiograph is one of the most important tools in making a diagnosis. Without radiograph, case selection, diagnosis and treatment would be impossible as it helps in examination of oral structure that would otherwise be unseen by naked eye.

Radiographs help to diagnose tooth related problems like caries, fractures, root canal treatment or any previous restorations, abnormal appearance of pulpal or peri-radicular tissues, periodontal diseases and the general bone pattern. Sometimes the normal anatomic landmarks like maxillary antrum, foraminas, tori, inferior alveolar canal, etc. may be confused with endodontic pathologies which may result in wrong diagnosis and thus improper treatment.

Periapical lesions of endodontic origin have following characteristic features
➡ Loss of lamina dura in the apical region
➡ Etiology of pulpal necrosis is generally apparent
➡ Radiolucency remains at the apex even if radiograph is taken by changing the angle.

Indications of dental radiographs
➡ Deep carious lesion
➡ Large restoration
➡ History of pain
➡ History of trauma
➡ History of root canal treatment
➡ History of periodontal therapy
➡ Family history of dental anomalies
➡ Impacted teeth
➡ Mobility of teeth
➡ Swelling in relation to teeth
➡ Presence of sinus/fistula
➡ Unusual tooth morphology
➡ Missing teeth with unknown reasons
➡ Growth abnormalities.

Disadvantages of radiographs

→ Radiograph gives two dimensional picture of a three dimensional object
→ Caries is always more extensive clinically when compared to radiograph

Radiographs help us in the following ways
- Establishing diagnosis
- Determining the prognosis of tooth
- Disclosing the presence and extent of caries (**Fig. 8.15**)
- Check the thickness of periodontal ligament
- To see presence or absence of lamina dura
- To look for any lesion associated with tooth (**Fig. 8.16**)
- To see the number, shape, length and pattern of the root canals (**Fig. 8.17**)

- To check any obstructions present in the pulp space
- To check any previous root canal treatment if done (**Fig. 8.18**)
- To look for presence of any intraradicular pins or posts (**Fig. 8.19**)
- To see the quality of previous root canal filling (**Figs 8.20 and 8.21**)
- To see any resorption present in the tooth
- To check the presence of calcification in pulp space (**Fig. 8.22**)
- To see rootend proximal structures
- Help in determining the working length, length of master gutta percha cone and quality of obturation (**Figs 8.23 to 8.25**).

Study Casts (Fig. 8.26)

Study casts are also used as adjunct to develop the proper treatment plan. Study casts help in study of the following
- To educate the patient
- Occlusal relationship
- Tilted or extruded teeth
- Cross bite

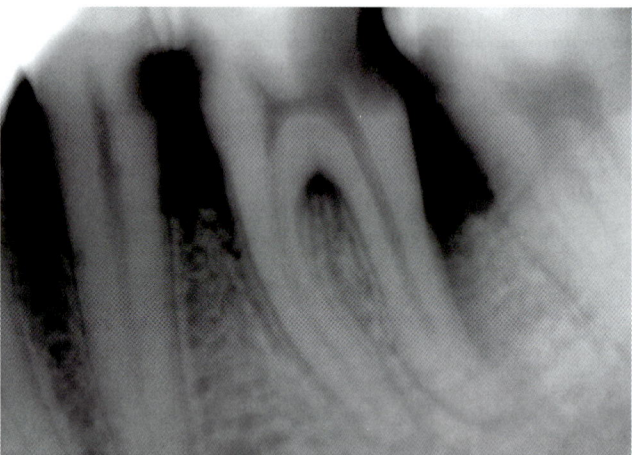

Figure 8.15: Radiograph showing extent of caries

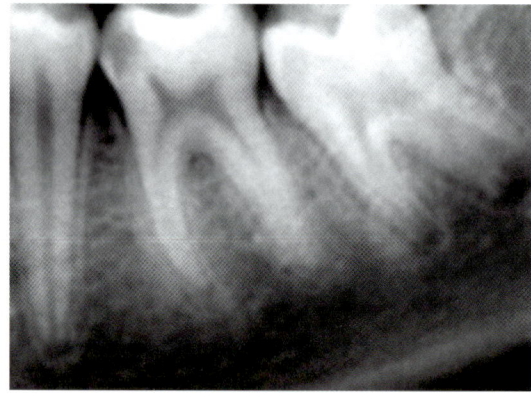

Figure 8.17: Radiograph showing number, shape and pattern of root canals

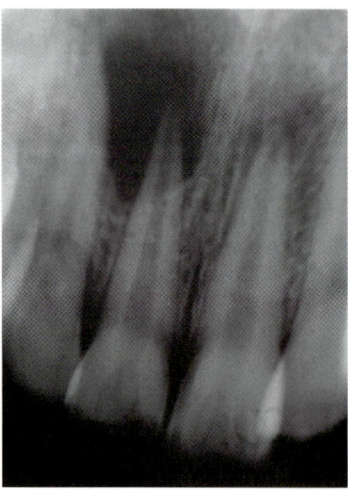

Figure 8.16: Radiograph showing periapical lesion associated with 11

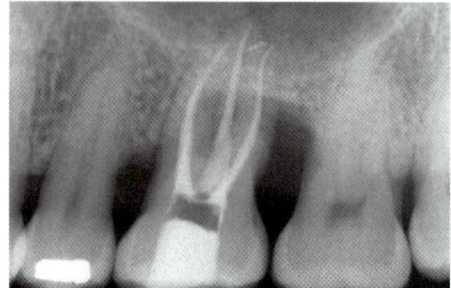

Figure 8.18: Radiograph showing obturation of 26

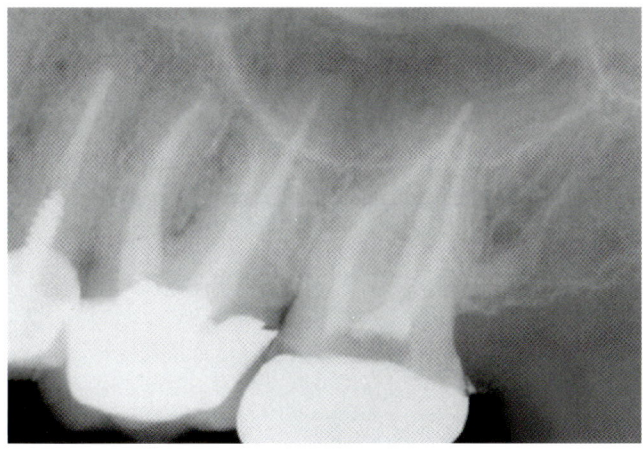

Figure 8.19: Radiograph showing teeth with post, gutta percha and crown

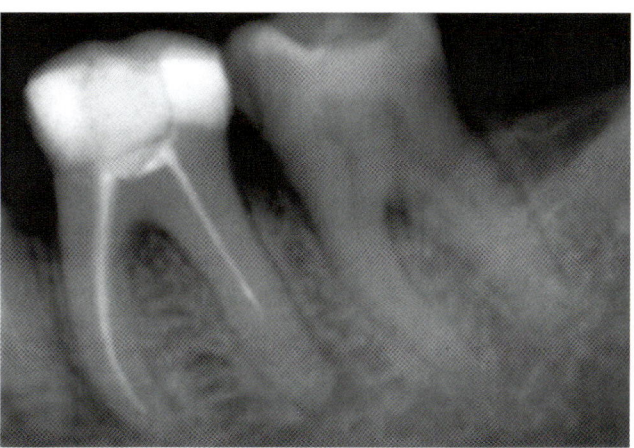

Figure 8.21: Radiograph showing quality of obturation in 46

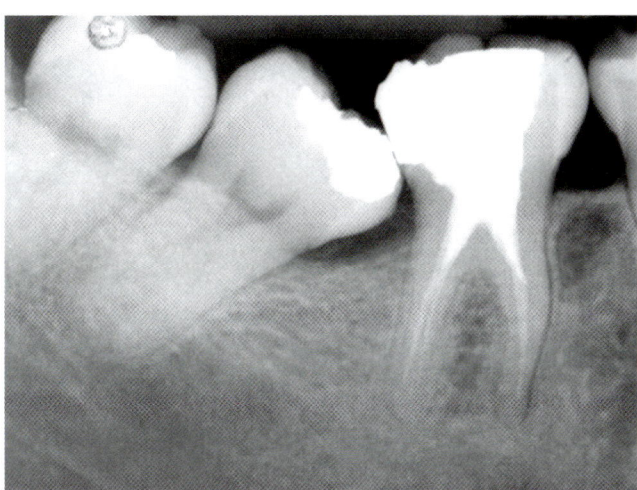

Figure 8.20: Radiograph showing improper obturation in 36

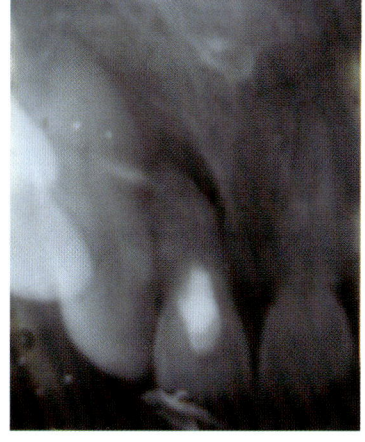

Figure 8.22: Radiograph showing calcified 21

- Plunger cusps
- Wear facet.

Laboratory Investigations

Most common laboratory investigations required are TLC, DLC, BT, CT, etc. including HIV test.

Occlusion Examination

Through occlusal examination one can identify the signs of occlusal trauma such as enamel cracks, tooth mobility and other occlusal abnormalities. During occlusal examination one should check presence of supraerupted teeth, spacing, fractured teeth and marginal ridge discrepancies. Teeth are examined for abnormal wear patterns, such as

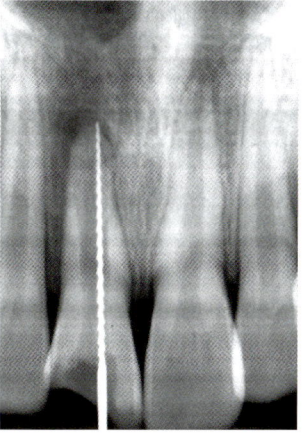

Figure 8.23: Working length X-ray

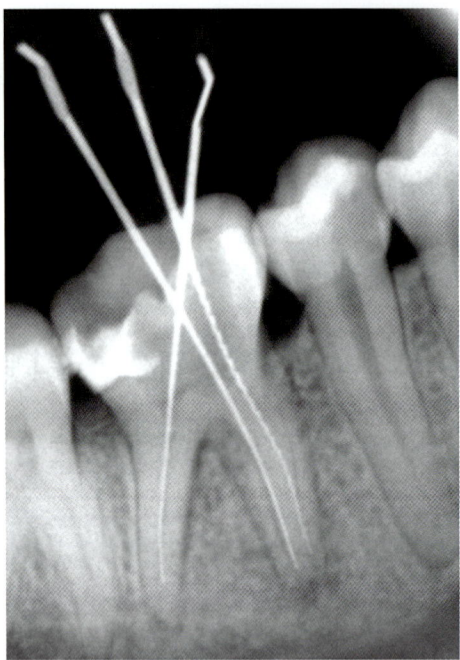

Figure 8.24: Working length X-ray while root canal treatment of 46

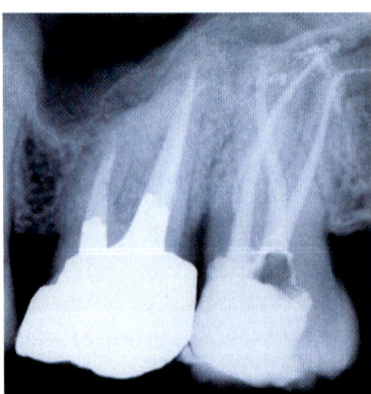

Figure 8.25: Radiograph showing obturation of 26 and 27

nocturnal bruxism or para-functional habits in addition to unfavorable occlusal relationships such as plunger cusp, which may result in food impaction. Dynamic relationship of teeth during forward, backward and lateral excursive movements should be done properly by articulating study casts. The occlusal examination should be considered for restorative treatment plan.

Pulp Vitality Tests

Pulp testing is often referred to as vitality testing. Pulp vitality tests play an important role in diagnosis because

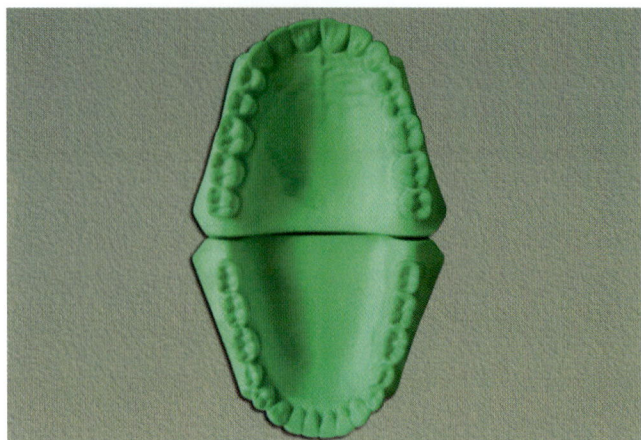

Figure 8.26: Study cast acts as adjunct in diagnosis

these tests not only determine the vitality of tooth but also the pathological status of pulp.

Various types of pulp tests performed are:
- Thermal test
  - Cold test
  - Heat test
- Electrical pulp testing
- Test cavity
- Anesthesia testing
- Bite test.

Thermal Test

In thermal test, the response of pulp to heat and cold is noted. The basic principle for pulp to respond to thermal stimuli is that patient reports sensation but it disappears immediately. Any other type of response, i.e. painful sensation even after removal of stimulus or no response are considered abnormal.

Cold test: The basic step of the pulp testing, i.e. individually isolating the tooth with rubber dam is mandatory with all types. Use of rubber dam is specially recommended when performing the test using the ice-sticks because melting ice will run on to adjacent teeth and gingivae resulting in false-positive result. Commonly used methods for performing cold pulp test are following
- Spraying cold air directed against the isolated tooth
- Application of cotton pellet saturated with ethyl chloride (**Fig. 8.27**)
- Spray of ethyl chloride after isolating tooth with rubber dam (The ethyl chloride evaporates so rapidly that it absorbs heat and thus, cools the tooth)
- Application of dry ice on the facial surface of the tooth after isolating the oral soft tissues and teeth with gauze or cotton roll. The frozen carbon dioxide (dry ice) is

available in the form of solid sticks having extremely low temperature. It should not come in contact with oral tissues because soft tissue burns may occur

- Wrap an ice piece in the wet gauze and apply to the tooth. The ice sticks can also be prepared by filling the discarded anesthetic carpules with water and placing them in refrigerator.

Heat test: It is most advantageous in the condition where patient's chief complaint is intense dental pain upon contact with any hot object or liquid. It can be performed using different techniques.

- The easiest method is to direct the *warm air* to the exposed surface of tooth and note the patient response.
- If a higher temperature is needed to illicit a response, then other options like heated stopping stick, hot burnisher, hot water, etc. can be used.

    Among these, *heated gutta percha stick* (**Fig. 8.28**) is most commonly used method for heat testing. In this method, tooth is coated with a lubricant such as petroleum jelly to prevent the gutta percha from adhering to tooth surface. The heated gutta percha is applied at the junction of cervical and middle third of facial surface of tooth and patient's response is noted.

- The other methods of heat testing is the use of *frictional heat produced by rotating polishing rubber disk* against the tooth surface.
- One more method of heat test is to *deliver warm water* from a syringe on to the isolated tooth to determine the pulpal response. This method is especially useful for teeth with porcelain or full-coverage restoration.

    The patient may respond to heat or cold test in following possible ways:

    Mild, transitory response to stimulation show normal pulp. Absence of response in combination with other tests indicates pulp necrosis. An exaggerated and lingering response indicate irreversible pulpitis.

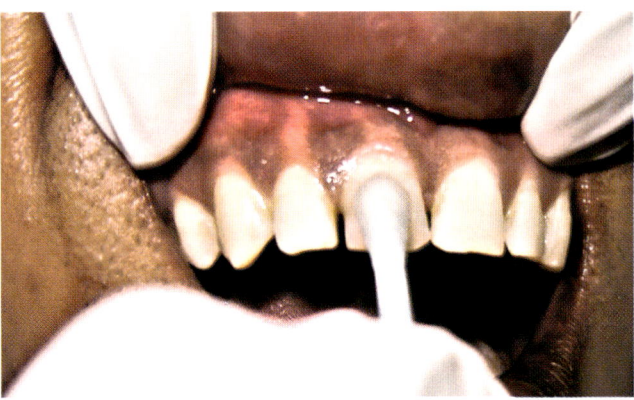

Figure 8.27: Cold test using a cotton pellet saturated with ethyl chloride

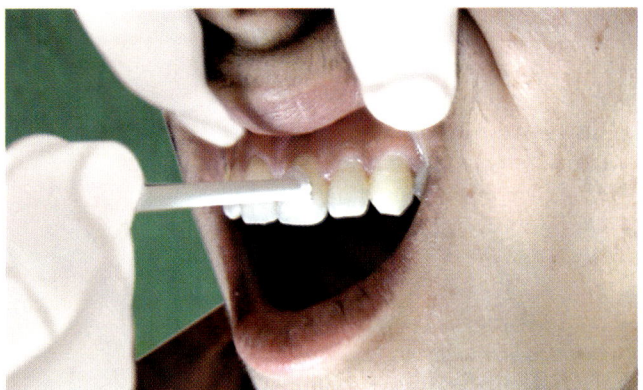

Figure 8.28: Heat test using heated gutta percha stick
[The preferred temperature for heat test is 150°F (65.5°C)]

There are certain *conditions which can give false negative response*, i.e. the tooth shows no response but the pulp could be possibly vital. These conditions can be

- Recently erupted teeth with immature apex
- Recent trauma—injury to nerve supply at the apical foramen or because of inflammatory exudates around the apex may interfere the nerve conduction
- Excessive calcifications may also interfere with the nerve conduction.

Electric Pulp Testing

Electric pulp tester is used for evaluation of condition of the pulp by electrical excitations of neural elements within the pulp. The pulp tester is an instrument which uses the gradations of electrical current to excite a response from the pulpal tissue. A positive response indicates the vitality of pulp. No response indicates nonvital pulp or pulpal necrosis.

Procedure

- Isolation of the teeth to be tested is one of the essential steps to avoid any type of false positive response.
- Apply an electrolyte on the tooth electrode and place it on the facial surface of tooth (**Fig. 8.29**).
- One should note that there should be a complete circuit from electrode through the tooth to the body of the patient and then back to the electrode. If gloves are not used, the circuit gets completed when clinician's finger contact with electrode and patient's cheeks. But with gloved hands, it can be done by placing patient's finger on metal electrode handle or by clipping a ground attachment onto the patient's lip.

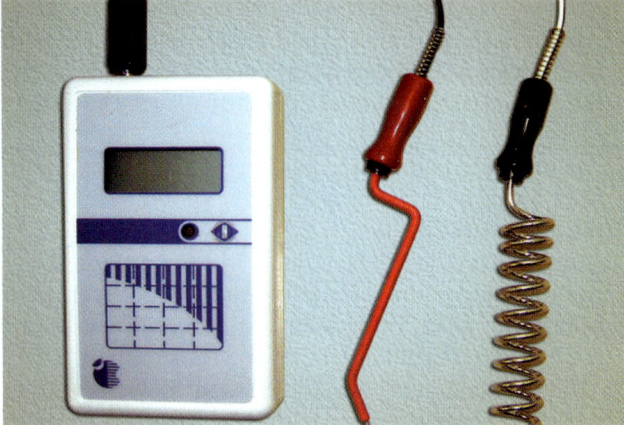

Figure 8.29: Electric pulp tester

- Once the circuit is complete, slowly increase the current and ask the patient to point out when the sensation occurs.
- Each tooth should be tested 2 to 3 times and the average reading is noted. If the vitality of a tooth is in question, the pulp tester should be used on the adjacent teeth and the contralateral tooth, as control.

Disadvantages of electric pulp testing: Following conditions can give rise to wrong results:
- In teeth with acute alveolar abscess.
- Electrode may contact gingival tissue thus giving the false positive response.
- In multirooted teeth, pulp may be vital in one or more root canals and necrosed in others, thus eliciting a false positive response.
- In certain conditions, it can give false negative response, for example:
  - Recently traumatized tooth
  - Recently erupted teeth with immature apex
  - Patients with high pain threshold
  - Calcified canals
  - Poor battery or electrical deficiency in plug of pulp testers
  - Teeth with extensive restorations or pulp protecting bases under restorations
  - Patients premedicated with analgesics or tranquilizers, etc.

Test Cavity

This method should be used only when all other test methods are inconclusive in results. Here, a test cavity is made with high speed number 1 or 2 round burs with appropriate air and water coolant. The patient is not anesthetized while performing this test. Patient is asked to respond if any painful sensation occurs during drilling. The sensitivity or the pain felt by the patient indicates pulp vitality. Here, the procedure is terminated by restoring the prepared cavity. If no pain is felt, cavity preparation may be continued until the pulp chamber is reached and later on endodontic therapy may be carried out.

Anesthesia Testing

When patient is not able to specify the site of pain and when other pulp testing techniques are inconclusive, the selective anesthesia may be used. The main objective of this test is to anesthetize a single tooth at a time until the pain is eliminated. It should be accomplished by using intraligamentary injection. Injection is administered to the most posterior tooth in the suspected quadrant. If the pain persists, even after tooth has been fully anesthetized, repeat the procedure to the next tooth mesial to it. It is continued until the pain disappears. If source of pain cannot be determined, repeat the same technique on the opposite arch.

Bite Test

This test helps if patient complains of pain on mastication. Tooth is sensitive to biting if pulpal necrosis has extended to the periodontal ligament space or if a crack is present in a tooth. In this, patient is asked to bite on a hard object such as cotton swab, tooth pick or orange wood stick with suspected tooth and the contralateral tooth (**Fig. 8.30**). Tooth sloth is another commercially available device for bite test. It has a small concave area on its top which is placed in contact with the cusp to be tested (**Fig. 8.31**). Patient is asked to bite on it. Pain on biting may indicate a fractured tooth.

Recent Advances in Pulp Vitality Testing

Recently available pulp vitality tests are
➡ Laser Doppler flowmetry (LDF)
➡ Pulp oximetry
➡ Dual wavelength spectrophotometry
➡ Measurement of temperature of tooth surface
➡ Transillumination with fiberoptic light
➡ Plethysmography
➡ Detection of interleukin—1-beta
➡ Xenon—133
➡ Hughes probeye camera
➡ Gas desaturation
➡ Radiolabeled microspheres
➡ Electromagnetic flowmetry.

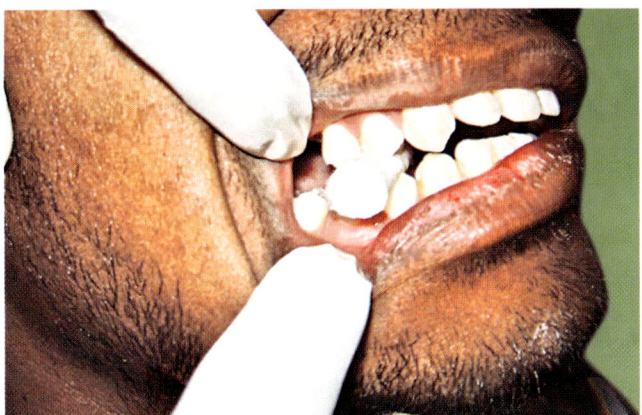

Figure 8.30: Patient is asked to bite on cotton swab or hard object for bite test

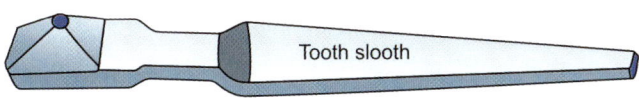

Figure 8.31: Tooth sloth

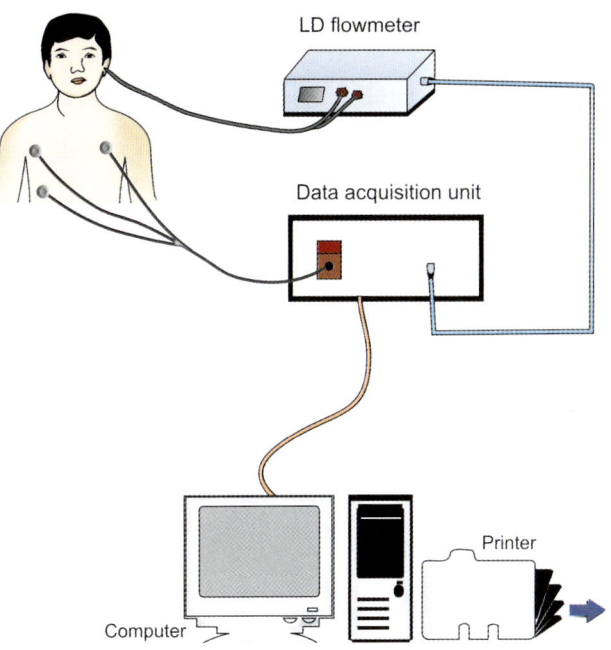

Figure 8.32: Working of LDF

Laser Doppler Flowmetry (LDF)

Laser Doppler flowmeter was developed by Tenland in 1982 and later by Holloway in 1983. The technique depends on Doppler principle in which a low power light from a monochromatic laser beam of known wavelength along a fiberoptic cable is directed to the tooth surface, where the light passes along the direction of enamel prisms and dentinal tubules to the pulp.

The light that contacts a moving object is Doppler shifted, and a portion of that light will be back scattered out of tooth into a photodetector. Some light is reflected off moving red blood cells in pulpal capillaries and as a consequence frequency broadened. The reflected light is passed back to the flowmeter where the frequency broadened light, together with laser light scattered from static tissue, is photodetected for strength of signal and pulsatility (**Fig. 8.32**).

Advantages of laser Doppler flowmetry

- An objective test
- Accurate to check vitality.

Disadvantages of laser Doppler flowmetry

- Medications used in cardiovascular diseases can affect the blood flow to pulp
- Requires higher technical skills
- Expensive.

Pulp Oximetry

The principle of this technology is based on modification of Beer's law and the absorbency characteristics of hemoglobin in red and infrared range.

Pulp oximetry is especially helpful in cases of traumatic injury to the teeth during which nerve supply of the pulp may be injured, but the blood supply stays intact.

Advantages of pulp oximetry

- Effective and objective method to evaluate pulp vitality
- Useful in cases of traumatic injuries where the blood supply remains intact but nerve supply is damaged
- Easy to reproduce pulp pulse readings
- Smaller and cheaper pulp oximeters are now available.

Disadvantage of pulp oximetry

Background absorption associated with venous blood.

Dual Wavelength Spectrophotometry

Dual wavelength spectrophotometry (DWLS) is a method independent of a pulsatile circulation. The presence of arterioles rather than arteries in the pulp and its rigid encapsulation by surrounding dentin and enamel make it difficult to detect a pulse in the pulp space. This method measures oxygenation changes in the capillary bed rather than the supply vessels and hence does not depend on a pulsatile blood flow.

Measurement of Surface Temperature of Tooth

This method is based on the assumption that if pulp becomes nonvital, the tooth no longer has internal blood supply, thus should exhibit a lower surface temperature than that of its vital counterparts.

Transillumination with Fiberoptic Light

It is a system of illumination whereby light is passed through a finely drawn glass or plastic fibers by a process known as total internal reflection.

By this method, a pulpless tooth that is not noticeably discolored may show a gross difference in translucency when a shadow produced on a mirror is compared to that of adjacent vital teeth.

TREATMENT PLANNING

Treatment planning consists of following phases:

- *Urgent phase*: In urgent phase, treatment mainly aims at providing the relief from symptoms, for example, incision and drainage of an abscess with severe pain and swelling, endodontic treatment of a case of acute irreversible pulpitis, etc.
- *Control phase*: In this phase, the treatment involves halting the progress of primary disease, i.e. caries or periodontal problem by removing etiological factors. Finally, the patient is made to understand the disease and its treatment which further increases his/her compliance to the treatment. This approach is beneficial for the long-term prevention of the dental caries and periodontal disease.
- *Holding phase*: It comes between control phase and the definitive phase. Thus, holding phase is a time between control phase and definitive phase that allows time for healing and analysis of inflammation. During this phase, patient is advised home care habits and motivated for further treatment. The initial treatment is re-evaluated before the definitive treatment.
- *Definitive phase*: The definitive phase may involve many procedures like endodontic, orthodontic, periodontic, oral surgical and operative procedures prior to further treatment.
- *Maintenance phase*: In maintenance phase, regular recall and examination of patient is done. This helps in prevention of the recurrence of the disease and maintenance of the previous treatment results. Recall visits for patients can vary from patient-to-patient, for example, patients who are at high-risk for dental caries should be examined more frequently than the patients at low risk for dental caries.

Phases of treatment planning
➡ Urgent phase
➡ Control phase
➡ Holding phase
➡ Definitive phase
➡ Maintenance phase.

TREATMENT RECORD

All the activities from the initial treatment plan to the final treatment plan that is examination, diagnosis and final treatment should be maintained in the form of record. Maintenance of the records also becomes a legal document in support of a particular action a dentist may take while rendering a treatment. This record must be dated, with the headings made chronologically.

 Key Points

- Diagnosis is defined as utilization of scientific knowledge for identifying a diseased process and to differentiate from other disease process. In other words, literal meaning of diagnosis is determination and judgment of variations from the normal.
- The diagnostic process actually consists of four steps
  First step: Assemble all the available facts gathered from chief complaints, medical and dental history, diagnostic tests and investigations.
  Second step: Analyze and interpret the assembled clues to reach the tentative or provisional diagnosis.
  Third step: Make differential diagnosis of all possible diseases which are consistent with signs, symptoms and test results gathered.
  Fourth step: Select the closest, possible choice.
- If a chief complaint is toothache but symptoms are too vague to establish a diagnosis, then analgesics should be prescribed to help the patient in tolerating the pain until the toothache localizes.
- The most common toothache may arise from either pulp or periodontal ligament. Pulpal pain can be sharp piercing if A-delta fibers are stimulated. Dull, boring or throbbing pain occurs if there is stimulation of C-fibers.
- Localization of pain also tells origin of pain since pulp does not contain proprioceptive fibers; it is difficult for patient to localize the pain unless it reaches the periodontal ligament.
- Clinical examination includes both extraoral and intraoral examination.

- Intraoral examination includes the examination of soft and hard tissue.
- The mobility of a tooth is tested by placing a finger or blunt end of the instrument on either side of the crown and pushing it and assessing any movement with other finger.

Mobility can be graded as
- Slight (normal)
- Moderate mobility within a range of 1 mm.
- Extensive movement (more than 1 mm) in mesiodistal or lateral direction combined with vertical displacement in alveolus.

The periapical lesions of endodontic origin have following characteristic features
- Loss of lamina dura in the apical region
- Etiology of pulpal necrosis is generally apparent
- Radiolucency remains at the apex even if radiograph is taken by changing the angle.
- In thermal test, the response of pulp to heat and cold is noted. The basic principle for pulp to respond to thermal stimuli is that patient reports sensation but it disappears immediately. Any other type of response, i.e. painful sensation even after removal of stimulus or no response are considered abnormal.

Commonly used methods for performing cold pulp test are following
- Spraying cold air directed against the isolated tooth.
- Application of cotton pellet saturated with ethyl chloride.
- Spray of ethyl chloride after isolating tooth with rubber dam (The ethyl chloride evaporates so rapidly that it absorbs heat and thus, cools the tooth).
- Application of dry ice on the facial surface of the tooth after isolating the oral soft tissues and teeth with gauze or cotton roll . The frozen carbon dioxide (dry ice) is available in the form of solid sticks having extremely low temperature. It should not come in contact with oral tissues because soft tissue burns may occur.
- Wrap an ice piece in the wet gauze and apply to the tooth. The ice sticks can also be prepared by filling the discarded anesthetic carpules with water and placing them in refrigerator.
- For heat test, the easiest method is to direct the warm air to the exposed surface of tooth and note the patient response.
- If a higher temperature is needed to illicit a response, then other options like heated stopping stick, hot burnisher, hot water, etc. can be used.
- The preferred temperature for heat test is 150°F (65.5°C).
- But there are certain conditions which can give false negative response, i.e. the tooth shows no response but the pulp could be possibly vital. These conditions are recently erupted teeth with immature apex, recent trauma and excessive calcifications.
- The pulp tester is an instrument which uses the gradations of electrical current to excite a response from the pulpal tissue. A positive response indicates the vitality of pulp. No response indicates nonvital pulp or pulpal necrosis.

QUESTIONS

1. Write short notes on:
   a. Treatment planning
   b. Recent advances in pulp vitality testing

BIBLIOGRAPHY

1. American Dental Association, American Academy of Orthopedic Surgeons. Antibiotic prophylaxis for dental patients with total joint replacements. J Am Dent Assoc 2003;134:895-9.
2. Anusavice K. Criteria for placement and replacement of dental restorations: an international consensus report. It Dent J. 1988;38:193-4.
3. Bader J, Shugars D. Systematic review of the performance of the DIAGNOdent device for caries detection. J Am Dent Assoc. 2004;135:1413-26.
4. Bader JD, Brown JP. Dilemmas in caries diagnosis. JADA. 1993;124: 48.
5. Bader JD, et al. A systematic review of selected dental caries diagnostic and management methods. Community Dent Oral Epidemio. 2001;l 29:399-41.
6. Bader JD, et al. A systematic review of the performance of methods for identifying carious lesions, J Public Health Dent. 2002;62:201-13.
7. Berg R, Morgenstern NE. Physiological changes in the elderly. Dent Clin North Am. 1997;41:651-68.
8. Brantley CF, et al. Does the cycle of rerestoration lead to larger restorations? J Am Dent Assoc. 1995;126:1407-13.
9. Brooks SL, Miles DA. Advances in diagnostic imaging in dentistry. DCNA. 1993;37:91.
10. Christensen GJ. Educating patients about dental procedures. J Am Dent Assoc. 1995;126:371-2.
11. Ettinger RL. The unique oral health needs of an aging population. Dent Clin North Am. 1997;41:633-49.
12. Fanibunda KB. Diagnosis of tooth vitality by crown surface temperature measurement: a clinical evaluation. J Dent 1986;14:160.
13. Guthrie RC, Difiore PM. Treating the cracked tooth with full crowns. JADA. 1991;122:71.
14. Homewood CI. Cracked tooth syndrome—Incidence, clinical findings and treatment. Aust Dent J. 1998;43:217.
15. Horner K, Shearer AC, Walker A. Radiovisiography: an initial evaluation. BDJ. 1990;168:244.

16. Howat AP. A comparison of the sensitivity of caries diagnostic criteria. Caries Res. 1981;15:331.

17. Ismail AI. Clinical diagnosis of precavitated carious lesions. Comm Dent Oral Epid. 1997;25:13.

18. Khocht A, et al. Assessment of periodontal status with PSR and traditional clinical periodontal examination, J Am Dent Assoc. 1995;126:1658-65.

19. Kidd EAM. Caries diagnosis within restored teeth. Oper Dent 1989;14:149.

20. Longbottom C, Pitts NB. CO_2 laser and the diagnosis of occlusal caries: in vitro study. J Dent 1993;21:234.

21. Lussi A. Validity of diagnostic and treatment decisions of fissure caries. Caries Res. 1991;25:296-303.

22. Narcisi EM, Culp L. Diagnosis and treatment planning for ceramic restorations. DCNA. 2001;45:127.

23. Newburn E. Problems in caries diagnosis. Int Dent J 1993;43: 133.

24. Sackett DL, et al. Evidence-based medicine: what it is and what it isn't. BMJ. 1996;312:71-2.

25. Sfikas PM: Informed consent and the law, AM Dent Assoc. 1998;129:1471-3.

26. Shugars DA, Bader JD. Practice parameters in dentistry: where do we stand? J Am Dent Assoc. 1995;126:1134-43.

27. Vissink A, et al: Aging and saliva: a review of the literature, Spec Care Dentist. 1996;16:95-103.

28. Winkler S, et al. Depressed taste and smell in geriatric patients. J Am Dent Assoc. 1999;130:1759-65.

Patient and Operator Position

CHAPTER 9

INTRODUCTION

The patient and operator position are important for the benefits of both individuals. A patient, who is comfortably seated in dental chair with right posture is going to experience less muscular strain, less fatigue and is more cooperative during the treatment. The same is the case with operator. If operator maintains proper position and posture during treatment, the operator is less likely to get strained, fatigued, be more efficient and has less chances of getting musculoskeletal disorders. Most of the restorative dental procedures can be completed while sitting (**Figs 9.1A and B**).

Following points should be kept in mind in relation to dental chair

- It should be able to provide comfort to the patient
- It should be able to provide total body support during working
- Headrest of chair should be attached for supporting patient's chin and reducing strain on chin muscles
- It should be able to provide maximum working area to the operator
- It should be placed at the convenient location with adjustable control switches
- Foot switches are preferred to improve infection control
- It is always preferred to have programmable operating position.

CHAIR AND PATIENT POSITIONS

Dental chair and patient positions are important aspect in restorative dentistry. Modern dental chairs are properly designed so as to provide total body support and comfort in any position (**Fig. 9.2**).

Patient should be seated so that all his body parts are well supported. The patient's head should always be supported by adjustable/articulated headrest. Preferably the patient's head should be in line with his back, whether the dental chair base is parallel or slightly at an angle to the floor. The dental chair should be designed in such a way that it should provide maximum working area to the operator. The foot switches are preferred than hand switches so as to improve infection control. And the adjustable control switches should be conveniently located.

The chair height should be kept low, backrest should be upright and armrest should be adjustable while making the patient to seat in the dental chair. Now, the chair can be adjusted to place the patient in reclining position. Patient position can vary with operator, type of procedure and area of the oral cavity.

For restorative dental procedures, the most preferred operating positions are

- Upright position
- Almost supine
- Reclined 45 degree.

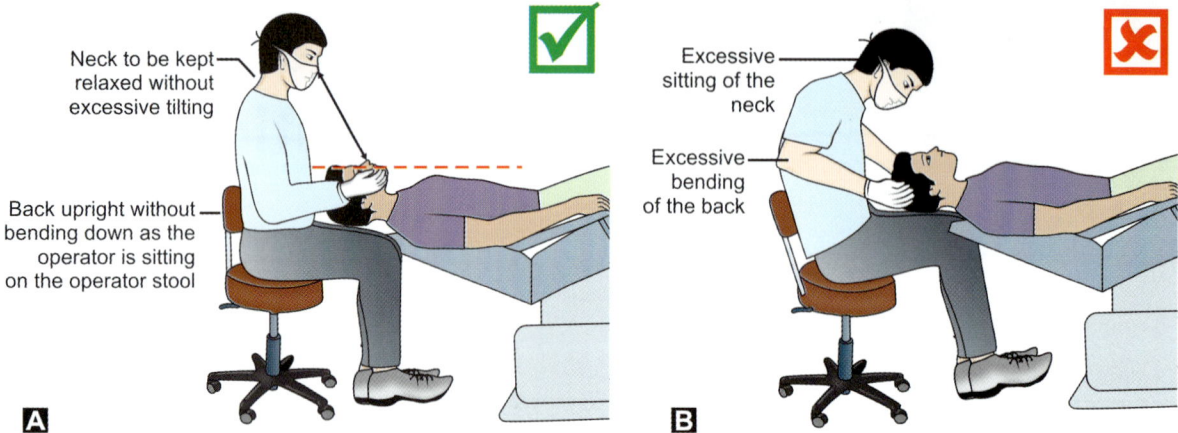

Figures 9.1A and B: Operator and the patient should maintain proper posture so as to have less muscular strain, less fatigue and more efficiency: (A) Correct posture; (B) Incorrect posture

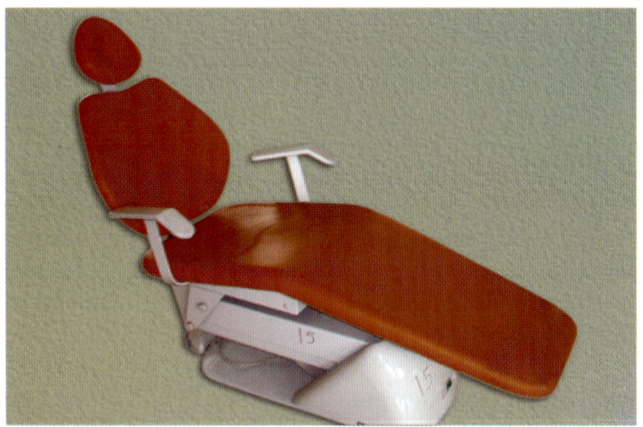

Figure 9.2: A dental chair should be ergonomically designed so as to provide total body support and comfort to the patient

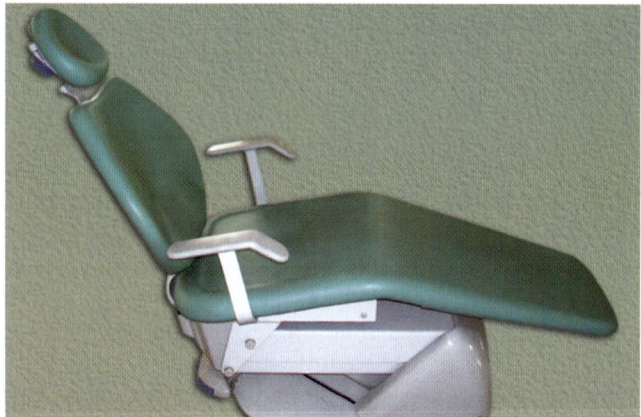

Figure 9.3: Upright position

Upright Position (Fig. 9.3)

This is the initial position of chair from which further adjustments are made.

Almost Supine (Fig. 9.4)

In this, chair position is such that:
- Patient's head, knees and feet are approximately at same level
- Patient is almost in a lying position as the name indicates
- Patient's head should not be lower than feet except in case of syncopal attack.

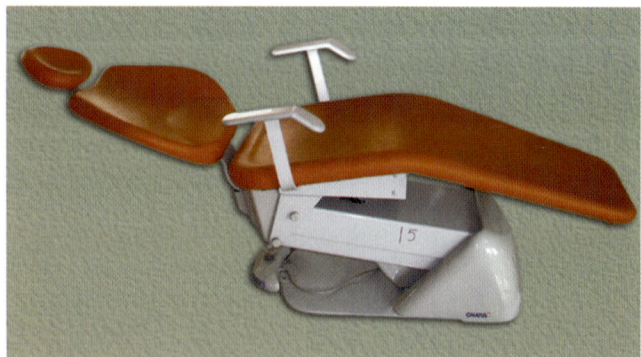

Figure 9.4: Almost supine chair position

Reclined 45 Degree (Fig. 9.5)

- In this position, chair is reclined at 45°
- Mandibular occlusal surfaces are almost at 45° to the floor.

After the treatment is done, chair can be brought back to upright position so that patient can leave the dental chair with ease.

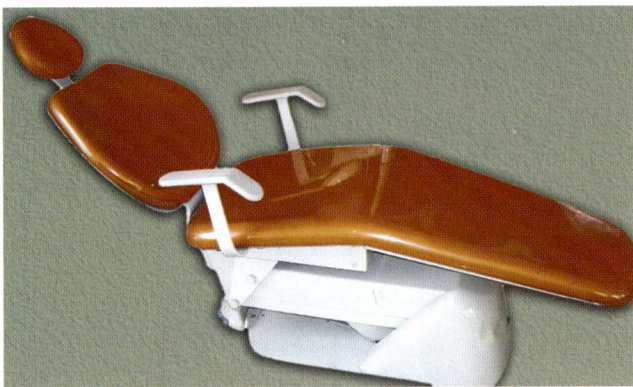

Figure 9.5: Reclined 45° chair position

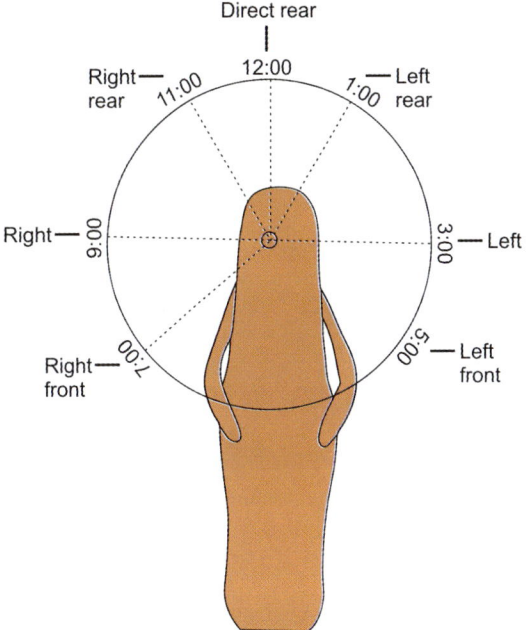

Figure 9.6: Sitting position of operator when related to clock

OPERATING POSITION

Accurate operating positions are essential while doing restorative work so as to increase the efficiency and to decrease physical strain. The position of the patient depends upon the procedure to be performed. Most of the dental procedures are performed with the patient in the supine position. Once the patient has been comfortably positioned, the dentist and the assistant should sit in the proper positions for treatment. Usually, sitting position is preferred in modern dentistry to relieve stress on operator's leg and support the operator's back. The level of teeth being treated should be same as that of operator's elbow.

For better understanding, sitting positions of operator are related to a clock. In this clock concept, an imaginary circle is drawn over the dental chair, keeping the patient's head at the center of the circle. Then the numbering to circle is given similar to a clock with the top of the circle at 12 o'clock.

Accordingly the operator's positions (right handed operator) can be 7 o'clock, 9 o'clock, 11 o'clock, and 12 o'clock and for left handed operator, it can be 5 o'clock, 3 o'clock and 1 o'clock (**Fig. 9.6**).

Right Front Position (7 o'clock) (Fig. 9.7)

- It helps in examination of the patient
- Working areas include
  - Mandibular anterior
  - Mandibular posterior teeth (Right side)
  - Maxillary anterior teeth
- To increase the ease and visibility, the patient's head may be turned towards the operator.

Right Position (9 o'clock) (Fig. 9.8)

- In this position, dentist sits exactly right to the patient
- Working areas include

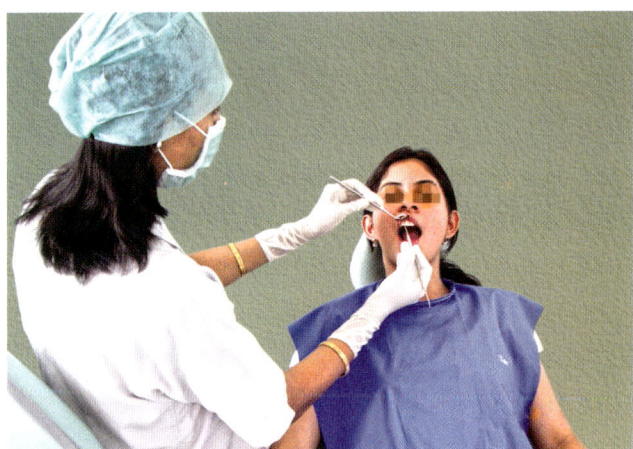

Figure 9.7: Right front position (7 o'clock position)

  - Facial surfaces of maxillary right posterior teeth
  - Facial surfaces of mandibular right posterior teeth
  - Occlusal surfaces of mandibular right posterior teeth.

Right Rear Position (11 o'clock) (Fig. 9.9)

- In this position, dentist sits behind and slightly to the right of the patient and the left arm is positioned around patient's head

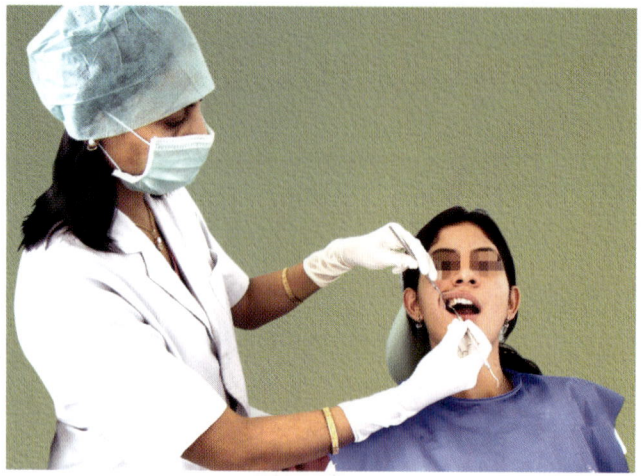

Figure 9.8: Right position (9 o'clock position)

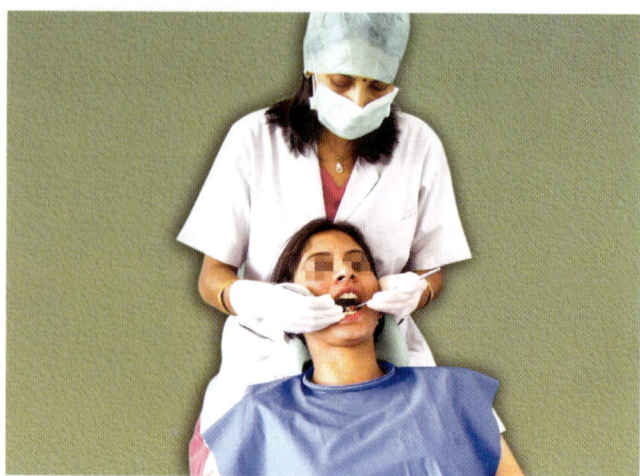

Figure 9.10: Direct rear position (12 o'clock position)

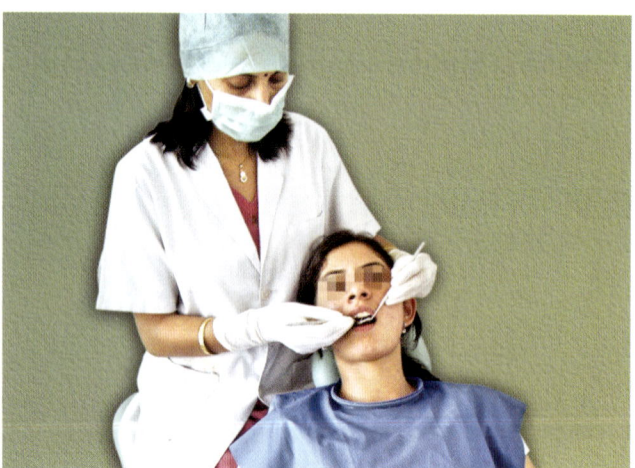

Figure 9.9: Right rear position (11 o'clock position)

- This is preferred position for most of dental procedures
- Most areas of mouth are accessible from this position either using direct or indirect vision
- Working areas include
  – Palatal and incisal (occlusal) surfaces of maxillary teeth
  – Mandibular teeth (direct vision).

Direct Rear Position (12 o'clock) (Fig. 9.10)

- Dentist sits directly behind the patient and looks down over the patient's head during procedure
- Working areas are lingual surfaces of mandibular teeth
- This position has limited application.

Preferred operator positions

Right handed operator–3 Preferred position	Left handed operator–3 Preferred position
Right front or 7 o'clock	Left front or 5 o' clock
Right or 9 o'clock	Left or 3 o'clock
Right rear or 11 o'clock	Left rear or 1 o'clock

CONSIDERATIONS FOR DENTISTS WHILE DOING PATIENT

- While doing work in maxillary arch, maxillary occlusal surfaces should be oriented perpendicular to the floor
- In mandibular arch, mandibular occlusal surface should be oriented 45° to the floor
- Patient's head can be rotated backward or forward or from side to side for operators ease and visibility while doing work
- Dentist should not sacrifice good operating posture as it will decrease visibility, accessibility and efficiency
- Maintain proper working distance during dental procedure. This will result in increased cooperation and confidence from the patient
- Another important point is to avoid minimize body contact with patient. Dentist should not rest forearms on the patient's shoulders and hands on the face of the patient
- Dentist should not use patient's chest as an instrument trolley
- The operator should leave left hand free during most of dental procedures for retraction using mouth mirrors or fingers of left hand
- Operator should keep changing position if procedure is of long duration to decrease the muscle strain and fatigue.

Operating Stool

Many types of operating stools are commercially available (**Fig. 9.11**). An operating stool should have some features like it should

- Has casters for mobility and easy movement
- Be sturdy and well balanced
- Has seat which is well padded with cushion
- Has adjustable backrest to provide full support to the dentist.

SITTING ARRANGEMENT OF OPERATOR AND ASSISTANT (FIG. 9.12)

- The dentist should sit on the back of the cushion rather than edges
- The dentist should sit on the stool such that
  - Spiral column is straight or slightly bent taking the advantage of backrest
  - Thighs are parallel to the floor
  - Lower legs are perpendicular to the floor.
- The patient should be lowered to a position that keeps the treatment site as close to the dentist's elbow level as possible. When the patient is properly positioned, the dentist's eyes should be 14 to 16 inches from the treatment site (**Fig. 9.13**).
- Nowadays, stools having backrest with curved extensions that provide additional body support are also available.
- If seat is positioned too high, the edges will cut off supply to user's legs resulting in more fatigue and stress.
- Assistant should sit as close as possible to the back of the patient's chair with feet directed towards the head of the chair.

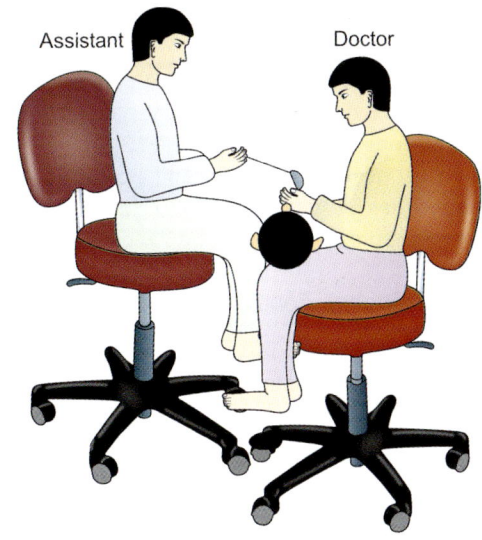

Figure 9.12: The stool height of assistant should be 4 to 6 inches above the dentist's eye level

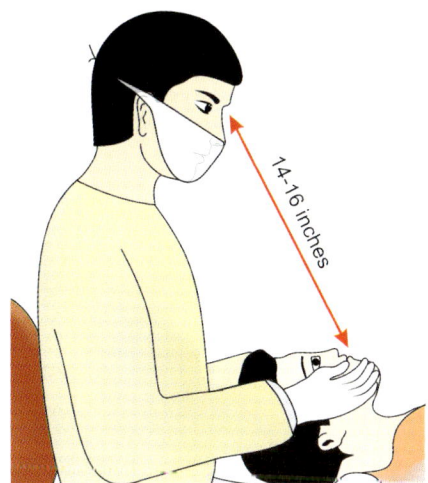

Figure 9.13: Patient should be seated at dentist's elbow level and dentist's eye should be 14-16 inches from the treatment site

- Stool height of assistant should be 4 to 6 inches above the dentist's eye level.
- The assistant should sit in an erect position with feet firmly placed on the foot-support ring at the base of the assistant chair.
- The instrument tray should be placed towards the head of the patient's chair, and positioned to allow easy access to the instruments and materials.
- Above positions can be adjusted according to specific needs.

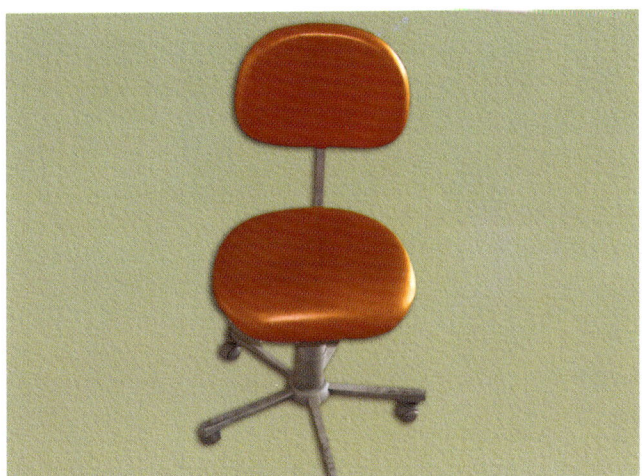

Figure 9.11: Operating stool

Zones of Working Area

Zones of working area
The working area is divided into four zones (**Figs 9.14A and B**) → Operator's zone (lies between 7 and 12 o' clock) → Assistant's zone (lies between 2 and 4 o'clock) → Static zone (lies between 12 and 2 o'clock) → Transfer zone (lies between 4 and 7 o'clock).

Instrument Exchange Zone

The efficient exchange of instruments between the operator and the dental assistant is fundamental to have an efficient and stress free dental practice. The transfer of instrument between the operator and assistant should occur in exchange zone which is below the patient's chin and several inches above the patient's chest. All instruments and materials are located in the assistant's zone. Static zone lies from 11 to 2 o'clock. It is a nontraffic area where other equipments can be placed. When an object or material is heavy or dangerous if held near the patient's face, it should be passed through the static zone.

Instrument Exchange

To increase efficiency, and reduce stress and fatigue of the dentist and the assistant, there should be cooperation from the both sides. To accomplish this, assistant should know the sequence of the treatment steps and have the required instruments and materials ready at the proper time. Ideally, the instrument transfer is accomplished with a minimum of motion involving movement only of fingers, wrist, and elbow. Assistant should be ready when signalled by the dentist to pass the next instrument and receive the used one in a smooth motion. The assistant should take the instrument from operator rather than operator dropping the instrument in assistant's hand. Instruments should be arranged in an orderly fashion for comfortable exchange. As a rule the instruments should be set from left to right, in the sequence in which they are to be used. After use, they should be returned to their original position in case they need to be reused.

Magnification

Another important aspect of the restorative procedure for increasing efficiency and visibility is magnification of working area. Several types of magnification devices are available

- Loupes
- Surgical telescopes
- Bifocal eyeglasses.

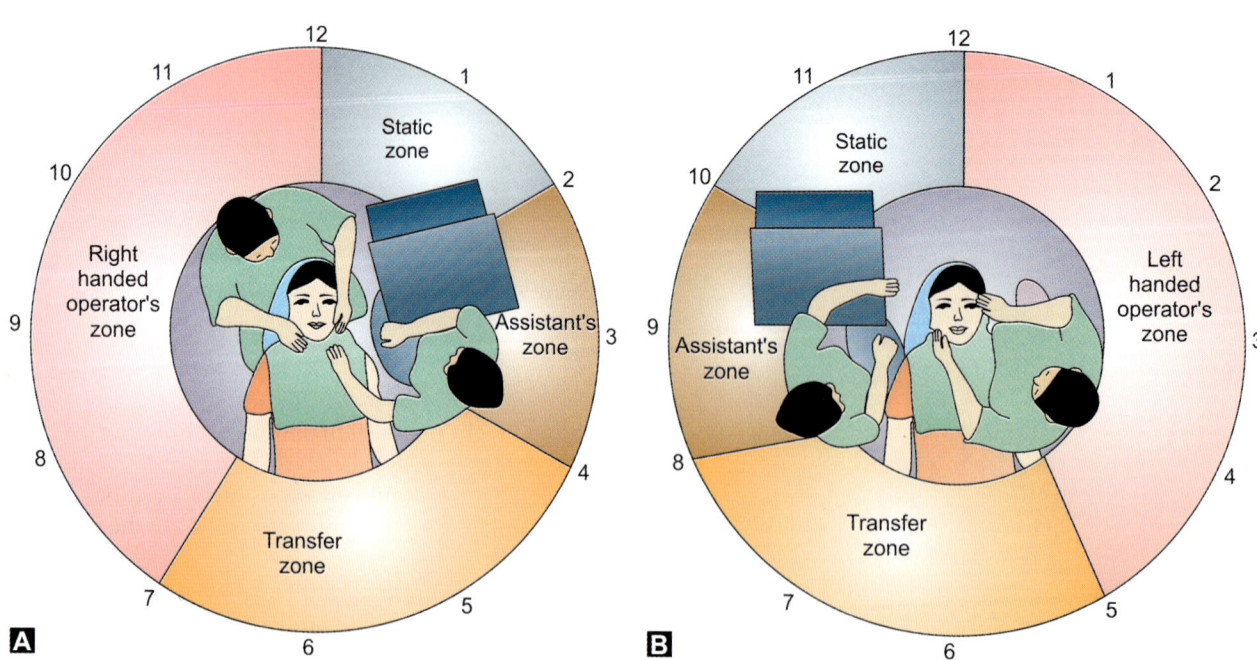

Figures 9.14A and B: Different zones of working area: (A) Right handed operator; (B) Left handed operator

Advantages of magnification

➠ Increase in the visibility of the working area
➠ Minute and delicate procedures can be easily carried out
➠ Increase in the operator's efficiency and success outcome
➠ Helps in getting good posture as using magnification maintains a constant working distance
➠ Provides protection to eye from injury.

Key Points

- Patient should be seated so that all his body parts are well supported. The patient's head should always be supported by adjustable/articulated.
- Upright Position is the initial position of chair from which further adjustments are made.
- Almost Supine position is such that patient's head, knees and feet are approximately at same level, patient is almost in a lying position. Patient's head should not be lower than feet.
- In reclined 45 degree, chair is reclined at 45°, and the mandibular occlusal surfaces are almost at 45° to the floor.
- For better understanding, sitting positions of operator are related to a clock. In this clock concept, an imaginary circle is drawn over the dental chair, keeping the patient's head at the center of the circle. Then the numbering to circle is given similar to a clock with the top of the circle at 12 o'clock.
- Accordingly the operator's positions (right handed operator) can be 7 o'clock, 9 o'clock, 11 o'clock, and 12 o'clock and for left handed operator, it can be 5 o'clock, 3 o'clock and 1 o'clock .

- In mandibular arch, mandibular occlusal surface should be oriented 45° to the floor.
- Stool height of assistant should be 4 to 6 inches above the dentist's eye level.
- The working area is divided into four zones
  - Operator's zone (lies between 7 and 12 o' clock)
  - Assistant's zone (lies between 2 and 4 o'clock)
  - Static zone (lies between 12 and 2 o'clock)
  - Transfer zone (lies between 4 and 7 o'clock)
- The transfer of instrument between the operator and assistant should occur in exchange zone which is below the patient's chin and several inches above the patient's chest. All instruments and materials are located in the assistant's zone.
- Static zone lies from 11 to 2 o'clock. It is a nontraffic area where other equipments can be placed. When an object or material is heavy or dangerous if held near the patient's face, it should be passed through the static zone.

QUESTIONS

1. Discuss in short about zones of working area.
2. What are the different operator positions for right handed dental surgeon?

BIBLIOGRAPHY

1. Paul E. A practical guide to assisted operating. 1. principles of assisted operating. Br. Dent J. 1972;133:258-61.
2. Paul JE. Four handed dentistry 1. Principles and techniques: a new look. Dent update. 1983;10:1557,159-60:162-4.

Isolation of the Operating Field

INTRODUCTION

The complexities of oral environment present obstacles to the operating procedures starting from diagnosis till the final treatment is done. In order to minimize the trauma to these surrounding structures and to provide comfort to the patient the clinician needs to control the operating field. While performing any operative procedure, many structures require proper control so as to prevent them from interfering with the operating field. These structures together constitute the oral environment.

COMPONENTS OF ORAL ENVIRONMENT

Following components of oral environment need to be controlled during operative procedures

- Saliva
- Moving organs
  - Tongue
  - Mandible
- Lips and cheek
- Gingival tissue
- Buccal and lingual vestibule
- Floor of mouth
- Adjacent teeth and restoration
- Respiratory moisture.

Saliva

Since it poses the maximum problem, it must be removed from the oral cavity while performing any procedure. Saliva can be reduced from operative field by:

- Evacuation
- Reducing salivary secretion
- Allowing the patient to swallow it
- Isolation of the operating field using cotton rolls, rubber dam.

One should always take care to control saliva while performing operative procedure because it obstructs proper vision and access, affect the physical properties of dental materials and may decrease the effect of medicaments.

Moving Organs

Tongue, mandible and head of the patient come under moving organs which need to be controlled during operative procedures. Moving tongue can interfere while a procedure is being performed so it should be retracted so as to minimize the interference and protect it from injury. Similarly head of patient should be kept stable and immobile so as to prevent unpredictable and unwanted injury to tissue while performing with the instruments.

Lips and Cheek

Lips and cheek may interfere during procedure so they need to be retracted for better access and visibility of the operating field.

Gingival Tissue

When the lesion extends to the root surface, gingival tissue can interfere with instrumentation and restoration. Thus, it is mandatory to retract gingival tissue so as to have better access, visibility, and prevent injury during procedure.

Buccal and Lingual Vestibules

They can reduce accessibility so need to be retracted while performing operative procedure.

Floor of Mouth

Floor of mouth usually does not interfere during an operative procedure, except in some cases, for example, while operating on cervical area on lingual surfaces of molars and incisors. These areas need to be isolated using cotton rolls, rubber dam or using mouth mirror.

Adjacent Teeth and Restoration

While performing operative procedure, harm can occur to the proximal surface of adjacent tooth. So it is always preferable to isolate the adjoining teeth using bands, wedges or other means.

Respiratory Moisture

Respiratory moisture can result in foggy appearance of mirror and other reflecting surfaces which obstructs visibility while performing an operative procedure. This can be prevented using antifogging solutions or isolation using rubber dam.

Sources of moisture in the clinical environment

- *Saliva*: From salivary glands
- *Blood*: It can come from
  - Inflamed gingival tissues
  - Iatrogenic damage to tissues.
- *Gingival crevicular fluid*: Specially from inflamed gingival tissues.
- *Water*: Water can come from
  - Rotary instruments during cutting
  - Air water syringe.
- *Dental materials* like etchants, irrigant solutions used during various procedures.

Advantages of Moisture Control

Patient Related Factors

- Provides comfort to the patient
- Protects patients from swallowing or aspirating foreign bodies
- Protects patient's soft tissues–tongue, cheeks by retracting them from operating field.

Operator Related Factors

The following are the operator related advantages of isolation of operating field:
- A dry and clean operating field
- Infection control by minimizing aerosol production.
- Increased accessibility to operative site
- Improved properties of dental materials, hence better results are obtained
- Protection of the patient and operator
- Improved visibility of the working field and diagnosis.
- Less fogging of the dental mirror.
- Prevents contamination of tooth preparation.
- Hemorrhage from gingiva does not enter operative site.

Methods of moisture control

- Comfortable position of patient
- Direct methods
  - Rubber dam
  - Aspiration
  - Air-Water Syringe
  - Absorbent materials
  - Gingival retraction cord
  - Electrosurgery.
- Local anesthetics
- Pharmacological methods
  - Antisialagogues
  - Antianxiety drugs
  - Muscle relaxants.

EQUIPMENT NEEDED FOR ISOLATION OF OPERATING FIELD

Different equipments and materials can be used for making isolation of operating field. These can be divided into following groups

- *Tissue retractors and protection devices*
  - Best tissue retractor and protector is rubber dam
  - Cheek and lip retractors are used to pull both lips and cheek backwards and outwards. They fit half of upper and lower lips including corners of the mouth held in grooved area of the device
  - Tongue depressors help in depressing the tongue during procedures
  - Tongue guards are used to create a wall between the tongue and operating field. They can be made-up of metal or plastic
  - Metallic band can also be used to protect the adjacent tooth while class II tooth preparation.
- *Equipment used for evacuation of fluids and debris*
  - Saliva ejectors/low volume ejectors are used to remove saliva and water coming from air rotor while working
  - High volume evacuators: These are attached to high volume suction unit.
- *Fluid absorbing materials*: These materials are used to absorb salivary secretion. They can be
  - Absorbent paper pads or wafers
  - Cotton rolls
  - Gauze pieces.

Isolation with Rubber Dam

Rubber dam was introduced by Barnum, a New York dentist in 1863.

Rubber dam can be defined as a flat thin sheet of latex/nonlatex that is held by a clamp and frame which is perforated to allow the tooth/teeth to protrude through the perforations while all other teeth are covered and protected by sheet (**Fig. 10.1**). The rubber dam eliminates saliva from the operating site, retracts the soft tissue and defines the operating field by isolation of one or more teeth from the oral environment (**Fig. 10.2**).

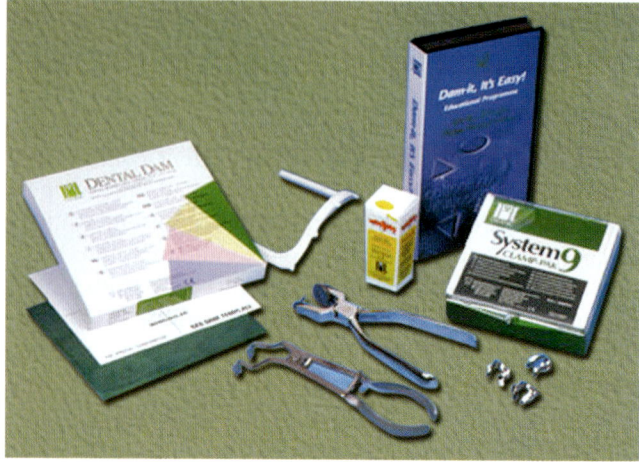

Figure 10.1: Rubber dam kit

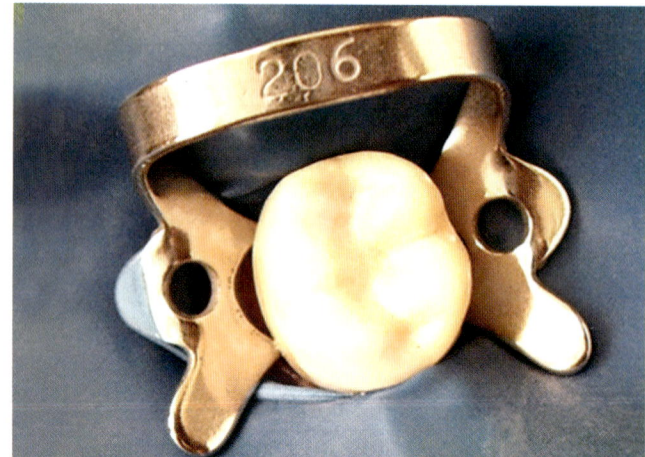

Figure 10.2: A tooth isolated using rubber dam

Advantages of using a rubber dam
➡ Acts as a raincoat for the teeth
➡ Complete, long-term moisture control
➡ Maximizes access and visibility
➡ Gives a clean and dry field while working
➡ Protects the lips, cheeks and tongue by keeping them out of the way
➡ Avoids unnecessary contamination through infection control
➡ Prevents accidental swallowing or aspiration of foreign bodies
➡ Improves the efficiency of the treatment
➡ Limits bacteria laden splash and splatter of saliva and blood
➡ Improves the properties of dental materials
➡ Protection of patient and dentist.

Disadvantages of using a rubber dam
➡ Takes time to be applied
➡ Communication with patient can be difficult
➡ Incorrect use may damage porcelain crowns/crown margins/traumatize gingival tissues
➡ Insecure clamps can be swallowed or aspirated.

Contraindications of use of rubber dam
→ Asthmatic patients
→ Allergy to latex
→ Mouth breathers
→ Extremely malpositioned tooth
→ Third molar (in some cases).

Rubber dam equipment
→ Rubber dam sheet
→ Rubber dam clamps
→ Rubber dam forceps
→ Rubber dam frame
→ Rubber dam punch.

Rubber dam accessories
→ Lubricant/petroleum jelly
→ Dental floss
→ Rubber dam napkin.

Rubber Dam Sheet (Fig. 10.3)

The rubber dam is available in size 6" × 6" squares and colors are usually green, blue or black. It is available in three thicknesses, i.e. light, medium and heavy. The middle grade is usually preferred as thin is more prone to tearing and thickest more difficult to apply. Latex free dam is necessary as number of patients are increasing with latex allergy. Flexi Dam is latex free dam of standard thickness with no rubber smell (**Fig. 10.4**).

Thickness of rubber dam sheet	
→ Thin	– 0.15 mm
→ Medium	– 0.2 mm
→ Heavy	– 0.25 mm
→ Extra heavy	– 0.30 mm
→ Special heavy	– 0.35 mm.

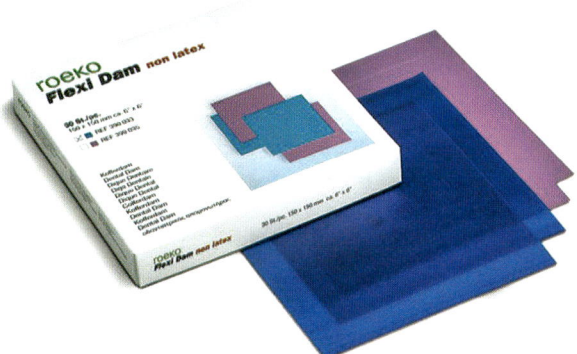

Figure 10.3: Rubber dam sheet

Rubber Dam Clamps

Rubber dam clamps, to hold the rubber dam on to the tooth are available in different shapes and sizes (**Fig. 10.5**).

Clamps mainly serve two functions
→ They anchor the rubber dam to the tooth
→ Help in retracting the gingivae.

Rubber dam clamps can be divided into two main groups on the basis of jaw design:
1. Bland
2. Retentive.

Bland clamps: Bland clamps are usually identified by the jaws, which are flat and point directly towards each other. In these clamps, flat jaws usually grasp the tooth at or above the gingival margin. They can be used in fully

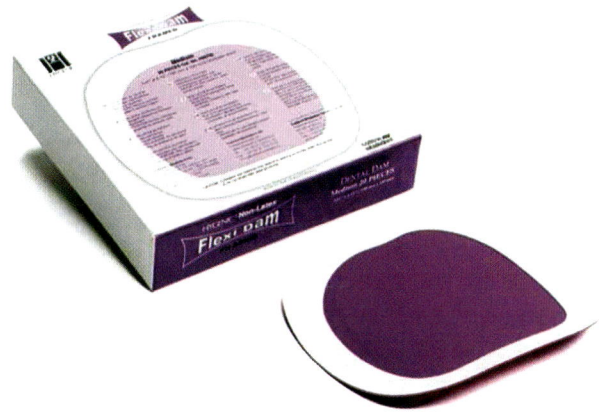

Figure 10.4: Flexi dam

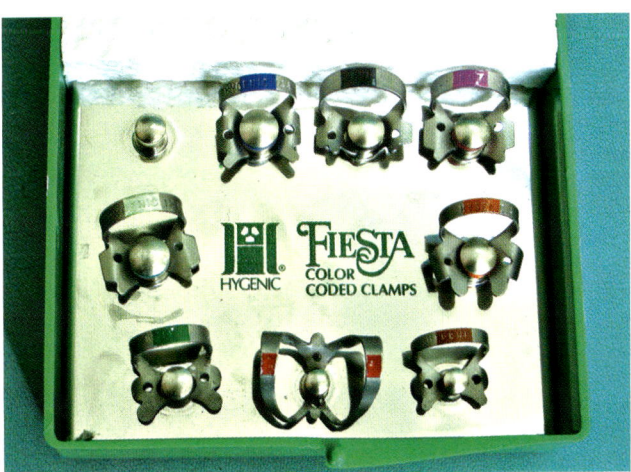

Figure 10.5: Rubber dam clamps

erupted tooth where cervical constriction prevents clamp from slipping off the tooth.

Retentive clasps: As the name indicates, these clasps provide retention by providing four-point contact with the tooth. In these, jaws are usually narrow, curved and slightly inverted which displace the gingivae and contact the tooth below the maximum diameter of crown (**Fig. 10.6**).

Both flanges are further subdivided into
- Winged
- Wingless
  Rubber dam clamp can also be divided on the basis of material used
- Metallic
- Nonmetallic.

Metallic: Traditionally, clamps have been made from tempered carbon steel and more recently from stainless steel.

Nonmetallic: Nonmetallic are made from polycarbonate plastic. An advantage of these clamps over metallic is radiolucency.

A good length of dental floss should always be passed through the holes in the clamp as a security in case it is dropped in the mouth or the bow fractures.

Rubber dam clamps
➡ # 22 Similar to # 207, but wingless
➡ # 27 Similar to # 206, but wingless, festooned
➡ # 29 For upper and lower bicuspids, with broad beaks
➡ # 206 For upper and lower bicuspids, with festooned beaks
➡ # 207 For upper and lower bicuspids, with flat beaks
➡ # 208 For bicuspids (large), with similar pattern to # 207
➡ # 209 For lower bicuspids, with flat beaks
➡ # 0 For small bicuspids and primary central incisors
➡ # 00 For very small bicuspids and primary central incisors
➡ # 1 For roots, with deep festooned beaks
➡ # 2 For lower bicuspids, with flat beaks
➡ # 2A Similar to # 2, but with large beaks
➡ # W2A Similar to # 2A, but wingless
➡ # P-1, # P-2 For children's first molars.

Rubber Dam Forceps (Fig. 10.7)

Rubber dam forceps are used to carry the clamp to the tooth. They are designed to spread the two working ends of the forceps apart when the handles are squeezed together (**Fig. 10.5**). The working ends have small projections that fit into two corresponding holes on the rubber dam clamps. The area between the working end and the handle has a sliding lock device which locks the handles in positions while the clinician moves the clamp around the tooth. It should be taken care that forceps do not have deep grooves at their tips or they become very difficult to remove once the clamp is in place.

Rubber Dam Frame (Figs 10.8 and 10.9)

Rubber dam frames support the edges of rubber dam (Fig. 10.6). They have been improved dramatically since the old style with the huge "butterflies". Modern frames have sharp pins which easily grip the dam. These are mainly designed with the pins that slope backwards.

Rubber dam frames serve following purposes
➡ Supporting the edges of rubber dam
➡ Retracting the soft tissues
➡ Improving accessibility to the isolated teeth.

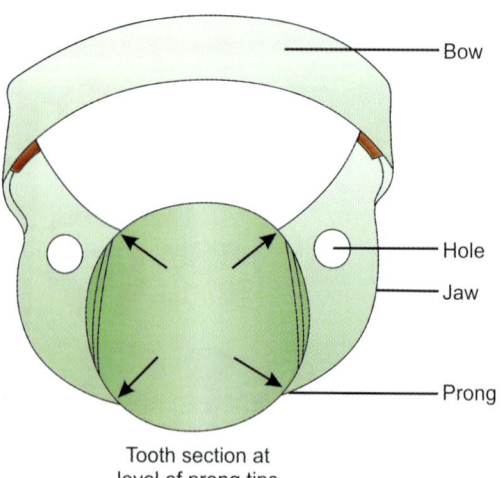

Bow

Hole

Jaw

Prong

Tooth section at
level of prong tips

Figure 10.6: A clamp should contact tooth from all sides

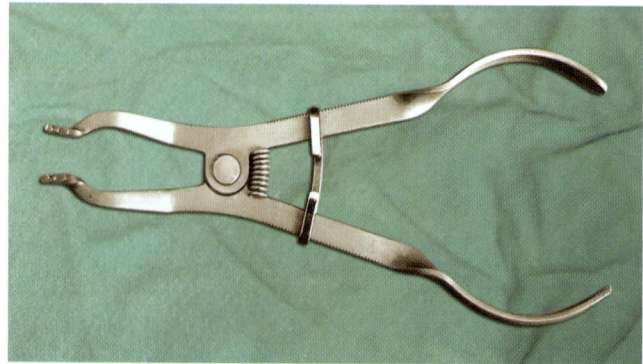

Figure 10.7: Rubber dam forceps

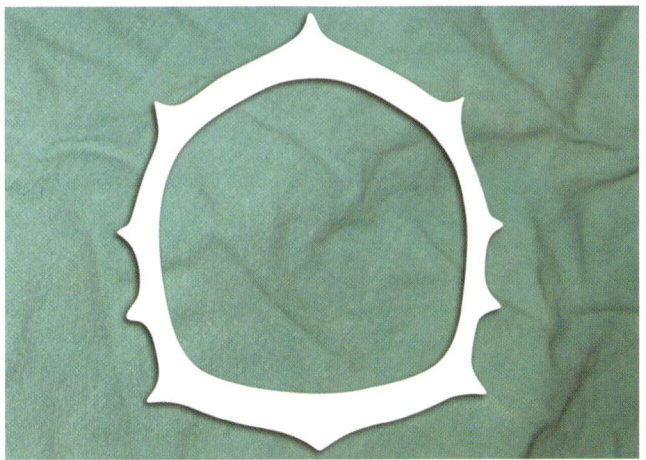

Figure 10.8: Rubber dam frame

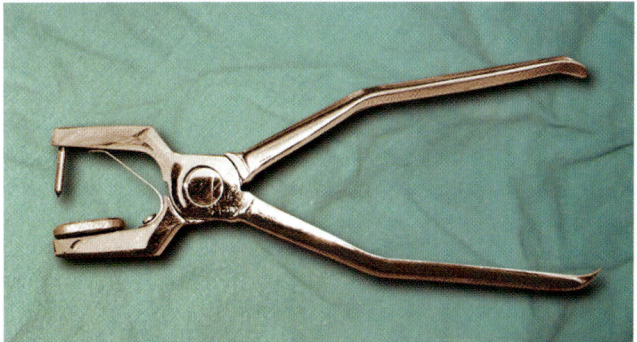

Figure 10.10: Rubber dam punch

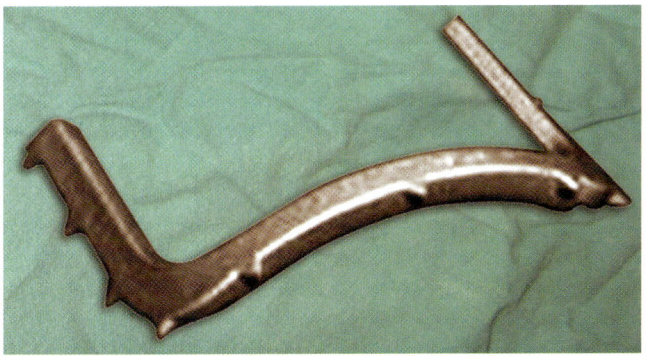

Figure 10.9: U-shaped rubber dam frame

Rubber dam frames are available in either metal or plastic. Plastic frames have advantage of being radiolucent.

When taut, rubber dam sheet exerts too much pull on the rubber dam clamps, causing them to become loose, especially clamps attached to molars. To overcome this problem, a new easy-to-use rubber dam frame (Safe-T-Frame) has been developed that offers a secure fit without stretching the rubber dam sheet. Instead, its "snap-shut" design takes advantage of the clamping effect on the sheet, which is caused when its two mated frame members are firmly pressed together. In this way, the sheet is securely attached, but without being stretched. Held in this manner, the dam sheet is under less tension, and hence, exerts less tugging on clamps—especially on those attached to molars.

Rubber Dam Punch (Fig. 10.10)

Rubber dam punch is used to make the holes in the rubber sheet through which the teeth can be isolated. The working end is designed with a plunger on one side and a wheel on the other side. This wheel has different sized holes on the flat surface facing the plunger. The punch must produce a clean cut hole every time. Two types of holes are made, single and multihole. Single holes are used in endodontics mainly. If rubber dam punch is not cutting cleanly and leaving behind a tag of rubber, the dam will often split as it is stretched out.

Rubber Dam Template (Fig. 10.11)

It is an inked rubber stamp which helps in marking the dots on the sheet according to position of the tooth. Holes should be punched according to arch and missing teeth.

Rubber Dam Accessories

A lubricant or petroleum jelly is usually applied on the undersurface of the dam. It is usually helpful when the rubber sheet is being applied to the teeth.
- ***Dental Floss (Figs 10.12 and 10.13)***
    - It is used as flossing agent for rubber dam in tight contact areas. It is usually required for testing interdental contacts.
- ***Wedjets (Fig. 10.14)***
    - Sometimes wedjets are required to support the rubber dam (**Fig. 10.9**).

Rubber Dam Napkin (Fig. 10.15)

This is a sheet of absorbent materials usually placed between the rubber sheet and soft tissues. It is generally not recommended for isolation of single tooth.

Recent Modifications in the Designs of Rubber Dam

Insti-Dam

It is recently introduced rubber dam for quick, convenient rubber dam isolation.

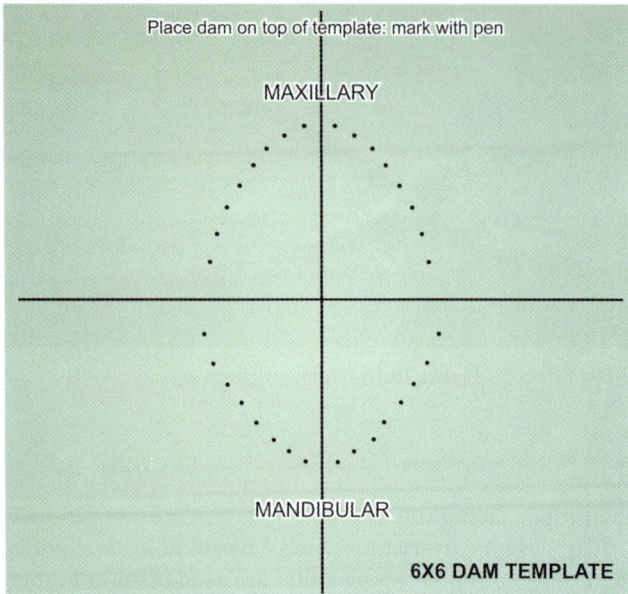

Figure 10.11: Rubber dam template

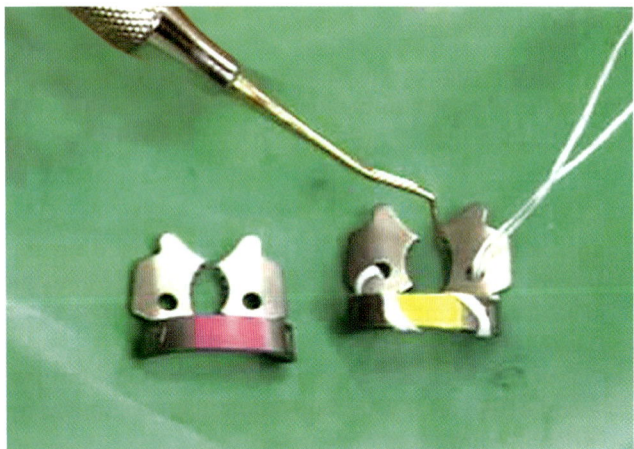

Figure 10.12: Floss tied on the clamp

Salient Features of Insti-Dam
- It is natural latex dam with prepunched hole and built-in white frame
- Its compact design is just the right size to fit outside the patient's lips
- It is madeup of stretchable and tear-resistant, medium gauge latex material
- Radiographs may be taken without removing the dam
- Built-in flexible nylon frame eliminates bulky frames and sterilization
- Off-center, prepunched hole customizes fit to any quadrant—add more holes if desired.

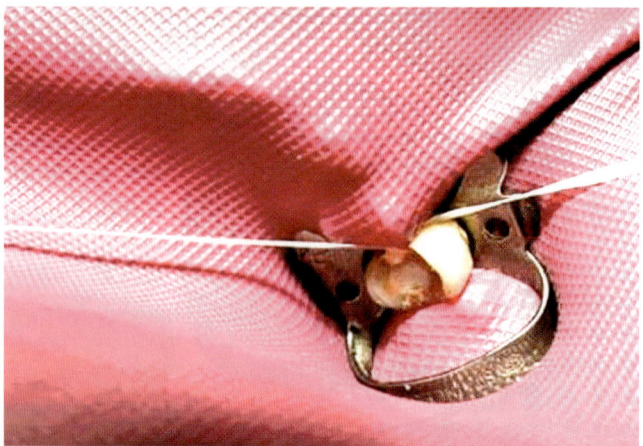

Figure 10.13: Floss is required to check interdental contacts

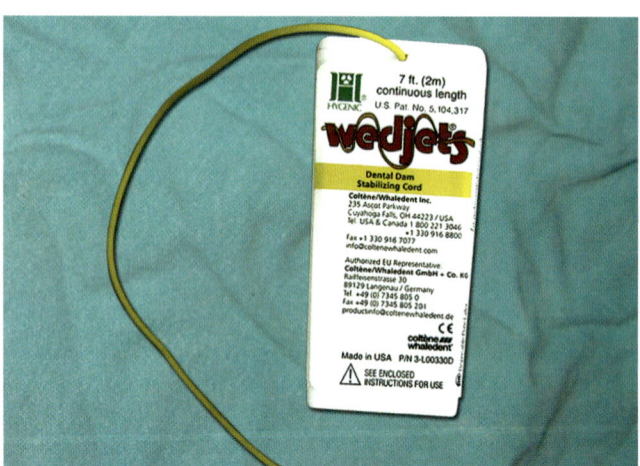

Figure 10.14: Wedjets

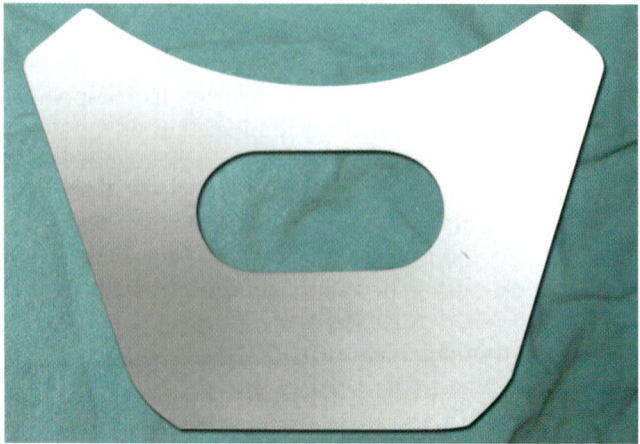

Figure 10.15: Rubber dam napkin

Handi Dam

Another recently introduced dam is Handi dam. This is preframed rubber dam, eliminates the need for traditional frame (**Fig. 10.16**).

Handi dam is easy to place and saves time of both patient as well as doctor. It allows easy access to oral cavity during the procedure.

Dry Dam

Another newer type of rubber dam is also available which does not require a frame 'dry dam'.

Placement of Rubber Dam

Before placement of rubber dam, following procedures should be done
- Thorough prophylaxis of the oral cavity
- Check contacts with dental floss
- Check for any rough contact areas
- Anesthetize the gingiva if required
- Rinse and dry the operating field.

Methods of Rubber Dam Placement

Method I—Clamp placed before rubber dam
(Figs 10.17A to C)
- Select an appropriate clamp according to the tooth size.
- Tie a floss to clamp bow and place clamp onto the tooth.
- Larger holes are required in this technique as rubber dam has to be stretched over the clamp. Usually two or three overlapping holes are made.
- Stretching of the rubber dam over the clamps can be done in the following sequence

– Stretch the rubber dam sheet over the clamp
– Then stretch the sheet over the buccal jaw and allow to settle into place beneath that jaw
– Finally, the sheet is carried to palatal/lingual side and released.

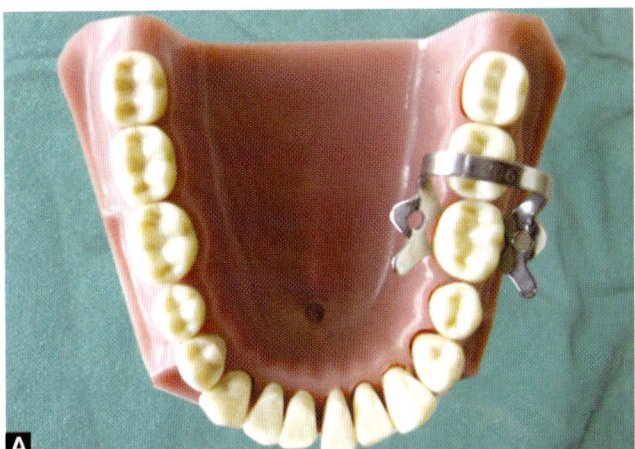

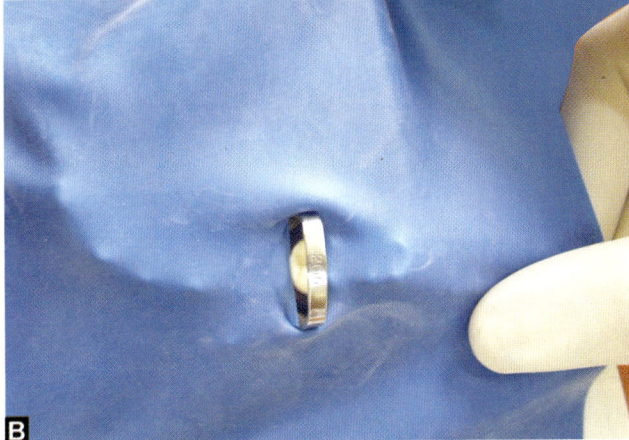

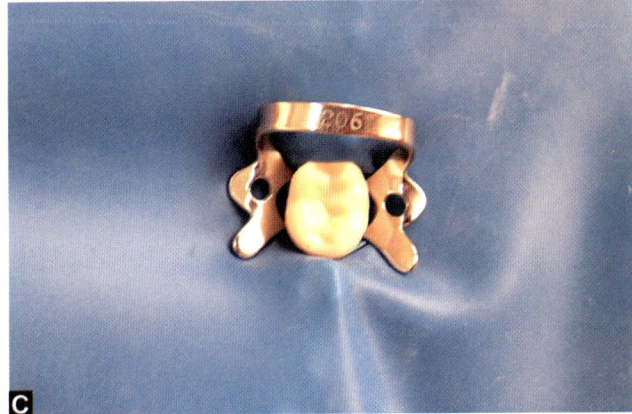

Figures 10.17A to C: Placement of rubber dam. (A) Placing clamp on selected tooth; (B) Stretching rubber dam sheet over clamp; (C) After complete stretching tooth is isolated

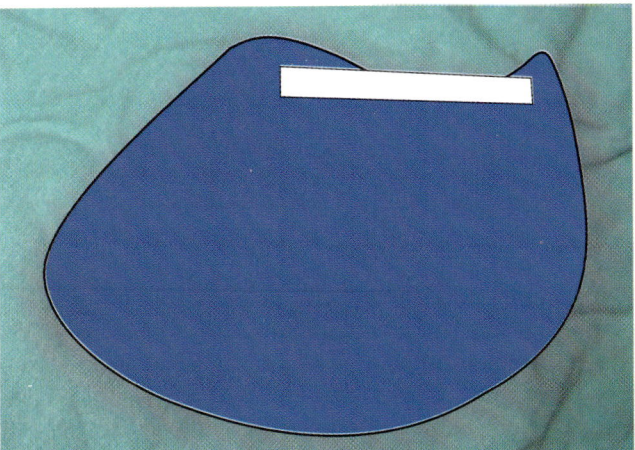

Figure 10.16: Handi dam

This method is mainly used in posterior teeth in both adults and children except third molar.

Method II—Placement of rubber dam and clamp together (Figs 10.18A to C)

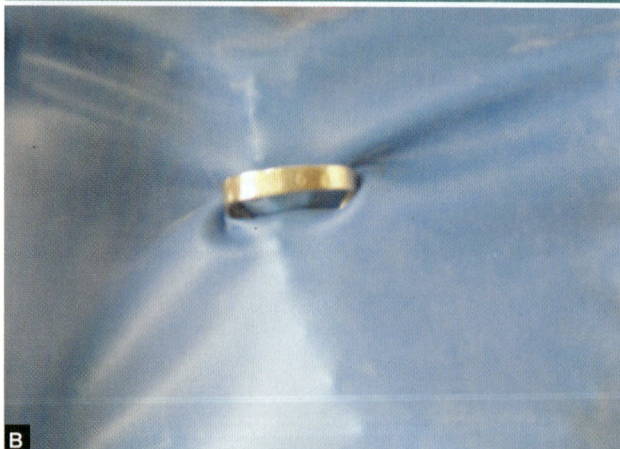

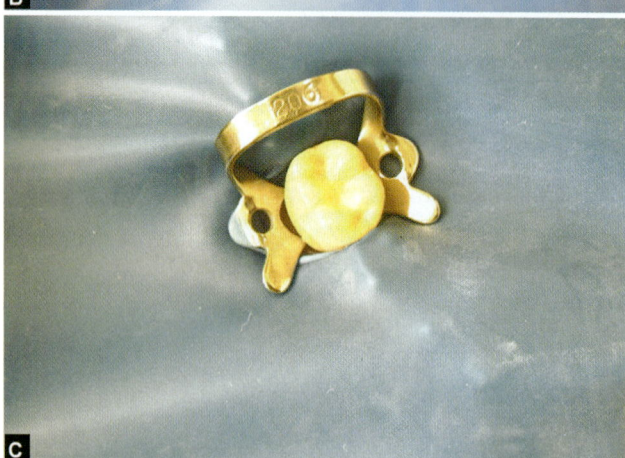

Figures 10.18A to C: (A) Punch hole in the rubber dam sheet according to selected tooth; (B) Clamp and its wings are inserted in the punched hole; (C) Carry both clamp and rubber dam over the crown and seat it

- Select an appropriate clamp according to tooth anatomy
- Tie a floss around the clamp and check the stability
- Punch the hole in rubber dam sheet
- Clamp is held with clamp forceps and its wings are inserted into punched hole
- Both clamp and rubber dam are carried to the oral cavity and clamp is tensed to stretch the hole
- Both clamp and rubber dam is advanced over the crown. First, jaw of clamp is tilted to the lingual side to lie on the gingival margin of lingual side
- After this, jaw of the clamp is positioned on buccal side
- After seating the clamp, again check stability of clamp
- Remove the forceps from the clamp
- Now, release the rubber sheet from wings to lie around the cervical margin of the tooth.

Method III—Split dam technique: This method is split dam technique in which rubber dam is placed to isolate the tooth without the use of rubber dam clamp. In this technique, two overlapping holes are punched in the dam. The dam is stretched over the tooth to be treated and over the adjacent tooth on each side. Edge of rubber dam is carefully teased through the contacts of distal side of adjacent teeth. This technique is indicated
- To isolate anterior teeth
- When there is insufficient crown structure
- When isolation of teeth with porcelain crown is required. In such cases placement of rubber dam clamp over the crown margins can damage the cervical porcelain.

Management of Difficult Cases

Malpositioned Teeth

To manage these cases, following modifications are done
- Adjust the spacing of the holes
- In tilted teeth, estimate the position of root center at gingival margin rather than the tip of the crown
- Another approach is to make a customized cardboard template
- Tight broad contact areas can be managed by
  - Wedging the contact open temporarily for passing the rubber sheet
  - Use of lubricant.

Extensive Loss of Coronal Tissue

When sound tooth margin is at or below the gingival margin because of decay or fracture, the rubber dam application becomes difficult. In such cases, to isolate the tooth
- Use retentive clasps
- Punch a bigger hole in the rubber dam sheet so that it can be stretched to involve more teeth, including the tooth to be treated.

- In some cases, the modification of gingival margin can be tried so as to provide supragingival preparation margin. This can be accomplished by gingivectomy or the flap surgery.

Crowns with Poor Retentive Shapes

Sometimes anatomy of teeth limits the placement of rubber dam (lack of undercuts and retentive areas). In such cases, following can be done
- Placing clamp on another tooth.
- By using clamp which engages interdental spaces below the contact point.
- By building retentive shape on the crown with composite resin bonded to acid etched tooth surface.

Teeth with Porcelain Crowns

In such cases, placing a rubber dam may cause damage to porcelain crown. To avoid this
- Clamp should be placed on another tooth.
- Clamp should engage below the crown margin.
- Do not place clamp on the porcelain edges.
- Place a layer of rubber dam sheet between the clamp and the porcelain crown which acts as a cushion and thus minimizes localized pressure on the porcelain.

Leakage

Sometimes leakage is seen through the rubber dam because of the accidental tears or holes. Such leaking gaps can be sealed by using cavit, periodontal packs, liquid rubber dam or oraseal. Now-a-days, the rubber dam adhesive can be used which can adhere well to both tooth as well as rubber dam. For sealing the larger gaps, the rubber dam adhesives in combination with orabase can be tried.

If leakage persists inspite of these efforts, the rubber dam sheet should be replaced with new one.

Depending upon clinical condition, isolation of single or multiple teeth can be done with the help of rubber dam. **Table 10.1** entails problems commonly encountered during application of rubber dam.

Single tooth isolation is done in following cases
➡ Class I and V restorations
➡ Endodontic treatment.

Isolation of multiple teeth is done in following conditions
➡ Class II restoration
➡ Quadrant dentistry
➡ Bleaching.

Removal of Rubber Dam

Before the rubber dam is removed, use the water syringe and high volume evacuator to flush out all debris that collected during the procedure. Cut away tied thread from the neck of the teeth. Stretch the rubber dam facially and pull the septal rubber away from the gingival tissue and the tooth. Protect the underlying soft tissue by placing a fingertip beneath the septum. Free the dam from the interproximal space, but leave the rubber dam over the anterior and posterior anchor teeth. Use the clamp forceps to remove the clamp. Once the retainer is removed, release the dam from the anchor tooth and remove the dam and frame simultaneously. Wipe the patient's mouth, lips, and chin with a tissue or gauze to prevent saliva from getting on the patient's face.

Check for any missing fragment after procedure. If a fragment of the rubber dam is found missing, inspect interproximal area because pieces of the rubber dam left under the free gingival can result in gingival irritation.

Table 10.1: Commonly encountered problems during application of rubber dam

Problem	Consequences	Correction
Excessive distance between holes	• Wrinkling of dam • Interference in accessibility	• Proper placement of holes by accurate use of rubber dam punch and template
Too short distance between holes	• Overstretching of dam • Tearing of dam • Poor fit	• Proper placement of holes by accurate use of rubber dam punch and template
Off-center arch form	• Obstructs breathing • Makes patient uncomfortable	• Folding of extra dam material under the nose • Proper placement of holes
Torn rubber dam	• Leakage • Improper isolation	• Replacement of dam • Use of cavit, periodontal packs or liquid rubber dam.

Absorbents (Cotton Roll and Cellulose Wafers) (Figs 10.19 to 10.22)

Cotton rolls, pellets, gauze, and cellulose wafers absorbents are helpful for short period of isolation, for example, in examination, polishing, pit and fissure sealant placement (**Fig. 10.19**). Absorbents play an essential role in isolation of the teeth especially when rubber dam application is not possible.

- Cotton rolls are usually placed in buccal or lingual sulcus specially where salivary gland ducts exit so as to absorb saliva. The maxillary teeth are isolated by placing a cotton roll in the buccal vestibule. Mandibular teeth are isolated by placing a small sized cotton roll in the buccal vestibule and a larger sized cotton roll in lingual vestibule.

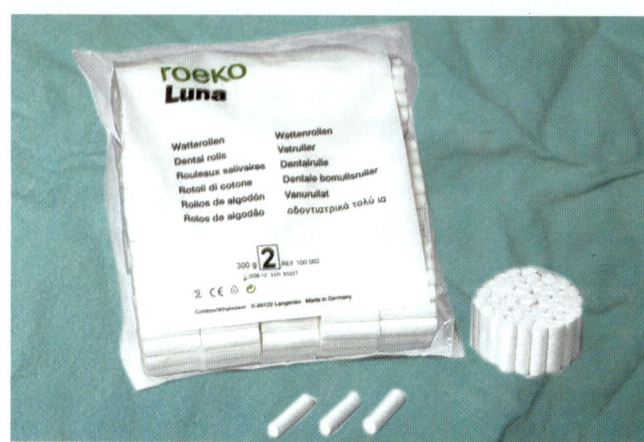

Figure 10.21: Cotton rolls

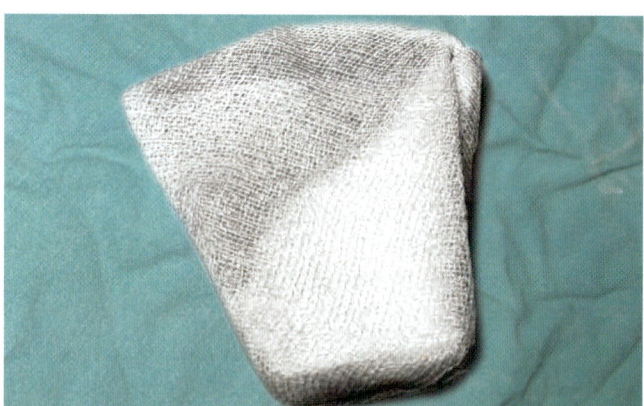

Figure 10.22: Gauze

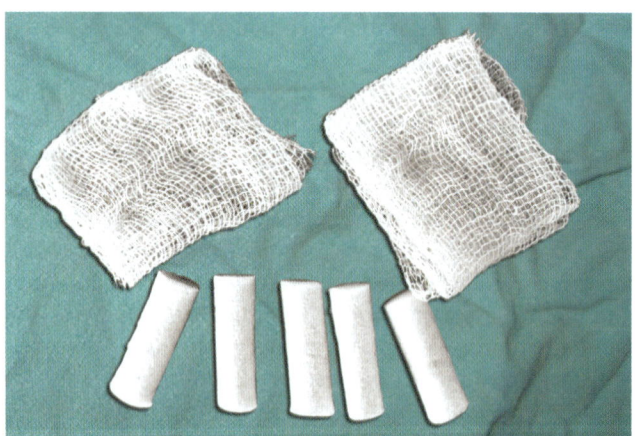

Figure 10.19: Cotton rolls and gauzes used for absorbing saliva and moisture

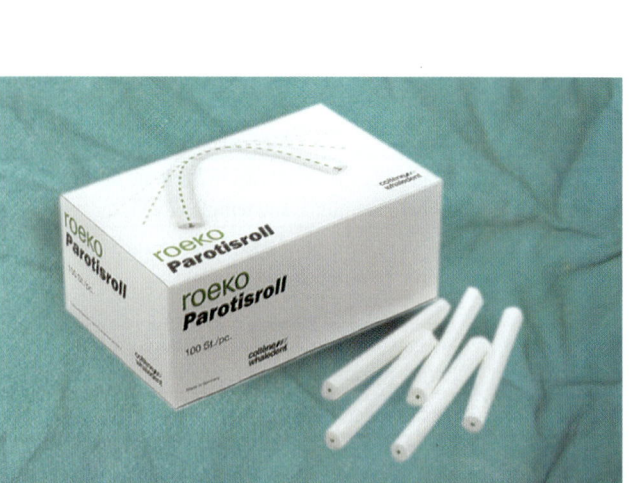

Figure 10.20: Cotton rolls

- Cotton rolls may be held in place with the help of cotton holder which has an added advantage of providing retraction of cheeks and tongue.
- Cellulose wafers are used in addition to cotton rolls and are placed in the buccal sulcus to retract the cheek. They are used to absorb saliva and other fluids for short periods of time, for example, during examination, fissure sealants, polishing.
- Other methods of moisture control, for example, saliva ejector may be positioned, after the cotton rolls or cellulose wafers are in place.
- One should take care while removing cotton rolls or cellulose wafers that they should be moist, to prevent inadvertent removal of the epithelium.

Advantages of absorbents

➡ Effective to control small amounts of moisture for short time periods
➡ Retract soft tissues at same time.

- Provide only short-term moisture control
- Ineffective if high volumes of fluid are present
- Shallow sulci and hyperactive tongue may make placement and retention difficult.

Low Volume Evacuator

Low volume evacuation is basically done using saliva ejectors. *Saliva ejector* is best used to remove small amounts of moisture and saliva collected in the oral cavity during clinical procedure. It can be used in conjunction with other methods of moisture control. Tip of saliva ejector should be smooth to prevent any tissue injury. It is better to have small diameter disposable tip (**Figs 10.23 and 10.24**). To avoid any interference with working, it can be bent to place in the required area of mouth. Saliva ejector with flexible

plastic tubing and protective flange provides an added advantage of retraction of tongue (**Fig. 10.25**).

Advantages of low volume evacuator

- Economical
- Easy to use
- Can be held by patient
- Can be placed under rubber dam
- Some have flanges attached which help in retraction of tongue and floor of mouth.

Disadvantages of low volume evacuator

- Hyperactive tongues can make its placement difficult
- Low volume aspirators do not remove solids well
- If used inappropriately, can be uncomfortable for patient
- May cause soft tissue damage by sucking in soft tissues into the tip.

Precautions to be Taken While Using Saliva Ejector

- Before using, mold the ejector so that its tip faces backward with upward curvature. In other words, floor of mouth should not directly contact the tip so as to avoid trauma.
- Sides of saliva ejector should not rub against surface of mouth to avoid injury
- When rubber dam is used, always make a hole so that ejector can pass through the dam instead of placing it under the dam.
- Always protect floor of mouth beneath the ejector using cotton rolls or gauze piece to avoid tissue injury.

High Volume Evacuator

It is used to remove water from airotor and large particulate matter with high suction speed (**Fig. 10.25**). It is best performed by double ended aspiration tip. One aspiration

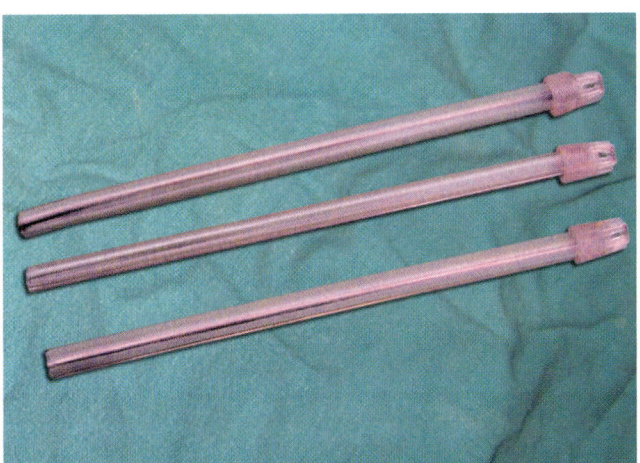

Figure 10.23: Disposable suction tips

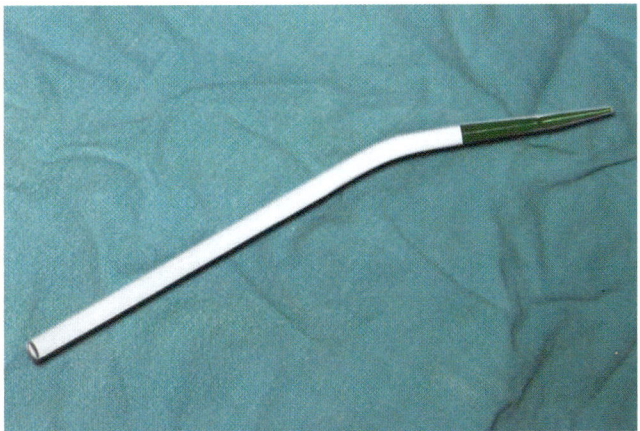

Figure 10.24: Suction tip

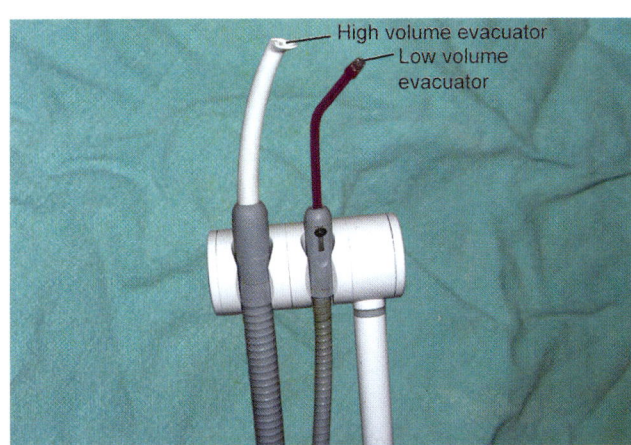

Figure 10.25: High volume evacuator and low

tip is kept on lingual side and another on the buccal side so as to aspirate from both sides. It also helps in retracting cheek and tongue. Tip used in high volume evacuator can be made-up of plastic or stainless steel.

Advantages of volume evacuator
It facilitates fast removal of
➡ Large particulate matter
➡ Water from high speed drills
➡ Air water spray
➡ Since clean field is achieved in less time, quadrant dentistry is made easy
➡ Added advantage of double ended aspiration tip is that if by chance one end gets clogged, another end can keep on aspirating.

Air-Water Syringe

By air-water syringe an air blast can be useful to dry tooth or soft tissues during examination or used during operative procedures (**Fig. 10.26**).

Advantage of air-water syringe
Easy to use.

Disadvantages of air-water syringe
➡ Can dehydrate dentin and cause pain and discomfort to patient
➡ Not effective if there are large volumes of moisture
➡ Does not remove the moisture from oral cavity, it can just transfer moisture from one tooth to the next.

Throat Shield

Throat shield is especially important when the maxillary tooth is being treated. In this, an unfolded gauze sponge is stretched over the tongue and posterior part of the mouth.

It is useful in recovering a restoration(inlay or crown), if it is dropped in the oral cavity.

Advantages of throat shield
➡ Avoids aspiration of restorations
➡ Economical
➡ Easy to use.

Disadvantage of throat shield
Not well tolerated by some patients as it can cause gagging.

Cheek Retractors

They are used to expand the mouth opening more in the vertical rather than horizontal direction (**Fig. 10.27**). This makes them ideal for use when working on the gingival border of upper and lower front teeth and for the adjustment of orthodontic bands.

Mouth Prop

A mouth prop should establish and maintain suitable mouth opening, thus help in tooth preparation of posterior teeth (**Fig. 10.28**). It is placed on the side opposite to treatment site, placed between mandibular and maxillary teeth. A mouth prop should have following features
- It should be easily positioned in the mouth without any discomfort
- It should be easily and readily removable by clinician or the patient in case of an emergency
- It should be either disposable or sterilizable
- It should be adaptable to all mouths.

Advantages of mouth prop
➡ Offers muscle relaxation for patient
➡ Provides sufficient mouth opening for long durations
➡ Easily positioned and removed.

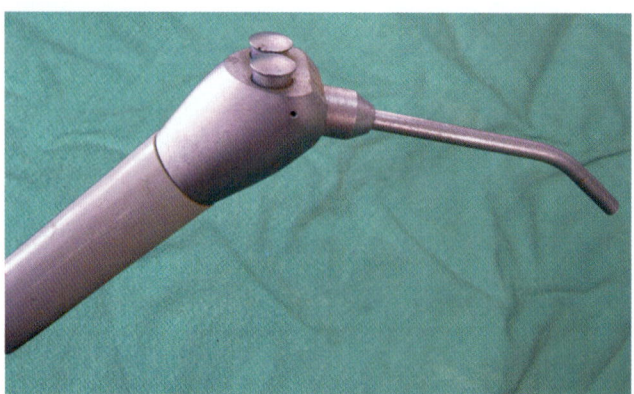

Figure 10.26: Air-water syringe

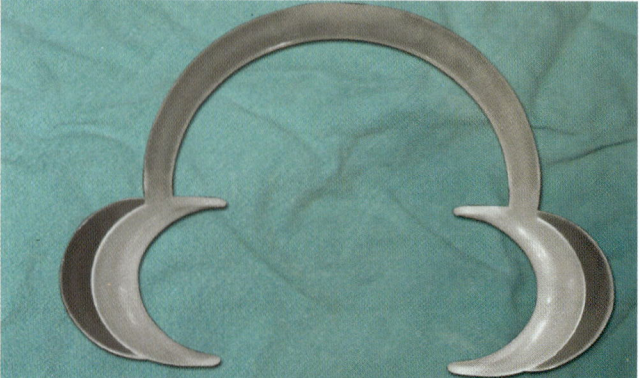

Figure 10.27: Cheek retractor

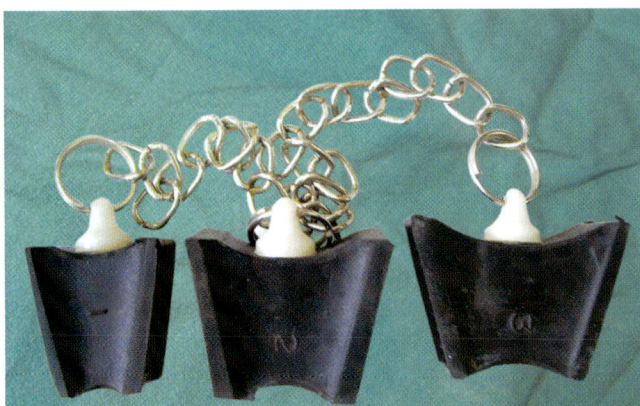

Figure 10.28: Mouth prop

PHARMACOLOGICAL METHODS

In this method, a chemical agent is administered orally 1 to 2 hours prior to the procedure which causes temporary dry mouth by acting on sympathetic nervous system.

Occasionally, atropine is the drug which is used in restorative dentistry in a dose of 0.3 to 1 mg, 1 to 2 hours prior to procedure. But since it has autonomic effects, atropine is contraindicated for nursing mothers and for patients with glaucoma.

Advantage of pharmacological methods
Controls salivary flow in case of hypersalivation when other methods are ineffective.

Disadvantage of pharmacological methods
Side effects; tachycardia, dilatation of pupils, urinary retention, sweat gland inhibition.

METHODS USED FOR GINGIVAL TISSUE MANAGEMENT

There are various methods available which can be used for effective gingival tissue retraction. These methods are
- Physicomechanical
- Chemical
- Chemomechanical
- Rotary curettage
- Electrochemical
- Surgical.

Physicomechanical Means

In this, different methods are used, which mechanically displace the gingiva both laterally and apically away from the tooth surface.

Before using these methods following requirements should be fulfilled
- Normal and healthy gingiva with good vascular supply.
- Adequate zone of attached gingiva
- Adequate amount of healthy bone without the sign of tooth resorption.

Methods for Physicomechanical Means
➡ Rubber dam
➡ Wooden wedges
➡ Gingival retraction cords
➡ Rolled cotton twills.

Methods for Physicomechanical Means

Rubber dam: Various type of rubber dam sheets such as heavy and extra heavy sheets provide adequate type of mechanical displacement of gingival tissue.

For additional retraction, Clamp No. 212 (cervical retainer) can be also used.

Wooden wedges: They are used interdentally to displace the gingival tissue, thus helping in retraction. Care should be taken while using wooden wedge as it can damage the interproximal tissue if inserted forcibly.

Gingival retraction cords (Fig. 10.29): Different types of retraction cords are available in the market which displace the gingiva both laterally and apically away from the tooth surface.

Retraction cord can be of cotton or synthetic and braided/nonbraided type.

Different sizes of retraction cords available in the market
➡ 000 – 1
➡ 00 – 2
➡ 0 – 3

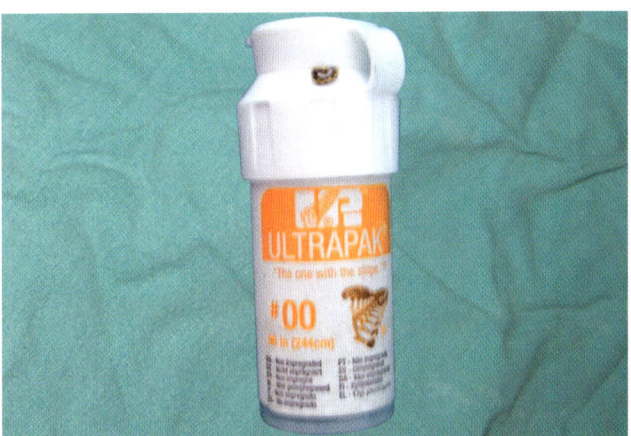

Figure 10.29: Retraction cord

Indications of gingival retraction

- Control of gingival flow or gingival bleeding—especially when the margins of restoration are close to gingiva, for example, restoration of class V preparation
- To provide esthetics for final restoration of fixed prosthesis by exposing the finish line
- To increase retention in case of indirect restorations where crown height is inadequate
- To extend the margins subgingivally in case of cervical caries extending below the gingiva
- For accurate recording of preparation margins while taking impressions
- For removing the hypertrophied gingiva, interfering with placement of preparation margins.

Placement and Removal of Retraction Cord
(Figs 10.30A to E)

- Anesthetize the area.
- Select the appropriate size of cord which can be placed into gingival sulcus without causing any injury/ischemia.
- Take the length of cord so that it extends 1 mm beyond the gingival width of the preparation or extends around the whole circumference of the tooth.
- Take an instrument for packing the cord. It should be blunt hatchet or hoe shaped (**Fig. 10.31**).
- Apply slight force laterally and slightly angulated towards the tooth surface. Avoid application of apical

pressure as it may harm the junctional epithelium (**Fig. 10.32**)

- Insert one end of the cord, stabilize it with blunt instrument and pack the rest of the cord. Avoid putting ends of the cord interproximally for better grip of the cord. Cord should end where interdental col has the maximum height.
- Remove the cord slowly and take care that it should not be dry. A dry cord may adhere to epithelium and on removal it may cause its abrasion.
- Check for any pieces of retraction cord immediately after its removal and remove if any, to avoid gingival irritation.

Rolled cotton twills: This is simplest and effective method which is used for lateral displacement of the gingival tissue by mechanically packing the cotton twills in the sulcus.

Cotton twills combined with zinc oxide eugenol (fast-setting) can also be used for gingival retraction.

Chemical Means (Fig. 10.33)

Chemical method is one of the oldest methods used in its retraction of gingiva. But its use is now abandoned because of its undesirable effects on the tissue.

Different types of chemicals used are:
- Trichloroacetic acid
- Sulfuric acid.

Trichloroacetic acid: This is only chemical which is used in some centers. Nowadays their use has been limited.

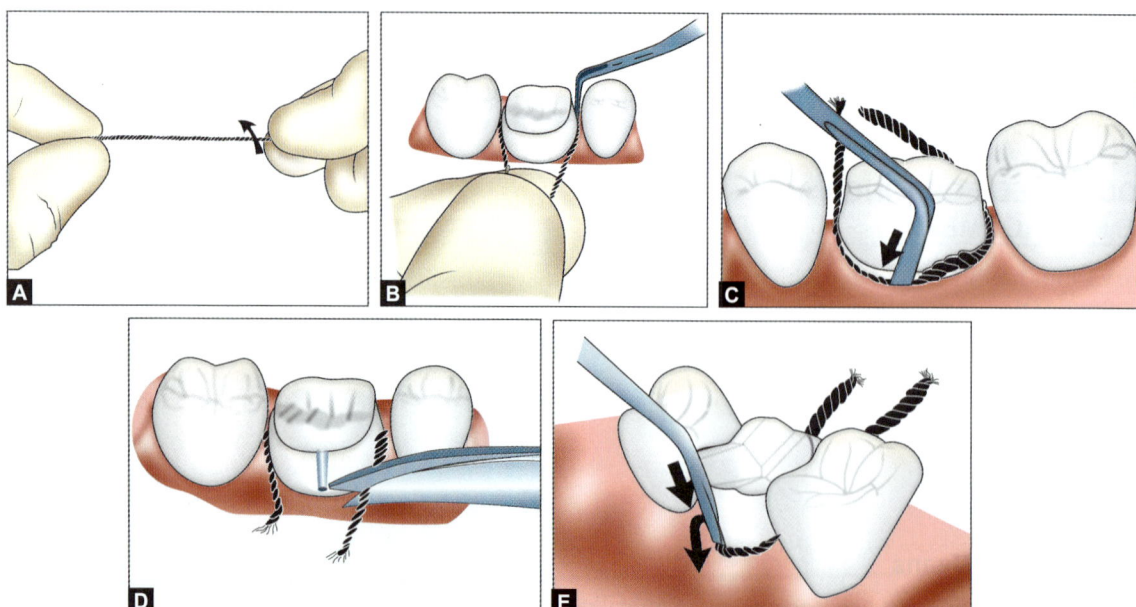

Figures 10.30A to E: Placement of retraction cord: (A) A two inch long cord is taken and twisted to make it tight; (B and C) Cord is placed around the tooth and pushed into the sulcus; (D) Extra cord is cut off; (E) Remaining cord piece is tucked into the sulcus

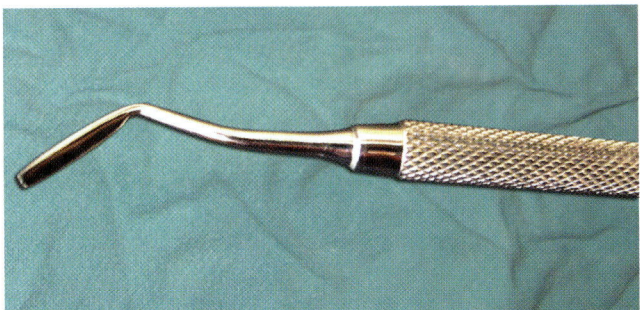

Figure 10.31: Cord tucking instrument

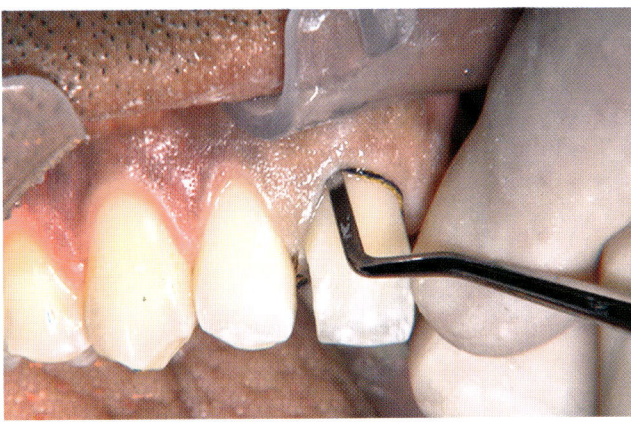

Figure 10.32: While tucking cord into the sulcus, apply slight force laterally and angulated towards tooth surface

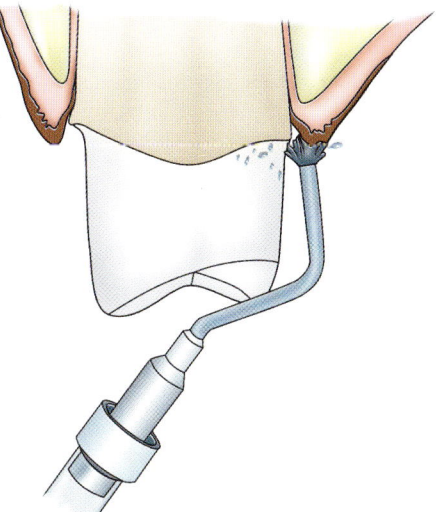

Figure 10.33: Application of chemical agent for management of gingival tissue

Advantages of trichloroacetic acid
Effectively controls the bleeding site.

Disadvantages of trichloroacetic acid
Caustic in nature—can cause soft tissue damage if accidently dropped on tissues.

Chemicomechanical Methods

This is the most common and popular technique used for gingival retraction and has been considered safe, also it provides adequate amount of gingival tissue displacement.

Different chemicals used are
➡ Vasoconstrictors ♦ Epinephrine ♦ Norepinephrine ➡ Astringents ♦ Alum (100%) ♦ Aluminum chloride (15–25%) ♦ Tannic acid (15–25%) ♦ Ferric sulphate (15–15.5%). ➡ Tissue coagulants ♦ Zinc Chloride ♦ Silver nitrate.

Vasoconstrictors

As the name indicates, these cause local vasoconstriction, reduce the blood supply and gingival fluid seepage.

Epinephrine and norephinephrine are included in this category.

But nowadays, their use has been declined because of systemic adverse effects.

Advantage of vasoconstrictors
Used as an adjunct to gingival retraction cord when gingival bleeding is present.

Disadvantages of vasoconstrictors
➡ Invasive procedure. ➡ Contraindicated in patients with cardiovascular disease, diabetes mellitus. ➡ Not effective if profuse bleeding is present.

Astringents (Biologic Fluid Coagulants)

As compared to vasoconstrictors, these chemicals are considered to be safe and have no systemic effects.

These chemicals coagulate blood and gingival fluid in the sulcus, thus forms a surface layer which seals against blood and fluid seepage.

Alum, aluminum chloride, tannic acid and feric sulphate are included in this category.

Tissue Coagulants

These chemicals or coagulants are not preferred because of its side effects. These agents usually act by coagulating the surface layer of sulcular and gingival epithelium. These chemicals form a nonpermeable film for underlying fluids.

Zinc chloride and silver nitrate are included in the tissue coagulants.

If applied for prolonged time, these chemicals can cause
- Ulceration
- Local necrosis
- Change in contour, size and position of free gingiva.

Rotary Curettage (Gingettage) (Fig. 10.34)

This is troughing technique which is used to remove minimal amount of gingival epithelium during placement of restorative margins subgingivally. This is usually done with high speed handpiece and chamfer diamond bur.

The main disadvantages of this technique are:
- Excessive bleeding
- Damage to gingiva.

Electrosurgical Methods (Fig. 10.35)

Electrosurgical method is preferred when approach to working area is not obtained by more conservative methods. One of the main advantage of electrosurgical method is minimal bleeding during surgery.

Before going into detail, one should have clear idea about principles of electrosurgery so that damage to tissue is minimal and desirable effects can be obtained.

Principles: Alternating electric current energy is used at high frequency. Concentrate this energy at tiny electrodes, producing localized changes in the tissues, limited only to 2 to 3 cell layers.

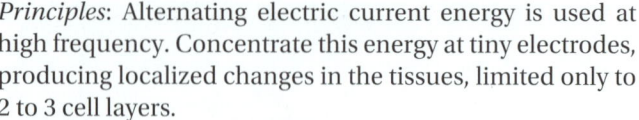

Advantages of electrosurgical Methods
➡ Easier to obtain bloodless area
➡ Healing by primary intention
➡ Rapid procedure
➡ Causes atraumatic cutting of tissue
➡ Sterilizes the wound

Four Types of Actions are done in this (Figs 10.36 and 10.37)

1. *Cutting*:
   - Most commonly used
   - Extremely precise in nature
   - Minimal involvement of tissue without any bleeding
   - Minimum after effects.

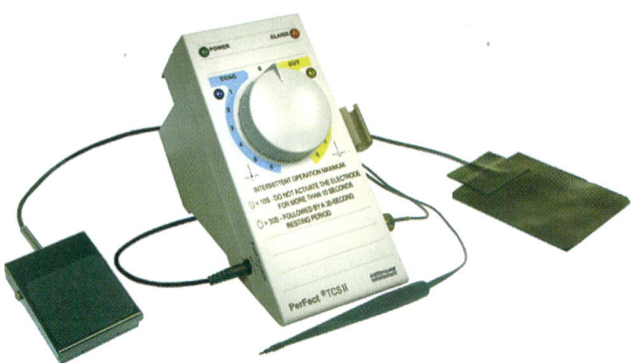

Figure 10.35: Electrosurgical unit

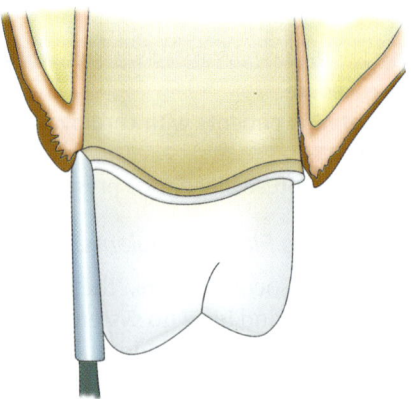

Figure 10.34: Rotary curettage

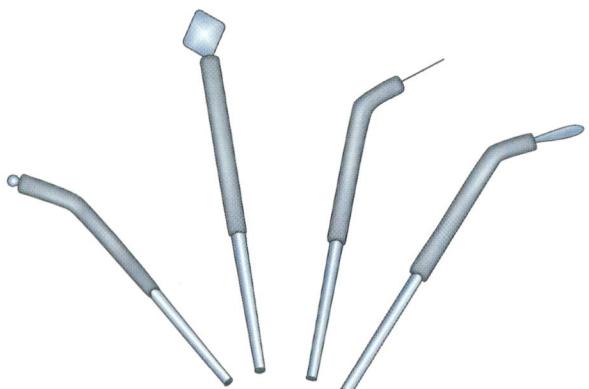

Figure 10.36: Different electrodes for different actions (cutting, coagulation, etc.)

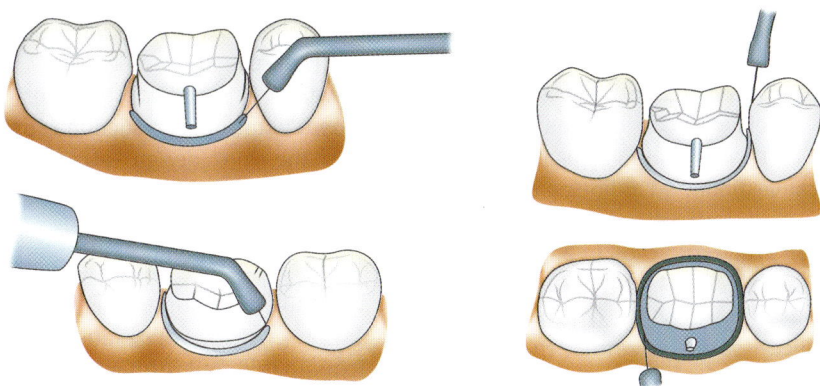

Figure 10.37: Electrosurgical management of excess gingival tissue

2. *Coagulation*:
   - Less commonly used
   - Surface coagulation of tissues, fluid and blood as greater heat is used
   - Overdose causes carbonization.
3. *Fulguration*:
   - Use of greater heat and energy than coagulation
   - Deeper tissue involvement
   - More after effects.
4. *Dessication*:
   - Most dangerous among four actions
   - Uncontrolled and unlimited in nature
   - Massive destruction of tissue
   - More after effects among four actions.

Rules for Electrosurgery

- Proper isolation of working site. Avoid excessive drying up of the tissues
- Use adequate current
- Use fully rectified, filtered current with minimum energy output for cutting action on tissues.

For cutting type of action:
- Use unipolar electrode either in probe or loop type
- Use with light touch, rapid and intermittent strokes
- Use electrode on the inner area of sulcus
- Avoid touching the gingival crest area as it may result in gingival recession.

For coagulation type of action:
- Use bulky unipolar electrode
- Use partially rectified current
- Place electrode close to the tissue
- Avoid touching the electrode to the tissue
- Avoid touching the metallic restorations with electrode to prevent short circuit

- Sparks during working indicates high energy output
- Always clean electrode tips with alcohol sponge after energy use.

Surgical Methods

This method is used to remove interfering gingival tissues with surgical blade.

Key Points

- Rubber dam was introduced by Barnum, a New York dentist in 1863.
- Rubber dam can be defined as a flat thin sheet of latex/nonlatex that is held by a clamp and frame which is perforated to allow the tooth/teeth to protrude through the perforations while all other teeth are covered and protected by sheet.
- Flexi dam is latex free dam of standard thickness with no rubber smell.
- Rubber dam clamps are used to hold the rubber dam on to the tooth and help in retracting the gingiva.
- Insti-Dam is natural latex dam with prepunched hole and built-in white frame.
- Handi dam eliminates the need for traditional frame. It allows easy access to oral cavity during the procedure.
- "Split dam technique" is that in which rubber dam is placed to isolate the tooth without the use of rubber dam clamp. Here two overlapping holes are punched in the dam, then the dam is stretched over the tooth to be treated and over the adjacent tooth on each side. Edge of rubber dam is carefully teased through the contacts of distal side of adjacent teeth. It is done to isolate anterior teeth, or when crown structure is insufficient and to isolate porcelain crown where placement of rubber

dam clamp over the crown margins can damage the cervical porcelain.

- Cotton rolls are usually placed in buccal or lingual sulcus specially where salivary gland ducts exit so as to absorb saliva. The maxillary teeth are isolated by placing a cotton roll in the buccal vestibule. Mandibular teeth are isolated by placing a small sized cotton roll in the buccal vestibule and a larger sized cotton roll in lingual vestibule.
- Cellulose wafers are used in addition to cotton rolls and are placed in the buccal sulcus to retract the cheek. They are used to absorb saliva and other fluids for short periods of time, for example, during examination, fissure sealants, polishing.
- Saliva ejector is used to remove small amounts of moisture and saliva collected in the oral cavity during clinical procedure.
- High volume evacuator is used to remove water from airotor and large particulate matter with high suction speed.
- Throat shield is especially important when the maxillary tooth is being treated. In this, an unfolded gauze sponge is stretched over the tongue and posterior part of the mouth. It is useful in recovering a restoration (inlay or crown), if it is dropped in the oral cavity.
- Occasionally, atropine is the drug which is used in restorative dentistry in a dose of 0.3 to 1 mg, 1-2 hours prior to procedure. But since it has autonomic effects, atropine is contraindicated for nursing mothers and for patients with glaucoma.
- Rotary curettage (Gingettage) is troughing technique which is used to remove minimal amount of gingival epithelium during placement of restorative margins subgingivally. This is usually done with high speed handpiece and chamfer diamond bur.

🕵 Want to Know More

Optra Dam
- It is recently introduced dam in which no metal clamps are required, resulting in fast and easy placement by one person and patient comfort. Both arches are fully exposed and a completely dry field is achieved simultaneously

Opti Dam
- It is anatomically designed frame and dam which provide better access and visibility. Because of preshaped dam and frame, the time consuming procedure of conventional rubber dam application is saved. Assembly and placement are easy and quick.

- Svedopter is a tongue retraction device, introduced by EC Moore.
- SweFlex Saliva Ejector reduces aerosols during treatment with superior suction capability. Its atomical "under-the-chin" design retracts tongue and stays there without hand support.

QUESTIONS

1. Why isolation of operating field is important? Enumerate various methods of isolation of operating field.
2. Explain in detail rubber dam.
3. Short notes:
   a. Gingival tissue management
   b. Rubber dam kit
   c. Problems during application of rubber dam.
4. Enumerate various methods of isolation of operating field. Discuss in detail about the rubber dam.
5. Enumerate various methods employed for isolation of operative field. Describe advantages and disadvantages of each method.
6. Define isolation. What is the importance of isolation in operative dentistry? List various methods of isolation and discuss rubber dam in detail.

BIBLIOGRAPHY

1. Barghi N, et al. Comparing two methods of moisture control in bonding to enamel: a clinical study. Oper Dent. 1991;16:130-5.
2. Barghi N, Knight GT, Berry TG. Comparing two methods of moisture control in bonding to enamel: a clinical study. Oper Dent. 1991;16:130.
3. Bowles WH, Tardy SJ, Vahadi A. Evaluation of new gingival retraction agents. J Dent Res. 1991;70:1447.
4. Christensen GJ. Using rubber dams to boost quality, quantity of restorative services. J Am Dent Assoc. 1994;125:81-2.
5. Cochran MA, et al. The efficacy of the rubber dam as a barrier to the spread of microorganisms during dental treatment. J Am Dent Assoc. 1989;119:141-4.
6. Cunningham PR, Ferguson GW. The instruction of rubber dam technique. J Am Acad Gold Foil Oper. 1970;13:5-12.
7. Heling I, et al. Rubber dam - an essential safeguard, Quintessence Int. 1988;19:377-8.
8. Jones CM, Reid JS. Patient and operator attitudes toward rubber dam. ASDC J Dent Child. 1988;55:452.
9. Medina JE. The rubber dam - an incentive for excellence. Dent Clin North Am. 1957;March, 255.
10. Medina JE. The rubber dam - an incentive for excellence, Dent Clin North Am. 1967;255-64.
11. Stibbs GD. Rubber dam. I Can Dent Assoc. 1951;17:311.
12. Wong RCK. The rubber dam as a means of infection control in an era of AIDS and hepatitis. J Indiana Dent Assoc. 67, 41, Jan./Feb. 1988.

Infection Control

RATIONALE FOR INFECTION CONTROL

The deposition of organisms in the tissues and their growth resulting in a host reaction is called infection. The number of organisms required to cause an infection is termed as "the infective dose". Factors affecting infective dose are:
- Virulence of the organism
- Susceptibility of the host.
- Age, drug therapy, or pre-existing disease, etc.

Microorganisms can spread from one person to another via direct contact, indirect contact, droplet infection and airborne infection **Flow chart 11.1**.

Direct contact occurs by touching soft tissues or teeth of patients. It causes immediate spread of infection by the source.

Indirect contact results from injuries with contaminated sharp instruments, needle stick injuries or contact with contaminated equipment and surfaces.

Droplet infection occurs by large particle droplets spatter which is transmitted by close contact. Spatter generated during dental procedures may deliver microorganisms to the dentist. Airborne infection involves small particles of < 5 μm size. These microorganisms remain airborne for hours and can cause infection when inhaled.

CROSS-INFECTION

Cross-infection is transmission of infectious agents among patients and staff within a clinical environment. This source of infection can be:
- Patients suffering from infectious diseases
- Patients who are in the prodromal stage of infections
- Healthy carriers of pathogens.

Different Routes of Spread of Infection

Different routes of spread of infection
→ Patient to dental health care worker (DHCW)
→ DHCW to patient
→ Patient to patient
→ Dental office to community
→ Community to patient.

Patient to Dental Health Care Worker

It can occur in following ways:

Flow chart 11.1: Chain of infection

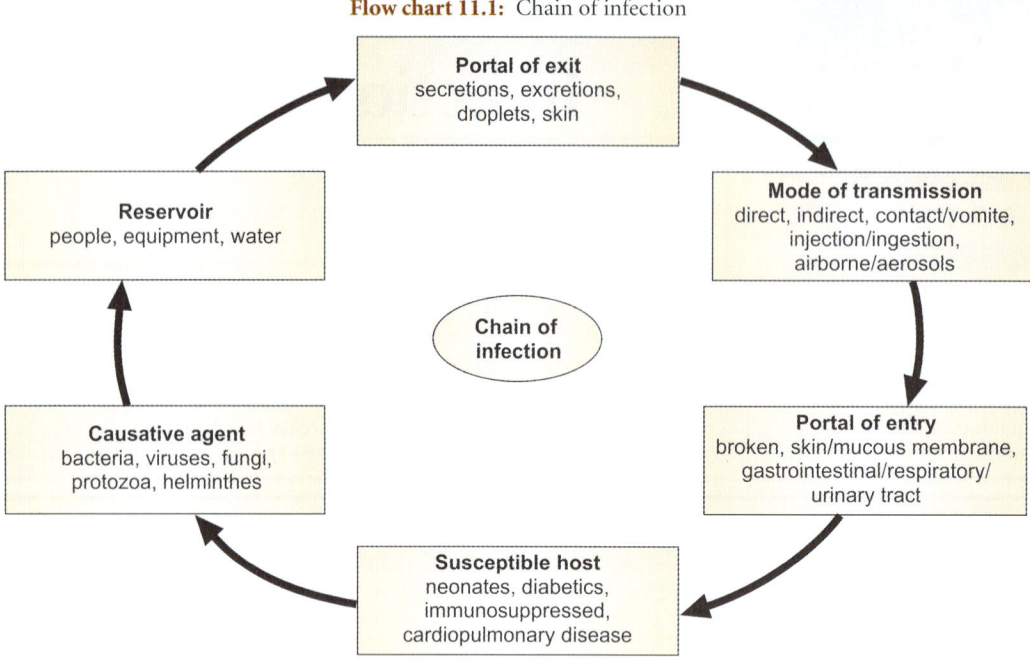

- Direct contact through break in skin or direct contact with mucous membrane of DHCW
- Indirect contact via sharp cutting instruments and needle stick injuries
- Droplet injection by *spatter* produced during dental procedures and through mucosal surfaces of dental team.

Dental Health Care Worker to the Patient

It occurs by:
- Direct contact, i.e. through mucosal surfaces of the patient
- Indirect contact, i.e. via use of contaminated instruments and lack of use of disposable instruments
- Droplet infection via inhalation by the patient.

Patient to Patient

It occurs by use of contaminated and nondisposable instruments.

Dental Office to the Community

It occurs:
- When contaminated impression or other equipments contaminate dental laboratory technicians
- Via spoiled clothing and regulated waste.

Community to the Patient

Community to the patient involves the entrance of microorganisms into water supply of dental unit. These microorganisms colonize inside the water lines and thereby form biofilm which is responsible for causing infection.

OBJECTIVE OF INFECTION CONTROL

The main objective of infection control is elimination or reduction in spread of infection from all types of microorganisms. It is the duty of a clinician for implementing effective infection control to protect other patients and all members of the dental team.

Basically two factors are important in infection control
➡ Prevention of spread of microorganisms from their hosts
➡ Killing or removal of microorganisms from objects and surfaces.

UNIVERSAL PRECAUTIONS

Some strategies have to be followed in order to reduce the risk of infection and transmission caused by blood borne pathogens such as HBV and HIV. It is always recommended to follow some basic infection control procedures for all patients, termed as "universal precautions". These are as follows:

- *Immunization:* All members of the dental team (who are exposed to blood or blood contaminated articles) should be vaccinated against hepatitis B.
- Use of personal protective barrier techniques, that is use of protective gown, face mask, protective eyewear, gloves, etc. These reduce the risk of exposure to infectious material and injury from sharp instruments.
- Maintaining hand hygiene.

Personal Protection Equipment

Barrier Technique

The use of barrier technique is very important, which includes gown, face mask, protective eyewear and gloves (**Fig. 11.1**).

Protective gown: Protective gown should be worn to prevent contamination of normal clothing and to protect the skin of the clinician from exposure to blood and body substances.

- The clinician should change protective clothing when it becomes soiled and if contaminated by blood.
- Gown can be reusable or disposable for use. It should have a high neck and long sleeves to protect the arms from splash and splatter.
- Protective clothing must be removed before leaving the workplace.
- Protective clothing should be washed in the laundry with health care facility. If it is not present, the gown should be washed separately from other clothing.

Facemasks (Fig. 11.2): A surgical mask that covers both the nose and mouth should be worn by the clinician during procedures. Though facemasks do not provide complete microbiological protection, they prevent the splatter from contaminating the face. In other words, face masks provide protection against microorganisms generated during various procedures and droplet spatter that contain bloodborne pathogens.

Points to remember regarding facemasks

- Masks should be changed regularly and between patients
- The outer surface of mask can get contaminated with infectious droplets from spray or from touching the mask with contaminated fingers, so should not be reused
- If the mask becomes wet, it should be changed between patients or even during patient treatment
- The maximum time for wearing masks should not be more than one hour, since it becomes dampened from respiration, causing its degradation
- In order to get greater protection against splatter, a chin length plastic face shield must be worn, in addition to face masks
- To remove mask, grasp it only by its strings, not by the mask itself (**Fig. 11.3**).

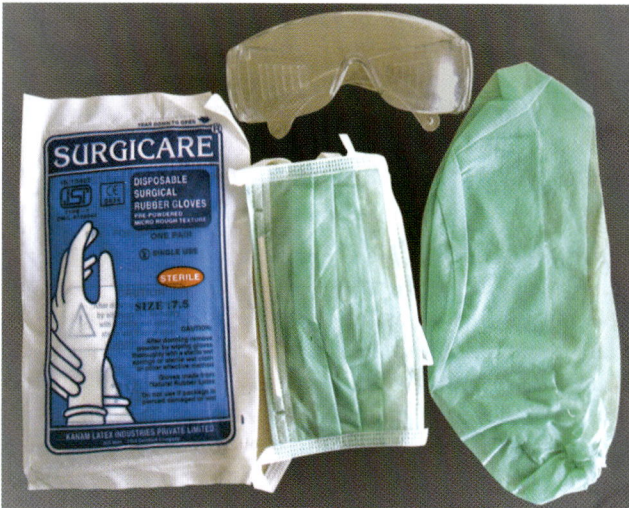

Figure 11.1: Personal protective equipment showing mouth mask, gloves, eye wear, head cap

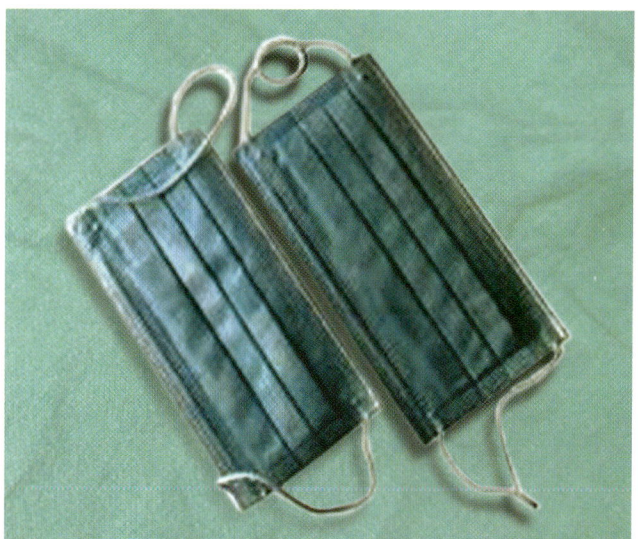

Figure 11.2: Facemask

Head caps: Hair should be properly tied. Long hair should be either covered or restrained away from face. To prevent hair contamination head caps must be used.

Protective eyewear: Clinician, helping staff and patient must protect their eyes against foreign bodies, splatter and aerosols which arise during operative procedures by using protective glasses. Eyewear protects the eyes from injury and from microbes such as hepatitis B virus, which can be transmitted through conjunctiva.

Eyewear with solid side-shields or chin-length face shields must be used for optimal protection. Contaminated glasses should be washed in soapy water and disinfected with a product that does not cause irritation to the eyes. Do not touch the eyewear with ungloved hands, because it can be contaminated with spatter of blood and saliva during patient care.

Gloves (Fig. 11.4): Gloves should be worn to prevent contamination of hands when touching mucous membranes, blood, saliva and to reduce the chances of transmission of infected microorganisms from clinician to patient. All persons with direct patient contact must wear nonsterile gloves routinely. They must be worn for all dental procedures including extra and intraoral examination and not only for those procedures where there is a possibility of bleeding. It has been shown that working with bare hands results in the retention of microorganisms, saliva and blood under the fingernails for several days.

Ideally gloves should be:

- Good quality, sterile for all types of surgical procedures and non-sterile for all clinical procedures and changed after every patient.
- Well fitted and nonpowdered since the powder from gloves can contaminate veneers and radiographs and can interfere with wound healing.
- Made up of 'low extractable latex protein' to reduce the possibility of allergy.

Some important points regarding use of gloves
➠ Gloves are manufactured as disposable items meant to be used for only one patient.
➠ A new pair of gloves should be used for each patient and may need to be changed during a procedure.
➠ Gloves should be changed between patients and when torn or punctured.
➠ Overgloves or paper towels must be used for opening drawers, cabinets, etc.
➠ Handwashing should be performed immediately before putting on gloves. Similarly, handwashing after glove removal is essential.
➠ Gloves must be worn when handling or cleaning materials or surfaces contaminated with body fluids.
➠ Some persons can show allergic reactions to gloves due to latex (polyisoprene) or antioxidants such as mercaptobenzothiazole. Ensure that latex free equipment and non latex gloves (polyurethane or vinyl gloves) are used on patients who have a latex-allergy.
➠ Person with skin problems (if related to use of glove) should be assessed properly.
➠ Latex gloves should be used for patient examinations and procedures and should be disposed off thereafter.
➠ Heavy utility gloves should be worn when handling and cleaning contaminated instruments and for surface cleaning and disinfection.

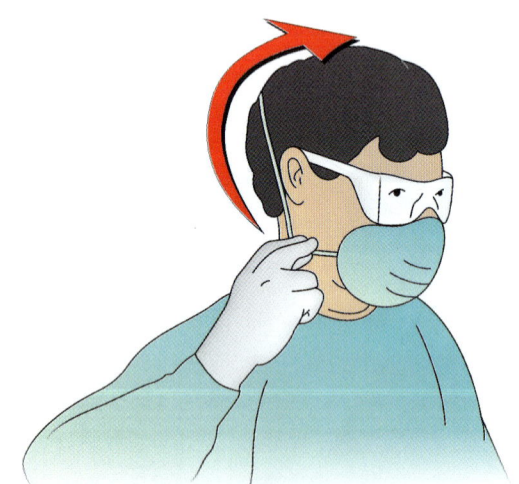

Figure 11.3: Removal of facemask should be done by grasping it only by its strings, not by mask itself

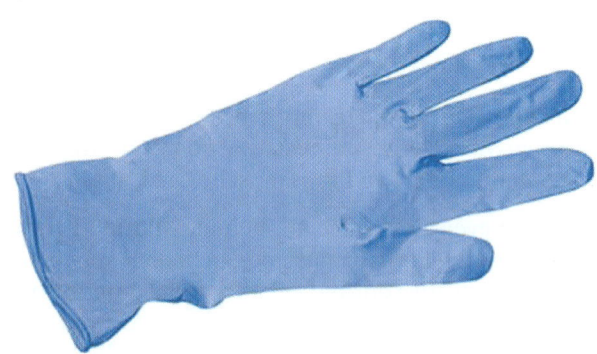

Figure 11.4: Gloves

Hand Hygiene

As in any clinical practice setting, hand hygiene plays a central role in the reduction of cross-contamination and in infection control. Hand hygiene significantly reduces potential pathogens on the hands and is considered as the single most critical measure for reducing the risk of transmitting organisms to patients and dentists. The microbial flora of the skin consist of transient and resident microorganisms.

Transient flora, which colonize the superficial layers of the skin, are easier to remove by routine handwashing. They are acquired by direct contact with patients or contaminated environmental surfaces. These organisms are most frequently associated with health-care–associated infections.

Resident flora attached to deeper layers of the skin are more resistant to removal and less likely to be associated with such infections.

The preferred method for hand hygiene depends on the type of procedure, the degree of contamination and the desired persistence of antimicrobial action on the skin. For routine dental examinations and nonsurgical procedures, handwashing and hand antisepsis is achieved by using either a plain or antimicrobial soap with water. If the hands are not visibly soiled, an alcohol-based hand rub is adequate.

The purpose of surgical hand antisepsis is to eliminate transient flora and reduce resident flora for the duration of a procedure to prevent introduction of organisms in the operative wound, if gloves become punctured or torn. Skin bacteria can rapidly multiply under surgical gloves if hands are washed with soap that is not antimicrobial. Thus, an antimicrobial soap or alcohol hand rub with persistent activity should be used before surgical procedures.

For the routine dental procedures washing hands with plain, nonantimicrobial soap is sufficient. For more invasive procedures, such as cutting of gum or tissue, hand antisepsis with either an antiseptic solution or alcohol-based handrub is recommended. If available, waterless alcohol handrub/gel could be used in place of handwashing if hands are not visibly soiled.

Types of hand scrubs
➡ **Alcohol-based hand rub:** An alcohol containing preparation help in reducing the number of viable microorganisms on the hands.
➡ **Antimicrobial soap:** A detergent containing an antiseptic agent.
➡ **Antiseptic:** It is a germicide used on living tissue for the purpose of inhibiting or destroying microorganisms.

Indications for Hand Hygiene

Handwashing should be done:
- At the beginning of patient
- Between patient contacts
- Before putting on gloves
- After touching inanimate objects
- Before touching eyes, nose, face or mouth
- After completion of case
- Before eating, drinking
- Between each patient
- After glove removal

- After barehanded contact with contaminated equipment or surfaces and before leaving treatment areas
- At the end of the day.

Handwash Technique (Figs 11.5A to F)

- Removal of rings, jewellery and watches
- Cover cuts and abrasions with waterproof adhesive dressings
- Clean fingernails with a plastic or wooden stick
- Scrub hands, nails and forearm using a good quality liquid soap preferably containing a disinfectant
- Rinse hands thoroughly with running water
- Dry hands with towel.

CLASSIFICATION OF INSTRUMENTS

The center for disease control and prevention (CDC) classified the instrument into critical, semicritical and noncritical depending on the potential risk of infection during the use of these instruments. These categories are also referred to as Spaulding classification *(by Spaulding in 1968)*.

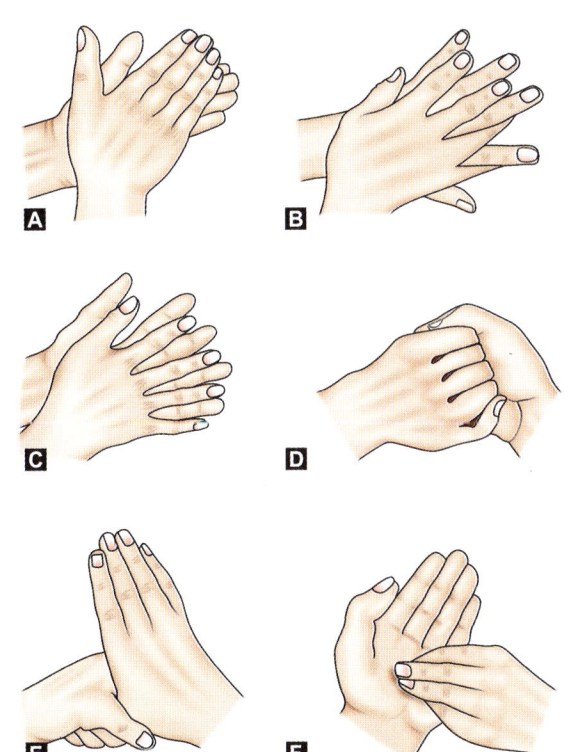

Figures 11.5A to F: Technique of Handwash: (A) Rub both palms; (B) Rub the back of both palms; (C) Rub palms again with fingers interlaced; (D) Rub back of interlaced fingers; (E) Wash back of thumbs; (F) Rub both palms with fingertips

Classification of instrument sterilization

Category	Definition	Examples
Critical	• Where instruments enter or penetrate into sterile tissue, cavity or blood stream	• Surgical blades and instruments • Surgical dental bur
Semicritical	• Which contact intact mucosa or nonintact skin	• Amalgam condenser • Dental handpieces • Mouth mirror • Saliva ejectors
Noncritical	• Which contact intact skin	• Pulse oximeter • Stethoscope • Light switches • Dental chair

For complete sterilization, rule of universal sterilization should be followed. It means that all reusable instruments and handpieces are sterilized (not disinfected) between use on patient.

CDC Recommends:
- Critical and semicritical instruments are to be heat sterilized
- Semicritical items sensitive to heat should be treated with high level disinfectant after cleaning
- Noncritical items can be treated intermediate to low level disinfectant after cleaning.

Definitions

- *Cleaning:* It is the process which physically removes contamination but does not necessarily destroy microorganisms. It is a prerequisite before decontamination by disinfection or sterilization of instruments since organic material prevents contact with microbes, inactivates disinfectants.
- *Disinfection:* It is the process of using an agent that destroys germs or other harmful microbes or inactivates them, usually referred to chemicals that kill the growing forms (vegetative forms) but not the resistant spores of bacteria.
- *Antisepsis:* It is the destruction of pathogenic micro-organisms existing in their vegetative state on living tissue.
- *Sterilization:* Sterilization involves any process, physical or chemical that will destroy all forms of life, including bacterial, fungi, spores and viruses.
- *Aseptic technique:* It is the method which prevents contamination of wounds and other sites, by ensuring that only sterile objects and fluids come into contact with them; and that the risks of air-borne contamination are minimized.
- *Antiseptic:* It is a chemical applied to living tissues, such as skin or mucous membrane to reduce the number of microorganisms present by inhibition of their activity or by destruction.

- *Disinfectant:* It is a chemical substance, which causes disinfection. It is used on nonvital objects to kill surface vegetative pathogenic organisms but not necessarily spore forms or viruses.

INSTRUMENT PROCESSING PROCEDURES

Instrument processing is the collection of procedures which prepare the contaminated instruments for reuse. For complete sterilization process, prevention of the disease transmission and instruments should be processed *correctly* and *carefully* **Flow chart 11.2**.

Steps of instrument processing

- Presoaking (Holding)
- Cleaning
- Corrosion control
- Packaging
- Sterilization
- Monitoring of sterilization
- Handling the processed instrument.

Presoaking (Holding)

It facilitates the cleaning process by preventing the debris from drying.

Procedure:
- Wear puncture resistant heavy utility gloves and personnel protective equipment.
- Place loose instruments in a perforated cleaning basket and then place the basket into the holding solution.

Holding solution can be

- Neutral pH detergents
- Water
- Enzyme solution.

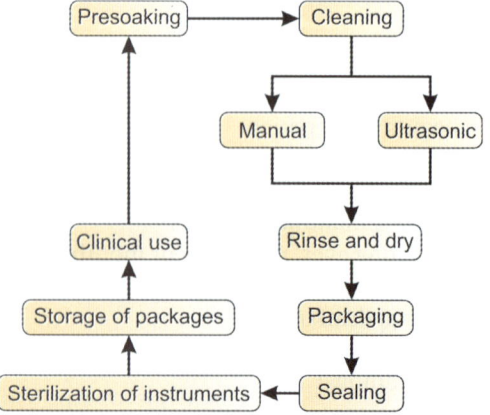

Flow chart 11.2: Instrument processing procedure

- Perforated cleaning basket reduces the direct handling of instruments. So, chances of contamination are decreased.
- Holding solution should be discarded atleast once a day or earlier if seems to be soiled.
- Avoid instrument soaking for long time as it increases the chances of corrosion of instruments.

Cleaning

It aids in the subsequent cleaning process by removing gross debris. It is considered as to be one of the important steps before any sterilization or disinfection procedure. The advantage of this procedure is that it reduces the bioburden, i.e. microorganisms, blood, saliva and other materials.

Methods used for cleaning
➡ Manual scrubbing
➡ Ultrasonic cleaning
➡ Mechanical – instrument washer.

Manual scrubbing: It is one of the most effective method for removing debris, if performed properly. Now-a-days, this method is not recommended because of the risk-factors involved.

Procedure

- Brush delicately all surfaces of instruments while submerged in cleaning solution.
- Use long-handled stiff nylon brush to keep the scrubbing hand away from sharp instrument surfaces.
- Always wear heavy utility gloves and personnel protective equipments.
- Use neutral pH detergents while cleaning.
- Instruments' surfaces should be visibly clean and free from stains and tissues.

Disadvantage: This procedure is not recommended as there are maximum chances of direct contact with instrument surfaces and also of cuts and punctures.

Ultrasonic cleaning (Fig. 11.6): It is excellent cleaning method as it reduces direct handling of instruments. So, it is considered as safer and more effective than manual scrubbing.

Procedure

- *Mechanism of action*: Ultrasonic energy generated in the ultrasonic cleaner produces billions of tiny bubbles which, in further, collapse and create high turbulence at the surface of instrument. This turbulence dislodges the debris.
- Maintain the proper solution level.
- Use recommended cleaning solution.

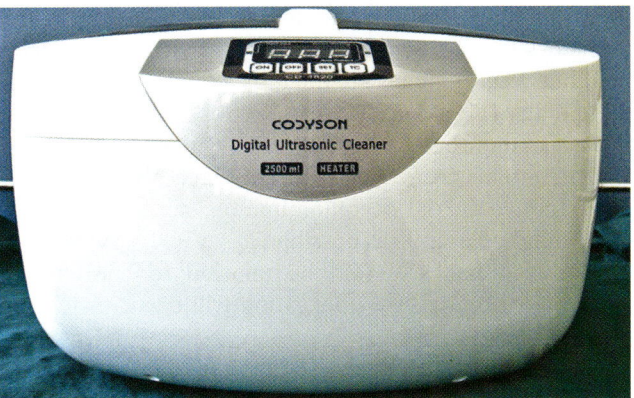

Figure 11.6: Ultrasonic cleaner

- Time may vary due to
  - Nature of instrument
  - Amount of debris
  - Efficiency of ultrasonic unit.
  Usually the time ranges vary from 4 to 16 minutes.
- After cleaning, remove the basket/cassette rack and wash under tap water. Use gloves while washing under tap water as the cleaning solution is also contaminated.
- Discard the solution daily.
- *Mechanical–instrument washer:* These are designed to clean instruments in hospital setup. Instrument washer has also the advantage that it reduces the direct handling of the instrument.

Control of Corrosion by Lubrication

It prevents damage of instruments because of drying. Some instruments or portions of instruments and burs (made up of carbon steel) will rust during steam sterilization, for example, grasping surfaces of forceps, cutting surfaces of orthodontic pliers, burs, scalers, hoes and hatchets.

For rust-prone instruments, use dry hot air oven/chemical vapor sterilization instead of autoclave. Use spray rust inhibitor (sodium nitrite) on the instruments.

Packaging

It maintains the sterility of instruments after the sterilization. Unpacked instruments are exposed to environment when sterilization chamber is opened and can be contaminated by dust, aerosols or by improper handling or contact with contaminated surfaces.

Packaging is the procedure in which cleaned instruments are organized in functional sets, thereafter with wrapping, these are placed in sterilization pouches or bags. One may also add chemical and biological indicators of sterilization in the pouches or bags.

Varieties of packaging materials are available in the market such as self-sealing, paper-plastic and peel-pouches. Peel-pouches are the most common and convenient to use (**Fig. 11.7**).

Packs should be stored with the following considerations:
- Instruments are kept wrapped until ready for use
- To reduce the risk of contamination, sterile packs must be handled as little as possible
- Sterilized packs should be allowed to cool before storage; otherwise condensation will occur inside the packs
- Sterile packs must be stored and issued in correct date order. The packs, preferably, are stored in UV chamber (**Fig. 11.8**) or drums which can be locked.

Methods of Sterilization

Sterilization is process by which an object, surface or medium is freed of all microorganisms either in the vegetative or spore state **Table 11.1**.

Classification of sterilizing agents

Physical agents:
- Sunlight
- Drying
- Cold
- Dry heat
  - Flaming
  - Incineration
  - Hot air oven
- Moist heat
  - Boiling
  - Steam under pressure
  - Pasteurization
- Filtration
  - Candles
  - Membranes
  - Asbestos pads
- Radiation

Chemical agents:
- Alcohols
  - Ethanol
  - Isopropyl alcohol
- Aldehydes
  - Formaldehyde
  - Gluteraldehyde
- Halogens
  - Iodine
  - Chlorine
- Dyes
  - Acridine
  - Aniline
- Phenols
  - Cresol
  - Carbolic acid
- Metallic salts gases
  - Ethylene oxide
  - Formaldehyde
  - Betapropiolactone
- Surface active agents

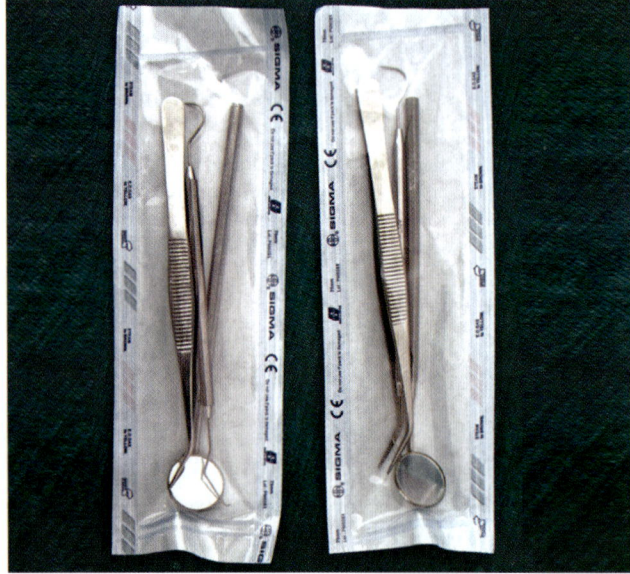

Figure 11.7: Peel-pouches for packing instruments

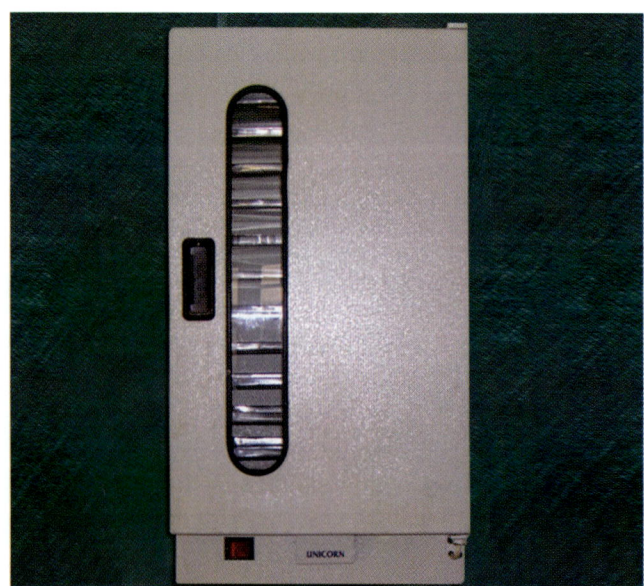

Figure 11.8: UV chamber for storage of sterile instruments

Table 11.1: Sterilization method and type of packaging material

Sterilization method	Packaging material
Autoclave	• Paper or plastic peel-pouches, wrapped cassettes • Plastic tubing (made up of nylon) • Thin clothes (Thick clothes are not advised as they absorb too much heat) • Sterilization paper (paper wrap)
Chemical vapor	• Paper or plastic pouches • Sterilization paper
Dry heat	• Sterilization paper (paper wrap) • Nylon plastic tubing (indicated for dry heat) • Wrapped cassettes

The accepted methods of sterilization in our dental practice are:
- Moist/steam heat sterilization
- Dry heat sterilization
- Chemical vapor pressure sterilization
- Ethylene oxide sterilization.

Moist/Steam Heat Sterilization

Autoclave: Autoclave provides the most efficient and reliable method of sterilization for all dental instruments. It involves heating water to generate steam in a closed chamber resulting in moist heat that rapidly kills microorganisms (**Fig. 11.9**).

Use of saturated steam under pressure is the most efficient, quickest, safest, effective method of sterilization because:

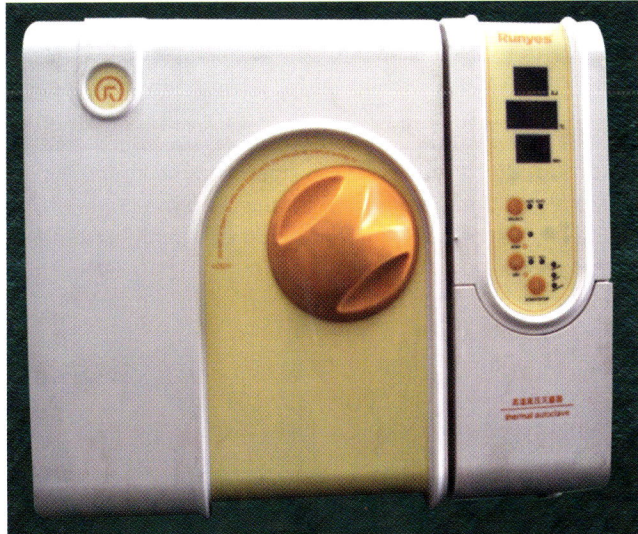

Figure 11.9: Autoclave for moist heat sterilization

- It has high penetrating power.
- It gives up a large amount of heat (latent heat) to the surface with which it comes into contact and on which it condenses as water.

Types of autoclaves: Two types of autoclaves are available:
1. Downward (gravitation) displacement sterilizer: This is nonvacuum type autoclave.
2. Steam sterilizers (autoclave) with pre and postvacuum processes.

Steam sterilizers (Autoclave) with pre and post vacuum processes: In this, the sterilization process is composed of three main phases:
1. *Pretreatment phase/heat-up cycle*: All air is virtually expelled by a number of pulses of vacuum and the introduction of steam, so that the saturated steam can affect the instruments during second phase.
2. *Sterilizing phase/sterilization cycle*: The temperature increases adequately up to the degree at which sterilization is to take place. Actual sterilizing period (also called "Holding Time") starts when the temperature in all parts of the autoclave chamber and its contents has reached the sterilizing temperature. This should remain constant within specified temperature throughout the whole sterilization phase.
3. *Posttreatment phase/depressurization cycle*: In this phase either the steam or the revaporized condensed water is removed by vacuum to ensure that the goods are dried rapidly.

Three main factors required for effective autoclaving:
1. *Pressure*: It is expressed in terms of psi or kPa.
2. *Temperature*: For effective sterilization the temperature should be reached and maintained at 121°C. As the temperature and pressure increases, superheated steam is formed. This steam is lighter than air, thus rises to the upper portion of the autoclave. As more steam is formed, it eliminates air from autoclave. The reason of complete elimination of air is to help superheated steam to penetrate the entire load in the autoclave and remain in contact for the appropriate length of time.
3. *Time*: A minimum of 20 to 30 minutes of time is required after achieving full temperature and pressure.
   Significance: Higher the temperature and pressure, shorter is the time required for sterilization.
   - At 15 psi pressure, the temperature of 121°, the time required is 15 minutes
   - At 126°C, time is 10 minutes
   - At 134°C, time is 3 minutes.

Wrapping instruments for autoclaving: Packing instruments before sterilizing prevents them from becoming contaminated after sterilization till it is opened and used. For wrapping, closed containers such as closed metal trays, glass vials and aluminium foils should not be used, since they stop the steam from reaching the inner part of the packs.

For packaging of autoclaving instruments, one should use porous covering so as to permit steam to penetrate through and reach the instruments. The materials used for packaging can be fabric or sealed paper or cloth pouches and paper-wrapped cassettes. Finally, the wrap is heat-sealed or sealed with tape.

If instruments are to be stored and not used shortly after sterilization, the autoclave cycle should end with a drying phase to avoid tarnish or corrosion of the instruments.

Advantages of autoclaves

- Time efficient
- Good penetration
- The results are consistently good and reliable
- The instruments can be wrapped prior to sterilization.

Disadvantages of autoclaves

- Blunting and corrosion of sharp instruments
- Damage to rubber goods.

Dry Heat Sterilization

It is alternative method for sterilization of instruments. This type of sterilization involves heating air which on further transfers energy from air to the instruments. In this type of sterilization, higher temperature is required than steam or chemical vapor sterilization.

Conventional hot air oven: The hot air oven utilizes radiating dry heat for sterilization as this type of energy does not penetrate materials easily. So, long periods of exposure to high temperature are usually required.

Packaging of instruments for dry heat: Dry heat ovens usually achieve temperature above 320°F (160°C). The packs of instrument must be placed at least 1 cm apart to air to circulate in the chamber. In conventional type of hot air, oven, air circulates, by gravity flow, thus it is also known as gravity convection. The type of packaging or wrapping material used should be able to withstand high temperature otherwise it may get char.

Packaging material requirements for dry heat

- Should not be destroyed by temperature used.
- Should not insulate items from heat.

Acceptable materials

- Paper and plastic bags
- Wrapped cassettes

- Paper wrap
- Aluminum foil
- Nylon plastic tubing.

Unacceptable materials: Plastic and paper bags which are unable to withstand dry heat temperatures.

Recommended temperature and duration of hot oven

Hot air oven			
Temp°C	Time	Temp°C	Time
141°C	3 hr	170°C	1 hr
149°C	2.5 hr	180°C	30 min
160°C	2 hr		

Mechanism of action: The dry heat kills microorganisms by protein denaturation, coagulation and oxidation It is very important that organic matter such as oil or grease film must be removed from the instruments as this may insulate against dry heat.

Instruments which can be sterilized in dry hot oven are glassware such as pipettes, flasks, scissors, glass syringes, carbon steel instruments and burs. Dry heat does not corrode sharp instrument surfaces. Also it does not erode glassware surfaces. Before placing in the oven, the glassware must be dried. The oven must be allowed to cool slowly for about 2 hours as glassware may crack due to sudden or uneven cooling.

Rapid heat transfer (forced air type): In this type of sterilizer, a fan or blower circulates the heated air throughout the chamber at a high velocity which, in turn, permits a more rapid transfer of heat energy from the air to instruments, thereby reducing the time.

Temperature/cycle recommended

- 370°F to 375°F – 12 minutes for wrapped instruments
- 370°F to 375°F – 16 minutes for unwrapped instruments

Advantages of dry heat sterilization

- No corrosion is seen in carbon-steel instruments and burs
- Maintains the sharpness of cutting instruments
- Effective and safe for sterilization of metal instrument and mirrors
- Low cost of equipment
- Instruments are dry after cycle
- Industrial forced draft types usually provide a larger capacity at reasonable price
- Rapid cycles are possible at higher temperatures.

Disadvantages of dry heat sterilization

- Poor penetrating capacity of dry heat
- Long cycle is required because of poor heat conduction and poor penetrating capacity

- High temperature may damage heat sensitive items such as rubber or plastic goods
- Instruments must be thoroughly dried before placing them in sterilization
- Inaccurate calibration and lack of attention to proper settings often lead to errors in sterilization
- Heavy loads of instruments, crowding of packs and heavy wrapping easily defeat sterilization
- Generally not suitable for handpieces
- Cannot sterilize liquids
- May discolor and char fabric.

Chemical Vapor Sterilization

Sterilization by chemical vapor under pressure is known as chemical vapor sterilization. In this, special chemical solution is heated in a closed chamber, producing hot chemical vapors that kill microorganisms.

The various modes of action are:
- Coagulation of protein
- Cell membrane disruption
- Removal of free sulphydryl groups
- Substrate competition.

Contents of chemical solution: The solution contains various ingredients which are as follows:
- Active ingredient – 0.23 percent Formaldehyde
- Other ingredient – 72.38 percent Ethanol + Acetone + Water and Other Alcohols

Temperature, pressure and time required for completion of one cycle is –270°F (132°C) at 20 lb for 30 minutes. Chemical vapor sterilizer is also known as chemiclave. Usually four cycles are required for this sterilizer which is as follows:
- Vaporization cycle
- Sterilization cycle
- Depressurization cycle
- Purge cycle (which collects chemicals from vapors in the chamber at the end of cycle).

Advantage of chemical solution
Eliminates corrosion of carbon steel instruments, burs and pliers.

Disadvantages of chemical solution
• The instruments or items which are sensitive to elevated temperature are damaged.
• Sterilization of liner, textiles, fabric or paper towels is not recommended.
• Dry instruments should be loaded in the chamber.

Precautions to be taken
- Use gloves and protective eyewear while handling the chemical solution.

- Use paper/plastic peel-pouches or bags recommended for use in chemiclave.
- Use system in ventilated room.
- Space should be given between the instruments that are to be sterilized in the chamber for better conduction and penetration.
- Water should not be left on the instruments.

Ethylene Oxide Sterilization (ETOX)

This sterilization method is best used for sterilizing complex instruments and delicate materials.

Ethylene oxide is highly penetrative, noncorrosive gas above 10.8°C with a cidal action against bacteria, spores and viruses. It destroys microorganisms by alkylation and causes denaturation of nucleic acids of microorganisms.

Since it is highly toxic, irritant, mutagenic and carcinogenic, thus should not be used on routine bases. It is suited for electric equipment, flexible-fiber endoscopes and photographic equipment.

The duration that the gas should be in contact with the material to be sterilized is dependent on temperature, humidity, pressure and the amount of material.

Advantages of ETOX
• It leaves no residue
• It is a deodorizer
• Good penetration power
• Can be used at a low temperature
• Suited for heat sensitive articles, e.g. plastic, rubber, etc.

Disadvantages of ETOX
• High cost of the equipment
• Toxicity of the gas
• Explosive and inflammable.

Irradiation

Radiations used for sterilization are of two types:
1. Ionizing radiation, e.g. X-rays, gamma rays and high-speed electrons.
2. Non-ionizing radiation, e.g. ultraviolet light and infrared light.

Ionizing Radiation

Ionizing radiations are effective for heat labile items. They are commonly used by the industry to sterilize disposable materials such as needles, syringes, culture plates, suture material, cannulas and pharmaceuticals sensitive to heat. High energy gamma rays from cobalt-60 are used to sterilize such articles.

Nonionizing Radiation

Two types of nonionizing radiations are used for sterilization, i.e. ultraviolet and infrared.

1. *Ultraviolet rays*: UV rays are absorbed by proteins and nucleic acids and kill microorganisms by the chemical reactions. Their main application is purification of air in operating rooms to reduce the bacteria in air, water and on the contaminated surfaces. Care must be taken to protect the eyes while using U-V radiation for sterilization.

2. *Infrared*: It is used for sterilizing a large number of syringes sealed in metal container, in a short period of time. It is used to purify air in the operating room. Infrared is effective, however, it has no penetrating ability.

Boiling Water

Boiling water produces a temperature of 100°C at normal atmospheric pressure. Usually 10 minutes exposure at this temperature is required to kill most of the bacteria and some viruses (including HIV and HBV). But even the prolonged time exposure does not kill many viruses. Thus, boiling water is not suggested for sterilization of tissue penetrating instruments.

Oil

Hot oil baths have been used for sterilization of metallic instruments. It requires at least 15 minutes of submersion at the temperature of 175°C for sterilization.

Disadvantages of using oil
➡ Poor penetration
➡ Poor sporicidal activity
➡ Fire hazard
➡ Difficult to remove from instruments.

Glass Bead Sterilizer (Fig. 11.10)

It is a rapid method of sterilization which is used for sterilization of instruments. It usually uses table salt which consists approximately of 1 percent sodium silico-aluminate, sodium carbonate or magnesium carbonate. So, it can be poured more readily and does not fuse under heat. Salt can be replaced by glass beads provided the beads are smaller than 1 mm in diameter because larger beads are not efficient in transferring the heat to endodontic instruments due to presence of large air spaces between the beads.

The instruments can be sterilized in 5 to 15 seconds at a temperature of 437 to 465°F (260°C) even when inoculated with spores.

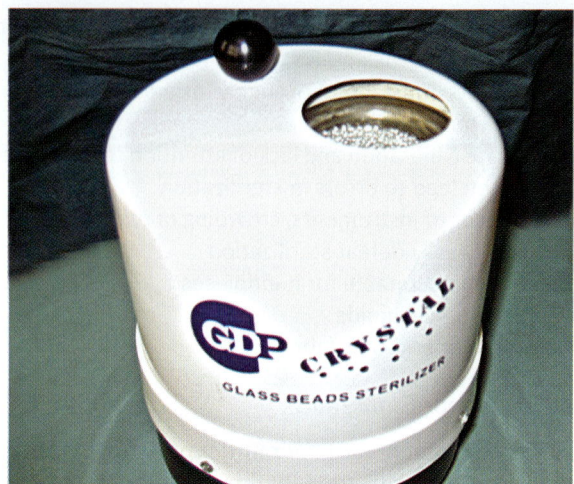

Figure 11.10: Glass bead sterilizer

The specific disadvantage of these sterilizers is that the handle portion is not sterilized and therefore these articles are not entirely 'sterile'. These are not recommended unless absolutely required.

Advantages of glass bead sterilizer
➡ Commonly used salt is table salt which is easily available and cheap.
➡ Salt does not clog the root canal. If it is carried into the canal, it can be readily removed by irrigation.

MANAGEMENT OF DENTAL EQUIPMENT

Handpieces

The internal surfaces of handpieces become contaminated with blood and debris, which can occur as source of infection. Limited access to internal surfaces limits its cleaning and disinfection, thus, surface disinfection is not adequate. Handpiece must be first cleaned and then sterilized after each patient. Cleaning can be done by using water and detergent or wiping the handpiece using a suitable disinfectant like alcohol (**Fig. 11.11**). Lubricate the handpiece prior to sterilization (**Fig. 11.12**) and finally sterilize it by autoclaving.

The handpieces which are not autoclavable should be treated by a disinfection regimen. For this, wrap the handpiece in gauze soaked with disinfectant and keep it in a sealed plastic bag for a specific time.

Dental Unit Water Systems (DUWSs)

The dental unit water systems (DUWSs) are the tubes which join high speed handpiece, air/water syringe and

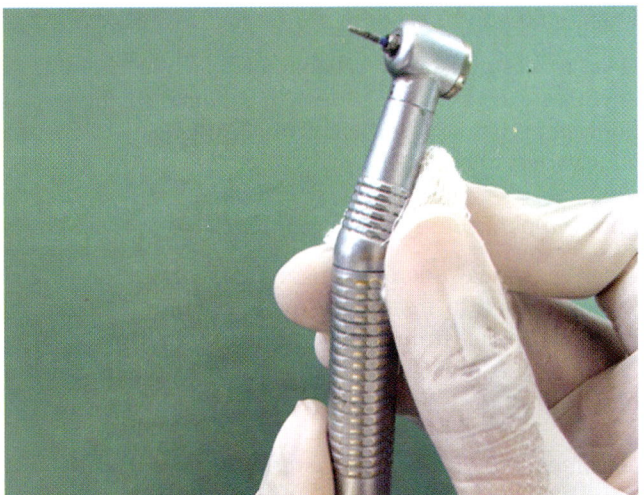

Figure 11.11: Clean handpiece by wiping it with a suitable disinfectant

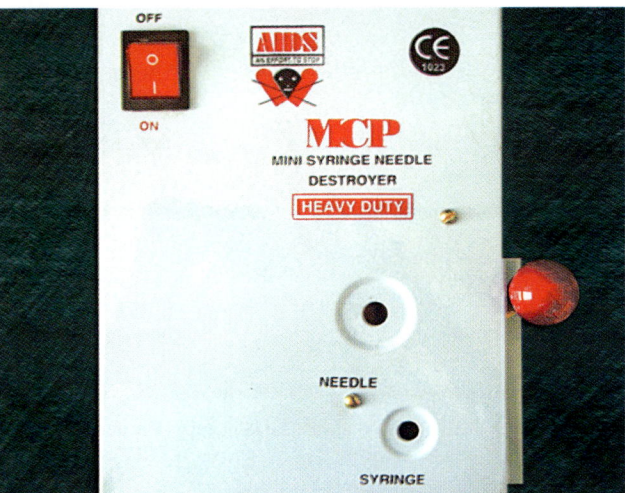

Figure 11.13: Needle Destroyer should be used for disposing used syringes

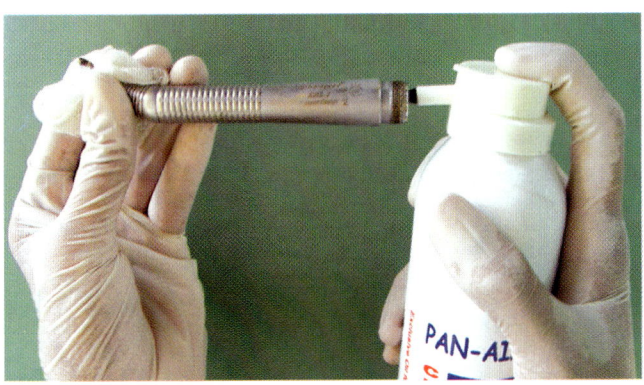

Figure 11.12: Lubricate handpiece before sterilization

ultrasonic scaler to the water supply. They have shown to house a wide range of microorganisms like bacteria, fungi and protozoas. These organisms can make an entry along with water. After the system is switched off, there is formation of negative pressure which causes retraction of water. The microorganisms colonize and replicate on the inner surfaces of the water-line tubings, resulting in microbial accumulations called as "biofilms". These biofilms act as a reservoir for floating microorganisms in the water exiting the water-lines. If dental unit waterlines systems are not cleaned properly, the microbial colonies can result in odors and visible particles of biofilm material exiting the system.

To solve this problem, following can be done:
- Use of antiretraction valves in the DUWSs. Retraction valves aspirate the infected material back into the handpiece and waterlines. Antiretraction valves are used to prevent aspiration and to prevent transfer of infected material.
- Bacterial filter fitted in water lines of handpieces and two-way syringe.
- DUWSs should be flushed with a disinfectant (sodium hypochlorite solution) to reduce bacterial population.
- Aspirators should be cleaned and flushed after every patient and at the end of the day, they should be flushed with a disinfectant.

NEEDLE STICK INJURY

Sharp instruments such as needles, blades, etc. should be considered as potentially infective and handled with care to prevent injuries. These should be disposed in puncture-resistant containers (**Fig. 11.13**). An uncapped needle and syringe should not be handled or passed from assistant to the clinician and vice-versa.

All clinicians should take care to:
- Prevent needle stick injuries.
- Manage needle stick injuries, if they occur.

Measures to Prevent Needle Stick Injuries

- Ensuring that the needles and surgical blades are sheathed/covered, when not in use (**Fig. 11.14**)
- If resheathing is used, single hand resheathing of needles should be followed
- Never handle sharp instruments by the working end
- Adequate retraction of tissues with appropriate instruments

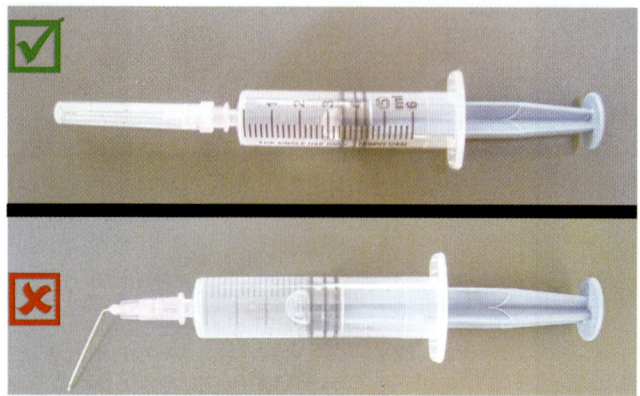

Figure 11.14: Needle should always be kept capped when not in use

- Placing needles in sharp safe box
- Taking care while handling with surgical sharps and wires
- Keeping full control of sharp instruments
- Keeping gloved fingers behind the cutting edges of surgical blades
- Needles should not be bent, sheared, broken, removed from disposable syringes by hand before disposal.

Management of needle stick injuries

- ➡ The victim should report the incident immediately
- ➡ Wash the area immediately under running water
- ➡ Make the wound bleed for three to four minutes, at the same time continue to wash the area
- ➡ Dry the area with paper towel
- ➡ Cover the wound with a water-impermeable plaster
- ➡ Take the blood sample of the source patient and test it for the presence of the blood borne viruses hepatitis B, hepatitis C and HIV
- ➡ Take the blood sample of victim to determine the hepatitis B antibody level
- ➡ Plan further treatment and follow-up of the victim.

DISINFECTION

It is the term used for destruction of all pathogenic organisms, such as, vegetative forms of bacteria, mycobacteria, fungi and viruses, but not bacterial endospores.

Methods of Disinfection

Disinfection by Cleaning

Cleaning with a detergent and clean hot water removes almost all pathogens including bacterial spores.

Disinfection by Heat

Heat is a simple and reliable disinfectant for almost anything except living tissues. Mechanical cleaning with hot water provides an excellent quality of disinfection for a wide variety of purposes.

Low Temperature Steam

Most vegetative microorganisms and viruses are killed when exposed to steam at a temperature of 73°C for 20 minutes below atmospheric pressure. This makes it a useful procedure to leave spoiled instruments safe to handle prior to sterilization.

Disinfection by Chemical Agents

They are used to disinfect the skin of a patient prior to surgery and to disinfect the hands of the operator.
Disadvantages of using chemicals:
- No chemical solution sterilizes the instruments immersed in it
- There is a risk of producing tissue damage if residual solution is carried into the wound.

Levels of Disinfectant

Alcohols Low Level Disinfectant

- Ethanol and isopropyl alcohols are commonly used as antiseptics
- Possess some antibacterial activity, but they are not effective against spores and viruses
- Act by denaturing proteins
- To have maximum effectiveness, alcohol must have a 10 minutes contact with the organisms
- Instruments made of carbon steel should not be soaked in alcoholic solutions, as they are corrosive to carbon steel
- Rubber instruments absorb alcohol thus their prolonged soaking can cause a reaction when material comes in contact with living tissue.

Phenolic Compounds—Intermediate Level, Broad Spectrum Disinfectant

Phenol itself is toxic to skin and bone marrow. The phenolic compounds were developed to reduce their side effects but are still toxic to living tissues. These compounds, in high concentration, are protoplasmic poison and act by precipitating the proteins and destroy the cell wall.

Lawrence and Block (1968) reported that their spectrum of activity includes lipophilic viruses, fungi and bacteria but not spores. The newer synthetic combinations seem to be active against hydrophilic viruses; hence these are approved by ADA for use as surface or immersion disinfectant.

These compounds are used for disinfection of inanimate objects such as walls, floors and furniture. They may cause damage to some plastics and they do not corrode certain metals such as brass, aluminium and carbon steel. It has unique action that is it keeps working for longer period after initial application, known as "Residual Activity".

Aldehyde Compounds—High Level Disinfectant

Formaldehyde
- Broad spectrum antimicrobial agent
- Flammable and irritant to the eye, skin and respiratory tract
- Has limited sporicidal activity
- Used for large heat sensitive equipment such as ventilators and suction pumps excluding rubber and some plastics
- Not preferred due to its pungent odor and because 18 to 30 hours of contact is necessary for cidal action.

Glutaraldehyde
- Toxic, irritant and allergenic
- A high level disinfectant
- Active against most vegetative bacteria, fungi and bacterial spores
- Frequently used for heat sensitive material
- A solution of 2 percent glutaraldehyde (Cidex), requires immersion of 20 minutes for disinfection; and 6 to 10 hours of immersion for sterilization
- Safely used on metal instruments, rubber, plastics and porcelain
- Activated by addition of sodium bicarbonate but in its activated form, it remains potent only for 14 days.

Antiseptics (Fig. 11.15)

Antiseptic is a chemical disinfectant that can be diluted sufficiently to be safe for application to living tissues like intact skin, mucous membranes and wounds.

Alcohols
- Two types of alcohols are used ethyl alcohol and isopropyl alcohol
- Used for skin antisepsis
- Their benefit is derived primarily in their cleansing action
- The alcohols must have a prolonged contact with the organisms to have an antibacterial effect
- Ethyl alcohol is used in the concentration of 70 percent as a skin antiseptic.
- Isopropyl alcohol is used in the concentration of 60 to 70 percent for disinfection of skin.

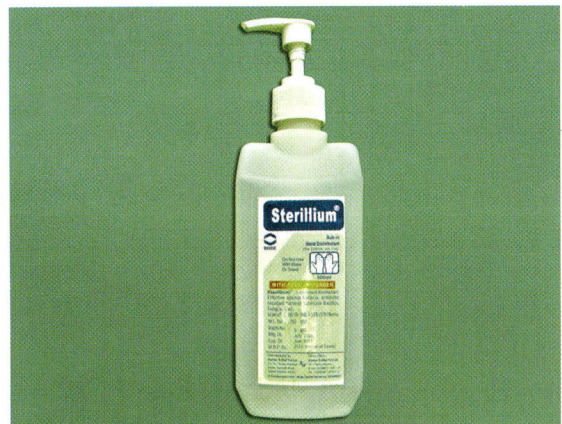

Figure 11.15: Hand disinfectant commercially available

Aqueous Quarternary Ammonium Compounds

Benzalkonium chloride (Zephiran) is the most commonly used antiseptic. It is well tolerated by living tissues.

Iodophor Compounds
- Used for surgical scrub, soaps and surface antisepsis
- Usually effective within 5 to 10 minutes
- Discolor surfaces and clothes
- Iodine is complexed with organic surface active agents such as polyvinyl-pyrrolidine (Betadine, Isodine). Their activity is dependent on the release of iodine from the complex
- Concentrated solutions have less free iodine. Iodine is released as the solution is diluted
- These compounds are effective against most bacteria, spores, viruses and fungi.

Chloride Compounds
- Commonly used are sodium hypochlorite and chlorine dioxide
- Sodium hypochlorite has rapid action
- A solution of 1 part of 5 percent sodium hypochlorite with 9 parts of water is used
- Chlorous acid and chlorine dioxide provides disinfection in 3 minutes.

Diguanides
- Chlorhexidine is active against many bacteria
- Gets inactivated in the presence of soap, pus, plastics, etc.
- Mainly used for cleaning skin and mucous membrane.
- As a 0.2 percent aqueous solution or 1 percent gel it can be used for suppression of plaque and postoperative infection.

Method	Effect	Method	Used for
Sterilization	Destroys all microorganisms including spores	Moist Heat, Dry heat, ETOX, glutaraldehyde, H_2O_2, glutaraldehyde with phenol	For critical and semicritical items
High level disinfection	Destroys all microorganisms but not necessarily spores	Glutaraldehyde, Hydrogen peroxide	Semicritical items
Intermediate level disinfection	Destroys most of bacteria, inactivate *Mycobacterium bovis* but does not kill spores.	Chlorine containing products, iodiophores, Quarternary ammonium compounds	Non critical surfaces
Low level disinfection	Destroys vegetative bacterias. Does not inactivate *Mycobacterium bovis*	Iodophores , quarternary ammonium compounds, phenols	Non critical surfaces

INFECTION CONTROL CHECKLIST

Infection Control During the Pretreatment Period

- Utilize disposable items whenever possible.
- Ensure before treatment that all equipment have been sterilized properly.
- Remove avoidable items from the operatory area to facilitate a thorough cleaning following each patient.
- Identify those items that will become contaminated during treatment, for example, light handles, X-ray unit heads, tray tables, etc. Disinfect them when the procedure is complete.
- Review patient records before initiating treatment.
- Place radiographs on the X-ray view box before starting the patient.
- Preplan the materials needed during treatment to avoid opening of the cabinets and drawers once the work is started.
- Use separate sterilized bur blocks for each procedure to eliminate the contamination of other, unneeded burs.
- Always keep rubber dam kit ready in the tray.
- Follow manufacturer's directions for care of dental unit water lines (DUWL).
- Clinician should be prepared before initiating the procedure, this includes the use of personal protective equipment (gown, eyewear, masks and gloves) and hand hygiene.
- Update patient's medical history.

Chairside Infection Control

- Treat all patients as potentially infectious.
- Take special precautions while handling syringes and needles.
- Use a rubber dam whenever possible.
- Use high volume aspiration.
- Ensure good ventilation of the operatory area.
- Be careful while receiving, handling, or passing sharp instruments.

- Do not touch unprotected switches, handles and other equipment once gloves have been contaminated.
- Avoid touching drawers or cabinets, once gloves have been contaminated. When it becomes necessary to do so, ask your assistant to do this or use another barrier, such as overglove to grasp the handle or remove the contaminated gloves and wash hands before touching the drawer and then reglove for patient treatment.

Infection Control During the Posttreatment Period

- Remove the contaminated gloves used during treatment, wash hands and put on a pair of utility gloves before beginning the clean up.
- Continue to wear protective eyewear, mask and gown during clean up.
- Dispose of blood and suctioned fluids which have been collected in the collection bottles during treatment.
- After disposing of blood and suctioned fluids, use a 0.5 percent chlorine solution to disinfect the dental unit collection bottle. Keep the solution in the bottle for at least 10 minutes.
- Clean the operatory area and disinfect all the items not protected by barriers.
- Remove the tray with all instruments to sterilization area separate from the operatory area.
- Never pick up instruments in bulk because this increases the risk of cuts or punctures. Clean the instruments manually or in an ultrasonic cleaner.
- Sterilize the hand pieces whenever possible. In general, hand piece should be autoclaved but the hand piece which cannot be heat sterilized, should be disinfected by the use of chemicals. Clean the handpiece with a detergent and water to remove any debris. Sterilize it.
- Waste that is contaminated with blood or saliva should be placed in sturdy leak proof bags.
- Handle sharps items carefully.
- Remove personal protective equipment after clean-up. Utility gloves should be washed with soap before removal.
- At the end, thoroughly wash hands.

Key Points

- Cross-infection is transmission of infectious agents among patients and staff within a clinical environment. This source of infection can be patients suffering from infectious diseases, patients who are in the prodromal stage of infections and healthy carriers of pathogens.
- The main objective of infection control is elimination or reduction in spread of infection from all types of microorganisms.
- "Universal precautions" are as follows:
  - Immunization: All members of the dental team (who are exposed to blood or blood contaminated articles) should be vaccinated against hepatitis B.
  - Use of personal protective barrier techniques that is use of protective gown, face mask, protective eyewear, gloves, etc. These reduce the risk of exposure to infectious material and injury from sharp instruments.
  - Maintaining hand hygiene.
- The barrier technique involves the use of gown, face mask, protective eyewear and gloves.
- Hand hygiene significantly reduces potential pathogens on the hands and is considered as the single most critical measure for reducing the risk of transmitting organisms to patients and dentists.
- The center for disease control and prevention (CDC) classified the instrument into critical, semicritical and noncritical depending on the potential risk of infection during the use of these instruments. These categories are also referred to as Spaulding classification (by Spaulding in 1968).
- For complete sterilization, rule of universal sterilization should be followed. It means that all reusable instruments and handpieces are sterilized between use on patient.
- CDC Recommends:
  - Critical and semicritical instruments are to be heat sterilized.
  - Semicritical items sensitive to heat should be treated with high level disinfectant after cleaning.
  - Noncritical items can be treated intermediate to low level disinfectant after cleaning.
- Instrument processing is the collection of procedures which prepare the contaminated instruments for reuse. The steps in instrument processing involve presoaking, cleaning, corrosion control, packaging, sterilization, monitoring of sterilization and handling the processed instrument.
- Autoclave provides the most efficient and reliable method of sterilization for all dental instruments. It involves heating water to generate steam in a closed chamber resulting in moist heat that rapidly kills microorganisms.
- Use of saturated steam under pressure is the most efficient, quickest, safest, effective method of sterilization because it has high penetrating power and it gives up a large amount of heat (latent heat) to the surface with which it comes into contact.
- For autoclaving instruments:
  - At 15 psi pressure, the temperature of 121°, the time required is 15 minutes.
  - At 126°C, time is 10 minutes.
  - At 134°C, time is 3 minutes.
- The dry heat kills microorganisms by protein denaturation, coagulation and oxidation. Instruments which can be sterilized in dry hot oven are glassware such as pipettes, flasks, scissors, glass syringes, carbon steel instruments and burs.
- Ethylene oxide sterilization (ETOX) is best used for sterilizing complex instruments and delicate materials. Ethylene oxide is highly penetrative, noncorrosive gas above 10.8°C with a cidal action against bacteria, spores and viruses. It destroys microorganisms by alkylation and causes denaturation of nucleic acids of microorganisms.
- Glass bead sterilizer uses table salt which consists approximately of 1 percent sodium silicoaluminate, sodium carbonate or magnesium carbonate. Salt can be replaced by glass beads. The instruments can be sterilized in 5 to 15 seconds at a temperature of 437 to 465°F (260°C) even when inoculated with spores.
- The specific disadvantage of these sterilizers is that the handle portion is not sterilized and therefore these articles are not entirely 'sterile'.
- Handpiece must be first cleaned and then sterilized after each patient. Cleaning can be done by using water and detergent or wiping the handpiece using a suitable disinfectant like alcohol. Lubricate the handpiece prior to sterilization and finally sterilize it by autoclaving.
- Disinfection is destruction of all pathogenic organisms, such as, vegetative forms of bacteria, mycobacteria, fungi and viruses, but not bacterial endospores.
- Antiseptic is a chemical disinfectant that can be diluted sufficiently to be safe for application to living tissues like intact skin, mucous membranes and wounds.

QUESTIONS

1. How will you maintain asepsis in operating field?
2. What is rationale of infection control?

3. Short notes on:
   a. Universal precautions of infection control
   b. Steps of instrument processing procedure
   c. Autoclave
   d. Glass bead sterilizer
   e. Disinfection.

BIBLIOGRAPHY

1. Ahtone J, Goodman RA. Hepatitis B and dental personnel: transmission to patients and prevention issues. J Am Dent Assoc. 1983;106:219-22.

2. Allen A, Bryan R. Occult blood accumulation under fingernails. J Am Assoc. 1982;105:358-62.

3. Association of Dental Schools. Recommended clinical guidelines for infection control in dental education institutions. J Dent Educ. 1991;55:621-30.

4. Autio KK, et al. Studies on cross-contamination in the dental office, J Am Dent Assoc. 1980;100:358-61.

5. Bagga BSR, et al. Contamination of dental unit cooling water with oral microorganisms and its prevention. J Am Dent Assoc. 1984;109:712-6.

6. Bentley CD, et al. Evaluating spatter and aerosol contamination during dental procedures. J Am Dent Assoc. 1994;125:579-84.

7. Burkhart NW, Crawford JJ. Critical steps after cleaning: removing debris after sonication. J Am Dent Assoc. 1997;128:456-63.

8. Christensen RP, et al. Antimicrobial activity of environmental surface disinfectants in the absence and presence of bioburden. J Am Dent Assoc. 1989;119:493-504.

9. Christensen RP, et al. Efficiency of 42 brands of facemasks and two face shields in preventing inhalation of airborne debris. Gen Dent. 1991;39:414-21.

10. Cochran MA, et al. The efficiency of the rubber dam as a barrier to the spread of microorganisms during dental treatment. J Am Dent Assoc. 1989;119:141-4.

11. Council on Dental Materials, Instruments and Devices, American Dental Association: Dental units and water retraction. J Am Dent Assoc. 1988;116:417-20.

12. Crawford JJ, Broderius C. Control of cross-infection risks in the dental operatory: prevention of water retraction by bur cooling spray systems. J Am Dent Assoc. 1988;116:685-7.

13. Crawford JJ, Broderius C. Evaluation of a dental unit designed to prevent retraction of oral fluids. Quintessence Int. 1989;21:47-51.

14. Crawford JJ. State of the art: practical infection control in dentistry. Proceedings of the National Symposium on hepatitis B and the dental profession, J Am Dent Assoc. 1985;110:629-33.

15. Hackney RW. Using a biological indicator to detect potential sources of cross-contamination in the dental operatory. J Am Dent Assoc. 1998;129:1567-77.

16. Lettau LA. The A, B, C, D, and E, of viral hepatitis: spelling out the risks for health care workers. Infect Control Hosp Epidemiol. 1992;13:77-81.

17. Lewis DL, Boe RK. Cross-infection risks associated with current procedures for using high-speed dental handpieces. J Clin Microbiol. 1992;30:401-6.

18. Martin MV. The significance of the bacterial contamination of dental unit water systems. Br Dent J. 1987;163:152-4.

19. Miller RL, Micik RE. Air pollution and its control in the dental office. Dent Clin North Am. 1978;22:453.

20. Peterson NJ, et al. Air sampling for hepatitis B surface antigen in a dental operatory. J Am Dent Assoc. 1979;99:65-7.

21. Raloff J. Successful hepatitis A vaccine debuts, Science News. 1992;142:103.

22. Reinthaler FF, et al. Serologic examination for antibodies against Legionella species in dental personnel. J Dent Res. 1988;67:942-3.

23. Shearer B. ADA statement on dental unit waterlines, J Am Dent Assoc. 1996;127:185-9.

Pain Control

Chapter Outline

INTRODUCTION

Pain management is an integral part of operative dentistry. Any operative procedure cannot be performed properly without pain control. In field of dentistry, dentist commonly faces the problems regarding pain, anxiety and infection. Accordingly, clinician has to be well-prepared to use drugs, which help to solve these problems. Pain enhances the chances of apprehension, anxiety, nervousness, syncope and shock during treatment. A patient who is not in a calm state may interfere with treatment and is prone to injury during treatment. All these lead to decreased work output and poor quality of work.

Pain control in operative dentistry though is not very difficult but sometimes it becomes almost impossible to control pain.

Sometimes patient may suffer from mild to severe apprehension regarding the treatment. Also, dental incident or the stories told by other persons about their dental experience causes further dental fear in patient's mind. When this reaches a degree that produces alteration of physiologic and psychological functions, preoperative sedation is required usually in the form of sedatives or tranquilizers. In the present day, pharmacological drugs are available that work directly against anxiety without much of side effects, making dental treatment easier for the patient and the practitioner, enabling more patients to receive optimal dental care.

METHODS OF PAIN CONTROL IN DENTAL CLINIC

Pain control in a dental clinic can be obtained by the following methods

- Anxiety control of the patient
- Local anesthesia
- Use of high speed rotary instruments with sharp burs and coolants
- Analgesia
- Hypnosis
- General anesthesia.

ANXIETY CONTROL

Certain patients enter the office in such a state of nervousness or agitation that they even find taking of radiographs almost unbearable. Some of them who outwardly appear normal may also be suffering from severe inner apprehension. A kind, supportive and understanding attitude together with suggestion for control of such feelings will be greatly appreciated and usually yield acceptable response.

A variety of techniques for management of anxiety are available. Together these techniques are termed as spectrum of pain and anxiety control. They represent a wide range from nondrug technique to general anesthesia.

On the whole there are two major types of sedation, first, requiring no administration of drugs (iatrosedation) and second, requiring administration of the drugs (pharmacosedation).

Iatrosedation

It is a nondrug technique of causing sedation. A relaxed and pleasant doctor-patient relationship has favorable influence on action of the sedative drugs. A patient, who is comfortable with doctor, responds well to the drugs than patient who is anxious about the doctor and treatment to be done. An effective effort should be done by all the members of dental clinic to help allay the anxiety of patients.

Pharmacosedation

Sedatives and tranquilizers are drugs that are CNS depressants and decrease cortical excitability. Both have similar actions reducing abnormal and excessive response to environmental situations that produce agitation, tension and anxiety.

Sedative is a drug that subdues excitement and calms the subject without inducing sleep but drowsiness may be produced. At higher doses sleep may occur.

Tranquilizers do not produce sleep and serves effectively to block intolerant and overly aggressive reactions. With tranquilizer use, no attendant is required to the clinic as driving is not contraindicated with tranquilizers. Tranquilizers themselves do not produce sleep but may relax the patient to such a degree that extreme drowsiness will develop.

Short acting barbiturates and their substitutes are excellent for use with operative procedures. Initial dose should be given the night before the appointment to ensure restful night, with another taken 30 min before the patient is seated for the treatment. Patients requiring sedatives should be seen in the morning.

Short acting barbiturates commonly used are:
- Butobarbitone
- Secobarbitone
- Pentobarbitone.

Benzodiazepines

Commonly used benzodiazepines for reducing anxiety are:
- Diazepam
- Chlordiazepoxide
- Oxazepam
- Lorazepam
- Alprazolam.

LOCAL ANESTHESIA (FIG. 12.1)

Definition

It is defined as a loss of sensation in a circumscribed area of the body caused by depression of excitation in nerve endings or an inhibition of the conduction process in peripheral nerves. Before administering local anesthesia evaluate patient's heart rate, blood pressure (BP) and pulse rate. Local anesthetic preparations contain 1:80,000 to 200,000 concentration of adrenaline and 2 percent local anesthetic salt. The increased concentration of adrenaline may cause increase in blood pressure, rise in heart rate and arrhythmia also. In cardiac patients local anesthetic solution without adrenaline should be used.

Classification of Local Anesthetic Agents

All local anesthetics except cocaine are synthetic. They are broadly divided into two groups, i.e. ester and amide (nonester) group.

Classification Based on Chemical Structure

Ester group
- Cocaine
- Benzocaine
- Procaine
- Tetracaine

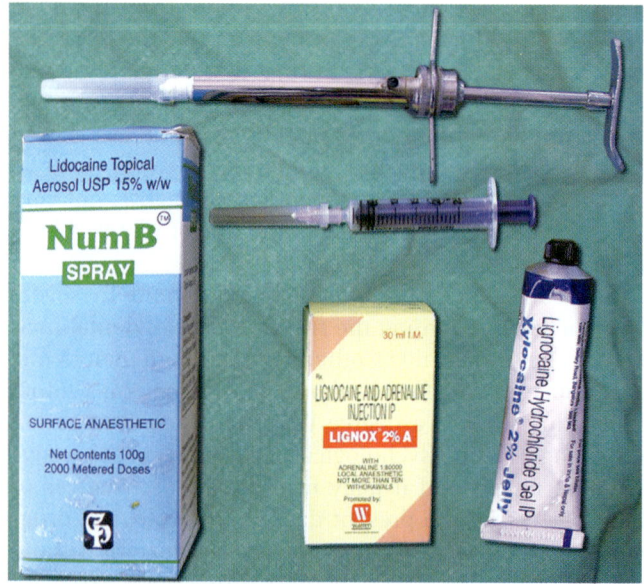

Figure 12.1: Commonly used local anesthetics in dental practice

Amide (Nonester group)

- Lidocaine
- Mepivacaine
- Prilocaine
- Etidocaine
- Bupivacaine

Classification Based on Duration of Action

- Short acting
  - Procaine
- Intermediate acting
  - Lidocaine
- Long acting
  - Bupivacaine.

The primary action of the local anesthetics agent in producing a nerve conduction block is to decrease the nerve permeability to sodium (Na^+) ions, thus preventing the inflow of Na^+ ions into the nerve. Therefore local anesthetics interfere with sodium conductance and inhibit the propagation of impulse along the nerve fibers (**Figs 12.2A and B**).

In tissues with lower pH, local anesthetics show slower onset of anesthesia while in tissues with higher pH, local anesthetic solution speeds the onset of anesthesia. This happens because at alkaline pH, local anesthetic is present in undissociated base form and it is this form, which penetrates the axon.

Composition of a local anesthetic agent

- Local anesthetic—salt form of lidocaine hydrochloride
- Vasoconstrictor—epinephrine
- Reducing agent—sodium bisulfite
- Isotonic solution—sodium chloride
- Preservative—methyl paraben
- Sterile water to make the rest of the volume

Following factors should be kept in mind prior to administration of local anesthesia:

Age: In very young and extremely old persons, less than the normal therapeutic dose should be given.

Allergy: Since it is life-threatening in most of the cases, proper history about allergy should be taken before administering local anesthesia.

Pregnancy: It is better to use minimum amount of local anesthetic drugs especially during pregnancy.

Thyroid disease: Patients with uncontrolled hyperthyroidism show increased response to the vasoconstrictor present in local anesthetics. Therefore, in such cases, local anesthesia solutions without adrenaline should be used.

Hepatic dysfunction: In hepatic dysfunction, the biotransformation cannot take place properly, resulting in higher levels of local anesthetic in the blood. So, in such cases low doses of local anesthetic should be administered.

Precautions to be taken before administration of local anesthesia:

- Patient should be in supine position as it favors good blood supply and pressure to brain
- Before injecting local anesthesia, aspirate a little amount in the syringe to avoid chances of injecting solution in the blood vessels
- Do not inject local anesthesia into the inflamed and infected tissues as local anesthesia does not work properly due to acidic medium of inflamed tissues
- Always use disposable needle and syringe in every patient. Needle should remain covered with cap till its use
- To make injection a painless procedure, temperature of the local anesthesia solution should be brought to body temperature
- Clean the site of injection with a sterile cotton pellet before injecting the local anesthesia
- Insert the needle at the junction of alveolar mucosa and vestibular mucosa. If angle of needle is parallel to long axis, it causes more pain
- Inject local anesthesia solution slowly not more than 1 ml per minute and in small increments to provide enough time for tissue diffusion of the solution
- Needle should be continuously inserted inside till the periosteum or bone is felt by way of slight increase in resistance of the needle movement. The needle is slightly withdrawn and here the remaining solution is injected
- Check the effect of anesthesia two minutes after injection
- Patient should be carefully watched during and after local anesthesia for about half an hour for delayed reactions, if any
- Discard needle and syringe in a leak-proof and hardwalled container after use.

Techniques of local anesthesia

- Local infiltration technique
- Nerve block technique.

Techniques of Local Anesthesia

Supraperiosteal/Local Infiltration Technique

It is also known as local infiltration and is most frequently used technique for obtaining anesthesia in maxillary teeth.

Technique: The needle is inserted through the mucosa and the solution is slowly deposited in close proximity to

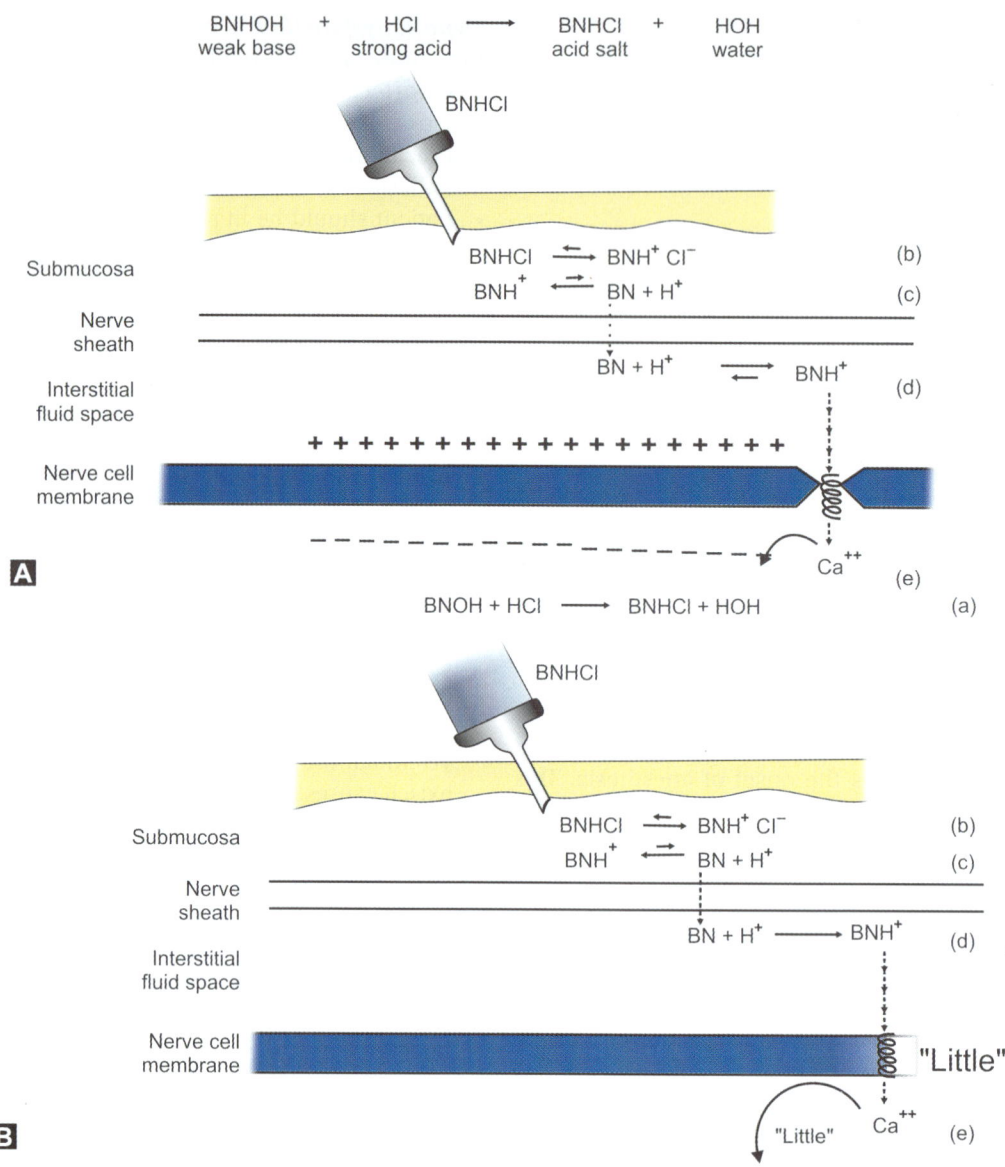

Figures 12.2A and B: Mechanism of action of local anesthetic

the periosteum, in the vicinity of the apex of the tooth to be treated (**Fig. 12.3**).

Advantage
It is simple to learn.

Disadvantage
Multiple injections are required for large area.

Regional Nerve Block

In this technique anesthetic solution is deposited near the nerve trunk at a distance from the working site. This is commonly used for mandibular teeth as for maxillary teeth usually the local infiltration works.

Various maxillary anesthesia techniques
➡ Supraperiosteal technique
➡ *Anterior and middle superior alveolar nerve block
➡ Posterior superior alveolar nerve block
➡ Greater palatine nerve block (anterior palatine nerve block)
➡ Nasopalatine nerve block
➡ *Maxillary nerve block
➡ Periodontal ligament injection.

*Both can be given intraorally and extraorally while all other are given intraorally only.

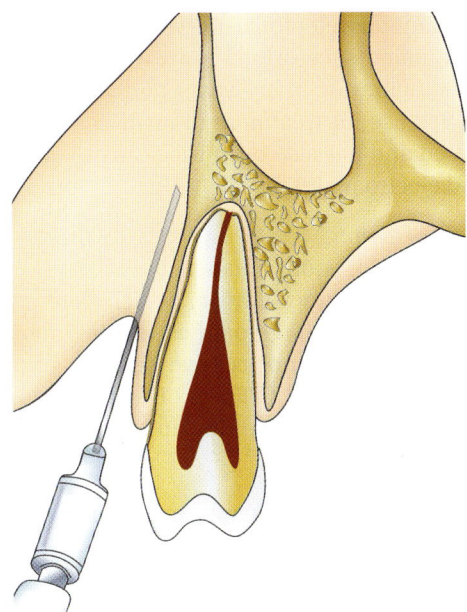

Figure 12.3: Supraperiosteal technique of local anesthesia

Various mandibular anesthesia techniques
➡ Inferior alveolar nerve block
➡ Long buccal nerve block
➡ Mandibular nerve block
➡ Vazirani-Akinosi closed mouth technique
➡ Mental nerve block.

Advantages of Local Anesthesia

Following are the main advantages of local anesthesia during dental procedure:
- Better patient co-operation by removing fear and apprehension of the patient
- Control of salivary flow by completely anesthetizing the tissues
- Control of bleeding due to presence of a vasoconstrictor, usually epinephrine or adrenaline which is added in local anesthesia mainly for increasing the period of anesthesia by decreasing flow of blood at the site of injection
- Increased operator's efficiency due to reduced blood flow in the vicinity of the injection site. It also increases the patient co-operation.

Recent Advances in Local Anesthesia

Many advances have been tried for making the experience of local anesthesia more comfortable and less traumatic. These advances are:
- Wand system of local anesthesia
- Comfort control syringe
- TENS local anesthesia

- Electronic dental anesthesia (EDA)
- Needle-less syringes.

Both Wand and comfort control syringe systems utilize computer technology for anesthesia. These two systems are based on the fact that more slowly the injection is given, less trauma is to the injection site and thus more comfortable the injection is to the patient.

Wand System of Local Anesthesia (Fig. 12.4)

Wand local anesthesia system is considered as the significant advancement in the delivery of local anesthetic system. This is computer-automated injection system which allows precise delivery of anesthesia at a constant flow rate despite varying tissue resistance.

It has been renamed CompuDent—featuring the Wand handpiece. This has been approved by US Food and Drug Administration (FDA) as local anesthesia delivery device.

CompuDent system consists of two main elements:
1. CompuDent computer
2. Wand handpiece.

Method: Topical anesthetic is first applied to freeze the mucosa and then a tiny needle is introduced through the already numb tissue to anesthetize the surrounding area. In this system, a disposable anesthetic cartridge is placed in a disposable plastic sleeve, which docks with the pump that delivers anesthetic solution through a microintravenous tubing attached to handpiece.

Uses: Considered as effective for all injections that can be performed using a standard aspirating syringe.

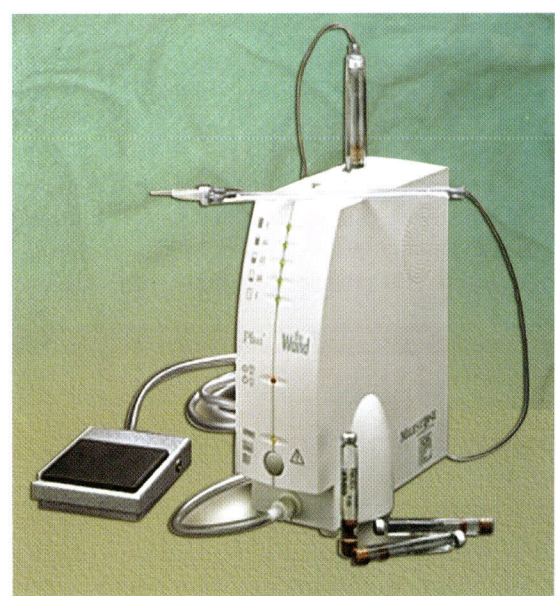

Figure 12.4: WAND system of local anesthesia

Advantages of wand system

- Reduced pain and anxiety
- More rapid onset of anesthesia
- Considered as more accurate than standard aspirating syringe
- Enables the operator to use pen grasp while injecting.

Disadvantages of wand system

- Unit is expensive
- Longer injection time
- Due to longer tubing attached to handpiece, only 1.4 ml of anesthetic solution is injected from cartridge
- System sometime requires to get accustomed
- System is operated by foot-pedal control and anesthetic cartridge is not directly visible.

Comfort Control Syringe

It is an electronic, preprogrammed delivery system for local anesthesia that dispenses the anesthetic in a slower, more controlled and more consistent manner than traditional manual syringe.

The comfort control syringe has two-stage delivery system in which injection begins at a very slow rate to decrease the discomfort associated with rapid injection. After ten seconds, comfort control syringe (CCS) automatically increases injection rate for the technique which has been selected. There are five different injection rates to choose from that are pre-programmed into CCS system. As a result, CCS can be adapted for any intraoral injection and still deliver an injection that can be less painful than with a manual syringe.

Advantages of comfort control syringe

- During the first-phase of injection, anesthetic is delivered at very slow rate. This minimizes pressure, tissue trauma and patient discomfort
- More rapid onset of anesthesia
- Enables the operator to use pen grasp while injecting
- It has anesthetic cartridge directly behind the needle, that as in traditional syringe and injection controls are on finger tip rather than on foot-pedal.

Disadvantages of comfort control syringe

- Longer injection time
- Unit is expensive
- Handpiece is bulkier than Wand system.

Transcutaneous Electrical Nerve Stimulation (TENS)

This is noninvasive technique in which a low-voltage electrical current is delivered through wires from a power unit to electrodes located on the skin.

Transcutaneous electrical nerve stimulation (TENS), has been applied successfully to treat acute and chronic pain in medicine for many years and more recently in dentistry. It's use for treatment of myofascial pain is well documented and has also been tried during simple restoration and electroanalgesia.

Mechanism of action
- Release of endogenous opiates
- Based on Gate's control theory, which states that stimulating input from large pain conducting nerve fibers closes the gate on nociceptive sensory phenomena from the A-delta and C-fibers. This prevents descendent motor activity (tightening up).

Indications
- Most commonly used in temporomandibular disorders (TMDs)
- Restorative dentistry
- In patients, allergic to local anesthesia
- In patients having needle phobia.

Contraindications
- Patients having cardiac pacemakers
- Patients having neurological disorders such as epilepsy, stroke, etc.
- Pregnant patients.

Technique
- Clean the surface by alcohol swab over the coronoid notch area
- Dry the area with gauze piece
- Apply electrode patches
- Make sure that TENS unit is off
- Attach electrode leads from patch to TENS unit
- Adjust the timer
- Adjust the controls to high bandwidth and high frequency
- Slowly adjust the amplitude so that patient feels a gentle pulsing sensation
- Adjust pulse width and pulse rate
- Proceed with dental procedure in usual manner
- At the completion of the procedure, disconnect the leads and remove the electrode patches from the patient.

Electronic Dental Anesthesia

Electronic dental anesthesia (EDA) was developed in mid-1960's for management of acute pain, but the use of electricity as therapeutic modality is not new in the field of medical and dental sciences.

Indications
- Most common use is in temporomandibular disorders (TMDs)

- Restorative dentistry
- Patients who are allergic to local anesthesia
- Patient having needle phobia.

Contraindications
- In patients with cardiac pacemakers
- Pregnant patients
- In patients with neurological disorders such as epilepsy, stroke, etc.
- Young pediatric patient
- Dental phobics (individuals afraid of every dental treatment)
- Very old patients with senile dementia.

Mechanism of EDA
This is explained on the basis of Gate control's theory. In this, higher frequency is used which causes the patient to experience a sensation described as throbbing or pulsing. It also causes stimulation of larger diameter nerve fibers (A-fibers) which are usually responsible for touch, pressure and temperature.

These large diameter fibers (A-fibers) are said to inhibit the central transmission of effects of smaller nerve fibers (A-delta and C-fibers) which in turn are stimulated during drilling at high speed and curettage. So, when no impulse reaches the central nervous system, there would be no pain.

Mechanism of EDA
➡ Based on Gate Control theory
➡ Uses higher frequency to experience a sensation
➡ Causes the patient to experience a sensation described as throbbing or pulsing
➡ Causes stimulation of large diameter nerves (A-fibers) which inhibit central transmission of effects of smaller nerve fibers basis.

Advantages of EDA
➡ No fear of needle
➡ No fear for injection of drugs
➡ No residual anesthetic effect after the completion of procedure
➡ Residual analgesic effects persists after completion of procedure.

Disadvantages of EDA
➡ Expensive
➡ Technique sensitive—requires training.

Needle-less Syringes

Needle-less syringe are especially designed syringes to administer anesthetic drugs which shoot a pinpoint jet of fluid through the skin at high speed.

USE OF HIGH SPEED ROTARY INSTRUMENTS WITH SHARP BURS AND COOLANTS

The use of high speed and ultrahigh speed rotary instruments with sharp burs and coolants result in elimination of pain. Even lengthy and complicated procedures are performed very quickly without any discomfort to the patient.

ANALGESIA

Inhalation sedation may be used for the patient who has a low threshold of pain and are very apprehensive. In these patients, nitrous oxide and oxygen increase threshold of pain. Inhalation sedation does not mean general anesthesia rather it is sometimes given along with local anesthetic injections to elevate threshold of pain. With this, patient is conscious of surrounding activities.

Pain control can be achieved through:
- Opioid drugs
- Nonopioid drugs.

Opioid Drugs

Generally narcotic (opioid) analgesics are used to relieve acute and severe to moderate pain. Clinician's therapeutic judgment determines which analgesic should be prescribed. He must decide the strength of the drug, whether it is to be used alone or in compound form, the frequency of use and side effects associated with it. The drugs used most often are the mild, nonopioid analgesics.

The opioid receptors are located at several important sites in brain, and their activation inhibits the transmission of nociceptive signals from trigeminal nucleus to higher brain regions. Opioids also activate peripheral opioid receptors.

Nonopioid Drugs

They act primarily on peripheral pain mechanism and also in CNS to raise pain threshold. In comparison to opioid drugs, they are weaker analgesics.

Nonopioid analgesics interfere with membrane phospholipid metabolism. Mild analgesics interfere with cyclooxygenase pathway and reduce synthesis of prostaglandin which result in the reduction or elimination of pain. More frequently used nonnarcotic analgesics are aspirin, acetaminophen, diflunisal, naproxen and ibuprofen, etc.

Selective COX-2 Inhibitors
- Rofecoxib
- Celecoxib
- Etocoxib, etc.

NSAIDs are very effective for managing pain of inflammatory origin and by virtue of binding to plasma proteins actually exhibits increased delivery to inflamed tissue.

HYPNOSIS

Hypnosis is also used to reduce or alleviate apprehension and pain. It is done through suggestion of relaxation. In other words, patient undergoing hypnosis feels relaxed and less fatigued, also the clinician remains in a more relaxed atmosphere. Before applying this technique, the clinician should have awareness about psychological, emotional and mental conditions of the patient.

Key Points

- Iatrosedation is a nondrug technique of causing sedation. A patient, who is comfortable with doctor, responds well to the drugs than to patient who are anxious about the doctor and treatment to be done.
- In pharmacosedation sedatives and tranquilizers drugs are used as CNS depressants and to decrease cortical excitability.
- The primary action of the local anesthetics agent in producing a nerve conduction block is to decrease the nerve permeability to sodium (Na^+) ions, thus preventing the inflow of Na^+ ions into the nerve. Therefore local anesthetics interfere with sodium conductance and inhibit the propagation of impulse along the nerve fibers
- In tissues with higher pH, local anesthetics acts faster because at alkaline pH, local anesthetic is present in undissociated base form and it is the form, which penetrates the axon.
- Wand local anesthesia system is computer-automated injection system which allows precise delivery of anesthesia at a constant flow rate despite varying tissue resistance.
- Comfort control syringe (CCS) is an electronic, preprogrammed delivery system for local anesthesia that dispenses the anesthetic in a slower, more controlled and more consistent manner than traditional manual syringe.
- The use of high speed and ultrahigh speed rotary instruments with sharp burs and coolants result in elimination of pain. Even lengthy and complicated procedures are performed very quickly without any discomfort to the patient.

QUESTIONS

1. How do you achieve pain control in operative dentistry?
2. Write short notes on:
   a. Recent advances in local anesthesia
   b. Wand system of local anesthesia.

Matricing and Tooth Separation

INTRODUCTION

Teeth and periodontium are designed in such a manner that mutually they significantly contribute to their own health and support. They are complimentary to each other. Proper form and alignment of teeth protect periodontium. During mastication, the contours of teeth as a unit protect the periodontium. A breach in the continuity of contacts of teeth give rise to diseases of periodontium resulting in loss of teeth.

Ideal tooth form of interproximal area is as follows (**Fig. 13.1**):

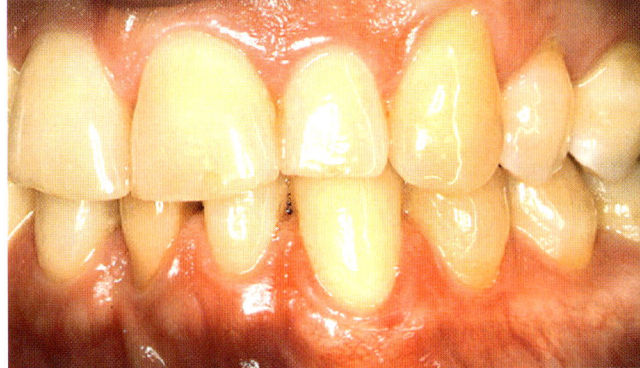

Figure 13.1: Photograph showing interproximal areas of the teeth

- Interproximal embrasures extend on all the four sides of a tooth with definite shape around each contact area. These four embrasures are gingival, occlusal, lingual, and facial.
- Anterior teeth have less pronounced embrasures than posterior teeth (**Fig. 13.2**).
- Interproximal space between the adjacent teeth is proper triangular in shape with apex at the contact area and base towards the outer surface (**Fig. 13.3**). This triangle increasingly widens out from the contact area in all the four directions, occlusal, lingual, gingival and facial.

Consequences of not restoring proximal areas

➡ Food impaction leading to recurrent caries (**Fig. 13.4**)
➡ Change in occlusion and intercuspal relations
➡ Rotation and drifting of teeth
➡ Trauma to the periodontium.

MATRICING

Restoration of a tooth requires great clinical acumen so as to reproduce the original contours and contacts of the tooth. In case of large missing wall of the tooth, support has to be provided while placing and condensing the

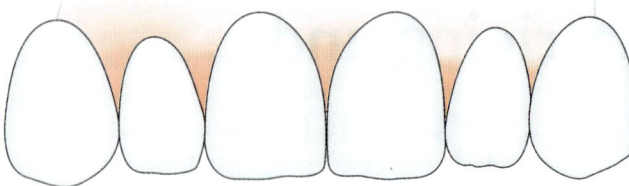

Figure 13.2: Interproximal spaces of anterior teeth

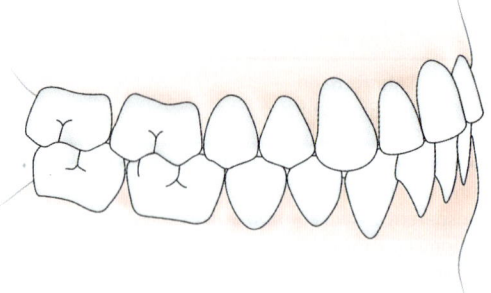

Figure 13.3: Interproximal spaces of posterior teeth

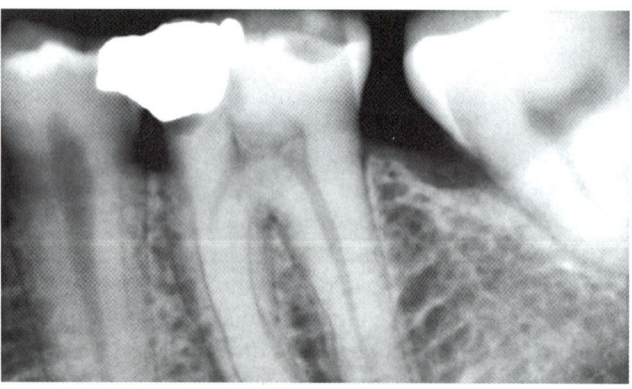

Figure 13.4: Radiograph showing faulty proximal restoration

restorative material. Usually, a metallic strip serves this function and is known as the matrix band. Matrix band which forms the temporary walls is held in its place by means of a matrix band retainer which may be a mechanical device, floss, wire, thread or impression materials, etc.

MATRICING: It is the procedure by which a temporary wall is built opposite to the axial wall, surrounding the tooth structure which has been lost during the tooth preparation.

MATRIX: It is an instrument which is used to hold the restoration within the tooth while it is setting.

Parts of Matrix

Retainer

It holds a band in desired position and shape.

Band

It is a piece of metal or polymeric material, intended to give support and form to the restoration during its insertion and setting.

Commonly used materials for bands are
➡ Stainless steel
➡ Polyacetate
➡ Cellulose acetate
➡ Cellulose nitrate.

Matrix band should extend 2 mm above the marginal ridge height and 1 mm below gingival margin of the preparation. Matrices range in width from 6.35 mm (1/4") to 9.525 mm (3/8") for permanent teeth and 3.175 mm (1/8") to 7.9375 mm (5/16") for deciduous teeth. Their thickness may range between 0.0381 mm (0.0015") to 0.0508 mm (0.002").

Functions of a matrix
➡ To confine the restoration during setting
➡ To provide proper proximal contact and contour
➡ To provide optimal surface texture for restoration
➡ To prevent gingival overhangs.

Requirements of a Matrix Band

To achieve an optimal restoration, matrix band should have following requirements:

- *Rigidity*: The matrix band should be rigid enough so as to withstand the pressure of condensation applied during restoration, placement and maintains its shape during hardening
- *Adaptability*: The matrix band should be able to match to almost any size and shape of tooth
- *Easy to use*: The band should be simple in design so that it does not cause any difficulty to the patient, or hindrance to the operator during restoration of the tooth
- It should be able to displace the gingiva and rubber dam for ease in working
- *Nonreactive*: It should be inert to tissues and the restorative material
- *Height and contour*: The matrix band should not extend more than 2 mm beyond the occlusogingival height of the crown of tooth. This facilitates vision and speeds up working

- *Application*: The matrix band should be such that it can be applied and removed easily
- *Sterilization*: It should be easy to sterilize
- *Inexpensive*: It should be inexpensive.

Classification of Matrices

Depending upon Their Method of Retention

- Mechanically retained, e.g. Ivory matrix retainers no.1 and 8, Tofflemire universal dental matrix band retainer.
- Self-retained, e.g. copper or stainless steel bands.

Depending upon Its Preparation

- Mechanical matrix, e.g. Ivory matrix retainers no.1 and 8
- Anatomic/custom made matrix, e.g. compound supported.

On the Basis of Transparency

- Transparent matrices, e.g. cellophane, celluloid
- Nontransparent matrices, e.g. stainless steel.

Depending upon the Tooth Preparation for Which They are Used

Type of preparation	Matrices and retainers
• Class II tooth preparation	• Ivory matrix number 1 • Nystrom's retainer
• Class II mesio-occluso-distal, (MOD) tooth preparation	• Ivory matrix number 8 • Tofflemire matrix • Steele's Siqveland self-adjusting matrix • Anatomical matrix band • 'T' shaped matrix band • Retainerless automatrix
• Class III tooth preparation	• 'S' shaped matrix band • Cellophane matrix strips • Mylar strips
• Class IV tooth preparation	• Plastic strips • Aluminium foil • Transparent crown form • Anatomic matrix
• Class V tooth preparation • Direct tooth colored and all other complex	• Custom made plastic matrix • Cellophane matrices • Anatomic matrices preparations • Aluminium or copper collars • Transparent plastic crown forms

Ivory Matrix Holder (Retainer) No. 1 (Figs 13.5 and 13.6)

Ivory matrix holder No. 1 is most commonly used matrix band holder for unilateral class II tooth preparations.

The matrix holder has a claw at one end with two flat semicircle arms having a pointed projection at the end (**Fig. 13.4**). On the other end of the matrix band holder, there is a screw which is when tightened, brings the ends of both the claws closer to each other. Band used with this matrix has one margin slightly projected in its middle part. This projected margin is kept towards the gingiva on the side of tooth preparation. The band of suitable size is selected and encircled around the tooth. Keeping the matrix band around the tooth, the screw of the retainer is tightened so that the band perfectly fits around the tooth. After this, wedge is placed which also helps in further adaptation of the matrix band to the tooth (**Fig. 13.7**).

Indication
For unilateral class II tooth preparations.

Advantages
➥ Economical ➥ Used for restoring class II tooth preparations ➥ Can be sterilized.

Disadvantage
Cumbersome to apply and remove.

Ivory Matrix Band Retainer No. 8 (Figs 13.8 and 13.9)

Ivory matrix band retainer holds the matrix band that encircles the tooth to provide missing walls on both proximal sides. The matrix band is made up of thin sheet of metal so that it can pass through the contact area of the unprepared proximal side of the tooth (**Fig. 13.8**). The circumference of the band can be adjusted using the screw present in the matrix band retainer.

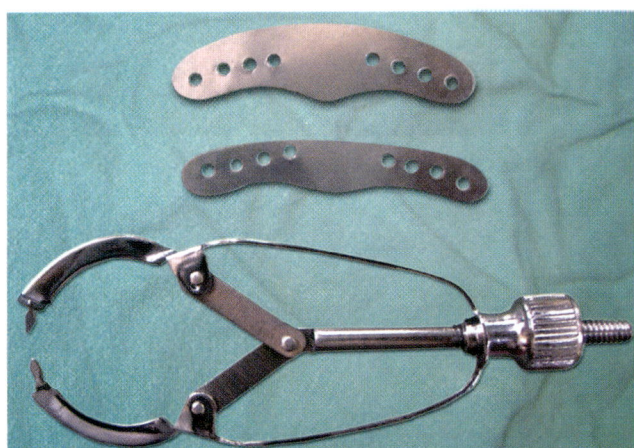

Figure 13.5: Ivory no. 1 matrix retainer and band

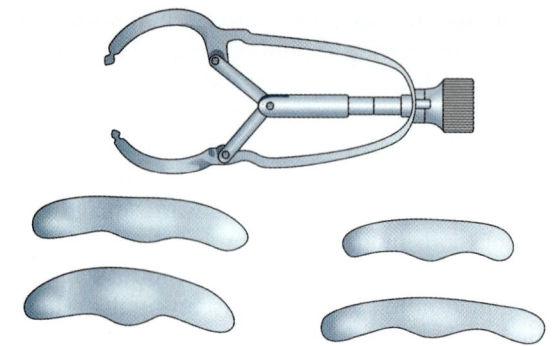

Figure 13.6: Diagrammatic representation of Ivory no. I retainer and band

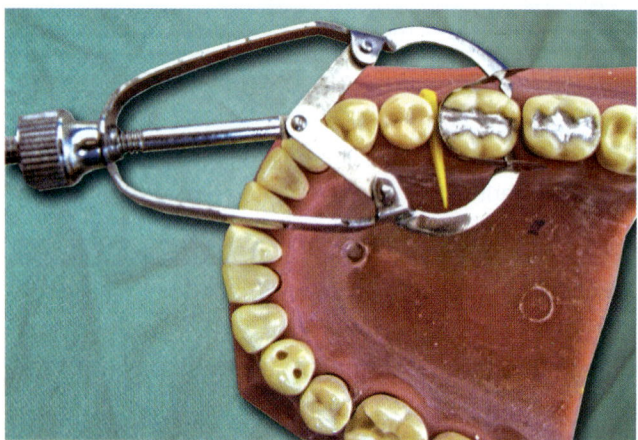

Figure 13.7: Matrix and band used in class II restoration

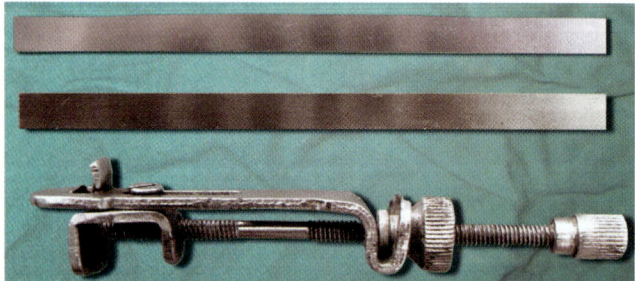

Figure 13.8: Ivory no. 8 matrix retainer and bands

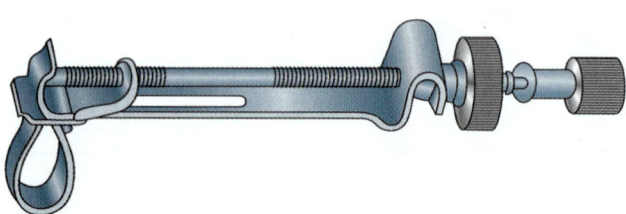

Figure 13.9: Diagrammatic representation of Ivory matrix retainer no. 8

Indications
➡ Unilateral or bilateral class II preparations (MOD).
➡ Class II compound tooth preparations having more than two missing walls.

Advantages
➡ Economical
➡ Can be sterilized.

Disadvantage
Cumbersome to apply and remove.

Tofflemire Universal Matrix Band Retainer (Fig 13.10)

It was designed by Dr BF Tofflemire. It is also well known as 'universal' matrix because it can be used in all types of tooth preparations of posterior teeth. In this, the matrix band is fitted onto the retainer and then fitted loosely over the tooth, which then can be tightened in position by means of the screw (**Fig. 13.10**).

Tofflemire matrix
➡ Also known as Universal matrix
➡ Design given by Dr. Tofflemire (Name based on inventor)
➡ Preferred for class II and compound amalgam restorations.

Indications
➡ Class I tooth preparations with buccal or lingual extensions
➡ Unilateral or bilateral class II (MOD) tooth preparations
➡ Class II compound tooth preparations having more than two missing walls.

Advantages
➡ Can be used both from facial as well as lingual side
➡ Economical
➡ Sturdy and stable in nature
➡ Provides good contact and contours
➡ Can be easily removed
➡ Can be sterilized.

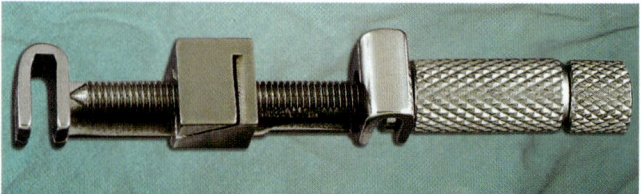

Figure 13.10: Tofflemire retainer

➡ Cannot be used in badly broken teeth
➡ Does not offer optimal results with resin restorations.

Types of Tofflemire Matrix

- Based on type of head
  - Straight (**Fig. 13.10**):
    i. Head of matrix system is straight
    ii. Placed only from buccal side
  - Contra-angle (**Fig. 13.11**):
    i. Head is angulated
    ii. Placed either from buccal or lingual side.
- Based on type of dentition
  - Standard—use in permanent dentition
  - Small—used in primary dentition.

Parts of Tofflemire Retainer (Fig. 13.12)

Head

- Uses slots for positioning of matrix
- U-shaped head with two slots in open side
- Open side of the head should be facing gingivally when the band is placed around the tooth (**Figs 13.13 and 13.14**).

Slide (Diagonal slot)

- Amount of band extending beyond the slot depends upon type of tooth to be treated.
- This portion is located near the head for installation of band in the retainer, helps in placement of band around the tooth.

Knurled nuts

- Two knurled knots in retainer
  - Large knurled nut—near the matrix band
  - Small knurled nut.

i. Large knurled nut (Also known as rotating spindle)
   a. Helps in adapting the loop of matrix band against the tooth.
   b. Helps in adjusting the size of loop of matrix band against the tooth.
ii. Small knurled nut—helps in tightening the band to retainer.

Assembly of retainer: When band and retainer are assembled, two ends of band must be of same length protruding from the diagonal slot (**Fig. 13.15**).

Loop extending from retainer can project in following ways (**Fig. 13.16**):

- Straight—used near anterior teeth
- Left/Right—used mostly in posterior areas of oral cavity.

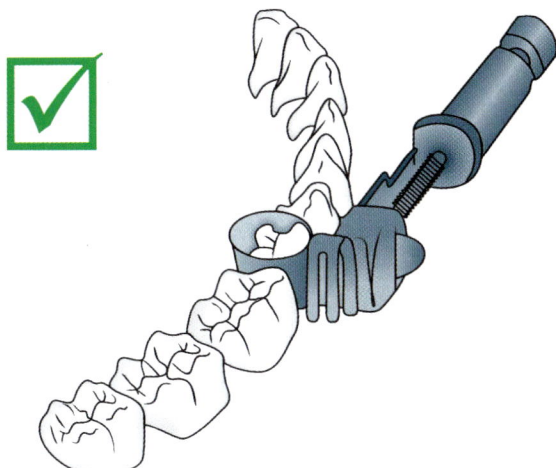

Figure 13.13: Slots of head should always be directed gingivally

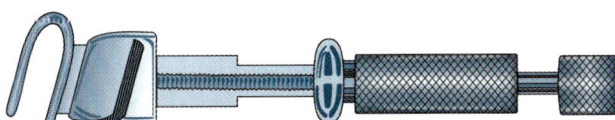

Figure 13.11: Angulated Tofflemire retainer

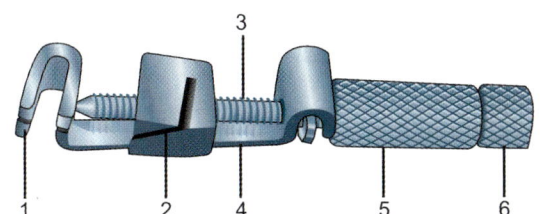

Figure 13.12: Parts of Tofflemire retainer: 1. Head; 2. Diagonal slot; 3. Rotating spindle; 4. Frame; 5. Small knurled nut; 6. Large knurled nut

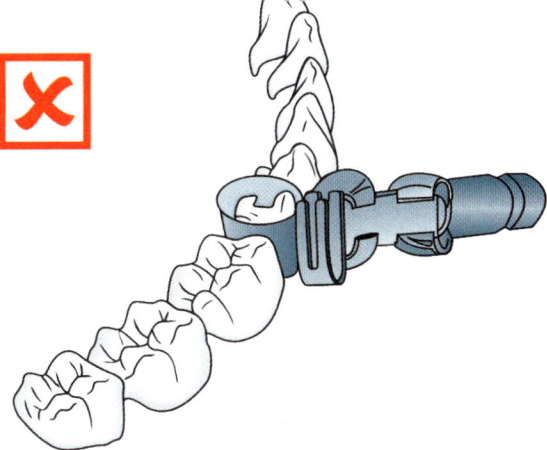

Figure 13.14: Slots should not be directed occlusally

While adapting the matrix band to retainer loop of the matrix, band appears as funnel shaped, i.e. one side of the opening has greater diameter than other (**Fig. 13.17**). Opening with greater diameter should be placed occlusally while with lesser diameter should be placed gingivally.

Types of bands

Two types of bands are usually used:
1. Flat Bands
2. Precontoured bands.

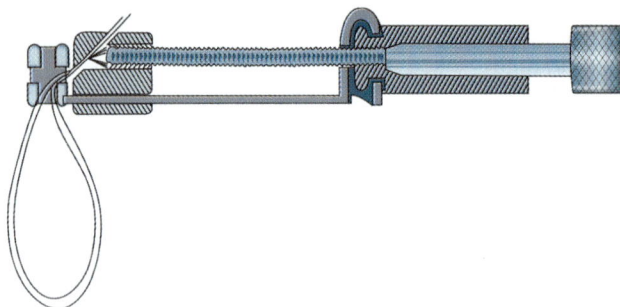

Figure 13.15: Assembled Tofflemire matrix band with retainer

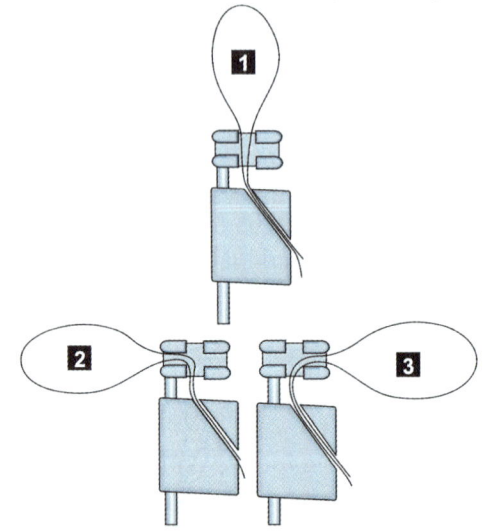

Figure 13.16: Loop from band can extend in straight, right or left direction

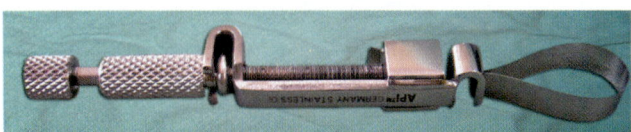

Figure 13.17: Tofflemire with band in place

1. Flat bands:
   - Available in two thicknesses
     - 0.0020 inches
     - 0.0015 inches
       Any of these thickness can be used, it depends upon operators preference.
   - According to shapes, three shapes of flat bands are available (**Fig. 13.18**)
     - No. 1 or universal band
     - No. 2 or (MOD band): It has two extensions projecting at gingival edge. It is commonly used in molars
     - No. 3: Similar to No. 2 band in design but narrower than No. 2.
   - Flat band need to be contoured before placing in retainer. Contouring of band can be done with the help of:
     - Ovoid burnisher
     - Spoon excavator (using its convex side).
2. Precontoured bands:
   They are also available but less commonly used. While removing these bands, one must take care of contour of band. Band should be rotated in such a way that its trailing end should not fracture the restoration.

Operative instruction for placement (**Figs 13.19A to D**)
- First open the large knurled nut so that slide is at least ¼ inches from the head (**Fig. 13.19A**).
- Hold the knurled nut (large) with one hand, open the small knurled nut in opposite direction (counter clock wise) for clearance of diagonal slot for reception of matrix band (**Fig. 13.19B**).
- Two ends of matrix band are secured together to form loop or either use preformed loop (**Fig. 13.19C**).
- Place the ends of band in diagonal slot.

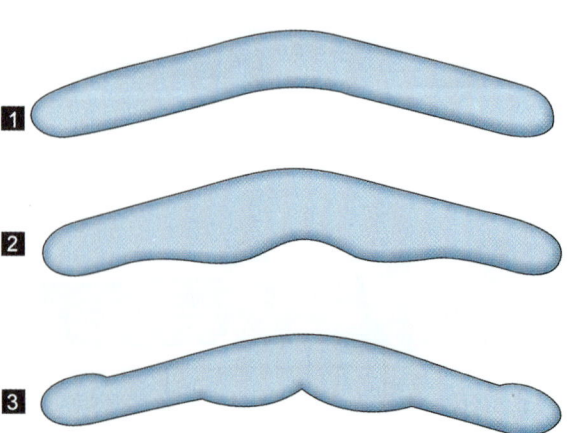

Figure 13.18: Three types of Tofflemire bands

- Then, small knurled nut is tightened to secure the band to the retainer.
- After securing the band tightly to the retainer, it is placed around the tooth to be restored.
- For final adaptation of matrix band to the tooth, tighten the large knurled nut (**Fig. 13.19D**).
- *Wedge placement*: Wedge should be placed after the retainer and band are snuggly fitted to the tooth. Always insert the wedge from widest embrasure area. Wedge helps in developing the adequate contact and contour despite the thickness of material.

Procedure for removal

This is usually accomplished in two steps:

1. Removal of retainer
2. Removal of band.

Removal of retainer

- Small knurled knot is moved counter clockwise to free the band from the retainer. While rotating the smaller knurled knot, hold the larger nut. Keep the index finger on occlusal surface of tooth to stabilize the band.

Removal of band

- Carefully remove the band from each contact point
- Support the occlusal surface of the restoration. While removing the band, a condenser can be held against the marginal ridge of the restoration
- Do not pull band in occlusal direction rather move the band in facial or lingual direction
- Band can be cut near to the teeth on the lingual side and then try to pull it from the buccal side.

Modification in Tofflemire retainer

Omni matrix
➡ Preassembled Tofflemire retainer
➡ One time use (disposable)
➡ Available with band thickness
  ♦ 0.0010 inch thick
  ♦ 0.0015 inch thick.

Advantage

Takes less time to use.

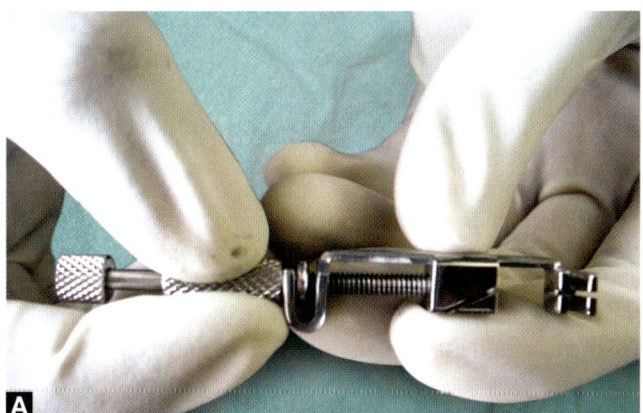
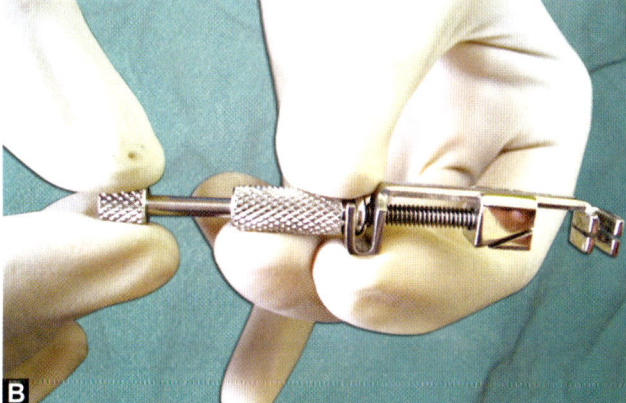
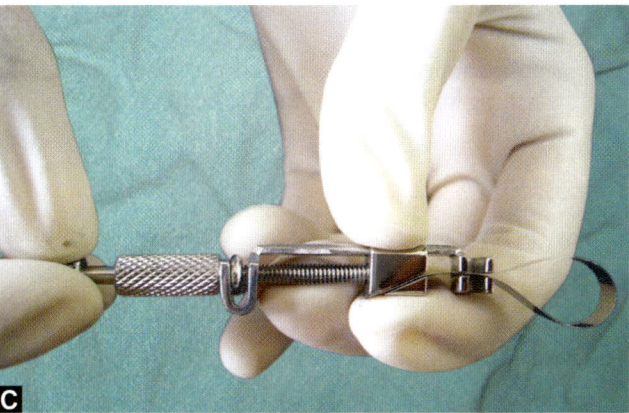
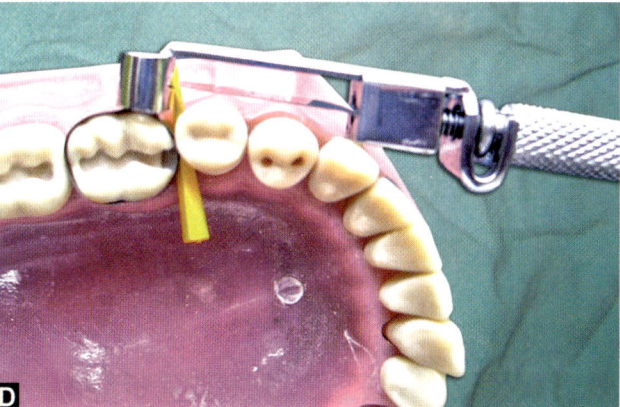

Figures 13.19A to D: Placement of Tofflemire retainer

Steele's Siqveland Self-adjusting Matrix Holder for Tapering Teeth (Fig. 13.20)

It is especially used when there is a significant difference between the diameters of the cervical and occlusal one-third of the tooth (**Fig. 13.16**). This matrix retainer can give two different diameters at the two ends of the matrix band. It is based on the principle of a movable slide which holds and tightens the band in the required position.

Indication

All types of compound and complex tooth preparations in posterior teeth.

Advantages

➡ Can adapt to tooth contour properly
➡ Due to Steele's siqveland self-adjusting matrix holder anatomic adaptation of the band is possible without the help of wedges.

Anatomical Matrix Band/ Compound Supported Matrix

It was described by Sweeney. It is adapted over the tooth with one healthy tooth on either side. To contour the band according to tooth, pliers are used, though precontoured anatomic matrix bands are also available. For further adaptation of the band to surface of the tooth, wedge is placed. Buccal and lingual embrasures are sealed with the help of selfcure acrylic or impression compound cones.

Indications

➡ Restoration of class II proximal tooth preparation involving one surface or both
➡ Large restoration, not supported by adjacent teeth.

Advantages

➡ Provides better contact and contour in restoring class II tooth preparation
➡ Adequate rigid and stable than other matrix system
➡ Easy to remove
➡ Little proximal carrying is required
➡ Recontouring can be easily done after compound placement.

Disadvantage

Time consuming.

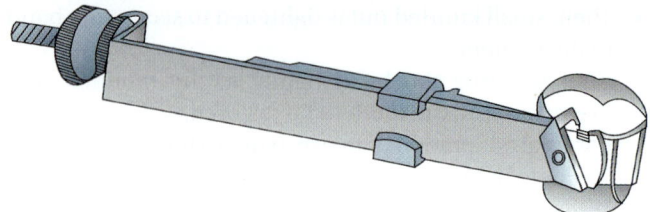

Figure 13.20: Siqveland matrix retainer

Materials Used

• Matrix band of width 5/16 inch (8 mm) and 0.002 inch (0.05 mm) thick stainless steel matrix band
• Impression compound or low fusing compounds.

Procedure

• Cut a sufficient length of matrix band so that it covers 1/3rd of facial and lingual surface along with prepared proximal tooth preparation
• Contour the band with egg-shaped burnisher in a back and forth motion to achieve desired proximal as well as facial and lingual contour of the tooth
• Check the contour of band occlusogingivally as well as facially and lingually
• Wedging should be done after securing the band in right position
• Heat one end of impression compound over flame for 5 to 10 seconds
• When compound starts drooping, carry it with dampened glove fingers into the oral cavity
• After the compound is pressed into desired place, cool and hardened it with air
• Recontouring of band can be easily done by pressing the warmed instrument to inside of matrix to soften the compound
• For extraretention and stability:
  – Compound can be carried over cusps of adjacent teeth
  – Staple shaped piece of metal can be inserted after warming for holding the facial and lingual compound together.

Removal

• Easy to remove
• Can be easily removed with sharp instrument such as enamel hatchet or hollenback carver.

Retainerless Automatrix System

This matrix system can be adjusted according to tooth shape and size. The bands are available in different sizes, and come in preformed and disposable form (**Fig. 13.21**). Height of bands vary from 3/16 to 5/16 inch. Thickness of bands can be 0.038 mm or 0.05 mm. The matrix is adapted over the tooth with the clip on the buccal aspect. To tighten the band, an automate mechanical device is used. Once the restoration is complete, the band is cut with the help of cutting pliers.

Indications

- In tilted and partially erupted teeth
- In patients who cannot tolerate retainers
- For complex amalgam restorations.

Advantages

- Simple to use
- Convenient
- Takes less time to apply
- No interference from retainer, therefore better visibility.

Disadvantages

- Unable to develop proper contours
- Costly
- Difficult to burnish because bands are flat.

T-Shaped Matrix Band

This is preformed brass, copper or stainless steel matrix bands without a retainer. In this band, the long arm of the T surrounds the tooth and overlaps the short arm of the T (**Figs 13.22A and B**). The band is adapted according to the tooth shape and size. Wedges and impression compound may be used to provide further stability to the band.

Indication

Unilateral or bilateral class II (MOD) tooth preparations.

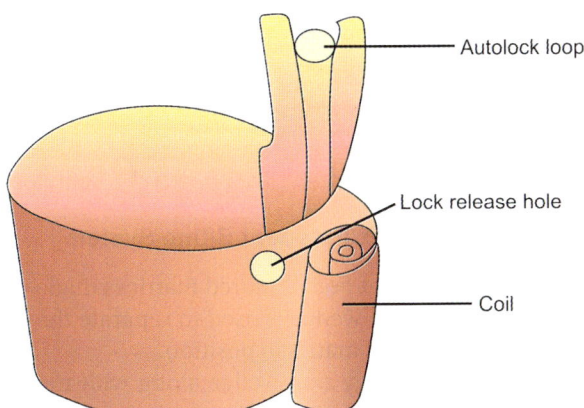

Figure 13.21: Automatrix band

Advantages

- Simple to use
- Economical.

Disadvantage

Not stable in nature.

S-Shaped Matrix Band

S-shaped matrix band is used for restoring distal part of canine and premolar. In this, stainless steel matrix band is taken and twisted like 'S' with the help of a mouth mirror handle. The contoured strip is placed interproximally over the facial surface of tooth and lingual surface of bicuspid (**Fig. 13.23**). To increase its stability, wedge and impression compound can be used.

Indications

- For restoring distal part of canine and premolar
- Class II slot restorations.

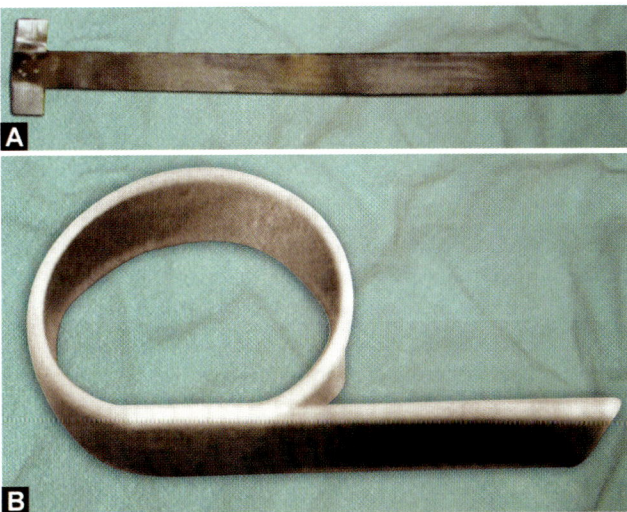

Figures 13.22A and B: (A) T-shaped band; (B) T-band matrix

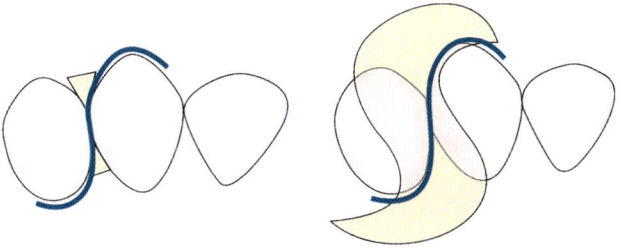

Figure 13.23: S-shaped matrix band

Advantage

Offers optimal contour for distal part of canine and premolar.

Disadvantage

Cumbersome to apply and remove.

Full Circle or Ring Bands

Copper or stainless steel full circle or ring bands are generally indicated for mesio-occlusodistal compound and complex tooth preparations. These are usually available in size ranging from 1 to 20. Band is selected according to required size, softened by heating it to the red hot state and then quenching in water. After all these steps, the band is contoured using pliers, trimmed by cutting pliers and finished by finishing stones. Occlusal height of the band is also adjusted accordingly. Proximal contact of the band may be thinned using a small round fine, grinding stone. Wedges and impression compound can also be used to further stabilize the band.

After condensation of restoration is done, the band can be cut by means of a bur at the same appointment or the next day.

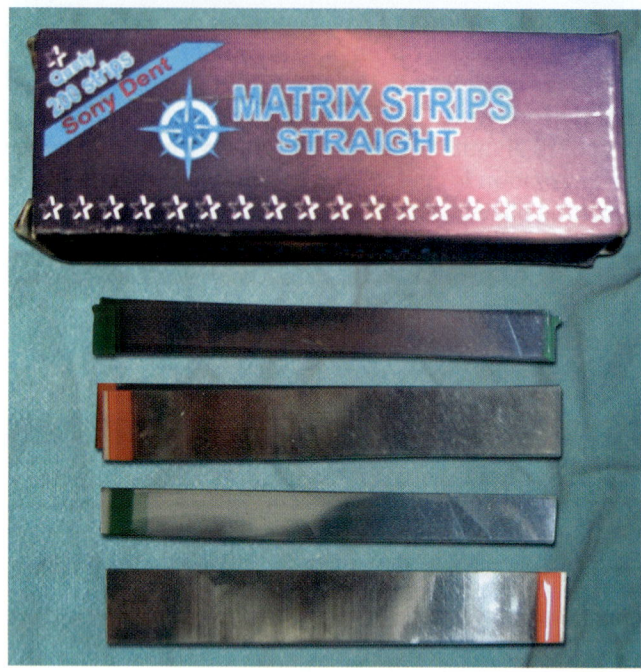

Figure 13.24: Mylar strips

Indications

➡ For restoring badly broken and mutilated teeth
➡ Mesio-occlusodistal compound tooth preparations and complex tooth preparations.

Advantage

Offers the optimal contour for damaged teeth.

Disadvantage

Time consuming to apply and remove.

Plastic Matrix Strips

These are transparent matrix strips used for tooth colored restorations. They can be of different types:
- Celluloid (Cellulose nitrate) strips are used for silicate cements
- Cellophane (Cellulose acetate) strips are used for resins
- Mylar strips used for composite and silicate restorations (**Fig. 13.24**).

For class IV tooth preparations, the strip is folded in 'L-Shape'. The matrix is measured and cut so that one side is as wide as the length of the tooth and the other side is as wide as the width of the tooth. The matrix strip is burnished over the end of a steel instrument (e.g. a tweezer handle) to produce a convexity in the strip. This convex contoured surface is positioned facing the proximal surface of the

tooth to be restored. A wedge is used for further stabilization and adaptation of the strip.

The preparation is filled to slight excess and one end of the strip is brought across the proximal surface of the filled tooth. The other end of the strip is folded over the incisal edge. The matrix is held with the thumb of the left hand till the initial setting or curing takes place.

Indication

For restoring class III and IV tooth preparations.

Advantages

➡ Simple and easy to use
➡ Economical.

Disadvantage

Lack of stability.

Precontoured Matrix/Palodent Bitine System

This system consists of precontoured matrices made up of soft metal. In this, the wedge is used to separate the teeth and hold the sectional matrix in position.

The 'BITINE' springy ring wedge along with matrix is shaped to provide the proximal contours of a posterior tooth (**Fig. 13.25**).

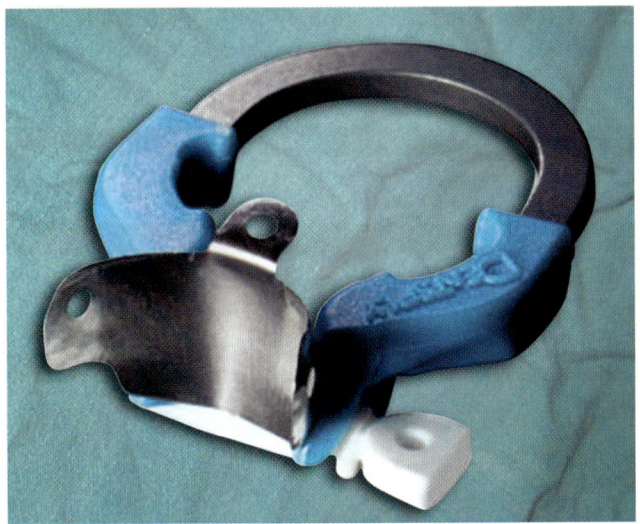

Figure 13.25: Precontoured matrix

Steps of Application and Removal

- Approximately 3 mm blob of impression compound is applied to each of its tips.
- The ring is held with rubber dam forcep.
- Impression compound is warmed quickly over the flame and carried into the oral cavity.
- Beaks are placed into the embrasures of the preparation side and ring is allowed to shrink. Ring tightly seals the sectional matrix band around the tooth due to spring action.
- The matrix band is properly contoured with a ball burnisher so as to adapt it to the tooth.
- After this gingival wedge is inserted under the contact area.
- After checking the fit of the matrix band, restoration is completed.
- Then the ring is widened apart and removed.
- The wedge is removed after this.

Indication
For restoring class II compound or complex tooth preparations.

Advantages
➡ Simple and easy to use ➡ Provides tooth separation ➡ Offers better contours with composite restorations.

Disadvantages
➡ Tight contacts may prevent insertion of the band ➡ Expensive.

Aluminum or Copper Collars

These are pre-shaped for class V restorations according to the gingival third of the buccal and lingual surfaces. They can be adjusted so as to cover 1 to 2 mm of the tooth surface circumferentially beyond the preparation margins (**Figs 13.26A and B**). After selecting appropriate size, they are mounted on the tip of a softened stick of compound which is being used as a handle. After the restoration is placed in preparation, apply the selected matrix onto the tooth till the initial setting is over (**Fig. 13.27**).

Indication
For restoring class V preparations

Advantages
➡ Simple and easy to use ➡ Offers better contours.

Disadvantage
Can not be used with resin restorations.

Transparent Crown Forms Matrices

These are 'Stock' plastic crowns which can be contoured according to tooth shape and size. These are specially used

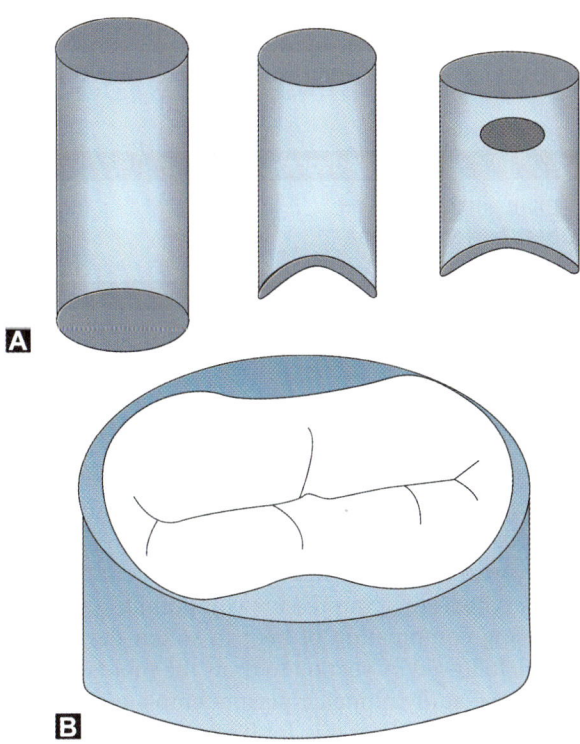

Figures 13.26A and B: (A) Copper band matrix; (B) Copper band matrix in place

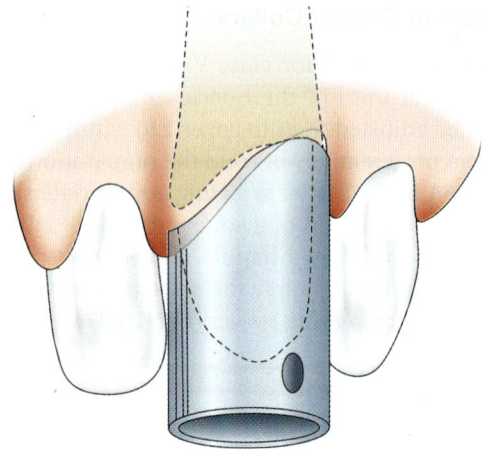

Figure 13.27: Copper collar in place

for bilateral class IV preparation. After selecting the appropriate crown form, it is trimmed to fit 1mm beyond the preparation margins. When composite restoration is loaded in this crown form, it is positioned over the prepared tooth and cured. After the restoration is completed, this crown form can be cut with the help of burs for its removal. For unilateral class IV, the plastic crown is cut incisogingivally to use one-half of the crown according to the side of restoration.

Indication
For restoring class IV tooth preparations and fractured teeth.

Advantages
➠ Simple and easy to use ➠ Offers better contours.

Disadvantages
➠ Time consuming ➠ Costly.

Anatomic Custom Made Matrix

This matrix offers best contours and contact for restoration of compound or complex class II tooth preparations. In this, the defective area is restored on study model to tooth anatomy with the help of heat resistant material like plasticine, acrylic resin or impression compound.

By using combination of heat to soften the template material, followed by suction to draw the moldable material onto the study model, a plastic template is made for the restored tooth. After this, for fitting on to the tooth this template is trimmed gingivally. Template should hold at least one sound tooth on each side. The restorative material

is loaded into the preparation, then the matrix filled with the material is inserted and properly seated over the tooth and cured.

Indication
For restoring class IV preparations and fractured teeth.

Advantages
➠ Simple and easy to use ➠ Offers better contours.

Disadvantages
➠ Time consuming ➠ Costly.

TOOTH SEPARATION

Separation of teeth is defined as the process of separating the involved teeth slightly away from each other or bringing them closer to each other and/or changing their spatial position in one or more dimensions.

Reason for Tooth Separation

Following are reasons for tooth separation:
- *Examination*: For examination of initial proximal caries which is usually not seen on the radiograph.
- *Preparation of teeth*: For providing accessibility to proximal area during preparation of class II and class III tooth preparations (**Fig. 13.28**).
- *Polishing of restorations*: Tooth separation helps in providing accessibility to the proximal area of class II and class III tooth preparations.
- *Matrix placement*: Matrix can be placed easily during restoration of class II preparation.
- *Removal of foreign bodies*: Foreign bodies and objects forced interproximally, can be removed using tooth separation.
- *Repositioning shifted teeth*: It also helps to some extent in repositioning of shifted teeth.

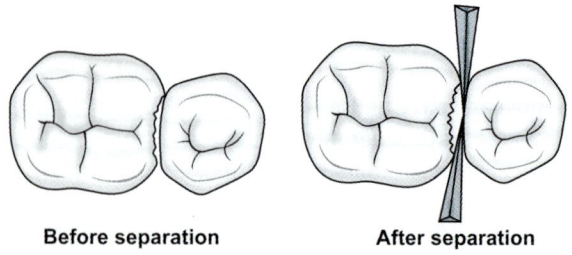

Before separation   **After separation**

Figure 13.28: Tooth separation provides accessibility to proximal area during class II and III preparations

Methods of Tooth Separation

Two methods used for tooth separation are

1. Slow or delayed separation
2. Rapid or immediate separation.

Slow or Delayed Separation

In this separation, teeth are slowly and gradually shifted apart by inserting some materials between the teeth. This separation usually takes long time, i.e from several days to weeks.

Indications

Tilted, drifted and rotated teeth in which rapid separation is not useful.

Advantages

One of the main advantage of slow tooth separation is that tooth repositioning occurs without damage to periodontal ligament fibers.

Disadvantages

➡ Time consuming
➡ May require many visits.

Methods for achieving slow separation

➡ Separating rubber ring/bands
➡ Rubber dam sheet
➡ Ligature wire/copper wire
➡ Gutta-percha stick
➡ Oversized temporary crowns
➡ Fixed orthodontic appliances.

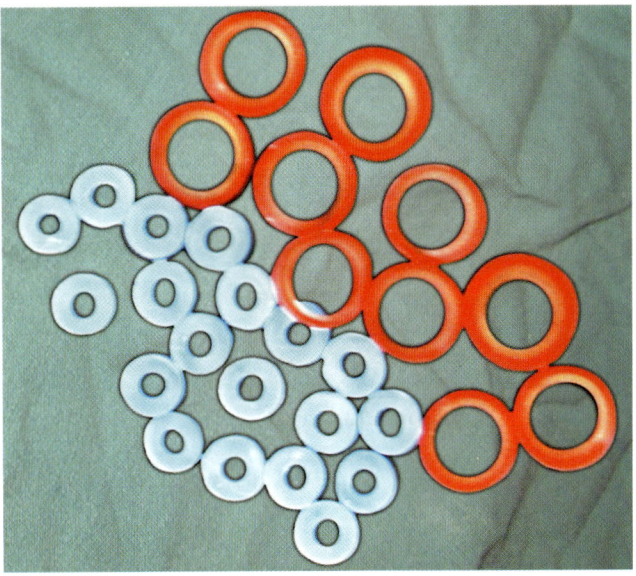

Figure 13.29: Separating rings

Seperating rubber ring/band (**Fig. 13.29**)
- Separating rubber band is usually used in orthodontic cases.
- It is stretched and placed interproximally between the two teeth to achieve separation.
- It may take 2 to 3 days to 1 week.

Rubber dam sheet (**Fig. 13.30**)
- It is stretched and placed interproximally between the teeth.
- Usually heavy or extra-heavy type is preferred due to thickness of sheet.
- Time for tooth separation may vary from 1 hour to 24 hours or more.
- In case of pain and swelling, a floss may be used to remove the sheet.

Ligature wire/copper wire (**Fig. 13.31**)
- Wire is passed beneath the contact area to form a loop.

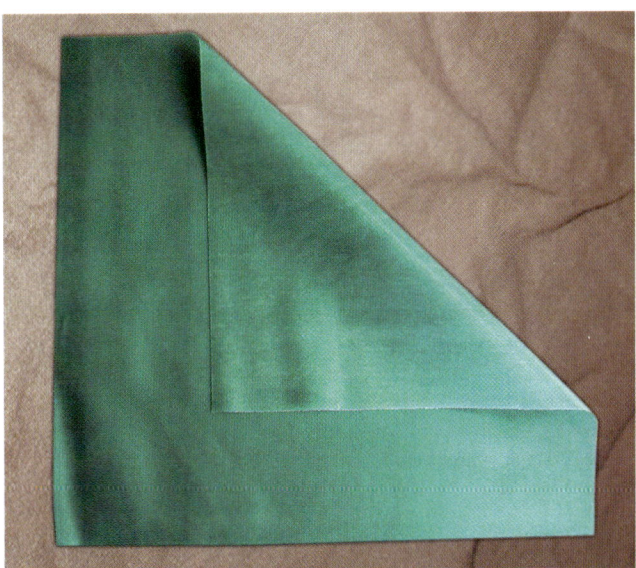

Figure 13.30: Rubber dam sheet

- Tightening of wire loop is done by twisting two ends together (**Fig. 13.32**). This causes increase in the separation.
- Separation is usually achieved in 2 to 3 days.

Gutta-percha stick
- It is softened with heat and packed into proximal area.
- Usually indicated for adjoining tooth preparation of posterior teeth.
- Tooth separation usually takes 1 week to 2 weeks.

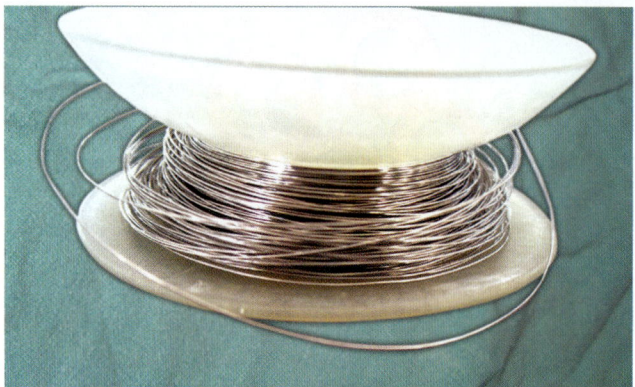

Figure 13.31: Ligature wire

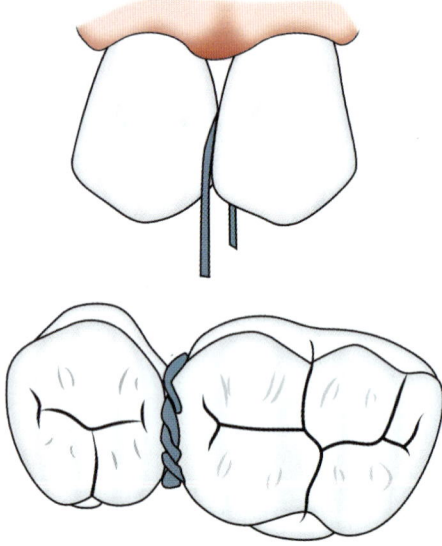

Figure 13.32: To separate the teeth, wire loop is passed beneath the contact area and loop is tightened by twisting the two ends

Oversized temporary crowns: Oversized temporary crowns is also one of the methods for slow separation.

In this, acrylic resin is periodically added in the mesial and distal contact area to increase the separation.

Fixed orthodontic appliances
- Indicated only in cases where extensive repositioning of teeth is required.
- Most predictable and effective method.

Rapid or Immediate Tooth Separation

Rapid separation is most frequently used method in which tooth separation can be achieved in very short span of time.

Advantages
➡ More useful and advantageous than slow separators
➡ Quicker than slow separators
➡ More predictable.

Principles used in rapid separator
➡ Traction principle
➡ Wedge principle.

Traction principle used for separation:

This type of principle always uses mechanical devices which engages the proximal area of the tooth with holding arms. These holding arms are moved apart to create the separation between the contacting teeth. Few devices are based on this principles which are:
- Ferrier double bow separator
- Noninterfering true separator.

Ferrier double bow separator (**Fig. 13.33**)
- As the name indicates, it has 2 bows.
- Each bow engages the proximal surface of the tooth just gingival to contact area (**Fig. 13.34**).
- A 'Wrench' system is used for turning the threaded bars, this helps in causing separation.

Advantages
- Stabilization of the separation throughout operation
- Separation is achieved at expense of both contacting teeth rather than one tooth.

  Uses: Tooth preparation and during finishing and polishing of class III direct gold restoration.

Noninterfering true separator
- As the name indicates, it is noninterfering type rapid separator
- It is used where continuous stabilized separation is required.

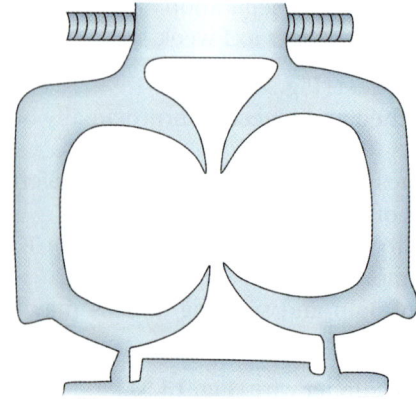

Figure 13.33: Ferrier double bow separator

Advantages
- Separation can be increased or decreased after stabilization
- Noninterfering in nature.

Wedge principle used for rapid separation: A pointed, wedge shaped mechanical device is inserted beneath the contact area of teeth, which in turn, produce the separation.

This is usually accomplished by 2 means:
1. Elliot separator
2. Wedges

1. Elliot separator (**Fig. 13.35**)
   - Also known as 'Crab claw' separator because of its design.

- Mechanical device consisting of:
   – Bow
   – Two holding jaws
   – Tightening screw.
- Two holding jaws are positioned gingival to contact area without damaging the interproximal area (**Fig. 13.36**)
- Clockwise rotation of tightening screw moves the contacting teeth apart
- The separation should not be more than thickness of periodontal ligament, i.e. 0.2 to 0.5 mm.
   Uses: Used for examination and final polishing of proximal restoration.

2. Wedges (**Fig. 13.37**): Wedges are devices which are usually preferred for rapid tooth separation. These are used for tooth preparation and restoration.

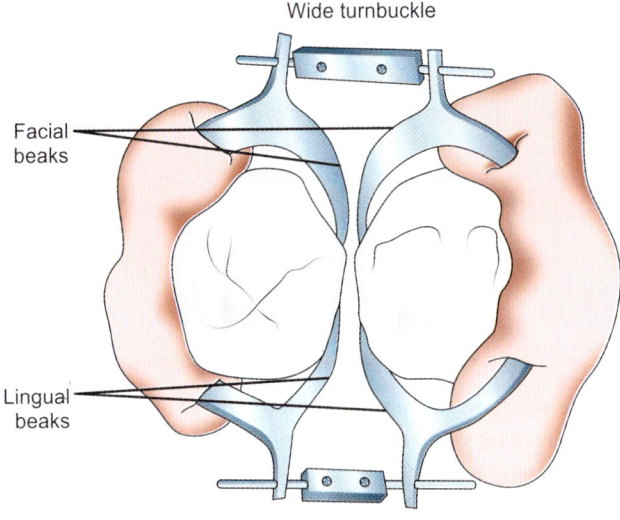

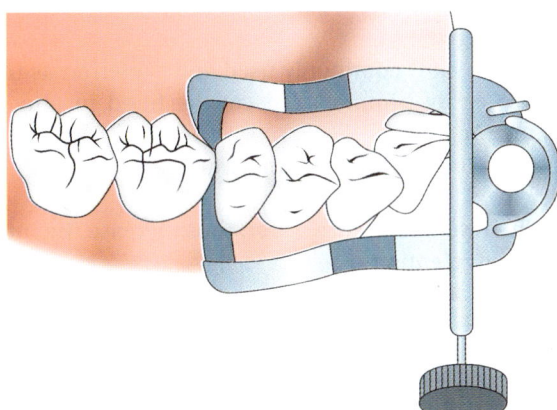

Figure 13.36: Here two holding jaws are positioned gingival to contact area

Figure 13.34: Two bows of Ferrier double bow separator engages the proximal surface of the tooth just gingival to contact area

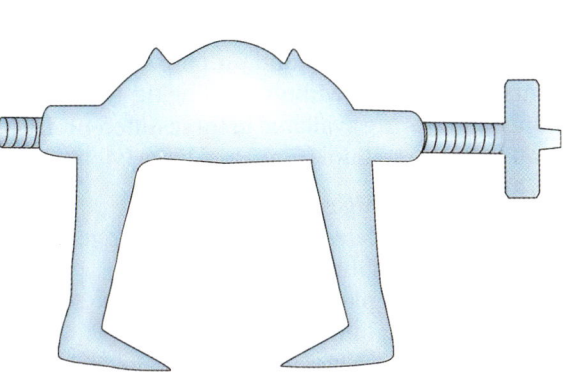

Figure 13.35: Elliot separator

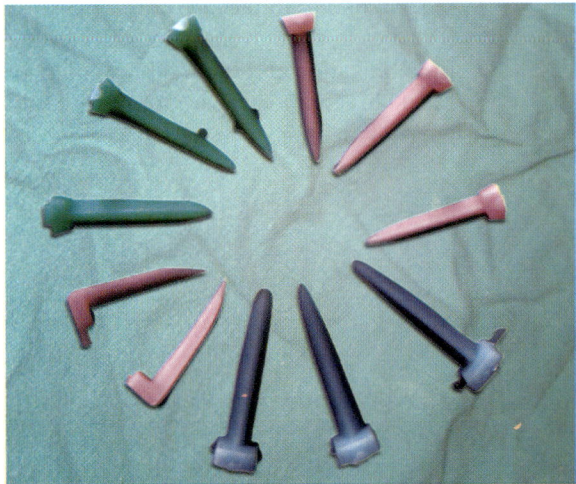

Figure 13.37: Wedges

Functions of wedges

➡ Help in rapid separation of teeth
➡ Prevent gingival overhang of restoration
➡ Provide space to compensate for thickness of matrix band
 ♦ Help in stabilization of retainer and matrix during restorative procedures **(Fig. 13.38)**
 ♦ Provide close adaptability in cervical portions of the proximal restorations, there by help in achieving correct contour and shape at cervical area
 ♦ Help in retracting and depressing the interproximal gingival area, thus help in minimizing trauma to soft tissue
 ♦ Help in depressing rubber dam in interproximal area.

Types of wedges:
• Wooden wedges
• Plastic wedges.

Wooden wedges:
• These are most commonly used and preferred as they can be easily trimmed and can be fitted in gingival embrasure.
• Adapt well in the gingival embrasure
• Easy to use
• Wooden wedges absorb water, thus increase the interproximal retention
• Provide stabilization to matrix band
• Available in two shapes **(Fig. 13.39)**:
 1. Triangular
 2. Round
  – Triangular wedge
   i. Most commonly used
   ii. It has two positions—apex and the base
   iii. Apex of the wedge usually lies in gingival portion of the contact area
   iv. Base lies in contact with gingiva. This helps in stabilization and retraction of gingiva
   v. Used in tooth preparations with deep gingival margins.

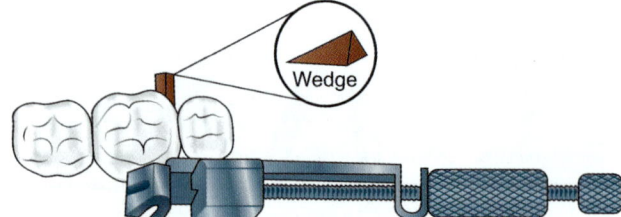

Figure 13.38: Wedge helps in stabilization of the retainer and the matrix band

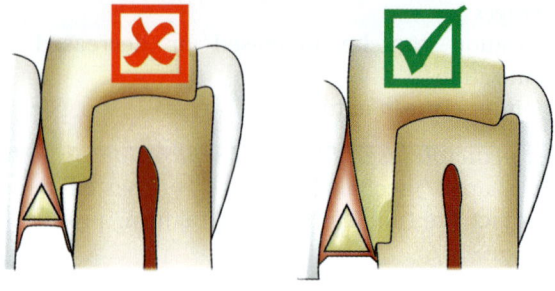

Triangular wedge application

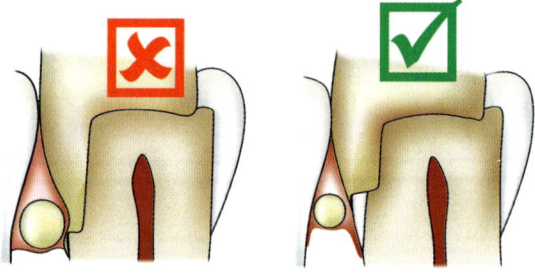

Round wedge application

Figure 13.39: Correct and incorrect placement of triangular and round wedge

  – Round wedge
   i. Not so commonly used
   ii. Made from wooden tooth picks by trimming the apical portion
   iii. It has uniform shape
   iv. Used in class II tooth preparation.

Plastic wedges: Though commercially available but they are not much preferred because:
• Trimming is difficult
• Adaptability is difficult in some cases.

Types of Plastic Wedge

• *Normal wedges:* They are similar to the wooden wedges in shape and use.
• *Wave shaped wedges **(Fig. 13.40)**:* Their curved shape helps in easy placement and proper seal of buccal and lingual embrasures without impinging gingiva. Wave shaped wedges are available in three different sizes, i.e. small (white), medium (pink) and large (violet) color.

Light transmitting wedges

• As the name indicates, these types of wedges transmit 90 to 95 percent of incident light
• They are a type of plastic wedges
• Transparent in nature
• Designed for use in cervical area of class II composite resin restoration.

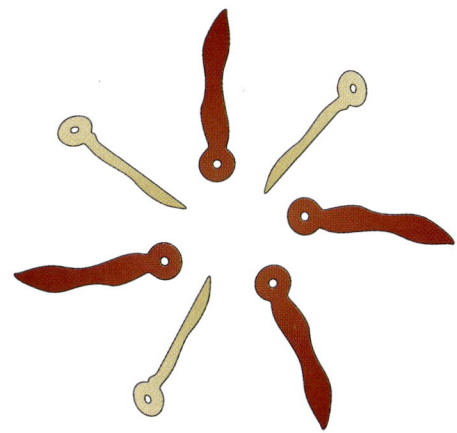

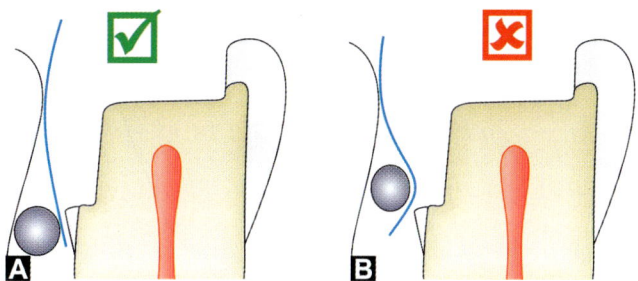

Figures 13.41A and B: Wedge in place: (A) Correct position; (B) Incorrect position

Figure 13.40: Wave shaped wedges

Advantages of light transmitting wedges over other wedges in composite restorations:
- Help in reducing the polymerization shrinkage because of light transmission
- Better adaptability.

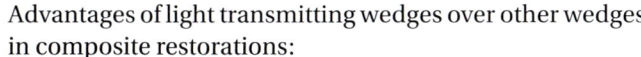

Important points regarding wedges

➡ Select the type and shape according to requirement. These are:
  ♦ Length of the wedge should be in the range of 1 to 1.2 cm
  ♦ It should not irritate tongue, cheek and gingival tissue
  ♦ Wedge should be inserted beneath the contact area in the gingival embrasure (**Figs 13.41A and B**)
  ♦ Usually inserted from lingual embrasure area as it is wider than buccal area. Sometimes when it irritates tongue; it can inserted from buccal area also
  ♦ Wedge should be firm and stable during restorative procedure
  ♦ Should not be forcibly inserted in the contact area leading to pain and swelling.

Type of wedge	Indications
Round wooden	Conservative class II preparations
Triangular wooden	Preparation with deep gingival margin
Plastic wooden	Preparation with deep gingival margin
Light transmitting wedge	Cervical portion of class II composite restoration

Modified Wedging Techniques

- Double wedging
- Wedge wedging
- Piggy back wedging.

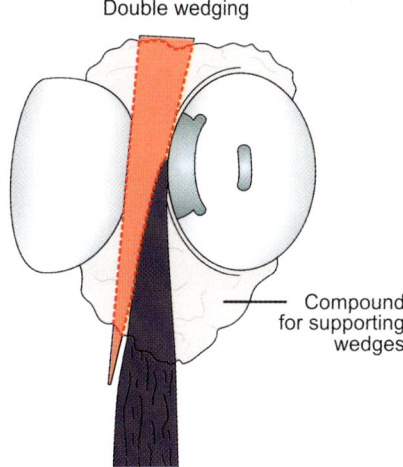

Figure 13.42: Double wedging technique

1. Double wedging (**Fig. 13.42**)
   - Two wedges are used:
     – One is inserted from buccal embrasure and another is inserted from lingual embrasure.
   - This technique is indicated in the following cases:
     – Spacing between adjacent teeth where single wedge is not sufficient
     – Widening of proximal box in buccolingual dimension.
2. Wedge wedging (**Fig. 13.43**):
   - In this technique, two wedges are used
   - One wedge is inserted from lingual embrasure area while another is inserted between the wedge and matrix band at right angle to first wedge
   - These are primarily indicated while treating mesial aspect of maxillary first premolar because of presence of flutes in root near the gingival area (**Fig. 13.44**)

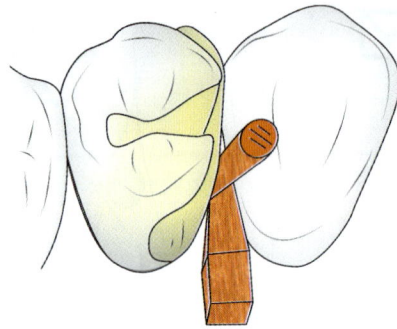

Wedge wedging

Figure 13.43: Wedge wedging technique

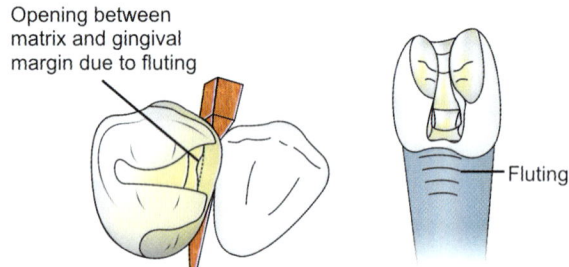

Opening between matrix and gingival margin due to fluting

Fluting

Figure 13.44: Fluting in the roots near gingival area

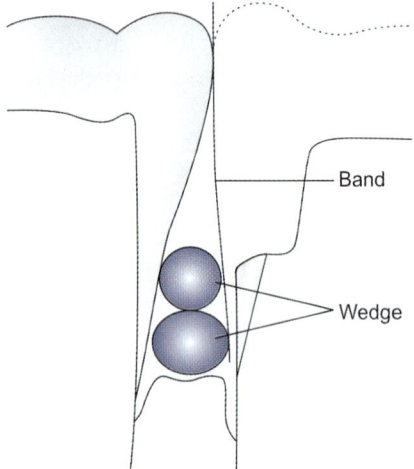

Band

Wedge

Figure 13.45: Piggyback wedging

3. Piggyback wedging (**Fig. 13.45**):
   • In this technique two wedges are used
   • One (larger) wedge is inserted as used normally, while the other smaller wedge (Piggyback) is inserted above the larger one

• It is indicated in cases of shallow proximal box with gingival recession
• This technique provides closer adaptation and contour of the matrix band.

🔑 Key Points

• During mastication, the contours of teeth as a unit protect the periodontium. A breach in the continuity of contacts of teeth give rise to diseases of periodontium resulting in loss of teeth.
• Interproximal space between the adjacent teeth is proper triangular in shape with apex at the contact area and base towards the outer surface. This triangle increasingly widens out in from the contact area of all the four directions, occlusal, lingual, gingival and facial.
• Matricing is the procedure by which a temporary wall is built opposite to the axial wall, surrounding the tooth structure which has been lost during the tooth preparation.
• Matrix is an instrument which is used to hold the restoration within the tooth while it is setting.
• The matrix band should not extend more than 2 mm beyond the occlusogingival height of the crown of tooth. This facilitates vision and speeds up working.
• Tofflemire universal matrix band retainer was designed by Dr BF Tofflemire. It is also well known as 'universal' matrix because it can be used in all types of tooth preparations of posterior teeth, though it is preferred for class II and compound amalgam restorations.
• Omni matrix is modified preassembled disposable tofflemire retainer. It is less time to use.
• Retainerless automatrix system can be adjusted according to tooth shape and size. The matrix is adapted over the tooth with the clip on the buccal aspect. To tighten the band, an automate mechanical device is used. Once the restoration is complete, the band is cut with the help of cutting pliers.
• S-shaped matrix band is used for restoring distal part of canine and premolar. In this, stainless steel matrix band is taken and twisted like 'S' with the help of a mouth mirror handle.
• Precontoured matrix/palodent bitine system consists of precontoured matrices made up of soft metal. In this, the wedge is used to separate the teeth and hold the sectional matrix in position.
• Transparent crown forms matrices are 'Stock' plastic crowns which can be contoured according to tooth shape and size. These are specially used for bilateral

class IV preparation. After selecting the appropriate crown form, it is trimmed to fit 1mm beyond the preparation margins.

- Separation of teeth is defined as the process of separating the involved teeth slightly away from each other or bringing them closer to each other and/or changing their spatial position in one or more dimensions.
- In slow separation, teeth are slowly and gradually shifted apart by inserting some materials between the teeth. This separation usually takes long time, i.e. from several days to weeks.
- Rapid separation is most frequently used method in which tooth separation can be achieved in very short span of time.
- Traction principle used for separation uses mechanical devices which engages the proximal area of the tooth with holding arms. These holding arms are moved apart to create the separation between the contacting teeth. Devices based on this principles are Ferrier double bow separator and noninterfering true separator.
- In Wedge principle used for rapid separation, a pointed, wedge shaped mechanical device is inserted beneath the contact area of teeth, which in turn, produce the separation. Elliot separator and wedges are used for this technique.
- Light transmitting wedge is a type of plastic wedge. It transmits 90 to 95 percent of incident light
- It is designed for use in cervical area of class II composite resin restoration. It helps in reducing the polymerization shrinkage as it transmits light.
- In double wedging technique, two wedges are used, one is inserted from buccal embrasure and another is inserted from lingual embrasure. It is done when single wedge is not sufficient.
- In wedge wedging technique, two wedges are used. One wedge is inserted from lingual embrasure area while another is inserted between the wedge and matrix band at right angle to first wedge. It is mainly indicated while treating mesial aspect of maxillary first premolar.

- In Piggyback wedging, one (larger) wedge is inserted as used normally, while the other smaller wedge (Piggyback) is inserted above the larger one. It is indicated in cases of shallow proximal box with gingival recession.

QUESTIONS

1. Define matricing. What are objectives of matricing?
2. Explain tooth separation in detail.
3. Short notes on:
   a. Tofflemire retainer
   b. Wedges and wedging techniques
   c. Elliot separator
   d. Anatomical matrix band
   e. Tooth separators
   f. Matrices and retainers
   g. Wedges
   h. Palodent Bitine system
   i. Modified wedging technique
   j. Double wedging technique
   k. Piggyback wedging technique
4. Write short note on matrices, retainers and wedges used in operative dentistry.
5. Write in short about the classification of matrices.

BIBLIOGRAPHY

1. Chan DCN. Custom matrix adaptation with elastic cords. Oper Dent. 2001;26:419.
2. Cunningham PJ. Matrices for amalgam restorations. Aust. Dent. J. 1968;13:139.
3. Harrington, WG Moon, PC, Crockett WD, Shepard, FE. Reinforced matrices for pin amalgam restorations reduce microleakage. JPD.1979;41:622.
4. Kaplan I, Schuman NJ. Selecting a matrix for class II amalgam restoration. JPD. 1986;56:25.
5. Kucey BK. Matrices in metal ceramics. JPD.1990;63:32.
6. Medlock JW, Re GJ. Contoured mylar matrices. JPD. 1984; 51:364.
7. Meyer A. Proposed criteria for matrices. J Can Dent Asso. 1987;53:851.
8. Qualtrough AJ, Wilson NH. Matrices: their development and in clinical practice. Dent Update. 1992;19:284.

CHAPTER 14

Pulp Protection

Chapter Outline

INTRODUCTION

By definition, pulp is a soft tissue of mesenchymal origin residing within the pulp chamber and root canals of teeth.

Some important features of pulp are as follows (Fig. 14.1)
➡ Pulp is located deep within the tooth, so defies visualization
➡ It gives radiographic appearance as radiolucent line
➡ Pulp is a connective tissue with several factors making it unique and altering its ability to respond to irritation
➡ Normal pulp is a coherent soft tissue, dependent on its normal hard dentin shell for protection and hence, once exposed, extremely sensitive to contact and te perature but this pain does not last for more than 1 to 2 seconds after the stimulus removed
➡ Since pulp is totally surrounded by a hard tissue, dentin limits the area for expansion and restricts the pulp's ability to tolerate edema
➡ The pulp has almost a total lack of collateral circulation, which severely limits its ability to cope with bacteria, necrotic tissue and inflammation
➡ The pulp possess unique cells the odontoblasts, as well as cells that can differentiate into hard-tissue secreting cells that form more dentin and/or irritation dentin in an attempt to protect itself from injury.

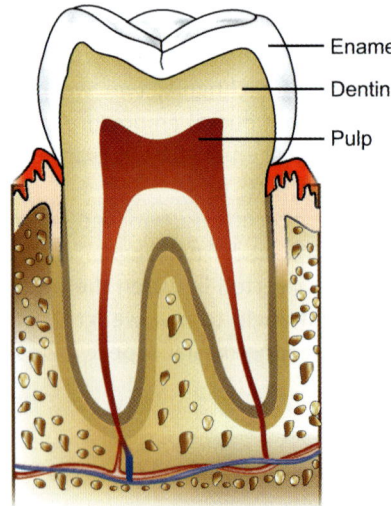

Figure 14.1: Diagrammatic representation of dental pulp

PULPAL IRRITANTS

Various pulpal irritants can be :
- *Bacterial irritants*: Most common cause for pulpal irritation are bacteria or their products which may enter pulp through a break in dentin from:

- Caries (**Fig. 14.2**)
- Accidental exposure
- Fracture
- Percolation around a restoration
- Extension of infection from gingival sulcus
- Periodontal pocket and abscess (**Fig. 14.3**)

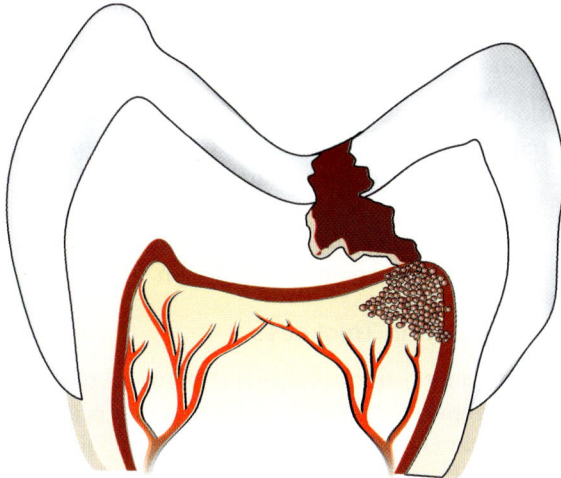

Figure 14.2: Bacteria from caries resulting in pulpal irritation

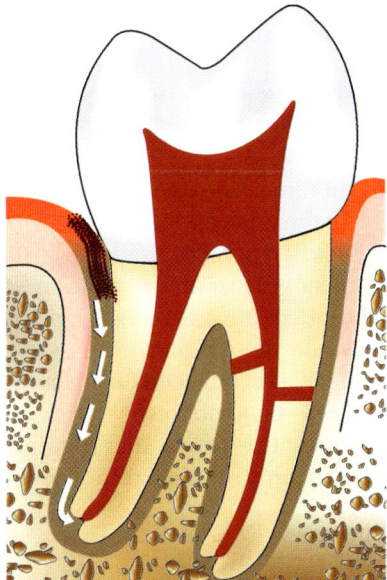

Figure 14.3: Involvement of pulp via periodontal pocket

- Anachoresis (Process by which microorganisms get carried by the bloodstream from another source localize on inflamed tissue).
- Traumatic
  - Acute trauma like fracture, luxation or avulsion of tooth
  - Chronic trauma including parafunctional habits like bruxism.
- *Iatrogenic*: Various iatrogenic causes of pulpal damage can be:
  - Thermal changes generated by cutting procedures, during restorative procedures, bleaching of enamel, microleakage occurring along the restorations, electrosurgical procedures, laser beam, etc. can cause severe damage to the pulp
  - Orthodontic movement
  - Periodontal curettage
  - Periapical curettage
  - Use of chemicals like temporary and permanent fillings, liners and bases and use of desiccants such as alcohol.
- Idiopathic
  - Aging
  - *Resorption*: Internal or external.

EFFECT OF DENTAL CARIES ON PULP

Dental caries is the most common route for causing irritation to the pulp. Dental caries is localized, progressive, decay of the teeth characterized by demineralization of the tooth surface by organic acids, produced by microorganisms. From carious lesion, the acids and other toxic substances penetrate through the dentinal tubules to reach the pulp.

The following defense reactions take place in a carious tooth to protect the pulp
➡ Formation of reparative dentin
➡ Dentinal sclerosis, i.e. reduction in permeability of dentin by narrowing of dentinal tubules
➡ Inflammatory and immunological reactions.

The rate of reparative dentin formation is related to rate of carious attack. More reparative dentin is formed in response to slow chronic caries than acute caries. For dentin sclerosis to take place, vital odontoblasts must be present within the tubules. In dentin sclerosis, the dentinal tubules are partially or fully filled with mineral deposits, thus reduce the permeability of dentin. Therefore dentinal sclerosis act as a barrier for the ingress of bacteria and their product (**Fig. 14.4**).

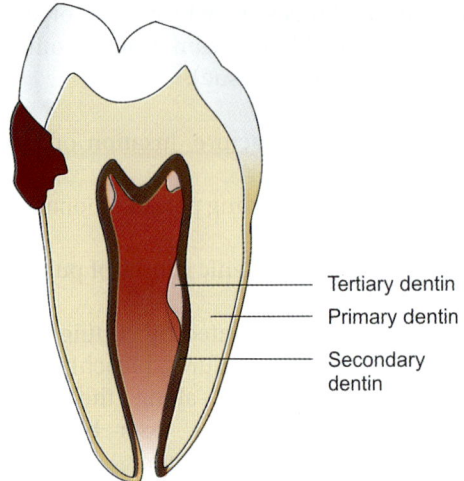

Figure 14.4: Formation of irritation dentin in response to caries

EFFECT OF TOOTH PREPARATION ON PULP

Factors affecting response of pulp to tooth preparation
➡ Pressure
➡ Heat
➡ Vibration
➡ Remaining dentin thickness
➡ Speed
➡ Nature of cutting instruments.

Pressure

The pressure of instrumentation on exposed dentin characteristically causes the aspiration of the nuclei of the odontoblasts or the entire odontoblasts themselves or nerve endings from pulp tissues into the dentinal tubules. This will obviously stimulate odontoblasts, disturb their metabolism and may lead to their complete degeneration and disintegration. This can occur by excessive pressure of hand or rotary instruments, especially in decreased effective depths.

Heat Production

Heat production is the second most damaging factor. If the pulp temperature is elevated by 11°F, destructive reaction will occur even in a normal, vital periodontal organ. That "heat" is a function of;

- *RPM*, i.e. more the RPM more is the heat production. In deep penetrations of dentin without using coolants, e.g. pin holes, the cutting speed must not exceed 3,000 rpm
- *Pressure:* It is directly proportional to heat generation. Whenever, the RPMs are increased, pressure must be correspondingly reduced

- *Surface area of contact:* It is related to the size and shape of the revolving tool. The more the contact between the tooth structure and revolving tool, the more is the heat generation
- *Desiccation:* If occurring in vital dentin, desiccation can cause aspiration of the odontoblasts into the tubules. The subsequent disturbances in their metabolism may lead to the complete degeneration of odontoblasts. Coolant sprays should be used even in nonvital or devitalized tooth structures, since the heat may burn the tooth structures.

Vibrations

Vibrations are measured by their amplitude or their capacity and frequency (the number/unit time). Vibrations are an indication of eccentricity in rotary instruments. Higher the amplitude, more destructive is the pulp response.

In addition to affecting the pulp tissues, vibration can create microcracks in enamel and dentin.

Remaining Dentin Thickness

Remaining dentin thickness (RDT) between the floor of the tooth preparation and the pulp chamber is one of the most important factor in determining the pulpal response. This measurement differs from the depth of tooth preparation since the pulpal floor in deeper preparation on larger teeth may be far from the pulp than that in shallow preparations on smaller teeth.

Remaining dentin thickness (RDT)
➡ In human teeth, dentin is approximately 3 mm thick
➡ Dentin permeability increases with decreasing RDT
➡ RDT of 2 mm or more effectively precludes restorative damage to the pulp
➡ At RDT of 0.75 mm, effects of bacterial invasion are seen
➡ When RDT is 0.25 mm, odontoblastic cell death is seen.

The amount of remaining dentin underneath the tooth preparation plays the most important role in the incidence of a pulp response. Generally, 2 mm of dentin thickness between the floor of the tooth preparation and the pulp will provide an adequate insulting barrier against irritants (**Fig. 14.5**). As the dentin thickness decreases, the pulp response increases. It is seen that response of cutting occurs only in areas beneath freshly cut dentinal tubules not lined with reparative or irregular dentin. In presence of reparative dentin only minimal response will occur.

Speed of Rotation

Ultra high-speed should be used for removal of enamel and superficial dentin. A speed of 3,000 to 30,000 rpm without coolant can cause pulpal damage. It should be

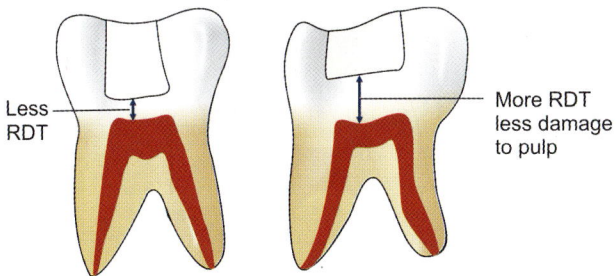

Figure 14.5: As dentin thickness decreases, the pulp response increases

kept in mind that without the use of coolant there is no safe speed. High speed without coolant can produce burning of dentin, which in turn affect the integrity of the pulp.

Nature of Cutting Instrument

Use of worn off and dull instruments should be avoided. Damaged cutting edges cause vibration and reduced cutting efficiency.

Use of dull instruments encourages the dentist to use excessive operating pressure, which results in increased temperature. This can result in thermal injury to pulp.

EFFECT OF CHEMICAL IRRITANTS ON PULP

The pulp is subjected frequently to chemical irritation from materials generally used in dentistry. Various filling materials produce some irritation ranging from mild-to-severe, as do various medicaments used for desensitization or dehydration of the dentin.

Properties of a material that could cause pulpal injury are its cytotoxic nature, acidity, heat evolved during setting and marginal leakage (**Fig. 14.6**).

Factors influencing the effect of restorative materials on pulp
➡ Acidity
➡ Absorption of water from dentin during setting
➡ Heat generated during setting
➡ Poor marginal adaptation leads to bacterial penetration
➡ Cytotoxicity of material.

PULP PROTECTION PROCEDURES

Pulp needs protection against various irritants as following (Fig. 14.7)
➡ Thermal protection against temperature changes
➡ Electrical protection against galvanic currents
➡ Mechanical protection during various restorative procedures
➡ Chemical protection from toxic components
➡ Protection from microleakage interface between tooth and the restoration.

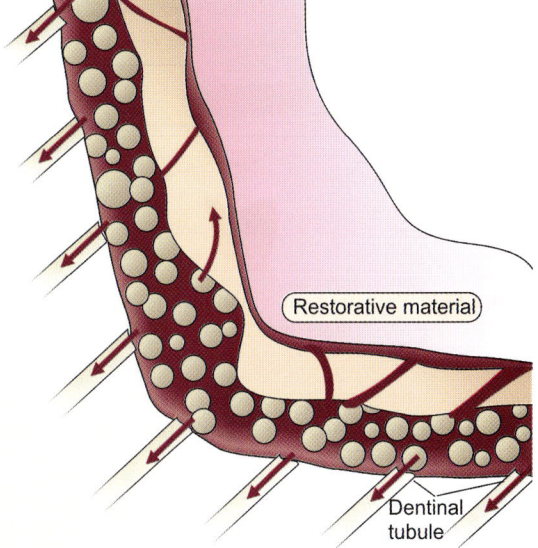

Figure 14.6: Pathways of marginal leakage

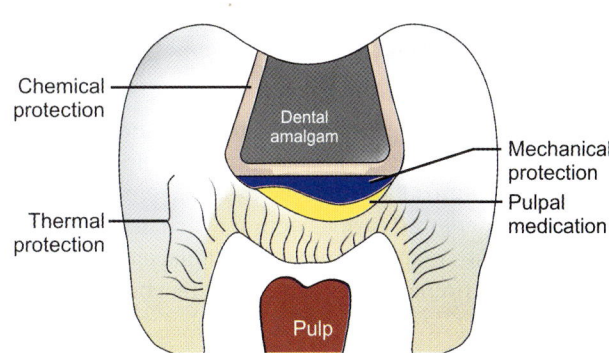

Figure 14.7: Need of pulp protection from various irritants

Pulp Protection in Shallow and Moderate Carious Lesions

In a moderate carious lesion, caries penetrates the enamel and may involve one half of the dentin, but not to the extent of endangering the pulp. In these cases, to protect the pulp, after tooth preparation, liner is applied to cover the axial and/or pulpal wall. Then, base material (zinc phosphate, zinc oxide eugenol, glass ionomer or polycarboxylate) is placed over the liner. After the base material hardens, permanent restoration is done (**Fig. 14.8**).

Pulp Protection in Deep Carious Lesions

In deep carious lesion, caries can reach very near or up to the pulp, so treatment of deep carious lesion requires precautions because of postoperative pulpal response.

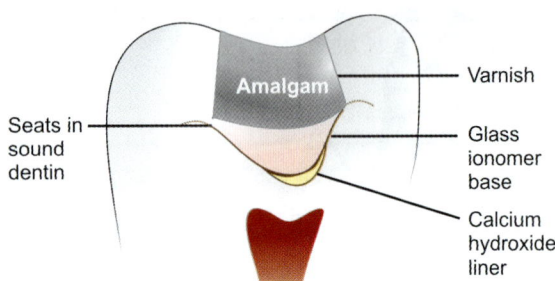

Figure 14.8: Pulp protection in moderate carious lesion using liner, base and varnish

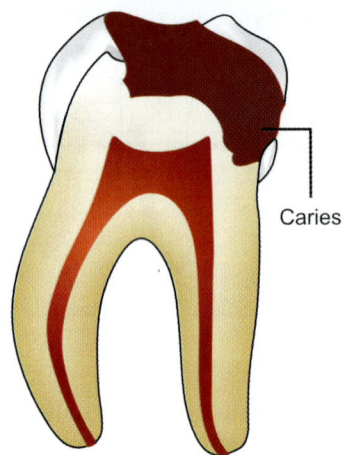

Figure 14.9: Tooth showing deep carious lesion adjacent to pulp

Depending upon the condition, following methods for pulpal protection are employed.

In Moderately Deep Carious Lesions

If hard dentin is present between carious lesion and the pulp and there is no threat to pulpal health after caries removal, give protective cement base and complete the permanent restoration as though it was a moderate lesion.

Indirect Pulp Capping

Indirect pulp capping is a procedure performed in a tooth with deep carious lesion adjacent to the pulp (**Fig. 14.9**). In this procedure, all the carious tissue is removed except the soft undiscolored carious dentin which lies adjacent to the pulp. Caries near the pulp is left in place to avoid pulp exposure and preparation is covered with a biocompatible material.

Indications
➟ Deep carious lesion near the pulp tissue but not involving it
➟ No mobility of tooth
➟ No history of spontaneous toothache
➟ No tenderness to percussion
➟ No radiographic evidence of pulp pathology
➟ No root resorption or radicular disease should be present radiographically.

Contraindications
➟ Presence of pulp exposure
➟ Radiographic evidence of pulp pathology
➟ History of spontaneous toothache
➟ Tooth sensitive to percussion
➟ Mobility present
➟ Root resorption or radicular disease is present radiographically.

Clinical technique
- Band the tooth if tooth is grossly decayed
- Anesthetize the tooth
- Apply rubber dam to isolate the tooth

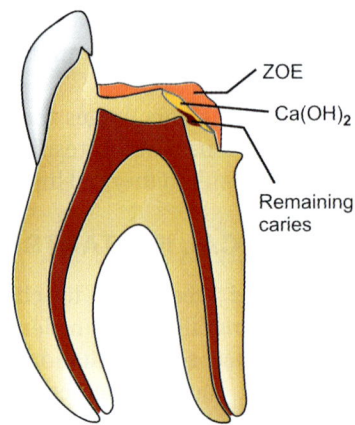

Figure 14.10: Placement of calcium hydroxide and zinc oxide eugenol dressing after excavation of soft caries

- Remove soft caries either with spoon excavator or round bur
- A thin layer of dentin and some amount of caries is left to avoid exposure
- Place calcium hydroxide paste on the exposed dentin
- Cover the calcium hydroxide with zincoxide eugenol base (**Fig. 14.10**)
- If restoration is to be given for a longer time, then amalgam restoration should be given
- Tooth should be evaluated after 6 to 8 weeks
- After 2 to 3 months, remove the cement and evaluate the tooth preparation. If due to remineralization and/or formation of secondary dentin, the soft dentin has become hard, then remove any residual soft debris and then finally give protective cement base and place the permanent restorative material.

The success of indirect pulp capping depends on the age of the patient, size of the exposure, restorative procedure and evidence of pulp vitality. In young patients, the potential for success is more due to large volume of pulp tissue and abundant vascularity.

Direct Pulp Capping

Direct pulp capping procedure involves the placement of biocompatible material over the site of pulp exposure to maintain vitality and promote healing.

When a small mechanical exposure of pulp occurs during tooth preparation or following a trauma, an appropriate protective base should be placed in contact with the exposed pulp tissue so as to maintain the vitality of the remaining pulp tissue (**Fig. 14.11**).

Indications

➡ Small mechanical exposure of pulp during
  ♦ Tooth preparation
  ♦ Traumatic injury.
➡ No or minimal bleeding at the exposure site.

Contraindications
➡ Wide pulp exposure ➡ Radiographic evidence of pulp pathology ➡ History of spontaneous pain ➡ Presence of bleeding at exposure site.

Clinical Procedure

- Administer local anesthesia
- Isolate the tooth with rubber dam

- When vital and healthy pulp is exposed, check the fresh bleeding at exposure site
- Clean the area with distilled water or saline solution and then dry it with a cotton pellet
- Apply calcium hydroxide (preferably Dycal) over the exposed area
- Give interim restoration such as zinc oxide eugenol for 6 to 8 weeks
- After 2 to 3 months, remove the cement very gently to inspect the exposure site. If secondary dentin formation takes place over the exposed site, restore the tooth permanently with protective cement base and restorative material. If favorable prognosis is not there, pulpotomy or pulpectomy is done.

The factors on which the success of direct pulp capping depends are as follows:

- *Age of the patient:* Due to vascularity of the pulp, young patients have greater potential for success than older ones
- *Type of exposure:* Mechanically done pulpal exposure has better prognosis than exposure caused by caries, due to less pulpal inflammation and deleterious effect of bacterial toxins on the pulp
- *Size of the exposure:* In large exposures, it is difficult to control the hemorrhage and tissue seepage. Small pinpoint exposures are easy to manage and have a greater potential for success
- *History of pain:* If previously pain has not occurred in the tooth, the potential for success is more.

MATERIALS USED FOR PULP PROTECTION (FIG. 14.12)

Various materials are used to:

- Insulate the pulp
- Protect the pulp in case of deep carious lesion

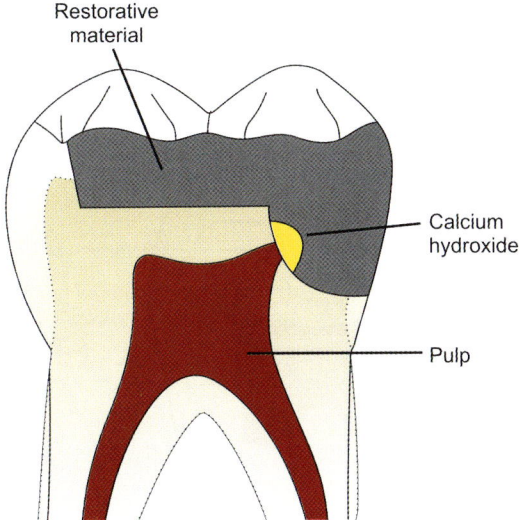

Figure 14.11: Direct pulp capping

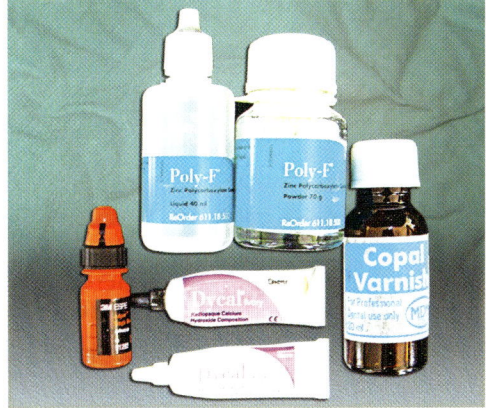

Figure 14.12: Different materials used for pulp protection

- Act as barriers to microleakage
- Prevent bacteria and toxins from affecting the pulp.

The term varnish, sealer, liner and base is applied for these materials.

Terminology of pulp protective materials according to thickness of material
→ *Solution liner (include varnish and adhesive sealer)*: Thin film of 2 to 5 μm thickness
→ *Suspension liner*: Relatively thin film of 20 to 30 μm thickness
→ *Cement liner*: Medium thickness of 100 to 500 μm thickness
→ *Cement base*: Thick film of 500 to 1000 μm thickness.
→ McCoy (1995) gave following definitions for these terms:
→ *Sealer*: Sealer provides a protecting covering the walls of tooth preparation and acts as barrier to leakage occurring at restoration tooth interface.
→ Sealer can be:
♦ *Varnish*: A varnish is an organic gum or rosin suspended in organic solutions like ether or chloroform
♦ *Adhesive sealer*: It helps in sealing and adhesion at the tooth-restoration interface. For example, dentin bonding agent and resin luting cements (**Fig. 14.13**).
→ *Liner*: Liner is applied in thin layer of less than 0.5 mm so as to attain a physical barrier to pulp and to provide therapeutic effect.
→ *Base*: Base is applied in an attempt to replace the lost dentin and to provide thermal, physical and therapeutic advantages to the pulp.

Varnish

A varnish is an organic copal or resin gum suspended in solutions of ether or chloroform (**Fig. 14.14**). When applied on the tooth surface the organic solvent evaporates leaving behind a protective film (**Fig. 14.15**).

Varnish liner is used for pulp protection and reduction of leakage. On drying, varnish acts as an inert plug between the tooth and restoration.

In case of amalgam restoration, varnish improves the sealing ability of the amalgam, reduces postoperative sensitivity and prevents discoloration of tooth by checking migration of ions into the dentin. If base is to be given or casting is to be cemented by zinc phosphate cement, varnish application is advantageous as it will block the seepage due to the available acid. Use of varnish is contraindicated under glass ionomers as it interferes the bonding of tooth to these cements. With restorative resins varnish is not used because the varnish liners dissolve in

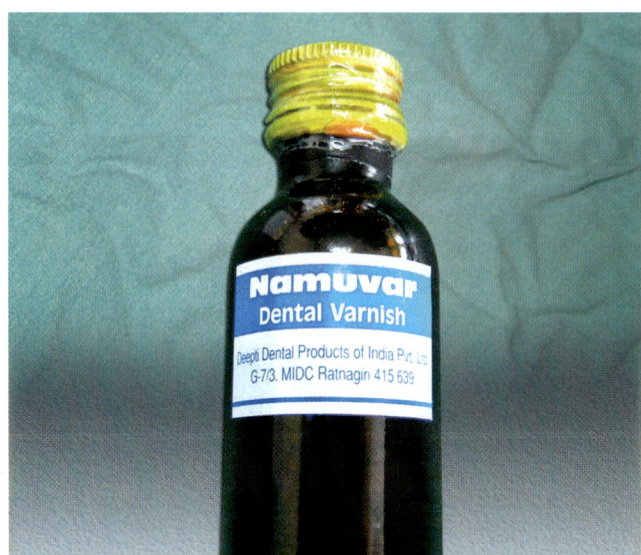

Figure 14.14: Varnish

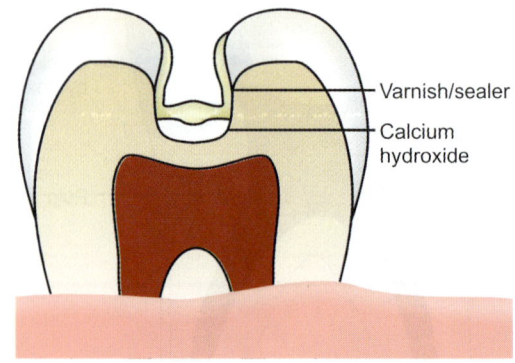

Figure 14.15: Varnish is applied on prepared tooth surface

Varnish/sealer
Calcium hydroxide

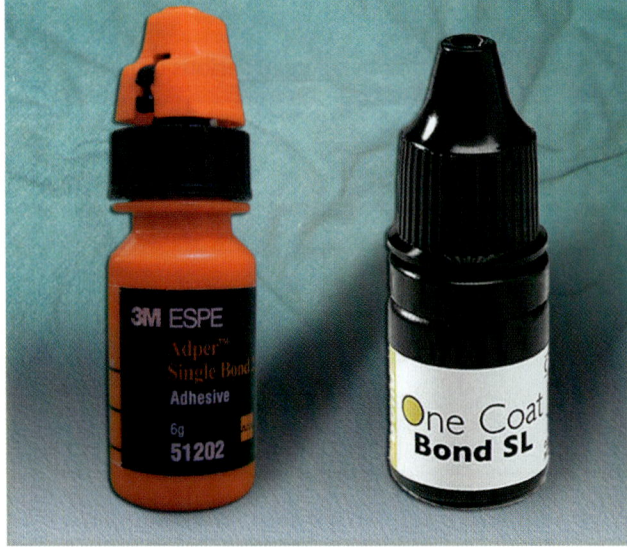

Figure 14.13: Dentin bonding agent to seal dentinal tubules

the monomer of the resin and it also interfere the polymerization of resins.

Indications for use of varnish

- To seal the dentinal tubules
- To act as barrier to protect the tooth from chemical irritants from cements
- To reduce microleakage around restorations.

Contraindications

Contraindicated under composite resin and glass ionomer restorations.

Adhesive Sealer

Indications for use of sealer

- To seal dentinal tubules
- To treat dentin hypersensitivity.

An adhesive sealer is commonly used under indirect restorations. For application, cotton tip applicator is used to apply sealer on all areas of exposed dentin.

Liners (Fig. 14.16)

Liners are typically fluid materials that, because of their rheology, can adapt more readily to all aspects of a tooth preparation. They can be used to create a uniform, even surface that aids in adaptation of more viscous filling materials such as amalgams or composites.

Liners usually do not have sufficient thickness, hardness and strength to be used alone in the deep preparation.

Indications of use of liners

- To protect pulp from chemical irritants by sealing ability
- To stimulate formation of reparative dentin.

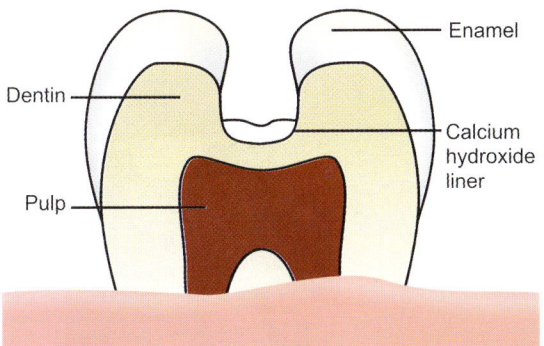

Figure 14.16: Calcium hydroxide linear is applied in an attempt to stimulate reparative dentin formation

Types of liners

Following materials are most commonly used as liners:
- Zinc oxide eugenol liners
- Calcium hydroxide
- Flowable composites
- Glass ionomers.

Zinc oxide eugenol liners (Fig. 14.17): Many dental materials containing eugenol and zinc oxide are used as liners. Eugenol is used to alleviate pain from mild-to-moderate inflammation of pulp. Though in low concentration, it acts as obtundant but in high concentration it acts as chemical irritant. When used as liner, there is release of eugenol for first few days of setting, therefore, this liner is not preferred especially in moderately deep tooth preparations.

Zinc oxide eugenol liner should not be used under composite restorations because it inhibits polymerization of bonding agent and composite.

Calcium hydroxide (Fig. 14.18): Calcium hydroxide has been used as liner in deep preparations because of its following features:

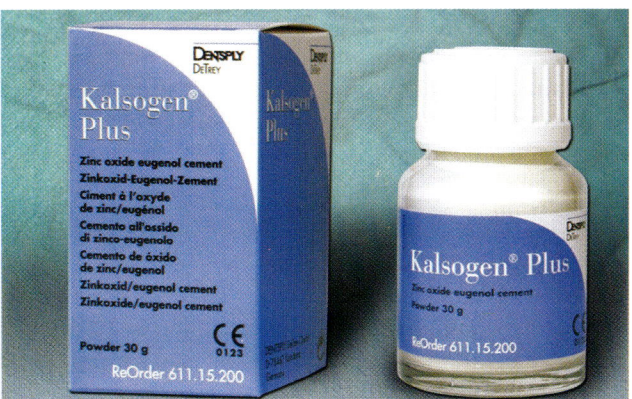

Figure 14.17: Zinc oxide eugenol liner

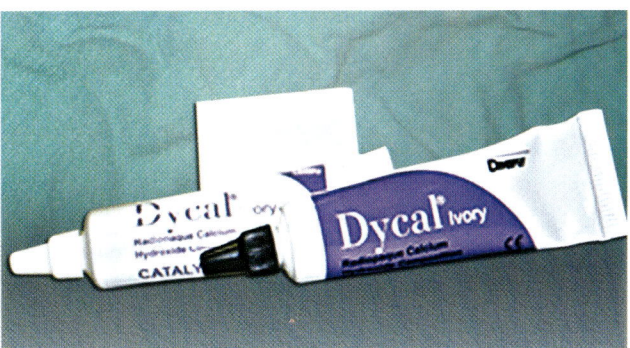

Figure 14.18: Calcium hydroxide liner

- It causes dentin mineralization by activating the enzyme ATPase
- It stimulates reparative dentin formation
- It forms a mechanical barrier, when applied to dentin
- Because of high pH, it neutralizes acidity of silicate and zinc phosphate cements
- Calcium hydroxide dissociates into Ca^{2+} and OH^- ions, the OH^- ions neutralize the (H^+) hydrogen ions from acids of cement
- Biocompatible in nature
- Bactericidal in nature.

Limitations: It has low strength, high solubility thus when it is exposed to the oral environment (e.g. due to leakage) it dissolves. This limits its use over only small areas requiring pulp protection. Sometimes glass ionomer or zinc phosphate base is applied over it to prevent its dissolution.

Flowable composites (Fig. 14.19): Flowable composites are the composites with a lower amount of filler. This reduced filler content allows more fluid consistency, less strength and lower modulus than fully filled composites.

They are primarily used under composite restorations and in crown and bridge preparations to block out undercuts prior to impression taking.

Advantages of using flowable composites as liners:
- Adaptation to preparation walls because of their flow
- Placement ease since the materials are injected directly into the preparation
- Esthetic
- Consistency.

Disadvantages of flowable composites:
- Technique sensitive
- Requires maintenance of contamination free field
- Polymerization shrinkage can result in gap formation at resin-tooth interface.

Glass ionomer cements (GIC): Glass ionomer (GI) or resin modified glass ionomer (RMGI) liners have been used as a renewable source of fluoride under restorations which has been shown to reduce the incidence of caries.

Advantages
- Bond to tooth structure
- Act as a thermal barrier
- Ability to bond in a moist environment
- Easy to use.
- Anticariogenic.

Light-cured resin-modified glass ionomers (RMGIs) (Figs 14.20 and 14.21): They provide good adhesion to both tooth structure and restorative materials along with strength, flexibility (because of low modulus of elasticity).

The RMGI materials have a dual-setting reaction—a light-activated, methacrylate crosslinking reaction and a slower, delayed, acid-base reaction that gives RMGIs an additional period of maximum flexibility to absorb stress from the adjacent shrinking composite.

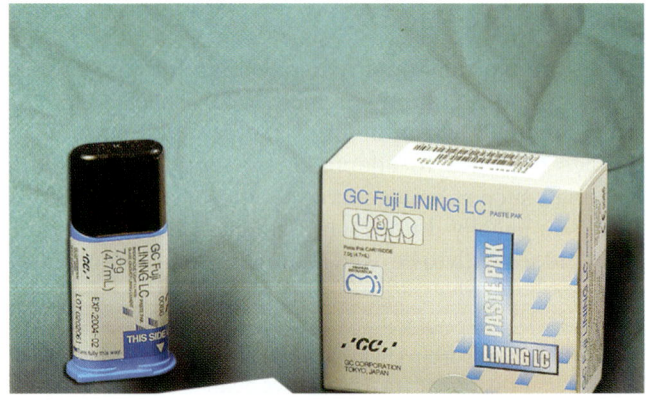

Figure 14.20: Light cured resin modified glass ionomer cement

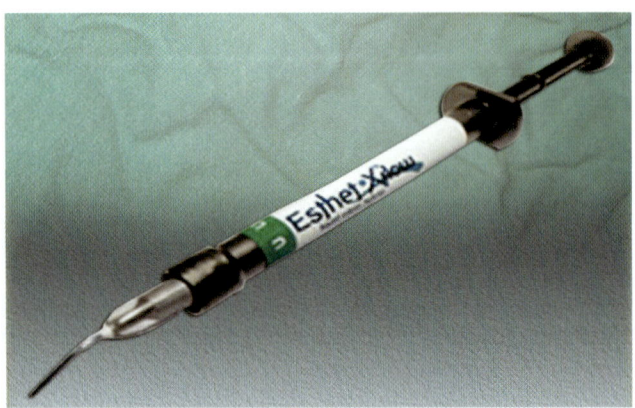

Figure 14.19: Flowable composite

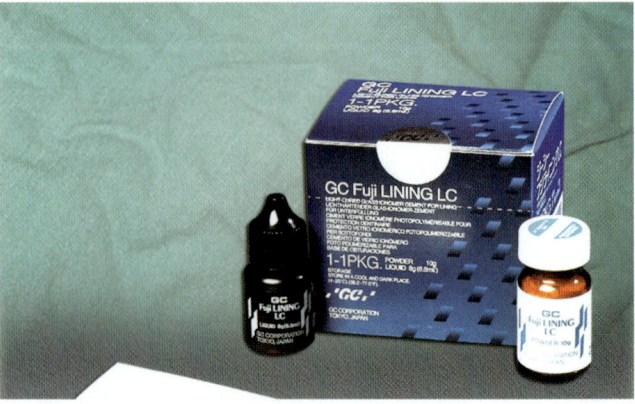

Figure 14.21: Resin modified glass ionomer cement

Bases (Fig. 14.22)

Bases are used as pulp protective materials since they provide thermal insulation, encourage recovery of injured pulp from thermal, mechanical or chemical trauma, galvanic shock and microleakage.

Bases should have sufficient strength so as to withstand forces of mastication and condensation of permanent restorations.

Bases can be classified as following
➡ *Protective bases*: They protect the pulp before restoration is placed
➡ *Sedative bases*: They help in soothing the pulp which has been irritated by mechanical, chemical or other means
➡ *Insulating bases*: They protect the tooth from thermal shock.
➡ Commonly used materials as base are zinc oxide eugenol, zinc phosphate cement, glass ionomer cement and calcium hydroxide.

Zinc Oxide Eugenol

It provides excellent sealing qualities and is bacteriostatic in nature. Zinc oxide eugenol is used as intermediatory base. Zinc oxide eugenol cement has anodyne effect, in other words it is helpful for relieving toothaches in case of deep preparations because of its sedative action. Zinc oxide eugenol cement should not be used with composite resins as it inhibits the polymerization of the resin.

Zinc Phosphate Cement

A thick creamy mix of zinc phosphate cement is used as base to reduce the thermal conductivity of metallic restorations and to block the undercuts in the preparation wall in case of cast restorations. Thick mixes should be used to minimize pulp irritation and marginal leakage. The thickness of the cement to provide effective thermal insulation should be at least between 0.50 to 1.0 mm. The cement should not cover on enamel wall or contact the cavo-surface margin. If required, shape the cement with slow speed fissure bur or sharp explorer.

Polycarboxylate Cement (Fig. 14.23)

Zinc polycarboxylate cement contains modified zinc oxide powder and an aqueous solution of polyacrylic acid. It chemically bonds to enamel and dentin and has antibacterial properties. Polycarboxylate cement is well tolerated by the pulp. Varnish should not be used with polycarboxylate cement because it would neutralize the adhesion potential of the cement.

Glass Ionomer Cement

Glass ionomer cements possess anticariogenic properties because of continuous release of fluoride throughout the life of restoration. Also these cements can bind to both enamel and dentin of the tooth via chemical bonding. They are also well tolerated by the pulp.

METHODS OF PULP PROTECTION UNDER DIFFERENT RESTORATIONS

Amalgam

Amalgam has been used in dentistry since ages. It is considered one of the safest filling materials with least irritating properties. It has been shown to produce discomfort due to its high thermal conductivity. So liners or bases are necessary to provide thermal insulation.

Effects of Amalgam on Pulp

- Mild-to-moderate inflammation in deep caries
- Harmful effects due to corrosion products
- Inhibition of reparative dentin formation due to damage to odontobalsts

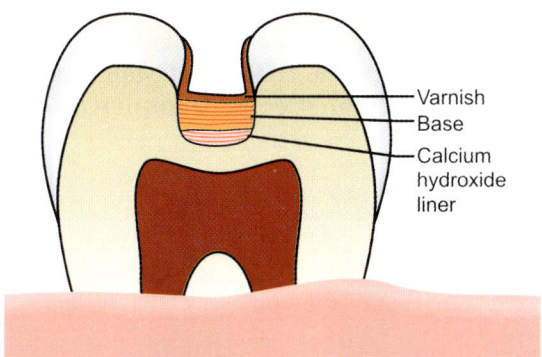

Figure 14.22: Base is applied over liner as pulp protective material in deep preparations

Varnish
Base
Calcium hydroxide liner

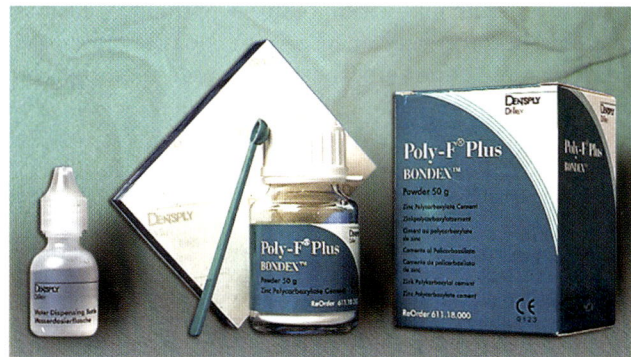

Figure 14.23: Zinc polycarboxylate cement

- Copper in high copper alloy is toxic
- High mercury content exerts cytotoxic effects on pulp
- Postoperative thermal sensitivity due to high thermal conductivity.

Precautions to be Taken While Using Amalgam as a Restorative Material

- Use of varnish or dentin bonding agent at the margins of restoration if more than 2 mm of remaining dentin thickness is present.
- Use of liner or base under the silver amalgam restoration when remaining dentin thickness is 0.5 to 2 mm.
- Use of calcium hydroxide as sub-base (0.5-1 mm) covered with a base material in preparations with less than 0.5 mm remaining dentin thickness.

PULP PROTECTION IN ACCORDANCE WITH DEPTH OF TOOTH PREPARATION

Restorative Resins

Restorative resins have been used in dentistry for past many years. Despite of having several advantages, they are not considered best materials because of their high coefficient of thermal expansion and polymerization shrinkage, which results in marginal leakage, subsequently the recu rent caries and ultimately the pulp damage. Monomer present in composite resins also acts as an irritant to the pulp.

Precautions to be Taken While Using Composite Resin as a Restorative Material

Use of liner is advocated under composite restorations in deep preparations. Liners containing calcium hydroxide have shown to provide good protection against bacteria. Zinc oxide eugenol liners should not be used with composite resins since they interfere with polymerization of composites.

Glass Ionomer Cements

Since it is compatible with pulp so nothing special is required except in very deep preparations (less than 0.5 mm remaining dentin thickness). In these cases, calcium hydroxide liner may be used for pulp protection.

Cast Gold Restorations

- If remaining dentin thickness is more than 2 mm, nothing is required
- If remaining dentin thickness is 0.5 to 2 mm, base is given below restoration
- If remaining dentin thickness is less than 0.5 mm, to protect pulp calcium hydroxide liner is placed over which base is applied.

DEFENSE MECHANISM OF PULP

Tubular Sclerosis

The peritubular dentin becomes wider gradually filling the tubules with calcified material progressing with the dentinoenamel junction pulpally. These areas are harder, denser, less sensitive and more protective to the pulp against subsequent irritation. Sclerosis resulting from aging is physiological dentin sclerosis and resulting from mild irritation is reactive dentin sclerosis.

Smear Layer

An amorphous debris layer consisting of both organic and inorganic constituents caused iatrogenically during operative procedures. Smear layer decreases both sensitivity and permeability of dentinal tubules. Smear layer is an iatrogenically produced layer that reduces permeability better than any of the varnishes.

Defense mechanism of the pulp
➡ Tubular sclerosis
➡ Smear layer
➡ Reparative dentin formation
♦ Healthy reparative reaction
♦ Unhealthy reparative reaction
♦ Destructive reaction.

Reparative Dentin Formation

- *Healthy reparative reaction*: This is the most favorable response and it consists of stimulating periodontal organ to form sclerotic dentin. It is followed by

Types of restoration	Shallow (RDT > 2.0 mm)	Moderately deep (RDT > 0.5–2 mm)	Deep (RDT < 0.5 mm)
Silver amalgam	Varnish	Base, e.g. zinc phosphate, zinc polycarboxylate	Calcium hydroxide as sub-base covered with base
Glass ionomer cement	Not required	Not required	Calcium hydroxide as liner
Composite resins	Dentin bonding agent	Dentin bonding agent	Calcium hydroxide as liner followed by glass ionomer as base
Cast gold restorations		Base	Calcium hydroxide as liner with base over it

normal secondary dentin containing dentinal tubules. Secondary dentin is different from primary dentin, in that the tubules of secondary dentin are slightly deviated from the tubules of the primary dentin. The healthy reparative reactions occur without any disturbances in the pulp tissues.

- *Unhealthy reparative reaction*: This response begins with degeneration of the odontoblasts. This is followed by the formation of the dead tract in the dentin and complete cessation in the formation of secondary dentin. The unhealthy reparative response is accompanied by mild pathological and clinical changes of a reversible nature in the pulp tissues, resulting in the formation of an irregular type of tertiary dentin. The tertiary dentin formation is considered to be the function of the pulp tissue proper. However, tertiary dentin has certain limitations. It is not completely impervious like the calcific barrier. Also, the rapid formation of tertiary dentin leads to the occupation of part of the pulp chamber with tissues other than those normally responsible for repair, metabolism and innervations. Thus tertiary dentin is said to "age the pulp", reducing its capacity for further defensive action against irritation. This is very important clinically, because if this reaction occurs as a result of a carious process, the restoration of this tooth may not be favorable, as received by the periodontal organ.

- *Destructive reaction*: This is the most unfavorable pulpal response to irritation. It begins with the loss of odontoblasts and the outer protective layer of the pulp which ultimately involves the pulp tissue proper, exceeding its reparative capacity. The resulting tissue reaction will be inflammation, which may progress to abscess formation, chronic inflammation and finally, complete necrosis of the pulp. In any event, the pulp tissue cannot recover from these pathologic changes and removal of these tissues or the whole tooth becomes necessary.

Prevention of pulpal damage due to operative procedure

To preserve the integrity of the pulp, the dentist should observe certain precautions while rendering treatment:

- Excessive force should not be applied during insertion of restoration
- Restorative materials should be selected carefully, considering the physical and biological properties of the material
- Excessive heat production should be avoided while polishing procedures
- Avoid application of irritating chemicals to freshly cut dentin
- Use varnish or base before insertion of restoration
- Patient should be called on recall basis for periodic evaluation of status of the pulp.

QUESTIONS

1. What are effects of tooth preparation on pulp?
2. Short notes:
   a. Remaining dentin thickness
   b. Pulp protection in deep carious lesion
   c. Role of liner and base
   d. Materials used for pulp protection
   e. Pulp protection in amalgam restoration.

BIBLIOGRAPHY

1. Bergenholtz G. Inflammatory response of the dental pulp to bacterial irritation. J Endod. 1981;7:100.
2. Brannstrom M, Lind PO. Pulpal response to early caries. J Dent Res. 1965;44:1045.
3. Brannstrom M, Nyborg H. Pulpal reaction to composite resin restoration. JPD. 1972;27:181.
4. Browne RM, Plant CG, Tobias RS. Quantification of the histologic features of pulpal damage. Int Endod J. 1980;13:104.
5. Cox CF, Waite KC, Ramus DL, Farmer JB. Reparative dentin: Factors affecting its deposition. Quint Int. 1992;23:257.
6. Cox CF, Suzuki F. Re-evaluating pulp protection: calcium hydroxide liner vs cohesive hybridization. IADA. 1994;125:823.
7. Dammascke T, Stratmann U, Mokrigs K. Histocytological evaluation of the reaction of rat pulp-tissue to carisolv. J Dent. 2001;29:283.
8. Fugaro JO, Nordahl I, Fugaro OJ, Matis BA, Six N. Pulp reaction to vital bleaching. Oper Dent. 2004;29:363.
9. Inokishi S, Iwaku M, Fusayama T. Pulpal response to a new adhesive restorative resin. JDR. 1982;61:1014.
10. Leidal TI, Eriksen HM. Human pulp response to composite resin restoration. Endo Dent Traumat. 1994;1:65.
11. Mjor IA. The importance of methodology in the evaluation of pulp reactions. Int Dent J. 1980;30:335.
12. Mjor IA, Sveen S, Ferrari M. Pulp dentin biology in restorative dentistry Part 1-6. Quint Int. 427, 537 and 611, 2001, 74, 28, 39, 2002.
13. Murray PE, About I, Lumlby PJ, Smith G. Post-operative pulpal and repair responses. JADA. 2000;131:321.
14. Stanley HR. Design of human pulp. O Surg, O Med, O Path. 1968;25:633-756.
15. Sulieman M, Rees JS, Addy M. Surface and pulp chamber temperature rise during tooth bleaching using a diode laser: a study *in vitro*. BDJ. 2006;11:631.
16. Suzuki S, Cox CF, White KC. Pulpal responses after complete crown preparation, dentinal sealing and provisional restoration. Quint Int. 1994;25:477.
17. Trowbridge. Pathogenesis of pulpitis resulting from dental caries. J Endod. 1981;7:52.
18. Tziafus D, Smith AJ, Lesot H. Designing new treatment strategies in vital pulp therapy. J Dent. 2000;28:77.
19. Wedenberg C, Bornstein R. Pulpal reactions in rat incisors to caridex. Aust Dent J. 1990;35:505.

Interim Restorations

Chapter Outline

INTERIM RESTORATION

Intermediary restorations/provisional restorations are used in the interval between tooth preparation and fitting a definitive restoration. They are temporarily used or inserted, cemented or filled until final restoration is permanently inserted or cemented. Intermediate restorations are used to protect or treat the pulp, dentin and enamel surfaces.

For example, with crown preparations intermediate restorations are usually essential to cover freshly cut dentin and prevent passive tooth movement. Also the intermediate restorations are placed to maintain the esthetics, functions and the relations of the tissues.

Objectives of interim restoration

- Maintains esthetics
- Acts as space maintainer
- Allows the tooth to function
- Acts as a diagnostic tool to determine occlusion
- Establishes function and phonetics
- Allows the development of the gingival contour
- Seals and insulate the prepared tooth from the oral environment, thereby protecting the underlying pulp
- Prevents passive tooth eruption and mesial drift.

Requirements of the Intermediate Restoration

All intermediate restorations/provisional restorations should:
- Have good marginal adaptation
- Have optimal strength and durability
- Maintain physiologic contours and embrasures
- Have smooth plaque resistant surface
- Be able to satisfy mechanical, biological and esthetic criteria
- Be economical
- Have easy and quick manipulation, placement and removal
- Be insoluble in oral fluids
- Be dimensional stable
- Be sedative to pulp and periodontium
- Be esthetically acceptable.

Purpose of Interim Restoration

- Protect the pulp by sealing and insulating the prepared tooth from the oral environment
- Sedative for hyperactive pulp due to tooth preparation
- Maintain tooth position and prevent occlusal changes
- Act as an indirect pulp cap as it creates a favorable biological environment
- Protect the gingival tissue inflammation
- Protect the tooth structure weakened during tooth preparation
- Maintain the esthetics.

MATERIALS USED FOR INTERIM RESTORATIONS

The materials used for intermediate restorations

For intracoronal preparation:
- Gutta-percha
- Zinc-oxide eugenol and its modifications
- Zinc phosphate cement
- Zinc silicophosphate cement
- Zinc polycarboxylate cement
- Glass ionomer cement
- Calcium hydroxide

For extracoronal preparations: Prefabricated crowns can be made from:
- Tooth colored polycarbonate crowns
- Aluminum cylinder
- Stainless steel crowns
- Celluloid crowns
- Indirect acrylic restorations.

Gutta-percha Stick

Gutta-percha is a dried coagulated extract which is derived from plants of Brazillian tree (Palaquium), belongs to Sapotaceae family. In India, these trees are found in Assam and Western Ghats.

Chemical Structure

Its molecular structure is close to natural rubber, which is also a cis-isomer of polyisoprene.

Composition of gutta-percha

- Matrix—gutta-percha 20% (Organic)
- Filler—zinc oxide 66% (Inorganic)
- Radio-opacifiers—heavy metal sulfates 11% (Inorganic)
- Plasticizers—waxes or resins 3% (Organic).

Chemically, pure gutta-percha exists in two different crystalline forms, i.e. α and β forms which differ in molecular repeat distance and single bond form. Natural gutta-percha coming directly from the tree is in α-form while the commercial available product is in β-form.

Manipulation

- Moisten the walls of tooth preparation with a solvent.
- Soften the gutta-percha stick over an alcohol lamp slowly. Do not overheat it, as it can cause burning and oxidation of its components.
- Insert it in the preparation in bulk or as pieces and condense it with ball burnisher.
- Remove the excess using warm instrument.
- Smoothen the surface using slightly warm instrument.

Advantages of gutta-percha

- Compactability allows it to be easily adaptable to preparation walls
- Inertness of this material makes it nonreactive
- Dimensionally stable
- Tissue tolerance
- Radiopacity makes it easily recognizable on radiograph
- Plasticity on heating, helps to mould it according to preparation walls.

Disadvantages

- Lack of rigidity
- Easily displaced by pressure
- Lacks adhesive quality.

ZINC OXIDE EUGENOL CEMENT (FIG. 15.1)

Zinc oxide eugenol cement is one of the oldest used cement. It has soothing action on pulpal tissues and eugenol has topical anesthetic properties, therefore it is also termed as an obtundent material. Though other cements are also used for temporization, but zinc oxide-eugenol cement is used most commonly because it is much less irritating to

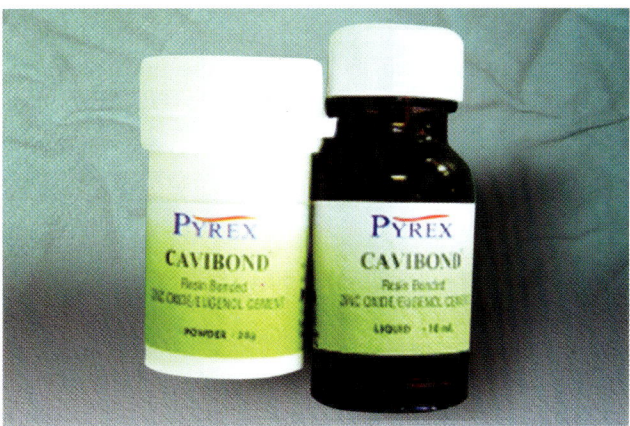

Figure 15.1: Zinc oxide eugenol cement

the pulp and produce better marginal seal than zinc phosphate. A thick mix of zinc oxide eugenol cement is used for small cavities but before placing the cement, the prepared cavity must be isolated and cleaned.

Zinc oxide eugenol is not used as base material especially when unfilled and filled resins are used as restorative materials because eugenol interferes with polymerization process of resins. In these cases, calcium hydroxide is used as a base material under resin restoration.

Composition
➡ Powder
◆ Zinc oxide (ZnO)—69.0%—Reactive ingredient
◆ White rosin—29.3%—Reduces brittleness
◆ Zinc stearate—1.0%—Catalyst
◆ Zinc acetate (acts as accelerator)—0.7%—Accelerator
➡ Liquid
◆ Eugenol—85.0%—Reactor
◆ Olive oil—15.0%—Plasticizer.

Setting Reaction of Zinc Oxide Eugenol Cement

On mixing powder and liquid, the zinc oxide hydrolysis and subsequent reaction takes place between zinc hydroxide and eugenol to form a chelate, zinc eugenolate. Within this matrix unreacted zinc oxide powder particles are embedded.

- First reaction
  $$ZnO + H_2O \rightarrow Zn(OH)_2$$
- Second reaction
  $$Zn(OH)_2 + 2HE \rightarrow ZnE_2 + 2H_2O$$
- Water is needed for the reaction and it is also byproduct of the reaction. So, reaction progresses more rapidly in humid conditions.
- Because zinc eugenolate rapidly hydrolyzes to form free eugenol and zinc hydroxide, it is one of the most soluble cements. To increase the strength of the set material, changes in composition can be made to the powder and liquid. For example, orthoethoxybenzoic acid can be added to the liquid or alumina or polymethyl methacrylate powder can be added to the powder. These modified zinc oxide-eugenol cements (**Fig. 15.2**) have the following compositions:

Alumina and orthoethoxybenzoic acid reinforced composition	
➡ Powder	
◆ Zinc oxide	70%
◆ Alumina	30%
or	
◆ Zinc oxide	70%
◆ Fused quartz and calcium	30%
➡ Liquid	
◆ Ortho-ethoxybenzoic acid	62.5%
◆ Eugenol	37.5%

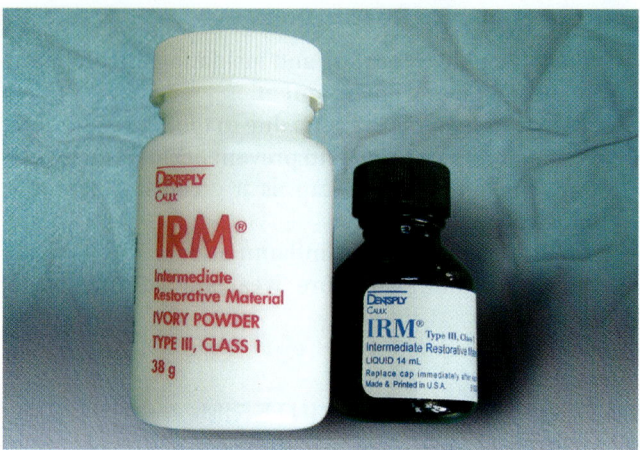

Figure 15.2: Modified zinc oxide eugenol cement (IRM)

EBA (Ortho-ethoxybenzoic acid) cement: In this cement, EBA chelates with zinc forming zinc benzoate. Addition of fused quartz, alumina and dicalcium phosphate has also shown to improve mechanical properties of cement.

Effect of EBA on eugenol cement
➡ Increase in compressive and tensile strength
➡ More powder can be incorporated to achieve standard consistency
➡ Decrease in setting time (if concentration is < 70 percent)
➡ EBA does not show adverse effects on pulp.

Polymer Reinforced Zinc Oxide	
➡ Powder	
◆ Zinc oxide	80%—Reactive ingredient
◆ Polymethyl methacrylate	20%—Increases strength
◆ Traces of zinc stearate, zinc acetate	
➡ Liquid	
◆ Eugenol	85%—Reactor
◆ Acetic acid	15%—Accelerator

Polymer reinforced zinc oxide eugenol cement: In this mixture, resin helps in improving strength, smoothness of the mix and decreasing flow, solubility and brittleness of the cement.

Manipulation of Zinc Oxide Eugenol (ZOE) Cement

ZOE cement is available as:
- Powder and liquid system
- Paste-paste system.

Manipulation of Powder and Liquid System

- Powder is measured and dispensed with a scoop where as liquid is dispensed as drops on glass slab

- Powder is dispensed at one end of glass slab, using cement spatula. The powder is divided in main bulk increment, followed by smaller increments (**Figs 15.3 and 15.4**). While dispensing liquid, bottle should be held 90° to the mixing pad. It lets the fluid fall under its own weight
- Start the mixing by incorporating half of the powder into the liquid with a heavy folding motion and pressure
- When powder particles are wet with the liquid, add the remaining powder to the mix and continue to use a heavy folding motion to attain a putty consistency
- For base, when mixing is done, bring the mix together and role it. One should be able to pick up the mix without deformation (**Fig. 15.5**)
- Pick-up a piece of mixed cement and place it into the preparation using a condenser
- If the mix sticks to the condenser, powder the condenser head with cement powder to prevent the instrument from sticking during condensation
- Use the condenser head and merge the restoration to the margin of the preparation

- For smoothening, clean up and hardening of the restoration, use a wet cotton pellet
- For luting consistency, "1 inch" string should be formed when flat surface of spatula is pulled from the mixed cement.

Paste-paste System

In this two pastes are dispensed in equal lengths on paper pad. Two pastes have different colors, mixing is done till a homogeneous color is obtained.

Working Time and Setting Time

These are usually not specified. In general, higher is the Powder: Liquid ratio, faster the materials sets. Cooling of glass slab slows down the setting reaction (unless the temperature is below the dew point). Setting time of this cement is long but since water accelerates the setting reaction, it sets faster in mouth than outside.

Advantages of ZOE cement
➡ Soothing effect on the pulp
➡ Good short-term sealing.

Disadvantages
➡ Highly soluble
➡ Low strength
➡ Long setting time
➡ Low compressive strength.

Biocompatibility of Zinc Oxide Eugenol Cement

ZOE is the best known obtundent. pH of cement is 7. This makes it least irritating cement. Because of this, it is considered as most palliative agent to the pulp.

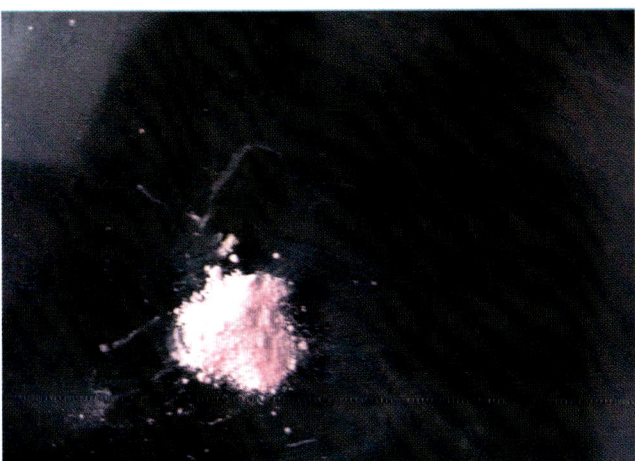

Figure 15.3: Dispense ZOE powder and liquid on glass slab

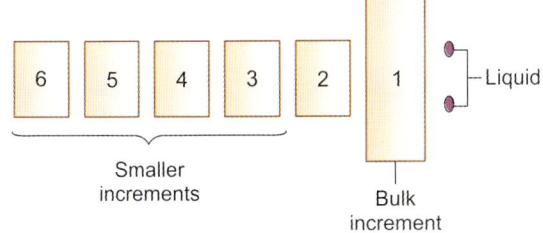

Figure 15.4: The powder is divided in main bulk increment, followed by smaller increment

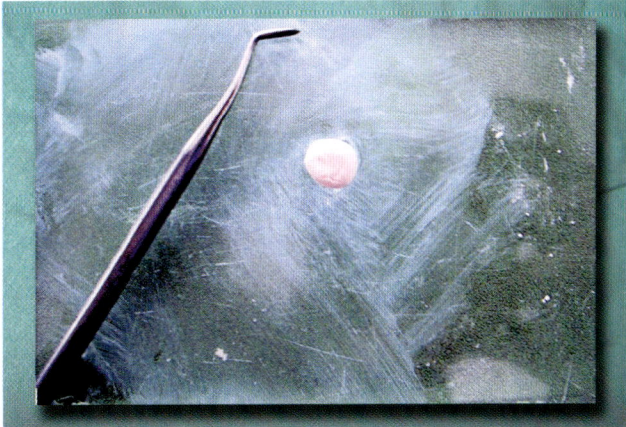

Figure 15.5: The final mix of ZOE cement should be such that one should be able to pick up the mix without deformation

ZINC PHOSPHATE CEMENT (FIG. 15.6)

One of the oldest and most widely used cements, zinc phosphate cement is the standard against which new cements are compared. It was first introduced in 1878 and still used today because of excellent clinical track record.

Two Types

Type I: Used for cementation. Specification requires the film thickness of less than 25 microns.

Type II: Used as a base and for luting. Specification requires a film thickness between 25 and 40 microns.

Composition

Powder: The primary ingredients of zinc phosphate cement powder are zinc oxide and magnesium oxide.

All the ingredients are sintered at temperatures between 1000°C and 1400°C into a cake that is subsequently ground into fine powder.

Liquid: The liquid is phosphoric acid and water in the ratio of two parts acid to one part water. It may also contain aluminum phosphate and zinc phosphate. The water content of the liquid is critical and should be controlled to provide an adequate setting time. When the liquid is exposed in open bottle, it absorbs moisture from the air in case of high humidity but in low humidity times, it will lose moisture. In case of very old liquids, the last 25 percent portion remaining in the bottle should be discarded because it is usually discolored or contaminated.

Composition of Zinc Phosphate cement
➡ Powder
◆ ZnO—90.2%.
◆ MgO—8.2%—condenses the ZnO during the sintering process
◆ SiO$_2$—1.4%—acts as an insert filler
◆ Bi$_2$O$_3$—0.1%—imparts smoothness to the mixed cement
◆ Miscellaneous—(BaO, Ba$_2$SO$_4$, CaO) – 0.1%.
➡ Liquid

◆ Phosphoric acid	– 38.2%
◆ Water	– 36.0%
◆ Aluminum or zinc phosphate	– 16.2%
◆ Zinc	– 7.1%
◆ Aluminum	– 2.5%

Both aluminum and zinc act as buffers to reduce the reactivity of the powder and liquid.

Setting Reaction

Phosphoric acid attacks surface of the particles and releases Zn ions into the liquid. Aluminum which already forms a complex with the phosphoric acid reacts with zinc and yields a zinc aluminophosphate gel.

The set cement consists of a zinc phosphate matrix in which unreacted zinc oxide powder particles are embedded. Crystals of tertiary zinc phosphate/ hopeite, are found on the surface of the cement (**Fig. 15.7**).

Manipulation of Cement

Manipulation of Zinc Phosphate Cement

* Working time ~ 5 minutes
* Setting time ~ 2.5 to 8 minutes

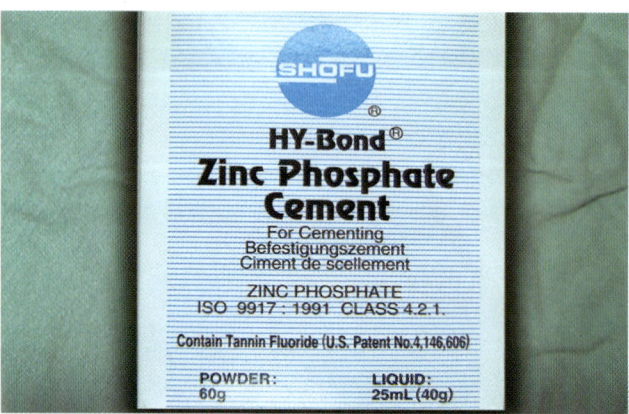

Figure 15.6: Zinc phosphate cement

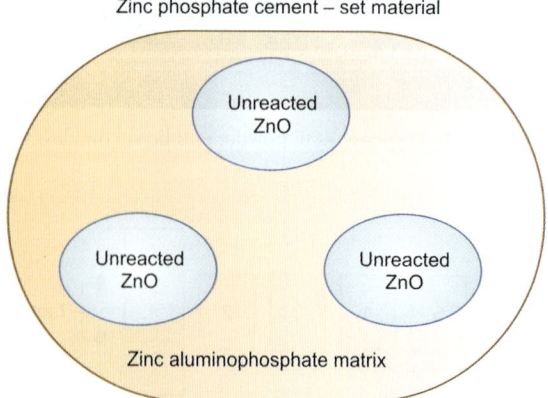

Figure 15.7: Set cement consists of zinc phosphate matrix in which unreacted ZnO powder particles are embedded

- Powder is measured and dispensed with scoop a liquid is dispensed as drops. Cement mixing should be done on cool glass slab with a narrow bladed stainless steel spatula. Lower the temperature of the slab during mixing, the longer will be the working time. This is advantageous because it allows incorporation of more powder into the liquid which results in greater compressive strength and lower solubility of the final cement.
- Some clinicians prefer to mix the cement using the "frozen slab" technique which greatly extends the working time and allows incorporation of more powder into the liquid. But this method has disadvantage of incorporating water into the mix.
- Since setting reaction is an exothermic type, the heat liberated while setting further accelerates the setting rate. So, it is very important to dissipate this heat which can be done by
  - Using chilled glass slab
  - Using smaller increment for initial mixing of cement
  - Mixing the large area of glass slab.
- Powder is divided into 5 to 8 increments (**Figs 15.8A and B**) in which initial two increments are smaller, third

and fourth increments are bigger one and after that increments are again smaller in size.
- Initial increments are smaller in size so as:
  - To achieve the slow neutralization of the liquid.
  - To control the reaction.
- Middle increments are larger in size so as to further saturate the liquid to form zinc phosphate. Because of presence of less amount of unreacted acid, this step is not affected by heat released from the reaction. In the end, the smaller increments of powder are added so as to achieve optimum consistency.
- After dividing powder, dispense liquid on the glass slab. While dispensing, the liquid bottle should be held vertical and close to the powder (**Fig. 15.9**). Repeated opening of the liquid bottle or early dispensing of the liquid prior to mixing should be avoided because evaporation of liquid can result in changes in water/acid ratio which can further result in decrease in pH and an increase in viscosity of the mixed cement.
- For luting, mixing is continued until a "1 inch string" is formed when spatula is pulled away from the glass slab (**Fig. 15.10**). For base, consistency should be such that it can be rolled into a ball without sticking (**Fig. 15.11**).
- While setting of cement is taking place, water contamination should be avoided because on moisture contamination, the phosphoric acid leaches out of the cement and solubility greatly increases.

Mechanical Properties

Strength of the cement is almost linearly depends on its powder to liquid ratio; zinc phosphate cement achieves 75 percent of its ultimate strength within 1 hour.

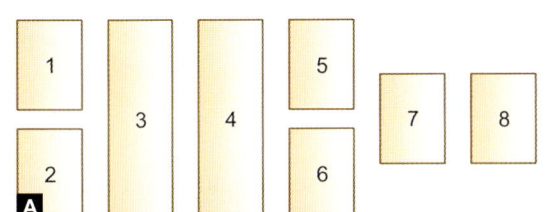

Zinc phosphate cement powder increments

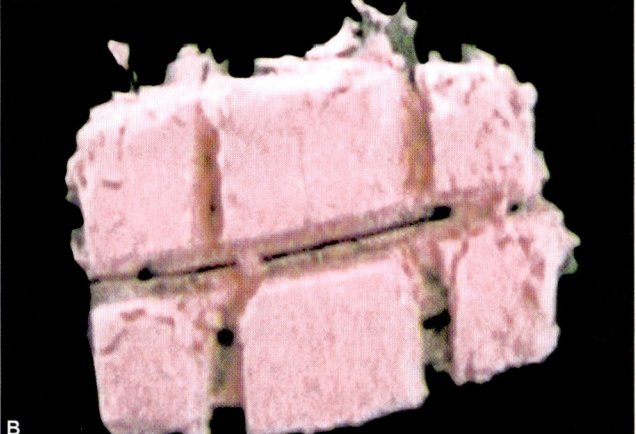

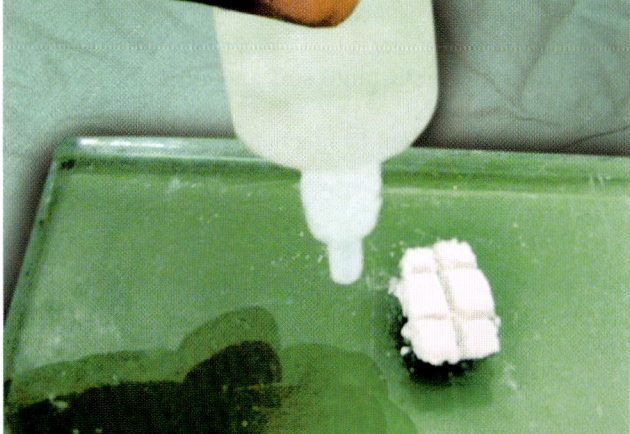

Figures 15.8A and B: The powder of zinc phosphate cement is divided in 5 to 8 increment in which initial 2 increments are smaller, 3rd and 4th are bigger in size and rest of increments are again smaller in size

Figure 15.9: While dispensing, the liquid, bottle should be held vertical and close to the powder

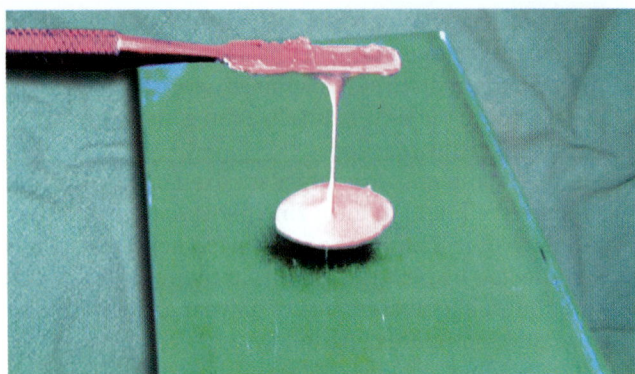

Figure 15.10: For luting, the consistency should be such that "1 inch" string should be formed when spatula is taken away from glass slab

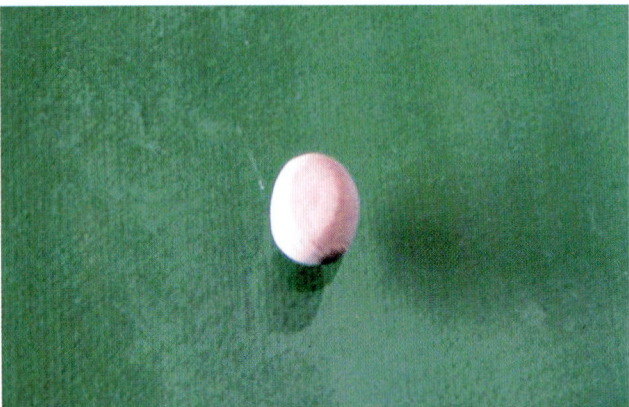

Figure 15.11: For base/restoration, consistency should be such that it can be rolled into the ball without sticking

- Compressive strength of cement is 104 Mpa
- Tensile strength - 5.5 Mpa
- Modulus of Elasticity is 13.7 gigapascals. This high MOE makes the cement quite stiff and resistant to elastic deformation.
- Retention of cement by mechanical interlocking is not chemical interaction.

Biocompatibility

Because of presence of phosphoric acid, acidity of cement is quite high making if irritable. pH of cement liquid is 2.0. Two minutes after mixing the pH is almost 2 and after 48 hours, it is 5.5.

Clinical Uses

It is used both as an intermediate base and as a cementing medium.

- *Intermediate base*: A thick mix of zinc phosphate cement is used as an intermediate base beneath a permanent metallic restoration.
- *Cementing medium*: It is used to cement crowns, inlays, orthodontic appliances and fixed partial dentures. A creamy mix of cement is applied to place the restoration.

It holds tooth and restoration together by mechanical interlocking, filling the space between the irregularities between the two.

Uses of zinc phosphate cement
➡ Luting agent for crowns, inlays
➡ Intermediate base
➡ Temporary restoration
➡ Luting orthodontics band.

Advantages
➡ Long record of clinical acceptability
➡ High compressive strength
➡ Thin film thickness.

Disadvantages
➡ Low initial pH
➡ Lack of an adhesion to tooth structure
➡ Lack of anticariogenic effect
➡ Soluble in water.

Zinc Silicophosphate Cements

Zinc silicophosphate cements (ZSPC) consist of a mixture of silicate glass and zinc phosphate cement.

Composition

Powder contains an acid soluble silicate, zinc and magnesium oxides. Liquid is phosphoric acid.

Properties of Zinc Silicophosphate Cements
➡ Translucent and more esthetic than zinc phosphate cement
➡ Anticariogenic because of fluoride release from this cement
➡ Has sufficient strength.

ZINC POLYCARBOXYLATE CEMENT (FIG. 15.12)

Zinc polycarboxylate cement is also known as zinc polyacrylate cement. It was one of the first chemically adhesive dental materials introduced in the 1960s. It sets by an acid-base reaction between a powder and a liquid. It bond to the tooth structure because of chelation reaction between the carboxyl groups of the cement and calcium present in the tooth structure. This implies that more mineralized the tooth structure, the stronger the bond.

acid 10-20%) for 10 to 20 sec, after this tooth is rinsed for 20 to 30 sec and dried.

Setting Reaction

When powder and liquid are mixed, hydrated protons formed from ionization of the acid, attack the zinc and magnesium powder particles. This results in release of zinc and magnesium ions which form polycarboxylates that crosslink the polymer chains. The final set consists of zinc polycarboxylate crosslinked polymer matrix in which unreacted zinc oxide particles are implanted.

Working Time and Setting Time

Working time ~ 2.5 minutes
Setting time ~ 6-9 minutes

Lowering the temperature increases working time. Since, cooling glass slab causes thickening of polyacrylic acid, this further increases viscosity so only powder should be refrigerated for increasing working time.

While setting, the cement passes through the rubbery stage which makes it difficult to remove the cement. If excess cement is removed at this stage, it can cause pulling of some cement leaving a void. So, the excess cement should be removed once it is set.

Bonding of Polyacrylate Cement to Tooth Structure

- The polyacrylic acid is believed to react with calcium ion via the carboxyl group
- The adhesion depends on the unreacted carboxyl group.

Mechanical Properties

Compressive strength ~ 55 to 67 MPa
Tensile strength ~ 2.4 to 4.4 MPa

Solubility

It is low in water. But in acidic environment with pH of less than 4.5, solubility increases. Reduction in P:L ratio also increases solubility.

Biological Considerations

pH of the liquid is 1.7 but increases rapidly after mixing. Zinc polycarboxylate cement shows excellent biocompatibility with the pulp because of the following reasons:
- The size of polyacrylic acid molecule is bigger, this makes it less favorable to disperse into the dentinal tubules
- The pH of the cement rises more rapidly when compared to that of zinc phosphate.

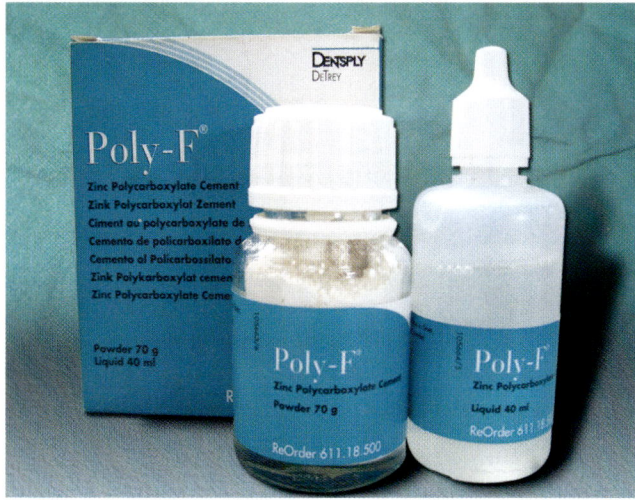

Figure 15.12: Zinc polycarboxylate cement

Composition

Powder: It is similar to that of zinc phosphate cement powder. Four percent (4%) stannous fluoride acts primarily as a strengthening agent. Fluoride does not exert an anticariogenic effect because zinc polycarboxylate cement leaches only 10 to 15 percent of the fluoride when compared to glass ionomer cement.

Liquid: Liquid is an aqueous solution of 32 to 43 percent high molecular weight polyacrylic acid.

The liquid has tendency to become viscous because it is a partially polymerized polyacrylic acid.

Even though it is quite viscous after mixing but it can attain a satisfactory film thickness because of pseudoplasticity and decrease in viscosity when sheared.

Manipulation of Zinc Polycarboxylate Cement

- Usually it is 1.5:1 powder to liquid ratio.
- Cement should be mixed on surface that will not absorb liquid like glass slab or paper pads.
- Liquid is dispensed just before mixing of the cement as the loss of water from liquid can result in increase in its viscosity.
- Mix first-half of powder to liquid to obtain the maximum length of working time.
- Mixed cement should be adapted to tooth till it is glossy in appearance. Loss of gloss makes it nonadhesive.
- Before application of cement on to the tooth, conditioning of prepared tooth surface is recommended. Conditioning is done with an organic acid (polyacrylic

Uses of zinc polycarboxylate cement

➡ Cement inlays or crowns
➡ Used as base
➡ Temporary restorations
➡ Lute the stainless steel crown.

Advantages

➡ Adhesion to tooth structure
➡ Rapid rise in pH upon cementation
➡ Lack of penetration of the large molecules into the dentinal tubules make this a biocompatible cement.

Disadvantages

➡ Short working time (2-3 minutes)
➡ Does not resist plastic deformation under high masticatory stresses.

Calcium Hydroxide

Calcium hydroxide has high alkaline pH (11 to 13). Its alkaline pH helps in neutralizing the acids produced by the microorganisms and irritating acidic component of restorative base and materials. Calcium hydroxide also provide antibacterial properties.

Calcium hydroxide can be used in:
- Powder form (**Fig. 15.13**)
- Quick setting paste form (Dycal) (**Fig. 15.14**).

Mixing Calcium Hydroxide Cement Armamentarium

- Calcium hydroxide mixing pad
- Calcium hydroxide applicator
- Spoon excavator
- Explorer

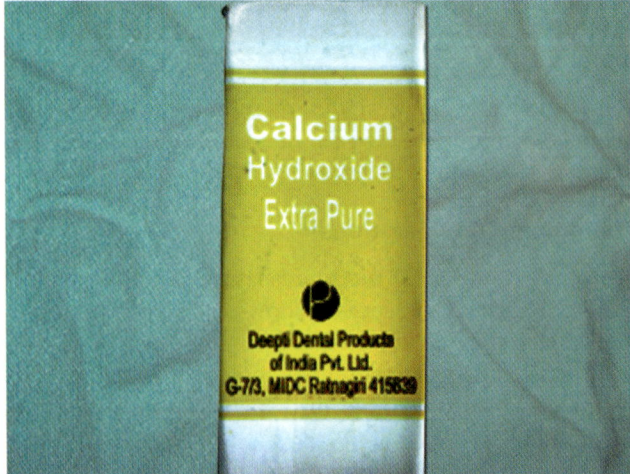

Figure 15.13: Powder form of calcium hydroxide

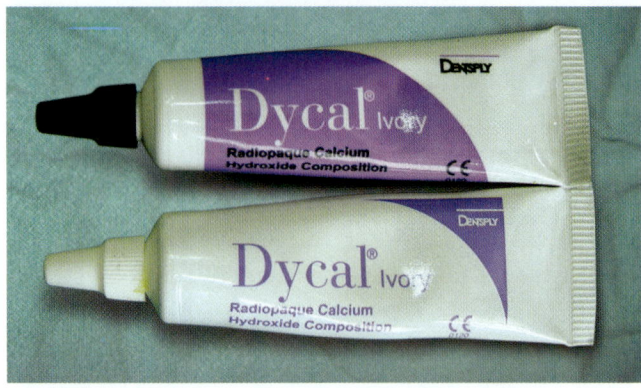

Figure 15.14: Paste form of calcium hydroxide

- Before placement of calcium hydroxide, check the dentin surface (it should be moist). Dispense 1 mm of base and 1 mm of catalyst onto the mixing pad
- For mixing the two pastes, use either the calcium hydroxide applicator or spoon excavator. Mixing should be done for 10 to 15 seconds until a uniform color is achieved. Take a small amount of the calcium hydroxide, place it in the deepest portion of the tooth preparation
- Check the setting of calcium hydroxide using the tip of an explorer with minimal pressure
- There should be no indentation.

FOR EXTRACORONAL PREPARATIONS

Various types of prefabricated crowns are available (made of plastic or metal), along with self-cured or light cured resins. Crown forms in anatomic shapes are most useful because their simulation to the tooth structure. For anterior teeth, transparent crowns are used and for posterior teeth, metal crowns can be used.

Crown Forms

Indications

➡ Extensive carious lesions undermining the cusps
➡ Failure of other available restorative materials
➡ Following pulpotomy or pulpectomy
➡ For fractured teeth.

Criteria of Using Crowns

- Surface of crown should be smooth and polished
- Crown margins should be closely adapted to the tooth
- There should be no excess cement
- Contact with adjacent teeth should be proper
- Crown should be in proper occlusion
- Crown should facilitate the patient to adequately maintain oral hygiene.

Materials

Preformed crowns: They are also called as proprietary shells. They are available in different sizes but for proper fitting they need to be adjusted. Plastic crowns are made from polycarbonate or acrylic material. Since they have good esthetics, therefore, they are commonly indicated in anterior teeth. Metal crowns are made of aluminum, stainless steel. They are commonly used on posterior teeth.

Cellulose acetate and polycarbonate crown forms:
- The crown is made up of soft, thin and transparent material
- Crows are available in diverse sizes and shapes
- Select the crown according to tooth
- Fill the crown with cold cure resin and seat it on prepared tooth
- Remove excess cement
- Adjust the occlusion
- Polish the crown.

Stainless steel crowns
- Commonly used for the posterior teeth.
- Select the crown according to the gingival diameter.

Aluminum shell crowns
- They are commonly used for posterior teeth.
- They are softer and weaker than stainless steel crowns.
- Take a crown and adapt it to the tooth.
- Place a luting cement to fix it.

Acrylic Restorations (Figs 15.15 and 15.16)

For making temporary restorations, self cure acrylic restorations have been used successfully. When used with direct technique, free monomer and the heat produced

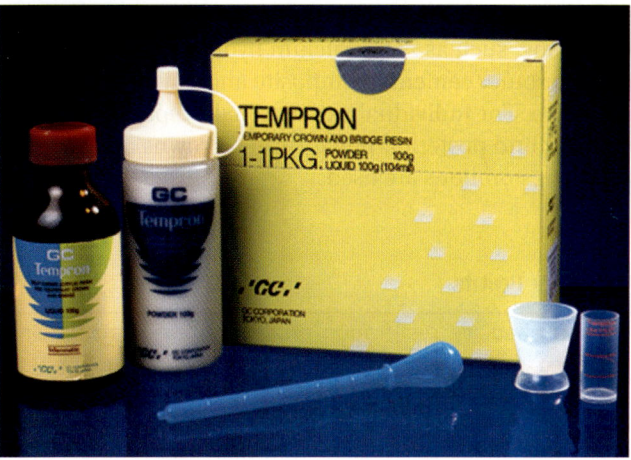

Figure 15.16: Self cure acrylic for temporary crowns

during exothermic reaction can harm pulp and the gingival tissues. To avoid this, indirect method is preferred.

Different materials available for direct or indirect technique are:
- Polymethyl-methacrylate
- Polyethyl-methacrylate
- Bis acryl-composite
- Urethane dimethacrylate.

Polymethyl-methacrylate has advantages of having high strength, good wear resistance and esthetics but it has three main disadvantages viz; polymerization shrinkage, exothermic heat produced during polymerization and free monomer release during setting.

Nowadays visible light cured resins have been made available. These are based on urethane-dimethacrylate. Since these are light cured, there is control over the working time of material.

Limitations of temporization
➡ Poor marginal adaptation is commonly seen with temporary restorations
➡ In intermediate restoration, discoloration may take place in long duration restorations
➡ Poor strength of temporary crowns may fracture in patients with bruxism or reduced interocclusal clearance
➡ Autopolymerizing resins may result in odor because of food accumulation
➡ Inadequate bonding between tooth and restoration may result their failure.

CONCLUSION

For the protection of pulp and to maintain the esthetics and function, interim restorations are given. Various

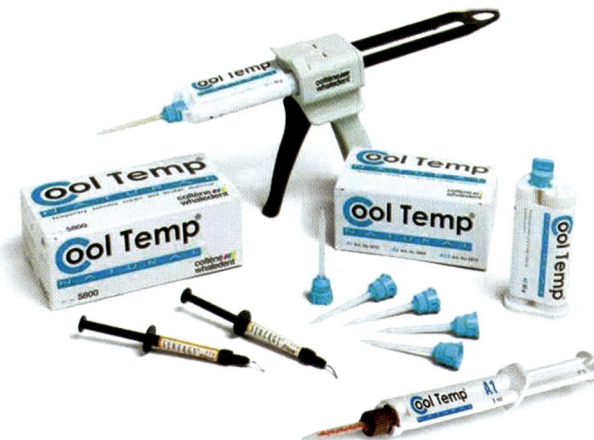

Figure 15.15: Self cure acrylic for temporary crowns

types of cements in one form or the other have been used since long, such as ZOE, calcium hydroxide preparations, glass ionomer cements, composite and pin retained silver amalgam. For individual extracoronal preparations, both anterior and posterior, prefabricated crowns and indirect acrylic restorations are used.

Key Points

- Intermediary restoration/provisional restorations are used in the interim between tooth preparation and fitting a definitive restoration. They protect the pulp by sealing and insulating the prepared tooth from the oral environment and maintain the tooth position and prevent occlusal changes.
- Zinc oxide eugenol cement is one of the oldest used cement. Though other cements are also used for temporization, but zinc oxide-eugenol cement is used most commonly because it is only mild irritant to the pulp, less soluble in oral fluids and produce better marginal seal than zinc phosphate.
- In EBA (Orthoethoxybenzoic acid) cement, EBA chelates with zinc forming zinc benzoate. Addition of EBA results in increase in compressive and tensile strength and decrease in setting time.
- In Polymer reinforced zinc oxide eugenol cement, resin helps in improving strength, smoothness of the mix and decreasing flow, solubility and brittleness of the cement. Olive oil acts as plasticizer and mask irritating properties of eugenol.
- The liquid of zinc phosphate cement is phosphoric acid and water in the 2:1 ratio.
- Repeated opening of the bottle containing the cement liquid or early dispensing of the liquid prior to mixing should be avoided because evaporation of liquid can result in changes in water/acid ratio which can further result in decrease in pH and an increase in viscosity of the mixed cement.
- For making temporary restorations, self-cure acrylic restorations have been used successfully. When used with direct technique, free monomer and the heat produced during exothermic reaction can harm pulp and the gingival tissues. To avoid this, indirect method is preferred.

QUESTIONS

1. What is the role of interim restorations? Enumerate different materials used as interim restorations.
2. Write short notes on:
   a. Materials used for interim restorations.
   b. Temporary restorations for extracoronal preparartions.
3. What are interim restorations? What are the requirements and purpose of interim restoration? Enumerate different materials used as interim restorations.

BIBLIOGRAPHY

1. Gilles JA, Hudget EF, Stone RC. Dimensional stability of temporary restorative. O Surg, O Med, O Path. 1975;40:796.
2. Gilson TD, Myres GE. Clinical studies of Dental Cement – II. Further investigation of the Zinc oxide eugenol cement for temporary restorations. JDR. 1972;48:366.
3. Grieve AR. A study of dental cements. BDJ. 1969;127:405.
4. Hume WR. The pharmacological and toxicological properties of zinc oxide eugenol. JADA. 1986;113:789.
5. Markowitz K, Moynihan M, Liu M, Kim S. Biologic properties of eugenol and zinc oxide eugenol. O Surg, O Med, O Path. 1992;73:729.
6. Meryon SD, Johnson SG, Smith AJ. Eugenol release and the cytotoxicity of different zinc oxide eugenol combination. J Dent. 1998;16:66.
7. Norman RD, Swartz ML, Phillips RW, Raibley JW. Direct pH determination of setting cements 2. The effects of prolonged storage time, powder/liquid ratio, temperature and dentin. JDR. 1966;45:1214.
8. Phillips RW, Swartz ML, Rhodes B. An evaluation of carboxylate adhesive cement J Am Dent Assoc. 1970;81:1353.
9. Servais GE, Cartz L. Structure of zinc phosphate dental cement. JDR. 1971;50:613.
10. Smith D C. A new dental cement. BDJ. 1968;5:381.
11. Smith DC. Dental cements, current status and future prospects. DCNA. 1983;6:763.
12. Wilson AD, Batchelor RF. ZnO eugenol cements II. Study of erosion and disintegration. JDR. 1970;49:593.
13. Wilson AD, Clinton DJ, Miller RP. Zinc oxide eugenol cements: IV Micro structure and hydrolysis JDR. 1973;52:253.
14. Wolcott RB, Kraske LM. A clinical evaluation of temporary restorative material. JPD. 1962;12:782.
15. Wudernabm FGM Eanesm WB, Serene TP. The physical and biological properties of Cavit. JADA. 1971;82: 378.

16 CHAPTER

Bonding to Enamel and Dentin

Chapter Outline

INTRODUCTION

The traditional "drill and fill" approach is fading now because of numerous advancements taking place in restorative dentistry. For a restorative material, adhesion is the primary requirement so that restorative materials can be bonded to enamel or dentin and without the need of extensive tooth preparation. The initial advancement was made in 1955, by a pedodontist, Buonocore, who developed acid etching of the enamel. He showed that when enamel is treated with a dilute acid for 30 seconds, it results in a microscopically roughened, porous surface into which the resin forms retentive tags. Dentin is different from enamel, it contains more than 25 percent organic material, which is mainly collagen and tissue fluid. The fluid present in dentinal tubules makes the bonding difficult. The adhesion to dentin requires decalcification of the dentinal surface to expose a layer of interlacing collagen fibrils and the entrances of the dentinal tubules. When resins are used, they form an intermediate layer with the exposed spongy collagen network which can be then bonded to the retentive inner surface of the restoration by means of a resin similar to that of enamel bonding.

The past decade has seen increased use of bonding agents in concurrence with traditional dental materials. The availability of adhesive techniques permits the placement of esthetic restorations like composite resins, esthetic inlays and veneers, etc. Though a wide range of adhesives is available, there are some requirements which a dental adhesive should possess.

ADHESIVE DENTISTRY

The following factors have shown to be responsible for the boost in adhesive dentistry

- ➡ The development of tooth colored restorative materials
- ➡ The introduction of new composite resins with superior properties
- ➡ Advances in the development of adhesive systems
- ➡ Increased concern among patients for esthetics and tooth colored restorations.

Indications for Use of Adhesives

- To treat carious and fractured tooth structure
- To restore erosion or abrasion defects in cervical areas

- To correct unesthetic contours, positions, dimensions, or shades of teeth
- To treat dentinal hypersensitivity
- For the repair of fractured porcelain, amalgam and resin restorations
- For pit and fissure sealants
- To bond composite restorations
- To bond amalgam restorations
- To lute crowns
- To bond orthodontic brackets.

Advantages of Bonding Techniques

→ Adhesion of composite resin restorations to enamel and dentin
→ Minimizes removal of sound tooth structure
→ Management of dentin hypersensitivity
→ Adhesion reduces microleakage at tooth restoration interface
→ As a part of resin cements for bonding cast restorations
→ Adhesion expands the range of esthetic possibilities
→ Bonding of porcelain restorations, e.g. porcelain inlays, onlays and veneers
→ Reinforces weakened tooth structure
→ Reduction in marginal staining
→ For repair of porcelain or composite
→ Bonding amalgam restorations to tooth
→ Repair of amalgam restorations
→ To bond orthodontic appliances.

History

→ 1955—Buonocore applied acid to tooth to render the tooth more receptive to adhesion
→ 1956—First commercially available bonding agent (NPG-GMA)
→ 1978—Second generation adhesives introduced
→ 1980's—Total etch concept gains acceptance
→ 1982—Hybrid layer concept by Nakabayashi
→ 1990's—Multistep and one step adhesive systems.

Definitions

→ *Adhesion or bonding*: The forces or energies between atoms or molecules at an interface that hold two phases together.
→ *Adherend*: The surface or substrate that is adhered (**Fig. 16.1**).
→ *Adhesive/adherent*: A material that can join substances together, resist separation and transmit loads across the bond (**Fig. 16.1**).
→ *Adhesive failure:* The bond that fails at the interface between the two substrates.
→ *Cohesive failure:* The bond fails within one of the substrates, but not at the interface.

Adhesion can occur by

→ Chemical means
→ Physical means
→ Mechanical means.

Mechanism of Adhesion (Figs 16.2A to C)

- *Physical means of adhesion* involve the:

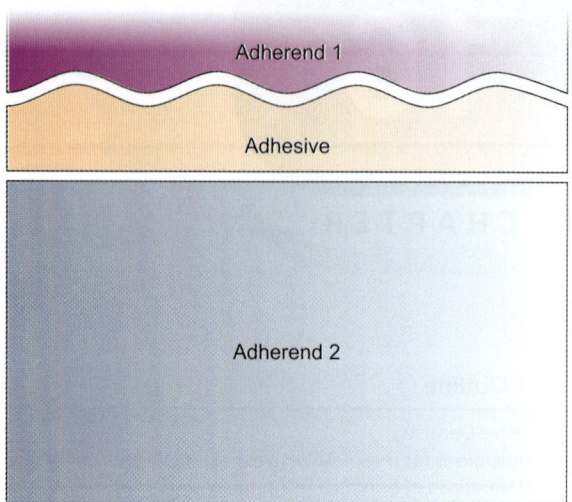

Figure 16.1: Diagrammatic representation of dental adhesive system, where Adherend 1 is enamel, dentin or both. Adhesive is bonding agent, Adherend 2 is composite resin

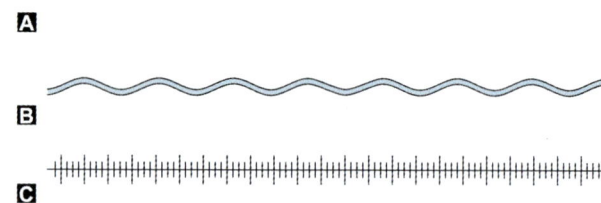

Figures 16.2A to C: (A) Physical bonding; (B) Mechanical bonding; (C) Chemical bonding

- *Van der Waals interactions*: Attraction between opposite charges on ions and dipoles.
- *Dispersion forces*: Interaction of induced dipoles
- *Hydrogen bond*: It is a particularly strong bond and can be included among physical forces.
- *Chemical means of adhesion* involves primary forces that is:
  - *Covalent bond*: It involves sharing electrons between two atoms or molecules. It represents strong bonds. Formation of a covalent bond liberates considerable energy. A covalent bond is present in all organic compounds.
  - *Ionic bond*: It involves an actual transfer of electrons from one atom to another. For example, the ion exchange adhesion mechanism in GICs.
  - *Metallic bond*: It is the chemical bond characteristics of metals in which mobile electrons are shared among atoms in a usually stable crystalline structure.

- *Mechanical means of adhesion*: Here the bonding occurs because of penetration of one material into another at the microscopic level. For example, in composite resins the bonding involves the penetration of resin into enamel and dentin and formation of resin tags.

Adhesion forces across different materials depend on
➡ Physical and chemical properties of both adhesive and the adherent
➡ Homogeneity
➡ Thickness of interface
➡ Oral environment with its moisture
➡ Chewing habits.

Factors Affecting Adhesion

Wetting

Wetting is an expression of the attractive forces between molecules of adhesive and adherent. In other words, it is the process of obtaining molecular attraction (**Fig. 16.3**). Wetting ability of an adhesive depends upon two factors:
- *Cleanliness of the adherend (Fig. 16.4):* Cleaner surface, greater adhesion.
- *Surface energy of the adherend:* More surface energy, greater adhesion.

Contact Angle (Fig. 16.5)

Contact angle refers to the angle formed between the surface of a liquid drop and its adherent surface. The stronger the attraction of the adhesive for the adherent, the smaller will be the contact angle. The zero contact angle is the best to obtain wetting.

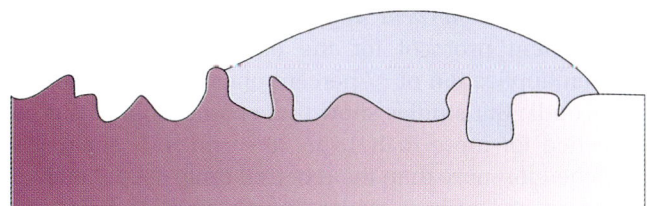

Figure 16.3: A good wetting ensures good adhesion

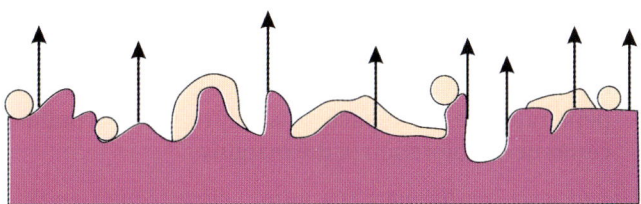

Figure 16.4: A clean surface increases the adhesion

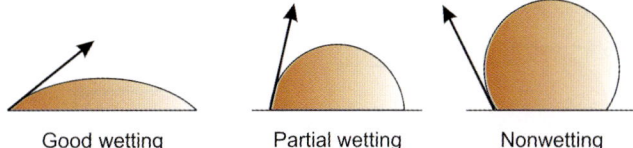

Good wetting   Partial wetting   Nonwetting

Figure 16.5: Lesser is the contact angle, better is the adhesion

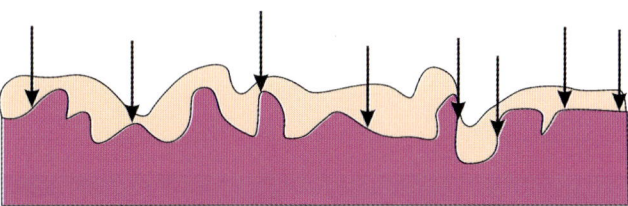

Figure 16.6: There should be intimate adaptation between two surfaces for optimal bonding

Surface Energy

The surface tension of the liquid and the surface energy of the adherend, ultimately determine the degree of wetting that occurs. Generally, the harder the surface is the higher the surface energy will be, which means the adhesive properties of the material will be higher.

Surface Contamination

The substrate surface should be clean as contamination prevents the adhesion. Adhesive should be able to fill the irregularities making the surface smooth allowing proper or intimate contact (**Fig. 16.6**).

Water

The higher the water content, the poorer is the adhesion. Water can react with both materials by the high polar group and hydrogen bond which can hamper the adhesion.

ENAMEL BONDING

Enamel, the hardest tissue in the human body consists of 95 percent mineralized inorganic substance, hydroxyapatite arranged in a dense crystalline structure and a small amount of protein and water (**Figs 16.7A and B**). To bond to enamel, it is very important to focus on the mineral component (hydroxyapatite) of enamel. Buonocore, in 1955, was the first to reveal the adhesion of acrylic resin to acid etched enamel. He used 85 percent phosphoric acid for etching, later Silverstone revealed that the optimum concentration of phosphoric acid should range between

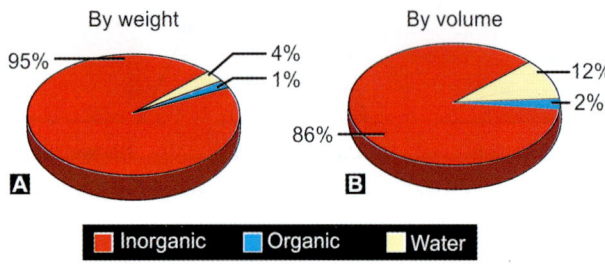

Figures 16.7A and B: Composition of enamel: (A) By weight; (B) By volume

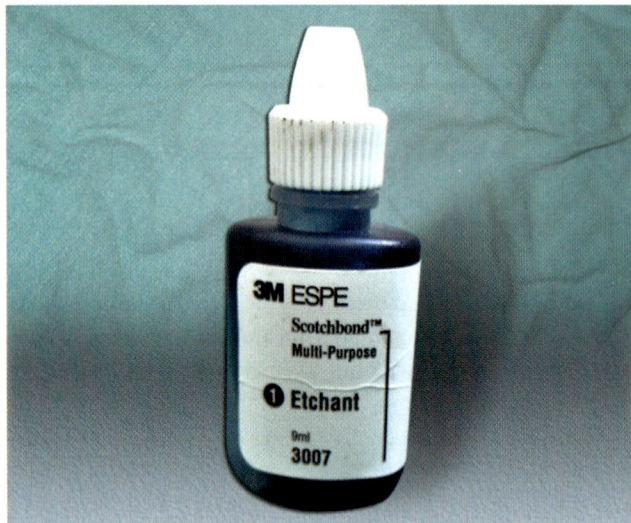

Figure 16.8: Etchant

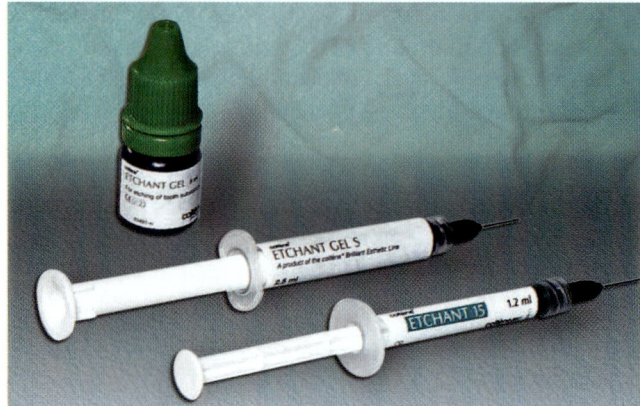

Figure 16.9: Etching gel provides greater control and precision in the etchant placement

ranges from 10 to 50 percent. Studies have shown no difference in etching of enamel using higher or lower concentrations of acid. Use of lower concentrations of phosphoric acid and reduced etching time has shown to give an adequate etch of the enamel while avoiding excessive demineralization of the dentin.

Abbreviations commonly used for resin chemicals	
Bis-GMA	Bisphenol glycidyl methacrylate
HEMA	2-Hydroxyethyl methacrylate
TGDMA/ TEGDMA	Triethylene glycol dimethacrylate
4-META	4-Methacryloxyethyl trimellitate anhydride
UDMA	Urethane dimethacrylate
PMDM	Pyromellitic acid diethylmethacrylate
NPG-GMA	N-phenylglycine glycidyl methacrylate
GPDM	Glycerophosphoric acid dimethacrylate
EDTA	Ethylene diamine tetra acetic acid

30 to 40 percent to get a satisfactory adhesion to the enamel. Usually 37 percent phosphoric acid is used for 15 to 30 seconds (**Fig. 16.8**). If the concentration is greater than 50 percent, then monocalcium phosphate monohydrate may get precipitated while at concentrations lower than 30 percent, dicalcium phosphate monohydrate is precipitated which interferes with adhesion.

Several changes have taken place regarding the acid etching of enamel surfaces. These include:

• *Development of phosphoric acid gels:* Gels provide the clinician a greater control and precision in the placement of etching agents (**Fig. 16.9**). Earlier most gel etchants used to contain silica as a thickening agent. But recently available gels employ polymeric thickening agents which have better wetting abilities and rinse-off more easily than silica containing gels.

• *Percentage of etchants used:* Currently used etchants employ the concentrations of phosphoric acid that

• *Decrease in the acid application time:* The standard treatment protocol for the etching of enamel has been application of 37 percent phosphoric acid for 60 seconds. But studies show that enamel should not be etched for more than 15 to 20 seconds. If enamel is etched for more than the required time, deeper etch of the enamel surface occurs. Since a bonding agent has a high viscosity, the surface tension effect of the agent would not allow full penetration of the etched enamel. This will result in a 'dead space' beyond the bonded area. When enamel bends, or the weak resin based bond breaks off, the dead space becomes exposed to oral fluids which has lower surface tension and thus penetrates the dead space. This may result in secondary caries or discoloration of the margins.

Use of acid conditioners (i.e. nitric, citric, oxalic, maleic acids) other than traditional phosphoric acid (Fig. 16.10):

Many acids have been developed recently for conditioning like nitric acid, citric acid and oxalic acids. These acids cause mild etching/conditioning, so for total etching it is advisable to use phosphoric acid.

Conditioning

It is the process of cleaning the surface and activating the calcium ions, so as to make them more reactive.

Etching

It is the process of increasing the surface reactivity by demineralizing the superficial calcium layer and thus creating the enamel tags. These tags are responsible for micromechanical bonding between tooth and restorative resin.

Steps for Enamel Bonding

- Perform oral prophylaxis procedure using nonfluoridated and oil less prophylaxis pastes.
- Clean and wash the teeth with water. Isolate to prevent any contamination from saliva or gingival crevicular fluid
- Apply acid etchant in the form of liquid or gel for 10 to 15 seconds. Deciduous teeth require longer time for etching than permanent teeth because of the presence of aprismatic enamel in deciduous teeth
- Wash the etchant continuously for 10 to 15 seconds
- Note the appearance of a properly etched surface. It should give a frosty white appearance on drying
- If any sort of contamination occurs, repeat the procedure
- Now apply bonding agent and low viscosity monomers over the etched enamel surface. Generally, enamel bonding agents contain Bis-GMA or UDMA with TEGDMA added to lower the viscosity of the bonding agent. The bonding agents due to their low viscosity, rapidly wet and penetrate the clean, dried, conditioned enamel into the microspaces forming resin tags. The resin tags which form between enamel prisms are known as Macrotags (**Fig. 16.11**)

- The finer network of numerous small tags are formed across the end of each rod where individual hydroxyapatite crystals were dissolved and are known as microtags. These microtags are more important due to their larger number and greater surface area of contact. The formation of resin micro and macro tags within the enamel surface constitute the fundamental mechanism of enamel-resin adhesion.

Mechanism of Etching

When seen microscopically, three types of enamel etching patterns are seen:

Type I Preferential demineralization of enamel prism core leaving the prism peripheries intact. Here corresponding tags are cone shaped.

Type II There is preferential removal of interprismatic enamel leaving the prism cores intact. The corresponding enamel tags are cup shaped.

Type III In this, the pattern is less distinct, including areas that resemble type I and II patterns and areas which bear no resemblance to enamel prism.

Basically, acid etching creates a 5 to 50 micron deep microporous layer into which adhesive resin flows. This result in a longlasting enamel bond achieved via micromechanical interlocking between the resin and enamel. Bond strength of etched enamel to composite resin usually varies between 15 and 25 mpa.

Etching of enamel produces a number of effects

- Cleanses debris from enamel
- Produces a complex three-dimensional microtopography at the enamel surface
- Increases the enamel surface area available for bonding
- Produces micropores into which there is mechanical interlocking of the resin (**Figs 16.12A to C**)
- Exposes more reactive surface layer, thus increasing its wettability.

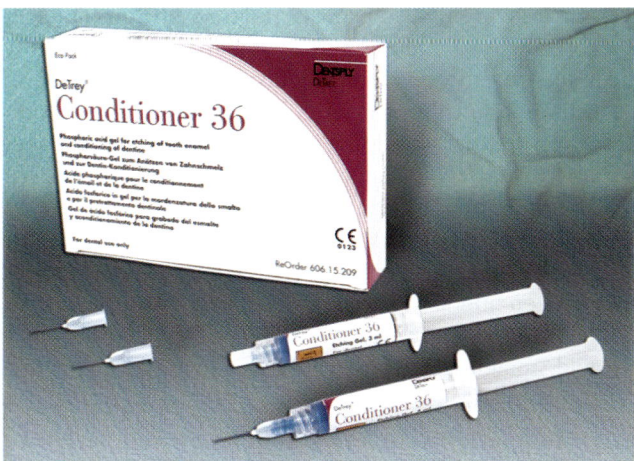

Figure 16.10: Phosphoric acid gel for etching enamel and conditioning of dentin

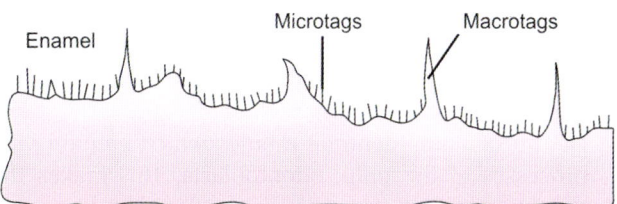

Figure 16.11: Formation of microtags and macrotags when bonding agent is applied to etched tooth surface

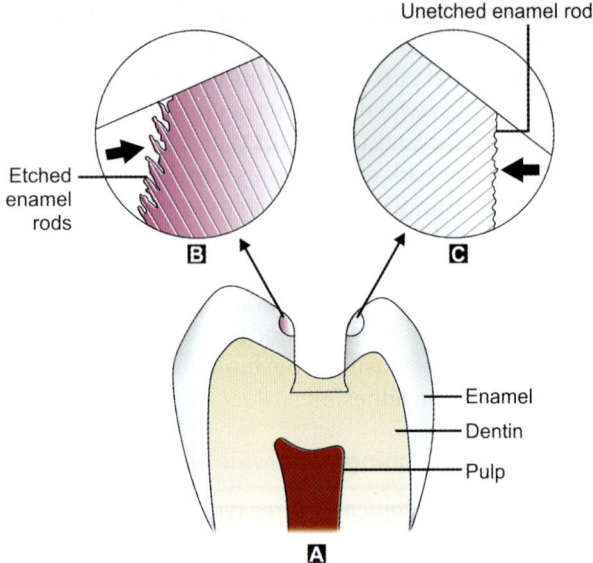

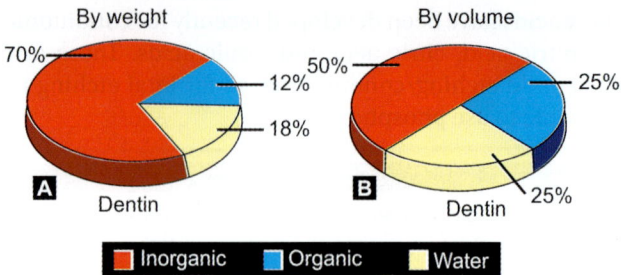

Figures 16.12A to C: Difference in appearance of etched and un-etched enamel rods

Figures 16.13A and B: Composition of dentin (A) By weight; (B) By volume

• Fluid present in dentinal tubules constantly flows outwards which reduces the adhesion of the composite resin.

Factors affecting effects of acid etching on enamel

➡ Type of acid used in either gel or liquid form
➡ Concentration of acid used and time of etching
➡ Type of acid used
➡ Chemical nature of enamel
➡ Whether enamel is fluoridated or demineralized
➡ Type of dentition, i.e. primary or permanent.

Among the factors that affect bonding of enamel are its fluoride content, arrangement of crystals and impurities, e.g. presence of magnesium and carbonates in the hydroxyapatite crystals.

DENTIN BONDING

Bonding to dentin has been proven more difficult and less reliable and predictable than to enamel. This is basically because of difference in morphologic, histologic and compositional differences between the two:

• In enamel, it is 95 percent inorganic hydroxyapatite by volume, in dentin it is 50 percent. Dentin contains more water than does enamel (**Figs 16.13A and B**)
• Hydroxyapatite crystals have a regular pattern in enamel whereas in dentin, hydroxyapatite crystals are randomly arranged in an organic matrix.
• The presence of the smear layer makes wetting of the dentin by the adhesive more difficult.
• Dentin contains dentinal tubules which contain vital processes of the pulp, odontoblasts. This makes the dentin a sensitive structure.
• Dentin is a dynamic tissue which shows changes due to aging, caries or operative procedures.

Dentin bond strength is quite variable because it is dependent upon the following factors

➡ Different quality of dentin including the number, diameter and size of dentinal tubules in deep and superficial dentin (Fig. 16.14). Dentin permeability is not uniform throughout the tooth, it is more permeable in coronal dentin than root dentin. There are differences within coronal dentin also. Since tubules are more numerous and wider near the pulp, there is more fluid and less intertubular dentin, this makes dentin bonding less effective in deeper dentin than superficial dentin.
➡ Amount of collagen: As dentin ages, there is an increase in mineralization, the ratio of peritubular/intertubular dentin and a decrease in the number of dentinal tubules which overall affects the adhesion quality of dentin.

Conditioning of Dentin

For removal or modification of the smear layer, many acids or/and calcium chelators are used:

• *Acids*: Commonly used acid for conditioning dentin is 37 percent phosphoric acid. It not only removes the smear layer but also exposes the microporous collagen network into which resin monomer penetrates. Usually, it forms exposed collagen fibrils which are covered with an amorphous layer, a combination of denatured collagen fibers and the collapsed residual collagen layer. This is collagen smear layer which is resistant to monomer penetration.

It is always preferred to maintain conditioned dentin in a moist state to prevent the collapse of unsupported collagen fibers.

Other acids used for dentin conditioning are nitric acid, maleic acid, citric acid, oxalic acid, and hydrochloric acid.

• *Calcium chelators*: These are used to remove and/or modify the smear layer without demineralizing the surface dentin layer. A commonly used chelator is ethylenediaminetetraacetic acid (EDTA).

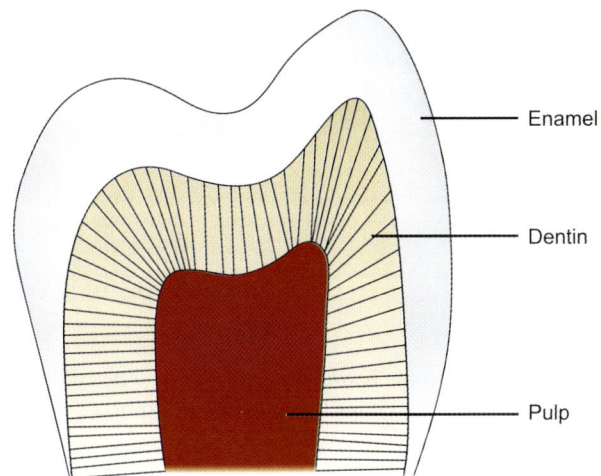

Figure 16.14: Difference in dimensions and quantity of dentinal tubules in deep and superficial dentin

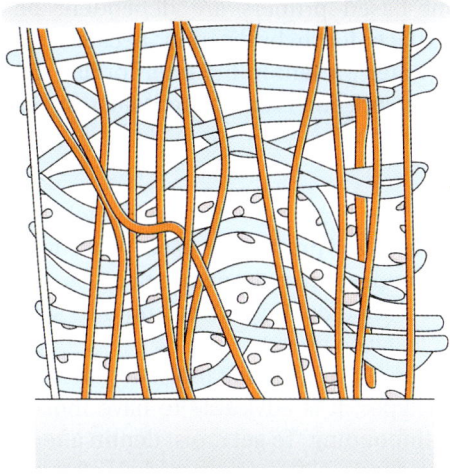

Figure 16.15: Etching of dentin causes exposure of collagen fibrils. interfibrillar water acts as plasticizer and keep the fibers open

Priming of Dentin

Primers are agents which contain monomers having a hydrophilic end with affinity for exposed collagen fibrils and a hydrophobic end with affinity for adhesive resin. Commonly used primers have HEMA and 4-META monomers, dissolved in organic solvents.

Primers are used to increase the diffusion of resin into moist and demineralized dentin and thus optimal micromechanical bonding. For optimal penetration of primer into demineralized dentin, it should be applied in multiple coats. Also it is preferred to keep the dentin surface moist, otherwise collagen fibers get collapsed in dry condition resisting the entry for primer and adhesive resin.

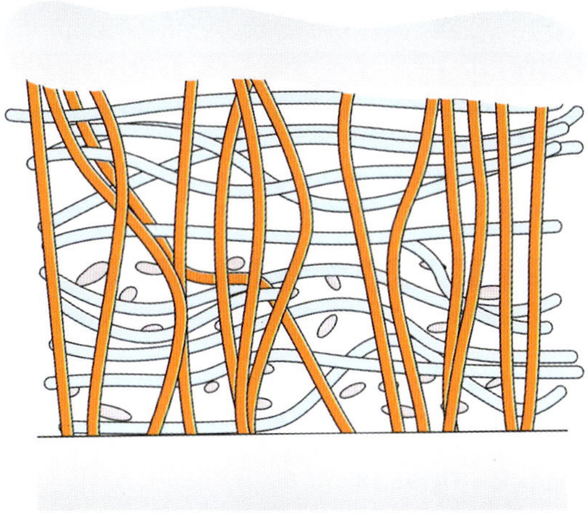

Moist vs Dry Dentin

By etching dentin, the smear layer and minerals from it are removed, exposing the collagen fibers (**Fig. 16.15**). Areas from where minerals are removed are filled with water. This water acts as a plasticizer for collagen, keeping it in an expanded soft state. Thus, spaces for resin infiltration are also preserved. But these collagen fibers collapse when dry and if the organic matrix is denatured (**Fig. 16.16**). This obstructs the resin from reaching the dentin surface and forming a hybrid layer.

Thus, the desired effect of acid etching, which is increased permeability, is lost. For this reason, presence of moist/wet dentin is needed to achieve successful dentin bonding. When primer is applied to wet/moist dentin, water diffuses from the primer to the organic solvent and the solvent diffuses along with the polymers into the

Figure 16.16: In dehydrated dentin, loss of water causes collapse of collagen fibrils which prevent penetration of monomer

demineralized dentinal matrix and tubules. Sensitivity to dry or moist dentin varies according to the type of solvent used for the primer resin.

Reasons for better bonding in moist dentin
→ The acetone trails water and improves penetration off the monomers into the dentin for better micromechanical bonding
→ Water keeps collagen fibris from collapsing, thus helping in better penetration and bonding between resin and dentin.

Wet Bonding

In this, primers consisting of hydrophilic resin monomers dissolved in water miscible organic solvents like ethanol and acetone are used.

Acetone-based primers are dependent on a moist dentin surface for hybridization because the acetone displaces water present in the interfibrillar spaces of the collagen network and carry hydrophilic resin alongwith it for hybridization.

Dry Bonding

In this, water-based primers are used. Water-based primers are not dependent on moist dentin because of their ability to self-wet a dried dentin surface and thus separating the collapsed collagen fibers.

Because we have seen that moist dentin is friendly with all primer types, it is advisable to have moist dentin for resin-dentinbonding. To get moist dentin after etching, do not dry the dentin with compressed air after rinsing away etchant. Instead use high-volume evacuation to remove excess water and then blot the remaining water present on the dentin surface using gauze or cotton to leave dentin optimally moist.

If the dentin surface is made too dry
➡ Collapse of the collagen fibers and demineralized dentin occurs (**Fig. 16.17**)
➡ This results in low bond strength because of ineffective penetration of the adhesive into the dentin.

If the dentin surface is too wet
➡ One cannot check for the "frosted" etch appearance of the enamel
➡ There is reduction in bond strength because:
◆ Presence of water droplets dilute resin primer and out-compete it for sites in the collagen network which prevents hybridization (**Fig. 16.18**)
◆ The phase changes occur in the ethanol or acetone based resins.

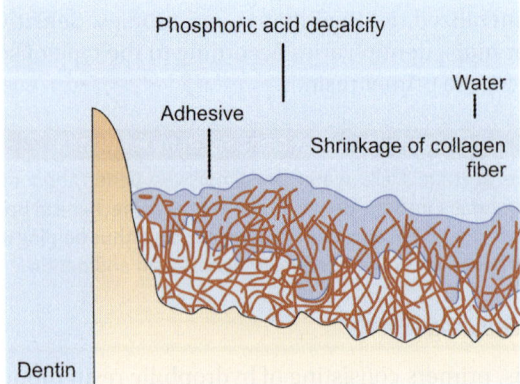

Figure 16.17: Overdrying of dentin causes collapse of collagen fibers and thus ineffective penetration of adhesive

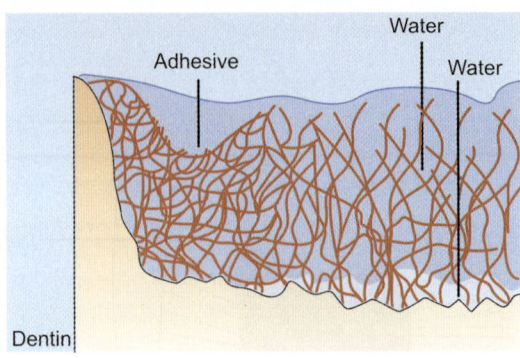

Figure 16.18: If dentin is overwet, presence of water dilutes the monomer and competes it for sites in collagen network. This lowers the bond strength

DENTIN BONDING AGENT

Mechanism of Bonding

The dentin adhesive molecule has a bifunctional structure:
$$M\text{————}R\text{————}X$$
Where,
M is the double bond of methacrylate which copolymerizes with composite resin.
R is the spacer which makes the molecule large.
X is a functional group for bonding which bonds to inorganic or organic portion of dentin.

Ideally a dentin bonding agent should have both hydrophilic and hydrophobic ends. The hydrophilic end displaces the dentinal fluid, to wet the surface. The hydrophobic end bonds to the composite resin.

Bonding to the inorganic part of dentin involves ionic interaction among the negatively charged group on X (for example, phosphates, amino acids and amino alcohols, or dicarboxylates) and the positively charged calcium ions. Commonly used bonding systems employ use of phosphates.

Bonding to the organic part of dentin involves interaction with Amino (–NH), Hydroxyl (–OH), Carboxylate (–COOH), Amide (–CONH) groups present in dentinal collagen. Dentin bonding agents have isocyanates, aldehydes, carboxylic acid anhydrides and carboxylic acid chlorides which extract hydrogen from the above mentioned groups and bond chemically.

Scientific classification of modern adhesives
➡ Based on generations
◆ First generation bonding agent
◆ Second generation bonding agent
◆ Third generation bonding agent
◆ Fourth generation bonding agent
◆ Fifth generation bonding agent
◆ Sixth generation bonding agent
◆ Seventh generation bonding agent.

- ➡ Based on smear layer treatment
  - ◆ Smear layer modifying agents
  - ◆ Smear layer removing agents
  - ◆ Smear layer dissolving agents.
- ➡ Based on number of steps
  - ◆ Three step
  - ◆ Two step
  - ◆ Single step.

First generation bonding agent
- ➡ Developed in 1960s
- ➡ Relied on adhesion to smear layer
- ➡ No. of steps involved were two; etching of enamel + application of adhesive
- ➡ Did not recommend dentin etching
- ➡ Low bond strength (2–3 MPa).

Evolution of Dentin Bonding Agents

Historically, DBAs have been classified based on chemistry and the manner in which they treat the smear layer.

First Generation Dentin Bonding Systems

The first step to achieve bonding to dentin was done by application of a coupling agent such as glycerol-phosphoric acid dimethacrylate as a primer and N-2-hydroxy-3-methacryloxypropyl and N-phenyl phenyl glycine (NPG-GMA) and silane coupling agents. The first dentin bonding agent to appear on the market was Cervident (SS White Co, King of Prussia, PA).

These products ignored the smear layer. The mechanism of adhesion was deep penetration of the resin tags into the exposed dentinal tubules after etching and the chelating component which could bond to the calcium component of dentin (**Fig. 16.19**). Since they could chelate with calcium ions of the tooth structure, they formed stronger bonds with enamel than dentin.

Problems with first generation bonding agents:

- Low bond strength, in the order of 2 to 3 MPa insufficient to retain the restorative material for extended periods of time.
- Loss in bond strength over time.
- Lack of stability of individual components during storage.

Second Generation Dentin Bonding Systems

They were introduced in the late 1970s. Most of the second generation bonding agents leave the smear layer intact when used but some of them employed the use of mild cleansing agents to remove the smear layer (**Fig. 16.20**). They achieved the bond strengths ranging from about 4.5 to 6 MPa. Three types of second generation products were made available:

1. *Etched tubule dentin bonding agents*: In these, bonding to dentin was attempted by etching the tubules with 25 percent citric acid and then making use of ethyl-methacrylate to mechanically interlock with the etched tubules.

2. *Phosphate ester dentin bonding agents*: This system made use of a mild cleanser to modify the smear layer. These bonding agents used analogs of Bis-GMA with attached phosphate esters. The phosphate group bonded with calcium present in the tooth structure while the methacrylate end of the molecule bonded to the composite resin. These bonding agents showed 10 to 30 percent increase in bond strength.

3. *Polyurethane dentin bonding agents*: These bonding agents were based on the isocyanate group of the polyurethane polymer which bonds to different groups present in dentin like carboxyl, amino and hydroxyl groups.

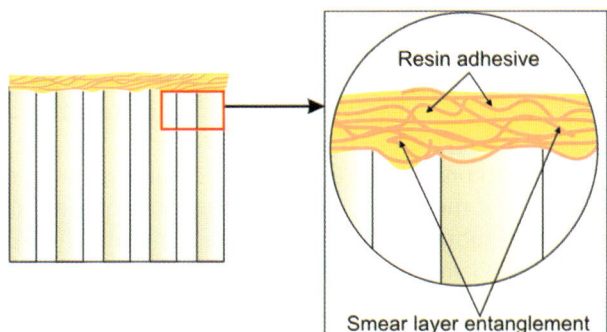

Figure 16.19: First generation bonding agents ignored the smear layer. The bonding occurred because of deep penetration of resin tags into open dentinal tubules

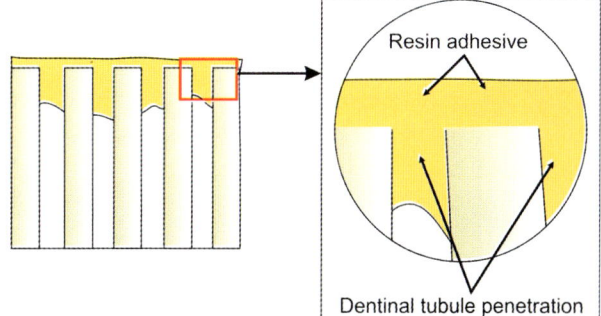

Figure 16.20: Second generation bonding agents involve complete removal of smear layer and penetration of resin in open tubules

Most of these agents used diisocyanates which simultaneously bonded to both the dentin and composite resin.

Since the setting reaction of polyurethane was not affected by the presence of fluid in the dentin tubules or smear layer, most of these systems left the smear layer intact, however some made use of hydrogen peroxide for cleansing of the smear layer.

Problems with second generation bonding agents:
- Low bond strength
- Unstable interface between dentin and resin because of the insufficient knowledge about the smear layer.

Second generation bonding agent
➡ Developed in 1970s
➡ Did not recommend dentin etching
➡ Low bond strength (4–6 MPa)
➡ Relied on adhesion to smear layer but some of them employed use of mild cleansing agent
➡ No. of steps involved were two; etching of enamel + application of adhesive

Third Generation Dentin Bonding Systems

In the late 1980s, the third generation DBA, two component primer/adhesive systems were introduced. In earlier used systems, a conditioning step on dentin was done in conjunction with the bonding agent, but in third generation bonding systems, chemistry is more diverse and various agents for modifying the dentin are used. These systems, employed the concept of conditioning and priming before application of bonding agent. In other words, in third generation systems, alteration or removal of the smear layer is done before bonding (**Fig. 16.21**). They attempted this in two different ways:
1. Removal of the smear layer without disturbing the smear plugs.
2. Modifying the smear layer to improve its properties.

The application of third-generation dentin bonding agents involves three steps: Etching with an acidic conditioner, priming with a bifunctional resin in a volatile

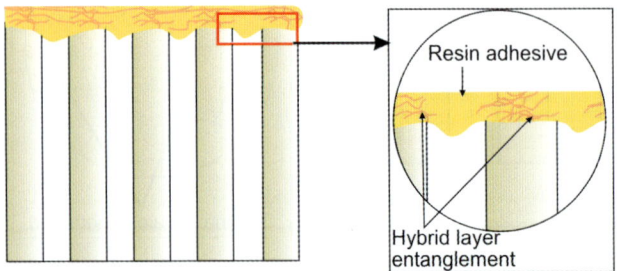

Figure 16.21: Third generation bonding agents involved alteration removal of smear layer by conditioning and priming before bonding

solvent and bonding with an unfilled or partially filled resin.

Advantages of third generation bonding agents over first and second generation bonding agents:
- Higher bond strengths (8–15 MPa)
- Reduced microleakage
- Form a strong bond to both sclerotic and moist dentin
- Reduced need for a retentive tooth preparation
- Can be used for porcelain and composite repairs
- Erosion, abrasion and abfraction lesions can be treated with minimal tooth preparation.

Drawbacks of third generation bonding agents:
- Decrease in bond strength with time
- Increase in microleakage with time.

Third generation bonding agent
➡ Employed the concept of conditioning and priming before application of bonding agent
➡ Involved removal or modification of smear layer
➡ Three steps application, i.e. Etching of enamel + Application of primer + Bonding agent application
➡ High bond strength and reduced microleakage.

Fourth Generation Dentin Bonding Agents

They were made available in the mid 1990s. Fourth generation bonding agents represent significant improvements in the field of adhesive dentistry. These agents are based on total etch technique and moist bonding concept.

Mechanism of bonding: The fourth "generation" is characterized by the process of hybridization at the interface of the dentin and the composite resin. Hybridization is the phenomenon of replacement of the hydroxyapatite and water at the dentin surface by resin. This resin, in combination with the collagen fibers, forms a hybrid layer. In other words, hybridization is the process of resin interlocking in the demineralized dentin surface (**Fig. 16.22**). This concept was given by Nakabayashi in 1982.

The fourth generation adhesives consist of:
1. *Conditioner (Etchant):* Commonly used acids are 37 percent phosphoric acid, nitric acid, maleic acid, oxalic acid, pyruvic acid, hydrochloric acid, citric acid or a chelating agent, e.g. EDTA.

   Use of conditioner/etchant causes removal or modification of the smear layer, demineralizes peritubular and intertubular dentin and exposes collagen fibrils.
2. *Primer:* Primers consist of monomers like HEMA (2-Hydroxyethyl methacrylate) and 4-META (4-Methacryloxyethyl trimellitate anhydride) dissolved in acetone or ethanol. Thus, they have both hydrophilic as well as hydrophobic ends which have affinity for the exposed collagen and resin respectively. Use

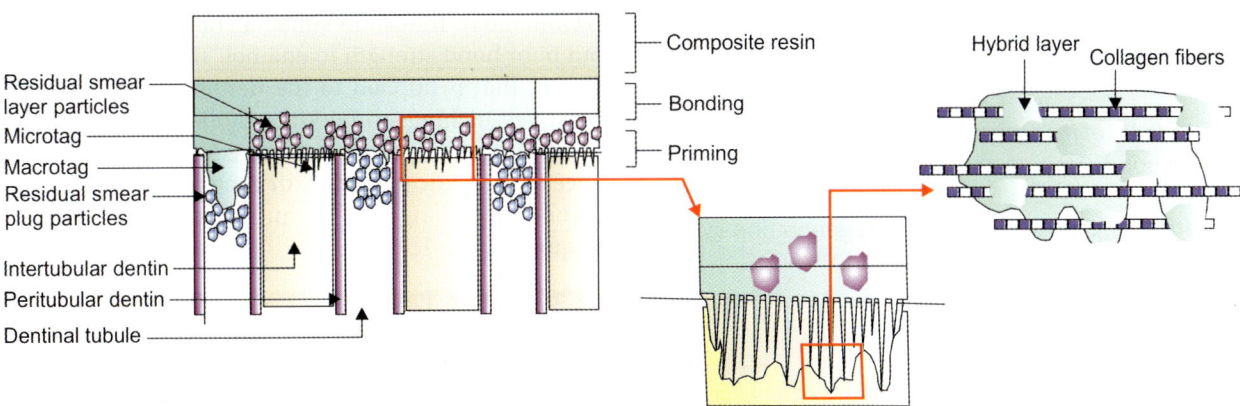

Figure 16.22: Fourth generation bonding agents show adhesion by formation of hybrid layer

of primer increases wettability of the dentin surface, bonding between the dentin and resin, and encourages monomer infiltration of demineralized peritubular and intertubular dentin.

3. *Adhesive:* The adhesive resin is a low viscosity, semi filled or unfilled resin which flows easily and matches the composite resin. Adhesive combines with the monomers to form a resin reinforced hybrid layer and resin tags to seal the dentin tubules.

The following are examples of the fourth generation DBA's:

1. All bond-2 (Bisco)
2. Scotch bond multipurpose (3M)
3. Optibond FL (Kerr)
4. Clearfil liner bond-2 (Kuraray).

Advantages of fourth generation bonding agents:

1. Ability to form a strong bond to both enamel and dentin.
2. High bond strength to dentin (17–25 MPa)
3. Ability to bond strongly to moist dentin
4. Can also be used for bonding to substrates such as porcelain and alloys (including amalgam).

Fourth generation bonding agent
➡ Developed in early 1990s
➡ Based on total etch technique and moist bonding concept
➡ Based on concept of hybridization and hybrid layer formation
➡ Three steps application, i.e. Total etching + Application of primer + Application of bonding agent
➡ High bond strength.

Fifth Generation Dentin Bonding Agents

Fifth-generation DBAs have been available since the mid-1990s. They are also known as "one-bottle" or "one-component" bonding agents. These products are distinguished from the fourth generation bonding agents by

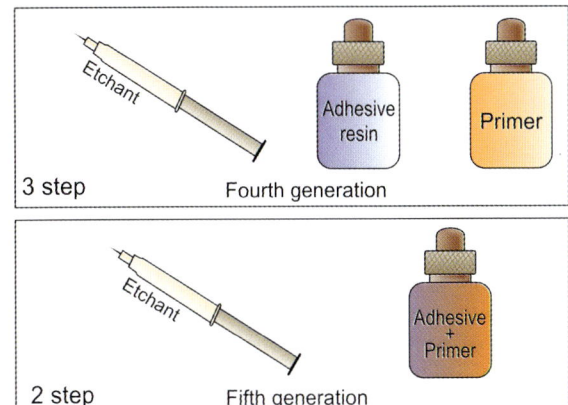

Figure 16.23: Fourth generation bonding system is available in two bottles, one primer and other adhesive resin, while in fifth generation bonding agents, primer and adhesive are combined in one bottle only

being one-step or one-bottle products. In these agents the primer and adhesive resin are in one bottle. The first product in this category was prime and bond. The basic differences between the fourth and fifth generation dentin bonding agents is the number of basic components of bottles. The fourth generation bonding system is available in two bottles, one consisting of the primer and the other the adhesive, the fifth generation dentin bonding agents are available in one bottle only (**Fig. 16.23**). This makes the fifth generation bonding agents simpler and faster than the fourth generation systems.

Advantages of fifth generation bonding agents:

1. High bond strength, almost equal to that of fourth generation adhesives, i.e. 20 to 25 MPa
2. Easy to use and predictable
3. Little technique sensitivity
4. Reduced number of steps

5. Bonding agent is applied directly to the prepared tooth surface
6. Reduced postoperative sensitivity.

Disadvantages of fifth generation bonding agents:
1. Lesser bond strength than fourth generation bonding agents.
   The following are some of the fifth generation systems in the market:
   – Prime and Bond (Dentsply)
   – Optibond solo (Kerr)
   – Single bond (3M) (**Fig. 16.24**).

Fifth generation bonding agent
➡ Developed in mid 1990s
➡ Uses two steps, i.e. Total etching + Application of primer and bonding agent
➡ Primer + Bonding agent are available in single bottle
➡ High bond strength
➡ Easy to use
➡ Reduced postoperative sensitivity.

Sixth Generation Dentin Bonding Agents

They have been available since 2000. These single bottle adhesives combine etching, priming and bonding in a single solution and as a single step. The fifth-generation bonding agent was made available in single bottle consisting of both the primer and the adhesive. Before applying it, tooth structure needed to be treated with etchant. Sixth generation, they are made available with self-etching primers which are used in place of the separate etchant (**Figs 16.25A to F**). Thus, etching as a separate step

is eliminated. They show sufficient bond strength to dentin but poor bond strength to enamel. These use an acidified primer that is applied to the dentin and not rinsed-off. Most self-etching primers are moderately acidic with a pH that ranges between 1.8 and 2.5. Because of the presence of an acidic primer, sixth generation bonding agents do not have a long shelf life and thus have to be refreshed frequently.

Sixth generation bonding agents are divided into two types
Self-etching primer and adhesive:
➡ Available in two bottles:
◆ Primer
◆ Adhesive
➡ Primer is applied prior to the adhesive
➡ Water is the solvent in these systems.
Self etching adhesive (Figs 16.26 and 16.27)
➡ Available in two bottles:
◆ Primer
◆ Adhesive
➡ A drop from each bottle is taken, mixed and applied to the tooth surface, for example, Prompt L-pop.

Mechanism of bonding: In these agents as soon as the decalcification process starts, infilteration of the empty spaces by the dentin bonding agent is initiated (see **Figs 16.25D to F**).

Advantages of Self Etching Primers

- Comparable adhesion and bond strengths to enamel and dentin
- Reduces postoperative sensitivity because they etch and prime simultaneously
- They etch the dentin less aggressively than total etch products
- The demineralized dentin is infiltrated by resin during the etching process
- Since they do not remove the smear layer, the tubules remain sealed, resulting in less sensitivity
- They form a relatively thinner hybrid layer than traditional product which results in complete infiltration of the demineralized dentin by the resin monomers. This results in increased bond strength
- Much faster and simpler technique
- Less technique sensitive as fewer number of steps are involved for the self etch system.

Disadvantages of Self Etching Primers

- pH is inadequate to etch enamel, hence bond to enamel is weaker as compared to dentin
- Bond to dentin is 18 to 23 MPa

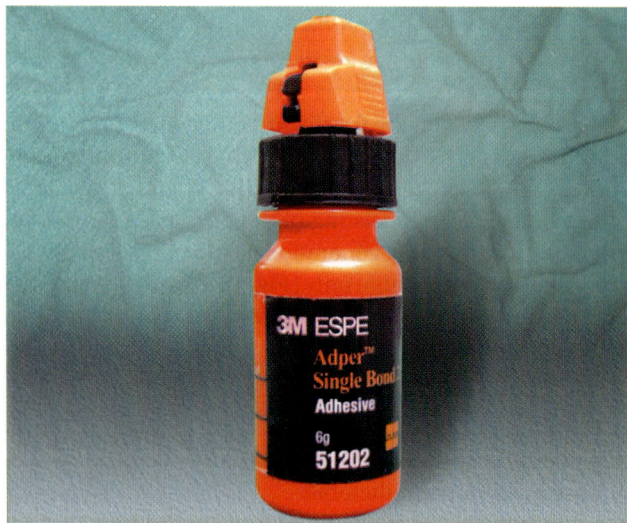

Figure 16.24: Fifth generation bonding agent

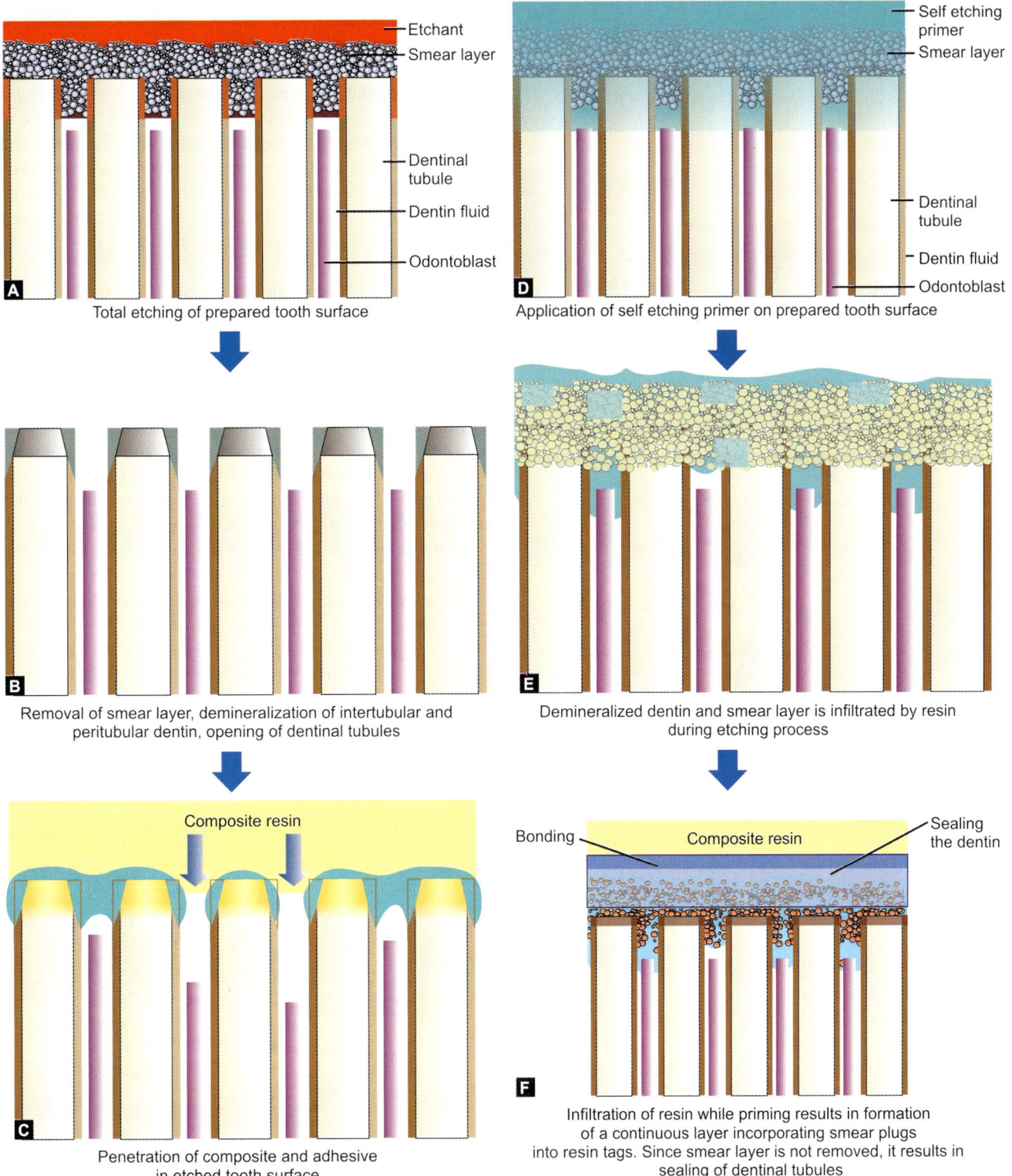

Figures 16.25A to F: Total etch vs self-etch systems

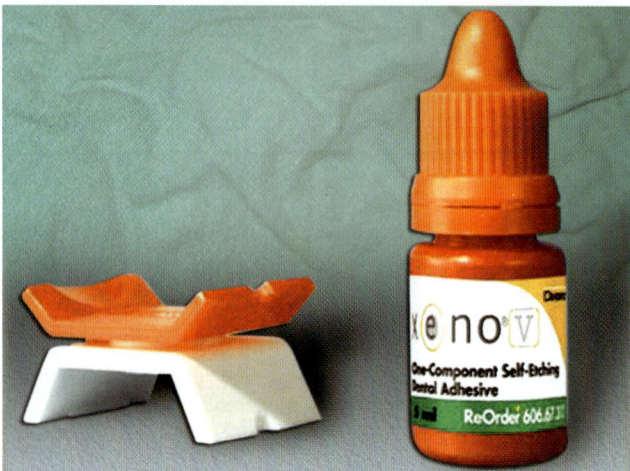

Figure 16.26: Self etching adhesive

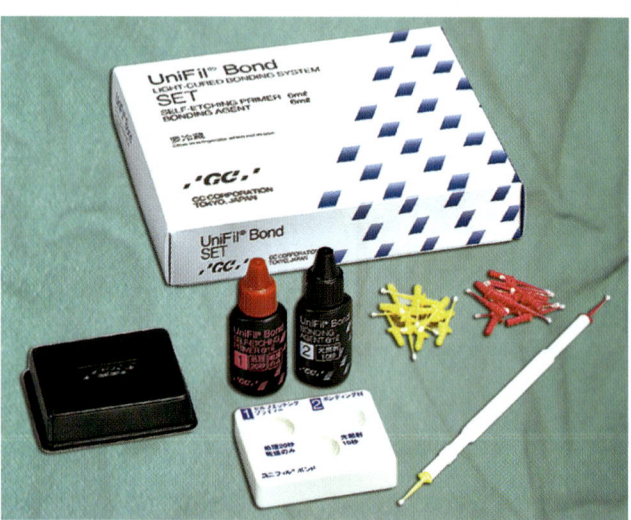

Figure 16.27: Self etching adhesive

- Since they consist of an acidic solution, they cannot be stored and have to be refreshed
- May require refrigeration
- High hydrophilicity due to acidic primers
- Promote water sorption
- Limited clinical data.

Sixth generation bonding agent

➡ Developed in early 2000s
➡ Etchant + Primer + Bonding agent are available in single bottle
➡ Use self etch primer
➡ Bond strength lower than fourth and fifth generation bonding agent
➡ Reduced postoperative sensitivity.

Total etch technique (see Figs 16.25A to C)

The total etch technique involves the complete removal of the smear layer by simultaneous acid etching of enamel and dentin. According to this, the smear layer is considered a hurdle to adhesion because of its low cohesive strength and its weak attachment to tooth structure. After total etching, primer and adhesive resin are applied separately or together. Acid removes the dentin smear layer, raises surface energy and modifies the dentin substrate so that it can be infiltrated by subsequently placed primers and resins.

Seventh Generation Bonding Agents (Fig.16.28)

They achieve the same objective as the sixth generation systems except that they simplified the multiple sixth generation materials into a single component, single bottle one-step self-etch adhesive, thus avoiding any mistakes in mixing. In other words seventh generation bonding consists of only one component. Seventh generation bonding agents also have disinfecting and desensitizing properties. They have attained consistently lower bond strengths than the fourth and fifth-generation adhesives.

Both the sixth and seventh generation adhesives are self etching, self priming adhesives which are minimum technique sensitive. The seventh generation DBAs have shown very little or no postoperative sensitivity. However, due to the complex mixed solution, they are prone to phase separation and formation of droplets within their adhesive layers. Example of a seventh generation bonding agent is 'i Bond'.

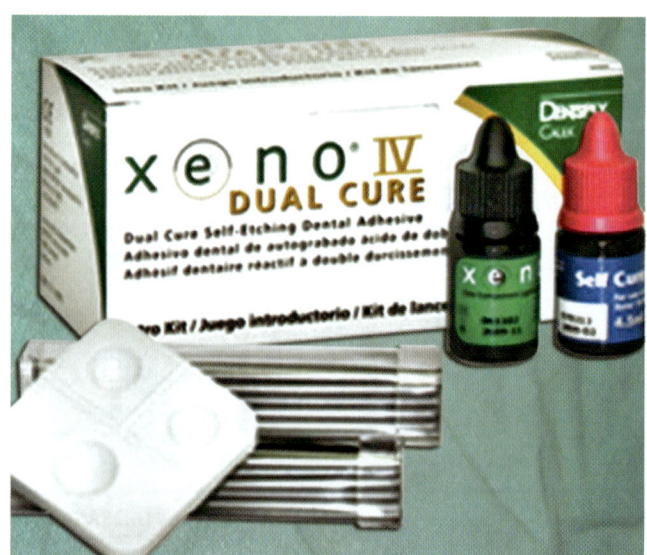

Figure 16.28: Seventh generation bonding agent

➔ Developed in late 2000s
➔ All in one concept, i.e. components available as single component
➔ Uses self etch primer
➔ Good bond strength
➔ No postoperative sensitivity.

Nanofilled Bonding Agents

These bonding agents contain extremely small filler particles. Bonding agents under this type are Prime and Bond NT (Dentsply/Caulk) (**Fig. 16.29**).

Prime and Bond NT contains 7-nanometer fillers, greater concentration of resin and a smaller molecular weight resin.

Advantages of Using Small Fillers

- Small fillers make the bonding agent tougher and stronger
- Covers dentin in one application
- Show better penetration in dentin
- Provides better marginal integrity
- Form low film thickness
- Satisfactory bonding to sclerotic and aged dentin.

Three-step Etch and Rinse Adhesives

Advantages

- Separate application of conditioner, primer, and adhesive resin
- Low technique sensitivity
- Better adhesion to enamel and dentin
- More effective and consistent results
- Possibility for particle-filled adhesive , acts as a "shock absorber".

Disadvantages

- Risk of overetching dentin because of presence of highly concentrated phosphoric acid etchants, resulting in incomplete resin infiltration
- Three-step application procedure
- Risk of surface contamination because postconditioning rinsing required
- Sensitive to overwet or overdry dentin surface conditions
- Weak resin-collagen interaction, this may result in nanoleakage and early bond degradatio.

<table>
<tr><th colspan="3">Comparison of number of clinical steps of different dentin bonding agents</th></tr>
<tr><th>Generation</th><th>No. of steps</th><th>Steps description</th></tr>
<tr><td>First</td><td>2</td><td>Etch enamel + Apply adhesive</td></tr>
<tr><td>Second</td><td>2</td><td>Etch enamel + Apply adhesive</td></tr>
<tr><td>Third</td><td>3</td><td>Etch enamel + Apply primer + Apply bonding agent</td></tr>
<tr><td>Fourth</td><td>3</td><td>Total etch + Apply primer + Apply bonding agent</td></tr>
<tr><td>Fifth</td><td>2</td><td>Total etch + Apply bonding agent</td></tr>
<tr><td>Sixth</td><td>1</td><td>Apply self etch adhesive</td></tr>
<tr><td>Seventh</td><td>1</td><td>Apply self etch adhesive</td></tr>
</table>

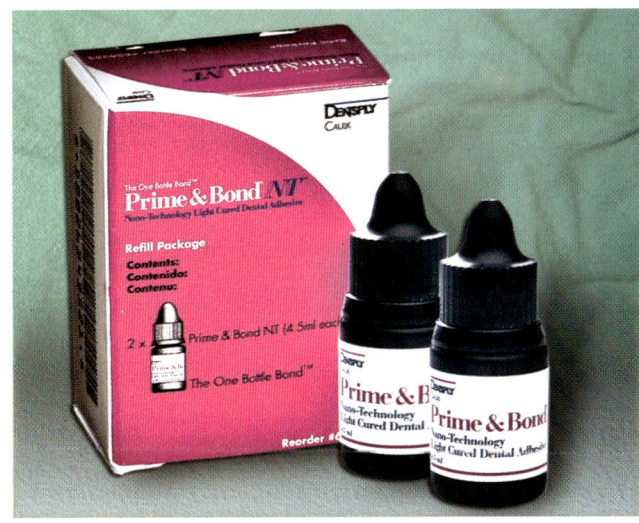

Figure 16.29: Nanofilled bonding agent

<table>
<tr><th colspan="6">Comparison of components of dentin bonding agents</th></tr>
<tr><th>Step</th><th>Fourth generation</th><th>Fifth generation</th><th>Sixth generation (self-etch primer)</th><th>Sixth generation (self-etch adhesive)</th><th>Seventh generation</th></tr>
<tr><td>1. Etching of enamel and dentin</td><td>Etchant</td><td>Etchant</td><td>Self etching, primer</td><td>Self etching, self priming sealer</td><td>self priming sealer</td></tr>
<tr><td>2. Priming of dentin</td><td>Primer</td><td>Self priming sealer</td><td>Selt etching primer</td><td>Same</td><td>Same</td></tr>
<tr><td>3. Bonding/sealing of enamel and dentin</td><td>Bonding agent</td><td>Self priming sealer</td><td>Bonding agent</td><td>Same</td><td>Same</td></tr>
</table>

Mild vs Strong self-etch adhesives

	Mild Self-etch adhesives (pH ≈ 2)	Strong Self-etch adhesives (pH ≈ 1)
Advantages	• Hydroxyapatite crystals available within the hybrid layer so better chemical interaction potential. • Good bond strength	Good enamel bonding
Disadvantages	Poor bonding to enamel	• No hydroxyapatite left throughout hybrid layer • Reduced shelf life • More hydrophilic • Lower dentin bond strengths • Incompatibility with autocuring composites

Two-step Etch and Rinse (one-bottle) Adhesives

Advantages
- Simpler application procedure
- Consistent and stable composition
- Hygienic application (to prevent cross contamination)
- Possibility for particle-filled adhesive, acts as "shock absorber".

Disadvantages
- More technique sensitive
- Risk of overetching because of presence of highly concentrated phosphoric acid etchants
- Risk of a bonding layer that is too thin
- Effects of etch and rinse technique
- Postconditioning rinse step is required, so chances of surface contamination
- Sensitive to dentin wetness and dryness
- Weak resin-collagen interaction
- Chances of collagen collapse due to overdried dentin
- Lower bonding effectiveness than for three-step etch- and rinse adhesives.

Self-etch Adhesives

One-step self-etch adhesives.

Advantages
- Easy and time-efficient application procedure
- No etching, postconditioning rinsing, or drying
- Possibility for single-dose packaging
- Consistent and stable composition
- Possibility for particle-filled adhesive, act as "shock absorber"
- Simultaneous demineralization and resin infiltration
- Less technique sensitivity.

Disadvantages
- Consists of both hydrophobic and hydrophilic components, together with water and high concentrations of solvents

- Prone to phase separation and entrapment of droplets in adhesive layer
- Most self-etch systems contain water, it influences polymerization badly.
- Reduced shelf life because of hydrolysis of monomers
- High hydrophilicity due to presence of acidic monomers
- Bonding effetiveness depends on composition of adhesive solution
- No long-term clinical evaluation
- Impaired durability
- Incompatibility with autocuring composites.

HYBRID LAYER AND HYBRIDIZATION

A dentin bonding agent is a low viscosity unfilled or semi-filled resin for easy penetration and formation of a hybrid layer. When a bonding agent is applied, part of it penetrates into the collagen network, known as intertubular penetration and the rest of it penetrates into dentinal tubules called intratubular penetration. In intertubular penetration, it polymerises with primer monomers forming a hybrid layer/resin reinforced layer (**Fig. 16.30**).

Hybridization (Given by Nakabayachi in 1982)

Hybridization is the process of formation of a hybrid layer. The hybrid layer is the phenomenon of formation of a

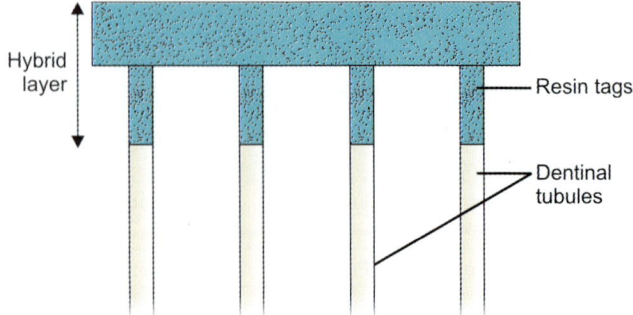

Figure 16.30: Diagrammatic representation of hybrid layer

resin interlocking in the demineralized dentin surface. The hybrid layer is responsible for micromechanical bonding between tooth and resin.

When dentin is treated with a conditioner, it exposes the collagen fibril network with interfibrillar microporosities. These spaces are filled with low viscosity monomers when primer is applied. This layer formed by demineralization of dentin and infiltration of monomer and subsequent polymerization is called the *hybrid layer*.

Hybridoid layer is that area of demineralized dentin into which resin fail to penetrate.

Zones of the Hybrid Layer (Fig. 16.31)

Hybrid layer has shown to have three different zones:
1. *Top layer:* Consists of loosely arranged collagen fibrils and interfibrillar spaces filled with resin.
2. *Middle layer:* Consists of interfibrillar spaces in which hydroxyapatite crystals have been replaced by resin monomer because of the hybridization process.
3. *Bottom layer:* Consists of almost unaffected dentin with a partly demineralized zone of dentin.

HEMA
➡ 2 Hydroxyethyl methacrylate
➡ Has both hydrophilic and hydrophobic ends
➡ Helps in increasing the wettability of hydrophobic agents
➡ Its low molecular weight infiltrates into the dentinal tubules
➡ Other monomers of same type are BPDM (biphenyl dimithacrylate), PMDMC (pyromellitic acid dimethacrylate and NTG - GMA (N-polyglycine glycidyl methacrylate)
➡ It retains water within adhesive formulations to decrease bonding
➡ It can polymerize only by linear polymerization so show weak polymerization in high concentrations.

META (By takeyama in 1978 as META/MMA-TBB)
➡ 4-methacryl-oxyethyl trimellitate anhydride
➡ Contains both hydrophilic and hydropholic ends
➡ Bonds to tooth due to excellant infilteration and chelation with Ca^{2+} ions as coupling agents
➡ Available as powder (containing PMMA) and liquid (containing MMA, META, TBB)
➡ Used as amalgam bonding agent and as a component in resin luting cement.

SMEAR LAYER

Unknown and unrecognized for years, the smear layer has become a factor to be considered. The advantages and disadvantages of the smear layer and whether it should be removed or not from a prepared tooth structure is still controversial. Boyde et al (1963) was the first to describe the presence of a smear layer on the surface of cut enamel.

Basically, when a tooth surface is altered using hand or rotary instruments, cutting debris are smeared on the enamel and dentin surface, this layer is called the smear layer (**Fig. 16.32**).

Structure

When viewed under a scanning electron microscope, the smear layer has an amorphous, irregular and granular appearance. Cameron (1983) and Mader (1984) described that smear layer consists of two separate parts:
1. One superficial and loosely attached to the underlying dentin
2. The other consisting of plugs of dentinal debris in the orifices of dentinal tubules (**Fig. 16.33**).

Depth

The smear layer has an average depth of 1 to 5 µm but in the dentinal tubules, it may go up to 40 µm. The depth of the smear layer depends on following factors:
• Dry or wet-cutting of the dentin
• Type of instrument used

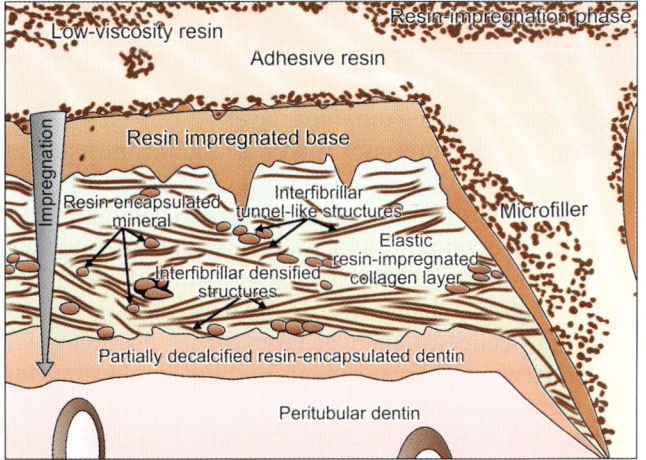

Figure 16.31: Diagrammatic presentation of different zones of hybrid layer

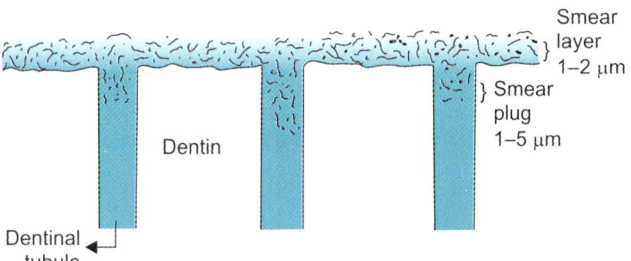

Figure 16.32: Smear layer and smear plugs

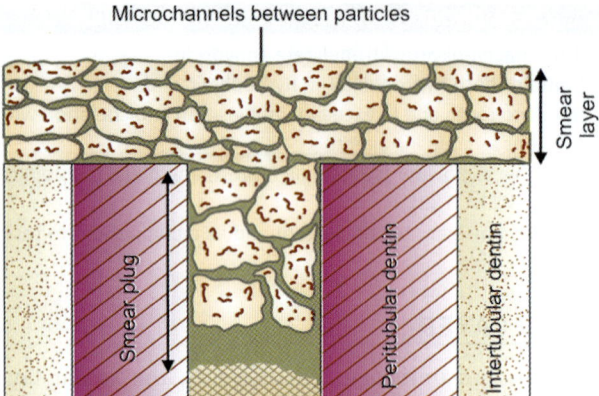

Figure 16.33: Magnified presentation of smear layer and plugs

- Chemical composition of irrigating solution when doing root canal treatment.

Dentin is composed of two different layers. Superficial dentin is dentin near the enamel. Deep dentin is near the pulp. Smear layers on deep dentin contains more organic material than superficial dentin because of greater number of proteoglycans lining the tubules and by the greater number of odontoblastic processes near pulp.

The adhesive strength of all cements is always 50 percent greater in superficial dentin. This may indicate that the quality and quantity of the smear layer found on superficial dentin may be greater than the smear layer produced on deep dentin.

Formation of the Smear Layer

When tooth structure is cut, instead of being uniformly sheared, the mineralized matrix shatters. Considerable quantities of cutting debris made-up of very small particles of mineralized collagen matrix are produced. Existing at the strategic interface between restorative materials and the dentin matrix, most of the debris is scattered over enamel and dentin surfaces to form what is known as the smear layer.

Because it is a very thin layer and is soluble in acid, the smear layer will not be apparent on routinely processed specimens examined with a light microscope. This may be why the smear layer received so little attention by restorative dentists.

Components of the Smear Layer

The smear layer consists of both organic and inorganic components.

The inorganic material in the smear layer is made-up of tooth structure and some nonspecific inorganic contaminants.

The organic components may consist of heated coagulated proteins (gelatin formed by the deterioration of collagen heated by cutting temperature), necrotic or viable pulp tissue and odontoblastic processes, saliva, blood cells and microorganisms.

A profile view of the specimen may show inconsistencies, disclosing fine particulate material, densely or loosely packed to various depths into dentinal tubules.

Role of the Smear Layer

The smear layer is apparently responsible for:
- Acting as a physical barrier for bacteria and bacterial products
- Restricting the surface area available for diffusion of both small and large molecules
- Resistance to fluid movement.

In vital teeth, the smear layer restricts the dentinal fluid from flushing the dentin surface. It also hinders the chemical process that produces the marginal seal.

In nonvital teeth, the marginal seal is improved because of the lack of moisture within dentinal tubules.

The initial sealing process occurring under amalgam restorations may be compromised because of the ability of the smear layer and its penchant for leaching under amalgam. This leaching process produces widening of the amalgam tooth microcrevice and ultimately weaking of the sealing mechanism.

Disadvantages of the Smear Layer

- Bonding to the smear layer forms a weak union because the smear layer can be torn away from the underlying matrix. Since this layer is nonhomogeneous and a weakly adherent structure, it may slowly disintegrate, dissolving around a leaking filling material, thus creating a void.

   Studies have shown that the bond strength of a glass ionomer cement to dentin can be increased significantly by removing the smear layer.
- Smear layers presence plays a significant part in increasing or decreasing in apical leakage which may be the cause of future failure of root canal fillings.
- Smear layer on root canal walls acts as an intermediate physical barrier and may interfere with adhesion and penetration of sealers into dentinal tubules.
- The prescence of a smear layer causes possibility for leakage of microorganisms and a source of substrate for bacterial growth.
- Presence of viable bacteria which may remain in the dentinal tubules and make use of the smear layer for sustained growth and activity.

Removal of the Smear Layer and its Antimicrobial Implications

Smear layer removal is a controversy that fluctuates with the various modalities of restorative dentistry.

In operative dentistry, it may depend on the type of dentin adhesive used or the use of glass ionomer.

In operative techniques, the concept of removing most of the smear layer over the tubules is an idea that is difficult to achieve clinically because of the complex geometry of many tooth preparations and the difficulty of achieving adequate success.

Inside the preparation, if the smear layer remains, it protects the pulp by plugging the tubules, preventing ingress of bacteria and their toxins as well as chemical toxins.

On the other hand, if it is removed, it allows absolute adaptation of the restoration to the true dentin surface, especially in the case of resins and amalgams. Microleakage is increased, if the smear layer remains, whereas dentin permeability is increased if the smear layer is removed.

The answer seems to lie in agents that clean the dentin surface yet leave tubules still plugged or better yet, completely clean the dentin and the tubuli orifices and then replug the tubules with a precipitate or a bonding agent.

Bonding or obturating to the smear layer must be considered a weak union because the smear layer can be torn away from the underlying matrix.

Role of the Smear Layer in Dentin Bonding

Smear layer may be deterrent to the bonding process, since it may serve as a barrier to the penetration of resin to the underlying dentin substrate.

Agents for Smear Layer Removal
➥ *Citric acid*: Acid etching dentin for 60 sec with 6 percent citric acid removed nearly all of the smear layer as well as the peritubular surface dentin. .
➥ *Polyacrylic acid*: It is used in combination with glass ionomer cement. An application of not more than 5 sec followed by a copious water rinse results in a cleaner surface.
➥ *Chelating agent, EDTA*: The use of chelating agents soften the smear layer allowing its successful removal. Although it is not bacteriocidal, it is considered to be antibacterial to the an extent since it eliminates the bacteria contaminated smear layer.
➥ *Maleic acid*: Maleic acid has been used as an acid conditioner in some adhesive systems.

Classification of Modern Adhesives

Basically, three adhesion strategies have been employed to modern dentin bonding agents on the basis of their interaction with the smear layer. These are:

- Smear layer modifying agents
- Smear layer removing agents
- Smear layer dissolving agents.

Smear Layer Modifying Agents

In this strategy bonding agents modify the smear layer and incorporate it in the bonding process. According to these, the smear layer acts as a natural protective barrier to the pulp, protecting it against bacterial penetration and also limiting the outflow of dentinal fluid which can hamper the bonding process.

Steps: In these, enamel is selectively etched with 37 percent phosphoric acid (taking care not to etch dentin). After washing and drying the tooth, primer and adhesive are applied separately or in combination. This results in micromechanical interaction of dentin and bonding system without exposure of collagen fibrils. For example, Prime and Bond.

Smear Layer Removing Dentin Adhesives

These bonding agents completely remove the smear layer employing the total etch concept. They work on the principle of hybrid layer and resin tags.

Steps: In these, enamel and dentin are etched simultaneously using an acid (preferably 37% phosphoric acid). After washing and drying the tooth surface, primer and bonding agent are applied either separately or in combination. For example:
- Scotch bond multipurpose
- Gluma.

Smear Layer Dissolving Adhesives

These agents partly demineralize the smear layer and the superficial dentin surface without removing the remnants of smear layer or the smear plugs. They make use of acidic primers also termed as self-etch primers or self-etch adhesives which provides simultaneous conditioning and priming of both enamel and dentin. After this, adhesive is applied without washing the tooth surface.

The basis for use of these systems is to condition the dentin and to simultaneously penetrate to the depth of demineralized dentin with monomers which can be polymerized. For example:
- Self-etch primer – Adper prompt
- Self-etch adhesive – Prompt – L – pop.

GLASS IONOMER BASED ADHESIVE SYSTEM

This is a new revolution in the adhesive dentistry where adhesive agents are based on resin modified glass ionomer technology. Glass ionomer based adhesives are resin diluted versions of resin modified glass ionomers where bonding occurs by interdiffusion of resin which forms the hybrid layer and then the chemical bonding takes place between tooth and the glass ionomer (**Fig. 16.34**).

Steps

Here both enamel and dentin are conditioned using poly-acrylic acid and washed. Polyacrylic acid conditions the tooth surface by removing the smear layer and exposing

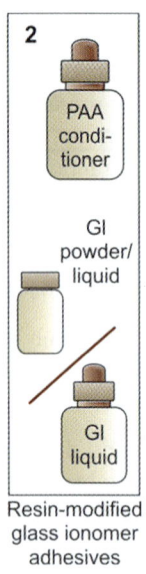

Figure 16.34: Glass ionomer based adhesives

the smear plugs. After this, adhesive is applied and light cured. For example, Fuji bond LC.

Advantages
- Easy and simple application
- Anticariogenicity because of fluoride release
- Dual bonding mechanism:
  - Micromechanical
  - Chemical.
- Adhesive filled with viscous particles, thus act as a shock absorber.

Disadvantages
- Adequate bonding requires smear layer removal
- Coarse particles present in the formulation may result in white lines around restoration
- Long-term clinical research not present.

FAILURE OF DENTIN BONDING (FIG. 16.35)

Reasons for failure of dentin bonding
Dentin can show poor bonding because of following reasons:
➡ Variable structure of dentin
➡ Contamination of dentin with sulcular fluid or saliva
➡ Structural changes of dentin close to the pulp make it difficult to bond
➡ Thickening of bonding agent because of evaporation of solvent. This reduces the penetration of the bonding agent.
➡ Contamination of tooth surface by lubricants used in hand-pieces
➡ Any contact of tooth surface with blood, can result in decrease in bond strength.

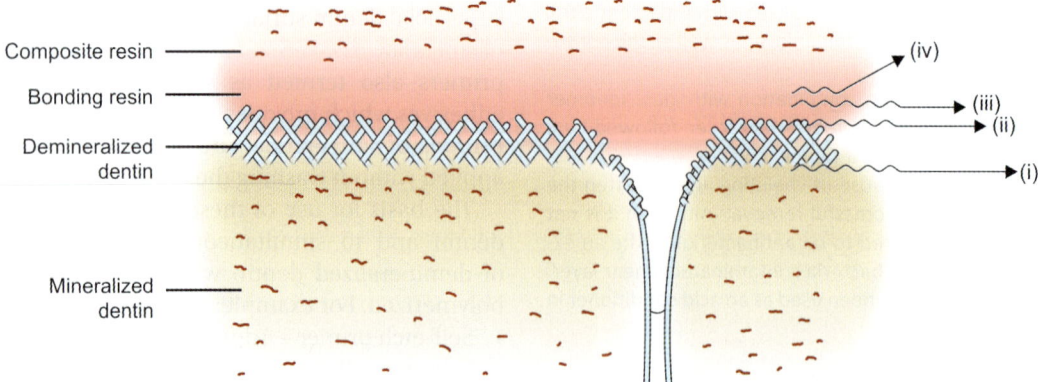

Figure 16.35: Failure of composite adhesive and tooth joint can occur between: (i) Mineralized and demineralized dentin; (ii) Bonding agent and dentin; (iii) Bonding agent; (iv) Composite and bonding agent

Key Points

- In 1955 Buonocore applied acid to tooth to render the tooth more receptive to adhesion.
- For enamel etching, 37 percent phosphoric acid is used for 15 to 30 seconds. If the concentration is greater than 50 percent, then monocalcium phosphate monohydrate may get precipitated while at concentrations lower than 30 percent, dicalcium phosphate monohydrate is precipitated which interferes with adhesion.
- Conditioning is the process of cleaning the surface and activating the calcium ions, so as to make them more reactive.
- Etching is the process of increasing the surface reactivity by demineralizing the superficial calcium layer and thus creating the enamel tags. These tags are responsible for micromechanical bonding between tooth and restorative resin.
- Primers are used to increase the diffusion of resin into moist and demineralized dentin and thus optimal micromechanical bonding. For optimal penetration of primer into demineralized dentin, it should be applied in multiple coats.
- Etching of dentin results in removal of smear layer and minerals from dentin structure, exposing the collagen fibers. Areas from where minerals are removed are filled with water. This water acts as a plasticizer for collagen, keeping them in an expanded soft state. Thus, spaces for resin infiltration are also preserved.
- If the dentin surface is made too dry, there will be collapse of the collagen fibers and demineralized dentin. This results in low bond strength because of ineffective penetration of the adhesive into the dentin.
- The basic differences between the fourth and fifth generation dentin bonding agents is the number of basic components of bottles. The fourth generation bonding system is available in two bottles, one consisting of the primer and the other the adhesive, the fifth generation dentin bonding agents are available in one bottle only. This makes the fifth generation bonding agents simpler and faster than the fourth generation systems.
- Because of presence of acidic primer, sixth generation bonding agents do not have a long shelf life and thus have to be refreshed frequently.
- Total etch technique involves the complete removal of the smear layer by simultaneous acid etching of enamel and dentin. After total etching, primer and adhesive resin are applied separately or together. Acid removes the dentin smear layer, raises surface energy and modifies the dentin substrate so that it can be infiltrated by subsequently placed primers and resins.

- Nanofilled bonding agents contain extremely small filler particles.
- Hybridization is the process of formation of hybrid layer. Hybrid layer is phenomenon of formation of resin interlocking in the demineralized dentin surface. Hybrid layer is responsible for micromechanical bonding between tooth and the resin.
- Bonding to the smear layer forms a weak union because smear layer can be torn away from the underlying matrix. Since this layer is nonhomogeneous and weakly adherent structure, it may slowly disintegrate, dissolving around a leaking filling material, thus creating a void.
- Glass ionomer based adhesives are resin diluted versions of resin modified glass ionomers where bonding occurs by interdiffusion of resin which forms the hybrid layer and then the chemical bonding takes place between tooth and the glass ionomer.

QUESTIONS

1. What is scope of adhesive dentistry? Discuss in detail about the mechanism and factors affecting adhesion.
2. Short notes on:
   a. Enamel bonding
   b. Moist vs dry dentin bobding
   c. Smear layer.
   d. Self etch primers
   e. Hybridization
3. Explain in detail dentin bonding agents.
4. Write in brief about the enamel etching and bonding agents.
5. Write short notes on:
   a. Acid etching technique
   b. Bonding system
6. Discuss in detail about the smear layer.
7. What are dentin bonding agents and discuss its different generations of dentin bonding agents. Also discuss the reasons for failure of dentin bonding agent.

BIBLIOGRAPHY

1. Abdalla AI, García-Godoy F: Bond strengths of resin-modified glass ionomers and polyacid-modified resin composites to dentin, Am J Dent. 1997;10:291-4.
2. Aida M, Hayakawa T, Mizukawa K. Adhesion of composite to porcelain with various surface conditions. JPD. 1995;73:464.
3. al-Salehi SK, Burke FJ: Methods used in dentin bonding tests: an analysis of 50 investigations on bond strength, Quintessence Int. 1997;28:717-23.
4. Armstrong SR, et al: Microtensile bond strength of a total-etch 3-step, total-etch 2-step, self-etch 2 step, and a self-etch

1-step dentin bonding system through 15-month water storage, J Adhes Dent. 2003;5:47-56.

5. Armstrong SR, et al: The influence of water storage and C-factor on the dentin-resin composite microtensile bond strengths and debond pathway utilizing a filled and unfilled adhesive resin, Dent Mater. 2001;17:268-76.

6. Asmussen E, Munksgaard EC: Bonding of restorative materials to dentine: status of dentine adhesives and impact on cavity design and filling techniques, Int Dent J. 1988;38:97-104.

7. Baier RE: Principles of adhesion, Oper Dent 5 (suppl): 1992;1-9.

8. Barkmeier WW, et al: Shear bond strength to dentin and Ni-Cr-Be alloy with the All-Bond universal adhesive system, J Esthet Dent. 1991;3:148-53.

9. Bastos PAM, et al: Effect of etch duration on the shear bond strength of a microfill composite resin to enamel, Am J Dent. 1988;1:151-7.

10. Belcher MA, Stewart GP: Two-year clinical evaluation of an amalgam adhesive, J Am Dent Assoc. 1997;128:309-14.

11. Ben-Amar A, et al: Long term sealing properties of Amalgambond under amalgam restorations, Am J Dent. 1994;7:141-3.

12. Bergenholtz G: Iatrogenic injury to the pulp in dental procedures: aspects of pathogenesis, management and preventive measures, Int Dent J. 1991;41:99-110.

13. Bertolotti RL, et al: Adhesive monomers for porcelain repair, Int J Prosthodont. 1989;2:483-9.

14. Bertolotti RL. Total etch – the rational dentine bonding protocol J Esthet Dent. 1991;1:1.

15. Blosser RL. Time dependence of 2.5% nitric acid solution as an etchant on human dentine and enamel Dent Mater. 1990;6:83.

16. Bouschlicher MR, et al: Surface treatment for resin composite repair, Am J Dent. 1997;10:2790-283.

17. Bowen RL, et al: Adhesive bonding of various materials to hard tooth tissue: forces developing in composite materials during hardening. J Am Dent Assoc. 1983;106:475-7.

18. Bowen RL, Rodriguez MS: Tensile strength and modulus of elasticity of tooth structure and several restorative materials, J Am Dent Assoc. 1962;64:378-87.

19. Bowen RL, Tung MS, Blosser RL, Asmussen E. Dentine and enamel bonding agents. IDJ. 1987;37:158.

20. Braem M, et al: Stifness increase during the setting of dental composite resing, J Dent Res. 1987;66:1713-6.

21. Brännström M, et al: movement of dentinal and pulpal fluid caused by clinical procedures, J Dent Res. 1968;47:679-82.

22. Brännström M, et al: The hydrodynamics of the dental tubule and of pulp fluid: a discussion of its significance in relation to dentinal sensitivity, Caries Res. 1967;1:310-7.

23. Brännström M: The effect of dentin desiccation and aspirated odontoblasts on the pulp, J Prosthet Dent. 1968;20:165-71.

24. Brewer JA, Pashley DH. Regional bond strengths of resins to human root dentine J Dent. 1996;24:435.

25. Browne RM, Tobias RS. Microbial leakage and pulpal inflammation. A review. Endod, Dent Traumatol. 1986;2:177.

26. Buonocore M, et al: A report on a resin composition capable of bonding to human dentin surfaces J Dent Res. 1956;35:846-51.

27. Burke FJT, McCaugthey AD. The four generations of dentine bonding Am J Dent. 1995;8:88.

28. Burke FJT, Watts DC: Fracture resistance of teeth restored with dentin-bonded crowns, Quintessence Int. 1994;25:335-40.

29. Burke FJT. Tooth fracture in vivo and in vitro: A review. J. Dent. 1992;20:131.

30. Causton BE. Improved, bonding of composite restorative to dentine. BDJ. 1984;156:93.

31. Chang J, et al: Shear bond strength of a 4-META adhesive system, J Prosthet Dent. 1992;67:42-5.

32. Chow LC, Brown WE: Phosphoric acid conditioning of teeth for piot and fissure sealants, J Dent Res. 1973;52:1158.

33. Christensen G: Preventing postoperative tooth sensitivity in Class I, II, and V restorations J Am Dent Assoc. 2002;133:229-31.

34. Christensen GJ. Bonding resin to dentin – Fact or facny. JADA. 1991;122:71.

35. Cooley RL, Dodge WW: Bond strength of three dentinal adhesives on recently extracted versus aged teeth, Quintessence Int. 1989;20:513-6.

36. Cooley RL, et al: Dentinal bond strengths and microleakage of a 4-META adhesive to amalgam and composite resin, Quintessence Int. 1991;22:979-83.

37. Davidson CL. et al: The competition between the composite-dentin bond strength and the polymerization contraction stress, J Dent Res. 1984;63:1396-9.

38. Diaz-Arnold AM, et al: Procelain repairs: an evaluation of the shear strength of three porcelain repair systems (abstract 806), J Dent Res. 1987;66:207.

39. Duke ES, Lindemuth J: Polymeric adhesion to dentin: contrasting substrates, Am J Dent. 1991;4:241-6.

40. Duke ES. Adhesion and its application with restorative materials. DCNA. 1993;37:329.

41. Eakle WS, et al: Mechanical retention versus bonding of amalgam and gallium alloy restorations, J Presthet Dent. 1994;72:351-4.

42. Eick JD, Robinson SJ, Byerley TJ, Chappelow CC. Adhesives and non-shrinking dental resins of the future. Quint Int. 1993;24:632.

43. Eliades G: Clinical relevance of the formulation and testing of dentine bonding systems, J Dent. 1994;22:73-81.

44. Erickson RL, Glasspoole EA. Bonding to tooth structure: A comparison of glass ionomer and composite resin systems J Esthet Dent. 1994;6:221.

45. Feilzer A, et al: Setting stress in composite resin in relation to configuration of the restoration, J Dent Res. 1987;66:1636-9.

46. Felton DA, et al: Evaluation of the desensitizing effect of Gluma dentin bond on teeth prepared for complete coverage restorations, Int J Prosthodont. 1991;4:292-8.

47. Ferrari M, et al: Clinical evaluation of a one-bottle bonding system for desensitizing exposed roots, Am J Dent. 1999;12:243-9.

48. Finger WJ, Uno S. Bond strength of Gluma CPS using the moist dentin bonding technique Am J Dent. 1996;9:27.

49. Freedman G, Goldstep F. Fifth generation bonding systems: State of the art in adhesive dentistry J Can Dent. Assoc. 1997;63:439.

50. Fuks AB, et al: Pulp response to a composite resin inserted in a deep cavities with and without a surface seal, J Prosthet Dent. 1990;63:129-34.

51. Fusayama T, Nakamura M, Kurosaki M, Iwaka M. Nonpressure adhesion of a new adhesive restorative resin. JDR. 1979;58:1364.

52. Gilpatrick RO, et al: Resin-to-enamel bond strengths with various etching times, Quintessence Int. 1991;22:47-9.

53. Gordan VV, et al: Effect of different liner treatments on post-operative sensitivity of amalgam restorations, Quintessence Int. 1999;30:55-9.

54. Gwinnett AJ, Buonocore MG: Adhesion and caries prevention: a preliminary report, Br Dent J. 1965;119:77-80.

55. Gwinnett AJ, García-Godoy F: Effect of etching time and acid concentration on resin enamel, Am J Dent. 1992;5:237-9.

56. Gwinnett AJ, Kanca J: Interfacial morphology of resin composite and shiny erosion lesions, Am J Dent. 1992;5:315-7.

57. Gwinnett AJ, Kanca JA: Micromorphology of the bonded dentin interface and its relationship to bond strength, Am J Dent 1992;5:73-7.

58. Gwinnett AJ. Moist versus dry dentin: its effect on shear bond strength, Am J Dent 1992;5:127-9.

59. Gwinnett AJ: Moist versus dry dentin: its effect on shear bond strength, Am J Dent. 1992;5:127-9.

60. Hansen EK, Asmussen E: Comparative study of dentin adhesives, Scand J Dent Res. 1985;93:280-7.

61. Hansen EK, Asmussen E: Improved efficacy of dentin-bonding agents, Eur J Oral Sci. 1997;105:434-9.

62. Hansen EK: Effect of Scotchbond dependent on cavity cleaning, cavity diameter and cavosurface angle, Scand J Dent Res. 1984;92:141-7.

63. Heymann HO, Bayne SC: Current concepts in dentin bonding: focusing on dentinal adhesion factors, J Am Dent Assoc. 1993;124:27-36.

64. Ito S, et al: Effects of multiple all-in-one adhesive coatings on dentin bonding (abstract 233), J Dent Res 83 (special issue A), 2004.

65. Mount GJ: Adhesion of glass-ionomer cement in the clinical environment, Oper Dent. 1991;16:141-8.

66. Murray PE, et al: Bacterial microleakage and pulp inflammation associated with various restorative materials, Dent Mater. 2002;18:470-8.

67. Nelson RJ, et al: Fluid exchange at the margins of dental restorations, J Am Dent Assoc. 1952;44:288.

68. Oliveira SS et al: The influence of the dentin smear layer on adhesion: a self-etching primer vs. a total-etch system, Dent Mater. 2003;19:758-67.

69. Olmez A, et al: Clinical evaluation and marginal leakage of Amalgambond Plus: three-year results, Quintessence Int. 1997;28:651-6.

70. Perdigão J Dentin bonding as a function of dentin structure, Dent Clin North Am. 2002;46:277-301.

71. Perdigão J, et al: Total-etch versus self-etch adhesive: effect on postoperative sensitivity, J Am Dent Assoc. 2003;134:1621-9.

72. Pilo R, et al: Cusp reinforcement by bonding of amalgam restorations, J Dent. 1998;26:467-72.

73. Prati C, et al: Shear bond strength and SEM evaluation of dentinal bonding systems, Am J Dent. 1990;3:283-8.

74. Reinhardt JW, et al: Effect of Gluma desensitization on dentin bond strength, Am J Dent. 1995;8:170-2.

75. Reinhardt JW, et al: Shear strengths of ten commercial dentin bonding agents, Dent Mater. 1987;3:43-5.

76. Retief DH. Adhesion to Dentine J Esthet Dent. 1991;3:106.

77. Sepetcioglu F, Ataman BA: Long-term monitoring of micro-leakage of cavity varnish and adhesive resin with amalgam, J Prosthet Dent. 1998;79:136-9.

78. Shupach P, et al: Closing of dentinal tubules by Gluma desensitizer. Eur J Oral Sci. 1997;105:414-21.

79. Staaford JW, Sabri Z, Jose S. A comparison of the effectiveness of dentin bonding agents. Int Dent J. 1985;35:139.

80. Taira Y, Imai Y. Primer for bonding resin to metal. Dent Mater. 1995;11:2.

81. Tani C, Finger WJ: Effect of smear layer thickness on bond strength mediated by three all-in-one self-etching priming adhesives, J Adhes Dent. 2003;16:340-6.

82. Tyas MJ. Clinical evaluation of five adhesive systems. Am J Dent. 1994;7:77.

17

CHAPTER

Composite Restorations

Chapter Outline

INTRODUCTION

An interpretation of esthetics is primarily governed by an individual's perception and varies from person to person. What is pleasing for one person, may not be satisfactory to another. Therefore, it is the clinician's responsibility to have knowledge of all restorative alternatives so as to present it to the patient and help him to reach at final decision about the choice of restorative material. The materials which have been used for aesthetic restorations are silicate cement, glass ionomer, acrylic resins, composites and fused porcelain. The modern history of tooth colored restorative materials started with silicate cement which was introduced by Fletcher in the year 1878 in England, and further encouraged by Steenback and Ashor in 1903. Silicate cements were discouraged later on because of their poor strength, irritation to pulp tissue and brittleness. Moreover tooth preparations for silicate cement need to be of the conventional type.

Self-curing acrylic resins were developed in 1930 in Germany, but they became popular in dentistry in late 1940s. They were used as veneers on the facial surface of metal restorations and as facings in crowns and bridges. But they too showed poor physical properties like high polymerization shrinkage and coefficient of thermal expansion (CTE), lack of wear resistance, poor marginal seal, irritation to pulp and dimensional instability.

In an attempt to improve their properties, R Bowen, in 1962 developed a polymeric dental restorative material reinforced with silica particles used as fillers. These materials were called 'composites'. Thus, we can say that composite resins have been introduced in operative dentistry to overcome the drawbacks of the acrylic resins that replaced silicate cements in the 1940s. Over the past two decades, there has been a substantial progress in the development and application of resin-based composites. Earlier composites were recommended only as a restorative material for anterior restorations, but now they have become one of the most commonly used direct restorative materials for both anterior and posterior teeth. This is because of better understanding of their application methods, including composite placement and curing and improvement of their physical and mechanical properties. The principal reasons for the shifting from dental amalgam to composites are the reduced need for preparation and the strengthening effect on the remaining tooth. Roeters et al. has said once that the introduction of resin composites is not just a change in materials and techniques but also a change in treatment philosophy. Nowadays, composite resins are considered as an economical and aesthetic alternative to other direct and indirect restorative materials. They can be used in different clinical conditions like diastema closures, veneers for anterior teeth and restorations for Class I, II, III, IV, and V conservative restorations. If properly manipulated, they can prove the success rate and longevity equal to those of other materials. Since composites do not have self-adhering property, an adhesive is required before their placement. Placement of a composite resin is very technique-sensitive than the placement of other restorations.

By definition, a composite is a compound composed of atleast two different materials with properties which are superior or intermediate to those of an individual component.

Dental composite resins have two primary components which are matrix phase and the filler phase and many secondary components like polymerization initiators, pigments for providing different shades and silane coupling agents. Though secondary components are required for every composite material, but most of the properties of material are dependent upon filler and matrix phases.

Although different composite materials have specific composition and distribution of the matrix and filler particles, but more often they are composed of bisphenol-A-diglycidylmethacrylate (Bis-GMA) or urethane dimethacrylate (UDMA) matrix polymers and glass filler particles. Both the amount and the size of the filler particles determine mechanical properties of different composites.

History of composite resins (From 1901–2007)
→ 1901 Synthesis and polymerization of methyl methacrylate
→ 1930 Use of PMMA as denture base resin
→ 1944 First acrylic filling material
→ 1951 Addition of inorganic fillers to direct filling materials
→ 1955 Acid etch technique introduced by Buonocore
→ 1956 Bowen investigated dimethacrylates (Bis-GMA) and silanized inorganic filler
→ 1962 Introduction of silane coupling agents
→ 1964 Marketing of Bis-GMA composites
→ 1968 Development of polymeric coatings on fillers
→ 1973 UV-cured dimethacrylate composite resins
→ 1976 Introduction of microfilled composites
→ 1977 Visible light cured dimethacrylate composite resins
→ 1996 Development of flowable composites
→ 1997 Development of packable composites
→ 1998 Development of fiber reinforced, ion releasing composites and ormocers.

COMPOSITION OF COMPOSITES

Composites are basically modified methacrylates or acrylates with other ingredients to produce different structures and properties. The *methacrylates are used because of their refractive index of* 1.3 which is close to tooth. This allows metamerism (chameleon effect). Since methacrylate shrinks on polymerization, to counter the effect of shrinkage, the inorganic inert filler particles of similar refractive index are added.

Dental composites are composed of following materials (Fig. 17.1)
➡ Organic matrix or organic phase
➡ Inorganic matrix
➡ Filler or dispersed phase
➡ An organosilane or coupling agent
➡ Activator-initiator system
➡ Inhibitors
➡ Coloring agents.

Composition of composites
Organic resins
➡ Bis-GMA (Bowen's resin)
➡ Dipentaerythritol pentaacrylate monophosphate
➡ Urethane dimethacrylate (UDMA)
➡ Urethane tetramethacrylate
➡ Hexamethylene diisocyanate
Fillers
➡ Fused or crystalline quartz
➡ Silicon dioxide
➡ Borosilicate/Lithium aluminosilicate glass
➡ Ceramics
➡ Ytterbium trifluoride
➡ Radiopaque silicates
➡ Organically modified ceramics (ORMOCERS)
Others
➡ Triethylene glycol dimethacrylate (TEGDMA)
➡ 2-hydroxylethyl methacrylate (HEMA)
➡ Camphoroquinone (CQ)
➡ META; phospherated esters
➡ Silane coupling agents
➡ Antibacterial monomers
➡ Benzoyl peroxide and amine activator

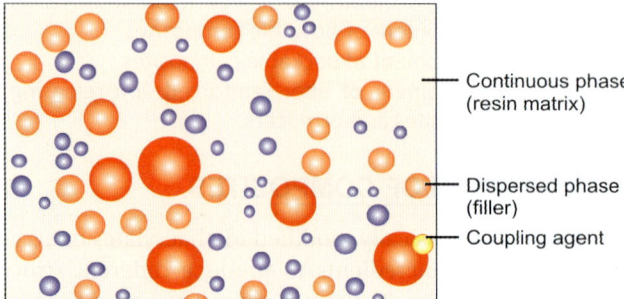

Figure 17.1: Composition of composite resin

Organic Matrix

The matrix base consists of polymeric mono-, di- or trifunctional monomers like Bis-GMA or UDMA. The monomer system represents as the backbone of the composite resin system. Most preferred monomer is Bis-GMA either alone or in conjunction with urethane dimethacrylate UDMA. Since this resin is very viscous, in order to improve clinical handling, it is diluted with low viscosity monomers to control the viscosity. These can be bisphenol A dimethacrylate (Bis-DMA), ethylene glycol dimethacrylate (EGDMA), triethylene glycol dimethacrylate (TEGDMA), methyl methacrylate (MMA). Bis-GMA and TEGDMA have been tried in the ratio of 1:1 and 3:1, later is preferred because an increase in TEGDMA increases the chances of polymerization shrinkage.

Fillers

The dispersed phase of composite resins is made up of an inorganic filler material. Since filler particles are added to improve the physical and mechanical properties of the organic matrix, the basic aim is always to incorporate high percentage of filler. Commonly used fillers are silicon dioxide, boron silicates and lithium aluminum silicates. The filler particles are silanated so that the hydrophilic filler can bond to the hydrophobic resin matrix. The wear of composite restorations depends on filler particle size, interparticle spacing and filler loading. Composites with smaller particles show decreased wear due to fewer voids and smaller interparticle spacing.

In composite resin, the addition of filler
➡ Reduces the coefficient of thermal expansion
➡ Reduces polymerization shrinkage
➡ Increases abrasion resistance
➡ Decreases water sorption
➡ Increases tensile and compressive strengths
➡ Increases fracture toughness
➡ Increases flexure modulus
➡ Provides radiopacity
➡ Improves handling properties
➡ Increases translucency

In some composites, the quartz is partly replaced with heavy metal particles like zinc, aluminum, barium, strontium or zirconium. Nowadays calcium metaphosphate has also been tried. Since these are less hard than glass, so they cause less wear on the opposing tooth.

Recently nanoparticles having the size of 25 nm and nanoaggregates of 75 nm, made up of zirconium/silica or nanosilica particles have also been introduced. The smaller size of filler particles results in better finish of the restoration.

Coupling Agents

Interfacial bonding between the matrix phase and the filler phase is provided by coating the filler particles with silane coupling agents. In other words, a coupling agent is used to bond the filler to the organic resin. This agent is a molecule with silane groups at one end (ion bond to SiO_2) and methacrylate groups at the other.

Functions of coupling agents
➡ Bonding of filler and resin matrix
➡ Transfer forces from flexible resin matrix to stiffer filler particles
➡ Prevent penetration of water along filler resin interface, thus provide hydrolytic stability
➡ Examples: Organic silane.
♦ r–methacryloxypropyltrimethoxysilane
♦ 10–methacryloxydecyltrimethoxysilane.

Coloring Agents

Coloring agents are used in very small percentage to produce different shades of composites. Mostly metal oxides such as titanium oxide and aluminum oxides are added to improve the opacity of composite resins.

Ultraviolet Absorbers

They are added to prevent discoloration, in other words they act like a "sunscreen" to composites. Commonly used UV absorber is benzophenone.

Initiator Agents

These agents activate the polymerization of composites. Most common photoinitiator used is camphoroquinone. Currently most recent composites are polymerized by exposure to visible light in the range of 410 to 500 nm.

Initiator varies with type of composites whether it is light cured or chemically cured.

Inhibitors

These agents inhibit the free radical generated by spontaneous polymerization of the monomers. For example, Butylated hydroxyl toluene (0.01%).

Difference between chemically cured and light cured composites

Chemically cured	Light cured
• Polymerization is central	• Polymerization is towards the source of light in the center
• Less color stability	• More than chemically cured
• Curing is done in single step, i.e. at one time	• Placement of material is done in increments
• Very less working time	• Adequate working time for insertion and contouring
• Setting time is long	• Sets after activation by light
• Less esthetics	• Esthetically good
• Economical	• Expensive
• More polymerization shrinkage	• Less polymerization shrinkage
• Less abrasion resistance	• More abrasion resistance

Initiator–activator system used in various types of composites

Type of composite	Initiator-activator system
• Chemically cured composite	• Benzoyl peroxide and 2% aromatic tertiary amine
• Ultraviolet light activated	• 0.1% Benzoin methyl ether composite
• Visible light cured composite	• 0.06% camphoroquinone and tertiary amine

Difference between visible light and ultraviolet light curing

Visible light curing	UV light curing
• Wavelength required for activation is 400-500 nm	• Wavelength required for activation is 360-400 nm
• Greater depth of curing is possible (up to 3 mm)	• Limited penetration (up to 1-2 mm)
• Intensity remains constant	• Intensity decreases with usage
• Less side effect to operator and patient's eye	• Harmful to operator and patient's eyes, can cause corneal burns
• Better color stability	• Less than visible light
• No warm up time required	• Units need warm up time of 5 minutes

CLASSIFICATION OF COMPOSITES

Composite resins can be classified according to filler size, percent filler loading, and the viscosity of the composite. With the expanded categories of composite resins, they can also be classified according to their uses.

Different classifications of composite:
- ***According to Skinner:***
  - Traditional or conventional composite—8-12 μm
  - Small particle filled composites—1-5 μm
  - Microfilled composites—0.4-0.9 μm
  - Hybrid composites—0.6-1 μm
- ***Philips and Lutz classification according to filler particle size:***
  - Macrofiller composites (particles from 0.1-100 μ)
  - Microfiller composites (0.04 μ particles)
  - Hybrid composites (fillers of different sizes).

- **According to the mean particles size of the major fillers:**
  - Traditional composite resins
  - Hybrid composite resins
  - Homogeneous microfilled composites—if the composite simply consists of fillers and uncured matrix material, it is classified as homogeneous
  - Heterogeneous microfilled composites—if it includes procured composites and other unusual filler, it is called as heterogeneous.
- **Classification according to Bayne and Heyman**

  Category   Particle size
  - Megafill   1-2 mm
  - Macrofill   10-100 μm
  - Midifill   1-10 μm
  - Minifill   0.1-1 μm
  - Microfill   0.01-0.1 μm
  - Nanofill   0.005-0.01 μm
- **Classification according to matrix compositions**
  - Bis-GMA
  - UDMA
- **Classification according to polymerization method**
  - Self-curing
  - Ultraviolet light curing
  - Visible light curing
  - Dual curing
  - Staged curing.

TYPES OF COMPOSITE RESINS

Though composites have been classified according to different characteristics, the most commonly followed classification is based on the type, distribution and filler phase of composites.

Composite resin can be divided into three types based on the size, amount and composition of the inorganic filler (**Figs 17.2A to C**):

1. Macrofilled composite resins
2. Microfilled resins
3. Hybrid composite resins.

Macrofilled Composite Resins

Average particle size of macrofill composite resins is from 5 to 25 micron. Filler content is approximately 75 to 80 percent by weight.

It exhibits a rough surface texture because of the relatively large size and extreme hardness of the filler particles. The surface becomes more rough as the resin matrix being less hard, wears at faster rate.

Due to roughness, discoloration and wearing of occlusal contact areas and plaque accumulation take place quickly than other types of composites.

Advantage of conventional composite
Physical and mechanical performance is better than unfilled acrylic resins.

Disadvantages
➡ Rough surface finish
➡ Poor polishability
➡ More wear
➡ More prone to staining.

Microfilled Composites Resins (Fig.17.3)

Microfilled composites were introduced in the early 1980s. Average particle size of microfilled resins ranges from 0.04 to 0.1 micrometer. Filler content of microfilled resins is 35 to 50 percent by weight. The small particle size results in smooth polished surface which is resistant to plaque, debris and stains.

But because of less filler content, some of their physical properties are inferior. They have low modulus of elasticity and high polishability, excellent translucency however, they exhibit low fracture toughness and increased marginal breakdown.

They are indicated for the restoration of anterior teeth and cervical abfraction lesions.

Advantages
➡ Highly polishable
➡ Good esthetic.

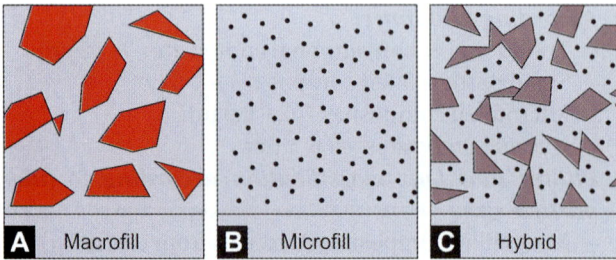

Figures 17.2A to C: Diagrammatic representation of different composites

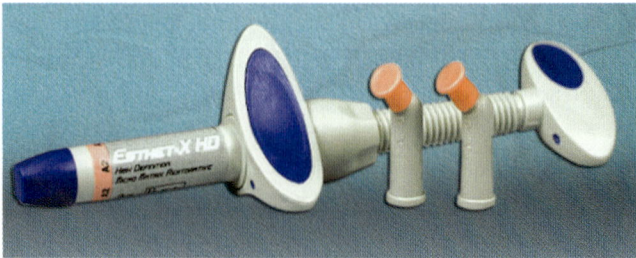

Figure 17.3: Microfilled composite resin

Disadvantages

- Poor mechanical properties due to more matrix content
- Poor color stability
- Low wear resistance
- Less modulus of elasticity and tensile strength
- More water absorption
- High coefficient of thermal expansion.

Hybrid Composite Resins

In order to combine the advantages of conventional and microfilled composites, hybrid composites were developed. Hybrid composites are named so because they are made up of polymer groups (organic phase) reinforced by an inorganic phase. Hybrid composites are composed of glasses of different compositions and sizes, with particle size diameter of less than 2 µm and containing 0.04 µm sized fumed silica. Filler content in these composites is 75 to 80 percent by volume. This mixture of fillers is responsible for their physical properties similar to those of conventional composites with the advantage of smooth surface texture.

Advantages of hybrid composites

- Availability in various colors
- Different degrees of opaqueness and translucency in different tones and fluorescence
- Excellent polishing and texturing properties
- Good abrasion and wear resistance
- Similar coefficient of thermal expansion
- Ability to imitate the tooth structure
- Decreased polymerization shrinkage
- Less water absorption.

Disadvantages of hybrid composites

- Not appropriate for heavy stress bearing areas
- Not highly polishable as microfilled because of presence of larger filler particles in between smaller ones
- Loss of gloss occurs when exposed to toothbrushing with abrasive toothpaste.

Two new generations of hybrid composite resins are:
1. Nanofill and nanohybrids
2. Microhybrids.
1. ***Nanofill and nanohybrid composites (Fig. 17.4):*** Nanofill and nanohybrid composites have average particle size less than that of microfilled composites.

The introduction of these extremely small fillers and their proper arrangement within the matrix results in physical properties equivalent to the original hybrid composite resins.

Advantages to nano composites

- Highly polishable
- Tooth like translucency with excellent esthetic
- Optimal mechanical properties
- Good handling characterstics.
- Good color stability
- Stain resistance
- High wear resistance
- Can be used for both anterior and posterior restorations and for splinting teeth with fiber ribbons.

2. ***Microhybrid composites (Fig. 17.5):*** Microhybrid composites have evolved from traditional hybrid composites.

Filler content in microhybrids are 56 to 66 percent by volume. The average particle size in these composites range from 0.4 to 0.8 µm.

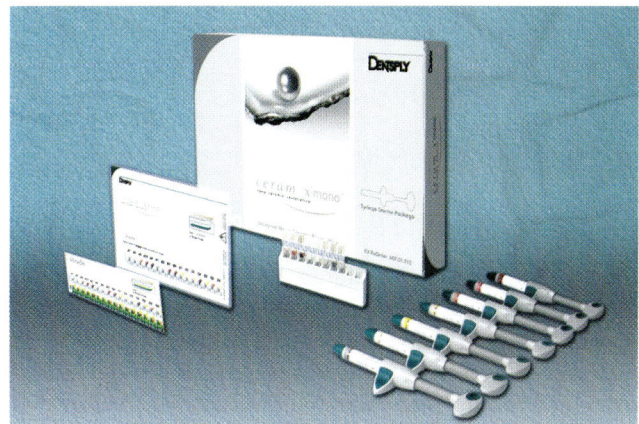

Figure 17.4: Nanofill composite resin

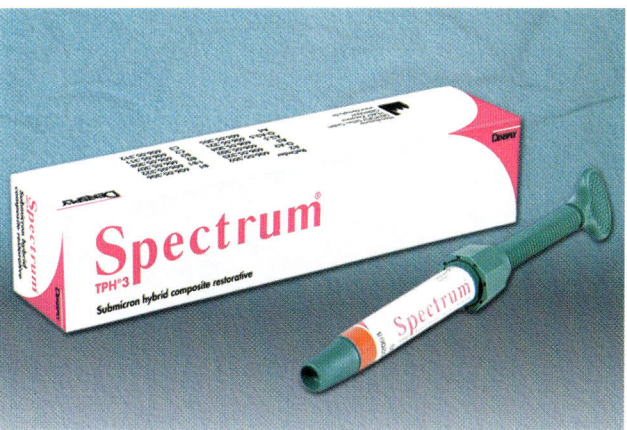

Figure 17.5: Microhybrid composite resin

Incorporation of smaller particles make them better to polish and handle than their hybrid counterparts. Because of presence of large filler content, microhybrid composites have improved physical properties and wear resistance than microfilled composites.

Advantages of microhybrid composites
➡ Better polish and surface finish
➡ Easy handling
➡ Improved physical properties
➡ Good wear resistance.

RECENT ADVANCES IN COMPOSITES

Recent Advances in Composites

- Flowable composite resin
- Condensable (packable) composites
- Giomers
- Compomers
- Ormocers
- Antibacterial/ion releasing composites
- Smart composites
- Expanded matrix resins composites.

Flowable Composite Resin (Fig.17.6)

They were introduced in the dentistry in late 1996. Filler content in flowable resins is 60 percent by weight. It is usually silica with particle size ranging from 0.02 to 0.05 µm. Low filler loading is responsible for decreased viscosity of composites, which allows them to be injected into small preparations, this makes them a good choice for pit and fissure restorations.

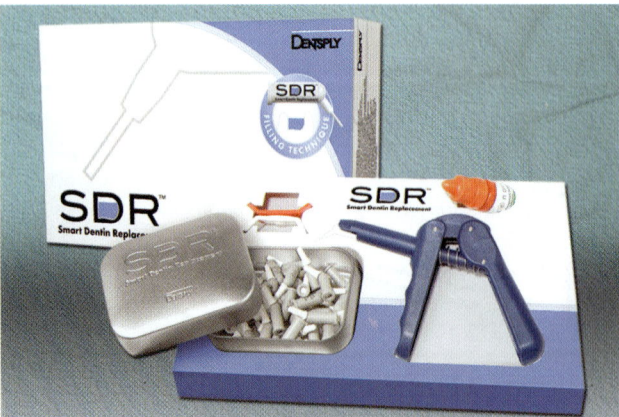

Figure 17.6: Flowable composite resin

But incorporation of lower filler content results in poor mechanical properties of these composites than conventional composites.

Advantages
➡ Low viscosity
➡ Improve marginal adaptation of posterior composites by acting as an elastic, stress absorbing layer over which composite is placed
➡ High wettability of the tooth surface
➡ High depth of cure
➡ Penetration into every irregularity of preparation
➡ Ability to form layers of minimum thickness, thus eliminate air entrapment
➡ High flexibility, so less likely to be displaced in stress concentration areas
➡ Radiopaque
➡ Availability in different colors
➡ Require minimally invasive tooth preparations
➡ For the pediatric patient to be used in narrow and deep pits and fissures.

Disadvantages
➡ More susceptible to wear in stress bearing areas
➡ Weaker mechanical properties
➡ More polymerization shrinkage
➡ Sticks to the instrument, so difficult to smoothen the surface.

Indications

- Preventive resin restorations
- Small pit and fissure sealants
- Small, angular Class V lesions
- For repairing ditched amalgam margins
- Repair of small porcelain fractures
- Inner layer for Class II posterior composite resin placement for sealing the gingival margin
- Resurfacing of worn composite or glass ionomer cement restorations
- For repair of enamel defects
- For repair of crown margins
- Repair of composite resin margins
- For luting porcelain and composite resin veneers
- Class I restorations
- Small Class III restorations
- As base or liner
- Tunnel restorations.

Condensable (Packable) Composites (Fig.17.7)

Condensable composites have been developed in an attempt to improve the compressive, tensile and edge strength and handling of the composite. The principle of

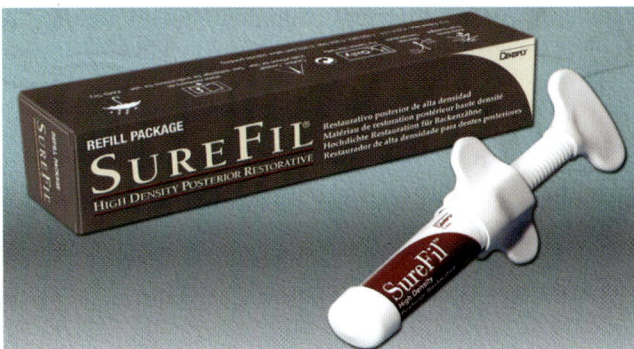

Figure 17.7: Packable composite resin

the high viscosity of packable composites is that they can be pushed into the posterior tooth preparation and has greater control over the proximal contour of Class II preparations. Their basis is polymer rigid inorganic matrix material (PRIMM). In this components are resin and ceramic inorganic fillers which are incorporated in silanated network of ceramic fibers. These fibers are composed of alumina and silicon dioxide which are fused to each other at specific sites to form a continuous network of small compartments. Filler content in packable composites ranges from 48 to 65 percent by volume. Average particle size ranges from 0.7 to 20 μm.

Packable composites posses improved mechanical properties because of presence of ceramic fibers. They have improved handling properties because of presence of higher percentage of irregular or porous filler, fibrous filler and resin matrix. The consistency of the condensable composites is like freshly triturated amalgam. Each increment can be condensed similar to amalgam restoration and can be cured to a depth of over 4 mm.

Indications

- Indicated for stress-bearing areas
- In class II restorations as they allow easier establishment of physiological contact points.

Advantages
➥ Increased wear resistance because of presence of ceramic fibers
➥ Condensability like silver amalgam restoration
➥ Greater ease in achieving a good contact point
➥ Produce better reproduction of occlusal anatomy
➥ Deeper depth of cure because of light conducting property of individual ceramic fibers
➥ High flexural modulus
➥ Decreased polymerization shrinkage because of presence of ceramic fibers

➥ Reduced stickiness
➥ Physical and mechanical performance is similar to that of silver amalgam.

Disadvantages
➥ Difficulty in adaptation of one composite layer with another
➥ Difficult handling
➥ Poor esthetics in anterior teeth.

Giomers

Giomer is hybrid of words "glass ionomers" and "composite". These are relatively new type of restorative materials. They are also known as PRG composites (Prereacted glass ionomer composites). Giomers have properties of both glass ionomers (Fluoride release, fluoride recharge) and resin composite (excellent esthetics, easy polishability, biocompatibility).

Chemistry

Giomers are hybrid esthetic restorative materials which employ the use of PRG technology, in other words, they are resin based materials which contain prereacted glass ionomer (PRG) particles. The particles are made of fluoroaluminosilicate glass that has been reacted with polyalkenoic acid before incorporating into the resin matrix. The prereaction may either involve the surface or full particle. Giomers are very much similar to compomers and composite materials in that they are light activated and require the use of bonding agent for adhesion to tooth structure.

Properties of giomers
➥ Easier to polish than glass ionomers
➥ Optimum fluoride release
➥ Excellent esthetics
➥ Better surface finish
➥ Chemical bonding to tooth structure
➥ Biocompatibility
➥ Sensitive to moisture and desiccation.

Indications

- Noncarious cervical lesions
- Root caries
- Deciduous tooth caries.

Compomers (Polyacid Modified Composite Resins) (Fig.17.8)

Compomers are class of dental materials that provide combined advantages of composites (term 'Comp' in their

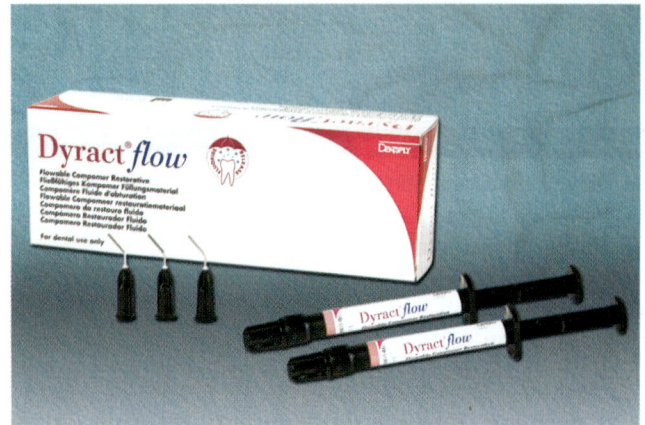

Figure 17.8: Compomer

name) and glass ionomer ('Omers' in their name). These materials consist of two components viz; dimethycrylate monomers with two carboxylic acid groups present. They are available in single paste, light enable material in syringe or compules.

History

The first compomer was introduced in 1993 under the name 'Dyract'. Initially the compomers were introduced as a type of glass-ionomers which offered fluoride release along with improved physical properties. But in terms of clinical use and proformance, it was considered as a type of composite resin.

Later on 'Compoglass' followed by Hytac was introduced.

Composition

- *Resin matrix:* Dimethacrylate monomers with two carboxylic group present in their structure
- *Filler:* Reactive silicate glass containing filler
- Photoinitiators and stabilizers
- There is no water in the composition and ion leachable glass is partially silanized to ensure bonding to matrix.

Setting Reaction

These materials set by free radical polymerization reaction. There are two stages in the polymerization reaction.

1. *Stage 1:* Typical light activated composite resin polymerization reaction occurs which helps in forming resin networks enclosing the filler particles. This reaction causes hardening of products.
2. *Stage 2:* It occurs after the initial setting of material. The restoration absorbs water and carboxyl groups present in the polyacid and metal ions in the glass ionomers show slow acid-base reaction. This results in formation

of hydrogel. It is like glass ionomer cement within the set resin structure. Slow release of fluoride also occurs here.

Properties

Their characteristics are very similar to composite resins:
- *Adhesion:* Adhesion to tooth structure is by micro-mechanical means and requires acid etching and use primer/adhesive.
- *Physical properties:* Physical properties such as strength, fracture toughness are very much similar to composites.
- *Bond strength:* It is similar to composite.
- Adaptation at cervical margin is similar to composite resins.
- *Fluoride release:* It is greater than composite resins but less than glass ionomer systems. They initially release high levels of fluorides but after some time the level falls rapidly to low level.
- Color matching and optical properties are superior to glass ionomer cements.

Advantages
→ Optimal esthetics
→ Easy to handle
→ Easy to polishing
→ Easy to place
→ Require no mixing
→ Bond strength is higher than glass ionomers.

Disadvantages
→ Require use of bonding agent
→ Technique sensitive
→ Limited fluoride release
→ Microleakage more than resin modified glass ionomers
→ Expansion of matrix due to water sorption
→ Physical properties decrease with time.

Clinical Usage

They are preferred in anterior proximal and cervical restorations as an alternative to composite and glass ionomer cements.

Difference between compomers and giomers
In compomers, variable amount of polyalkenoic acid is incorporated into the resin matrix and acid does not react with glass until the water uptake occurs into restoration, while in giomers, fluoroaluminosilicate glass particles are reacted with polyalkenoic acid in water prior to their incorporation into the resin matrix.

Organically Modified Ceramic (ORMOCER)

ORMOCER is an organically modified nonmetallic inorganic composite material. It is three dimensionally cross-linked copolymer. First time, it was introduced as dental restorative material in 1998.

Composition (Fig.17.9)

Organic modified ceramics have both organic as well as inorganic networks. They are characterized by presence of three main units:
- Organic molecules segment having methacrylate groups which form a highly cross-linked matrix.
- Inorganic condensing molecules to make three dimensional network which is formed by inorganic polycondensation. This forms the backbone of ORMOCER molecules.
- Fillers are further added to this complex.

Properties
➡ More biocompatible than conventional composites
➡ Higher bond strength
➡ Polymerization shrinkage is least among resin based filling material
➡ Highly esthetic, comparable to natural tooth
➡ High compressive (410 MPa) and transverse strength (143 MPa).

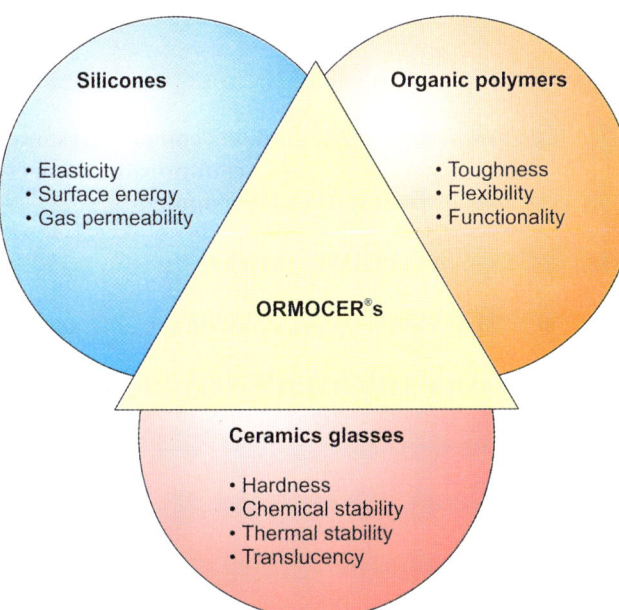

Figure 17.9: ORMOCER: Consist of both organic (organic polymers) and inorganic (ceramic glasses) network, having advantages of both

Indications

- Restoration for all type of preparations
- For esthetic veneers.
- As orthodontic bonding adhesive.

Antibacterial Composites/Ion Releasing Composites

Since composites show more tendency for plaque and bacteria accumulation in comparison to enamel, attempts have been made to develop caries resistant antibacterial composites. For this, following have been tried to incorporate in the composites:

Chlorhexidine

Though chlorhexidine has shown antibacterial properties but its addition to composites has been unsuccessful because of the following reasons:
- Weakening of the physical properties of composites.
- Release chemicals which show toxic affects.
- Temporary antibacterial activity.
- Shift in microorganisms and plaque to adjacent areas of the tooth.

Methacryloxydecyl Pyridinium Bromide (MDPB)

Use of methacryloxydecyl pyridinium bromide (MDPB) was recommended by Imazato in 1994. It has following features:
- Its antibacterial property remains constant and permanent.
- It has shown to be effective against streptococci.
- It does not have adverse effect on the physical properties of Bis-GMA based composites.
- On polymerization, it forms chemical bond to the resin matrix, therefore no release of any antibacterial component takes place.

Silver

Addition of silver ions in the composites has also been suggested so as to make antibacterial composites. Silver ions cause structural damage to the bacteria. In these composites, the antibacterial property is due to direct contact with bacteria and not because of release of silver ions. Addition of silver into composite without silica gel does not affect its physical properties like depth of cure, compressive strength, tensile strength, color stability and polymerization.

Silver ions can be added in any of the following methods:
- Incorporation into inorganic oxide like silicone dioxides.

- Incorporation into silica gel and then films are coated over the surface of composites.
- Hydrothermally supported into the space between the crystal lattice network of filler particles.

Smart Composite

In smart composites the micron size sensor particles are embedded during manufacturing process into composite. These sensors interact with resin matrix and generate quantifiable anions. This type of composites was introduced in 1998 under the name Ariston pHc (Vivadent).

It releases fluoride, hydroxyl and calcium ions if the pH falls in the vicinity of the restoration. The fall in pH value is attributed to the deposition of plaque in that area. Smart composites work based on the recently introduced alkaline glass fillers which inhibit the bacterial growth and thereby reduce formation of secondary caries. The paste of smart composites contain barium, aluminum fluoride and silicate glass fillers with silicon dioxide, ytterbium trifluoride and calcium silicate glass in dimethacrylate monomers. Filler content in these composites is 80 percent by weight.

The fluoride release from smart composites is higher than that of compomers but less than conventional glass ionomers.

Expanding Matrix Resins for Composites

As we know, composites show polymerization shrinkage on curing which can result in marginal leakage, postoperative sensitivity and secondary caries. Therefore, slight expansion of the composite during polymerization is desired to reduce these effects. It has been tried to add Spiro orthocarbonates (SOCs) in composites as these show expansion on polymerization.

Epoxy resin contract 3.4 percent and SOCs expand 3.6 percent. Both are mixed to achieve desired expansion.

PROPERTIES OF COMPOSITE RESTORATIVE MATERIALS

Coefficient of Thermal Expansion

Coefficient of thermal expansion of composites is approximately three times higher than normal tooth structure. This results in more contraction and expansion than enamel and dentin when there are temperature changes, and this can result in loosening of the restoration (**Fig. 17.10**). This can be reduced by adding more filler content. Microfill composites show more coefficient of thermal expansion because of presence of more polymer content.

Water Absorption

Composites have tendency to absorb water which can lead to the swelling of resin matrix, filler debonding and thus restoration failure. Composites with higher filler content exhibit lower water absorption and therefore better properties, than composites with lower filler content.

Factors Affecting Water Absorption of Composites

- More is the filler content, less is the water sorption
- Lesser degree of polymerization causes more sorption
- Type and amount of monomer and dilutent also affect water sorption. For example, UDMA based composites show less sorption and solubility.

Wear Resistance (Fig. 17.11)

Composites are prone to wear under masticatory forces or use of toothbrushing and abrasive food (**Fig. 17.12**). Wear resistance is a property of filler particles depending on their size and quantity. The site of restorations in dental arch and occlusal contact relationship, size, shape and content of filler particles affect the wear resistance of the composites.

Wear in Composites

Two principal modes of wear are:
- ***Two body wear***: When there is direct contact of restoration with opposing tooth or adjacent proximal surface of tooth, it leads to high stress development.

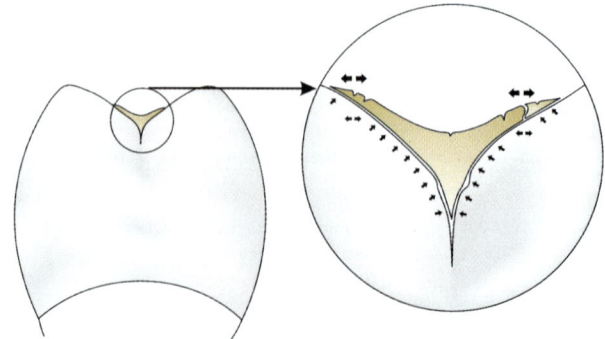

Figure 17.10: Coefficient of thermal expansion can result in dimensional change in restoration which can cause gap between tooth and the restoration

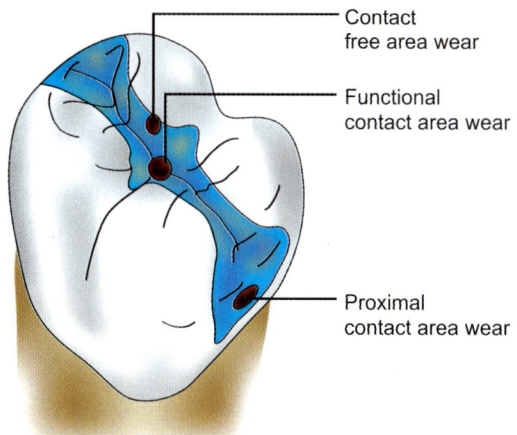

Figure 17.11: Wear in composite resin

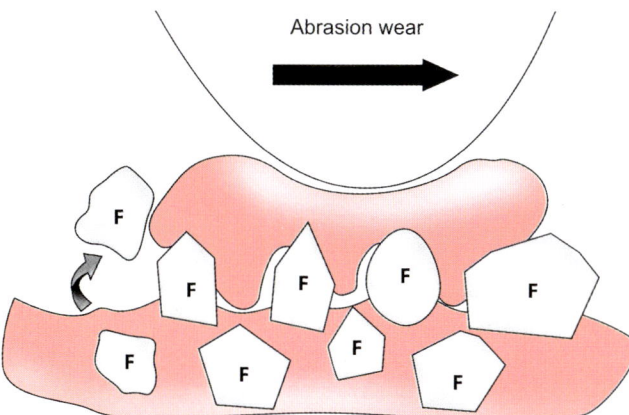

Figure 17.12: Abrasive wear in composite restoration causes exposure of filler-particles which get removed from the surface of composite restoration

- **Three body wear**: Three body wear is caused due to contact with the food bolus as it is forced across the occlusal surface. This type of wear depends upon, degree of monomer conversion, filler loading, type of filler particles and stability of silane coupling agent.

  Wear of composites leads to fracture or loss of the restoration. Different theories explaining wear are:
- **Microfracture theory**: Microfractures occur in composites because higher modulus filler particles are compressed into weaker matrix during occlusal loading
- **Hydrolysis theory**: Silane particles get unstable and debonded leading to loss of surface filler particles
- **Protection theory**: Erosion of weaker matrix occur between the particles.
  - *Microprotection theory*: If filler content is high and densely packed, the intervening matrix is protected.

Therefore in microfilled composites, even if filler loading is low but since it is densely packed, it helps in resisting wear of contact free area.
  - *Macroprotection theory*: If composite restoration is very small, the stresses are taken up by the tooth structure.
- **Chemical degradation theory**: Material from saliva and food are absorbed into the matrix resulting in its degration and sloughing from the surface.

Factors affecting degradation/wear of composites
➡ Lesser is the polymerization, more is the degradation
➡ Microfilled composites show less of degradation
➡ Hydrolytic degradation of strontium or barium glass fillers can result in pressure built up at resin filler junction. This may cause cracks and fracture of composite restoration
➡ Sudden temperature change can result in disruption in silane coating and thus bond failure between matrix and filler

Surface Texture

The size and composition of filler particles determine the smoothness of the surface of a restoration. Microfill composites offer the smoothest restorative surface. This property is more significant if the restoration is in close approximation to gingival tissues.

Radiopacity

Resins are inherently radiolucent. Presence of radiopaque fillers like barium glass, strontium and zirconium makes the composite restoration radiopaque.

Modulus of Elasticity

Modulus of elasticity of a material determines its rigidity or stiffness. Microfill composites have greater flexibility than hybrid composite since they have lower modulus of elasticity.

Solubility

Composite materials do not show any clinically significant solubility in oral fluids. Water solubility of composites ranges between 0.5 and 1.1 mg/cm^2.

Creep

Creep is progressive permanent deformation of material under occlusal loading. More is the content of resin matrix, more is the creep. For example, microfilled composites show more creep since they contain more of resin matrix.

Polymerization Shrinkage

Composite materials shrink while curing which can result in formation of a gap between resin based composite and the preparation wall (**Fig. 17.13**). It accounts for 1.67 to 5.68 percent of the total volume.

Polymerization shrinkage
→ In light cured composites, about 60 percent polymerization occurs within 60 seconds, further 10 percent in next 48 hours; remaining resin does not polymerize. Since the material nearest to the light sets first. Shrinkage in light cured composites occurs in the direction of light (**Figs 17.14A and B**).
→ For chemical cured composites shrinkage occurs slowly and uniformly towards the center of restoration (**Fig. 17.15**).

Polymerization shrinkage can result in
→ Postoperative sensitivity
→ Recurrent caries
→ Failure of interfacial bonding
→ Fracture of restoration and tooth (**Fig. 17.16**).

Polymerization shrinkage can be reduced by
→ Decreasing monomer level
→ Increasing monomer molecular weight
→ *Improving composite placement technique:* Placing successive layers of wedge-shaped composite (1–1.5 mm) decreases polymerization shrinkage (**Fig. 17.17**)
→ *Polymerization rate:* "Soft-start" polymerization reduces polymerization shrinkage.

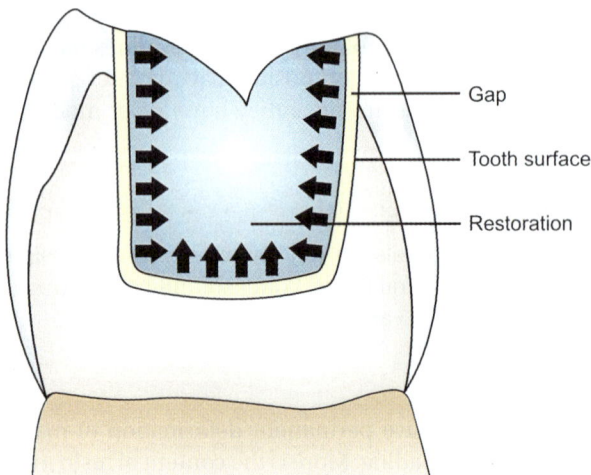

Figure 17.13: Polymerization shrinkage can result in gap between restoration and the tooth surface

Configuration or C-factor

The cavity configuration or C-factor was introduced by Professer Carol Davidson and his colleagues in 1980s. The configuration factor (C-factor) is the ratio of bonded surface of the restoration to the unbonded surfaces. The higher the value of 'C'-factor, the greater is the polymerization shrinkage (**Fig. 17.18**).

Evaluation of C-factor in different tooth preparations

S.no	Type of preparation	$C = \dfrac{Bonded}{Unbonded}$	Value
1.	Class I and V (five walled preparation)	$C = \dfrac{5}{1}$	5
2.	Class II (four walled preparation)	$C = \dfrac{4}{2}$	2
3.	Class III (three walled preparation)	$C = \dfrac{3}{3}$	1
4.	Class IV (two walled preparation)	$C = \dfrac{2}{4}$	0.5
5.	Smooth surface restoration (one walled preparation)	$C = \dfrac{1}{5}$	0.2

Therefore, three-dimensional tooth preparations (Class I) have the highest (most unfavorable) C-factor and thus are at more risk to the effects of polymerization shrinkage. C-factor plays a significant role when tooth preparation extends up to the root surface causing a 'V' shaped gap formation between the composite and root surface due to polymerization shrinkage.

Esthetics of Composites

Composites have shown good esthetics because of their property of translucency. Composites are available in different opacities and shades so they can be used in different places according to esthetic requirements. But due to oxidation, moisture and exposure to ultraviolet light, etc. some chemical changes can occur in the resin matrix which results in discoloration of composite with time. But improvements in composites like increase in filler content, decrease in tertiary amines and improvement in light curing techniques have shown more stability in composite shade.

Microleakage and Nanoleakage
→ Microleakage is passage of fluid and bacteria in microgaps (10–6 m) between restoration and tooth. It can result in damage to the pulp. Microleakage can occur due to:

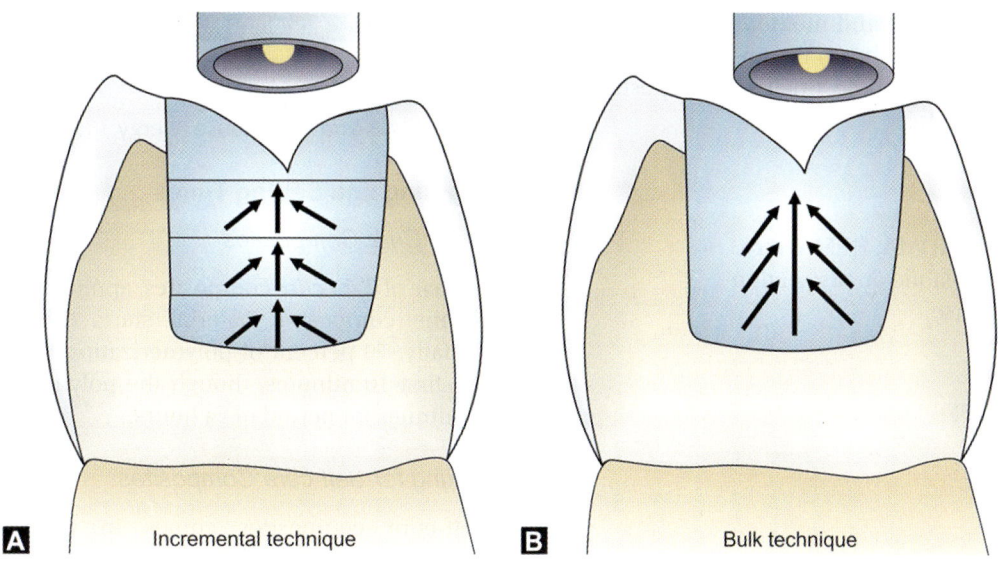

Figures 17.14A and B: In light cured composites, shrinkage occurs towards source of light

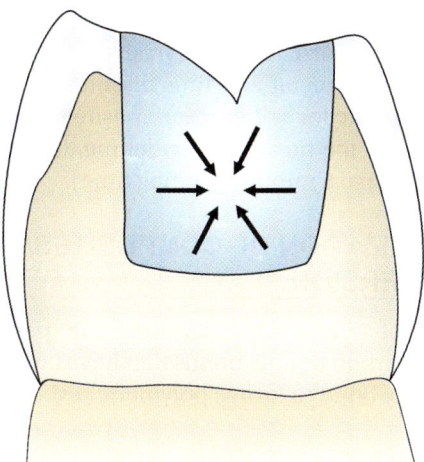

Figure 17.15: In chemical cured composites, shrinkage occurs towards center of restoration

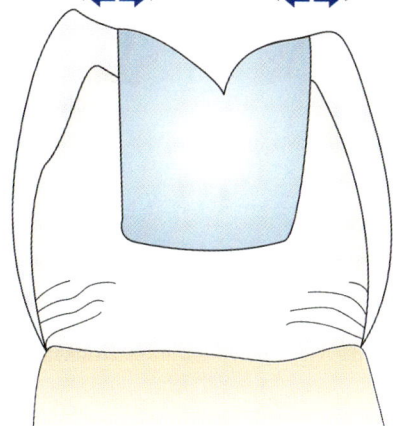

Figure 17.16: Polymerization shrinkage can pull cusps together and can result in fracture

♦ Polymerization shrinkage of composites
♦ Poor adhesion and wetting
♦ Thermal stresses
♦ Mechanical loading
   Microleakage can result in bacterial leakage which can further cause discoloration, recurrent caries and pulpal infection.
➡ *Nanoleakage:* It is passage of fluid/dissolved species in nanosized (10–9 m) gaps. These nanosized porosities occur within hybrid layer. These can occur because of:
   ♦ Inadequate polymerization of primer before application of bonding agent.

♦ Incomplete resin infiltration.
♦ Polymerization shrinkage of maturing primer resin.
♦ Nanoleakage can result in sensitivity during occlusal and thermal stresses.

Biocompatibility

Since composites are made from petrochemical products, studies have shown that the major components are cytotoxic if used in pure state. Further biological liability of composite depends upon release of these components from the polymerized composite, which further depend upon type of composite and method used to polymerize it. These products have shown to cause contact allergy in those who regularly handle uncured composite. These have shown to cause:

- Inflammation
- Toxicity
- Mutagenicity
- Leaching of TEGDMA, HEMA, etc.
- Deposition of plaque on restoration
- Allergic response
- Genotoxicity
- Mutagenicity
- Carcinogenicity.

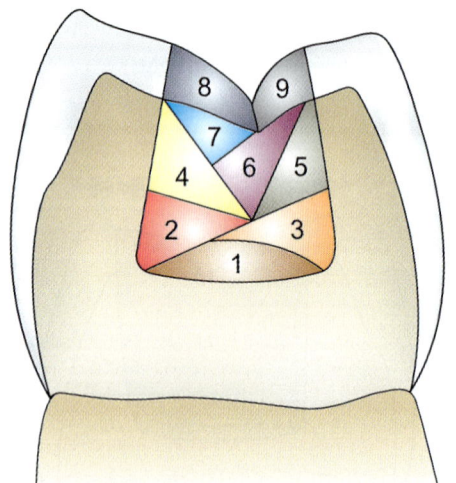

Figure 17.17: Incremental build-up of restoration results in decreased polymerization shrinkage

Biocompatibility of composites

- Unpolymerized monomers are responsible for toxic effects of composites
- HEMA is known to cause allergy.

Working and Setting Times

Light Cure Composites

In case of light cure composites, application of light source to the composite material starts the polymerization. Usually, 70 percent of polymerization takes place during the first 10 minutes, though the polymerization reaction continues for period of 24 hours.

Mixing for Self-cure Composites

Self-cure composites comes in two syringes. One syringe contains the peroxide initiator or catalyst while other syringe contains the amine accelerator. They are dispensed in equal amounts and then thoroughly mixed for 20 to 30 seconds. For mixing, plastic or wooden spatulas are preferred. Use of metal spatula is avoided because inorganic filler particles are abrasive, they can abrade small amount of metal and thus discolor the composite. The working time for self-cure composite resins is 1 to 1½ minutes. Once the mix starts hardening, it should not be disturbed for 4 to 5 minutes (setting time).

POLYMERIZATION OF COMPOSITES/DEGREE OF CONVERSION

- Degree of conversion measures the percentage of carbon-carbon double bonds that have been converted into single bond to form a polymeric resin.

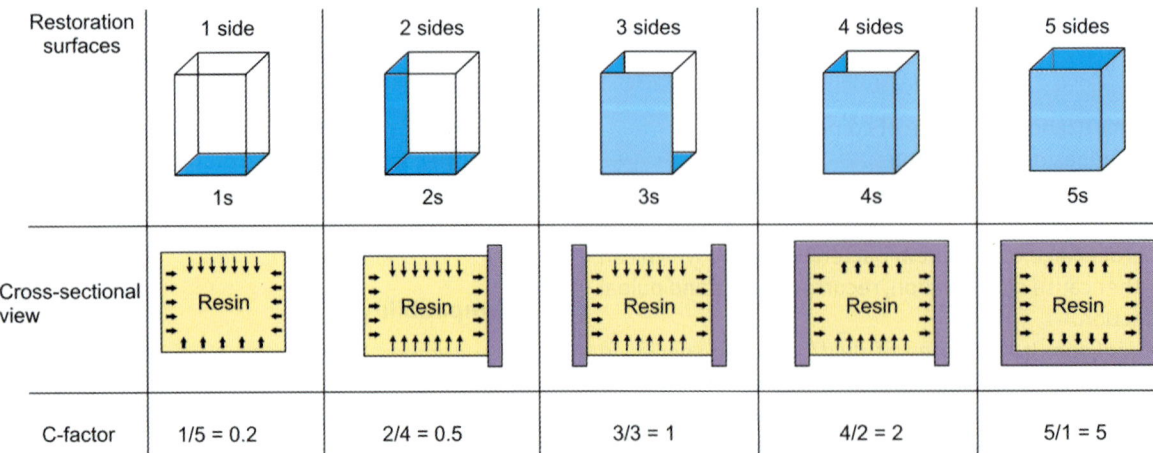

Figure 17.18: Configuration factor of different tooth preparations

- Complete polymerization of the composite is determined by degree of conversion of monomers into polymers.
- Strength of resin is directly linked to the degree of conversion.

Degree of conversion of the composite is dependent on following factors:

Curing Time

Curing time depends on different factors like shade of the composite, intensity of the light used, temperature, depth of the preparation, thickness of the resin, curing through tooth structure, composite filling.

Shade of Composite

It has been seen that darker composite shades polymerize slower when compared to lighter shades.

Distance and Angle between Light Source and Resin

The recommended distance between light source and resin is 1 mm. Intensity of light decreases as the distance is increased. If the cavity is deep, then use highpower density lamp (about 600 mW/cm^2) so that deeper layer is also cured (**Fig. 17.19**). Polymerization can also be achieved in tooth preparation with deep proximal box by curing from proximal surface (**Fig. 17.20**). The angle of source should be at 90° to the resin. If angle diverges from 90°, intensity of light decreases.

Temperature

Composite curing would be less if it is taken out immediately from refrigerator. Composite should be atleast kept at room temperature 1 hour before use.

Resin Thickness

Resin thickness is also one of the main factors for its curing. It should be ideally 0.5 to 1.0 mm for optimum polymerization of resin.

Inhibition of Air

Oxygen in the air also affects the polymerization of the resin.

Intensity of Curing Light

Intensity of curing light usually decreases as the lamp ages. Decrease in intensity of light affect the properties of composites significantly.

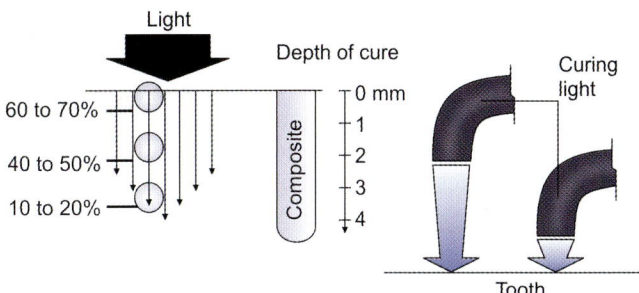

Figure 17.19: As the distance between light source and tooth increases, polymerization decreases

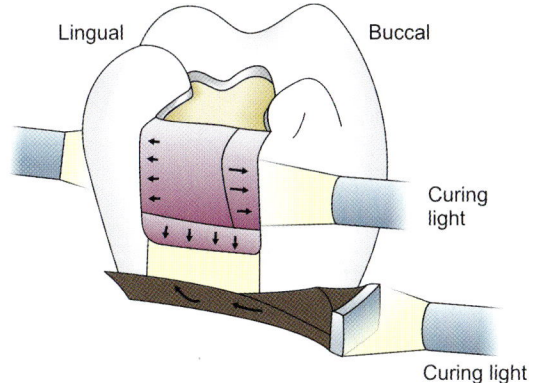

Figure 17.20: Polymerized light should be directed from all sides of proximal box so as to have complete polymerization

For optimal results, wavelength of light should range between 400 and 500 nm. To make it sure that 400 mW/cm reaches the first increment of the restoration, a power density of 600 mW/cm is needed (**Fig. 17.21**).

Type of Filler

Microfine composites are more difficult to cure than heavily loaded composites.

INDICATIONS OF COMPOSITE RESTORATIONS

- For restoration of mild to moderate class I and class II tooth preparations of all teeth.
- Restoration of class III, IV and V preparations of all teeth especially when esthetics is important (**Figs 17.22 to 17.26**) .
- Restoration of class VI preparations of teeth where high occlusal stress is not present.
- Esthetic improvement procedures:
  - Laminates
  - Partial veneers

- Full veneers
- Treatment of tooth discolorations
- Diastema closures (**Figs 17.27A and B**)
- To restore erosion or abrasion defects in cervical areas of all the surfaces of premolars, canines and incisors where esthetics is the main concern.

- For restoration of hypoplastic or other defects on the facial or lingual areas of teeth.
- As core build up for grossly damaged teeth and endodontically treated teeth.
- For cementation of indirect restorations like inlays, onlays and crowns.
- As a pit and fissure sealants
- For periodontal splinting of weakened teeth or mobile teeth
- For repair of fractured ceramic crowns
- For bonding orthodontic appliances.

CONTRAINDICATIONS OF COMPOSITES

- When isolation of operating field is difficult.
- Where very high occlusal forces are present.
- Class V lesions where esthetics is not the prime concern.
- When clinician does not possess the necessary technical skill for the restoration.
- When lesion extends up to the root surface.
- Small lesions on distal surface of canines where metallic restoration is treatment of choice.
- Patients with high caries susceptibility.
- When preparation extends subgingivally.
- Patients with poor oral hygiene.

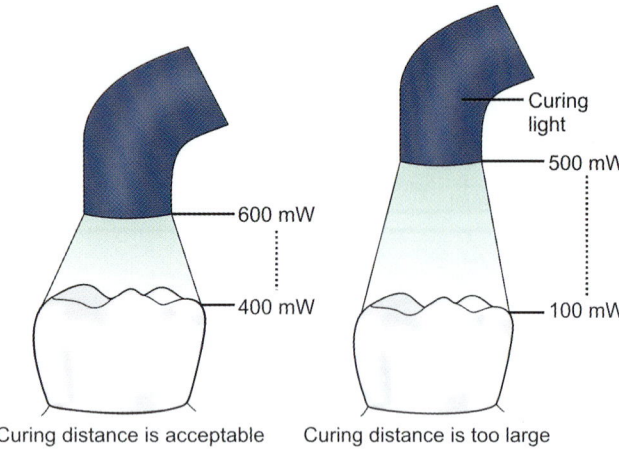

Figure 17.21: As the distance between light source and the restoration increases, the intensity of light decreases

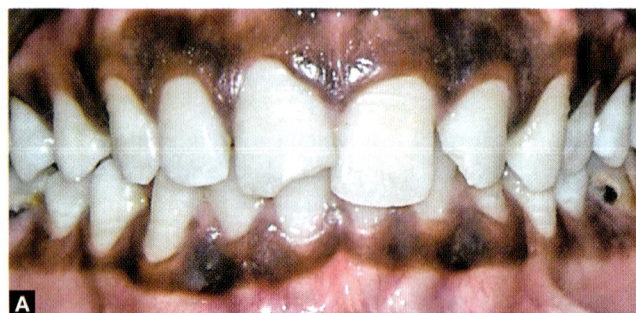
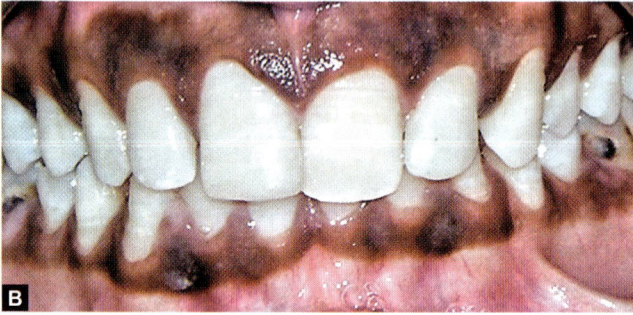

Figures 17.22A and B: Composite restoration of fractured 11

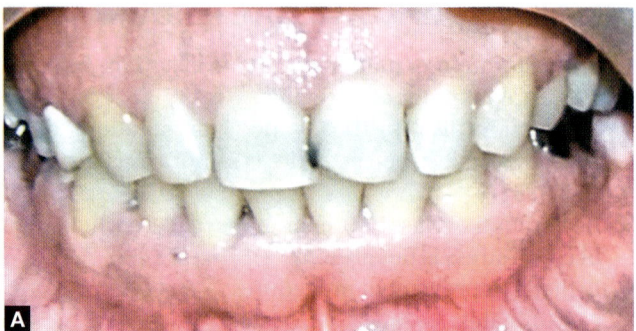
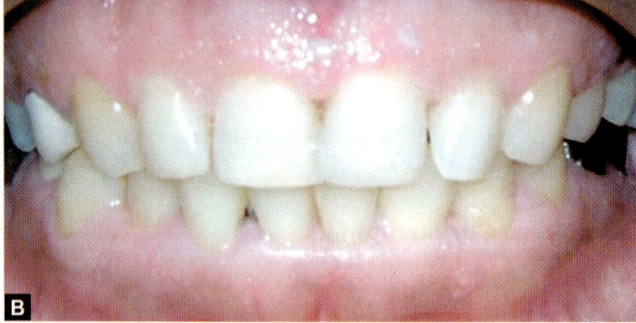

Figures 17.23A and B: Composite restoration of class III caries in 11

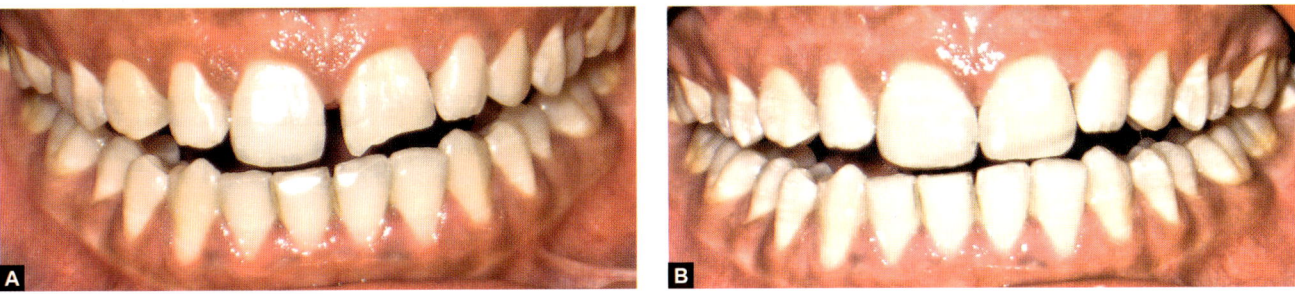

Figures 17.24A and B: Composite build up for restoration of fractured 21 and diastema closure

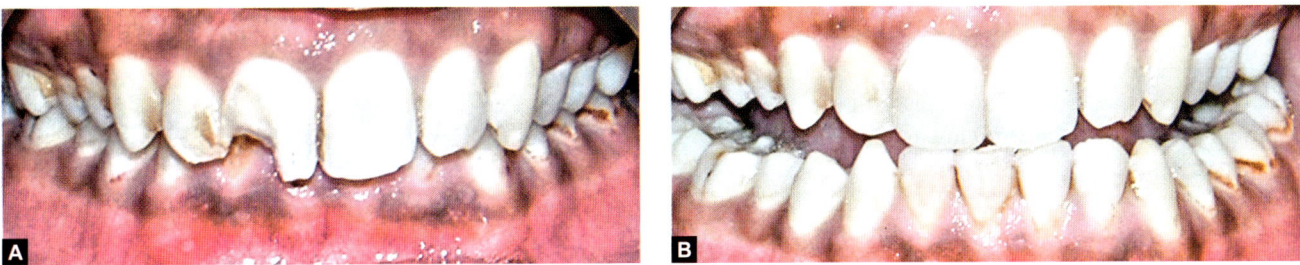

Figures 17.25A and B: Composite restoration of fractured 11

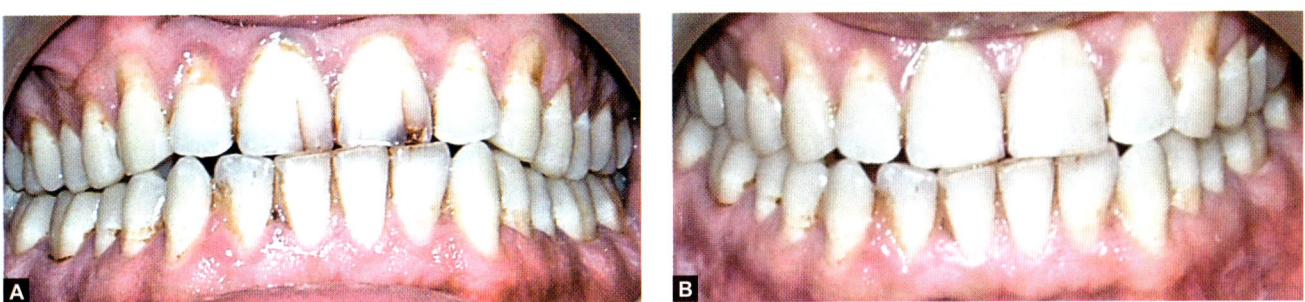

Figures 17.26A and B: Composite restoration of carious 11 and 21

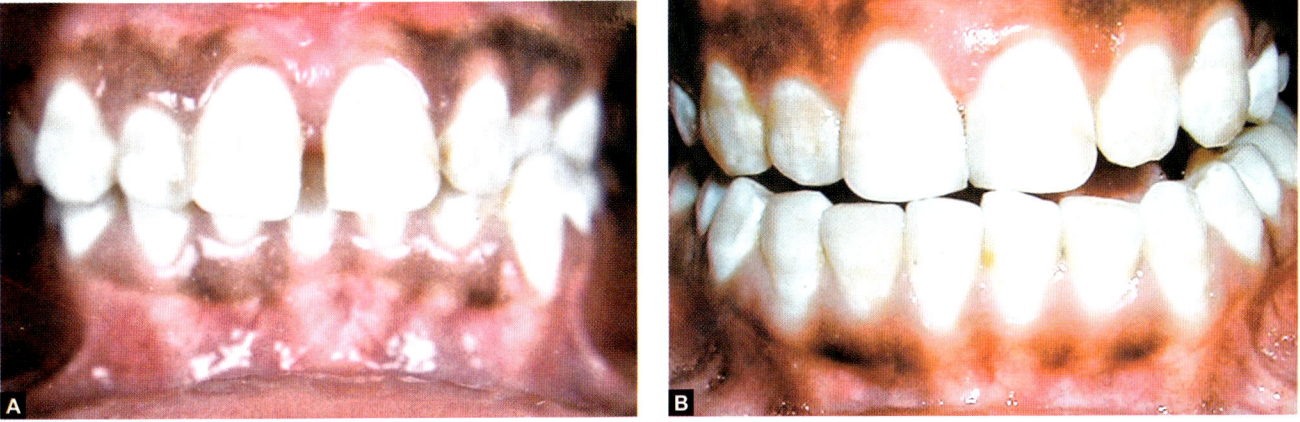

Figures 17.27A and B: Diastema closure using composite resin

Advantages of composites

- Since composite restoration requires minimal tooth preparation, maximum conservation of tooth structure is possible.
- Esthetically acceptable.
- Less complex tooth preparation is required.
- Composite resin can be used in combination with other materials, such as glass ionomer, to provide the benefits of both materials.
- Composites have low thermal conductivity, thus no insulation base is required to protect underlying pulp.
- Restorations are bonded with enamel and dentin, hence show good retention.
- Restoration with composite resins can be finished immediately after curing.
- It can be repaired rather than replaced.
- Composite restoration show low microleakage than unfilled resins.
- It can be used almost universally.
- They have extended working time, this makes their manipulation easier.
- Restoration can be completed in one dental visit.
- Composite restorations can bond directly to the tooth, making the tooth stronger than it would be with an amalgam filling.
- Indirect composite fillings and inlays are heat-cured, increasing their strength.
- No galvanism because composite resins do not contain any metals.
- Composite resins have adequate radiopacity to enable their detection in radiographs.

Disadvantages of composites

- Because of polymerization shrinkage, gap formation on margins may occur, usually on root surfaces. This can result in secondary caries and staining.
- More difficult, time consuming.
- Expensive than amalgam.
- More technique sensitive.
- Low wear resistance.
- Postoperative sensitivity due to polymerization shrinkage.
- High LCTE may results in marginal percolation around composite restorations.
- In large preparation, composites may not last as long as amalgam fillings.

CLINICAL PROCEDURES

For achieving optimal results, thorough examination, diagnosis and treatment plan should be finalized before initiating composite restoration. Following steps are undertaken for composite restoration:

Steps of clinical proceduring for composite restoration

- Local anesthesia
- Preparation of operating site
- Composite selection
- Shade selection
- Isolation
- Tooth preparation
- Bonding
- Composite placement
- Polymerization of composite resins
- Final contouring, finishing and polishing of composite restoration

Local Anesthesia

As and when required, local anesthesia is given in many cases since it makes the procedure pleasant, time saving and reduces the salivation.

Preparation of the Operating Site

Operating site is cleaned using slurry of pumice in order to remove plaque, calculus and superficial stains prior to the procedure.

Composite Selection

Composite selection is dependent on:

- *Position of the tooth preparation:* For restoration requiring high mechanical performance, like class IV preparations, large class I, II and class VI, choice of composite is that with the highest inorganic load. For restorations of anterior teeth, esthetics is the main concern. So, composites with submicronic fillers or nanoparticles are preferred in these cases. Composites which are highly polishable are preferred for cervical lesions both in the posterior and in the anterior areas to avoid plaque accumulation on them.
- *Esthetic requirements:* In special cases where esthetics is the main concern like treatment of defective shape, discolored teeth, diastemas, malpositioned teeth and for caries in anterior teeth, opacity and the translucency of the composites are to be kept in mind for attaining optimal results.

Shade Selection

For posterior composite restorations, shade selection is not as critical as for anterior restorations. Sometimes more than one shade is needed to attain optimal esthetics. The number of shades to be used depends on the:

- Complexity of the restoration
- Polychromatic characteristics of the tooth to be restored
- Relationship with adjacent teeth.

In cases where the dentin is to be replaced, composites having dentin shade and opacity are preferred while when enamel is to be replaced, composite that has enamel shade and translucency is preferred.

Initial Shade Selection

The following guidelines are followed for shade matching:
- Teeth and shade guide should be wet to simulate the oral environment.
- Shade matching should be carried in natural daylight (**Fig. 17.28**).
- The dentin shade is usually selected from the cervical third of the tooth, whereas the enamel shade is selected from its incisal third.
- To confirm the final shade, a small increment of selected composite is placed adjacent to the area to be restored and then light cured for matching.

Isolation

To achieve the optimal results of composite restoration, moisture and salivary contamination must be prevented, in other words isolation is must. Contamination of etched enamel or dentin by saliva results in a decreased bond strength and contamination of the composite material during insertion results in degradation of its physical properties. Isolation is best done by using rubber dam, though it can be done using cotton rolls, saliva ejector and retraction cord.

Tooth Preparation

Following features are to be kept in mind while doing tooth preparation for direct composite restorations.
- Tooth preparation is limited to extent of the defect, that is extension for prevention, including proximal contact clearance, is not necessary unless it is required to facilitate proximal matrix placement.
- To facilitate bonding, tooth surface is made rough using diamond abrasives.
- Pulpal and axial walls need not to be flat.
- Enamel bevel is given in some cases to increase the surface area for etching and bonding.
- Cavosurface present on root surfaces has butt joint.

Designs of Tooth Preparation for Composites

The following three types of designs or their combination are most commonly prepared for composites
➡ Conventional
➡ Beveled conventional
➡ Modified (conservative).

1. *Conventional:* Conventional design is similar to the tooth preparation for amalgam restoration, except that there is less outline extension and in tooth preparation, walls are made rough.

Indications for conventional tooth preparation
- Preparations located on root surface.
- Moderate to large class I or class II restorations.

Features (Fig. 17.29)
- Prepared enamel margins should be 90 degree or greater.

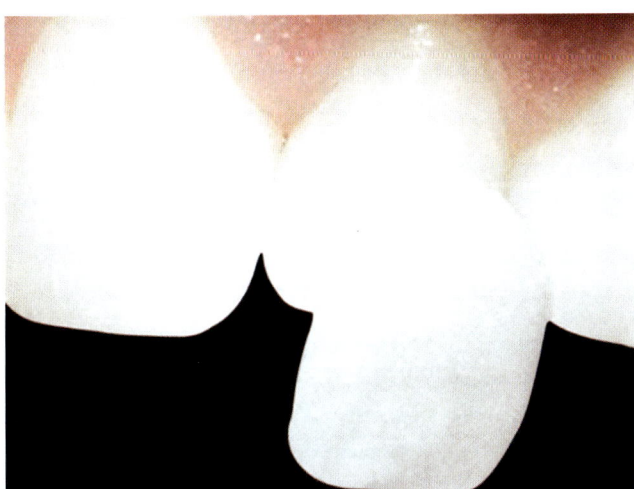

Figure 17.28: Shade matching should be done in natural light before isolating the tooth

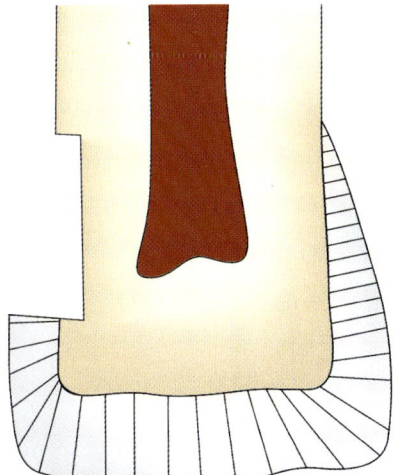

Figure 17.29: Conventional tooth preparation for composite restoration

- Butt joint cavosurface margin is made on root surfaces.
- The prepared tooth surface is roughened to increase the bonding.

2. *Beveled conventional tooth preparation:* This design is almost similar to conventional design but some beveled enamel margins are incorporated (**Fig. 17.30**).
   Indications
   - When restoration is being used to replace an existing restoration exhibiting a conventional design.
   - To restore a large preparation and especially indicated for classes III, IV, V and VI restorations.

3. *Modified (conservative tooth preparation):* It is more conservative in nature since retention is achieved by micromechanical bonding to the tooth (**Fig. 17.31**).
   Indications: For initial or small carious lesions.
   Features
   - Preparation has scooped out appearance.
   - It does not have specified wall configuration or pulpal and axial wall depth.
   - Extent and depth of the preparation depends upon the extent and the depth of carious lesion.
   - In combination preparations, that is part of the preparation is on crown and part is on root, the root surface is prepared as conventional preparation and enamel surface portion is prepared as beveled conventional preparation where enamel margin is beveled.

Bonding

Adhesion of composites to tooth structure can be attained with any of following methods:

- Total-etch involving 3-step adhesives that is etching, priming and bonding.
- Total-etch involving 2-step adhesives that is etching and bonding.
- Self-etch primers involving 2-step adhesives, that is priming and bonding.
- Self-etch adhesives involving single step of bonding.

Composite Placement

Instruments Used for Composite Insertion

Following instruments are used for the placement of composites in the prepared tooth.

Hand instruments: Hand instruments used for placing composites are usually made up of coating with Teflon so as to avoid sticking of composite to the instrument (**Fig. 17.32**). These instruments are simple and easy to use but

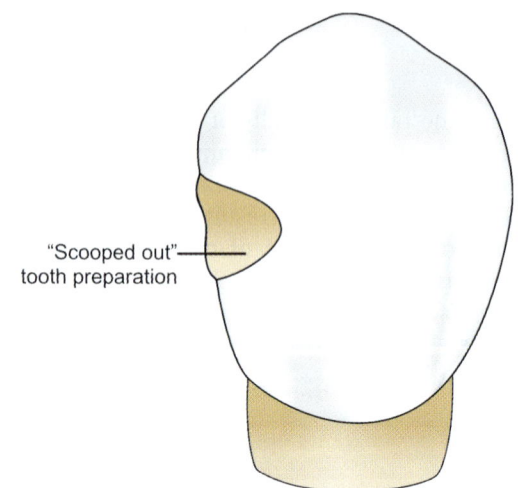

Figure 17.31: Modified tooth preparation for composites

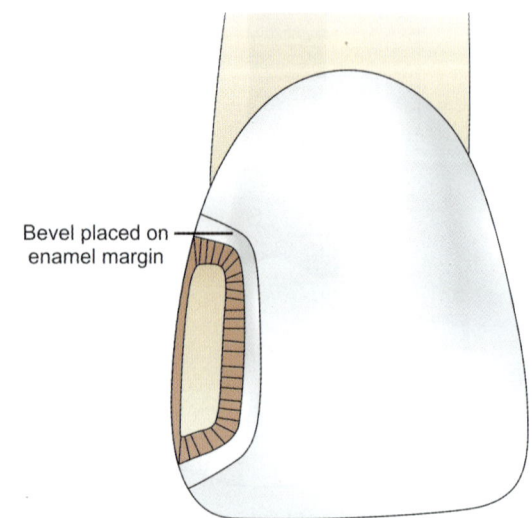

Figure 17.30: Beveled preparation for composite restoration

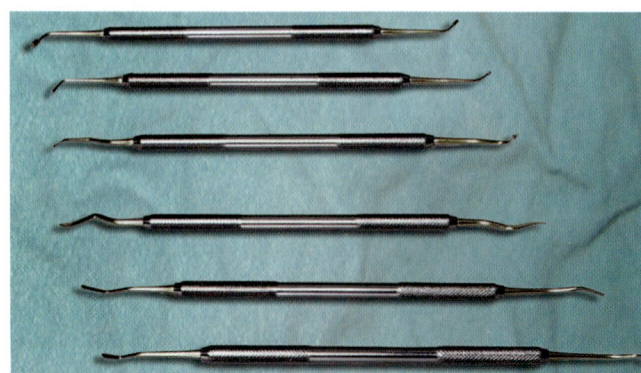

Figure 17.32: Teflon coated instruments used for composite placement

the problem of air trapping during insertion of composite can occur.

Composite gun: Composite gun is made up of plastic. It is commonly used with composite filled ampules. For use composite compules are fitted in the gun and the pressure is applied so that composite comes out from the ampule (**Fig. 17.33**).

Syringe: Composite syringe usually carries the low viscosity composite which can easily flow through needle (**Fig. 17.34**). This technique has advantage of providing an easy way for placement of composite with decreased chances of air trapping.

Irrespective of the location of the restoration, composites should be placed and polymerized in increments. This ensures complete polymerization of the whole composite mass and aids in the anatomical build-up of the restoration. Each increment should not be more than 2 mm in thickness, thickness of more than 2 mm is difficult to cure and result in more polymerization shrinkage stress.

Incremental Layering Technique (Fig. 17.35)

• Advocated for use in medium to large posterior composite restorations to avoid the limitation of depth of cure
• This technique is based on polymerization of resin-based composite layers of less than 2 mm thickness
• It helps to attain good marginal quality
• It prevent deformation of the preparation wall
• It ensures complete polymerization of the resin-based composite
• Incremental layering of dentin and enamel composite creates layers with high diffusion which allow optimal light transmission within the restoration, thus increasing esthetics.

Horizontal Technique (Fig. 17.36)

• In this, occlusogingival layering is done.
• It is usually indicated for small restorations.
• This technique increases the C-factor.

U-shaped Layering Technique (Fig. 17.37)

• First increment in the form of U-Shape is placed at the base, both gingival and occlusal.
• Over that place horizontal and oblique increments to pack the preparation.
• Then, curing is carried out from all the sides.

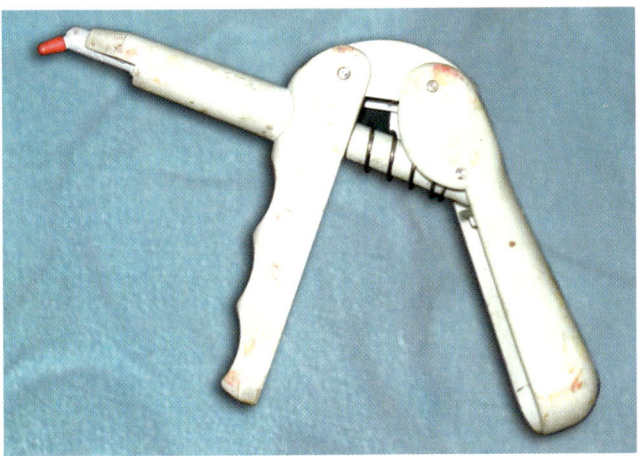

Figure 17.33: Composite gun used for composite compules

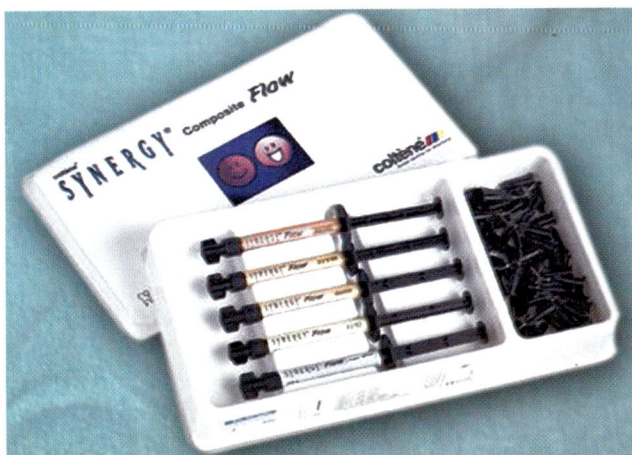

Figure 17.34: Composite syringe carries the low viscosity composite which can easily flow through the needle tip

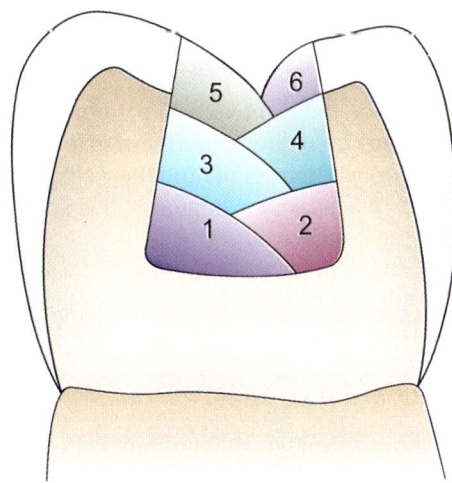

Figure 17.35: Incremental layering technique

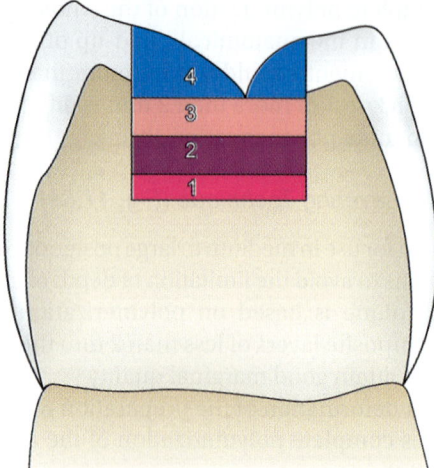

Figure 17.36: Horizontal technique

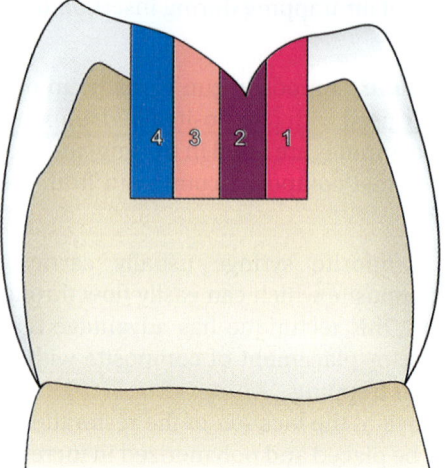

Figure 17.38: Vertical layering technique

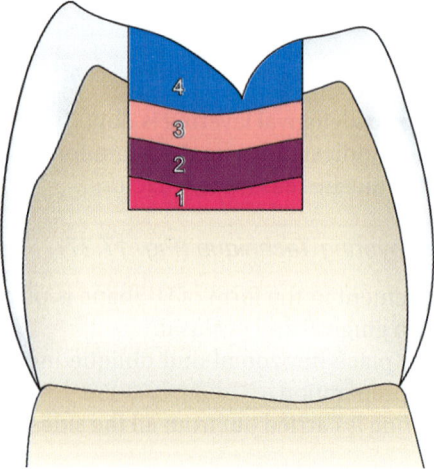

Figure 17.37: U-shaped layering technique

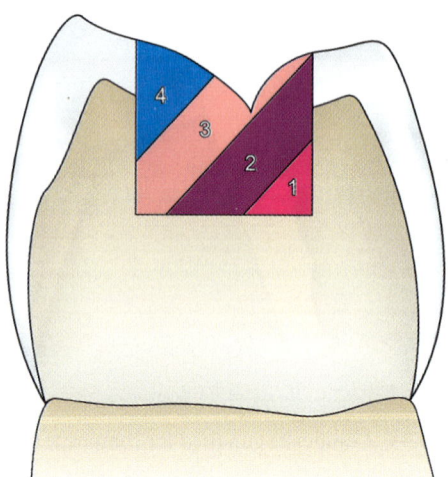

Figure 17.39: Oblique technique

Vertical Layering Technique (Fig. 17.38)

- Place small increments in vertical pattern starting from one wall, i.e. buccal or lingual and carried to another wall
- Start polymerization from behind the wall, i.e. if buccal increment is placed on the lingual wall, it is cured from outside of the lingual wall
- Reduces gap at gingival wall which is formed due to polymerization shrinkage, hence postoperative sensitivity and secondary caries.

Oblique Technique (Fig. 17.39)

- In this technique, wedge-shaped composite increments are placed to prevent deformation of preparation walls.
- It reduces the C-factor.

- In this technique, polymerization is started first through the preparation walls and then from the occlusal surface
- This technique directs the vectors of polymerization toward the adhesive surface, this is indirect polymerization technique.

Three-site Technique (Fig. 17.40)

- In this technique, polymerization vectors are directed towards the gingival margin
- This technique uses clear matrix and reflective wedges.

Successive Cusp Build-up Technique

- The first composite increment is applied to a single dentin surface without contacting the opposing preparation walls

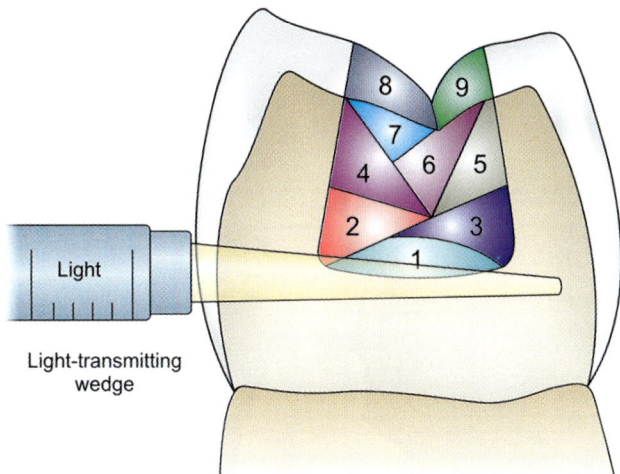

Figure 17.40: Use of light transmitting wedges for better curing at gingival margins

- After this restoration, built up is done by placing wedge-shaped composite increments
- This technique minimizes the C-factor in three dimensional tooth preparations.

Bulk Technique

- It is done to reduce stress at the cavosurface margins
- It is usually recommended with packable composites.

Polymerization of Composite Resins

According to polymerization method, the composite resins can be divided into two main categories:
1. Self-curing composites
2. Light-activated composites.

Self-curing Composite Resin

The earliest self-curing composite resins were mixed as a powder and liquid. Soon after, the composite resins were made available in paste/paste mixed system in form of a catalyst and a base material. One part of this consists of an organic tertiary amine accelerator and the other part consists of benzoyl peroxide initiator. Catalyst and base materials are mixed in a ratio of about 1:1. On mixing, their polymerization process is chemically activated. These chemicals showed poor color stability.

Light-activated Composite Resins

In the late 1960s and early 1970s, ultraviolet (UV) light cured composite resins were introduced. These composite resins tried to overcome some of the problems of self-cured composites but the problem with UV light polymerization was the limited depth of cure.

In late 1970s, visible light curing of composites replaced the UV light curing. Light activation in visible light curing ranges between 460 and 470 nm wavelength. On activation, photoinitiator (camphoroquinone) combines with amine accelerator and releases free radicles which start the polymerization. Since this reaction eliminated the need for tertiary amines, visible light cured composite resins showed improvement in the color stability of composite resins.

Curing Lamps

Several techniques have been used for curing of light cure composite resins. The various types of light used in curing of composite are:
- Tungsten-quartz halogen (TQH) curing unit
- Plasma arc curing (PAC) unit
- Light emitting diode (LED) unit
- Argon laser curing unit.

Tungsten-quartz Halogen Curing Unit (Figs 17.41 and 17.42)

Tungsten-quartz halogen (QHL) curing unit is conventional and most commonly used curing light for composite resins. It is incandescent lamp which uses visible light in the wavelength in the range of 410 to 500 nm. Halogen bulbs have limited effective lifetime of around 100 hours. At the start of curing cycle, this light emits a low power density (400-900 mW/cm^2). It means, there is lesser

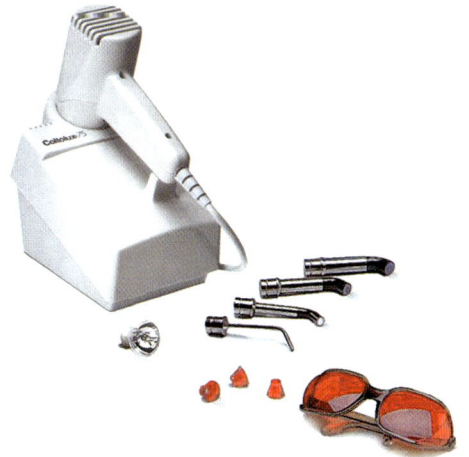

Figure 17.41: Tungsten-quartz halogen curing unit

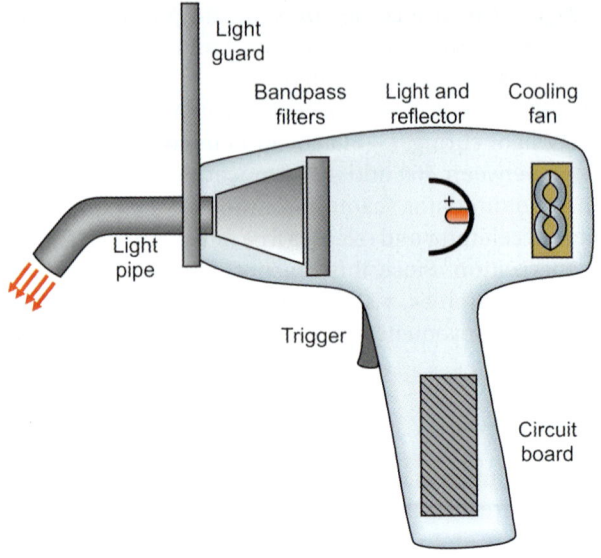

Figure 17.42: Diagramatic representation of light curing lamp

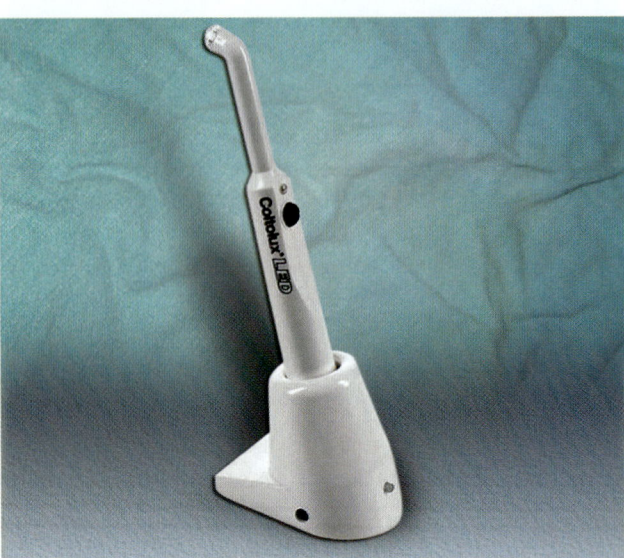

Figure 17.43: LED unit

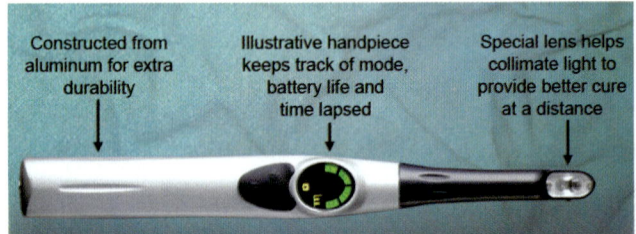

Figure 17.44: LED unit

polymerization at the start of cycle and maximum polymerization at the end of cycle.

Disadvantages of this technique are:
- Limited bulb life, i.e. 100 hours.
- Intensity of bulb decreases with time.
- Time consuming.

Plasma Arc Curing (PAC) Unit

In late 1990's, this system has been introduced as a means of rapid light curing.

Mechanism: In this, high frequency electrical field is generated using high voltage. This field ionizes the xenon gas into a mixture of ions, electrons and molecules, thereby releasing energy in the form of plasma.

Light guide helps in filtering the light to spectrum of visible light (450-500 nm) for peak absorption of camphoroquinone. PAC produces high intensity light more than 1800 mW/cm² curing cycle in PAC is 6 to 9 seconds.

Disadvantages of this technique are:
- Expensive
- Large size.

Light Emitting Diode Unit (Figs 17.43 and 17.44)

Light emitting diode (LED) unit usually have long life and emits powerful blue light. This light falls in narrow wavelength range of 400 to 500. This corresponds to range of camphoroquinone photoinitiator found in most of composite resins.

Advantages
- Low power consumption
- It can be used with batteries also
- It does not require filter
- Long life, i.e. 10,000 hours (approximately)
- Minimal changes in light output over time.

Disadvantage
- Only suitable for camphoroquinone based composites (because it has limited wavelength spectrum).

Argon Laser Curing Unit

Nowadays, composite resins are being cured with argon laser. Argon laser light has a wavelength of 470 nm which is monochromatic in nature. It produces intensity of 200 to 300 mW.

Advantages
- Polymerization is uniform, not affected by distance
- Greater depth of curing achieved with this light

• Degree of polymerization is higher with dark shades as compared to conventional halogen lights.

Disadvantages
• May affect adjacent restorations
• Chances of damage to pulp can occur due to rise in temperature.

Final Contouring, Finishing and Polishing of Composite Restorations

For composite restorations, the amount of contouring required after final curing can be minimized by careful placement technique. Always take care to remove the some composite excess which is almost always present.

The decreased need of contouring of the cured composite ensures that margins and surface of the composite restoration remain sealed and free of micro-cracks that can be formed while contouring.

The main objectives of contouring, finishing and polishing of final restoration are to:
• Attain optimal contour
• Remove excess composite material
• Polish the surface and margins of the composite restoration.

For removal of composite excess, usually burs and diamonds are used (**Fig. 17.45**). Surgical blade is used to remove proximal overhangs in the accessible area. For areas which have poor accessibility, composite strips can be used (**Figs 17.46 and 17.47**).

Final finishing and polishing of a composite restoration can be done with finishing diamond points. Polishing is done using rubber polishing points, abrasive discs or pumice impregnated points.

Contact areas may be finished by using a series of abrasive finishing strips threaded below the contact point so as not to destroy the contact point (**Fig. 17.48**) .

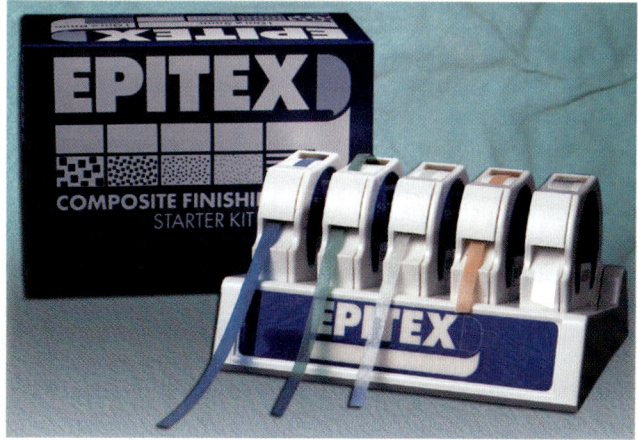

Figure 17.46: Finishing strips for interproximal areas

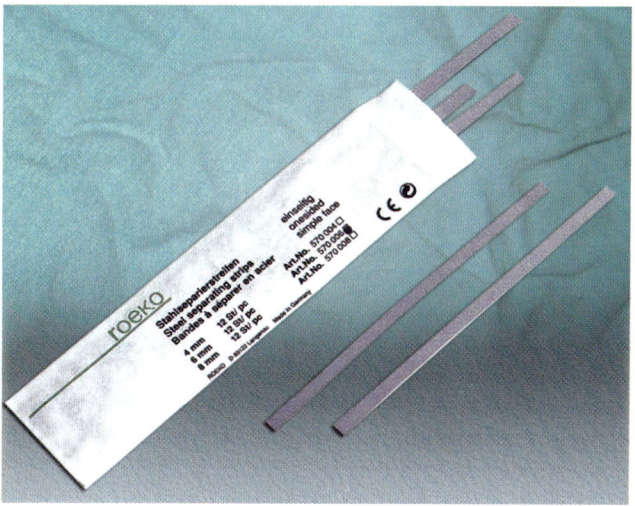

Figure 17.47: Finishing strips

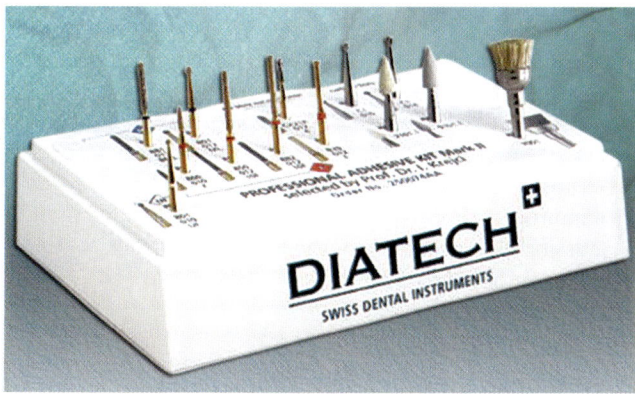

Figure 17.45: Abrasive diamonds for removal of excess composite material

FAILURES IN COMPOSITE RESTORATIONS

Composite restorations may show failure because of

➡ Incomplete removal of carious lesion
➡ Incomplete etching or incomplete removal of residual acid from tooth surface
➡ Excess or deficient application of bonding agent
➡ Lack of moisture control
➡ Contamination of composite with finger/saliva
➡ Following bulk placement technique during polymerization of composite
➡ Improper polymerization method
➡ Incomplete finishing and polishing of composites
➡ Inadequate occlusion of restored tooth.

Following failures are commonly seen in composite restorations with time

→ Discoloration, especially at the margins (**Fig. 17.49**)
→ Fracture of margins
→ Secondary caries
→ Postoperative sensitivity
→ Gross fracture of restoration
→ Loss of contact after a period of time
→ Accumulation of plaque around the restorations.

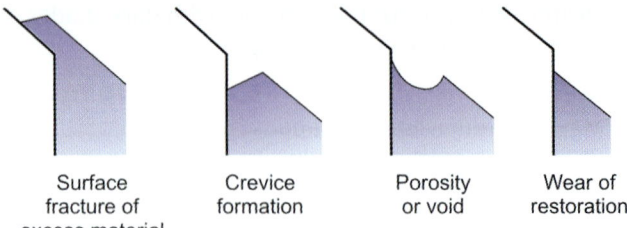

Surface fracture of excess material   Crevice formation   Porosity or void   Wear of restoration

Figure 17.50: Curing unit

Marginal Defects in Composite Restorations (Fig. 17.50)

Marginal defects in composites can occur in following forms:

• Surface fracture of excess material
• Voids in restoration because of air entrapment during placement

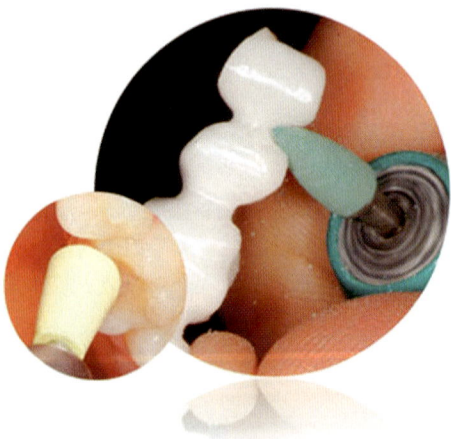

Figure 17.48: Contact area is finished by using series of abrasive stones below the contact point so as not to destroy it

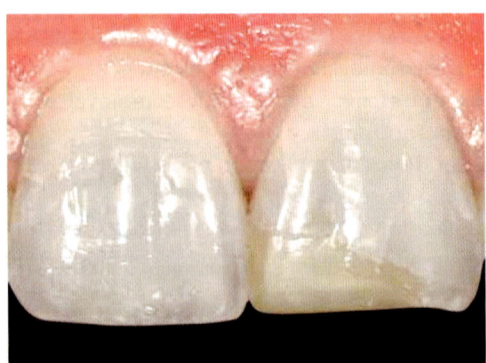

Figure 17.49: Discoloration of composite restoration of 21

• Composite wear resulting in progressive exposure of axially directed wall
• Gap formation.

Certain guidelines should be followed which can minimize the chances of composite failure:

• The tooth preparation should be kept as small as possible since composite in bulk lead to failure
• Avoid sharp internal line angles in tooth preparation, which increases stress concentration
• Deeper preparations should be given base of calcium hydroxide or glass ionomer cement
• Strict isolation regime is to be followed
• Avoid inadequate curing, since it lead to hydrolytic breakdown of composites
• Use small increments, holding each increment with Teflon coated instruments.
• Fill proximal box separately and create proper contact areas
• Composite, especially at the beveled areas, should be finished and polished properly.

INDIRECT COMPOSITE RESTORATIONS

Indirect restorations have been developed to overcome the disadvantages of the direct adhesive restorations like technique sensitivity, poor anatomic form, polymerization shrinkage, wear and interproximal contacts.

Classification of Indirect Composite Restorations

Classification of indirect composite resins systems

→ Classification based on method of fabrication:
  ♦ Direct
  ♦ Indirect.
→ Classification based on method of curing:
  ♦ Conventional cured
  ♦ Secondary cured
  ♦ Super cured.
→ Classification based on evolution:
  ♦ First generation
  ♦ Second generation.

Classification Based on Method of Fabrication

- *Direct:* These are directly made on the prepared tooth. In direct composite resin inlay system, after making preparation a suitable separating media and matrix system is applied on the tooth. Then, composite resin is built up in the preparation, extraorally cured, finished and polished.
- *Indirect:* These are made on a die of the prepared tooth in laboratory or at chair side.

Classification Based on Method of Curing

- *Conventional cured:* In this technique, curing is done on die of prepared tooth by use of light only
- *Secondary cured:* In this technique, curing is done in two cycles. Initial curing is done at room temperature using light followed by additional curing using heat and light
- *Super cured:* In this technique, curing is done in one step only. Curing is done under very high temperature and pressure in one stage only.

Classification Based on Evolution

- *First generation:* The first generation of indirect restorations was composite based, introduced in the early 1980. These materials were developed in an attempt to overcome the polymerization shrinkage and wear seen with direct composite restorations. But these also had poor physical properties because of low filler and high matrix load.

  They include SR Isosit system, Coltene Brilliant system and Kulzar system.

Advantages
→ Improved esthetics
→ Improved anatomy and interproximal contact
→ Chairside repair
→ Ease of fabrication.

Disadvantages
→ Low modulus of elasticity
→ Low resistance to wear abrasion
→ Low flexural strength
→ Fracture of restoration and debonding because of poor bonding between restoration and the cement.

- *Second generation:* They were introduced after mid 1990s so as to have better properties than first generation indirect restorations. They contained ceromers.

  In ceromers there are ceramic fillers which are silanized. Commonly used filler in these materials is barium silica. Second generation materials have a high filler load (70–80% by weight) and lower resin load.

Advantages
→ Low polymerization shrinkage
→ Increased modulus of elasticity
→ Increased the degree of conversion
→ Improved the fracture toughness.

Disadvantage
→ High wear rate.

Fiber Reinforced Composite

In 1998, this type of technique was introduced in the composite resin. In this, silane treated glass fiber or plasma treated polyethylene are added to resin matrix during the manufacturing process. Advantages of addition of polyethylene fibers are that they strengthen the restoration and increase its toughness (**Fig. 17.51**). Vectris (Ivoclar Williams, Amherst, Ny) is recent material which has been built from fiber reinforced technology.

Advantages of fiber reinforced composites
→ High flexure strength
→ Increased compressive strength
→ Increased hardness
→ Increased tensile strength
→ Increased resistance to crack propagation
→ Biocompatibility
→ Better in maintaining contact areas
→ Strength-to-weight ratios are superior when compared to most alloys
→ Noncorrosiveness
→ Good translucency
→ Satisfactory bonding properties
→ Ease of repair
→ Offer the potential for chair side and laboratory fabrication.

Indication for Use of Fiber Reinforced Composites

- Conservative tooth preparation
- Metal-free dentistry

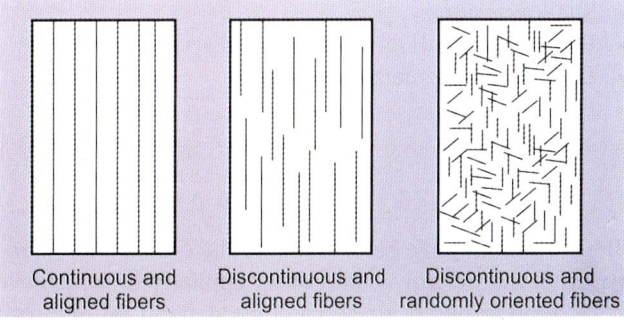

Figure 17.51: Fiber orientations in fiber reinforced composites

- Esthetics
- Splinting
- Postendodontic restorations.

Contraindications for Use of Fiber Reinforced Composites

- Patients with bruxism/clenching habit
- When opposite restoration is made up of porcelain
- In patients with high caries risk
- In long span partial dentures
- When moisture control is difficult.

Ceromers (Ceramic Optimized Polymer)

It is advanced type of composite material which also utilized the properties of ceramic fillers (metal oxides). The inclusion of ceramic fillers enhances the physical properties of composites such as ease in handling, improvement in wear and esthetic properties. Whenever filler is added to the composite, it increases the stiffness. To overcome this stiffness, organically layered silicate as rheological modifier is added in these materials. This system also incorporate a catalyst system which renders the material less sensitive to ambient light.

Composition

Ceromers consist of fine particle ceramic fillers which are closely packed and embedded in advanced organic polymer matrix. This material consists of paste containing barium glass, ytterbium trifluoride and silicon dioxide in dimethacrylate monomers.

Advantages
➡ Ease of final adjustment
➡ Excellent polishability
➡ Low degree of brittleness, hence less chances of fracture
➡ Good abrasion resistance
➡ Optimum esthetic properties.

Indications

- Shallow lesions
- Deep lesion with minimal occlusal access
- Large cervical defects
- Pulp capping
- Splinting.

RESIN CEMENTS (FIGS 17.52A AND B)

These cements have been available since 1952 for cementation of inlays, crowns and other appliances. To achieve high bond strength, these cements depend on acidetch technique with dentin conditioning, similar to composite restorations. Resin cements are marketed under different commercial names by manufacturers: Panavia Ex, Rely X, ARC–Resin cements, Scotchbond resin cement, Porcelite dual cure, etc.

Uses

- For cementation of inlays/onlays:
  - Metal
  - Porcelain
  - Precured composite.
- For cementation of crown and bridge
- For bonding amalgam restorations
- For cementation of orthodontic brackets
- For cementation of endodontic posts.

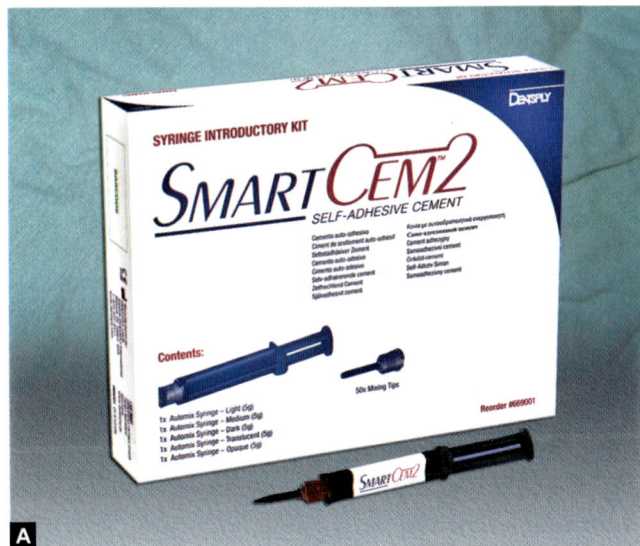

A

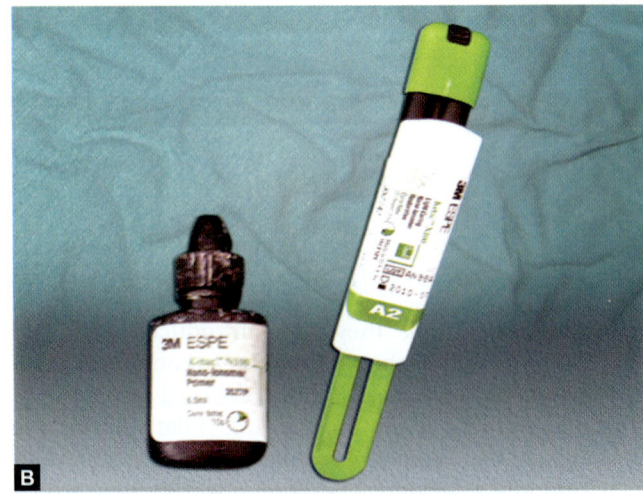

B

Figures 17.52A and B: Resin cements

Types of Resin Cements

- Unfilled resin cements.
- Filled resin cements.

Available in the form of:

- Powder and liquid system.
- Dual cure—two paste system.
- Supplied as single paste with accelerator in bonding agent.

Composition

- *Unfilled resin cements:* It is not used nowadays. It is based on methylmethacrylate and comonomers.

  Accelerator and initiator are tertiary amine and peroxide setting reaction is accomplished by liberation of heat and shrinkage of polymer.
- *Filled resin cements:* These are almost identical to resin based composite restorative materials.

Powder

- Resin matrix:
  - Bis-GMA
  - TEGDMA
- Inorganic filler:
  - Colloidal silica
  - Zirconia filler
- Coupling agent: Organosilane
- Chemical/photoinitiators and activators: For improving the rheology of material and handling.

Liquid

- Adhesive monomer
  - HEMA
  - 4-META
  - MDP (10-metha)
- Initiator: Benzoyl peroxide
- Inorganic fillers
  - Zirconia
  - Silica

Polymerization can be achieved by any means:

- Conventional chemical cure system
- Light activation
- Dual cure system.

Technique for Using Resin Cements

- Isolate the area, preferably with rubber dam.
- Apply etchant, wait for 15 seconds, rinse for 10 seconds with distilled water. Remove excess water, leaving tooth surface moist.

- Apply adhesive to enamel and dentin, dry for 5 seconds and light cure for 10 seconds.
- Roughen the bonding surface of restoration using air abrasion/diamond. In case of ceramic, apply ceramic primer such as organosilanes to etched porcelain and roughened metal surfaces. Dry for 5 seconds.
- Dispense appropriate amount of cement on mixing pad and mix for 10 seconds.
- Apply thin layer of cement on bonding surface of restoration.
- Seat the restoration, remove excess of cement and light cure for 40 seconds.

 Key Points

- The modern history of tooth colored restorative materials was started with silicate cement (Fletcher 1878).
- Composites are basically modified methacrylates or acrylates with other ingredients to produce different structures and properties.
- The methacrylates are used because of their refractive index of 1.3 which is close to tooth. This allows metamerism (chameleon effect) giving the effect of similar color.
- The matrix base consists of polymeric mono-, di- or trifunctional monomers like Bis-GMA or UDMA. Since this resin is highly viscous, to improve clinical handling, it is diluted with low viscosity monomers like bisphenol A dimethacrylate (Bis-DMA), ethylene glycol dimethacrylate (EGDMA), triethylene glycol dimethacrylate (TEGDMA), and/or methyl methacrylate (MMA).
- The filler particles are added to improve the physical and mechanical properties of the organic matrix. Commonly used fillers are silicon dioxide, boron silicates and lithium aluminum silicates.
- Recently nanoparticles having the size of 25 nm and nanoaggregates of 75 nm, made up of zirconium/silica or nanosilica particles have been tried as fillers.
- A coupling agent is used to bond the filler to the organic resin. This agent is a molecule with silane groups at one end (ion bond to SiO_2) and methacrylate groups at the other.
- The average particle size of macrofill composite resins is from 5 to 25 micron with filler content ranging from 75 to 80 percent by weight. It exhibits a rough surface texture because of the relatively large size and extreme hardness of the filler particles.
- Average particle size of microfilled resins ranges from 0.04 to 0.1 micrometer with filler loading of 35 to 50 percent by weight. The small particle size results in smooth polished surface which is resistant to plaque, debris and stains. But because of less filler content, some of their physical properties are inferior.

- Hybrid composites are composed of glasses of different compositions and sizes, with particle size diameter of less than 2 µm and containing 0.04 µm sized fumed silica and filler content of 75 to 80 percent by volume. This mixture of fillers is responsible for their physical properties similar to those of conventional composites with the advantage of smooth surface texture.
- Flowable composite resin has lower filler content (41 to 53% by volume and 60% by weight) with average particle size of 0.02 to 0.05 µm. Low filler loading is responsible for decreased viscosity and poor mechanical properties of these composites.
- The principle of the packable composites is that they can be packed into the tooth preparations. Their basic principle is polymer rigid inorganic matrix material (PRIMM). Here the components are resin and ceramic inorganic fillers which are incorporated in silanated network of ceramic fibers. These fibers are composed of alumina and silicon dioxide which are fused each other at specific sites to form a continuous network of small compartments. Filler content in packable composites ranges from 48 to 65 percent by volume. Average particle size ranges from 0.7 to 20 µm.
- Giomer is hybrid of words "glass ionomers" and "composite". Also known as PRG composites (Prereacted glass ionomer composites), they have properties of both glass ionomers (Fluoride release, fluoride recharge) and resin composite (excellent esthetics, easy polishability, biocompatibility).
- Compomers consist of 2 components viz; dimethacrylate monomers with two carboxylic acid groups present and reactive silicate glass containing filler. They are available in single paste, light enable material in syringe or compules.
- ORMOCER is an organically modified non metallic inorganic composite material. ORMOCERS have organic molecules segment (methacrylate groups) forming a highly cross-linked matrix, inorganic molecules to make three-dimensional network forming backbone of ORMOCER molecules.
- Composites exhibit polymerization shrinkage which accounts for 1.67 to 5.68 percent of the total volume.
- Since the material nearest to the light sets first, shrinkage in light cured composites occurs in the direction of light and for chemical cured composites shrinkage occurs slowly and uniformly towards the center of restoration.
- The cavity configuration or C-factor was introduced by Professor Carol Davidson and his colleagues in 1980s.
- The configuration factor (C-factor) is the ratio of bonded surface of the restoration to the unbonded surfaces. The higher the value of C-factor, the greater is the polymerization shrinkage.

- Microleakage is passage of fluid and bacteria in microgaps (10^{-6} m) between restoration and tooth. It can result in damage to the pulp.
- Nanoleakage is passage of fluid/dissolved species in nanosized (10^{-9} m) gaps. These nanosized porosities occur within hybrid layer.
- For optimal polymerization of composites wavelength of light should range between 400 and 500 nm.
- Conventional design for composite restoration is similar to that of amalgam restoration, except that there is less outline extension and in tooth preparation, walls are made rough. It is indicated specially when preparations are located on root surface.
- Beveled conventional tooth preparation is almost similar to conventional design but some beveled enamel margins are incorporated. It is indicated for large preparations (specially for classes III, IV, V and VI restorations).
- Modified (conservative tooth preparation) has scooped out appearance in which extent and depth of the preparation depends upon the extent and the depth of carious lesion.
- In the late 1960s, ultraviolet (UV) light cured composite resins were introduced, but they showed the problem of limited depth of cure.
- In late 1970s, visible light curing of composites came in which light activation ranges from 460 to 470 nm wavelength. On activation, photoinitiator (camphoroquinone) combines with amine accelerator and releases free radicles which start the polymerization.
- The indirect composite restorations were developed to overcome the disadvantages of the direct composite restorations like technique sensitivity, poor anatomic form, polymerization shrinkage, wear and interproximal contacts.
- The first generation of indirect restorations was composite based, introduced in the early 1980. They showed improvement in polymerization shrinkage but had poor physical properties because of low filler and high matrix load.
- Second generation of indirect restorations were introduced to have better properties than first generation. They contained ceromers in which silanized ceramic fillers were used. They showed low polymerization shrinkage, increased modulus of elasticity and improved the fracture toughness.
- In 1998, fiber reinforced composite was introduced. In this, silane treated glass fiber or plasma treated polyethylene is added to resin matrix during the manufacturing process to increase the flexure strength, tensile strength, and fracture toughness.

QUESTIONS

1. What is composition of composites? Explain importance of filler in composites.
2. Classify composites. Explain hybrid composite resins.
3. Short notes on:
   a. Flowable composites
   b. Packable composites
   c. Ormocers
   d. Smart composites
   e. C-factor
   f. Degree of conversion
   g. Composite placement techniques
   h. Indirect composite restorations.
   i. Resin cements
   j. Fiber reinforced composite
4. Write short notes on:
   a. Microfilled resin.
   b. Light cure composite
5. What are indications, contraindications, advantages and disadvantages of composite restoration. Write in detail about the clinical technique for direct class III composite restoration.

BIBLIOGRAPHY

1. Althoff O, Hartung M. Advances in light curing. Am J Dent. 2000;13:77.
2. Asmussen E. Composite restorative resins. Composition versus wall to wall polymerization contraction. Acta Odont Scand. 1975;33:337.
3. Baratieri LN, Monteiro S Jr, Correa M, Ritter AV. Posterior resin composite restorations: A new technique. Quint Int. 1996;27:733.
4. Bausch JR, DeLange K, Davidson CL, Peters A, DeGee, AJ. Clinical signification of polymerization shrinkage of composite resins. JPD. 1982;48:59.
5. Bayne SC, Heymann IIO, Swift EJ. Update on dental composite restorations. JADA. 1994;125:687.
6. Bayne SC, Thompson JY, Swift EJ, Stamatiades P, Wilkerson M. A characterization of first generation flowable composite. JADA. 1998;129:567.
7. Besnault C, Attal JP. Simulated oral environment and microleakage of Class II resin-based composite and sandwich restorations. Am J Dent. 2003;16:186-90.
8. Bryant RW. Direct posterior composite resin restorations: A review. II. Clinical technique. Aust Dent J. 1992;37:161.
9. Bryant RW. Posterior composite resin restorations—a review of clinical problems. Aust Dent J. 1987;1:41.
10. Buonocore M, et al. A report on a resin composition capable of bonding to human dentin surfaces. J Dent Res. 1956;35:846.
11. Collins CJ, et al. A clinical evaluation of posterior composite resin restorations. 8-year findings. J Dent. 1998;26:311-7.
12. Covey DA, Tahaney SR, Davenport JM. Mechanical properties of heat-treated composite resin restorative materials. JPD. 1992;68:458.
13. Craig RG. Chemistry, composition and properties of composite resins. Dent Clin North Am. 1981;25:219.
14. Farah JW, Dougherty EW. Unfilled, filled, and microfilled composite resins. Oper Dent. 1981;6:95.
15. Feilezer AJ, et al. Setting stress in composite resin in relation to configuration of the restoration. J Dent Res. 1987;66:1636-9.
16. Mazer RB, Leinfelder KF. Clinical evaluation of a posterior composite resin containing a new type of filler particle. J Esthet Dent. 1988;1:66-70.
17. Mazer RB, Leinfelder KF. Evaluating a microfill posterior composite resin. A five year study. J Am Dent Assoc. 1992;123:33-8.
18. McCune RJ, et al. Clinical comparison of anterior and posterior restorative materials (abstract no. 482). Int Assoc Dent Res. 1969;161.
19. McCune RJ, et al. Clinical comparison of posterior restorative materials (abstract no. 546). Int Assoc Dent Res. 1967;175.
20. Murray PE, et al. Bacterial microleakage and pulp inflammation associated with various restorative materials. Dent Mater. 2002;18:470-8.
21. Sanares AM, et al. Adverse surface interactions between one-bottle light-cured adhesives and chemical-cured composites. Dent Mater. 2001;17:542-56.
22. Simonsen RJ. Preventive resin restoration. Quintessence Int. 1978;9:69-76.
23. Sockwell CL. Clinical evaluation of anterior restorative materials. Dent Clin North Am. 1976;20:403.
24. Torstenson B, Brännström M. Composite resin contraction gaps measured with a fluorescent resin technique. Dent Mater. 1988;4:238-42.
25. Volker J, et al. Some observations on the relationship between plastic filling materials and dental caries. Tufts Dent Outlook. 1944;18:4.

Tooth Preparation for Composite Restorations

18

CHAPTER

Chapter Outline

Prerequisites for tooth preparation to receive composite restoration

➡ Use rubber dam for optimal isolation of the working area

➡ Use yellow filter for the operating light or to keep it on low intensity so as to avoid the premature polymerization of the composite

➡ Take proper precautions to protect eyes from glare. For this use safety specs or hand-held shield

➡ Use, teflon coated composite filling instrument so as to prevent the composite resin from sticking and 'pulling back'.

CLASS III TOOTH PREPARATION

Depending upon the type of dental tissues involved, the tooth preparation for the composites can be done in three designs: conventional, beveled conventional and modified.

Conventional Class III Tooth Preparation (Figs 18.1A and B)

- Indication for conventional tooth preparation is the lesion present on the root surfaces.
- Usually most of the lesions occur partly on the root and partly on the crown. The tooth preparation on the root is done in conventional method whereas on the crown it is prepared in beveled conventional or modified type (**Figs 18.2A and B**).
- The extent of lesion determines the outline of tooth preparation. For penetration into lesion, usually the direction for entry of bur is from lingual side except for a few cases (**Fig. 18.3**). This lingual approach helps in preservation of esthetics.

➥ Involvement of labial enamel.
➥ In cases of rotated teeth where lingual approach is difficult.
➥ In cases of malaligned teeth.

- When the damage is present only on the root surface, then the conventional preparation is made only on the root with 90 degree cavosurface margins. In the crown

portion of the preparation, the retention is mostly achieved by adhesive bonding to enamel and dentin.
- The external walls are made perpendicular to the root surface.
- While preparing, there should be adequate removal of caries, old restoration or defective tooth structure. The external walls of the preparation should be located on the sound tooth structure with a cavosurface angle of 90 degree for butt joint relation.
- If the carious lesion is not deep, the depth of the preparation is kept 0.75 mm. After this, it is deepened wherever caries is present.

➥ Roughening of the preparation surface
➥ Parallelism or convergence of opposing external walls
➥ Giving retention grooves and coves (**Fig. 18.4**).

- Grooves can be placed continuous or isolated. Continuous groove is placed in external walls, parallel to tooth surface. It should be located at least 1 mm from the tooth surface and at least 0.5 mm deep into dentin.

Beveled Conventional Class III Tooth Preparation

➥ For replacing an existing defective restoration on crown portion of an anterior tooth.
➥ For restoration of large preparations.

Steps

- Approach the area lingually with a no. ½, 1 or 2 round bur. Penetrate the lesion and move the bur in incisogingival direction.
- Entry angle of the bur should be such that it places the neck portion of the bur far into the embrasure.

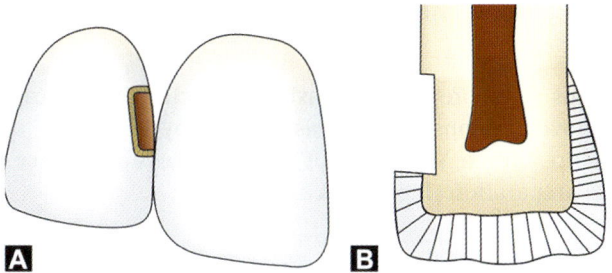

Figures 18.1A and B: Conventional class III tooth preparation for composites

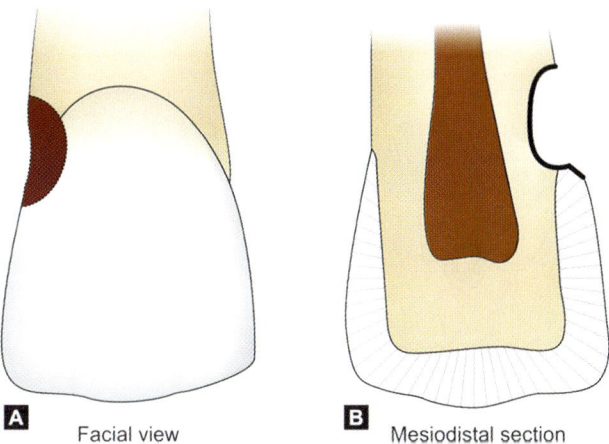

Facial view   Mesiodistal section

Figures 18.2A and B: When caries extend to root surface: (A) Conventional tooth preparation is made on root; (B) Bevelling is done in coronal portion

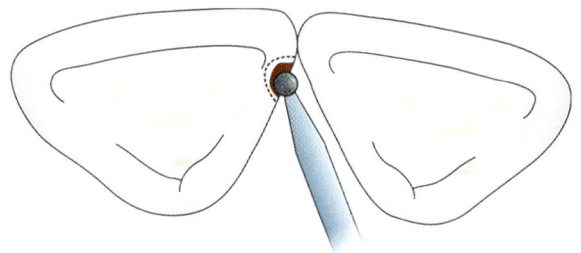

Figure 18.3: For initial penetration, entry into tooth should be made from the palatal side so as to preserve esthetics

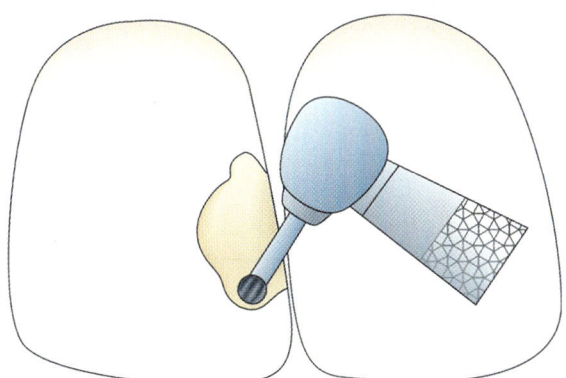

Figure 18.4: Making grooves in class III preparation for retention

- Shape of the tooth preparation should be identical to the shape of existing carious lesion or the restoration.
- One should take care to include any secondary caries, friable tooth structure and defects while placing the external walls on the sound tooth structure.
- Initial depth of the axial wall should be 0.75 mm deep gingivally and 1.25 mm deep incisally. This results in the axial wall depth of 0.2 mm into the dentin (**Fig. 18.5**).
- Shape of the axial wall should be convex outwardly, that is, it should follow the contour of the tooth.
- In final tooth preparation, remove all the remaining infected dentin or defective restoration using spoon excavator or slow speed round bur.
- For pulp protection, place a calcium hydroxide liner if indicated.
- Keep external walls of the tooth preparation perpendicular to the enamel surface with all enamel margins beveled (**Fig. 18.6**). Prepare the bevels using flat end tapering fissure diamond bur at cavosurface margins in the areas of centric contacts. The bevel should be about 0.2 to 0.5 mm wide at an angle of 45 degree to the external tooth surface (**Figs 18.7A and B**).
- Bevels are not given in areas bearing heavy occlusal forces or on cemental cavosurface margins.

- If required, prepare retentive grooves and coves along gingivoaxial line angle and incisoaxial line angle, respectively, with the help of no. 1/4 or 1/2 round burs. Depth of these grooves should be 0.2 mm into the dentin.

Modified (Conservative) Class III Tooth Preparation

It is the most conservative type of tooth preparation used for composites.

> Indication for modified preparation is small to moderate class III lesion.

In this tooth preparation, basically infected carious area is removed as conservatively as possible by "scooping" out. This results in 'scooped-out' or 'concave' appearance of the preparation (**Figs 18.8A and B**).

Steps

- Make initial entry through the palatal surface with a small round bur in the air rotor handpiece. It is always preferred to use the lingual approach since it conserves labial tooth structure which is more esthetic.

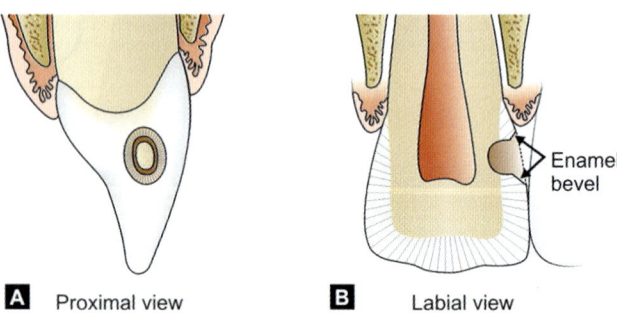

Figures 18.7A and B: Proximal and labial view of beveled class III tooth preparation for composites

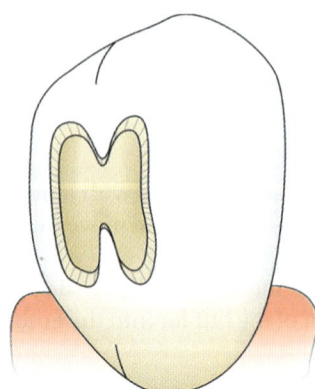

Figure 18.5: Completed class III tooth preparation for composites

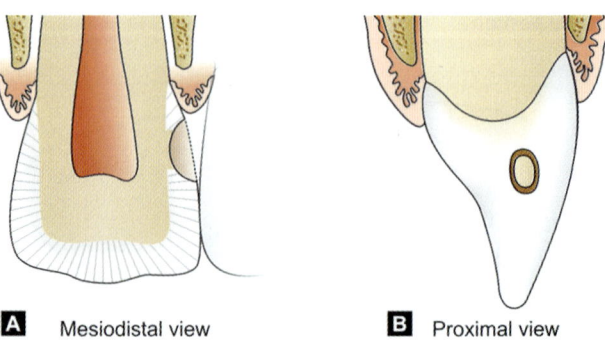

Figures 18.8A and B: Saucer shaped class III tooth preparation (A) Mesiodistal view; (B) Proximal view

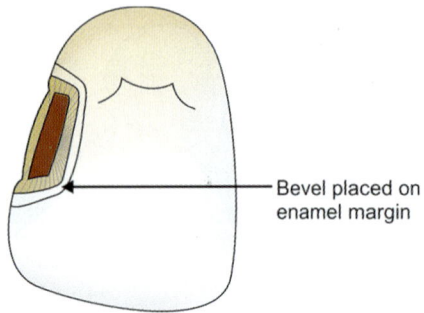

Figure 18.6: Beveled class III tooth preparation for composites

- The bur should be kept rotating when being entered into the tooth and should not stop rotating until being removed
- The design and extent of the preparation is determined by the extent of the carious lesion (**Fig. 18.9**)
- Keep all the internal line angles round to decrease internal stresses. It can be done using a half round bur head
- This type of preparation may not have any definite axial wall depth and the walls may diverge externally from axial depth in a scoop shape.
- In the final stage, remove the remaining infected dentin using slow speed round bur or spoon excavator.
- Then, finally check the preparation after cleaning with water and air spray and provide pulp protection.

CLASS IV TOOTH PREPARATION

Class IV restoration is required when anterior tooth has got incisal angle fracture because of trauma or caries.

Tooth Preparation for Conventional Class IV Preparation (Fig. 18.10)

Conventional type of class IV design is primarily indicated in those areas that have margins on root surface and where restoration is to be placed in high stress bearing area.

> **Features of conventional class IV preparation for composites**
> - Box like preparation with facial and lingual walls parallel to long axis of tooth.
> - Retention obtained by means of dovetail or grooves placed gingivally and incisally in the axial wall using number 1/4 round bur.

Beveled Conventional Class IV Preparation

A beveled conventional preparation is indicated for treatment of a large lesion. The initial axial wall depth should be kept 0.5 mm into dentin. Bevels are prepared at 45 degree angle to tooth surface with a width of 0.25 to 2 mm, depending on the amount of retention required. All internal angles should be rounded to avoid any stress concentration points (**Fig. 18.11**).

The success of a class IV restoration depends upon achieving retention other than found within the preparation itself. *Various modes of gaining retention are placing grooves, coves, undercuts, flares, bevels and pins. These methods help in providing the additional retention, however the use of pins for anterior resins has decreased significantly because of the following reasons:*
- *Risk of perforation either into the pulp or through the external surface.*
- *Pins do not enhance the strength of the restorative material.*
- *Pins may corrode because of microleakage of the restoration, resulting in discoloration of the tooth and restoration.*

Modified (Conservative) Class IV Preparation

Modified class IV preparation is done in small class IV lesions or for treatment of small traumatic defects. Objectives, technique, procedure and instrument used for this preparation are identical to class III preparation. Preparation for modified class IV preparation should be

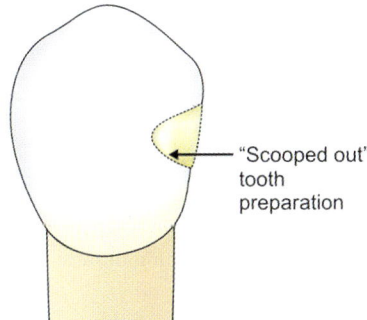

"Scooped out" tooth preparation

Figure 18.9: Extent of preparation is determined by extent of caries

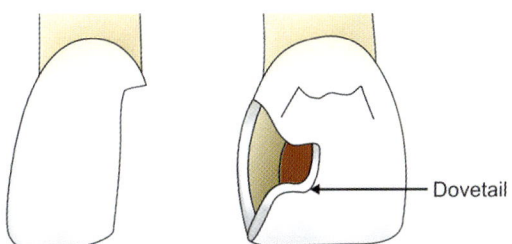

Dovetail

Figure 18.10: Conventional class IV tooth preparation for composites

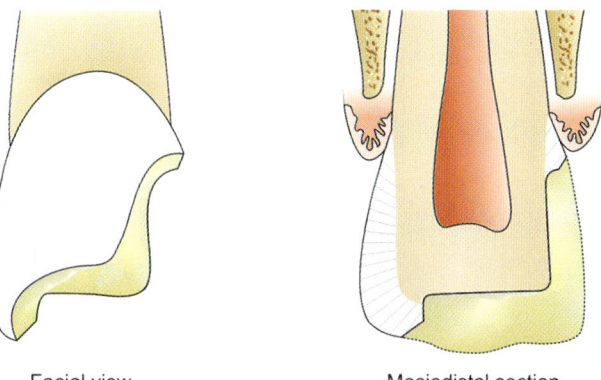

Facial view   Mesiodistal section

Figure 18.11: Beveled class IV tooth preparation for composites

done conservatively without removing the normal tooth structure (**Fig. 18.12**).

CLASS V TOOTH PREPARATION

Composites are material of choice for restoration of class V lesions which are esthetically prominent. Among composites, microfill composites are material of choice because they provide better and more smooth surface and have sufficient flexibility to resist stresses caused by cervical flexure, when tooth flexes under heavy occlusal forces.

Conventional Class V Preparation

Conventional class V preparation is indicated if it is present completely or mainly on root surface (**Fig. 18.13**). If the lesion is partly on crown and partly on root, then the crown portion is prepared using beveled conventional or modified preparation design and the root surface lesion is prepared in conventional method.

In conventional class V tooth preparation, shape of the preparation is a "box" type. Isolate the area well and use a tapered fissure (no. 700 or 701) bur to make entry at 45 degree angle to tooth surface initially. After this, keep long axis of bur perpendicular to the external surface in order to get a cavosurface angle of 90 degree.

During initial tooth preparation, keep the axial depth of 0.75 mm into the dentin.

After achieving the desired distal extension, move the bur mesially, incisally (occlusally) and gingivally for placing the preparation margins onto the sound tooth surface while maintaining a cavosurface margin of 90 degree.

The axial wall should follow the contour of facial surface incisogingivally and mesiodistally.

During the final tooth preparation, remove any remaining infected dentin, restoration material using spoon excavator or slow speed round bur.

For pulp protection, use calcium hydroxide liner, if necessary.

If additional retention is required, place retention grooves all along the whole length of incisoaxial and gingivoaxial line angles using a no. 1/4 or 1/2 round bur 0.25 mm deep into the dentin (**Fig. 18.14**). At this stage, all the external walls appear outwardly divergent. Finally, clean tooth preparation with water and air dry it (**Fig. 18.15**).

Beveled Conventional Class V Tooth Preparation

Beveled conventional class V preparation is indicated for replacing defective existing restoration or for restoring a large, carious lesion.

The initial axial wall depth should be limited to only 0.25 mm into the dentin, when retention grooves are not placed and 0.5 mm when a retention groove is placed. Place a mechanical retention groove inside the gingival cavosurface margin.

After this, bevel the enamel margins at an angle of 45 degree to the external surface and to a width of 0.25 to 0.5 mm (**Fig. 18.16**). When the class V carious lesion is large

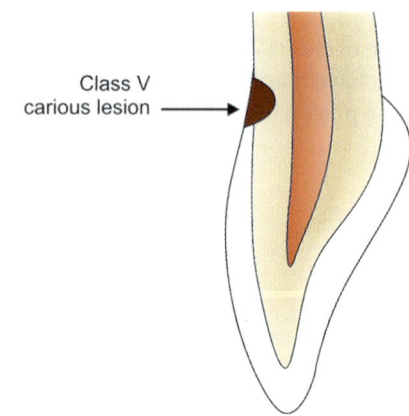

Figure 18.13: Conventional tooth preparation is indicated if caries are present mainly on root surface

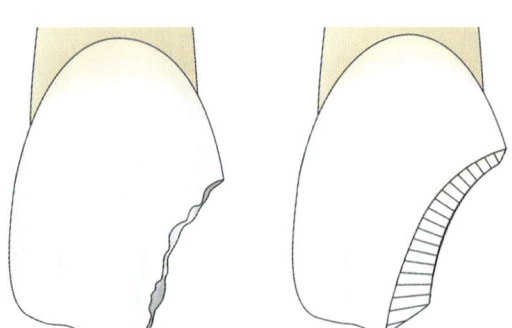

Figure 18.12: In case of fracture of teeth or small carious lesion, only removal of defect and beveling is required

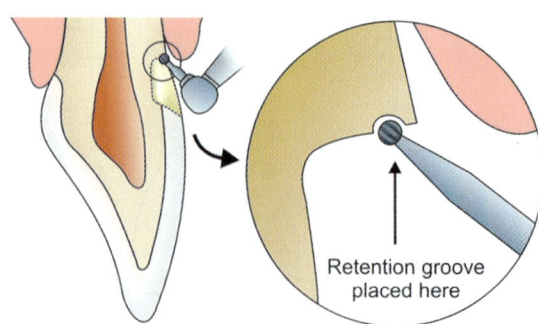

Figure 18.14: Placing retention grooves in class V preparation

enough to extend onto the root surface, the gingival part is prepared in the conventional class V tooth preparation design with the initial axial depth of 0.75 mm. Beveling is done only on enamel cavosurface margins (**Fig. 18.17**).

Roughen the dentin with a medium size diamond bur to provide mechanical retention and thus increasing the bond strength.

Modified (Conservative) Class V Tooth Preparation

Modified class V design is indicated for

→ Restoration of small and moderate carious lesions and defects.

→ Small enamel defects like decalcified and hypoplastic areas present in cervical third of the teeth (**Figs 18.18A and B**).

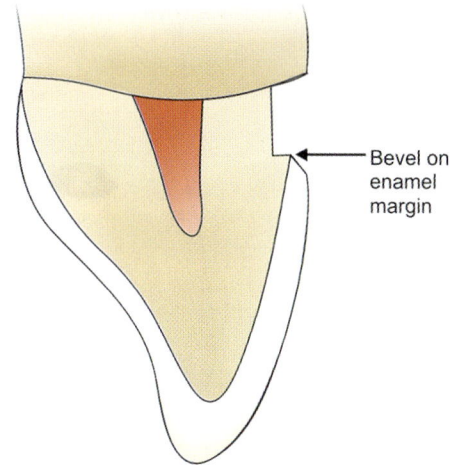

Bevel on enamel margin

Figure 18.17: Beveling is done on enamel surface

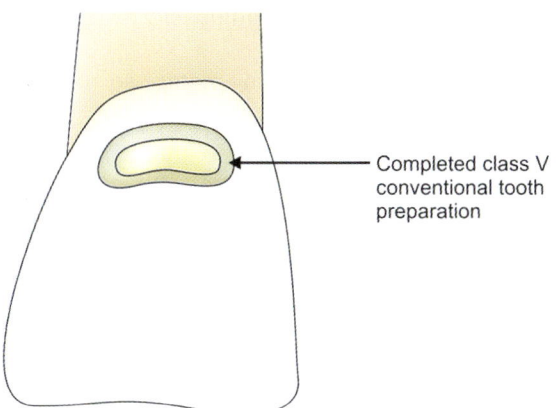

Completed class V conventional tooth preparation

Figure 18.15: Conventional class V tooth preparation

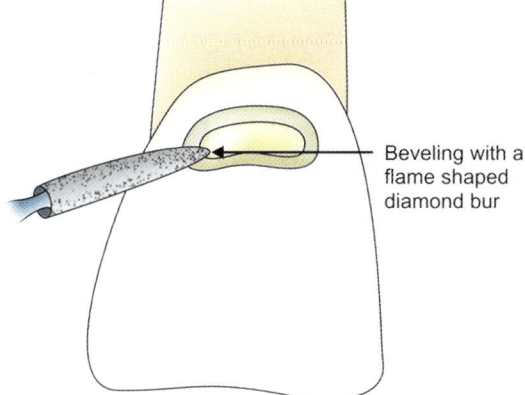

Beveling with a flame shaped diamond bur

Figure 18.16: Beveling of preparation using a flame shaped bur

Modifed class V, tooth is prepared as discussed in the previous modified preparation.

The final tooth preparation should have 'scooped out' appearance with divergent walls and axial wall either in enamel or dentin (**Fig. 18.19**).

TOOTH PREPARATION FOR POSTERIOR COMPOSITE RESTORATION

Indications for Use of Composites for Class I, II and VI Preparations

→ Small to moderate sized lesions in posterior teeth.
→ Incipient lesions.
→ In premolars and first molars where esthetics is the main concern.
→ When moisture control of operating site is possible.
→ When tooth being restored, does not experience occlusal stresses.
→ In patient with low caries risk.
→ As a core foundation for full crown restoration.

Contraindications for Use of Posterior Composite Restorations

→ When it is difficult to achieve moisture control.
→ When large lesion is present extending onto the root surface.
→ When restoration is subjected to high occlusal stresses.
→ When heavy contacts are present on the restoration.
→ In patients with high caries risk and poor oral hygiene.
→ In patients with parafunctional habits like clenching and bruxism.

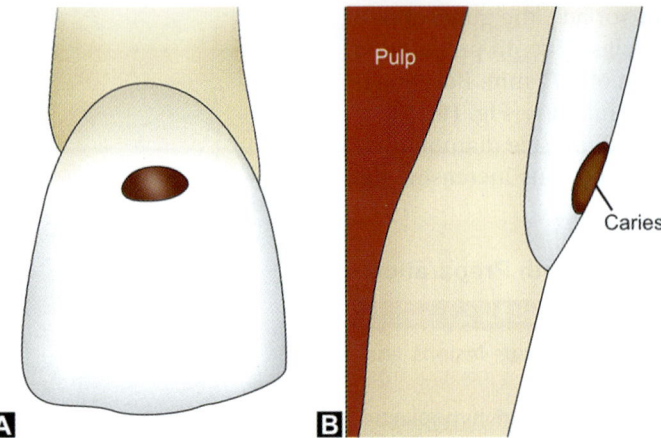

Figures 18.18A and B: Modified class V tooth preparation is indicated only in cases when small lesion is present in cervical third of the teeth

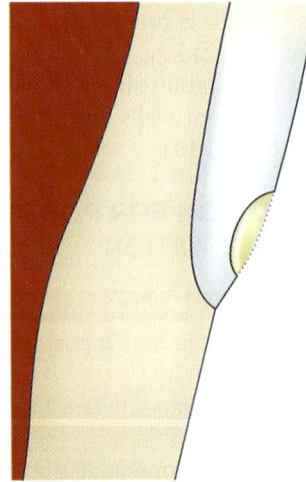

Figure 18.19: Scooped out appearance of tooth preparation

Advantages of Posterior Composite Restoration

- Good esthetics.
- Conservation of tooth structure because of adhesive tooth preparation.
- Low thermal conductivity of composites provide insulation to thermal changes.
- Because of their micromechanical bonding, tooth preparation is easier, simple and less complex.
- Economically cheap when compared to indirect restorations and crown forms.
- Because of adhesion to tooth, there is increased retention and strengthening of remaining tooth structure.

- Composites have adequate radiopacity to be seen in the radiographs.
- Since it does not contain metal, so no risk of galavanism.

Disadvantages

- Polymerization shrinkage occurring after polymerization of composites can lead to:
  - Postoperative sensitivity
  - Secondary caries
  - Discoloration.
- More technique sensitive than amalgam.
- Less resistance to wear especially the microfilled composites.
- Takes more time for placement.
- Expensive in comparison to amalgam restoration.

CLASS I TOOTH PREPARATION

Composite is preferred in small pit and fissure lesions in conservative modified preparations. Concept of ultra-conservative restoration, also known as 'conservative composite restoration' was given by Simonsen in 1978. It is also referred to as 'preventive resin restorations'. This preparation precede diagnosis of cavitation, instead of frank carious lesion.

Depending on the extent of preparation to be restored, there are three designs:
1. Conventional
2. Beveled conventional
3. Modified.

Conventional Design for Class I Tooth Preparation

For moderate sized lesions, conventional design is preferred for composite restorations. Fundamentals of tooth preparation are similar to that of amalgam except for few differences. Gain entry into lesion with small round bur keeping the bur parallel to tooth structures and then extend the preparation using flat fissure bur, keep the minimal depth (1.5 mm) throughout the preparation (**Figs 18.20A to C**).

Differences from Tooth Preparation for Amalgam
➡ Faciolingual dimension of preparation are kept as small as possible (¼th of intercuspal distance).
➡ No need to prepare dovetail or other retention features
➡ Preparation floor need not be kept perpendicular.

Modified Design for Class I Tooth Preparation (Fig. 18.21)

Features of modified preparation design for class I composite restoration:
- Preparation has scooped out appearance extended to only the extent of caries. Preparation is done using rounded corner inverted cone bur so as to:
  – Prepare walls converging occlusally.
  – Prepare rounded line angles.
  – Provide flat floor.
  – Produce minimal width faciolingually.
  – Provide occlusal marginal configuration.

The initial enamel depth of preventive resin restoration is kept as 1 mm. Flame shaped diamond instruments are used to bevel the enamel cavosurface margins approximately. Usually the cavosurface bevel is 0.5 mm wide and placed at an angle of 45 degrees to the external enamel surface. If the marginal ridge is not supported by dentin, remaining weakened enamel may be left, provided there is no heavy centric contact on this area (**Fig. 18.22**). The unsupported marginal ridge will be strengthened by composite restoration. Shallow fissures radiating from pits and fissures are treated by enameloplasty.

Beveling of the enamel margin results in
➡ Increased retention (beveling increases the surface for bonding)
➡ Reduction in microleakage
➡ Improvement in esthetics since bevel enables the restoration to blend more esthetically with surrounding tooth structure
➡ Increase in bond strength
➡ Conservation of tooth structure since the need for grooves for additional retention can be avoided.

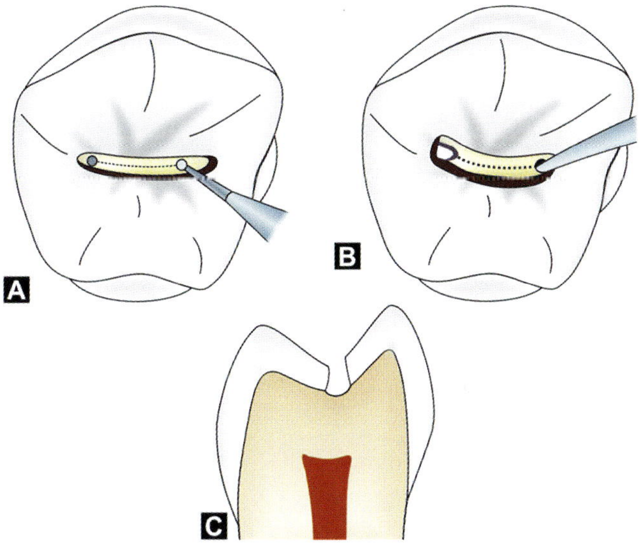

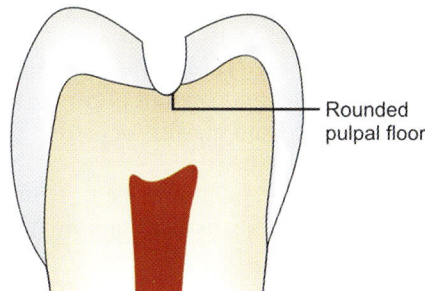

Figure 18.21: Modified class I tooth preparation for composite restorations

Rounded pulpal floor

Figures 18.20A to C: Conventional class I tooth preparation for composite restoration (A) Preparation of outline using round bur; (B) Excavation of caries, keeping the pulpal floor shallow; (C) Completed class I tooth preparation

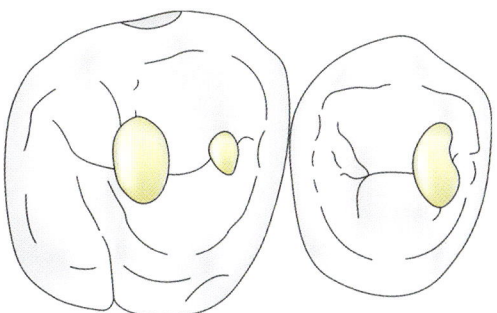

Figure 18.22: Modified class I preparation

CLASS II TOOTH PREPARATION

Composites if manipulated properly can be successfully used in Class II restorations.

The advantages of using composites in class II are
• Better esthetics
• Conservative tooth preparation
• Strengthening of remaining tooth structure
• Bonding of tooth by composite.

Problems with Composites for Use in Class II Restorations
➡ Difficult to achieve moisture control
➡ In deep subgingival extension cases
➡ In teeth with heavy occlusal contact on the composites.

Although features for class II restoration are similar to those used for amalgam preparations were suggested in the past, but nowadays, a more conservative tooth preparation is commonly recommended today.

Before initiating tooth preparation for composite, proper isolation of the operating field by means of rubber dam placement is compulsory. Since composites bond better to enamel than to dentin, there is no need to prepare into dentin if lesion has not penetrated.

Steps

- Prepare the occlusal part of the tooth preparation similar to class I (**Fig. 18.23**) but the proximal box preparation depends upon extent of caries, contour of the proximal surface and masticatory stresses to which restoration will be subjected.
- For proximal box preparation, extend the occlusal preparation using straight fissure bur onto the marginal ridge (**Fig. 18.24**). Keep the bur perpendicular to the pulpal floor.
- Thin out the marginal ridge and deepen the preparation towards the gingival direction as to give proximal ditch cut. This will form the width of 1.0 to 1.5 mm (**Fig. 18.25**).
- For small carious lesion, proximal walls can be left in the contact but for large carious lesion, contact area is broken.
- Keep the gingival floor flat with butt joint cavosurface angle. Whether or not to give gingival beveling, depends on location and the width of gingival seat. If gingival seat is supragingival and above cementoenamel junction, beveling can be done but if gingival seat is close to cementoenamel junction, beveling is avoided so as to preserve the enamel present in this area (**Fig. 18.26**).
- The final conventional tooth preparation for composite is more conservative than for traditional amalgam restoration (**Fig. 18.27**).

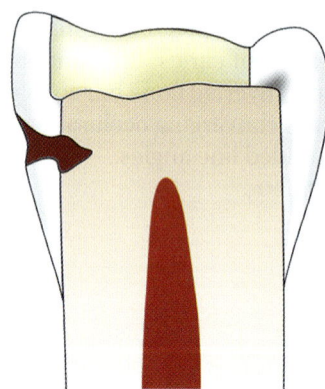

Figure 18.24: Extension of occlusal step to the marginal ridge

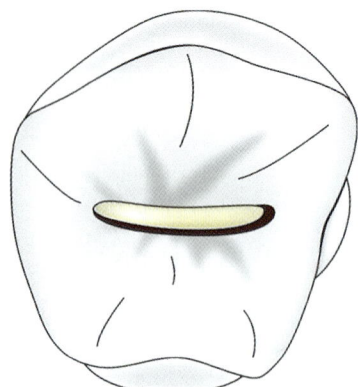

Figure 18.23: Make the occlusal outline as done for class I tooth preparation

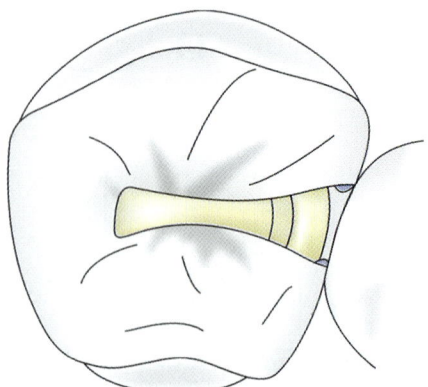

Figure 18.25: Completed class II tooth preparation for composites

Modification for Class II Composite Restoration

- When minimal caries are present, saucer shaped class II preparation is done. Here, the preparation is deepened only to the extent where caries are present. The scooped out preparation does not have uniform depth (**Fig. 18.28**).
- When caries are present only on proximal surface, box only preparation is indicated. In this, proximal box is prepared without the need of secondary retention features (**Fig. 18.29**).
- When proximal caries can be approached from facial or lingual side rather than occlusal surface, slot preparation is indicated (**Figs 18.30A and B**). In this, bur is

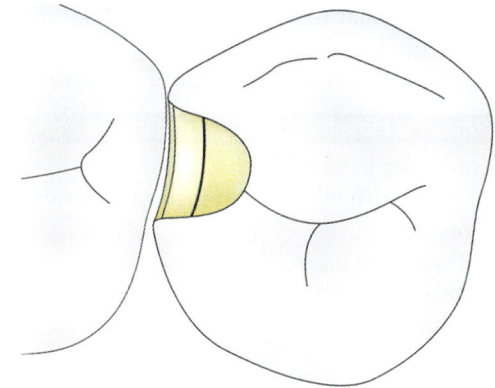

Figure 18.28: Saucer shaped class II tooth preparation

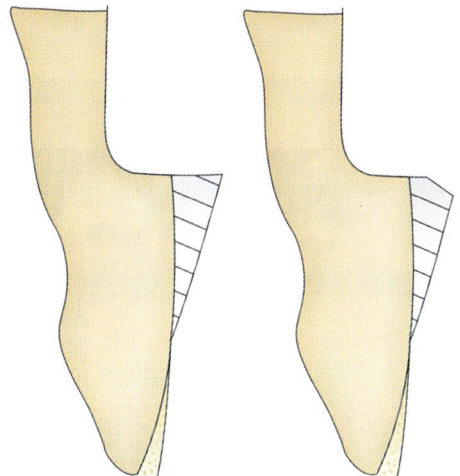

Figure 18.26: If sufficient enamel is present, the beveling can be done so as to increase the composite seal

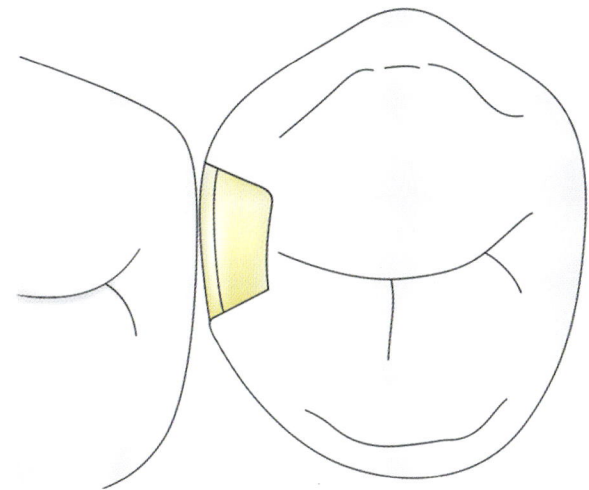

Figure 18.29: 'Box shaped' tooth preparation

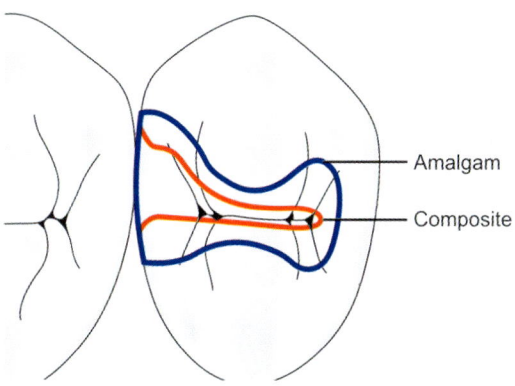

Figure 18.27: Conservative outline of composite resin in comparison to traditional amalgam restoration

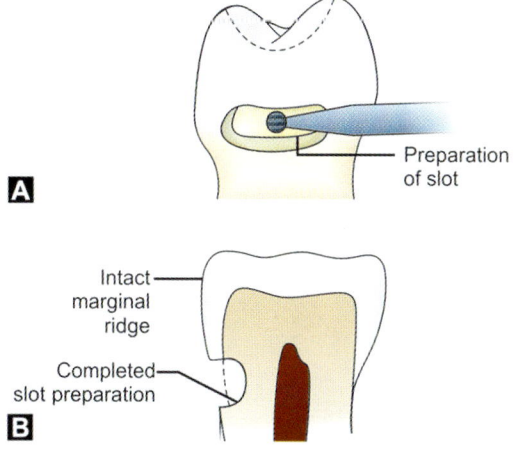

Figures 18.30A and B: Slot preparation

kept perpendicular to long axis of the tooth and entry to lesion is made through facial or lingual surface. Here preparation has cavosurface angle of 90 degree.

Features of class II composite tooth preparation
➡ Tooth preparation for class II has decreased pulpal depth of axial wall which allows greater conservation of tooth structures.
➡ Occlusal and proximal walls converge occlusally and provide additional retention form.
➡ Proximal box preparation has cavosurface angle at right angles to the enamel surface facially and lingually.
➡ Bevels on occlusal surface are optional due to direction of enamel rods whereas on proximal surface, beveling must be done prudently.
➡ Gingival floors should clear the contact apically and they should be butt joined.

RESTORATIVE TECHNIQUE FOR COMPOSITES (FIGS 18.31A TO R)

Matrix Application

A matrix helps in confining the excess restorative material and in development of appropriate axial tooth contours. It also helps in isolation of the prepared tooth. The matrix should be applied and stabilized by a wedge before applying etchant, primer and adhesive to protect the adjacent teeth from being etched and bonded. The matrix should extend 1 mm beyond the incisal and gingival cavosurface margins.

Matrix used for composite resin
➡ Mylar strip matrix
➡ Compound supported metal matrix.

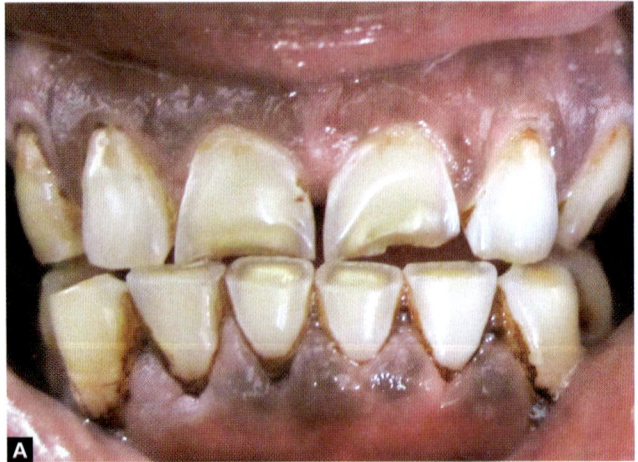
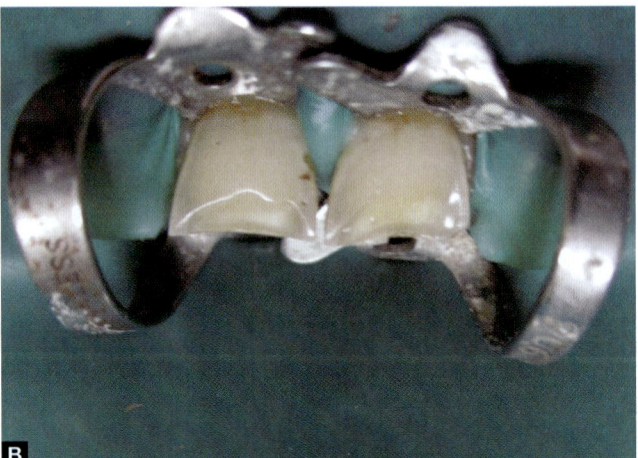
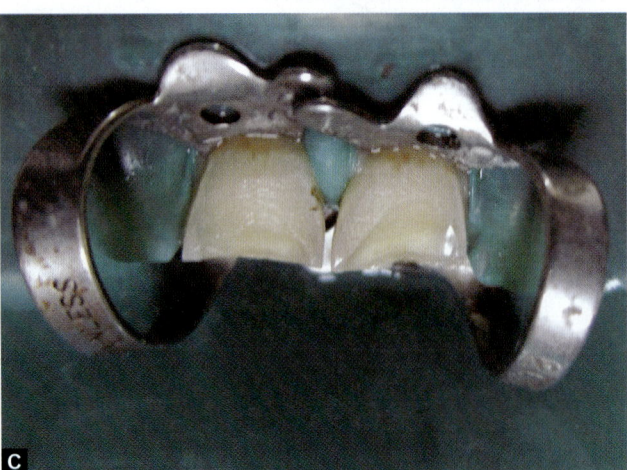
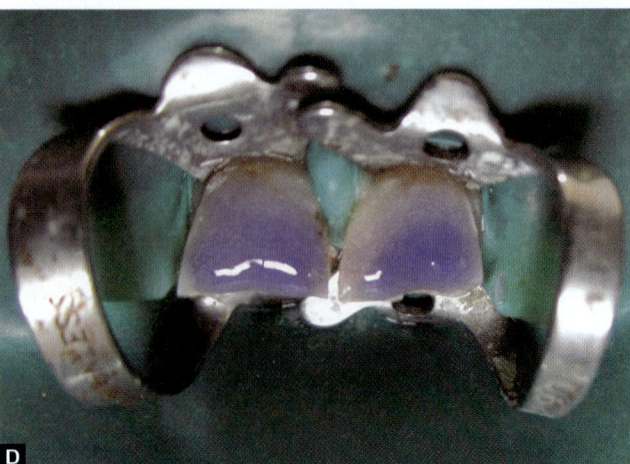

Figures 18.31A to D

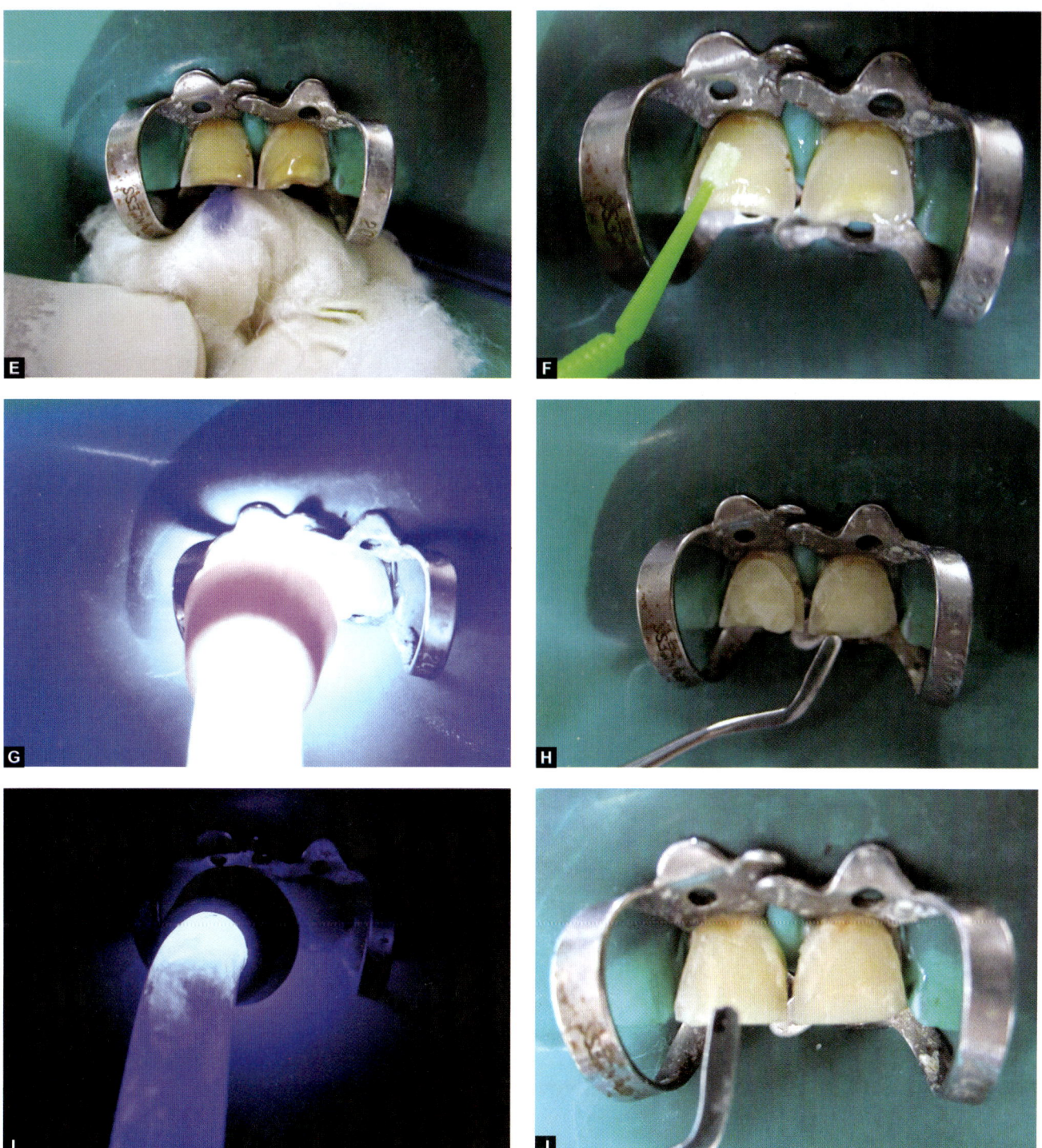

Figures 18.31E to J

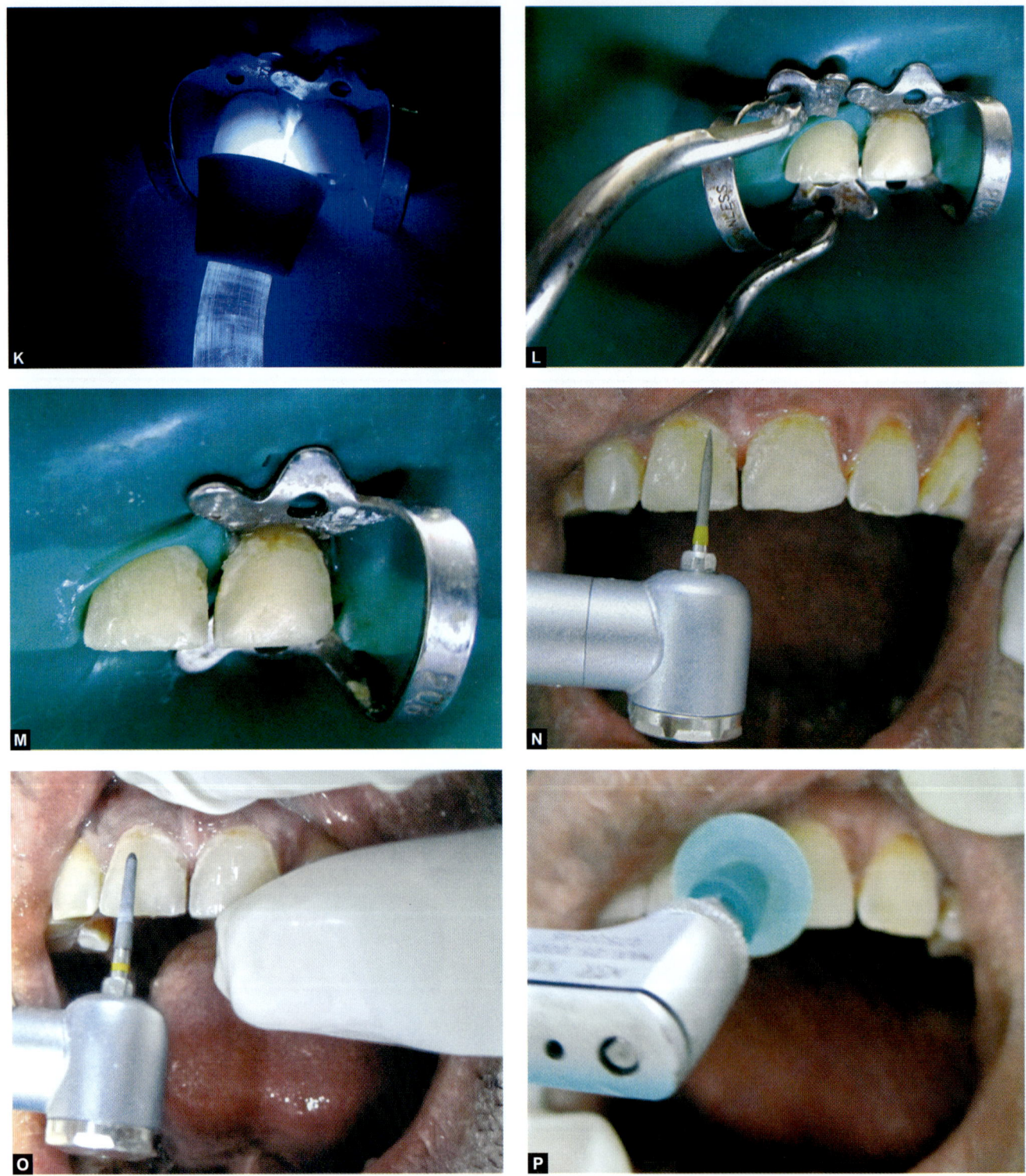

Figures 18.31K to P

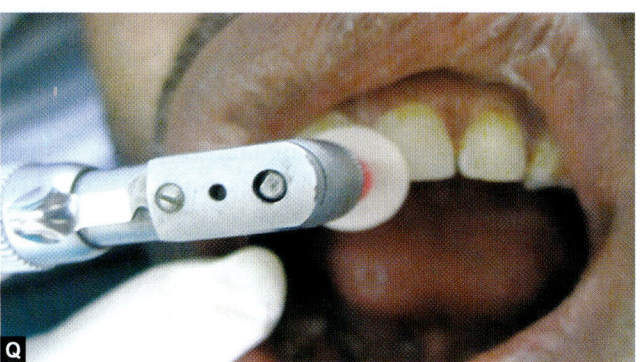

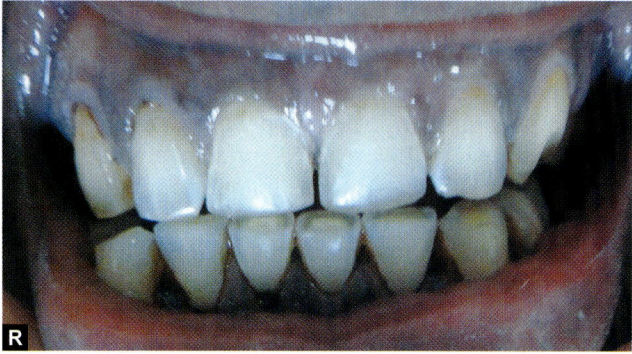

Figures 18.31Q and R

Figures 18.31A to R: Restorative technique for composites: (A) Abrasion of 11 and 21; (B) Isolation of teeth with rubber dam; (C) Complete the tooth preparation; (D) Apply etchant on the prepared surface; (E) Clean and dry the surface; (F) Apply bonding agent; (G) Cure it; (H) Apply dentin shade; (I) Cure the dentin shade; (J) Apply enamel shade; (K) Cure the enamel shade; (L) Remove the rubber dam; (M) Remove the rubber dam; (N) Finish the prepared tooth with diamond point; (O) Finish the preparation using silicon carbide; (P) Finish the preparation with super snap green; (Q) Finishing of preparation with super snap pink; (R) Postoperative photograph

For class III restoration, a properly contoured wedge supported, clear polyester strip matrix is used (**Fig. 18.32**). For small sized class IV preparations, a flexible polyester matrix strip should be placed and wedged. The strip should be folded at the position of lingual line angle to prevent undercontoured restoration in this area (**Fig. 18.33**). Incisally, it should not protrude more than 1 to 2 mm beyond incisal edge. For large class IV preparation, an impression compound supported metal matrix should be used.

Mylar strip serves the following purpose

- Contains the material
- Restores the proximal contact
- Reduces flash
- Reduces oxygen contact with the surface of the composite so ensures more complete polymerization.

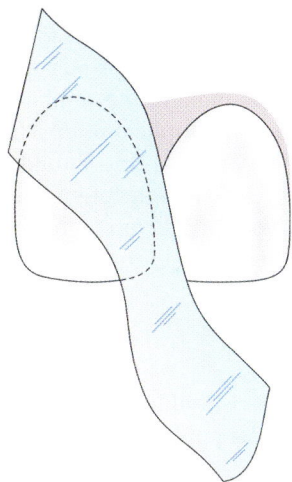

Figure 18.32: For class III restoration, a properly contoured mylar strip is used

One of the major drawback with the use of composite in class II restoration is the difficulty to achieve a convex proximal contour. For this, one should use ultra-thin, contoured metallic bands. A good matrix is the precontoured sectional matrix of about 0.0015 inch thickness. To place it, properly proximal box should have sufficient clearance from the adjacent tooth. If the proximal box is conservative, a very soft 0.001 inch circumferential band should be used.

Purpose of using wedge is to

- Seal the gingival margin
- Hold the band into position
- Provide slight separation of teeth
- Prevent the gingival overhang of the material
- Push the proximal dam and tissue gingivally and open the gingival embrasure.

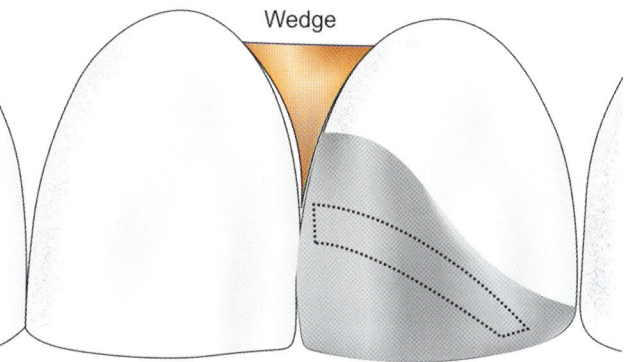

Figure 18.33: Matrix and wedge applied in class IV restoration

Etching of the Tooth Preparation

First of all, proximal surface of adjacent unprepared tooth should be protected from involuntary etching by covering it with a polyester strip. Then apply a gel etchant with a syringe or brush to the prepared surfaces, approximately 0.5 mm beyond the cavosurface margins onto the unprepared tooth surface. Usually 37 percent buffered phosphoric acid is used to provide the optimal etch pattern having ground glass or frosted appearance. Etching is done for generally 15 to 20 seconds. After this, rinse the etched area for at least 15 seconds with copious amounts of water. Dry the area if only enamel has been etched but leave it moist if only dentin is involved in the tooth preparation. If by chance dentin has been dried, rewet it with water saturated applicator tip.

Application of Adhesive System

After etching, a primer and an adhesive are applied according to the instructions provided. Though bonding systems are available in different forms, but current bonding systems combine the primer and adhesive into a single bottle, thus making the application easier. Use disposable brushes or applicator tips for applying the adhesive agents (**Fig. 18.34**). One should avoid collection of these resins in corners and line angles. If the system does not contain both primer and adhesive, then bonding adhesive is applied after the primer and polymerized with curing light.

Pulp Protection

Zinc oxide eugenol should not be used as a subbase because it inhibits the polymerization of resins.

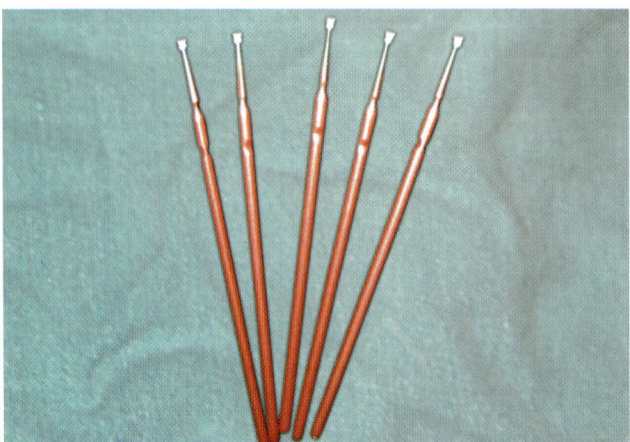

Figure 18.34: Disposable applicator tips for application of adhesive resins

If the intermediatory basing has been applied, then all dentinal walls and floors should be covered with powdered calcium hydroxide, before etching is carried out. This calcium hydroxide should be removed after etching. If the tooth preparation is deep, that is, it has less than 1 mm distance from the pulp, it is preferable to use a glass ionomer base before acid etching because of the following reasons:

- There is compromised resin bond strength in the areas of partially demineralized or deep dentin areas which results in a gap formation between restoration and the tooth. Since glass ionomer cements undergo minimum polymerization shrinkage during the setting reaction, this tends to preserve the bonded interface
- For restoration in future, the presence of the white opaque surface of glass ionomers make them easily distinguishable from the tooth surface
- Anticariogenicity property because of fluoride release from glass ionomer cement
- Use of glass ionomer cement decreases postoperative sensitivity.

Apply glass ionomer liner, etch the preparation, wash and gently air dry it. Then apply bonding agent and cure it.

Composite Placement

Placing Self-Cured Composite

Mix the base and accelerator paste for bonding adhesive on a pad and immediately apply to etched enamel and primed dentin with a microbrush. Simultaneously, mix the base and catalyst paste of selected composite on mixing pad for 30 seconds and place it into the preparation. Use hand instrument to spread the composite material uniformly and plugger to condense it. If two or three increments are needed for packing the preparation, they should be placed in less than one minute for insertion. Slightly overfill the preparation so that condensing pressure can be applied with matrix strip. Remove gross excess using sharp spoon excavator. Close the lingual end of strip over the composite followed by the facial and tighten the matrix using pressure from fingers holding the strip. Hold the matrix for approximately three minutes, until polymerization is complete and the composite hardens. After the composite has hardened, remove the wedge and matrix strip.

Placing Light-Cured Composites

As we know that greater the bulk of material, the greater is the shrinkage and, thus more is the resultant stress on bonded interfaces. Therefore, composite restoration should be placed in small increments to reduce polymerization shrinkage (4-7% shrinkage) (**Fig. 18.35**). Place the first increment of composite using a plastic instrument and pack.

After its insertion, cure it for 20 to 30 seconds by holding the light source close to but not in contact with the restorative material. Longer exposure to light is required for darker and opaque shades. Each increment is added and cured till the complete preparation is filled.

Serious consideration should be at the gingival margin in a class II situation (**Fig. 18.36**). If decay is to reoccur, it is likely to do so at this junction; to that end, apply a very thin (1 mm) layer of composite at the gingival margin of the proximal box and light cure for a 20 seconds. After this, build the whole of proximal box up to the level of the pulpal floor in increments. Now restore the remainder of the preparation in one or two increments according to size

of preparation. It is always preferred to contour the restoration before curing using hand instruments with rounded tips so as to achieve a proper anatomical form.

Remove the matrix and wedge and give an additional 20 second cure lingually and facially for complete curing (**Fig. 18.37**).

Final Contouring, Finishing and Polishing of Composite Restoration

- For composite restorations, the amount of contouring required after final polymerization of the composite can be reduced by careful placement technique. Minimizing contouring retains the sealed margins of the restoration. It also helps minimizing microcracks which can be formed by using abrasives on the surface of restoration.
- Remove flash with a sharp hand instrument. Any excess material can be trimmed with sharp scalpel blade no. 11, composite finishing diamond bur and/or multi-bladed tungsten carbide finishing bur. Use a coolant/lubricant in gross reduction to reduce production of heat and friction.
- Gross contouring of proximal restoration can be done using a small and thin disk rotating from 90 degrees towards the facial surface (**Fig. 18.38**).
- Contact areas may be finished by using a series of abrasive finishing strips threaded below the contact point so as not to destroy the contact point (**Fig. 18.39**). In class III restoration, to avoid any damage to contact point, the finishing strip should be used in S-shaped pattern. If strip is pulled on same side it can lead to open contact points (**Fig. 18.40**).
- Final contouring, finishing and polishing of a composite restoration is done with finishing diamond points (**Figs**

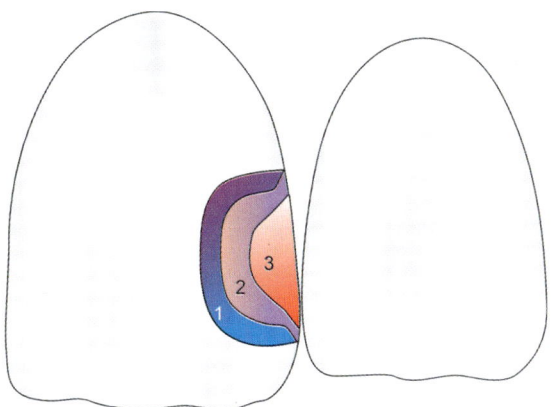

Figure 18.35: Composite should be placed in small increments so as to reduce polymerization shrinkage

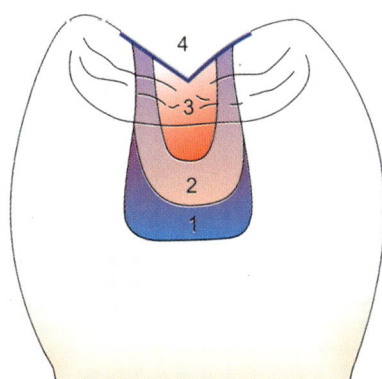

Figure 18.36: During restoration of a class II preparation, proximal box should be filled before rest of the preparation. Complete restoration should be done in increments

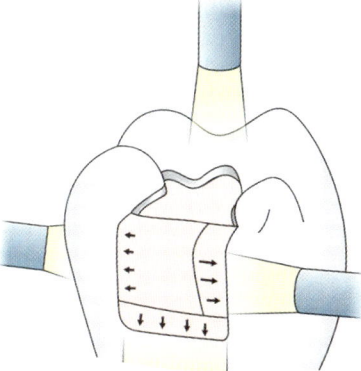

Figure 18.37: After removing the band and matrix, give additional curing lingually and facially for complete polymerization

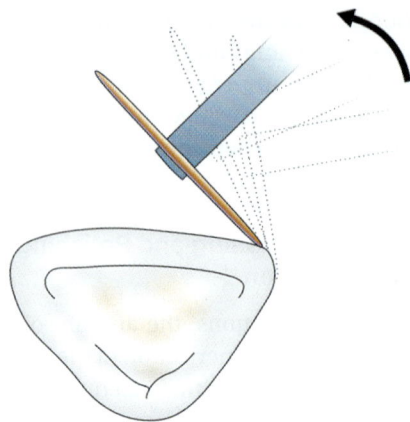

Figure 18.38: Gross proximal contouring of restoration can be done using small thin disc rotating from 90° towards the facial surface

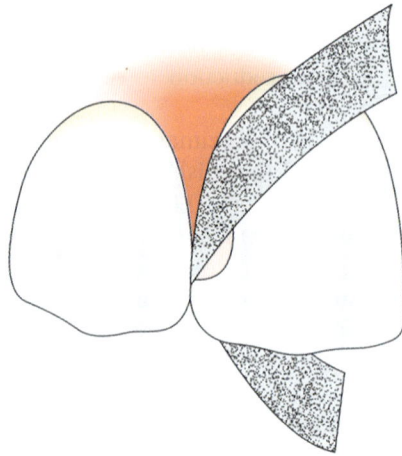

Figure 18.39: Contact area is polished with the help of abrasive finishing strips

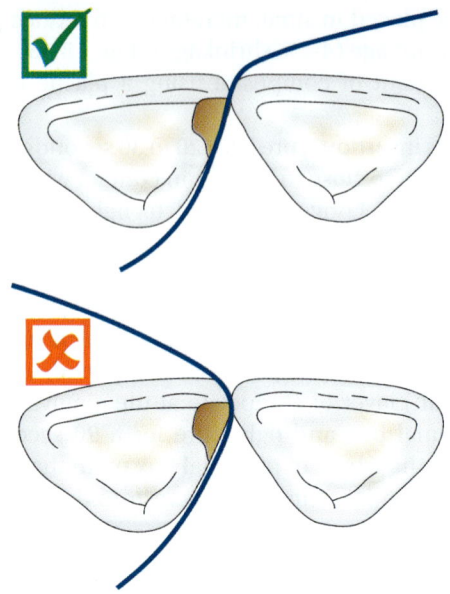

Figure 18.40: In class III restoration, to avoid damage to contact point, finishing strip should be used in S-shaped pattern. Pulling of strip on same side can lead to open contact points

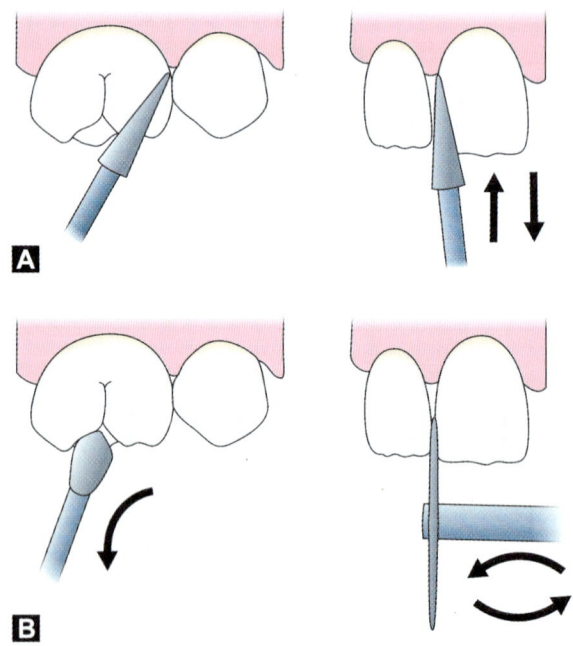

Figures 18.41A and B: Final contouring, finishing and polishing of restoration is done with the help of finishing diamond points

18.41A and B). Polishing is done using rubber-polishing points, abrasive disks or pumice-impregnated points.

Check the contours and margins on proximal area with explorer and dental floss. A sharp no. 12 surgical blade in BP handle or gold finishing knife contouring, is used for contouring and finishing of composite filling at gingival margin. It is specially important to avoid creating a ledge cervically as it is difficult to remove excess from this area.

Checking the Occlusion

After contouring of restoration, occlusion is evaluated in centric position and during various mandiular movements for proper contacts. If occlusion is not proper further adjustments are made and restorations are finished with fine rubber abrasive points or disks.

Glazing

The surface smoothness and shine of a composite restoration can be increased by a "glazing". Glazing is the process

Tooth preparation–amalgam vs composites

Features	Amalgam	Composite
Outline form tended	• Include all pits and fissures (**Figs 18.42A and** B) and adjacent suspicious areas. • For class II tooth preparation, proximal contact has to be broken	• Include faults but need not to be extended to adjacent pits and fissures. • For class II tooth preparations, proximal contact need not to be broken in all the cases
Pulpal depth	• Should be maintained uniform (**Figs 18.43A and B**) • Depth–1.5 mm (Minimum)	• Need not to be uniform • Depth–1–2 mm (usually)
Axial depth	• Should be uniform • Depth–0.2-0.5 mm inside DEJ	• Not necessarily uniform • Depth–to extent of the defect
Cavosurface margin	90° at margin	Equal to and greater than 90° at margin
Nature of prepared walls	Smooth	Rough
Primary retention form	Occlusal convergence	Etching, priming and bonding
Bevels	Not indicated in large preparations	Bevels indicated
Resistance form	Box shaped preparation (**Figs 18.44A and B**) Flat pulpal and gingival floor	Not indicated For small to moderate preparations
Secondary retention	Grooves, Coves, slots, pins, locks and bonding	Indicated only for extensive preparations
Pulp protection and base	By use of varnish, liner	Varnish not indicated
	Base: GIC, calcium hydroxide liner	

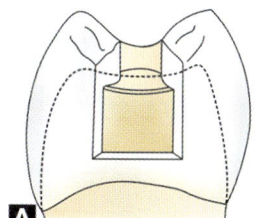 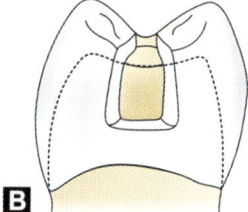

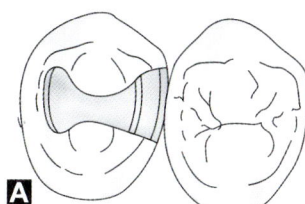

Figures 18.42A and B: (A) Box shaped involvement of all fissures for class II preparation of amalgam; (B) Conservative tooth preparation for composite

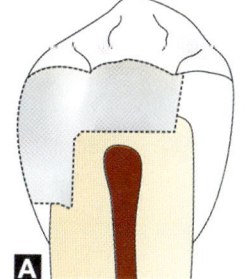 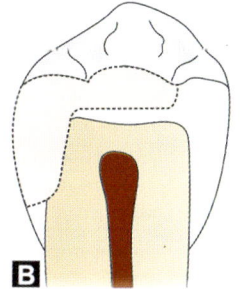

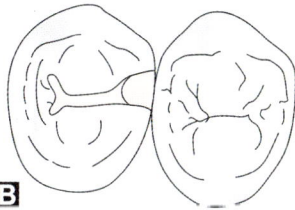

Figures 18.44A and B: (A) Box shaped tooth preparation for amalgam; (B) Conservative tooth preparation for composites

Figures 18.43A and B: (A) Uniform pulpal floor depth for amalgam restoration; (B) Pulpal floor depth need not be uniform for composite restoration

for few weeks. Since it lacks the abrasive resistance and adhesion, with time the surface is abraded away during function. To improve the adhesion of glaze, before glazing the restoration, surface should be etched with low concentration of hydrofluoric acid.

of placing of a thin layer of unfilled resin over the finished composite resin. This is then light cured. The resultant surface is very smooth and shiny initially but it lasts only

Glazing serves the following purposes

➡ Improves esthetics.
➡ Creates a smooth glossy surface, resistant to plaque retention.
➡ Fills surface porosity.

REPAIR OF COMPOSITE RESTORATIONS

When the area to a defective restoration is accessible, for repair, the old restoration is roughened with a diamond stone and the enamel margins are etched. After this, primer and adhesive are applied and finally composite is placed, finished and polished. In case, when the defective restoration is in area which is difficult to access, the defective restoration should be exposed by tooth preparation. After this, place a matrix and wedge and etch the enamel margins. Apply primer and bonding agent and finally place composite. Cure it and do the final finishing and polishing.

INDIRECT COMPOSITE INLAYS AND ONLAYS

Tooth colored restorations which are fabricated outside the oral cavity are called as indirect tooth colored restorations. These are prepared on a replica of a prepared tooth.

Direct posterior composite restorations do not perform optimally especially when a large lesion is present. In these cases, indirect restorations in the form of inlay and onlay have shown better reproduction of contacts and contour, more strength, hardness and reduced polymerization shrinkage.

Indications

Wide defects: In preparations, which are wide faciolingually and require cuspal coverage.
Esthetics: When more esthetics is required, because by indirect method, better esthetics is attained.

Contraindications

Heavy occlusal forces: These restorations may fracture in the patients with bruxing or clenching habits.

Problems, causes and treatments associated with composite restorations

Problems	Causes	Treatments
Pain due to pressure at a point over the restored dentin	Presence of small air bubble in restoration. On pressure, due to resiliency, the composite is slightly pressed and air bubble is also pressed. On being pressed, air bubble enters the exposed dentinal tubules thereby pressing the nerve endings resulting into pain.	Restoration with more care to avoid entrapment of any air bubble
Incorrect shade	• Inappropriate shade selection • Tooth is dry during shade selection • Selection of wrong shade.	• Use of natural light for shade selection • Selection of shade before isolation • Understand the typical zones of different shades of natural teeth
White line around the margin of restoration	• Improper contouring or finishing technique • Inadequate etching or bonding • High intensity light curing technique.	• Use atraumatic finishing technique • Apply primer and bond the area • Use slow start polymerization.
Poor surface of restoration	• Poor technique • Deep gingival preparation where isolation is difficult • Repeated etching, priming and adhesive placement	• Better technique • Use of matrix • Use of microfilled restorative material
Weak or missing proximal contacts	• Inadequately contoured matrix bands • Inadequate wedging • Movements of matrix band during composite insertion • Use of too thick matrix band • Composite pulling away from matrix contact area.	• Use of thin matrix band • Use of proper wedging technique • Matrix band should contact the adjacent tooth • Hold the matrix against the adjacent tooth while polymerization.
Voids	• Faulty mixing of self cured composites • Space left between increments • Composite with large filler particles.	• Follow proper technique • Repair of marginal voids by microfilled composite
Improper contouring and finishing	• Injury to adjacent unprepared tooth structure • Overcontoured restoration • Undercontoured restoration • Inadequate anatomic tooth form	• Careful use of rotary instruments • Use of proper matrix system • Use of proper instruments for anatomic contouring
Poor retention	• Inadequate tooth preparation • Contamination of operating site • Poor bonding technique from different system.	• Place bevels, flares or secondary retentive features • Proper isolation of site • Do not intermingle bonding materials from different system.

Difficult in moisture control: When isolation of operative field is not possible, cementation becomes difficult.

Deep subgingival preparations: Impression taking and finishing of preparations with deep subgingival margins is difficult.

Difference between ceramic and composite inlays

Ceramic inlays	Composite inlays
Excellent esthetics	Good esthetics
Better marginal fit, thus less leakage	Poor marginal fit, thus more leakage
Good adhesion to resin cements	Poor adhesion to resin cements
Does not stain	May stain with time
Expensive	Relatively less expensive than ceramic
Complex laboratory steps	Simple laboratory steps
Intraoral finishing and polishing is time consuming	Intraoral finishing and polishing easier
Fragile and brittle so, prone to fracture while seating	Easier adjustment and seating
Abrasive to opposing enamel	Not abrasive to opposing enamel
Intraoral repair is not possible	Intraoral repair is possible

Advantages

Indirect tooth colored restorations have the following advantages:

- Less chairside time is required due to laboratory fabrication
- Much more wear-resistant than direct composite restorations
- Show less polymerization shrinkage, hence reduced microleakage and postoperative sensitivity
- Indirect restorations have improved physical properties
- More biocompatible with better tissue response.
- Achieve better contacts and contours
- Strengthens remaining tooth structure
- Extraoral polishing is easy.

Disadvantages

Indirect restoration has the following disadvantages:

- Requires more number of patient appointment
- Highly technique sensitive
- Restorations requires high level of operator skill
- Ceramics abrade opposing dentition and restorations.
- There is need for temporary restoration.
- More expensive than direct composites.
- Difficult repair with ceramics.
- Weak bonding of indirectly made composite restorations to composite cement. Thus, they require mechanical abrasion and/or chemical treatment for proper adhesion to cement.

Tooth Preparation for Composite Inlays and Onlays (Figs 18.45A and B)

Give local anesthesia and isolate the tooth using rubber dam for visibility and moisture control. Before applying the rubber dam, mark and assess the occlusal contact relationship with articulating paper.

Outline Form

- Outline form is usually guarded by the existing restorations and caries and is grossly similar to that for cast metal inlays and onlays except that there are no bevels or secondary flares. For the creation of round internal angles, use tapered fissure bur with round tip. Hold the bur parallel to long axis of the tooth. The outline form should result in smooth curves surrounding the cusps. There should be central groove reduction following the anatomy of the unprepared tooth rather than a monoplane. This provides the additional bulk for the restoration.
- Always remove undermined or weakened enamel properly.
- To facilitate passive seating of the inlay, facial and lingual walls should have 6 to 8 degrees of divergence.
- The outline should avoid occlusal contacts. Areas to be restored using inlay or onlay need 1.5 mm of clearance in all excursions to prevent fracture.
- Isthmus of tooth preparation should be wide to prevent fracture of restoration. Axial wall should be kept 1.5 mm deep from external tooth surface.
- Extend the proximal box to allow a minimum of 0.5 to 1 mm of proximal clearance for proper finish of these margins and impression making.
- Use a 90 degree butt joint for all cavosurface margins. Bevels are contraindicated because bulk is needed to prevent fracture.

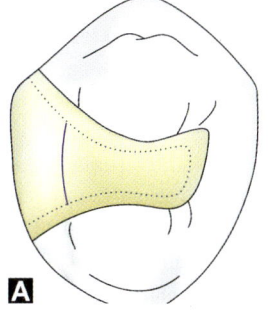 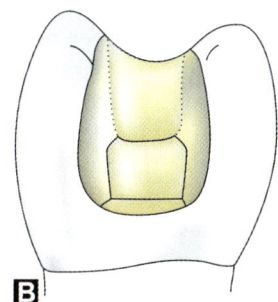

Figures 18.45A and B: (A) Occlusal view of tooth preparation for composite inlay; (B) Proximal view of inlay preparation

- Any undercut if present should be removed or blocked by glass ionomer lining.
- The margin of restoration should be kept supragingival, which will make isolation during the cementation easier and improve access for finishing.
- Remove any remaining caries (not included in the outline form) using an excavator or a slow speed round bur.
- For pulp protection place a resin-modified glass ionomer cement base if indicated.
- Redefine the preparation margins using finishing burs and hand instruments.
- Check the final tooth preparation after the removal of rubber dam. There should be 1.5 mm clearance to prevent fracture in all excursions.

Laboratory Technique of Composite Inlays and Onlays

Composite restorations show improved physical properties when processed free of contamination and when maximum polymerization of resin matrix has occurred.

Proper polymerization of composite restoration is best done in dental laboratories, which polymerize the composite under pressure, light, heat or vacuum or in combinations.

An accurate elastomeric impression is taken to form a replica of the tooth, on to which composite restoration is made. Before placing composite, apply separating media. Composite is initially light cured for one minute on each surface. Successive layers are added and polymerized till full contour is built. Final curing of restoration is achieved by inserting the die and/or restoration into curing oven which exposes the composite to additional light and heat for 8 to 10 minutes and allow it to cool and then final trimming and finishing is done.

Key Points

- Conventional tooth preparation is mainly indicated for lesion present on the root surface.
- Here, preparation depend upon extent of the lesion but external walls of the preparation should be located on sound tooth structure with a 900 cavosurface angle for butt joint relation.
- Beveled tooth preparation is indicated for replacing an existing defective restoration if a large carious lesion is present. Here, keep the external walls of the tooth preparation perpendicular to the enamel surface with all enamel margins beveled. The bevel should be about 0.2 to 0.5 mm wide at an angle of 45 degrees to the external tooth surface.

- In modified tooth preparation, only infected carious area is removed as conservatively as possible by "scooping" out. This results in 'scooped-out' or 'concave' appearance of the preparation.
- Class I preparation for composite is different from amalgam in that faciolingual dimension of preparation is kept as small as possible, and there is no need to prepare dovetail for retention of composite.
- Beveling of the enamel margin results in increased retention, reduction in microleakage, improvement in esthetics and increase in bond strength.
- One of the major drawback with the use of composite in class II restoration is the difficulty to achieve a convex proximal contour. For this, one should use ultra-thin, contoured metallic band (like precontoured sectional matrix of about 0.0015 inch thickness). To place it, proximal box should have sufficient clearance from the adjacent tooth. If the proximal box is conservative, a very soft 0.001 inch circumferential band should be used.
- 37 percent buffered phosphoric acid is used to provide the optimal etch pattern having ground glass or frosted appearance. Etching is done for generally 15 to 20 seconds. After this, rinse the etched area for at least 15 seconds with copious amounts of water.
- Zinc oxide eugenol should not be used as a sub-base because it inhibits the polymerization of resins.
- If the tooth preparation is deep, that is, it has less than 1 mm distance from the pulp, it is preferable to use a glass ionomer base before acid etching because of compromised resin bond strength in the areas of partially demineralized or deep dentin areas which results in a gap formation between restoration and the tooth. Since glass ionomer cements undergo minimum polymerization shrinkage during the setting reaction, this tends to preserve the bonded interface.
- To place self cured composite, mix the base and accelerator paste on a pad and apply to etched enamel and primed dentin with a microbrush. Use hand instrument to spread the composite material uniformly and plugger to condense it. If two or three increments are needed for packing the preparation, they should be placed in less than one minute for insertion.
- Composite material should be placed in small increments to reduce polymerization shrinkage (4-7% shrinkage).
- The surface smoothness and shine of a composite restoration can be increased by a "glazing".
- Glazing is the process of placing of a thin layer of unfilled resin over the finished composite resin, and then curing it using light.
- For repair of an old and defective restoration, if area is accessible for repair, the restoration is roughened with

a diamond stone and the enamel margins are etched, and primed. Then adhesive is applied and composite is placed.
- If the defective restoration is in area which is difficult to access, the defective restoration should be exposed by tooth preparation. Then etch the enamel margins, apply primer and bonding agent and finally place composite.
- Indirect tooth colored restorations are indicated in preparations which are wide faciolingually and require cuspal coverage.

QUESTIONS

1. What are the different designs for a class III tooth preparation for composite restoration?
2. How will you design tooth preparation for composite restoration of a class V lesion extending to the root surface of 11?
3. Differentiate the tooth preparation for amalgam and composite.
4. What are various problems and their remedies associated with composite restorations?
5. Discuss the difference between ceramic and composite inlays.

BIBLIOGRAPHY

1. Andersson-Wenckert IE, et al. Modified Class II open sandwich restorations: evaluation of interfacial adaptation and influence of different restorative technique. Eur J Oral Sci. 2002;110:270-5.
2. Barnes DM, et al. A 5- and 8-year clinical evaluation of a posterior composite resin. Quintessence Int. 1991;22:143-51.
3. Bayne SC, et al. Long-term clinical failures in posterior composites (abstract no. 32). J Dent Res. 1989;68:185.
4. Ben-Amar A, Metzger Z, Gontar G. Cavity design for class II composite restoration JPD. 1987;58:5.
5. Besnault C, Attal JP. Simulated oral environment and microleakage of Class II resin-based composite and sandwich restorations. Am J Dent. 2003;16:186-90.
6. Browning WD, Dennison JB. A survey of failure modes in composite resin restorations. Oper Dent. 1996;21:160.
7. Bruke FJT, Watts DC, Wilson NHF. Effect of cuspal coverage on fracture resistance of teeth restored with composite inlays. JDR. 1991;70:701.
8. Chuang SF, Liu JK, Jin YT. Microleakage and internal voids in class II composite restorations with flowable composible linings. Oper Dent. 2001;26:193.
9. Dietschi D. Free-hand bonding in the esthetic treatment of anterior teeth: creating the illusion. J Esthel Dent. 1997;9:156-64.
10. Ehrnford L, Derand J. Cervical gap formation in Class II composite resin restorations. Swed Dent J. 1984;8:15-9.
11. Jendresen MD. Clinical performance of a new composite resin for Class V erosion (abstract 1057). J Dent Res. 1978;57:339.
12. Liberman R, et al. The effect of posterior composite restorations on the resistance of cavity walls to vertically applied loads. J Oral Rehabil 1990;17:99-105.
13. Loguercio AD, et al. Microleakage in Class II composite resin restorations: total bonding and open sandwich technique. J Adhes Dent. 2002;4:137-44.
14. Lorton L, Brady J. Criteria for successful composite resin restorations. Gen Dent. 1981;29:234.
15. Mair LH. Ten-year clinical assessment of three posterior resin composite and two amalgams. Quintessence Int. 1998;29:483-90.
16. Murray PE, et al. Bacterial microleakage and pulp inflammation associated with various restorative materials. Dent Mater. 2002;18:470-8.
17. Ogata M, et al. Effect of self-etching primer vs phosphoric acid etchant on bonding to bur-prepared dentin. Oper Dent. 2002;27:447-54.
18. Opdam NJ, et al. Class I occlusal composite resin restorations: *in vivo* post-operative sensitivity, wall adaptation, and microleakage. Am J Dent. 1998;11:229-34.
19. Ritter AV, Swift EJ. Current restorative concepts of pulp protection. Endod Topics. 2003;5:41-8.
20. Tani C, Finger WJ. Effect of smear layer thickness on bond strength mediated by three all-in-one self-etching priming adhesives. J Adhes Dent. 2003;16:340-6.
21. Torstenson B, Brännström M. Composite resin contraction gaps measured with a fluorescent resin technique. Dent Mater. 1988;4:238-42.
22. Welk DA, Laswell HR. Rationale for designing cavity preparations in light of current knowledge and technology. Dent Clin North Am. 1976;20:231.
23. Wilson NHF, et al. Five-year findings of a multiclinical trial for a posterior composite. J Dent.1991;19:153-9.
24. Yoshikawa T, et al. Effects of dentin depth and cavity configuration on bond strength. J Dent Res. 1999;78:898-905.

Esthetics and Operative Dentistry

Chapter Outline

INTRODUCTION

Esthetic means pertaining to a sense of the beautiful.

As we know that the main aim of operative care is achieved by attaining health, function and esthetics. It is also known as health, function and aesthetic triad (HFA) (**Fig. 19.1**).

The sequence of this triad is achievement of health, followed by function and then by esthetics.

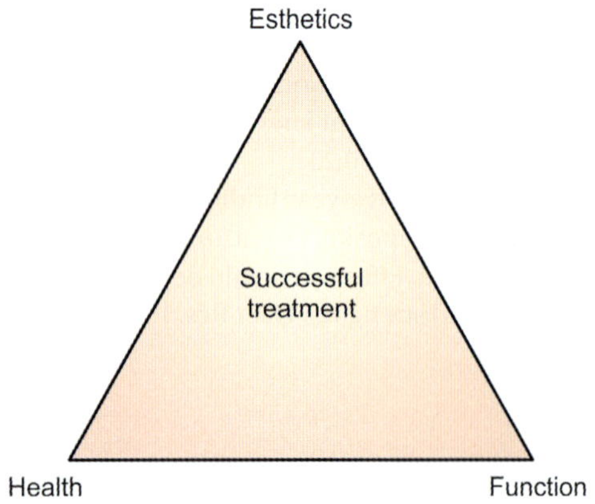

Figure 19.1: HFA triad for achieving optimal treatment

Dental esthetics can be divided into four components
➡ Facial composition
➡ Dentofacial composition
➡ Dental composition
➡ Gingival composition.

Smile analysis is generally defined in terms of
➡ Vertical placement of the anterior teeth to the upper lip at rest and on smile
➡ Smile arc characteristics
➡ The vertical relationship of gingival margins to each other
➡ Transverse smile dimension (buccal corridors).

Tooth Proportionality (Height and Width)

Dental esthetics comprises the touch of contour and color characteristics of individual teeth. The contour of a tooth can be analyzed in three-dimensional view: from the facial, interproximal, and incisal. The "face" of a tooth is defined as the reflective area inside the transitional line angles of the facial surface. It consists of size and shape of teeth along with their interarch and intra-arch relationship.

Size of tooth: It is determined by dividing cervicoincisal length of tooth to mesiodistal width, i.e.

Size of tooth = Width/length ratio (**Fig. 19.2**)

To have optimal dimension, width/length ratio of central incisor should range from 0.75 to 0.8 (**Figs 19.3A to C**).

- Ideal ratio 0.75 to 0.8
- < 0.75 – Narrower tooth
- > 0.8 – Wider tooth

Size of body is visible according to the light reflected from it. It controls width and length which appears to a viewer. When a tooth is highlighted upon direct light, then area of depression is shadowed and not very prominent. The tooth size which is to be appeared can be changed by creating different types of facial prominence. These illusions are useful for creating apparent size of a tooth which appears different from actual size. These concepts are important in many cases like correction of diastema in which composite are placed in such a way that apparent total width of teeth appears unchanged.

Shape of upper anterior teeth: It is determined by age, sex and personality of the individual.

For example, a young and feminine smile shows teeth with rounded incisal angles, open incisal and facial embrasure (**Fig. 19.4**), while a masculine smile shows closed incisal embrasures with prominent incisal angles (**Fig. 19.5**).

If in females slightly broader teeth are present, then they sometimes require conservative minor modification to produce better esthetics. This is called 'cosmetic contouring'. In this to create younger and more feminine smile, incisal angles are rounded and incisal embrasures are opened.

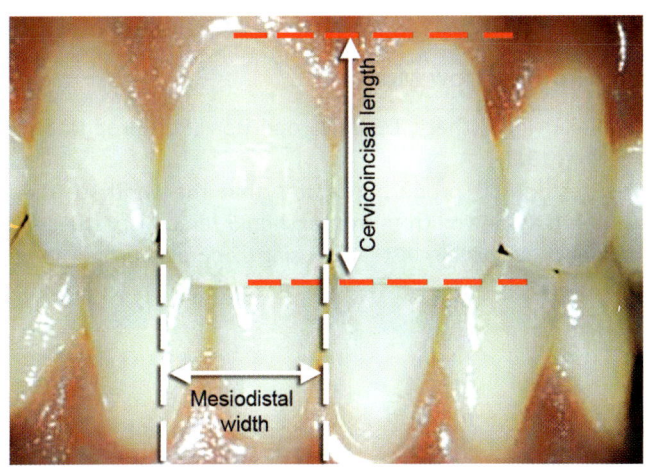

Figure 19.2: Size of tooth is determined by dividing cervicoincisal length to mesiodistal width

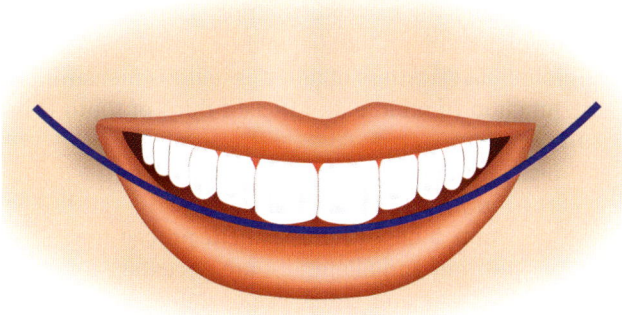

Figure 19.4: Young feminine smile shows teeth with rounded incisal angles, open incisal and facial embrasures

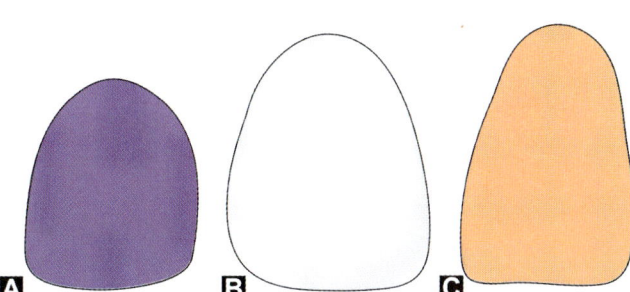

Figures 19.3A to C: Width/Length ratio: (A) >0.8 wider tooth; (B) 0.75-0.8 Normal tooth; (C) ≤ 0.75 Narrower tooth

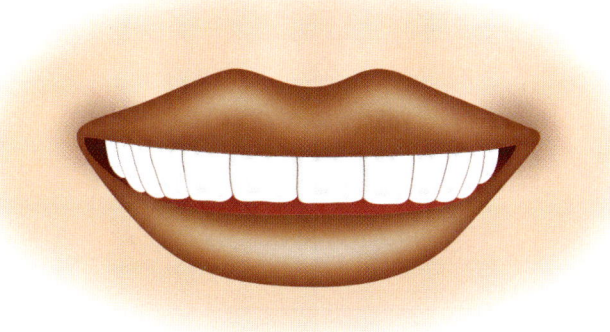

Figure 19.5: Masculine smile shows close incisal embrasures with prominent incisal angles

Intra-arch relationship:

- It is given by rule of golden proportion (**Fig. 19.6**). This concept was given by Lombardi and Levin. According to it, for an object to be proportional to one another the ratio of 1:1.618 is esthetically pleasing. As a normal rule, if apparent size of each tooth is seen from frontal view, 62 percent tooth size anterior to it relationship is considered esthetically pleasing. For example, for maxillary central incisor the apparent width is 1.618, for lateral incisor it is one and for canine it is 0.618. But many studies have shown that golden proportion is not always present in natural dentition, yet an esthetically pleasing smile can be there. So rather than having specific ratio a dentition should have repeating proportion.

- *Axial inclination of the tooth*: A line extending from the height of the tooth from the free gingival margin to the center of the incisal edge implies the alignment of the axis of each tooth. The maxillary anterior teeth ideally display mesial axial inclination, with the central incisors appearing to be the almost vertical and the lateral incisors and canines each tipping more toward the midline. After the canines, the posterior teeth display an inclination that is parallel to the canines.

- Labiolingual thickness of anterior teeth is measured at the junction of middle and incisor third of tooth (**Fig. 19.7**).
  - Ideally it should be between 2.5 and 3.5 mm
  - If > 3.5 mm, it is overcontouring
  - If < 2.5 mm, it necessitates esthetic procedures.

Proper position and alignment are necessary for good appearance of face and smile. Major defects in position

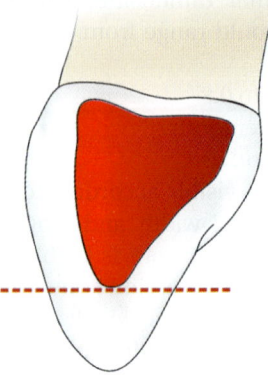

Figure 19.7: Labiolingnal width of a tooth is measured at the junction of middle and incisal third

and alignment are corrected by orthodontic treatment, but minor positional defects can be treated by composites or facial veneers.

Want to Know More

- Recurring Esthetic Dental Proportion (Red Proportion) (**Fig. 19.8**)
- Preston-RED proportion states that the width of the teeth as viewed from frontal should remain constant as one move distally instead of using 62 percent proportion.

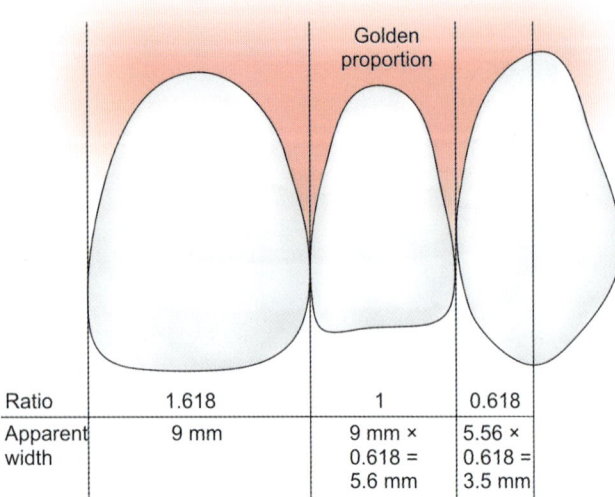

Ratio	1.618	1	0.618
Apparent width	9 mm	9 mm × 0.618 = 5.6 mm	5.56 × 0.618 = 3.5 mm

Figure 19.6: Rule of golden proportion

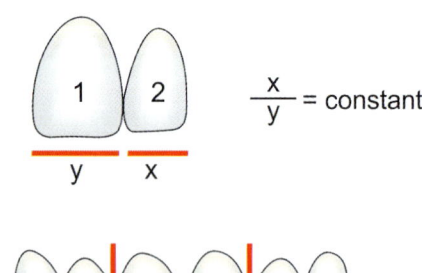

$$\frac{x}{y} = constant$$

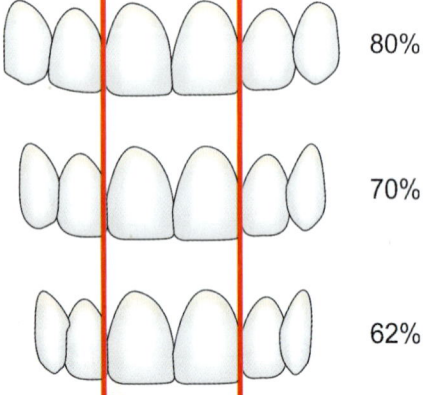

Figure 19.8: RED proportion

Contacts, Connectors and Embrasures

The exact place where the teeth touch is called a contact. The place where the incisors and canines "appear" to touch is defined as the connector (also referred to as the interdental contact area). As the teeth proceed from the midline to the posterior, the contact points progress apically. The connector height diminishes from the central to the posterior teeth and is greatest between the central incisors. The triangular space incisal to the contact defined as embrasures. Embrasure area gets larger as the teeth progress posteriorly (**Fig. 19.9**).

Gingival Esthetics—Gingival Shape and Gingival Contour

The cementoenamel junction and the osseous crest determine the curvature of the gingival margin of the tooth. This curvature of the gingival margin of the tooth is called gingival shape. The mandibular incisors and the maxillary laterals should display a gingival shape of symmetrical half oval or half – circular shape and that of the maxillary centrals and canines a gingival shape that is more elliptical (**Fig. 19.10**). The gingival zenith represents the most apical point at which each tooth emerges from the free gingival margin (**Fig. 19.11**). For an esthetically pleasing smile, it should be positioned distally to the center of each tooth within the maxillary anterior segment. The distal position gradually increases from the central incisor to the canine (**Fig. 19.12**). The gingival zenith of the maxillary laterals and mandibular incisors should coincide with their longitudinal axis.

Facial Proportions

Facial composition is measured by analyzing the face from frontal and sagittal aspect. From frontal aspect, many

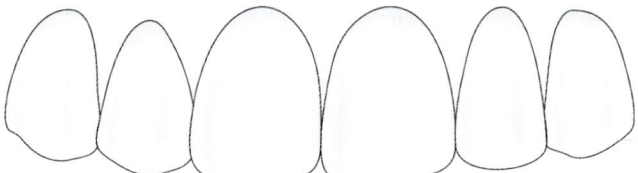

Figure 19.10: Gingival shape of incisors and canine

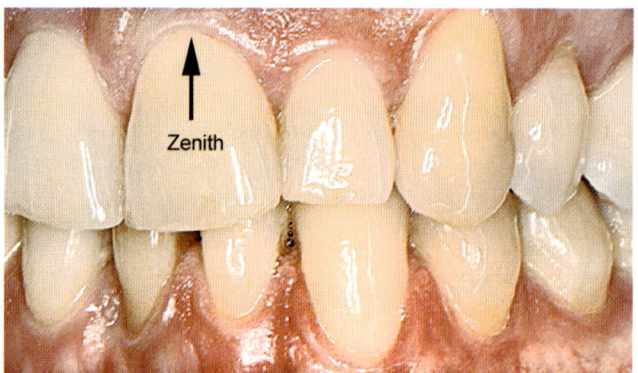

Figure 19.11: Gingival zenith is the most apical point at which each tooth emerges from free gingival margin

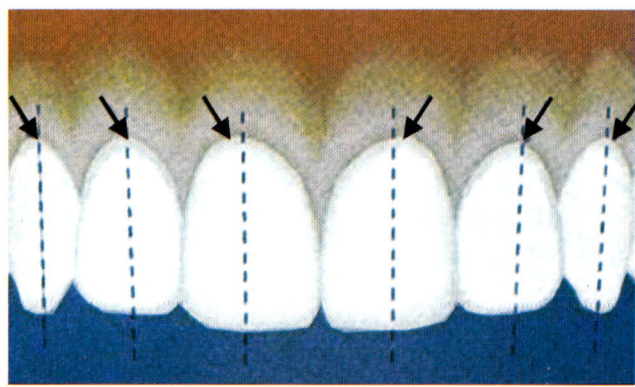

Figure 19.12: Zenith point should be located distal to the center of each tooth. Distal position gradually increases from the central incisor to the canine

landmarks are used to determine esthetics (**Figs 19.13 and 19.14**). Many horizontal lines are drawn horizontally from upper to lower part of face, these are hair ophriac, interpupillary, interalar and commissural lines. Parallelism of these lines results in horizontal symmetry of the face.

From sagittal aspect, two reference points are used that is nasolabial angle and Rickett's E-plane.

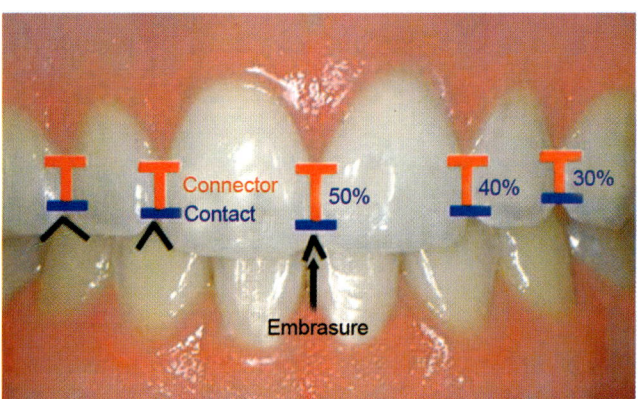

Figure 19.9: Contact, connector and embrasure

Nasolabial angle is formed by intersection of two lines using nose and lips as reference points (**Fig. 19.15**). Normal value of nasolabial angle for males is 90 to 100° and for females is 100 to 105°.

Rickets E-plane is line drawn from tip of nose to chin prominence (**Fig. 19.16**).

Using these two reference points, protrusion or retrusion of maxilla can be evaluated.

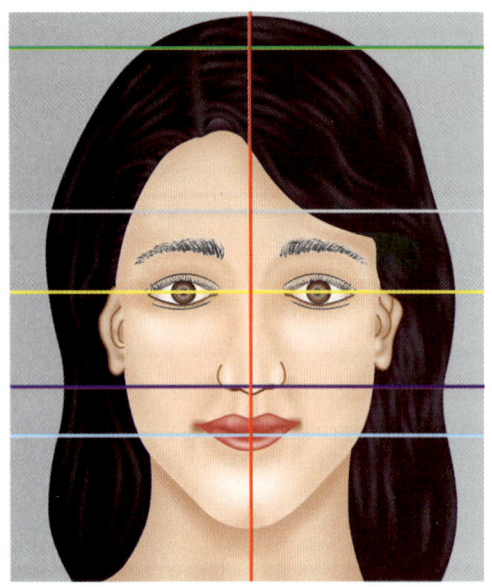

Figure 19.13: Horizontal lines to determine facial esthetics

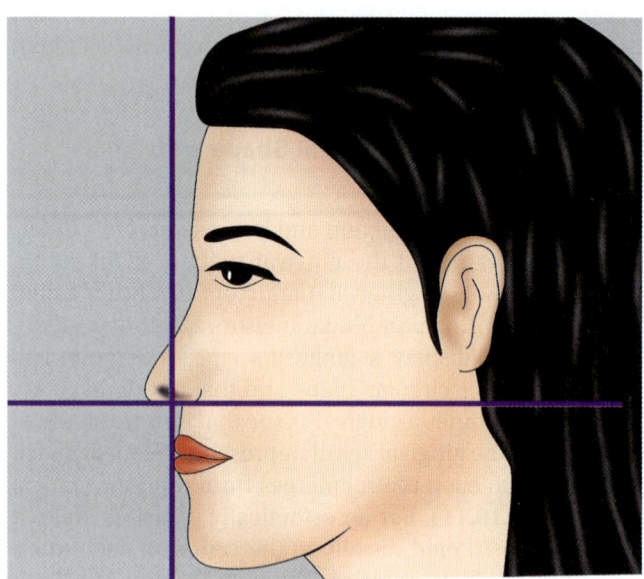

Figure 19.15: Nasolabial line angle

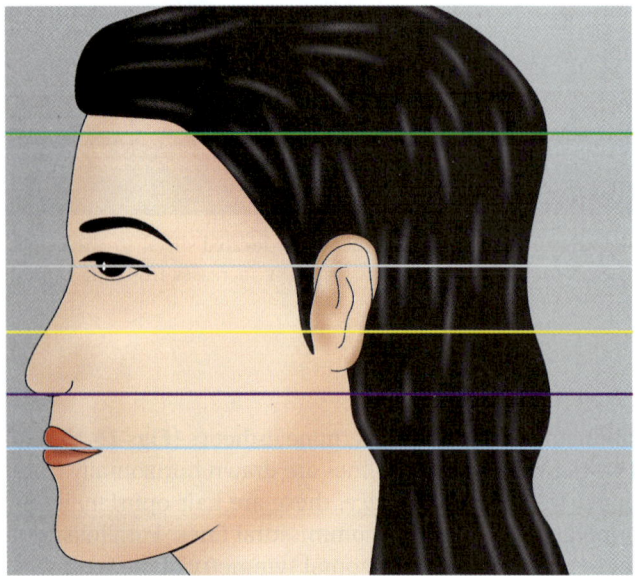

Figure 19.14: Lateral view of horizontal lines to determine facial esthetics

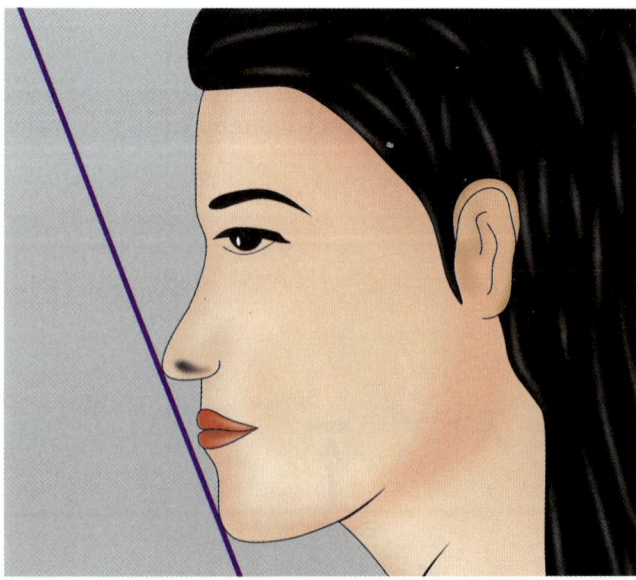

Figure 19.16: Ricket's E-plane

PRINCIPLES OF ORGANIZATION

Visual Forming (Ordering)

Both our eye and mind arrange different parts of a picture into a combined whole, trying to generate an order out of chaos. The bold and dominant elements seek the attention of our eye at first. Then it is drawn along visual channels through the entire work, following lines of color and texture in carefully planned order.

Harmony and Variety

The contrasts are held together by harmony, which is developed with rhythm and repetition. It is the repetition of lines, colors, shapes, and textures that brings harmony. A beautiful smile is the result of repeating lines. The repeating lines referred to as the smile line is formed by the incisal edges of the upper teeth and the border of the lower lip. It is this repetition that imparts harmony and unity to the smile and the repetition of vertical lines separating each tooth and the parallelism of the upper gingival line and lower border of the upper lip. Variety is integrated by subtly varying color within each tooth and between teeth. Varied arrangement is subtle rotations and the positioning of teeth out of the ideal.

Balance (Fig. 19.17)

The optical equilibrium in a composition is referred to as balance. The eye pauses momentarily at significant parts as it travels over a picture. These parts represent moving and directional forces that must counterbalance one another, so that controlled tension results. An artwork looks unfinished, unplanned, and full of tension when unbalanced.

Dominance

The dominant part of the face is the teeth as it occupies an important position, the dominant role being played by the maxillary central incisors.

ESTHETICS AND OPERATIVE DENTISTRY

There are number of problems which can alter the esthetics of anterior teeth.

Many treatment options are available which can be employed to improve the esthetics of affected tooth/teeth. Though not all of these treatment options give perfect effects, but alternatives can be explained to the patient for better results.

Commonly seen problems with anterior teeth which affect esthetics of these teeth are
- Caries
- Tooth discoloration because of trauma, hypoplasia and other factors
- Tooth malformations
- Diastema between teeth
- Malalignment of teeth
- Fracture of tooth
- Cervical lesions like erosion, abrasion and abfraction
- Attrition of teeth
- Ectopic eruptions.

Following treatment options are available for correction of these conditions. More than one option can be advocated in some cases so as to achieve optimal results
- Ameloplasty/enameloplasty
- Bleaching of teeth
- Restorations with composite resins
- Orthodontic treatment
- Veneering
  - Composite
  - Porcelain
  - Metal ceramic.
- Full coverage crown.

Ameloplasty/Enameloplasty

- It helps in improving minor changes in contour of tooth by removal of enamel

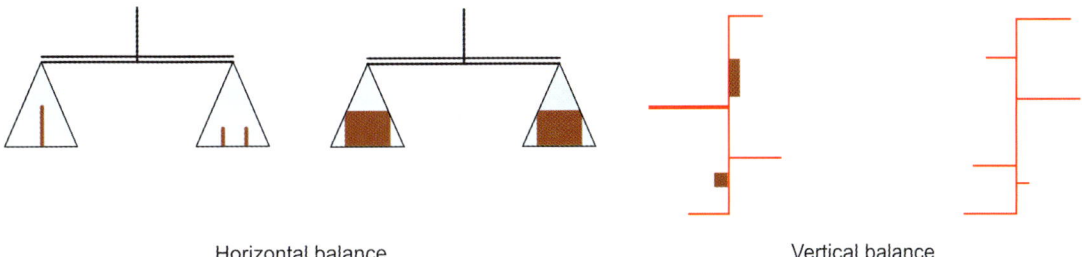

Horizontal balance   Vertical balance

Figure 19.17: Diagram showing horizontal and vertical balance

- It is commonly used to smoothen the roughened enamel margins, fractured tooth surfaces and to soften interproximal angles
- Tooth is polished after ameloplasty so as to have fine scratch proof appearance.

Bleaching

Refer to chapter No. 27 for details of bleaching.

Restorations with Composite Resins

Composite resins are indicated for treatment of minor defects present on incisal edges or labial surfaces of teeth like caries, fracture of teeth and for the modification of anatomy and morphology of teeth like correction of diastema, peg shaped laterals, etc.

Composite resins have advantages of being esthetic, noninvasive, inexpensive, simple to use but they tend to discolor and wear with time.

Technique of Using Composite Resins

- Do conservative tooth preparation or just roughen the enamel surfaces
- Do etching, rinsing and drying of the tooth
- Apply dentin bonding agent and cure it
- Apply composite of selected shade to the prepared tooth surface and cure it
- Finally do finishing and polishing of the restoration.

Orthodontic Treatment

Orthodontic treatment is done to improve functional relationship of arches and to align the teeth properly for enhancing esthetics. Orthodontic treatment is usually opted for correction of malaligned teeth, diastema, ectopic eruptions especially when patient is young and dentition is more amenable to rearrangement.

Veneers

Veneer can be described as a layer of tooth colored material which is applied on the tooth surface for esthetic purpose. They are used to mask the localized, generalized defects and intrinsic discolorations.

Indications

- Damaged, defective and malformed facial surface
- Discolored facial surface
- Discolored restorations.

Types of Veneers

- Based on method of fabrication
  - Direct technique
  - Indirect technique.
- Based on extent of coverage
  - Partial veneers are used for the localized damage, defect and discoloration of the tooth, i.e. they involve only a portion of the tooth crown
  - Full veneers are used when majority of facial surface or whole of the crown of a tooth is discolored.

Types of Full Veneers

- Full veneer with incisal overlapping
- Full veneer with window preparation.

Direct Veneer Technique

Direct partial veneers are placed on localized discolorations or defects which are surrounded by sound enamel (**Fig. 19.18**).

Indications

- Localized discoloration (**Figs 19.19A and B**)
- When entire facial surface is not defective (**Figs 19.20A and B**).

Procedure

- Cleaning of teeth which are to be veneered
- Selection of the shade
- Isolation of the teeth with cotton roll or rubber dam

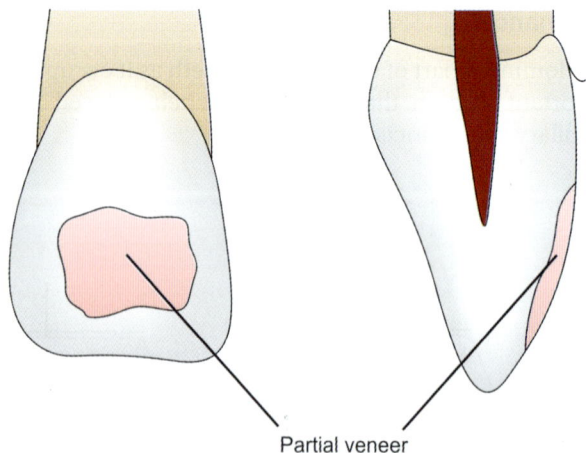
Partial veneer

Figure 19.18: Partial veneer is indicated to correct localized defect

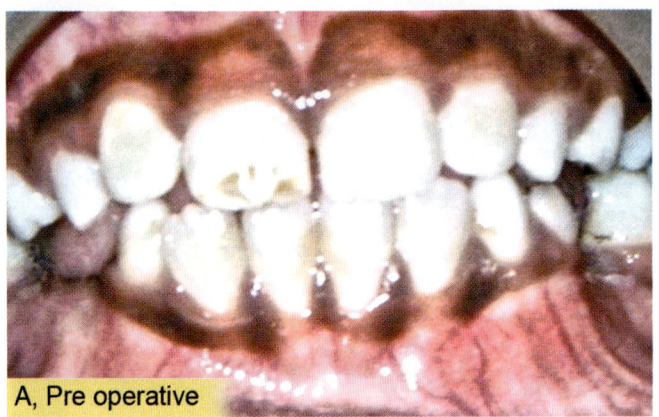
A, Pre operative

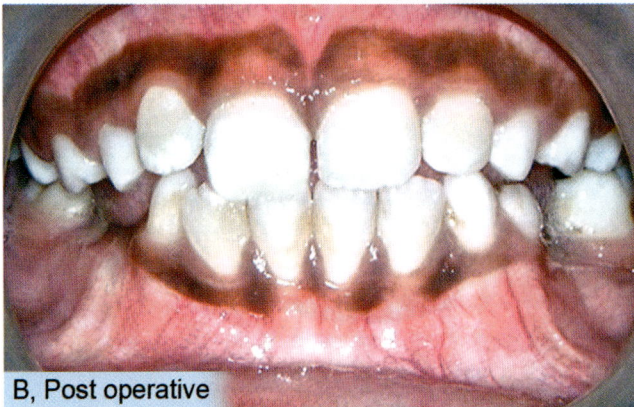
B, Post operative

Figures 19.19A and B: Partial veneer

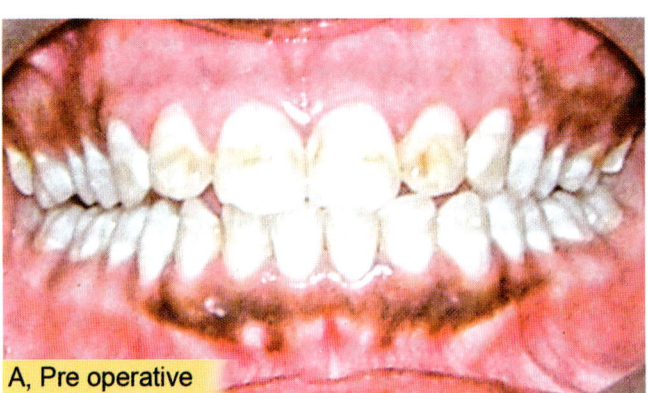
A, Pre operative

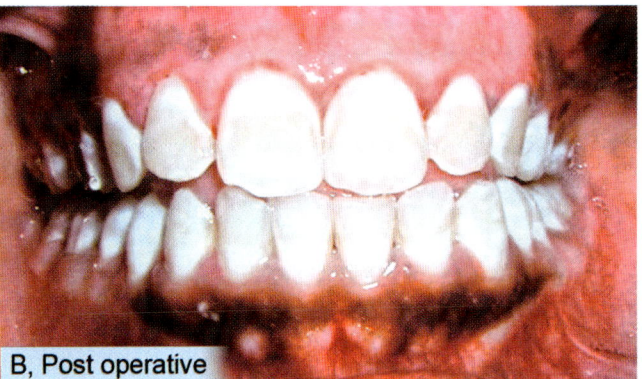
B, Post operative

Figures 19.20A and B: Partial veneer

- Removal of the defect and tooth preparation. The preparation should extend on some sound enamel also
- Application of composite as usual, i.e. first acid etching and then application of primer and bonding agent followed by placement of composite.

Advantages
- Single appointment
- Useful for young patients
- Useful for localized defects
- Economical.

Disadvantages
- More chair side time
- Require more labor.

Direct Full Veneers

Indications
- Diastema closure (**Figs 19.21A and B**)
- Tetracycline stained teeth (**Figs 19.22 and 19.23**)

- Grossly stained and pitted teeth (**Figs 19.24A and B**)
- Gross enamel hypoplasia of anterior teeth (**Figs 19.25A and B**).

Procedure (Figs 19.26A to C)
- Cleaning of the teeth
- Selection of the shade
- Tooth isolation and retraction of gingiva using retraction cords
- Reduction of tooth using coarse round end diamond bur. At the proximal side, the preparation should be facial to the contact point (**Fig. 19.27**). Heavy chamfer at the gingival margin is preferable
- Acid etching, washing and drying followed by application of bonding agent
- Placement of composite in increments. When adding composites, care should be taken to create proper physiological contour, contact point, and smooth surfaces.

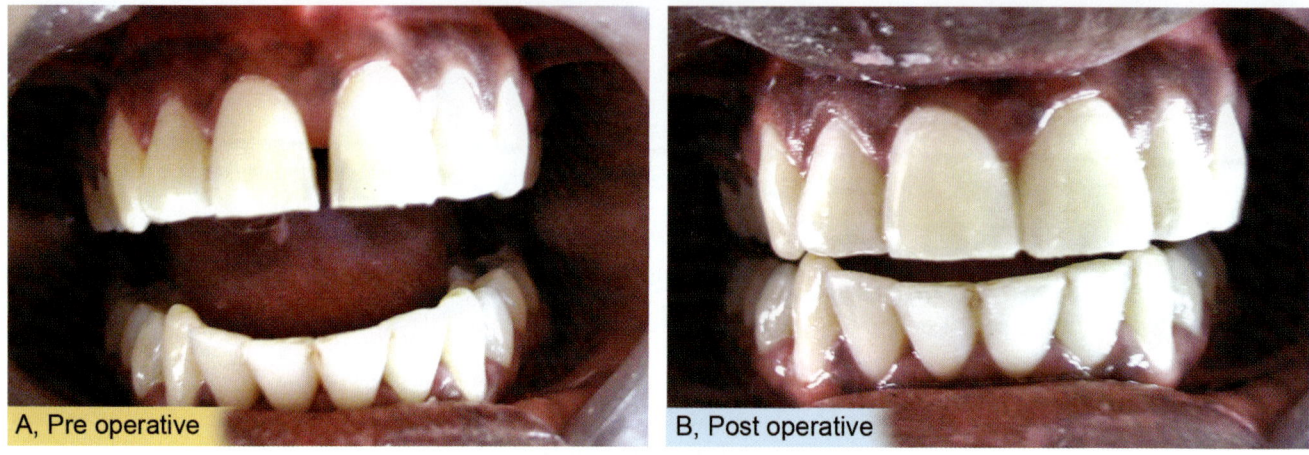

A, Pre operative

B, Post operative

Figures 19.21A and B: Diastema closure by full veneer

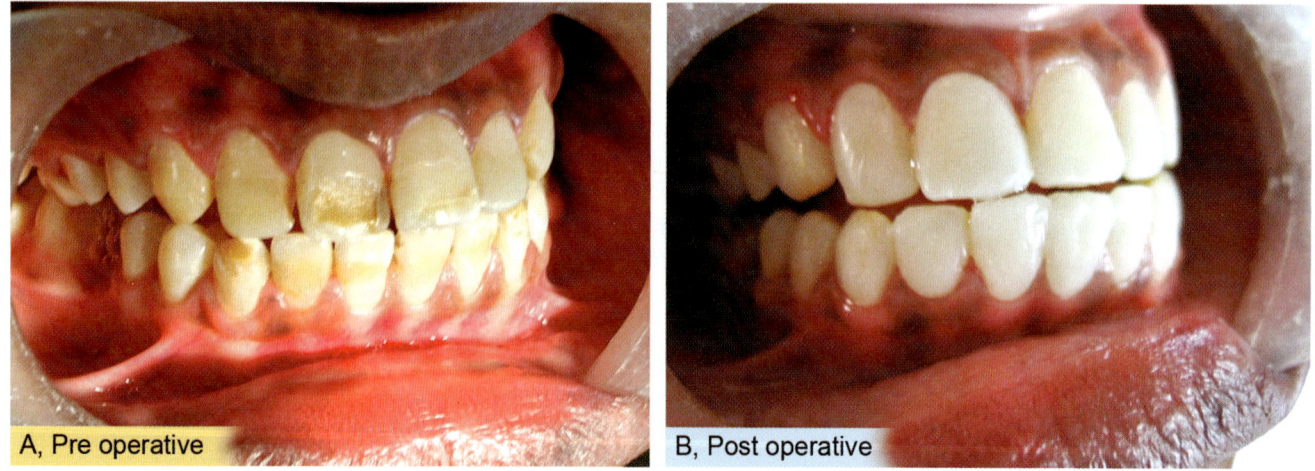

A, Pre operative

B, Post operative

Figures 19.22A and B: Treatment of tetracyclin stains by full veneers

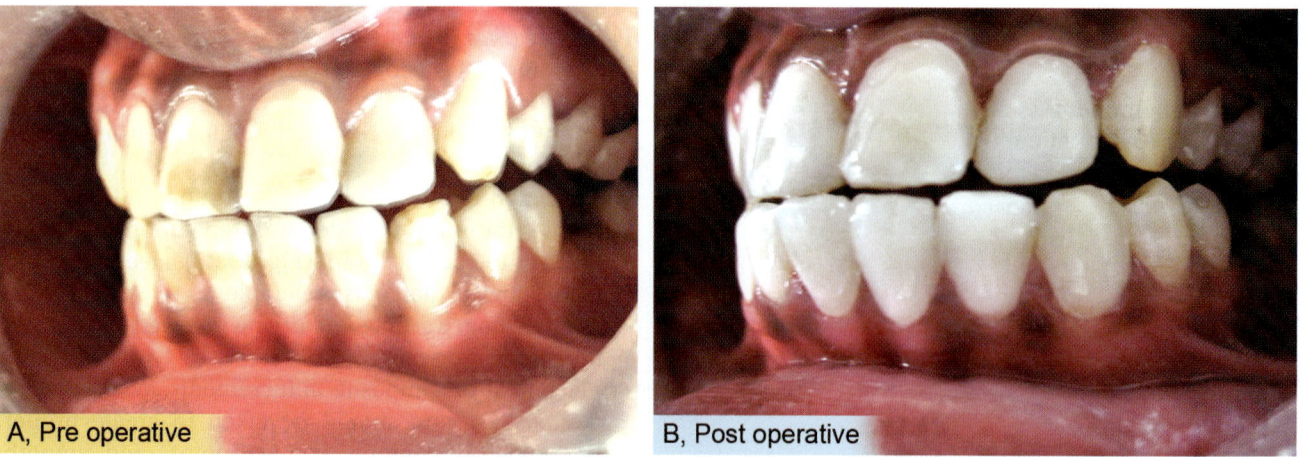

A, Pre operative

B, Post operative

Figures 19.23A and B: Treatment of stained teeth by full veneers

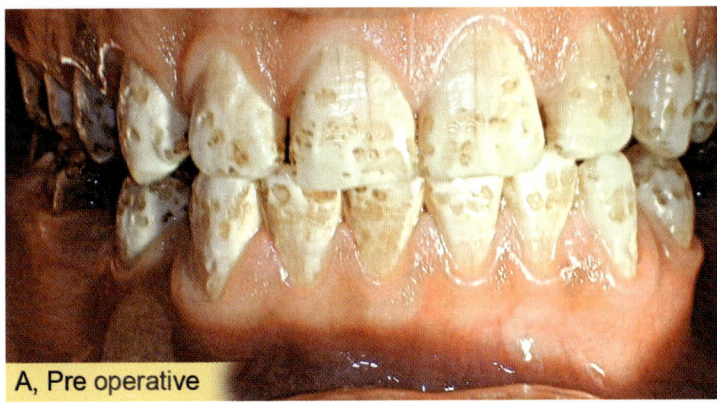

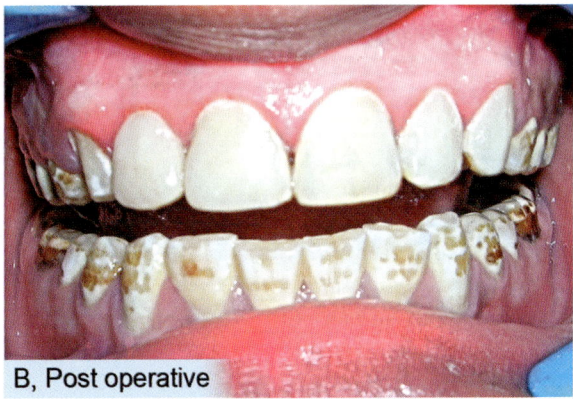

Figures 19.24A and B: Management of unesthetic, pitted teeth by full veneers

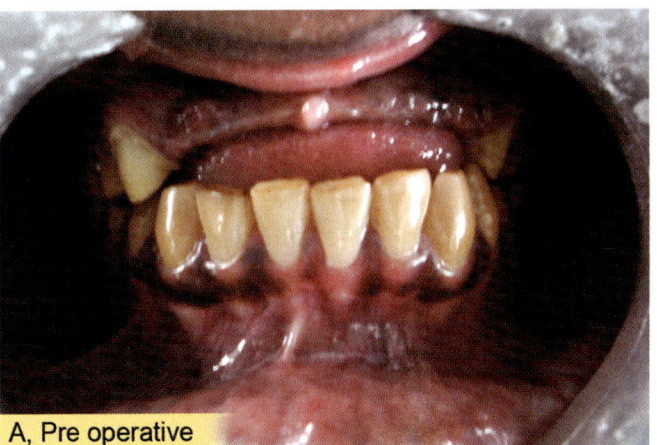

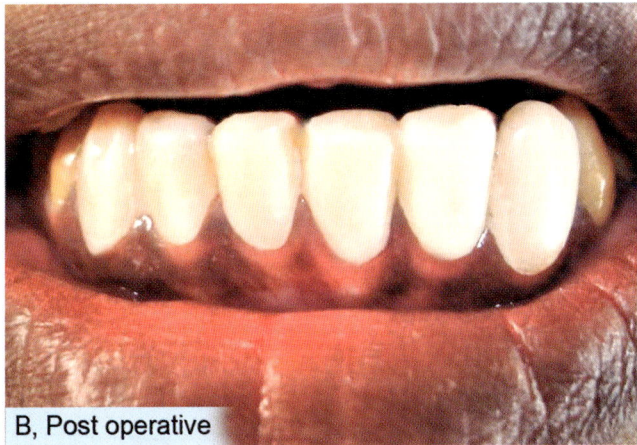

Figures 19.25A and B: Management of amelogenesis imperfecta case by full veneers

Advantages
- Less technique sensitive
- Last longer
- Effective for multiple veneers

Disadvantages
- Expensive
- Require special tooth preparation.

Tooth preparation for full veneers is of two types:

Window Preparation (Fig. 19.28)

Indications
- To preserve functional lingual and incisal surfaces of anterior teeth
- To prepare maxillary canines in patients with canine guided occlusion
- In patients with high occlusal stresses.

Advantages
- Saves the functional lingual and incisal surfaces of anterior teeth.
- It does not extend subgingivally or involve incisal edge.
- Decreases the chances of wear of opposing teeth.

Incisal Lapping Preparation (Fig. 19.29)

Indications
- When crown length is to be increased
- When incisal defect is severe and restoration is necessary.

Advantages
- As tooth preparation is within the enamel, hence no temporary restoration is given
- Improved esthetics along incisal edge.

Indirect Veneer Technique

It is done in two appointments. It has following advantages:

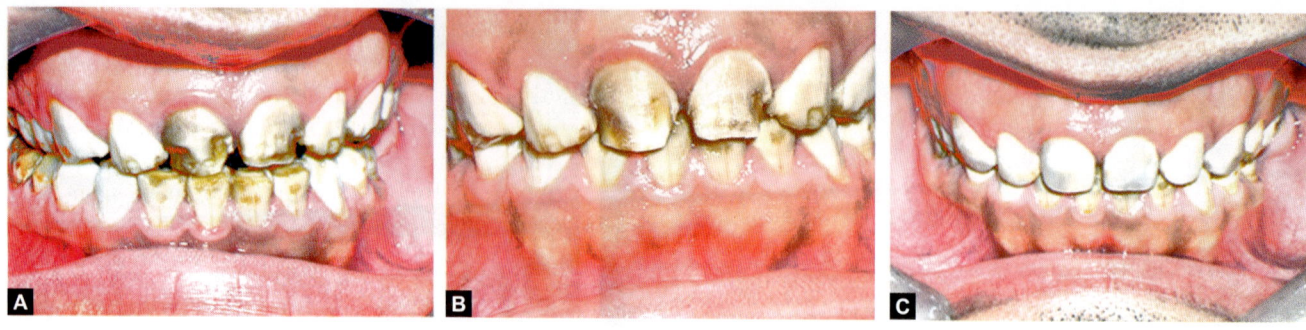

Figures 19.26A to C: Procedure of direct full veneer technique

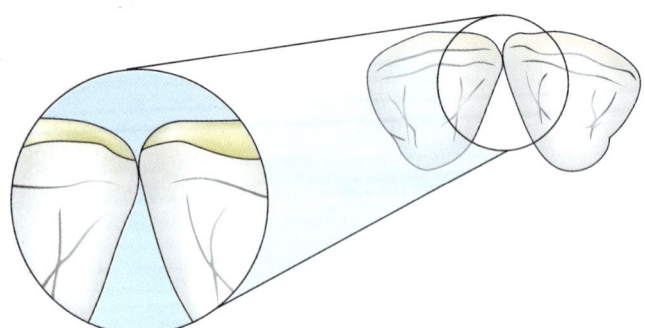

Figure 19.27: Tooth preparation should be facial to contact area

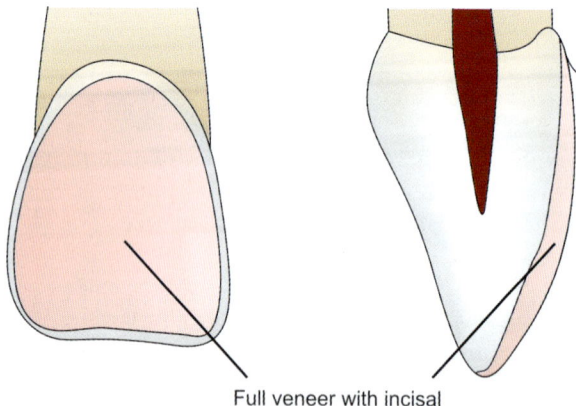

Full veneer with incisal
lapping preparation design

Figure 19.29: Incisal lapping preparation

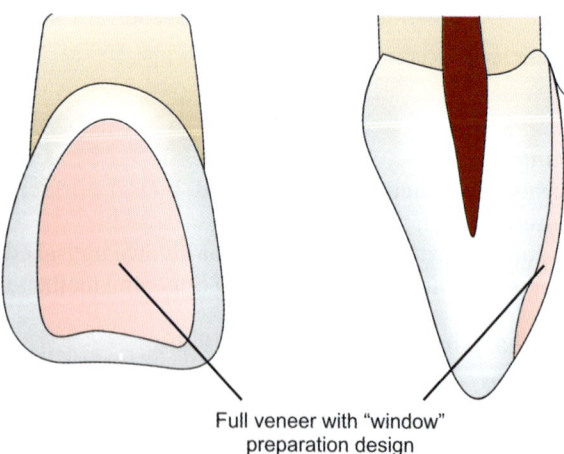

Full veneer with "window"
preparation design

Figure 19.28: Window preparation

- Less technique sensitive than direct veneers
- Multiple teeth can be done in less time
- Chair time required for indirect veneer is less

- Indirect veneers produce better contour, contacts and shade
- These veneers have longer life than direct veneers. Indirect veneers are commonly made-up of following:
  - Processed composite
  - Etched porcelain
  - Castable ceramic.

Processed Composite Veneers

Advantages
- Superior physical and mechanical properties
- Can be bonded to the teeth with a bonding agent
- Easy to finish and polish
- Can be easily repaired
- Processed veneers are made in the cases which show attrition of anterior teeth due to occlusal stress.

Steps of veneer placement
- Processed composites have less potential to form chemical bond with bonding medium, thus additional

micromechanical features are added by surface conditioning or sandblasting

- After this, bonding agent is applied to the tooth enamel
- Veneer is placed by using fluid resin bonding medium
- After placement, finishing and polishing is done.

Etched Porcelain Veneers

In these porcelain veneers, internal surface is acid etched which forms stronger bond with etched surfaces of tooth.

Advantages
- Better retention
- Less prone to stains
- Good esthetics
- Less prone to fractures than other types of veneers.

Steps
- After cleaning and shade selection, the isolation of teeth is done
- Tooth surfaces are prepared with round end diamond bur. Preparation should be incisal capping veneer type
- Impression is taken with rubber base impression material and sent to laboratory for veneer formation
- A completely finished veneer should be seated on clean, dry and isolated prepared tooth
- Internal surfaces of porcelain veneers are conditioned with silane primer
- After setting, excess cured resin is carefully removed by BP knife
- Recontouring and trimming is done, if required.

Castable Ceramic Veneers

- Commonly used castable ceramic is 'Dicor'. The traditional veneer is made of feldspathic porcelain and is still used today. A newer material which is commonly used today is a pressable ceramic.
- These are fabricated for only light to moderate discolorations because it is very translucent material.
- Formed by lost wax technique.
- Preparation of tooth and bonding are like etched porcelain veneers.
- These veneers are not finished with rotary instruments as rotary instruments cause loss of surface coloration.

Veneer for Metal Restoration

Sometimes, veneer is placed on the facial surface of tooth which has been restored with metal.

Steps of making veneers
- Cleaning of the teeth followed by shade selection is done
- Isolation of the area is carried out

- Preparation is done by removing metal and enamel. Butt joints are made at the cavosurface margin. Preparation should not extend on the occlusal surface. Grooves are made along the gingivoaxial and linguoaxial angles. Enamel surface is beveled to improve esthetics
- Acid etching of the preparation and then drying is done
- Placement of composite is done in usual manner
- Finishing and polishing of the restoration is carried out.

Repair of Veneers

Repair of veneers may be of two types:
- Veneers on tooth surface
- Veneers on the metal restoration.

Repair of veneer on tooth surface
- *Repair of direct composite veneers*: It is done with the same material with which it has been prepared. After cleaning, preparation of retentive grooves and roughening the surface, composite is applied in usual manner, i.e. etching, bonding and composite placement.
- *Repair of indirect processed veneers*:
  - *Composite*: These are repaired like direct composite veneers.
  - *Porcelain*:
    i. Acid etching with 10 percent hydrofluoric acid (HF)
    ii. Isolation of the tooth
    iii. Application of coupling agent
    iv. Application of resin bonding agent
    v. Placement of composite, curing and then finishing.

Repair of veneer on metal restoration
- Cleaning of the tooth
- Shade selection
- Isolation of the area
- Preparation of the facial surface by removing the remaining material
- Making chamfer finish line and retentive grooves on metal surface
- Application of acid on the metal surface (to clean the metal surface) followed by rinsing and drying
- Placing polyester strips and wedges interproximally to obtain proper contours
- Application of opaque resin with a brush on the metal surface
- For additional retention and masking effect, 4-META is used
- Placing and curing of composite material is done first on the cervical area in small increments followed by on entire tooth in small increments till the desired contour and esthetic is obtained.

Full Coverage Crowns

Crown

A crown completely covers the crown of the tooth. It can cover the tooth completely or partially. In partial crown a part of the coronal surface remains uncovered and rest of the coronal tooth surface is covered like three-quarter crown and seven-eighth crown.

Basically full coverage restorations are required to increase the esthetics. These restorations can result in change in shape, size, contour and remarkably change self image of the patient.

Indications of crown: Crown are indicated in following conditions:
- In areas with a high esthetic requirement where a more conservative restoration would be inadequate
- In teeth with proximal and/or facial caries that can not be restored with composite resin
- Teeth with extensive decay and when there is insufficient remaining tooth structure
- Teeth with extensive wear
- Fractured teeth
- Malformed teeth
- Extruded teeth
- Teeth with short clinical crowns.

Crowns are contraindicated in conditions where
- A more conservative restoration can be used
- Sufficient enamel is not present to provide adequate support.

Problems with full coverage restorations
- Chances of poor tissue response
- Limited life expectancy of crown, it depends upon type of material used, fit and maintenance done by the patient
- Difficulty in detecting secondary caries under full coverage restorations.

Patient should be explained about these problems and should be explained advantages, disadvantages of the full coverage restoration and the importance of immaculate home-care and oral hygiene maintenance.

The choice of material for restoration depends upon the esthetic and functional demands that will be placed upon it. Studies have shown that functionally all cast crowns were the most successful followed by metal ceramic restoration. But these restoration showed the problem of dark and opaque nature of the metal core resulting in decreased esthetics. The metal core casts a shadow that prevents light transmission into the root. For attaining more esthetics, the color of the core material has to be optically masked. For this the tooth preparation dimensions must necessarily be deep to allow space for masking techniques and materials. To overcome this problem the pressed ceramic systems were developed as an esthetic restorative alternative. They provide enhanced cohesive strength to expand the amount of unsupported restorative material that can augment the contours of teeth without the need for a metal core.

Because of elimination of internal metal coping, excessive opacity is reduced, and thus esthetics is more readily achieved.

Also the ability to etch the ceramic interface allows adhesion for restoration retention, thus the preparation design can be more conservative. But these restorations have their own limitations. Though they are more conservative than metal ceramic restorations, minimum preparation depth is still required to meet the physical constraints of the material itself.

Studies have shown that tooth flexure increases with the degree of tooth structure removed. Since the ultimate strength of a restoration is directly dependent on the strength of the underlying tooth structure, increased tooth flexure can result in increased ceramic fracture.

To overcome this problem, alumina and zirconia-based materials have been developed which provide a densely sintered crystalline structure with physical properties similar to metal-based systems.

In these, even though preparation depth requirements are the similar to metal ceramic restorations, the white ceramic core is rather easier to mask.

CONCLUSION

The contemporary concept of esthetics is revolutionizing the way dentists diagnose, treat, and communicate with patients. The techniques for achieving esthetics have improved and expanded the use of photography to analyze existing esthetic problems and communicate possible treatment alternatives. Patient satisfaction is achieved when the clinician meets or exceeds the patient's expectations. Satisfaction is attained only through a balance in diagnosis, effective communication, and evidence-based planning and proper treatment options which can be done for the delivery of excellence in cosmetic dental treatment.

 Key Points

- As we know that the main aim of operative care is achieved by attaining health, function and esthetics. It is also known as health, function and aesthetic triad (HFA).
- Smile analysis is generally defined in terms of vertical placement of the anterior teeth to the upper lip at rest

and on smile, smile arc characteristics, the vertical relationship of gingival margins to each other and transverse smile dimension (buccal corridors).

- Size of tooth = Width/length ratio
- For example, a young and feminine smile shows teeth with rounded incisal angles, open incisal and facial embrasure while a masculine smile shows closed incisal embrasures with prominent incisal angles.
- Rule of golden proportion was given by Lombardi and Levin. According to it, for an object to be proportional to one another the ratio of 1:1.618 is esthetically pleasing. As a normal rule, if apparent size of each tooth is seen from frontal view, 62% tooth size anterior to it relationship is considered esthetically pleasing.
- As the teeth proceed from the midline to the posterior, the contact points progress apically.
- The gingival zenith represents the most apical point at which each tooth emerges from the free gingival margin. For an esthetically pleasing smile, it should be positioned distally to the center of each tooth within the maxillary anterior segment. The distal position gradually increases from the central incisor to the canine.
- Veneer can be described as a layer of tooth colored material which is applied on the tooth surface for esthetic purpose.
- Tooth preparation for full veneers is of two types; window and incisal lapping preparation.
- Window preparation is done to preserve functional lingual and incisal surfaces of anterior teeth.
- Incisal lapping preparation is indicated when crown length is to be increased and when incisal defect is severe and restoration is necessary.

- Indirect veneers are commonly made up of processed composite, etched porcelain and castable ceramic.

QUESTIONS

1. What are characteristic features of a good smile? Enumerate various options available for smile designing.
2. Discuss in detail about veneers. What are indications, contraindications, advantages and disadvantages of window and incisal lapping designs?
3. Short notes:
   a. Rule of Golden proportions
   b. HFA triad
   c. Indirect veneer materials and technique.
   d. Repair of veneers.

BIBLIOGRAPHY

1. Daniel H Ward. Proportional smile design using the recurring esthetic dental (RED) proportion – DCNA, Vol 45, Jan 2001.
2. David M Sarver. Principles of cosmetic dentistry in orthodontics: part 1. Shape and proportionality of anterior teeth – American Journal of Orthodontics and Dentofacial Orthopedics, Vol 126, No.6, 2004.
3. Gurel G. The science and art of porcelain laminate veneers- London: Quintessence; 2003.
4. Morley J Eubank J. Macroesthetic elements of smile design- J Am Dent Asoc. 2001;132:39-45.
5. Thomas S Valo. Anterior esthetics and the visual arts: beauty, elements of composition, and their clinical application to dentistry-Cosmetic dentistry.

20

CHAPTER

Amalgam Restorations

INTRODUCTION

The first form of silver mercury mixture was given by M Taveau in 1826 at Paris. Crawcour brothers in US introduced dental amalgam to the dentistry in 1833. Since 1850, dental amalgam has been used more than any other restorative material. The dental amalgam alloys consist of silver and other alloys like tin, copper and small amounts of zinc which are mixed with mercury.

HISTORICAL DEVELOPMENT OF AMALGAM

- Silver paste was used to restore a tooth in as early as 659 AD in China
- Renowned physician Ambroise Paré (1510–1590) had used lead or cork to fill teeth
- In 1603, a German named Tobias Dorn Kreilius described a process for creating an amalgam filling by dissolving copper sulfide with strong acids, adding

mercury, bringing to a boil, and then pouring onto the tooth
- In France, D'Arcet's Mineral Cement was popular but it had to be boiled into a liquid before being poured onto a patient's tooth
- Louis Regnart added mercury to the mixture, lowering the temperature required significantly, and known as the "Father of Amalgam"
- Gold, platinum, silver, tin, lead, and alloys of these substances were highly preferred to Amalgam around the 1840s
- The Crawcour Brothers, two Frenchmen, brought Amalgam to the United States in 1833, and in 1844 it was reported that 50 percent of all dental restorations placed in upstate New York consisted of Amalgam
- 1843, the American Society of Dental Surgeons (ASDS), the only US dental association at the time, declared the use of dental amalgam to be malpractice and forced all of its members to sign a pledge to abstain from using it. This was the beginning of what are known as the Amalgam Wars
- The position against Amalgam led to the decline of the ASDS, as dental amalgam was much cheaper than gold, easier to apply, and less painful, as it was not boiled. In 1850, the ASDS rescinded its antiamalgam resolution, and in 1856 it disbanded. The American Dental Association was founded a few years later in 1859, placing its focus on the mechanical aspects of dentistry
- In 1895, GV Black published a Dental Amalgam Formula that provided for the most clinically acceptable performance
- In 1959, Dr. Wilmer Eames suggested a modification to the mercury-to-amalgam ratio, recommending it be dropped from 8:5 to 1:1
- The standard formula was again changed in 1963, when a superior amalgam consisting of a high-copper dispersion alloy was introduced.

Historical development of amalgam	
➡ 1650 Stocker	Copper amalgam
➡ 1818 Dr Louis Regnart	Father of amalgam
➡ 1959 Dr Wilmer Eames	1:1 ratio of mercury: alloy
➡ 1963 Innes and Youdelis	High copper alloy (Admixed type)
➡ 1974 Asgar	Single composition high copper alloy
➡ 1980 Showell	Amalgapin

- Alloy: Alloy is a union of two or more metals
- Amalgam: Amalgam is an alloy in which mercury occurs as a main constituent
- Dental amalgam: The dental amalgam is an alloy of mercury with silver, tin, and varying amounts of copper, zinc and other minor constituents.

COMPOSITION OF AMALGAM POWDER

Amalgam consists of amalgam alloy and mercury. Amalgam alloy is composed of silver-tin alloy with varying amounts of copper, zinc, indium and palladium (**Fig. 20.1**). Dental amalgam alloys are mainly of two types, low copper and high copper alloys.

Low copper alloys contain copper upto 6 percent by weight. In high copper alloys, the copper content lies between 6 to 30 percent.

In general, amalgam alloy consists of silver 40 percent minimum, tin 32 percent maximum, copper 30 percent maximum, zinc 2 percent maximum, and sometimes traces of indium or palladium. In preamalgamated alloys, mercury 3 percent is used which reacts more rapidly when mixed with silver tin alloy. Mercury used for dental amalgam is purified by distillation.

COMPOSITION OF AMALGAM ALLOYS (TABLE 20.1)

Effects of Constituent Metals on the Properties of Amalgam

Silver: It has the following effects on the properties of amalgam.
- Increases strength
- Increases setting expansion
- Reduces setting time
- Resists tarnish and corrosion
- Decreases flow.

Tin: Tin helps in formation of a silver/tin compound (AgSn). This is the gamma phase which readily undergoes an amalgamation reaction with mercury. Tin causes following effects:
- Increases setting time
- Retards the reaction
- Reduces strength, hardness, and setting expansion

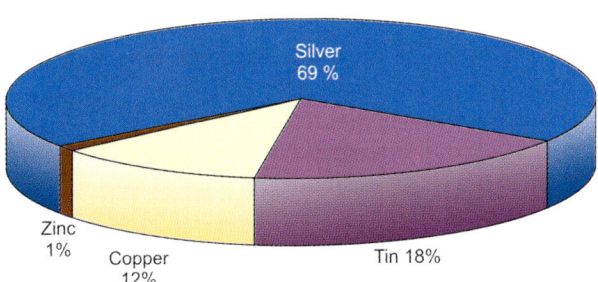

Figure 20.1: Composition of amalgam powder

Table 20.1: Percentage of elements by weight

Alloy	Particle	Silver	Tin	Copper	Zinc	Palladium	Indium
• Low copper	Lathecut or Spherical	65 to 77	26 to 28	2 to 5	0 to 2	0	0
• High copper							
– Admixed	Lathecut	40 to 70	26 to 30	13 to 30	0 to 1	0	0
	Spherical	40 to 70	0 to 30	20 to 30	0	0	0
– Unicompositional	Spherical	40 to 60	22 to 30	15 to 30	0 to1	0 to 4	0

Copper: It has the following effects on the properties of amalgam.

- Reduces tarnish and corrosion
- Reduces creep
- Strengthening effect on the set amalgam
- Helps in uniform comminution of the alloy.

Zinc: Its presence is not essential. It may vary from 0 to 2 percent by weight. It has the following effects on the properties of amalgam:

- Scavengers the available oxygen to impede oxidization of Ag, Sn or Cu during alloy ingot manufacturer.
- If zinc containing alloys are contaminated with moisture, Zn gives rise to delayed or secondary expansion.

Palladium (0 to 1% by weight): Improves the corrosion resistance and the mechanical properties.

Indium (0 to 4 % by weight): It decreases the evaporation of mercury and the amount of mercury required to wet the alloy particles.

Proportioning

Usually alloy/mercury ratio ranges between 5:8 and 10:8. But to achieve optimum properties of the amalgam, mercury should be less than 50 percent. For lathe cut alloys, it is 45 percent. For spherical alloys, it is 40 percent Hg. Disposable capsules containing preproportioned aliquots of mercury are available (**Figs 20.2 and 20.3**). To prevent any amalgamation during storage mercury and alloy are physically separated from each other.

Classification of Amalgam

There are different ways of classifying amalgam alloys. These are:

- ***Based on shape of particles***
  - *Irregular:* In this, shape of particles is irregular, may be in the shape of spindles or shavings.
  - *Spherical:* In this, shape of particle is spherical with smooth surface.
  - *Spheroidal:* In this, shape of particle is spheroidal with irregular surface.

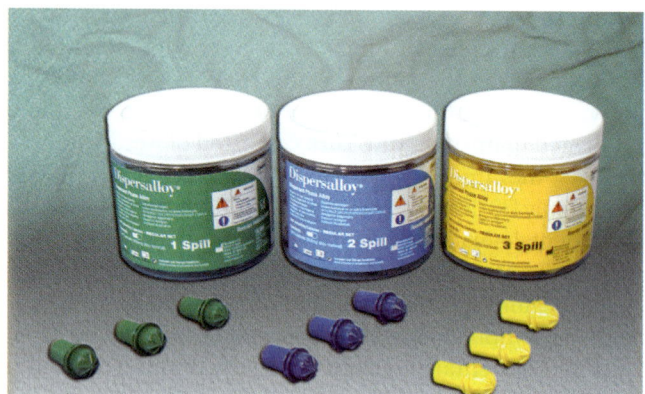

Figure 20.2: Disposable capsules containing silver alloy and mercury

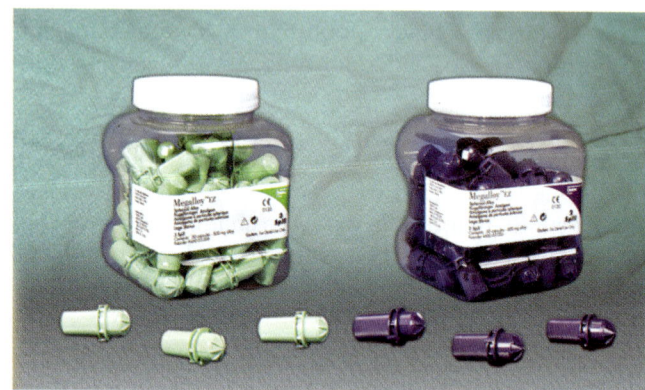

Figure 20.3: Silver alloy capsules

- ***Based on copper content***
  - *Low copper alloy:* Copper is in range of 2 to 6 percent
  - *High copper alloy:* Copper is in range of 6 to 30 percent
- ***Based on zinc content***
  - *Zinc containing alloys:* Zinc is in range of 0.01–1 percent
  - *Zinc free alloys:* Zinc is in range of < 0.01 percent
- ***Based on the presence of Noble metals***
  - *Binary alloys:* Contains two metals, i.e. silver and tin.

- *Ternary alloys:* Contain three metals, i.e. silver, tin and copper
- *Quaternary alloys:* Contains four metals, i.e. silver, tin, copper and zinc.

Out of these, Quaternary alloys are most acceptable.

Generations of dental amalgam
➡ Class–I Silver and Tin in ratio (8:1)
➡ Class–II Silver, Tin, Copper (4%), Zinc
➡ Class–III Silver eutectic alloy added to original alloy
➡ Class–IV Copper content increased to 29 percent
➡ Class–V Indium added to mixture of silver, tin and copper
➡ Class–VI Noble metals added such as palladium.

Difference between high copper and low copper alloys

	High copper alloys	*Low copper alloys*
Copper content	6–30%	<6%
Mercury required for amalgamation	Less	More
Setting reaction	Fast setting	Slow setting
Amalgamation speed and energy	Require high-speed and energy for amalgamation since copper has low solubility in mercury	Require less speed and low energy for amalgamation
Dormant phase	It is Cu_6Sn_5, i.e. η phase	It is Ag_2Hg_3, i.e. $\eta1$ phase
Tarnish and corrosion	It is due to copper rich phase, i.e. Cu_6Sn_5.	It is due to gamma 2 phase, i.e. $Sn_{7-8}Hg_3$
Creep	Less creep (<1%)	More creep (1–8%)
Compressive strength	High (250–500 Mpa)	Low (150–350 Mpa)
Dimensional change	Less (1–9 µm/cm)	More (10–20 µm/cm)

Setting Reaction of Amalgam

For Lathe-cut Low Copper Alloys

On mixing amalgam alloy with mercury, the alloy particles get dissolved in the mercury. In the initial reaction, mercury reacts with tin and silver without involving copper and zinc. Mercury reacts with alloy particles to form two products, i.e. the silver mercury phase and tin mercury phase. After this reaction, the unreacted particles are embedded in the matrix of reaction products with mercury. The reaction is as following:

$$Ag_3Sn + Hg \rightarrow Ag_2Hg_3 + Sn_{7-8}Hg_3 + Ag_3Sn$$
$$(\gamma) \qquad\qquad (\gamma_1) \qquad (\gamma_2) \qquad (\gamma)$$

In lathe-cut low copper amalgams both γ_1 and γ_2 form a continuous network. Since γ_2 phase is least corrosion resistant phase, its distribution in reaction product is important.

For Admixed High Copper Alloys

For high copper alloys, the reaction is different. It occurs in two phases. The initial reaction is similar to that of low copper alloys, i.e.

$$Ag_3Sn + Ag\text{-}Cu + Hg \rightarrow Ag_2Hg_3 + Sn_{7-8}Hg_3 + Ag_3Sn + Ag\text{-}Cu$$
$$(\gamma) \quad (eutactic) \qquad (\gamma_1) \qquad (\gamma_2) \qquad (\gamma) \ (unreached)$$

The second phase of reaction involves the silver copper phase (Ag-Cu).

It reacts with γ (Ag_3Sn) and mercury to form Ag_2Hg_3, $Sn_{7-8}Hg$ and Cu_6Sn_5 phase. The mercury released from $Sn_{7-8}Hg$ (γ_2 phase) reacts with silver to form Ag_2Hg_5 (γ_1) phase.

$$Sn_{7-8}Hg + Ag\text{-}Cu \rightarrow Cu_6Sn_5 + Ag_2Hg_3 + Ag\text{-}Cu$$
$$(\gamma_2) \qquad (eutectic) \qquad (\eta) \qquad (\gamma_1)$$

This reaction goes on. After one week, the γ_2 phase reacts completely with eutectic and replace all the γ_2 phase by γ and γ_1 phase.

For Unicompositional Silver Alloy

The difference in admix type and the unicompositional alloys is that in latter the eutectic phase, i.e. Ag-Cu phase is absent and the reaction is directly with silver, copper and tin phases. In these only silver reacts with mercury and the tin remains bound to copper.

$$Ag\text{-}Sn\text{-}Cu + Hg \rightarrow Ag_2Hg_3 + Cu_6Sn_5 + (Unconsumed$$
$$(alloy\ particles) \qquad (\gamma_1) \qquad (\eta) \qquad alloy\ particles)$$

The final phase formed is Cu_6Sn_5 (η) phase and there is no Ag_2Hg_3 (γ_2) phase.

Structure of Set Amalgam

The set amalgam mass consists of unreacted alloy particles surrounded by a matrix of the reaction products (**Figs 20.4 and 20.5**).

Advantages of silver amalgam
➡ Ease of manipulation
➡ Satisfactory marginal adaptation
➡ Wider range of application
➡ Physical characteristics of amalgam are comparable to enamel and dentin.
➡ Less technique sensitive
➡ Self-sealing

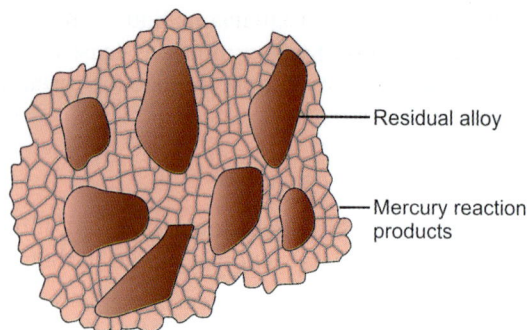

Figure 20.4: Microstructure of amalgam

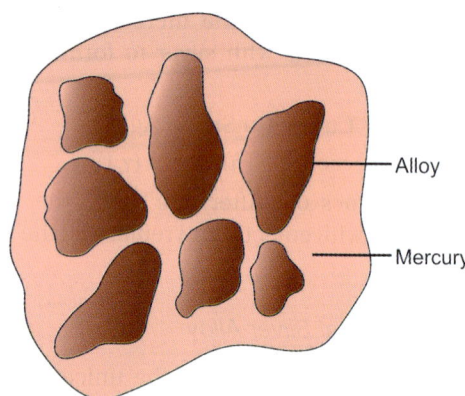

Figure 20.5: Structure of set amalgam

- Biocompatible
- Good wear resistance
- Low cost
- Can be completed in one dental visit
- Bonded amalgam restorations can also bond to tooth structure.

Disadvantages of silver amalgam

- Less esthetic
- Extensive preparation to hold an amalgam filling
- Amalgam fillings can corrode or tarnish overtime, causing discoloration
- Does not bond to tooth
- Being metallic restoration, it is noninsulating
- Marginal degradation is seen in low copper alloys
- Amalgam is not strong enough to reinforce the weakened tooth structure
- Poor tensile strength making it a brittle material

→ Results in galvanic current in association with gold restoration or even in same restoration with non-uniform condensation
→ Oral lichen planus is also seen with amalgam restoration.

INDICATIONS OF AMALGAM RESTORATION

- Moderate to large class I preparation.
- Class II preparations in which there is:
  - Heavy occlusion
  - Extension on the root surface
  - Problem of isolation.
    It is indicated in heavy occlusion because amalgam has greater wear resistance than composites. Minor contamination during the amalgam placement has less adverse effects as compared to composite restorations.
- Class V preparations in which:
  - Esthetic is not a problem
  - Preparation is entirely on root surface
  - Isolation is difficult.
- Class VI preparations
- Class III preparations (sometimes) where isolation is difficult
- Used as a foundation in cases of grossly decayed teeth while planning for cast restoration
- Used as a postendodontic restoration
- Teeth having no definitive pulpal prognosis—used as type of interim restoration before assessment of pulpal status of the tooth
- Tooth having fractured cusp can be restored with the help of amalgam using pin and slot.

CONTRAINDICATIONS OF AMALGAM RESTORATION

- *Esthetics*: Use of amalgam is avoided in esthetic areas of oral cavity. So, preparations class III, IV, V usually are not indicated except in certain cases.
- Small to moderate class I and class II preparations should be restored with composite rather than amalgam as former results in more conservative tooth preparation.

Indications

- Moderate to large class I and II preparations
- Class V preparations (some cases)
- Class VI preparation
- Class III preparation (some cases)
- Used as foundation
- Used as postendodontic filling
- Tooth having no definitive pulpal prognosis
- Tooth having fractured cusp.

➡ When esthetics is the prime concern
➡ Small to moderate class I and class II preparations.

Phases of silver amalgam

Code	Component
(γ) gamma	Ag_3Sn (Silver Tin phase)
(γ_1) gamma 1	Ag_2Hg_3 (Silver Mercury phase)
(γ_2) gamma 2	$Sn_{7-8}Hg_3$ (Tin Mercury phase)
(ε) epsilon	Cu_3Sn (Copper Tin phase)
(η) eta	Cu_6Sn_5 (Copper Tin phase)

TYPES OF AMALGAM POWDER

Lathe-cut is made by cutting fillings of alloy from a prehomogenized ingot which was heat treated at 420°C for many hours. The fillings are then reheated at 100°C for 1 hour for aging of the alloy.

Spherical (spheroidal) alloy is formed when molten alloy is sprayed into a column filled with inert gas, this molten metal solidifies as fine droplets of alloy.

Admixed alloy is that when different size or shape of amalgam powder is mixed together to increase filling efficiency.

Single composition is that alloy in which every particle of alloy is having same shape, size and composition.

Dispersion modified, high copper alloys is that in which high copper alloy is mixed with conventional alloy.

PHYSICAL PROPERTIES OF AMALGAM

Dimensional Change

Small amount of contraction occurs in the first half an hour after trituration because mercury diffuses into the silver and tin and the mix dissolves in the mercury. After this, expansion occurs because of crystallization of the new phases. According to ADA specification no. 1 dimensional change should be limited to 20 microns/cm measured between 5 minutes and 24 hours after trituration.

Factors Affecting Dimensional Changes of Amalgam

- *Type of alloy being used*, for example, single composition spherical alloys contract more than single composition lathe cut or admixed alloys.
- *Condensation technique*, i.e. more mercury removed from the alloy, the more it will contract.
- *Trituration time*, overtrituration causes contraction.
- *Presence of zinc:* If zinc containing amalgam comes in contact with moisture or saliva during condensation or

trituration, it can result in delayed expansion after 3 to 5 days of restoration, This occurs due to formation of zinc oxide and hydrogen gas when zinc react with water. This expansion can result in extrusion of restoration beyond preparation margins and pulpal pain.

MERCUROSCOPIC EXPANSION

The term "mercuroscopic expansion" was proposed by Jorgenson. This expansion occurs in amalgam restorations.

Phenomenon

Initially, there is volumetric contraction due to reduction in volume of various elements. But with time, crystallization of various phases occurs leading to expansion due to impinging of crystals over each other. Corrosion of amalgam leads to mercury release from γ_2 phase (Sn_8Hg), which rereacts with unreacted γ phase (AgSn), causing further expansion. This is termed mercuroscopic expansion.

Consequences of Mercuroscopic Expansion

Mercuroscopic expansion of amalgam leads to "shabby" edges that "catch", leading to a small unsupported ledge of amalgam which is broken off during function. Amalgam protrudes from the space and this chemical stress leads to increase in creep.

Difference between primary and secondary expansion?

Expansion that occurs due to reaction of Hg with alloy components is termed primary expansion or mercuroscopic expansion. Expansion that occurs after 1 to 7 days due to moisture contamination during trituration or condensation before the amalgam mass is set, is termed secondary expansion or delayed expansion.

Factors leading to mercuroscopic expansion:
- Increased Hg: alloy ratio
- Failure to squeeze out excess Hg
- Inadequate condensation pressure.

Strength

- Strength of amalgam develops slowly. It takes 24 hours to reach maximum. In the first hour, only 40 to 60 percent of its maximum compressive strength is achieved
- According to ADA specification no. 1, amalgam should have minimum 1 hour compressive strength of 11,600 psi (80 MPa)
- Amalgam has much higher compressive strength than tensile or shear strength making it brittle material

- Compressive strength of amalgam is seven times more than its tensile strength. Being a brittle material, it is weak in thin sections, thus unsupported edges of restoration fracture frequently. To avoid this, a 90° butt joint angle of amalgam is required at the margins
- Spherical alloys are harder and stronger when compared to lathe cut alloys because they require less mercury during trituration, thus less of the weak matrix portion forms.

Plastic Deformation (Creep) (Fig. 20.6)

- Creep is the time dependent response of an already set material to stress. This response is in the form of plastic deformation. It can be of two types depending on the stresses involved viz; static and dynamic
- By ADA specification no. 1, creep is limited to 3 percent in a set amalgam
- Creep/flow usually occurs near the melting temperature of the material. In amalgam, creep happens because gamma 1 is a fine grained structure and the particles "slide" across each other resulting in slipping of grain boundaries
- Creep is unfavorable to amalgam because it causes amalgam to flow out over margins where the thin amalgam fractures. This results in marginal deterioration.

Factors affecting creep:
- Low copper alloys have higher creep than high copper alloys because in later, copper binds the tin and forms eta phase, and this prevents formation of gamma 2 phase. Crystals of eta phase interlock and check slippage at gamma 1 grain boundaries, resulting in less creep.

- Higher the residual mercury levels, more is the creep.
- Increased condensation pressure reduces creep because it reduces residual mercury level.
- Marginal areas show more creep because they have higher levels of residual mercury.
- A delay between trituration and condensation increases creep.

Corrosion

- Amalgam restoration shows corrosion and tarnish over a period of time. Though corrosion causes decrease in strength of a restoration by 50 percent in five years, the advantageous fact of corrosion is that its by-products seal the preparation margin, resulting in self-sealing of amalgam (**Fig. 20.7**).
- In low copper amalgams, the most corrosion prone phase is gamma 2 ($Sn_{7-8}Hg_3$). In these alloys, corrosion products are tin oxides and tin chlorides. Here, the corrosion proceeds from outer surface to interior of restoration making it porous and spongy.
- In high copper amalgams, corrosion products are similar to that of low copper alloys. In addition, there is formation of copper chloride which corrode slower than low copper amalgams. High copper alloys corrode slower because they contain little or none of gamma 2

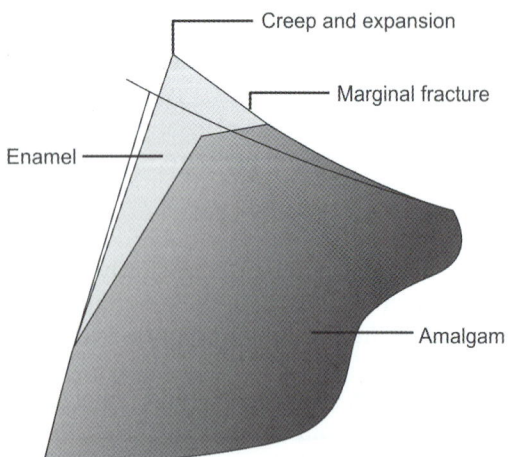

Figure 20.6: Creep and expansion results in marginal fracture of amalgam restoration

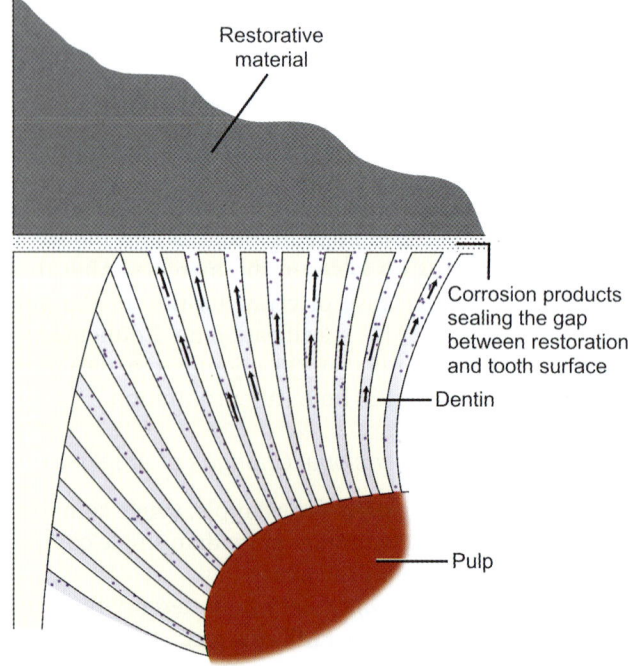

Figure 20.7: Sealing of restorative margins because of corrosion products of amalgam

phase. Also the corrosion is not of penetrating type as in low copper alloys. In high copper alloys, the most corrosion prone phase is the eta phase.

Biocompatibility

Though there has been a great debate related to mercury toxicity, if careful handling of mercury is taken, amalgam has proved to be a biocompatible material.

Thermal Conductivity

Because of good thermal conductivity, amalgam can transmit temperature changes readily to the pulp. Hence, its closeness to pulp should be avoided without adequate pulp protection.

Coefficient of Thermal Expansion

It is three times more in amalgam than that of dentin. This large difference is responsible for microleakage.

Microleakage in Amalgam

Microleakage occurs when there is 2 to 20 micron wide gap between the amalgam and tooth structure.

Following factors are responsible for microleakage in amalgam:
- Poor condensation techniques that cause marginal voids
- Lack of corrosion byproducts which are necessary for sealing of margins
- High coefficient of thermal expansion of amalgam
- Use of single composition spherical alloys which show more, leakage than lathecut or admixed alloys.

> **Microleakage can lead to (Figs 20.8A and B)**
> - Pulpal inflammation
> - Tooth discoloration
> - Postoperative sensitivity
> - Restoration failure.

RECENT ADVANCES IN AMALGAM

Mercury Free Direct Filling Alloy

The American dental association, in combination with national institute on standard and technology (ADA-NIST) patented a mercury free direct filling alloy which is based on Ag coated Ag-Sn particles that can be self-welded by compaction to create a restoration. To keep the surface of alloy particles clean, a fluoroboric acid solution is used. These alloys can be condensed in the same manner as direct filling gold restoration.

Low Mercury Alloy

In this approach, alloy particles are carefully selected so that they can be packed well. By this, it is possible to reduce the need of mercury content for mixing to the 15 to 25 percent. However, the clinical properties of these alloys are not yet known.

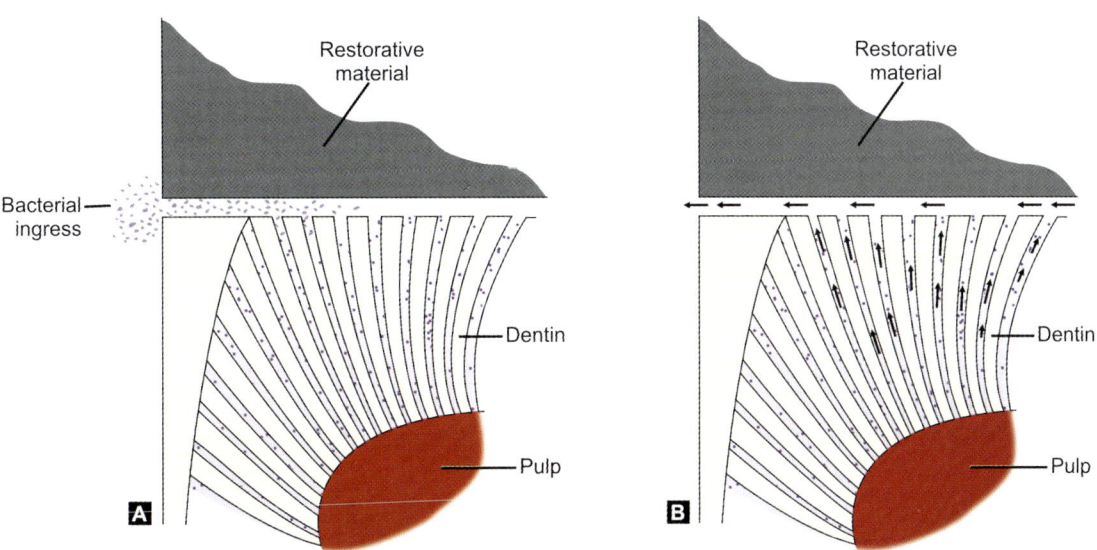

Figures 20.8A and B: (A) Bacteria can pass into the marginal gap causing pulpal inflammation;
(B) The dentinal fluid can come out of the marginal gap causing pain and sensitivity

Bonded Amalgam System

One of the major disadvantage of the amalgam is that it does not adhere to the preparation walls. To conquer this problem, bonding systems to bond the amalgam to tooth structure have been developed. In the bonded amalgam technique, a dentin bonding system is used along with a viscous resin liner which physically mixes with the amalgam and forms a micromechanical union to increase amalgam's retention to tooth structure.

Since amalgam is hydrophobic, and tooth is hydrophilic, therefore to achieve optimal wetting, bonding systems must have dual properties. For this, monomer molecule having hydrophilic and hydrophobic ends are used, for example 4-methyloxy ethyl trimellitic anhydride (4-META).

Indications of Bonding

- When remaining tooth structure, after tooth preparation is weak
- In extensively carious posterior teeth where it acts as cost effective alternative for cast metal and metal ceramic restorations
- In deep bite cases where short clinical crown is present, and pin retained restoration is not possible. In these cases, bonding provides auxiliary retention
- As core for foundation of cast crown restoration.

Advantages of using bonded amalgam system
➡ Adequate dentin sealing
➡ Increased resistance form
➡ Increased retention
➡ Conservative tooth preparation
➡ Improved marginal seal
➡ Elimination of use of retention pins and other modes of retention
➡ Reduction in microleakage, secondary caries and postoperative sensitivity
➡ Cost effective for extensively carious tooth
➡ Can be done in single appointment.

Disadvantages of amalgam bonding
➡ Reduction in bond strength over years because of repeated thermocycling in the oral cavity
➡ Technique sensitive system. Amalgam must be condensed over wet adhesive resin
➡ Expensive than nonbonded amalgam restoration.

Technique of Bonded Amalgam

Bonding agents used in amalgam bonding system: Although many products are available for adhesion to enamel and dentin, most of these are meant to be used with resin composites. Adhesives which have metal bonding capabilities can be used for amalgam bonding. These are amalgambond plus with HPA (High performance additive) powder (Parkell), optibond 2 (Kerr), all bond 2 (Bisco), Panavia EX and Panavia 21 (Kuraray).

Bonding interface (Figs 20.9A and B): The bonding interface constitutes tooth, amalgam and adhesive resin present between them.

The bonding interface may consist of the following:
- Tag formation
- Precipitates on pretreated dentin surfaces to which adhesive resin binds mechanically or chemically
- Formation of hybrid layer of reinforced dentin
- Chemical binding to the inorganic and organic components of dentin and enamel.

Technique of placing bonded amalgam
- Isolate the tooth with rubber dam
- Do the conservative preparation, i.e. conventional retention and resistance forms are not strictly followed.
- Remove all the carious portion and unsupported enamel rods

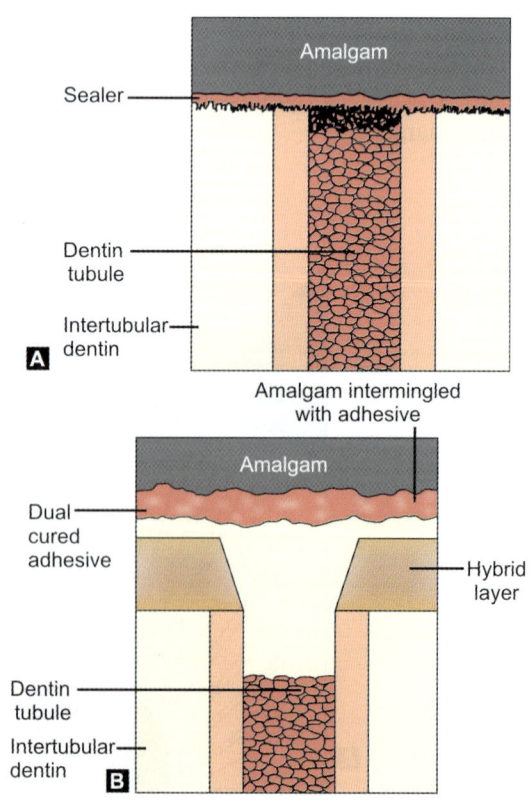

Figures 20.9A and B: Bonding interface of amalgam and tooth: (A) Conventional amalgam restoration; (B) Bonded amalgam restoration

- In deep preparation, protect the pulp with suitable liner and base
- Place matrix and wedges properly
- Etch the enamel and dentin walls of the preparation with 10 percent citric or phosphoric acid gel for 15 to 20 seconds. Wash and dry the preparation
- Apply adhesive primer to the conditioned dentin and then evenly apply dentin bonding agent
- Before the bonding agent gets dried, condense freshly triturated high copper amalgam into the preparation
- Carve, finish and polish the final restoration as usual.

Future of Bonded Amalgam Restoration

Bonded amalgam restoration has advantages of conservative tooth preparation, good qualities of amalgam, better marginal seal along with improved retention and resistance.

But since, there are very few comparative studies done on bonded amalgam restorations, hence exact conclusion cannot be made about their prognosis and future use. However, most of the workers have good hope about their future and expect that very soon bonded amalgam be routinely used in place of conventional unbonded amalgam restorations.

Gallium in Place of Mercury in Amalgam

To conquer the harmful effects of mercury, gallium metal which has second lowest melting point (next to mercury) has been tried in mercury free amalgam restoration. Use of alternative containing gallium, instead of mercury, was first suggested in 1928 in Germany.

Advantages of gallium amalgam
⇒ Gallium amalgam can be manipulated with same instruments used for silver amalgam
⇒ Its strength is almost equal to silver mercury amalgam, and like latter its strength also increases with time
⇒ The creep resistance complies with ISO requirements
⇒ Since gallium amalgam expands after trituration, it provides better marginal seal than silver amalgam
⇒ Setting time is less than silver mercury amalgam, therefore can be finished and polished after one hour
⇒ Most of the physical and mechanical properties of gallium alloy are similar to high copper mercury amalgam.

Disadvantages of gallium amalgam
⇒ Corrosion resistance of gallium amalgam is very low
⇒ Handling of gallium alloy is difficult because it has tendency to stick to the instruments. This sticking problem

can be reduced by adding a drop of absolute alcohol to the mix before trituration. Alcohol slowly evaporates and thus does not adversely affect the properties of the amalgam
- ⇒ Extremely technique sensitive, any moisture contamination during placement results in alloy expansion
- ⇒ Shows expansion after setting. Excessive expansion can produce stresses sufficient to crack the tooth.

Composition
⇒ Powder
♦ Silver (Ag)   - 55 to 65%
♦ Tin (Sn)   - 20 to 30%
♦ Copper (Cu)   - 10 to 16%
♦ Palladium (Pd) - 10 to 15%
⇒ Liquid
♦ Gallium (Ga)   - 57 to 67%
♦ Indium (In)   - 15 to 25%
♦ Tin (Sn)   - 15 to 25%

Setting reaction: The reaction between powder AgSn particles and liquid gallium results into the formation of AgGa phase and a pure tin phase

$$AgSn + Ga \rightarrow AgGa + Sn$$

Properties of Gallium Amalgam Restorations

- ***Compressive strength:*** Gallium alloys have sufficient strength for small restoration.
- ***Setting expansion:*** In initial stages, controlled expansion occurs but if contaminated, uncontrolled expansion can result. This excessive expansion can cause cuspal fracture, and postoperative sensitivity.
- ***Creep value:*** In gallium alloys, creep value is less.
- Gallium amalgam has very high wetting ability, hence the final restoration is highly resistant to microleakage.
- ***Time consuming:*** Since their handling is difficult because of being sticky, it takes more time for condensation and matrix band has to be removed very carefully to avoid fracture of restoration.
- ***Expensive:*** Gallium amalgam is about 16 times costlier than the silver mercury amalgam.

Conclusion

Gallium amalgam restorations have been developed in an attempt to provide a mercury free amalgam restoration. If meticulous attention is paid to moisture control, these restorations can function well for short-time. But since they are prone to tarnish and corrosion, long-term effects are unknown. To prevent excessive expansion, restoration should be sealed with a hydrophobic resin sealant. Since there is a demand for less technique sensitive alternative to silver amalgam than resin composite, for difficult and larger posterior situations, gallium alloys do not provide the answer.

Consolidated Silver Alloy

It is a recently introduced amalgam developed at National Institute of Standards and Technology. It uses fluoroboric acid solution for keeping the surface of silver alloy particles clean. The alloy is condensed in the preparation similar to direct filling gold. The main limitation of using this material is that alloy hardens due to repeated burnishing. This makes it difficult to compact in preparation. For good adaptation of material and to avoid voids in the final restoration, an excessive force is required for compaction.

PRINCIPLES OF TOOTH PREPARATION FOR AMALGAM RESTORATIONS

Amalgam Restoration for Class I Tooth Preparations

The basic principles of tooth preparation are as follows

➡ Initial tooth preparation:
    ♦ Outline form
    ♦ Primary resistance form
    ♦ Primary retention form
    ♦ Convenience form.
 ➡ Final tooth preparation:
    ♦ Management of remaining caries
    ♦ Secondary resistance and retention form
    ♦ Pulp protection, if required
    ♦ Finishing of enamel margins
    ♦ Final inspection of the preparation.

Outline Form

The outline form means extending the preparation margins to the place they will occupy in the final preparation. Following facts, must be kept in mind while making outline form:

- Removal of all carious and defective pits and fissures to healthy tooth structure
- Removal of all unsupported enamel rods
- To avoid ending preparation margins in high stress areas like cusp tip and crest of the ridges
- Placing margins on sound tooth structure.

Steps

- With the help of no. 245 bur, establish the external outline form to extend all margins into sound tooth tissue.

- Bur should be kept parallel to long axis of the tooth to make a ditch in the carious portion of the tooth and it should be rotating when applied to the tooth and should not stop rotating until removed.
- Maintain the initial depth of 1.5 mm, this is approximately one-half of the length of the cutting bur. This should be, at least 0.2 to 0.5 mm in dentin to provide adequate strength to resist fracture due to occlusal forces (**Fig. 20.10**). While maintaining the same depth and bur orientation, move the bur to extend the outline to include the central fissure. The margins of preparation not only extend into sound tooth tissue but also involve adjacent deep pits and fissures in the preparation.
- Extend the margin mesially and distally but do not involve marginal ridges. These walls should have dovetail shape to provide retention to the restoration (**Figs 20.11A and B**).
- While working towards mesial and distal surface, orient the bur towards respective marginal ridge. This will result in slight divergence of mesial and distal walls which helps to provide dentinal support for marginal ridges (**Figs 20.12A to C**).
- The isthmus width should be as narrow as possible, it should not be wider than the intercuspal distance.
- The deep pit and fissure defects less than 0.5 mm apart should be included within the outline form.
- The external outline form should have smooth curves, straight lines and rounded angles. All unsupported and demineralized enamel should be removed.
- Enameloplasty is the careful removal of sharp and irregular enamel margins by 'rounding' or 'saucering' it and forming a easily cleansable area. The enameloplasty should not extend the outline form. The use of enameloplasty should be done in ends of fissures whenever needed.

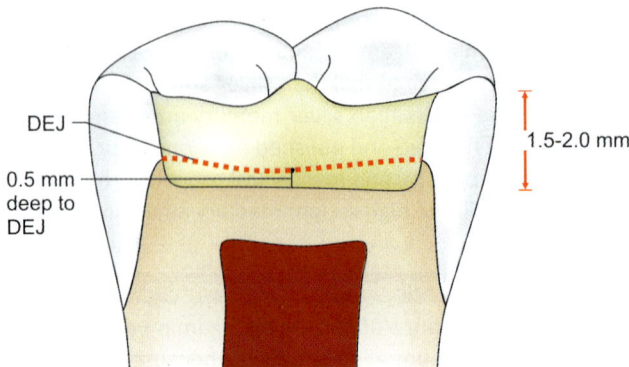

Figure 20.10: Initial depth of 1.5 mm should be maintained while preparing outline form

Primary Resistance Form

Resistance form is that shape given to a preparation planned to afford such a seat for the restoration so as to best enable it to withstand the occlusal stresses. Primary resistance form should have following features:

- Shape of the preparation should be like a box with flat floor (**Fig. 20.13**). This helps the tooth to resist occlusal masticatory forces without any displacement. Though it should be flat, at the same time it should follow the contour of occlusal surface (**Fig. 20.14**)
- To provide adequate thickness of amalgam, keep the minimum occlusal depth of 1.5 mm

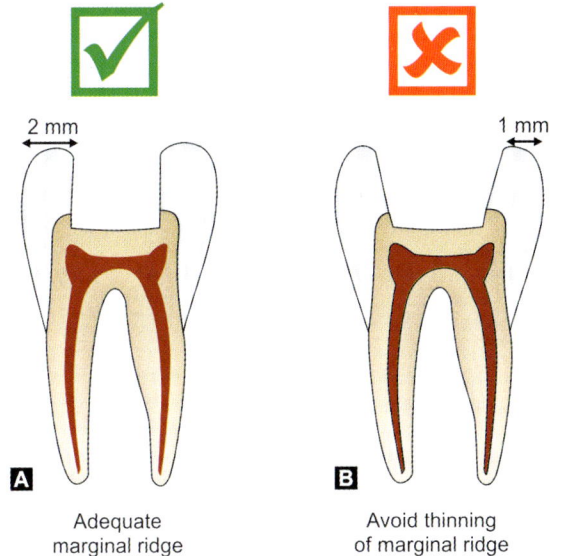

A Adequate marginal ridge

B Avoid thinning of marginal ridge

Figures 20.11A and B: (A) Sufficient marginal ridge; (B) Overcutting of marginal ridge causes thinning

- Provide the cavosurface angle of 90° (**Fig. 20.15**)
- Restrict the extension of external walls so as to have strong marginal ridge areas with sufficient dentin support
- Include all the weakened tooth structure
- Round off all the internal line and point angles (**Figs 20.16A and B**)
- Consider capping of cusp for preserving cuspal strength.

Primary Retention Form

Primary retention form prevents the restoration from being displaced.

Retention can be increased by the following:

- Occlusal convergence (about 2 to 5%) of buccal and lingual walls (**Fig. 20.17**)
- Giving slight undercut in dentin near the pulpal wall (**Figs 20.18A and B**)
- Conserving the marginal ridges
- Occlusal dovetail.

Convenience Form

The convenience form of the preparation facilitates and provides sufficient visibility, accessibility and ease of operation in preparation and restoration of the tooth. For amalgam restoration, it is the form or shape that also permits access of condensing and carving instruments.

Final Tooth Preparation

Removal of Remaining Carious Dentin

In this, remaining caries, old restorative material and adjacent deep pits and fissures are also removed and involved in the preparation.

In the large preparations with soft caries, the removal of carious dentin is done with spoon excavator or slow speed

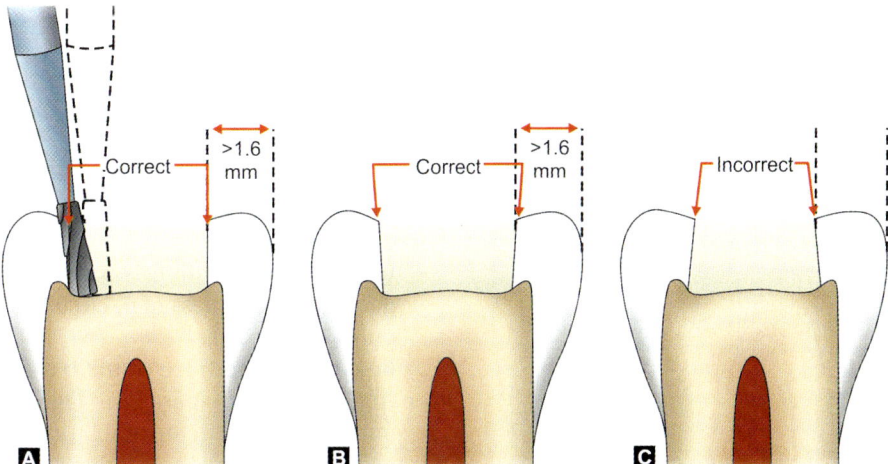

Figures 20.12A to C: Sometimes slight divergence of mesial and distal wall is done so as to have dentinal support of marginal ridges

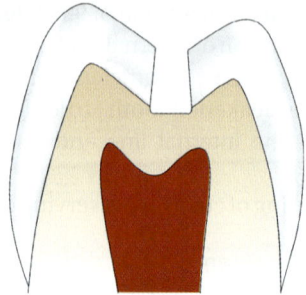

Figure 20.13: Box shaped preparation to provide resistance form

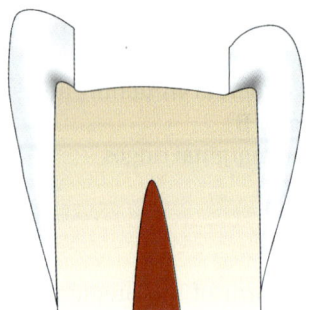

Figure 20.14: Though pulpal floor is flat but it should follow the contour of occlusal surface

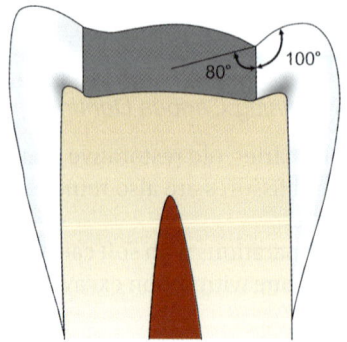

Figure 20.15: Amalgam-tooth interface should have butt joint

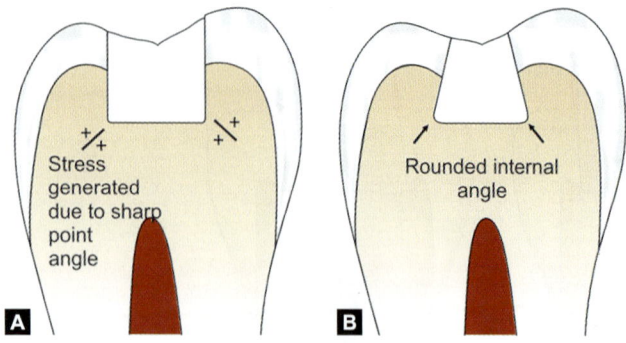

Figures 20.16A and B: Internal angles of preparation should be round (A) Sharp angles lead to stress concentration; (B) Rounded internal angle

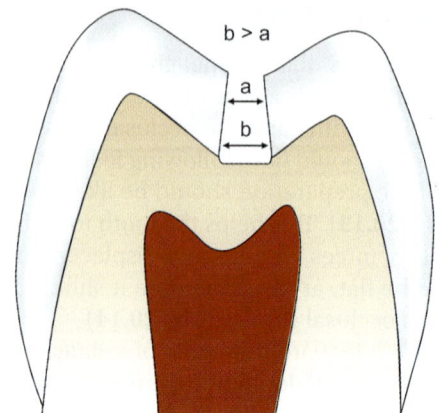

Figure 20.17: Convergence of walls to provide retention to amalgam restoration

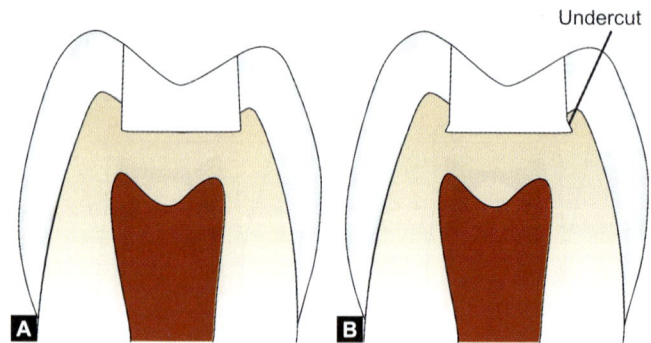

Figures 20.18A and B: Undercuts in dentin wall to provide retention of restoration

round bur (**Figs 20.19A and B**). In this, two-step pulpal floor is made, i.e. only portion of tooth which is affected by caries is removed, leaving the remaining, floor untouched (**Figs 20.20A to C**).

Protection of Pulp if Needed

Use of pulp protective materials depends upon following factors:

- A base is not required in shallow preparations, as it compromises thickness and thus compressive strength of amalgam
- In a deep preparation, a base is placed in the deepest part in the thickness of 0.5 to 0.75 mm, so as to protect pulp (**Fig. 20.21**).

Be sure that no trace of the base material remains on enamel walls of preparation (**Fig. 20.22**), as this would eventually dissolve in the oral fluids leaving a gap between the restoration and the tooth resulting in microleakage and recurrent caries.

The selection of base for amalgam restorations is based on two factors:
- It should have sufficient strength to support the forces of amalgam condensation
- It should be able to strengthen the restoration under masticatory stresses.

The strength of the bases depends upon the size, thickness and mechanical properties of base along with preparation design, position and amount of occlusal load.

Finishing of the Enamel Walls and Margins

Finishing of walls and margins is guided by the knowledge of dental histology. At this stage all unsupported enamel is removed. Cavosurface angle, i.e. angle between enamel wall and amalgam interface should be made 90° butt joint type. This provides bulk to restoration, which in turn provides maximum strength.

Final Cleaning and Inspection of the Preparation

The final stage of tooth preparation is to clean the preparation thoroughly with water and air spray. Then dry it with moist air and inspect it for final approval.

Tooth Preparation on Occlusal Surface of Different Teeth (Figs 20.23 to 20.25)

Tooth Preparation on Occlusal Surface with Buccal or Lingual Extension (Fig. 20.26)

- For removal of caries from buccal or lingual pits and fissures, slight modification in preparation is needed
- In this, extend the pulpal floor in the same plane to include the caries
- Make a box type preparation with mesial and distal walls parallel
- Place retention grooves in the mesial and distal walls
- Remove all the unsupported enamel by using slow speed bur
- Finally, inspect the preparation to evaluate the need of additional cleaning and additional finishing.

Class II Tooth Preparation for Amalgam Restoration

Class II restoration involves the proximal (mesial or distal) surfaces of premolars and molars.

Class II preparation is initiated same as Class I preparation, i.e. entrance through occlusal surface.

Outline of proximal preparations is controlled by the following factors
→ Caries susceptibility of the patient
→ Age of the patient
→ Position of gingiva
→ Extent of the caries on the proximal side
→ Dimensions of the contact area
→ Masticatory forces
→ Esthetic requirement of the patient.

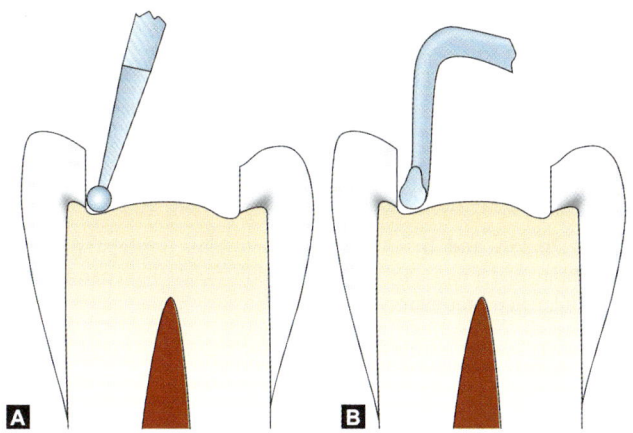

Figures 20.19A and B: (A) Removal of remaining caries using round bur; (B) Removal of caries using spoon excavator

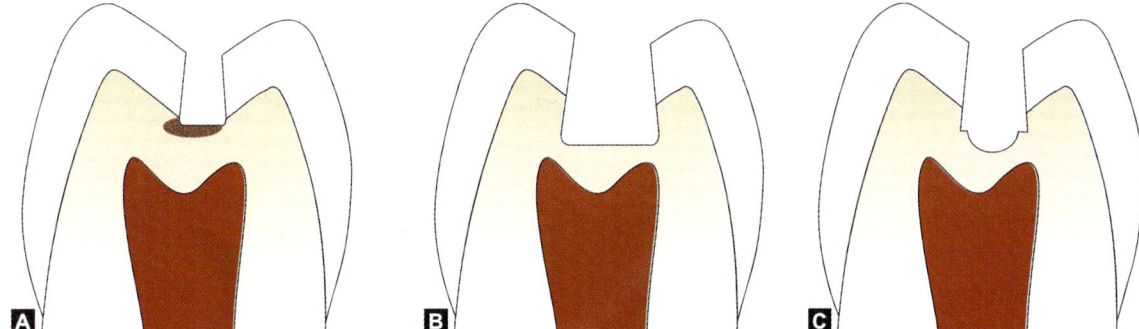

Figures 20.20A to C: (A) Caries present beyond tooth preparation; (B) Overpreparation of tooth in an attempt to involve caries; (C) Stepped pulpal floor to involve carious lesion

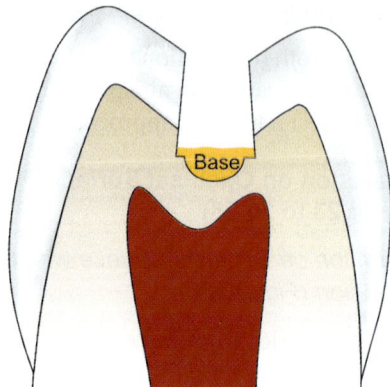

Figure 20.21: In deep preparations, base is applied on pulpal floor so as to protect pulp

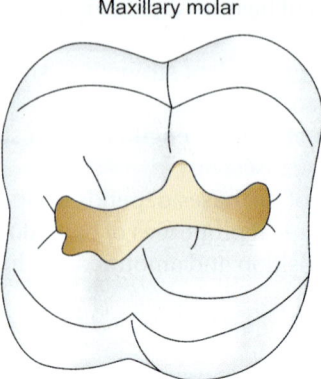

Maxillary molar

Figure 20.24: Conventional tooth preparation of maxillary first molar involving oblique ridge

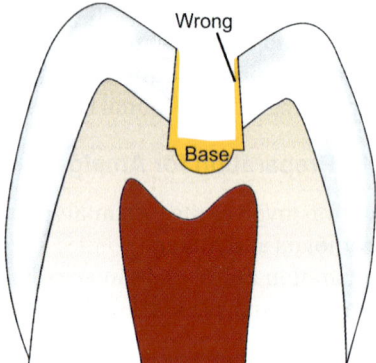

Figure 20.22: Do not place base on walls as it would ultimately dissolve in oral fluids, leaving a gap between tooth and restoration

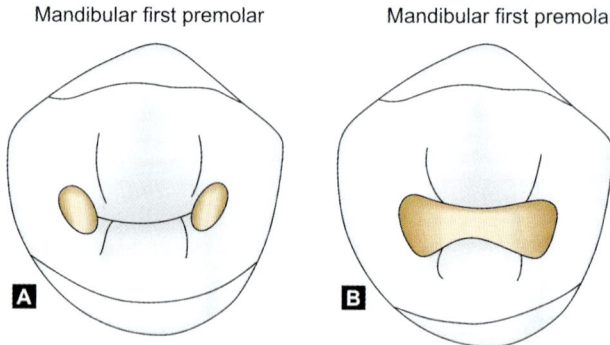

Mandibular first premolar   Mandibular first premolar

Figures 20.25A and B: (A) Conservative class I preparation of mandibular first premolar; (B) Conventional class I preparation of mandibular first premolar

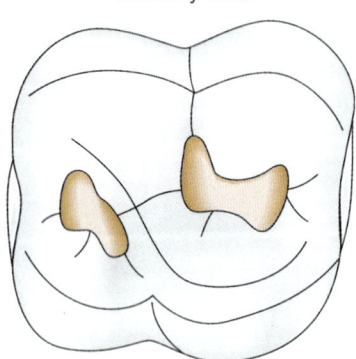

Maxillary molar

Figure 20.23: Conservative tooth preparation on occlusal surface of maxillary first molar showing preservation of oblique ridge

Outline form: The outline form for occlusal portion follows the same principles as given for pit and fissure lesions except that the external outline is extended proximally toward defective proximal surface.

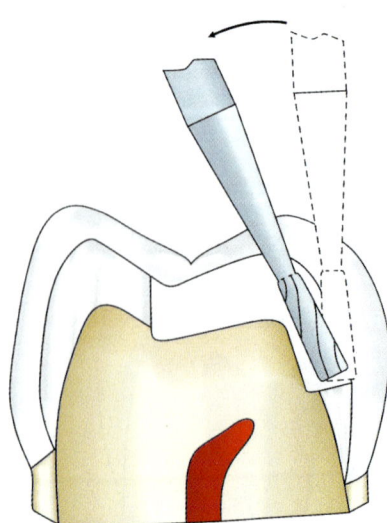

Figure 20.26: Tooth preparation on occlusal surface with buccal or lingual extension

- Using high-speed bur with air water spray, enter the pit on occlusal surface which is nearest to the involved proximal surface. Keep long axis of the bur parallel to the long axis of the tooth and maintain the initial depth of 1.5 to 2.0 mm (**Fig. 20.27**)
- Extend the outline to include the central fissure while maintaining uniformity in depth of pulpal foor (**Fig. 20.28**)
- Make isthmus width as narrow as possible, not wider than one fourth the intercuspal tip distance

- Give slight occlusal convergence to facial, lingual and proximal walls (in caries free side), this provides favorable retention for amalgam
- Consider enameloplasty wherever required to conserve tooth structure
- Visualize the proximal box relative to contact area before extending into proximal marginal ridge, this will prevent the over extension of the occlusal outline form.
- Outline form in the proximal area is primarily determined by the faciolingual position of the contact area and the extent of carious lesion. External outline form on the occlusal portion is extended to just break contact with the adjacent tooth.
- While maintaining the established pulpal depth and with the bur held parallel to the long axis of the tooth, extend the preparation towards the contact area of the tooth, ending short by 0.8 mm of cutting through the marginal ridge (**Fig. 20.29**). The proximal cutting is sufficiently deep into the dentin (0.5-0.6 mm) so that retentive locks are prepared into axiolingual and axiofacial line angles (**Fig. 20.30**).
- Widen the preparation faciolingually to just clear the contact areas. The proximal cut is diverged gingivally. In other words, faciolingual dimension at the gingival surface is greater than the occlusal surface, this provides good retention and conservation of marginal ridge (**Fig. 20.31**).
- Keep a small slice of enamel at the contact area to prevent accidental damage to the adjacent tooth (**Fig. 20.32**). If there is any doubt that accidental damage to

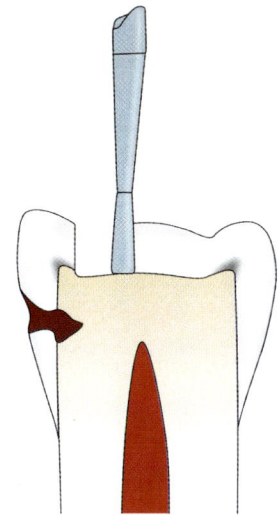

Figure 20.27: Extend the bur keeping it parallel to the long axis of tooth

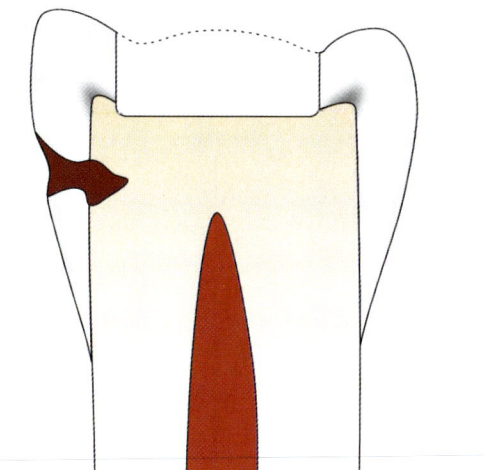

Figure 20.28: Make the occlusal box with the uniform depth of pulpal floor

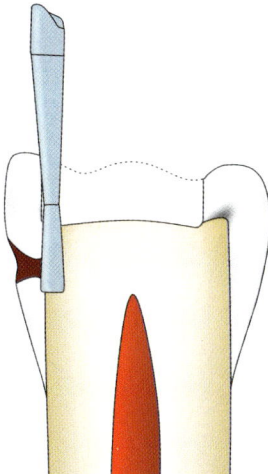

Figure 20.29: Extend the preparation ending short by 0.8 mm of cutting through marginal ridge

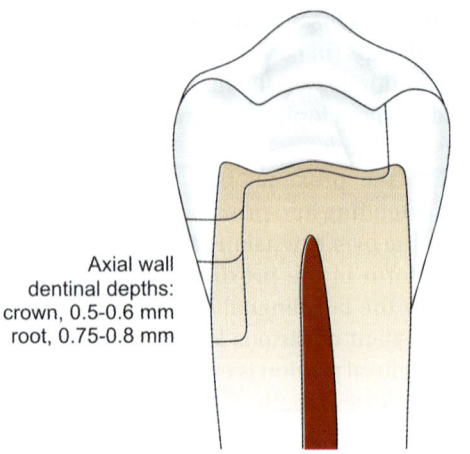

Figure 20.30: Proximal cutting should be sufficiently deep into dentin

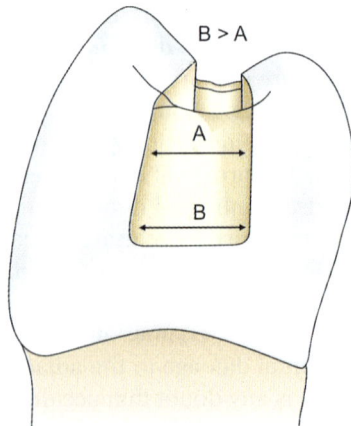

Figure 20.31: Faciolingual dimension of proximal box are more at gingival surface than at occlusal

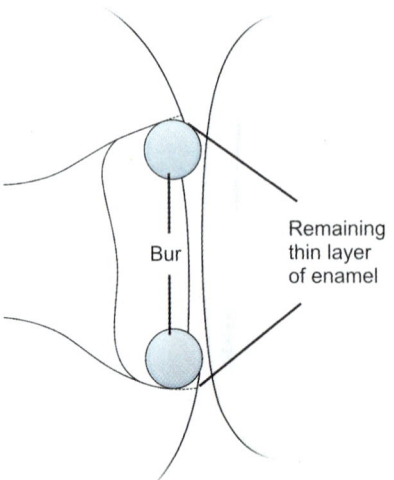

Figure 20.32: A small slice of enamel is kept at contact area so as to prevent accident damage to adjacent tooth

the adjacent tooth can occur, use a metal matrix band interdentally. This will offer some protection to the adjacent tooth.

- Fracture the slice of enamel in the region of the contact area with a small chisel or enamel hatchet.
- Proximal margins should have a cavosurface angle of 90° and when completed, the walls of the proximal box should converge occlusally (**Fig. 20.33**).
- It is important to conserve the tooth tissue so that the tooth remains as strong as possible and occlusal forces placed on the amalgam are as small as possible.
- Ideal clearance of facial and lingual margins of the proximal box should be 0.2 to 0.5 mm from the adjacent tooth (**Figs 20.34 and 20.35**).

The directions of the buccal and lingual proximal walls are affected by morphology of tooth, anatomy and relationship with the adjacent tooth.

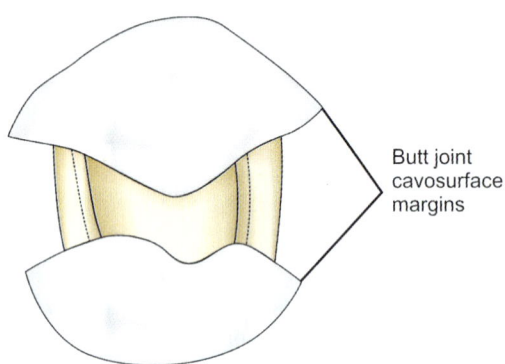

Figure 20.33: The cavosurface margins should be 90° with occlusal convergence

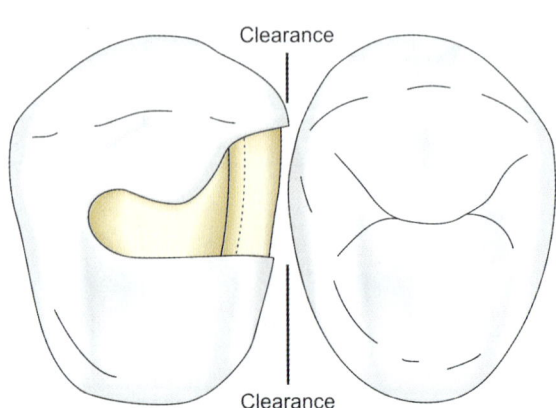

Figure 20.34: The ideal clearance of facial and lingual margins of proximal box should be 0.2 to 0.5 mm from adjacent tooth

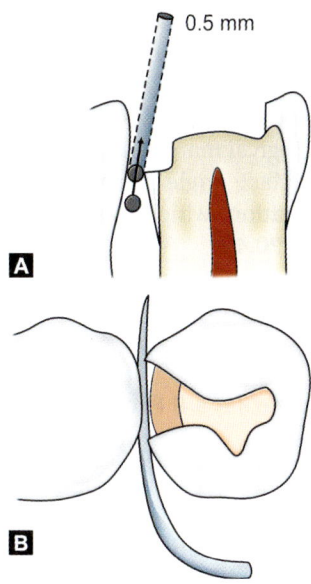

Figures 20.35A and B: (A) Gingival floor should have clearance of 0.5 mm from the adjacent tooth; (B) The clearance can be tested by passing the explorer

In this buccal and lingual proximal margins are extended:
- To include all the defects
- To break contact with the adjacent tooth so to provide convenience form and accessibility.

Reverse Curve

In the preparation of a class II amalgam restoration, extension of the preparation in the proximal area is important for elimination of caries and breaking proximal contacts. But in teeth with broader contacts, reverse-S shape curve is given to both widen the box yet remove less tooth structure. Reverse curve is given to the proximal walls by curving them inwards towards the contact area (**Fig. 20.36**). If excessive flare is given in these teeth, proximal walls will end past the axial angle of tooth through the cusps resulting in weakening of tooth structure and fracture of restoration.

Advantages of reverse curve
- Conserves the sound tooth structure
- Preserves the triangular ridge of the affected cusp
- Flare of the proximal wall leaves the tangent to that outer tooth surface at 90° angle, this causes further increase in resistance for both tooth and restoration.

Primary Resistance Form

This can be obtained by incorporating following features in the preparation:
- Shape of the preparation like a box with flat pulpal and gingival floor

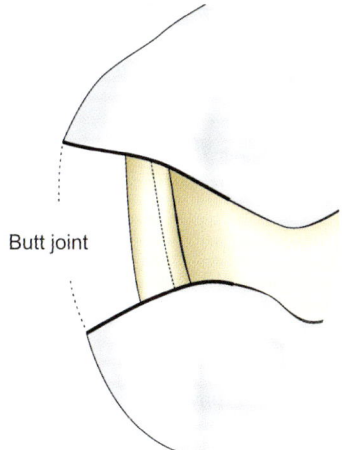

Figure 20.36: Reverse curve is given to the proximal walls by curving them towards the contact area

- Cavosurface angle of 90°
- Include all the weakened tooth structure
- Maintain minimal width of the preparation so as to preserve tooth structure
- Round off all the internal line and point angles
- Consider capping of cusp for preserving cuspal strength.

Primary Retention Form

Primary retention form prevents the restoration from being displaced.
Retention can be increased by the following:
- Occlusal convergence (about 2 to 5%) of buccal and lingual walls (**Fig. 20.37**).
- Occlusal dovetail.

Final Tooth Preparation

- During final preparation of tooth, clean it with air/water spray or with cotton pellet and inspect it for detection and removal of debris and examine for correction of all cavosurface angles and margins.
- Remove remaining caries, old restorative material and adjacent deep pit and fissure involved in the preparation as done in class I preparation.
- In the large preparations with soft caries, the removal of carious dentin is done with spoon excavator or slow speed round bur. In this, two step pulpal floor is made, i.e. only portion of tooth which is affected by caries is removed, leaving the remaining preparation floor untouched (**Figs 20.38A and B**).

Secondary retention and resistance form
- Placing retention grooves and locks in the proximal box (**Figs 20.39A and B**)

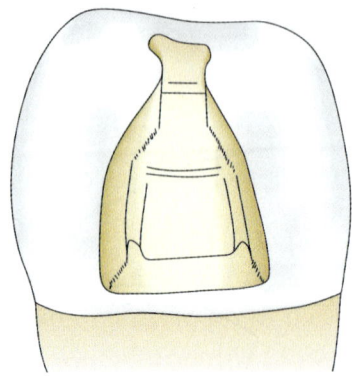

Figure 20.37: Occlusal convergence of buccal and lingual walls provide retention to amalgam restoration

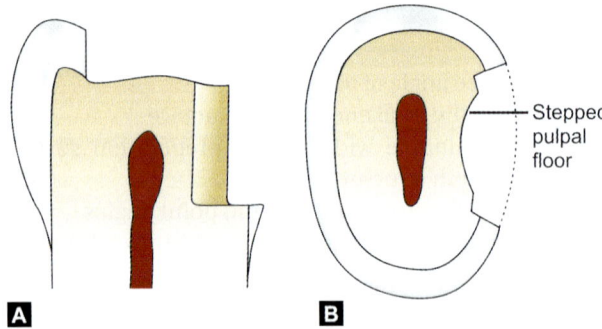

Stepped pulpal floor

Figures 20.38A and B: (A) Caries in axial wall extending towards pulp; (B) Removal of carious dentin only, resulting in stepped pulpal floor

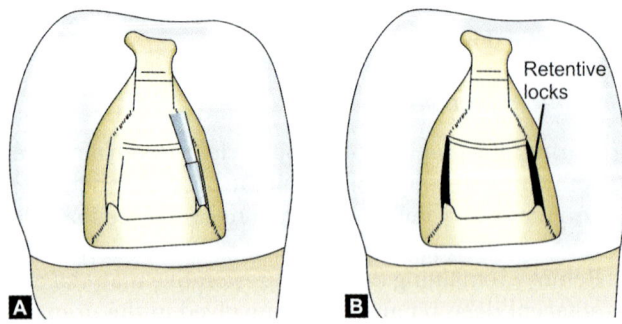

Retentive locks

Figures 20.39A and B: Retention locks in the proximal box (A) Preparation of locks using fissure bur; (B) Completed locks in proximal box

- 'Slots' and 'Pot holes' in the gingival floor may be given to provide additional retention.

Pulp protection
- Use pulp protective materials whenever needed as in class I restoration (**Fig. 20.40**)

- Finally finishing of walls and margins is done by removing all unsupported enamel. Beveling of enamel portion of gingival wall is done with the help of gingival marginal trimmer. This helps to have full length enamel rods at the gingival margin (**Figs 20.41A and B**)
- Make cavosurface angle 90° butt joint type to provide bulk to restoration, which in turn provides maximum strength (**Fig. 20.42**).
- The final stage of tooth preparation is to clean the preparation thoroughly with water and air spray. Then dry it with moist air.

Modifications in Class II Preparation Design

Sometimes depending upon following factors, various modifications are made in class II tooth preparation:
- *Extent of caries:* In extensive caries, there can be need for complex amalgam restorations as full coverage restorations. In case of small proximal caries, instead of making ideal class II preparation, only proximal box can do.

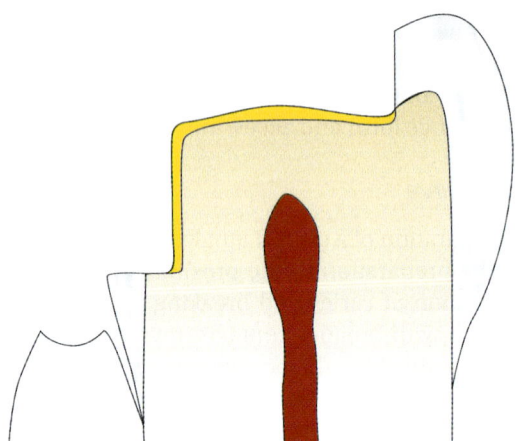

Figure 20.40: Base is applied on pulpal and axial wall in class II preparation

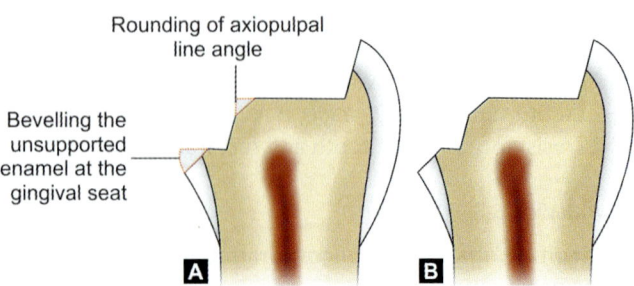

Rounding of axiopulpal line angle

Bevelling the unsupported enamel at the gingival seat

Figures 20.41A and B: Rounding of axiopulpal line angle and bevelling of unsupported enamel is done with the help of GMT

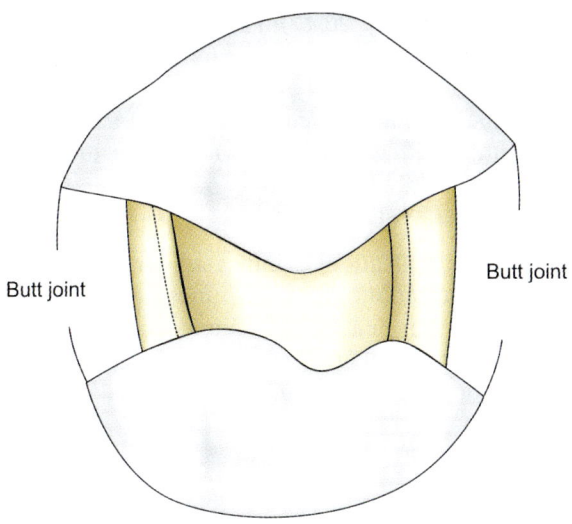

Figure 20.42: 90° cavosurface margin for amalgam restoration

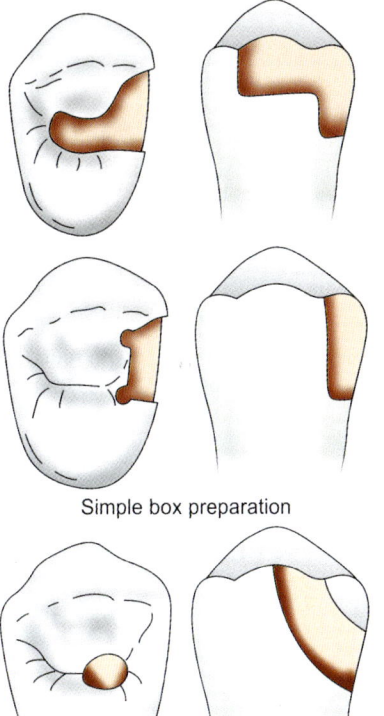

Simple box preparation

Tunnel preparation

Figure 20.43: Modifications of class II designs

- *Esthetic requirement:* In maxillary premolars, for aesthetics reasons, minimal facial extension is suggested so as to display less of amalgam.
- *Relationship with adjacent tooth:* If adjacent tooth is missing, slot preparations are made for treating proximal caries
- *Requirements for abutment teeth for partial dentures:* Here modifications are done for providing retention to the prosthesis without compromising class II amalgam restoration.
- *Rotated teeth:* Here preparation is modified according to contact with adjacent tooth.

Factors affecting class II preparation design
→ Extent of caries
→ Aesthetic requirement
→ Relationship with adjacent tooth
→ Requirement for abutment tooth
→ Rotated teeth.

Modifications in class II design (Fig. 20.43)
→ Slot preparation
→ Simple box preparation
→ Aesthetic considerations
→ Rotated teeth
→ Unusual outline form
→ Conservative preparation for mandibular first premolar and maxillary molar
→ Adjoining restoration
→ Modification for abutment teeth.

Slot Preparation

Indications of slot preparation
→ Proximal root caries in geriatric patients with gingival recession
→ When adjacent tooth is missing
→ When isolation is difficult in treating cervical one-third root caries.

Design features: It is similar to class V tooth preparation. Preparation is normally approached from the facial aspect. It is done with round bur no. 2 or no. 4 to a limited depth axially, i.e. 0.75 to 1.25 mm (**Fig. 20.44**). When occlusal margins are in enamel, go 0.5 mm inside the dentin. Prepare 90° cavosurface margins, give retention grooves at axio-occlusal and axiogingival line angles 0.2 mm inside the DEJ (**Figs 20.45 and 20.46**).

Simple Box Preparation

Indications of simple box preparation
• Small proximal caries, not involving the occlusal surface
• Proximal surface caries with narrow proximal contact
• Proximal caries in attrited teeth.

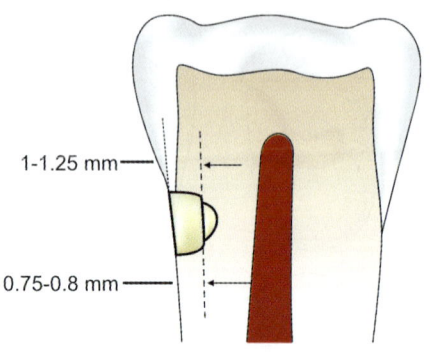

Figure 20.44: The preparation is done with round bur keeping the axial wall depth 0.75 to 1.25 mm

1-1.25 mm

0.75-0.8 mm

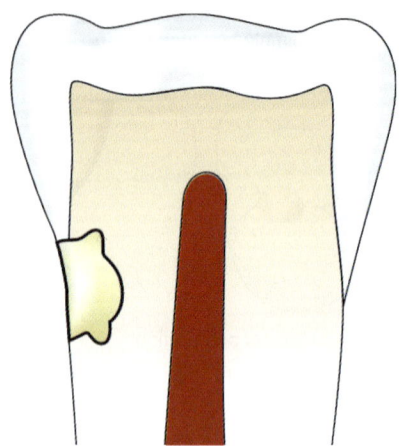

Figure 20.45: 90° cavosurface margins and retention grooves at axio-occlusal and axiogingival line angle of slot preparation

Design features (Fig. 20.47): Prepare proximal box only with minimum facial and lingual extensions. For retention, converge facial and lingual extensions. Proximal retention locks are made for added retention in proximal box. These have 0.5 mm depth gingivally and 0.3 mm occlusally.

Esthetic Considerations

Sometimes modification is indicated for maxillary first premolar restoration to avoid unesthetic display of amalgam. Design feature for mesio-occlusal preparation, is that facial wall of proximal box is prepared straight parallel to long axis of the tooth.

For Rotated Teeth

Design features: They are same as that of normally aligned teeth except that preparation depends on area of tooth which is in contact with adjacent tooth (**Fig. 20.48**).

Unusual Outline Form

If fissures are separated by 0.5 mm or more, restore the tooth with individual amalgam restorations. Until or unless fissure is emanating from occlusal surface, dovetail is not required.

Conservative Preparation for Mandibular First Premolar and Maxillary Molar

Conservative design in these teeth helps in the preservation of oblique ridge or the transverse ridge which protects the cuspal strength.

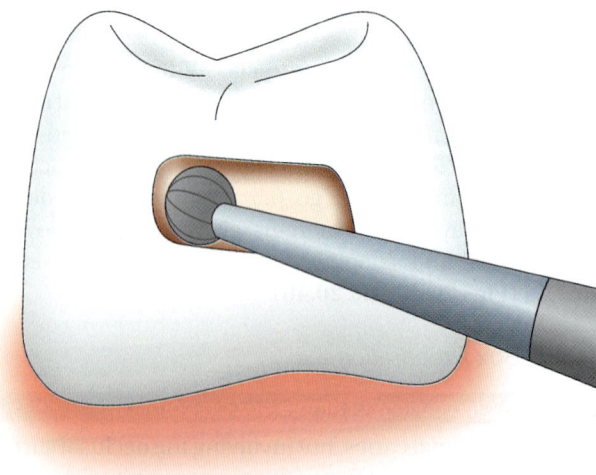

Figure 20.46: Slot preparation

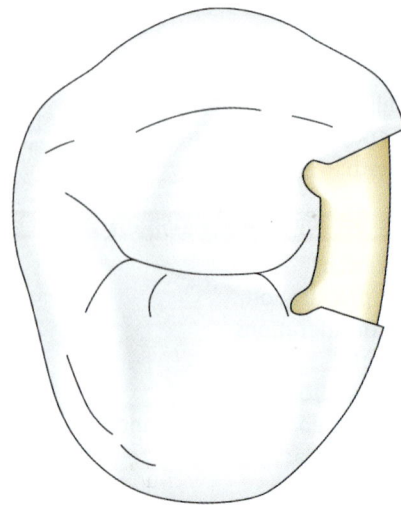

Figure 20.47: Box preparation

Design features (Fig. 20.49): For maxillary first molar, mesio-occlusal and disto-occlusal preparations are made independently without oblique ridge. For mandibular first premolar, transverse ridge is not involved in proximal preparation (**Fig. 20.50**). Also because of high facial pulp horn, pulpal floor should have facial inclination (**Figs 20.51 and 20.52**).

Adjoining Restoration

If proximo-occlusal restoration is already present and a new restoration is required adjoining it, then care should be taken while preparing the tooth for second restoration without weakening the margins of previous restoration. The intersecting margins of two restoration should be perpendicular to each other (**Fig. 20.53**).

If a tooth has continuous class II and class V preparation, then prepare and restore class II lesion before class V.

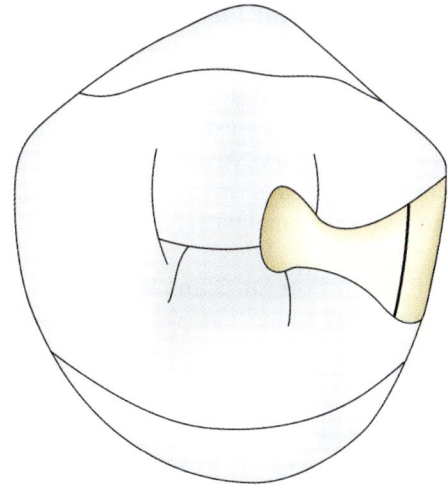

Figure 20.50: Conservative class II preparation in mandibular first premolar not involving transverse ridge

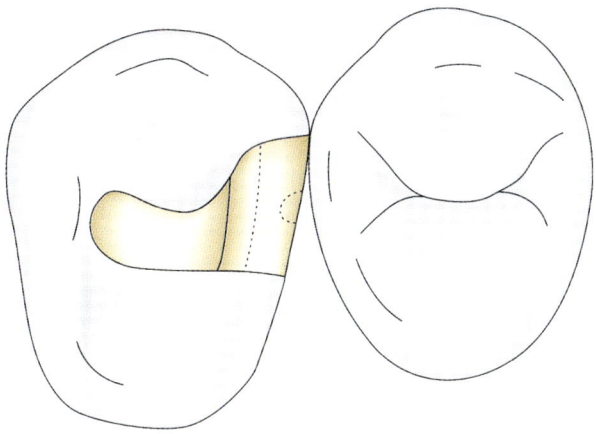

Figure 20.48: Class II tooth preparation for rotated teeth

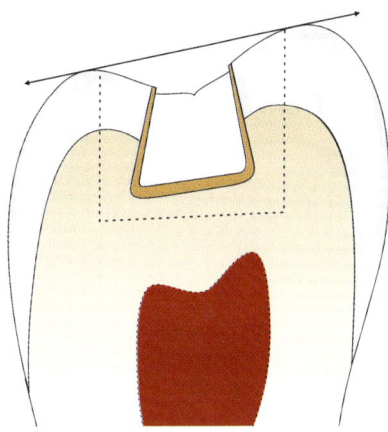

Figure 20.51: Because of high facial pulp horn, pulpal floor should have facial inclination so as to avoid exposure

Maxillary molar

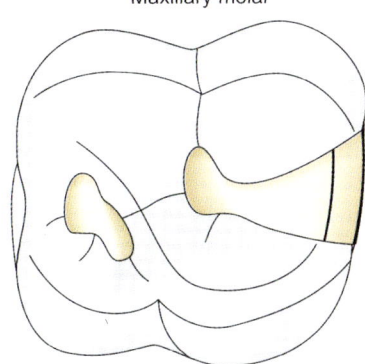

Figure 20.49: Conservative class II preparation in maxillary first molar. Here mesio-occlusal and distobuccal preparations are made independently without involving oblique ridge

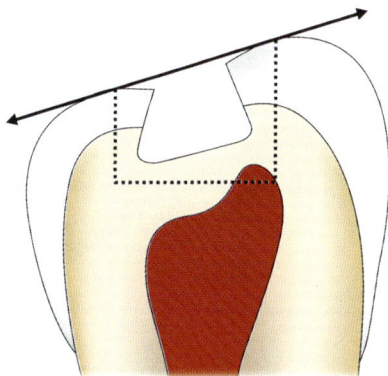

Figure 20.52: If proper inclination is not given in the pulpal floor, it may result in pulp exposure

Modification for Abutment Teeth

For abutment tooth, additional extension is required if rest seat is planned for partial denture. For abutment teeth, facial and lingual walls are extended more for providing space rest seat (**Fig. 20.54**). Also pulpal floor is deepened 0.5 mm more in the area of rest seat so as to provide sufficient thickness for the amalgam (**Fig. 20.55**).

Amalgam Restoration for Class III Tooth Preparation

Since amalgam is not esthetic restoration, it is not indicated for proximal surface of incisors and mesial surface of canines. Amalgam for class III restoration is indicated in the distal surface of maxillary and mandibular canines especially, if:

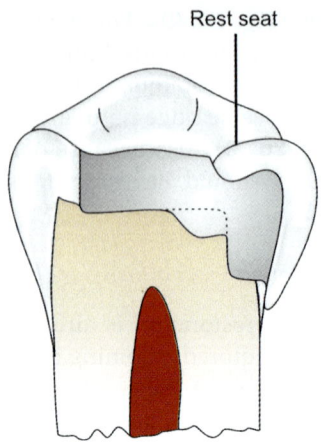

Figure 20.55: Class II restoration showing rest seat and deepening of pulpal wall in the area of rest seat so as to provide sufficient amalgam bulk

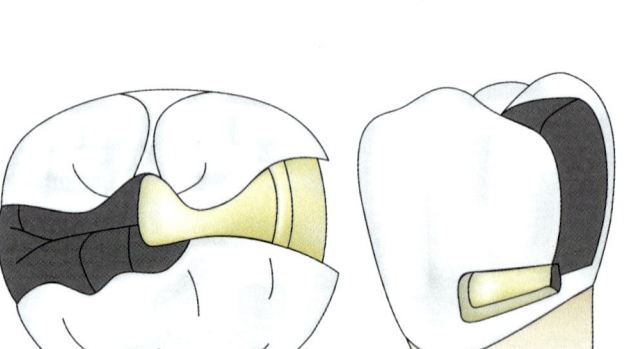

Figure 20.53: New amalgam restoration should be placed adjacent to old restoration such that the intersecting margins of two restorations are perpendicular to each other

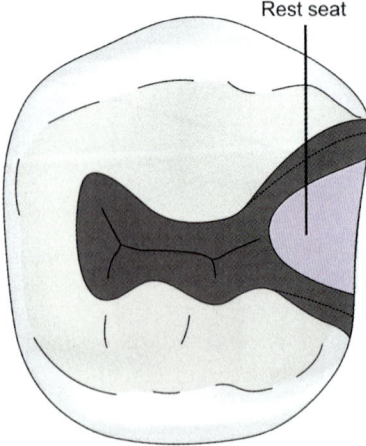

Figure 20.54: For abutment teeth, facial and lingual walls are extended for providing rest seat

- Caries do not undermine distal slopes of canines
- Labial axial angle is intact
- Even after removal of caries, sufficient tooth structure is present
- Restoration will not be directly loaded with occlusal forces.

Initial Tooth Preparation

- Outline form includes only the proximal surface. Shape of preparation is like a triangle with round corners. Labial side of triangle conforms more to the anatomy than with lingual side
- A no. 2 round bur is penetrated through enamel on distolingual marginal ridge (**Fig. 20.56**). Preliminary shaping of preparation is completed with inverted cone bur with long axis of bur keeping perpendicular to the lingual surface of the tooth
- Outline form is completed when facial, gingival and lingual walls are formed (**Fig. 20.57**)
- Lingual wall should meet the axial wall at obtuse angle
- Depth of bur should be 0.5 mm into the dentin
- Cavosurface angle should be about 90° at all margins
- Lingual margins should be in confines of lingual embrasure except for incisal and gingival turn extension, later is indicated when lingual embrasure is not sufficiently wide to aid instrumentation.

Final Tooth Preparation

- Removal of any remaining infected dentin is done using a slow speed round bur or/and spoon excavator

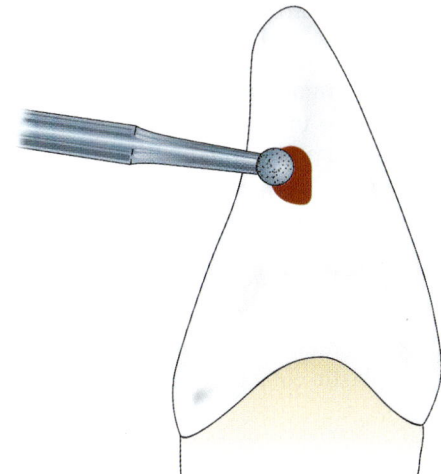

Figure 20.56: Entry of lesion is made through lingual side with the help of round bur

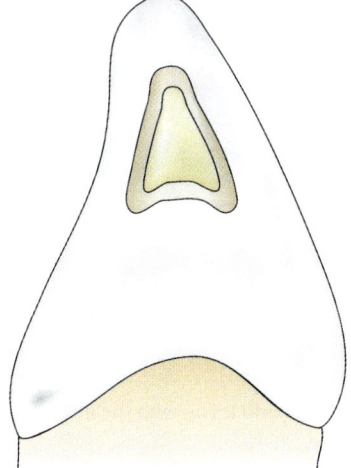

Figure 20.58: Class III preparation with retention grooves

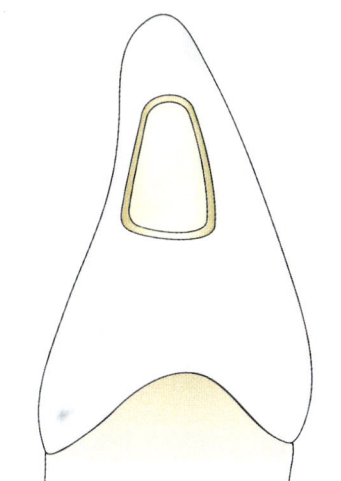

Figure 20.57: Outline of class III preparation

- Pulp protection is by using base or liner
- Secondary resistance and retention form is achieved by butt joint, rounded internal angles and sufficient bulk of amalgam. Retention is obtained by placing retention groove with a small round bur in the axiofaciogingival point angle and lingual dovetail (**Fig. 20.58**). Lingual dovetail is not required for small sized class III preparation. It is needed for large preparations. Lingual dovetail is prepared only when the preparation of proximal portion is complete because otherwise tooth structure needed for isthmus between proximal portion and dovetail might be removed when the proximal outline form is prepared.

- Finishing the external walls is done to remove all unsupported enamel and to make cavosurface angle 90°. For rounding of junctions between different retentive grooves, angle former or GMT can be used.
- Final cleaning and inspection of the preparation is done by cleaning the preparation thoroughly with water and air spray and then drying it with moist air.

Class V Tooth Preparation for Amalgam Restoration

Class V lesion is present on the gingival third of facial and lingual surfaces of all teeth. Amalgam is not indicated for anterior teeth except when esthetics is of no concern, for example in very aged patients.

Initial Tooth Preparation

- The outline form of class V lesions is dictated by the extension of caries process. Like in others, prepare the tooth in normal manner, i.e. breaking down the undermined enamel and extending the preparation to the sound tooth structure. This is accomplished by using inverted cone bur held perpendicular to the long axis of tooth (**Fig. 20.59**)
- Initial axial wall depth should be 0.5 mm into the dentin. Axial wall depth at the occlusal wall should be more than at the gingival wall (**Fig. 20.60**). This on will result in a curved axial wall which to conforms to the contour of the tooth
- Prepare the mesial and distal wall surfaces perpendicular to the outer tooth surface, paralleling the direction of enamel rods.

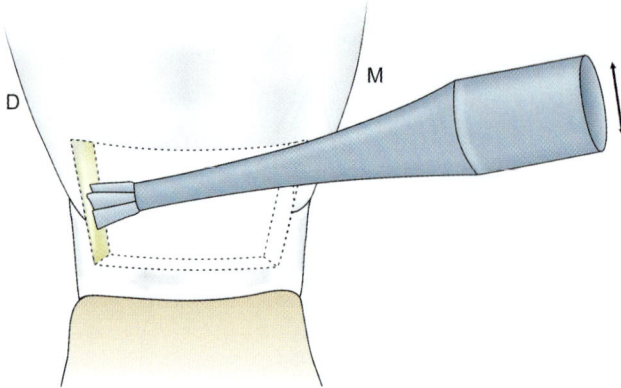

Figure 20.59: Entry into lesion with the help of inverted cone bur

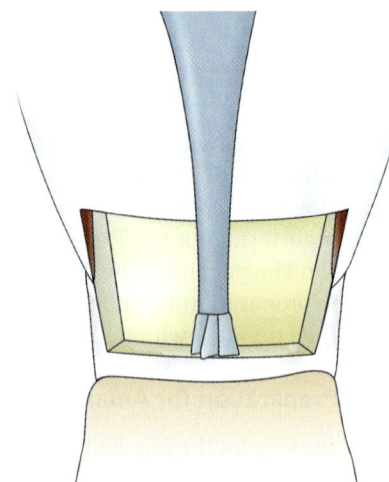

Figure 20.60: Preparation of gingival wall

Final Tooth Preparation

- Remove any remaining caries using a round bur
- Since preparation walls diverge towards the facial aspect, retention is mandatory in these preparations. Retention is made by giving grooves incisally and gingivally along axioincisal and axiogingival line angles using an inverted cone bur
- To prevent secondary caries, extend the preparation close to but not to axial angles of the tooth. In young patients, it is extended under free margins of gingiva and in older patients, it is determined by extent of the lesion
- Finally, hoes and chisels are used to finish the mesial, distal and gingival walls (**Fig. 20.61**)
- In the last, inspect the preparation using clean air and water spray followed by drying.

Class VI Tooth Preparation for Amalgam Restoration

Class VI tooth preparation involves restoration of incisal edge of anterior teeth or the cusp tip of posterior teeth. For class VI preparations in anterior teeth, amalgam is usually not filled because of poor esthetics. For posterior teeth it is indicated because of its satisfactory wear resistance.

Indications of restoration of class VI lesions with amalgam:

- In teeth where because of too much wear, enamel is gone and the underlying dentin has become carious, commonly seen in geriatric patients.
- In the hypoplastic cusp tip as these are more prone to caries.

Steps of Tooth Preparation (Fig. 20.62)

- Penetrate the enamel with a small tapered fissure bur extending to the depth of 1.5 mm.
- Prepare a 90° cavosurface margin on enamel.
- Make small undercuts along the internal line angles to provide retention.

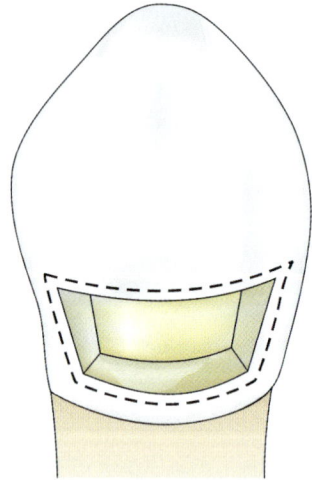

Figure 20.61: Completed class V preparation

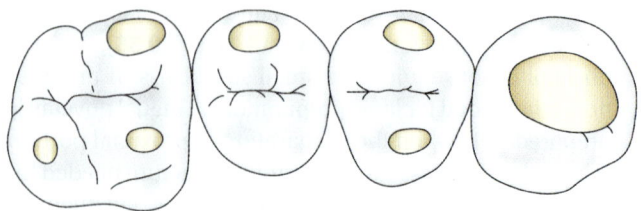

Figure 20.62: Class VI preparation for amalgam restoration

Steps of amalgam restoration

- Selection of amalgam alloy
- Mercury—alloy ratio
- Trituration
- Mulling
- Application of matrix bond
- Insertion of amalgam
- Condensation
- Burnishing
- Carving
- Finishing and polishing.

STEPS OF AMALGAM RESTORATION

Selection of Amalgam Alloy

Following factors are considered while selecting an alloy for restoration:
- Type of alloy:
  - High copper or low copper alloys
  - Zinc free or zinc containing alloys
  - Size and shape of the particles.
- If restoration undergoes high occlusal stresses, choose amalgam with high resistance to marginal fracture
- Patients with psychological problems or other diseases, requiring early disposal, indicate the use of fast setting alloy
- In wider and broader preparations, alloy with low creep values is preferred
- If it is difficult to control moisture it is preferred to use zinc-free alloy to avoid delayed expansion.

Mercury Alloy Ratio (Fig. 20.63)

For success of the restoration, mercury ratio should be specific and accurate are according to type of alloy used. Mercury is basically required to wet the alloy particles before they can react. Eames has preferred 1:1 ratio of alloy/mercury for best results. Generally, it is 5:8 or 5:7, if mercury content is more than required amount, resultant mix will be weaker, but if it is less, it might not sufficiently wet the alloy particles. Lathecut amalgam alloys require more (45%) of mercury to wet than the spherical alloys (40%).

Trituration

The purpose of trituration is to remove oxide layers from the alloy particles so as to coat each alloy particle with mercury, resulting in a homogeneous mass for condensation. Trituration can be done by hand or mechanical means. Mechanical method is done with the help of automatic amalgamator (**Figs 20.64 and 20.65**) and hand

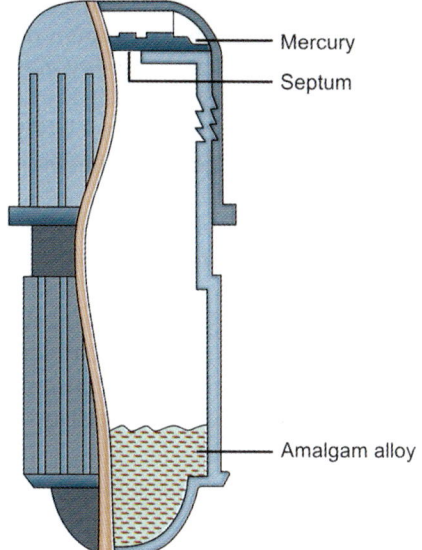

Figure 20.63: Amalgam capsule

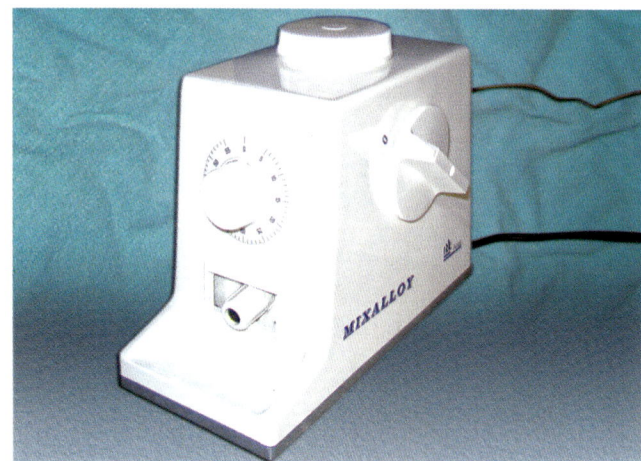

Figure 20.64: Amalgamator used for mechanical trituration

method of trituration is done with the help of mortar and pestle (**Fig. 20.66**).

Objectives of trituration

- Achieve a workable mass of amalgam within minimum time
- Increase direct contact between the particle and mercury by removing oxides from powder
- Reduce particle size of powder so that fast and more complete amalgamation can be done
- Help in dissolving the particles of powder in mercury
- Reduce the amount of gamma-1 and gamma-2.

Time for which the trituration is carried out, speed and force applied for trituration, affect the quality of trituration.

Signs of a good mix amalgam is shiny, homogeneous mass that adheres together (**Fig. 20.67**). Undertrituration results in a crumbly mix that is very weak (**Fig. 20.68**). It causes decrease in the tensile and compressive strength values and increase in creep.

Overtrituration results in a mix that is warm and has a shiny surface. This overtriturated mix sticks to the capsule which is difficult to remove. There occurs fast setting because the amalgam mass becomes heated. Overtrituration causes increase in contraction, creep, tensile and compressive strength values for lathe-cut alloys, decrease in tensile and compressive strengths for spherical alloys.

Test for trituration
➡ Normal trituration
◆ Good shiny mix
◆ Homogeneous mass, adheres together.
➡ Over trituration
◆ Mix is 'warm'
◆ Difficult to remove from capsule
◆ Shiny wet and soft.
➡ Under trituration
◆ Dry mix
◆ Crumbled mix that is very weak.

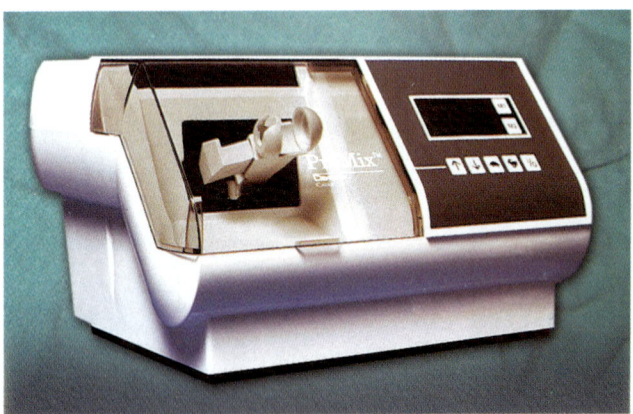

Figure 20.65: Amalgamator

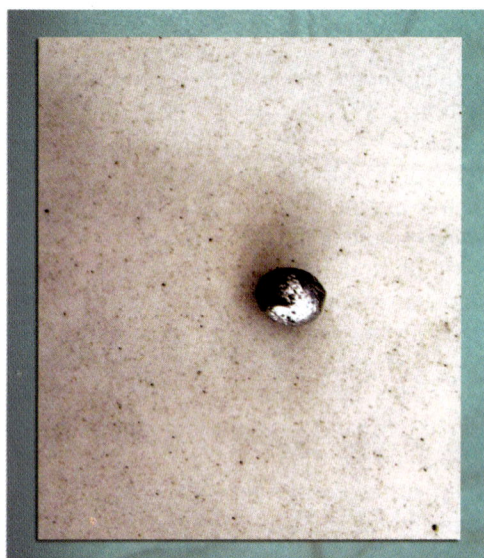

Figure 20.67: Properly mixed amalgam should be shiny, cohesive homogeneous mass

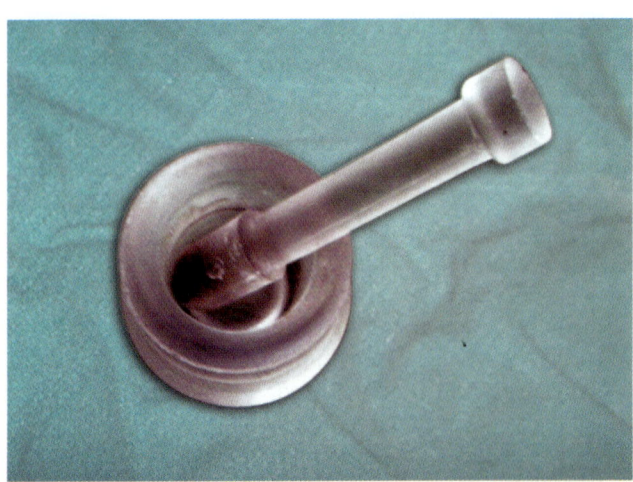

Figure 20.66: Mortar pestle used for hand trituration

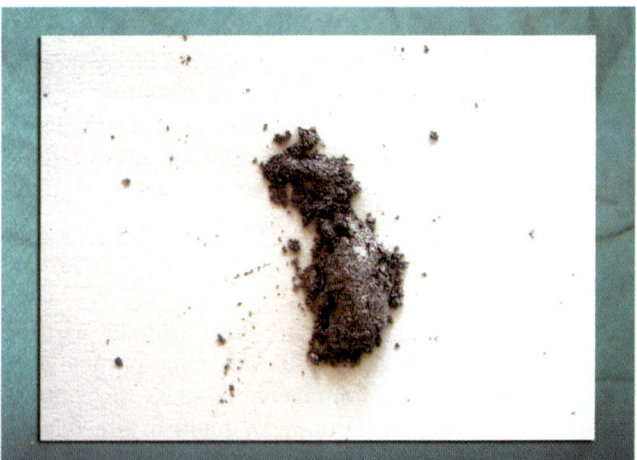

Figure 20.68: Undertriturated amalgam mix appears dry and crumbled

Mulling

Mulling is done so that all alloy particles are properly coated with mercury, in other words, it is continuation of the trituration. Mulling of the amalgam can be done manually or mechanically. By hand, it can be done by squeezing the freshly mixed amalgam collected in the chamois skin. Mulling should not be done by bare hands as it can be contaminated by moisture. Mechanical mulling is done in the amalgamator by triturating it for one to two seconds.

Application of Matrix Band

Using a rigid matrix to support the lingual portion of the restoration during condensation is necessary. A matrix is helpful to prevent "land-sliding" during condensation and to ensure marginal adaptation and strength of the restoration. The Tofflemire matrix retainer is used to secure a matrix band to the tooth. Place the matrix band in the matrix retainer. Pass the matrix band between the contact points so that its lower edge comes just over the cervical margin of the preparation. Tighten the band and stabilize it using wedges (**Fig. 20.69**). It is very important not to overtighten the band because this will flex the cusps, resulting in postrestoration sensitivity, and failure of the restoration. Finally, burnish the contact area of the band against the adjacent tooth.

Barton technique
In case of lingual preparation, toffelmire band does not intimately adapt to the lingual groove area of the tooth, so an additional step is generally required to firmly adapt the band on the lingual portion of the tooth preparation. In this, cut a piece of stainless steel matrix band, approximately [0.05 mm] thick, [8 mm] wide. This will fit between the lingual surface of the tooth and the band already in place. Place the gingival margin of this piece of band slightly gingival to the gingival edge of the band. To secure the band, take approximately 1/2 inch long toothpick. Heat the stick of compound and cover the end of the tooth-pick wedge. Immediately insert the compound-coated wedge between the Tofflemire band and the cut piece of matrix band. While the compound is still soft, with the help of burnisher press the compound gingivally. The main advantage of lingual matrix is its ability to respond to require change in contour by pressing a warmed, metal instrument against the band from the preparation side. The heat is transferred through the matrix material to the compound, which may then be reshaped to provide the proper contour. This matrix for the occlusolingual amalgam restoration is referred to as the Barton matrix.

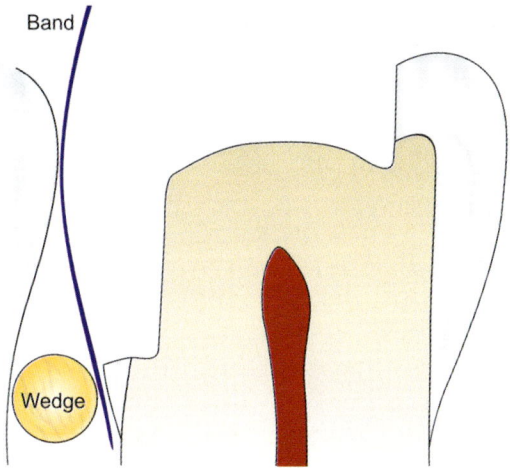

Figure 20.69: Placement of band and wedge

Insertion of Amalgam (Figs 20.70A and B)

Pick a small amount of amalgam alloy with the help of amalgam carrier and transfer it to the preparation. Proximal box should be filled before the occlusal part of the preparation.

Place the first increment of amalgam in the deepest proximal part of the preparation and condense it with flat surface of condenser.

Apply firm pressure on the amalgam mass for adequate condensation. After it, add next increment and again condense it.

When the level of amalgam reaches the preparation margins, continue the packing of preparation to allow an excess to build up for better finishing.

Condensation (Fig. 20.71)

Various shapes (triangular, round, elliptical, trapezoidal and rectangular) and sizes of condensers are used for amalgam condensation. Working end of a condenser is usually serrated (**Fig. 20.72**). Since the force delivered to the amalgam depends upon the area of condensing tips and selection of condenser depends on the outline form of tooth preparation.

Rules of condensation
➡ Start condensation within three minutes of trituration
➡ Condense continuously
➡ Condense laterally as well as apically
➡ Apply adequate force for condensation
➡ Have a constant supply of amalgam.

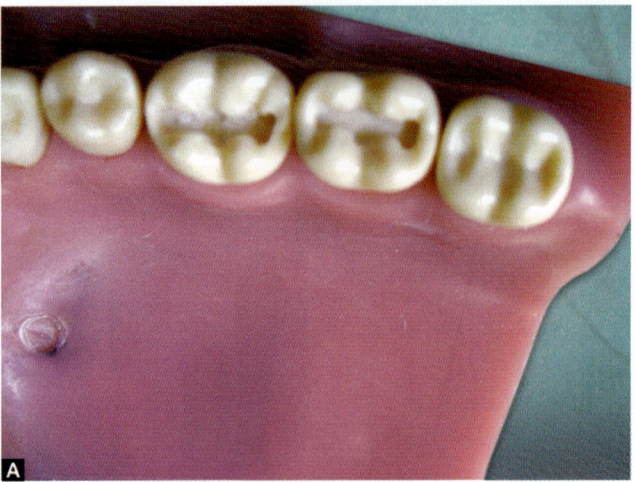
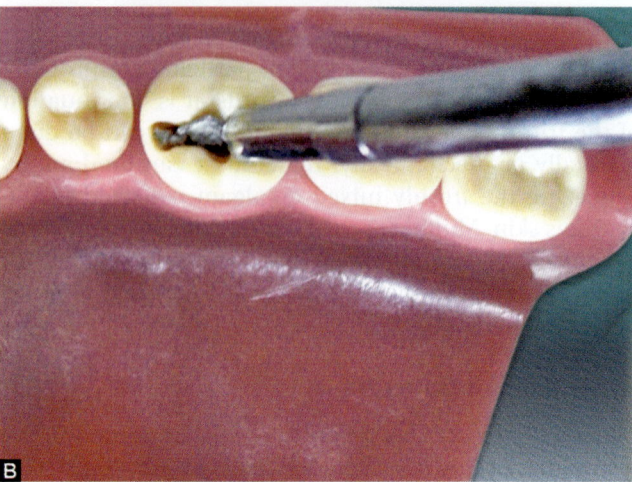

Figures 20.70A and B: (A) Class I preparation in 46, 47; (B) Insertion of amalgam into the preparation

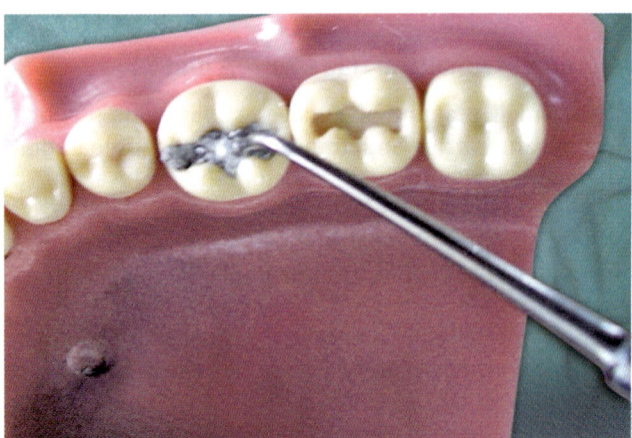

Figure 20.71: Condense amalgam with the help of flat surface of condenser

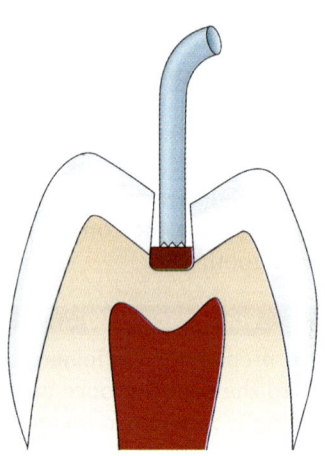

Figure 20.72: Working end of condensor should be serrated

Objectives of condensation

➜ Brings excess mercury on the surface of restoration
➜ Reduces the number and size of voids in the restoration
➜ Prepares the surface of restoration for carving
➜ To adapt amalgam to the preparation walls and floors.

Condensation Depends upon Following Factors

- Plasticity of the mass
- *Size of the amalgam increment*: A larger mass results in incomplete condensation
- *Condenser size*: The smaller the condenser working end, the greater the force
- Direction of force
- Amount of force

- *Type of alloy*: Use larger condensers when condensing spherical alloys because smaller condenser will displace the spherical particles rather than condensing them.

Choice of condenser depending upon type of amalgam alloy
(Figs 20.73A and B)

Type of alloy	Type of condenser
Lathecut alloy	Small condenser
Blended alloy	Small condenser
Spherical alloy	Large condenser

Burnishing

Precarve burnishing is done after condensation. It is the process of rubbing, generally done to make the surface

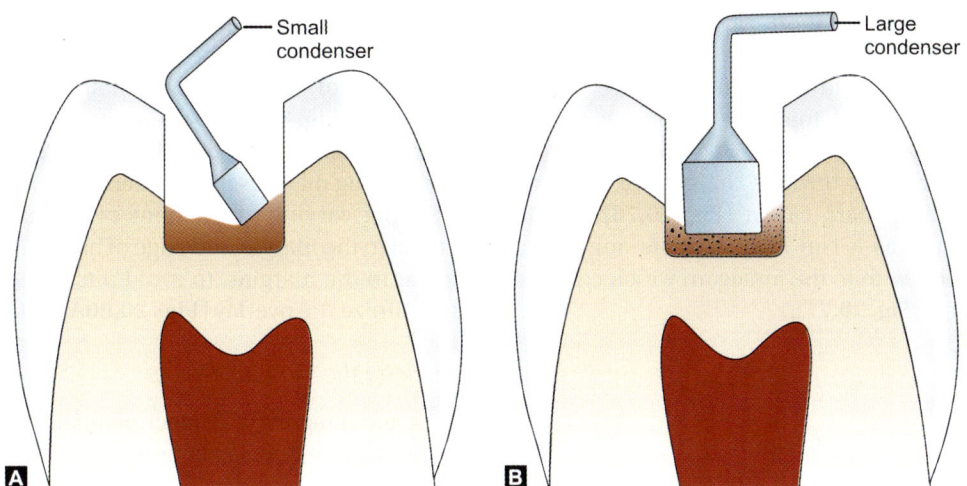

Figures 20.73A and B: (A) Condensation of nonspherical alloy using small condenser; (B) Condensation of spherical alloy with large condenser

shiny. Amalgam is overfilled and burnished immediately with heavy strokes so as to improve marginal adaptability of the restoration and remove excess mercury from over-packed amalgam (**Fig. 20.74**).

Advantages of precarve burnishing

- Improves the marginal integrity of restoration
- Shapes the restoration according to contours and curvatures of the tooth
- Helps in reducing the mercuric content of amalgam.

Postcarve burnishing

It is done after completion of carving with the help of small sized burnishers using light strokes.

Advantages of postcarve burnishing

- Reduces number of voids on surface of restoration
- Produces denser amalgam at margins
- Improves marginal seal
- Increases surface hardness
- Decreases rate of corrosion.

Carving

Amalgam should not be carved until it is sufficiently firm. For adequate carving, it is preferable to overpack the preparation and then carve it to the margins. Carving causes removal of mercury rich surface layer. For proper carving, occlusal anatomy should be kept low to preserve bulk of the alloy at the margins. The carving instruments should

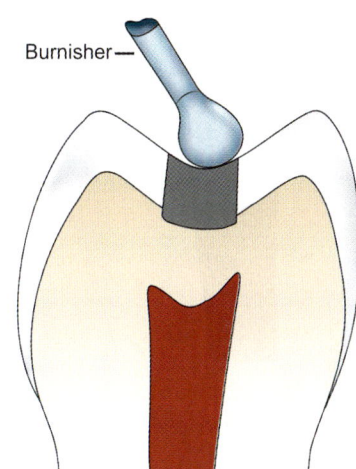

Figure 20.74: Precarve burnishing improves marginal adaptation of amalgam and removes excess mercury from amalgam

have discoid and cleiod blade design (**Fig. 20.75**). Larger instrument is used first, followed by smaller instruments.

Objectives of carving are to achieve restoration with

- No over and under hangs
- Proper size, location and good interproximal contact
- Adequate marginal ridges
- Proper contours
- Optimal occlusal anatomy
- Adequate embrasures
- Enhancing the health of periodontium.

In proximal tooth preparation, carving of the cervical margins should begin following the removal of matrix band. Loosen the band and then wedge before carving because axial and cervical margins become accessible after removal of band.

Trim the axial margins towards the gingiva in downward direction with a sharp carver (**Fig. 20.76**). Do not over carve amalgam as it can lead to acute angles and stress concentration with in the amalgam which can fracture the restoration (**Fig. 20.77**).

Carve the occlusal surface with a sharp carver like hollenback. Held it in the way so that its blade lies across the margin of the restoration, half on tooth and half on restoration (**Fig. 20.78**). Define marginal ridge and occlusal embrasure using a sharp explorer (**Fig. 20.79**). Remove any overhanging margins in the interdental region, if present.

During carving, movement of instrument should be parallel to the margin and edge of blade should be perpendicular to the margins, to avoid ditching of the metal and to minimize the overlay (**Figs 20.80A and B**).

Checking the Contact Points

Check the integrity of contact points using dental floss by passing it buccally, palatally and gingivally (**Figs 20.81A to C**).

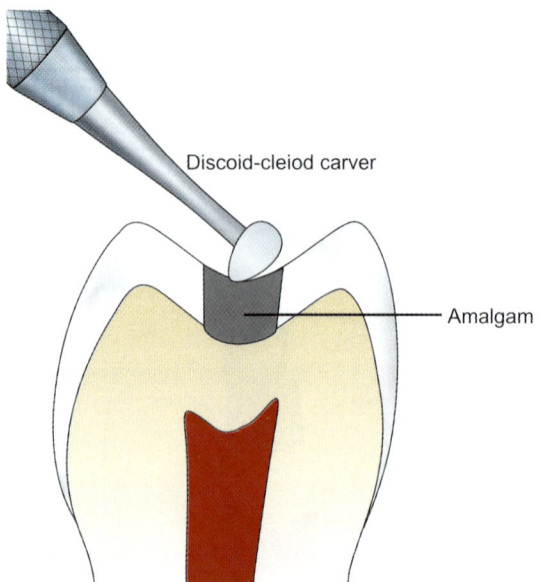

Figure 20.75: Use of discoid-cleoid carver for carving occlusal surface

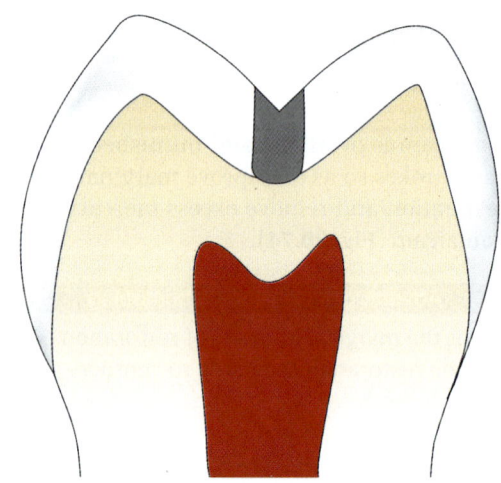

Figure 20.77: Overcarving of amalgam can cause fracture of restoration

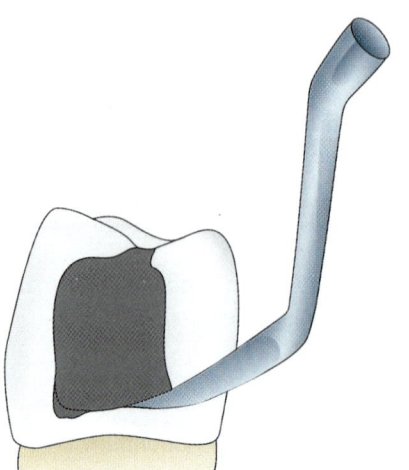

Figure 20.76: Trim the axial margins towards gingiva with sharp carvers

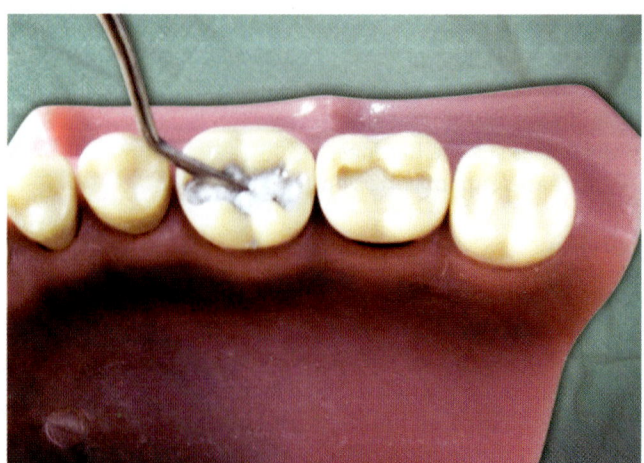

Figure 20.78: Carving amalgam restoration

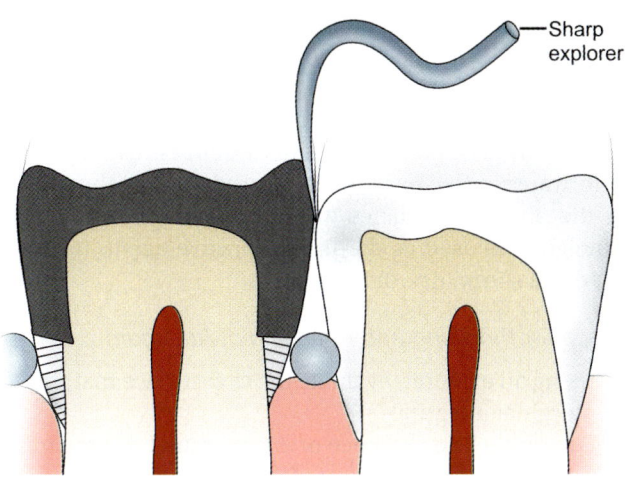

Figure 20.79: Sharp explorer is used to define marginal ridge

Checking the Occlusion

It is done after carving so as to remove any areas left high in the final restoration. Ask the patient to close the mouth so that the teeth meet lightly.

Use articulating paper to localize any high spots, if the restoration is high, it indicates the premature contacts which are carefully removed. Then carving is carefully done. The process of light closure is repeated and carving is finally done until the teeth are in their prerestoration occlusion.

Burnish the finished restoration. Finally, smoothen the restoration with a cotton pledget.

Postcarve burnishing: It is done after carving with suitable size of burnisher to improve the smoothness with shiny appearance. It helps in reducing the surface roughness

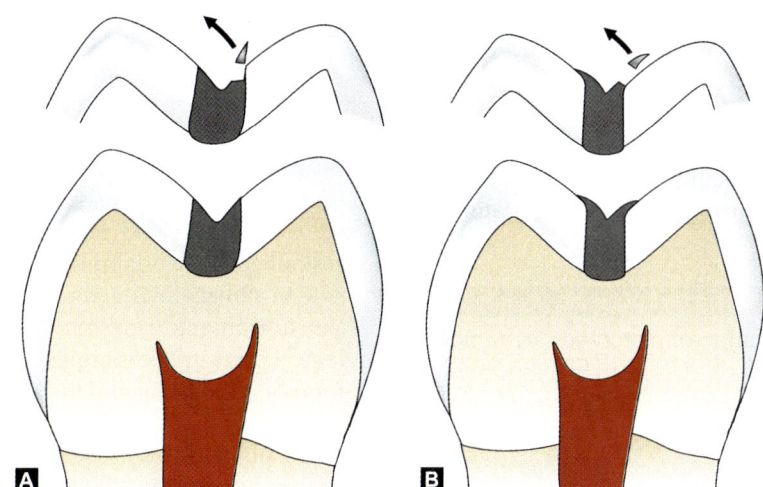

Figures 20.80A and B: Improper carving can result in; (A) Ditching of restoration; (B) Restoration overlay

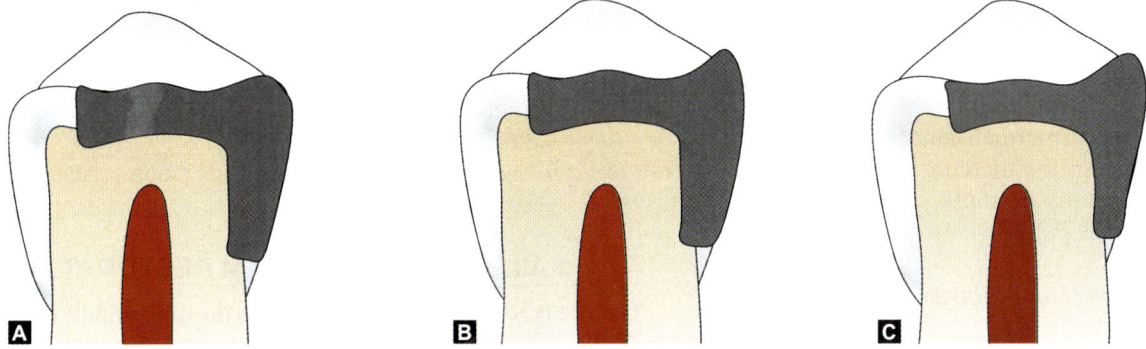

Figures 20.81A to C: (A) Optimal proximal contour; (B) High marginal ridge and improper occlusal embrasure form; (C) Too high contact and improper occlusal embrasure form

produced by carving. In high copper amalgam restoration postcarve burnishing has no significant effect on the clinical performance but in low copper amalgam, postcarve burnishing produces denser amalgam at the margins.

Finishing and Polishing

Finishing amalgam restorations involves removal of marginal irregularities, defining anatomical contours, and smoothening the surface roughness of the restoration. Polishing is done to achieve a smooth, shiny luster on the surface of the amalgam. Finishing is done before polishing by use of abrasive agents that are coarse enough to remove the bulk from the surface. Polishing requires mildly abrasive materials for producing smooth and shiny surface of amalgam restoration.

Finishing and polishing of the restorations should be done atleast 24 hours after the placement of the amalgam. Premature finishing and polishing will interfere with the crystalline structure of the hardening amalgam. The result will be a weakened restoration. Polishing may not be essential for restorations with high-copper alloys because they have a tendency of self-polishing.

The clinician should check the margins and proximal contacts of the restoration initially using metal filling strip to remove any roughness or overhand of the restoration in the proximal area.

Advantages of finishing and polishing
⇢ Improves marginal adaptation of restoration by removing flash
⇢ Reduces tarnish and corrosion
⇢ Polished surface is plaque resistant
⇢ Polished surface is smoother and easier to clean
⇢ Prevention of recurrent decay
⇢ Prevention of amalgam deterioration
⇢ Maintenance of periodontal health
⇢ Prevention of occlusal problems.

One of the most important precautions to be taken while doing finishing and polishing is the minimization of heat production. Heat generated during the polishing procedure is potentially dangerous because:
- It can cause thermal damage to the pulp
- Heat brings the mercury to the surface of the restoration resulting in a dull, cloudy surface, and makes it more susceptible to corrosion.

To Minimize Heat Production

- Use light, intermittent pressure with rotary instruments
- Use slow speed with rotary instruments
- Use abrasive agents that are wet rather than dry.

The most commonly rotary instruments used are abrasive stones, disks and finishing burs available in a different shapes, sizes, degrees of abrasiveness, and in either high-speed or slow speed. Pumice and tin oxide are two commonly used polishing agents. Pumice is usually mixed with water to decrease the heat produced by the friction of the abrasive particles during polishing. Tin oxide or Amalgloss is used as the finest abrasive agent. It can be used in a slurry, dry, or both forms.

Steps for Finishing and Polishing of Amalgam

- Using an explorer, evaluate the cavosurface margins for marginal integrity
- Determine the presence of any marginal discrepancies and evaluate the contour of the restoration
- Identify the occlusal pattern. Mark the occlusal contacts in centric occlusion and excursive movements. Areas that need to be reduced are identified by darker markings on the restoration. Establish proper occlusion by grinding
- Smoothen the margins by using a round bur moving it along all cavosurface margins. This procedure is done to blend the tooth structure to amalgam
- Use a large round finishing bur to eliminate scratches and graininess from the amalgam
- Using the side of the finishing bur, smoothen the occlusal surface and marginal ridges. Move the bur mesiodistally, overlapping each stroke, then do the same in a buccolingual direction
- Use a finishing strip for smoothening and polishing of the gingival cavosurface margins and interproximal space
- Smoothen the facial and lingual surfaces with finishing disks
- Finally polish the surface by using progressively finer abrasive agents (**Fig. 20.82**)
- Rinse and clean out all debris completely
- Evaluate all margins and surfaces of the restoration (**Fig. 20.83**).

A polished amalgam restoration should have following features
⇢ Surface is smooth with no scratches or graininess
⇢ Surface is lustrous, with a mirror like shine
⇢ There is no break between margins and the tooth surface
⇢ Restoration has proper contact and contour
⇢ There is no damage to the restoration or adjacent tooth structure

FAILURES OF AMALGAM RESTORATIONS

Since 1860, amalgam has been the most widely used restorative material in posterior teeth. But after 1970, because of development of newer restorative materials and mercury toxicity, its use has been limited.

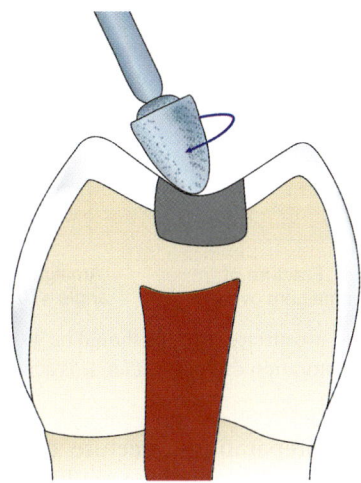

Figure 20.82: Final polishing of amalgam restoration using abrasive stones

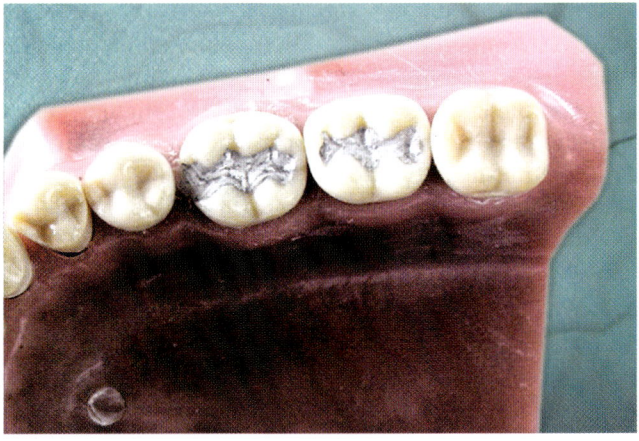

Figure 20.83: Completed amalgam restoration

Studies have shown that the life of a properly manipulated and restored silver amalgam restoration is about 10 to 12 years. With time, the restoration may show some changes like tarnish, corrosion, recurrent marginal caries, discoloration of teeth, fracture of restoration or tooth and ultimately loss of restoration.

Most common failures associated with dental amalgam restoration

➡ *At microscopic level*:
- ◆ Pain after amalgam restoration
- ◆ Periodontal tissue injury due to proximal overhangs
- ◆ Pulpal involvement
- ◆ Tarnish and corrosion
- ◆ Internal stresses due to excessive masticatory forces.

➡ *At macroscopic level*:
- ◆ Bulk fracture of restoration
- ◆ Tooth fracture
- ◆ Marginal fracture of amalgam
- ◆ Secondary or recurrent caries commonly takes place due to marginal leakage.
- ◆ Dimensional changes especially in zinc containing amalgam
- ◆ Discoloration of restoration
- ◆ Discoloration of tooth.

Reasons for Failure of Amalgam Restorations

The reasons for failure of amalgam restorations can be divided under following headings:

➡ Poor case selection
➡ Defective tooth preparation
➡ Defective amalgam manipulation
➡ Defective matrix adaptation
➡ Postrestorative failures.

Poor Case Selection

For long-term success of the amalgam restorations, a careful selection of case is very important. Since amalgam requires sufficient sound tooth structure to provide sufficient resistance and retention form for the amalgam, selecting teeth with extensive caries, abnormal habits like bruxism and heavy masticatory forces can result in restoration failure. Amalgam should be placed in small to moderate size carious lesions.

Defective Tooth Preparation

This is one of the major cause of failure of amalgam restorations. The following defects usually occur during tooth preparation.

- *Inadequate occlusal extension:* Insufficient extension to include adjacent deep pits and fissures increases chances for secondary/recurrent caries. This is specially seen in patients with high caries index. One should involve all susceptible pits and fissures in the preparation margins.
- *Under extension of the proximal box:* To prevent occurrence of secondary caries, walls of the proximal box of class II preparation must be extended to self-cleansing areas. If the proximal margins of the filling are not adequately extended into the embrasures, they are not open to cleaning by mastication and brushing resulting in secondary caries. On the other hand, over extension into the embrasure areas makes the preparation walls weak specially in lower bicuspids and on distal sides of maxillary and mandibular first molars.

Therefore, one should avoid overextension of the margins of the restoration into the embrasures.

- **Overextended tooth preparation (Fig. 20.84):** Ideally the faciolingual width of the preparation at isthmus for amalgam restoration should be less than one fourth of the intercuspal distance. If the faciolingual width of the preparation is more than half of the intercuspal distance, cusp capping should be considered. Cusp capping becomes necessary if the tooth preparation involves more than two-third of the intercuspal distance. Though for cusp capping, onlay cast restoration is preferred. If amalgam is to be used for capping, it should be atleast 2 mm thick over the functional cusp and 1.5 mm over nonfunctional cusp to prevent its fracture over the cusps under masticatory load.
- **Depth of preparation:** Minimum depth of preparation should be 1.5 to 2 mm so as to provide bulk which can prevent its fracture under masticatory load.
- There should be flat pulpal floor of the preparation to avoid fracture of amalgam and the tooth. Curved floor for restoration acts as a wedge, which can result tooth fracture
- The tooth and amalgam joint, i.e. cavosurface angle should be a butt joint especially where the masticatory stresses are present. If cavosurface angle is acute, enamel margins may fracture under load. But if cavosurface angle is obtuse, marginal amalgam may fracture under masticatory stresses (**Fig. 20.85**)
- Presence of unsupported enamel rods can result in fracture and thus secondary caries because of gap formation. They should be removed properly

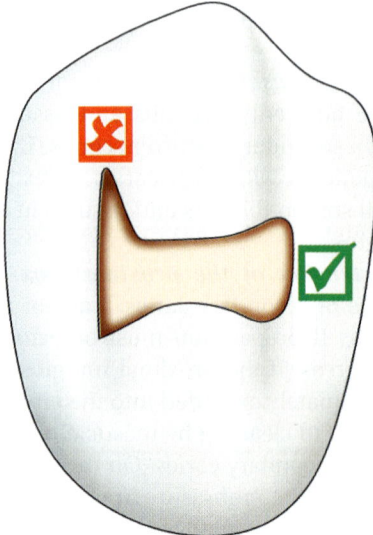

Figure 20.84: One should avoid excessive removal of cuspal inclines

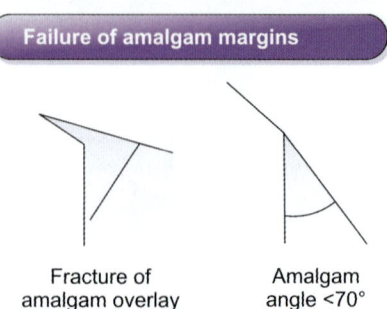

Figure 20.85: Cavosurface margins should be 90° for amalgam fracture of restoration can occur if angle is acute or obtuse

- In proximal preparations, fracture of amalgam can occur because of inadequate width and depth of isthmus or insufficient proximal retention form
- Fracture of amalgam restoration may occur because of sharp axiopulpal line angle because of concentration of stresses in that area. So these angles should be rounded
- Wherever additional retentive forms and devices are used for additional retention, they should be prepared entirely in dentin
- Incomplete removal of the defective enamel before restoration can also result in fracture of the restoration under masticatory load
- Postoperative pain may occur due to pulpal hyperemia. To avoid, this one should make use of effective cooling, sharp burs and intermittent cutting.

Defective Amalgam Manipulation

Defective amalgam manipulation may occur in the following forms.

Inappropriate condensation: The purpose of condensation is to adapt amalgam to the preparation walls and floors and to express excess mercury from the amalgam. An ideal amalgam mix should have mercury content below 55 percent, this can be achieved during condensation.

Following points should be kept in mind while condensing amalgam
➡ Small increments of amalgam should be used to make sure proper condensation
➡ Use of adequate condensation pressure
➡ Avoid delay between trituration and condensation
➡ Amalgam mix should be used within three minutes of its trituration.

Incorrect mercury alloy ratio: Ideally in amalgam, the mercury content should be less than 55 percent. If it is more than 55 percent, there is decrease in strength of the amalgam. If large amount of mercury is used in trituration, the excess removal of mercury becomes difficult by mulling and condensation. Hence, before trituration, proper proportion of alloy and mercury should be used.

Contamination during manipulation: While manipulation of amalgam if the amalgam gets contaminated with moisture, there occurs reduction in strength of amalgam. In zinc containing alloys, contamination with moisture causes delayed expansion resulting in pain, weakness at the margins, tarnish, and corrosion.

Faulty finishing and polishing: Excessive heat production during polishing may result in pulpal trauma. Heavy pressure applied during polishing results in spur like overhangs, which fracture under mastication causing leaky margins and prone to secondary caries.

Overcarving of deep pits and fissures results in reduced thickness of amalgam, this can cause fracture of the restoration. Improper polishing results in rough surface which is prone to tarnish, corrosion, pitting, plaque accumulation and gingival irritation.

To reduce these while polishing, temperature at the surface should be maintained below 65°C. Excessive heat production can be minimized by use of adequate coolant and polishing should be done with very light pressure.

Defective Matrix Adaptation

- As we know variety of matrices are available, proper matrix and retainer should be selected according to requirement. Matrix should be properly contoured according to the tooth type and stabilized using a wedge
- If wedge is not used, excess material can go into gingiva and thus irritate the periodontium
- Before condensation of amalgam, matrix should be properly made stable to avoid distortion of the restoration
- It matrix band is removed prematurely before the restoration is set, it may fracture the restoration.

Postrestorative Failures

Postrestorative pains: It can occur because of following reasons:
- High points in amalgam restoration can result in apical periodontitis or, fracture of the filling or tooth and pain
- In zinc containing alloys, delayed expansion can cause fracture of filling or tooth and pain
- If the patient has restoration placed adjacent or opposite to gold restoration, in presence of saliva, there is production of galvanic currents. This can also result in pain after amalgam restoration

- Extreme changes in temperature in oral cavity may cause pulpal hyperemia resulting in pain. Because of good thermal conductivity, insufficient pulp protection may give rise to pain. Thus it is advisable to use pulp protective materials beneath amalgam restoration.

Premature fracture of restoration: If patient bites the restoration soon after its placement and before final setting of amalgam takes place, restoration may fracture. Therefore, postoperative instructions must be clearly explained to the patient.

MERCURY HYGIENE

Mercury has been used in dentistry from a very long time. It is considered as major component in amalgam restorations and also used in medicines such as skin, antibacterial ointment and laxatives.

Mercury has been considered to be hazardous if not managed properly. Mercury vapors present in the dental office are toxic if they cross the threshold limit. So, management of free mercury is very important.

History of conflicts regarding amalgam use	
→ 1920	(First Amalgam war)—War between the dentists using gold foil and dental amalgam.
→ 1980	Dr Hal Huggins—amalgam responsible for cardiovascular and nervous problem.
→ 1991	NIH-NIDR and Food and Drug Administration (FDA) (National Institute of Health-National Institute for Dental Research) Several experts concluded that amalgam is not considered as a significant health hazard.

Mercury is present in the environment which is taken into the body through water, air and food, daily in one or another form.

The mercury usually enters into the body everyday no matter what type of restorative filling is present in oral cavity. Very low amount of mercury is usually released from set amalgam as compared to daily intake.

It has been found that health hazards from the amalgam use are mainly to dental and its associated staff in dental office than patient because of the long-term contact with mercury usage.

Forms of mercury

Exists in three chemical forms:
- → Elemental mercury
  - ♦ Most volatile
  - ♦ Exist in liquid/vapor form

- Inhaled and absorbed into lungs (80%) and GIT (0.01%)
- Most common form of entry in human body during amalgam restoration
- Exposure to this form can occur due to accidental spillage of mercury in dental office.
→ Inorganic mercury
  - Normally mined as inorganic sulfide ore
  - Mainly in liquid form
  - Can also exist in other forms than sulfides
  - Potentially toxic
  - Irritating in nature
  - Main route of entry is through lungs (80%).
→ Organic mercury
  - Mainly in the form of methyl mercury
  - Main route of entry is absorption through GIT (95-98%) through food
  - Used in fungicide and pesticide
  - Found in vegetables, fruits and grains
  - Toxic in nature.

Committee of International Toxicology experts classified mercury and its compounds according to their order of decreasing toxicity—Methyl and Ethyl mercury (Organomercury), Mercury vapor (Elemental mercury), Inorganic salts and a number of additional Organic forms such as phenyl mercury salts.

Mercury Exposure in Dental Office

In the dental office, mercury exposure can occur from the following sources (**Fig. 20.86**):
- Storage of amalgam raw materials for use
- Mixed but unset amalgam during trituration, insertion and intraoral hardening
- Amalgam scrap containing insufficient alloy for consuming mercury completely
- Finishing and polishing of restoration
- Removal of old restoration.

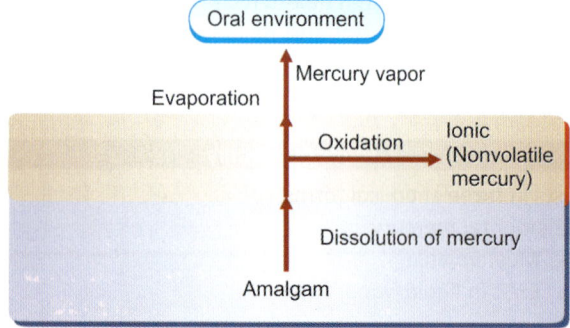

Figure 20.86: Sources of mercury in oral environment

Steps to Reduce Mercury Exposure in the Dental Clinic

- **Storage of mercury:** Storage of mercury is considered difficult because it:
  - Is very mobile
  - Has high diffusion rate
  - Can penetrate extremely fine spaces
    Therefore, one should take care while storage of mercury is concerned.
  - Precapsulated alloys should be preferred for avoiding mercury spill
  - If bulk mercury is purchased, store it in tight container with tight lid in closed cabinets.
  - Location of storage should be near the window/exhaust vent.
- **Trituration of amalgam**
  - Use precapsulated alloy in amalgamator
  - Avoid manual mixing
  - High vibrations during mixing can create aerosols of liquid droplets and these vapors may extend up to 6-12 ft from the amalgamator. So, to minimize the risk, small covers are used over the amalgamator to contain the aerosol in that area
  - Air flow should be reasonably high in dental office to minimize air contamination
  - Avoid direct exposure of the mercury with skin as it may cause hypersensitivity reactions.
- **Designing of office:** Office should be designed so as to reduce mercury contamination. Following points are to be kept in mind while designing:
  - Proper ventilation of the dental office
  - Avoid carpeting/floor coverings in dental office as there is no way of removing mercury from the carpet.
- Insertion and condensation of amalgam
  - After mixing, the unhardened mixture releases mercury vapors in air and causes air pollution. Proper ventilation of the area should be done
  - Proper aseptic techniques such as use of mouth masks, gloves and protective eyeglasses should be done
  - Avoid direct exposure of mercury with skin
  - Use rubberdam to isolate the tooth
  - Use high volume evacuation system to control the mercury level in air.
- **Polishing of amalgam:** The mercury is tightly bound when amalgam is set. Polishing should be done with coolant to decrease heat and vapors present in atmosphere
- **Disposal of scrap amalgam:** Scrap amalgam during insertion and condensation should be carefully collected and stored under water, glycerin or spent X-ray fixer solution in tightly capped jar.

Spent X-ray fixer is preferred for storage of amalgam scrap because it is source of both silver and sulfide ions which react with mercury present in scrap amalgam to form solid product and decrease the mercury vapor pressure.

- ***Disposal of mercury contaminated waste:*** Disposal of spent capsules, mercury contaminated cotton rolls and paper napkins should be done properly. These items should be disposed in tightly closed plastic container/ plastic bag which can be placed into sanitary landfill for disposal
- ***Removal of old amalgam restorations:*** Certain points should be kept in mind while removing amalgam restoration:
  - Rubberdam and high volume evacuator should be used to decrease mercury vapor
  - Watercooling should also be used as high rotary instruments used without water increase the temperature of filling and increase the mercury vapors in that area.
- ***Cleaning of mercury contaminated instruments***
  - Clean the mercury contaminated instrument used during insertion, finishing and polishing and during removal of restoration as amalgam material left on the instrument surface, heated during sterilization can release mercury vapor in atmosphere
  - Isolation of the area along with proper ventilation of sterilization area is preferred.
- ***Monitoring of mercury vapors:*** The accepted threshold limit for exposure to mercury vapor for a 40-hour work per week is 50 µg/m³ (given by OSHA).

Periodical monitoring of mercury vapor in dental office should be done and carefully recorded.

Dental Mercury Hygiene Recommendations in Dental Office

- Follow aseptic technique, i.e wear protective clothing, protective masks, gloves and glasses to prevent exposure to mercury vapors
- Dental personnel's involved in handling of mercury and dental amalgam products should follow proper mercury hygiene practice
- Dentists and dental assistants should have proper knowledge of amalgam disposal and their handling
- Proper ventilation of the working space should be there, to reduce mercury levels in the atmosphere
- Periodically check the working area to analyze the mercury vapor pressure using dosimeter badges
- Avoid carpet/floor coverings in dental office; floor coverings should be easy to clean, nonabsorbent and seamless

- Mercury should be stored in unbreakable closed container in isolated area
- Use precapsulated alloy for mixing
- Instead of manual/hand mixing, use amalgamator with completely closed arm
- Polish amalgam restoration under coolant to decrease the mercury vapor pressure
- Avoid direct contact of mercury with skin
- Use high volume evacuation and rubberdam during insertion, condensation and polishing of restoration
- Store scrap amalgam in water, glycerine or spent fixer solution in closed container
- Precapsulated alloys, mercury contaminated cotton rolls should be disposed in closed plastic container
- Clean the spilled mercury using trap bottles or freshly mixed amalgam
- Remove professional clothing, gloves, masks before leaving operating area.

Mercury Toxicity (Fig. 20.87)

Mercury toxicity is mainly seen because of chronic exposure of mercury which can be in form of food, restorations or other sources. Since too many factors are involved, it takes time for symptoms to appear. Usually mercury gradually accumulates in the body over a period of time, contributes to chronic mercury poisoning.

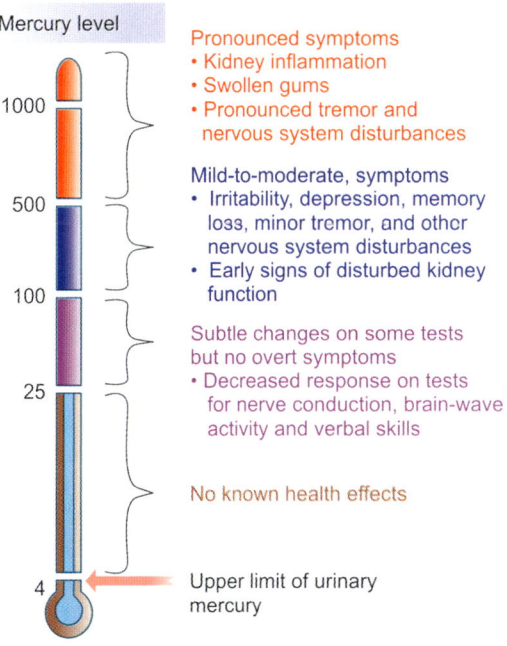

Figure 20.87: Mercury thermometer depicting different levels of mercury toxicity

Toxic effects of mercury depend upon following factors

- Amount of exposure
- Length of exposure
- Location of mercury accumulation in body
- Amount of accumulated mercury
- Overall health of the patient (for detoxification).

Acute Mercury Poisoning

It occurs when there is sudden exposure of high levels of mercury especially from elemental mercury or organic mercury. It results in immediate and severe symptoms requiring urgent medical attention.

Toxic levels of mercury are measured in micrograms. The following table compares the effects of different levels of mercury present in urine.

Levels of Hg toxicity

- At level of 4 µg: This level is attributed as the upper limit in urine when extensive restoration of amalgam is present in patient's month
- At level 0 to 25 µg: No known health hazards are detected
- At level 25 to 100 µg: Decreased response on tests done for brain conduction. Decreased response related to verbal skills
- 100 to 500 µg: Mild-to-moderate effects can be seen:
  - Irritability – Memory loss
  - Depression – Tremors
  - Nervous system disturbances.
- 500 to 1,000 µg: Pronounced symptoms
  - Inflammation of kidney
  - Tremors and pronounced nervous system disturbances
  - Swollen gums.

IS DENTAL AMALGAM SAFE?

- Dental amalgams are still widely used by the dental profession in most parts of the world
- Some countries, like Sweden, Canada and Germany, UK have either banned or imposed serious limitations on amalgam usage
- In the 1990s, several governments evaluated the effects of dental amalgam and concluded that the most likely health effects would be due to hypersensitivity or allergy
- In 2004, the Life Sciences Research Office analyzed studies related to dental amalgam. They took mean urinary mercury concentration (µg of Hg/L in urine, HgU) as the most reliable estimate of mercury exposure. 95 percent of study participants showed µg HgU below 4 to 5

- Chewing gum, particularly for nicotine, along with more amalgam, seemed to pose the greatest risk of increasing exposure. However, the World Health Organization states mercury levels in biomarkers such as urine, blood, or hair do not represent levels in critical organs and tissues
- The American Dental Association Council on Scientific Affairs has concluded that both amalgam and composite materials are considered safe and effective for tooth restoration.

 Key Points

- The first form of silver mercury mixture was given by M Taveau in 1826 at Paris.
- Dental amalgam is an alloy of mercury with silver, tin, and varying amounts of copper, zinc and other minor constituents.
- In preamalgamated alloys, mercury 3 percent is used which react more rapidly when mixed with mercury.
- On mixing amalgam alloy with mercury, the alloy particles get dissolved in the mercury. In the initial reaction, mercury reacts with tin and silver without involving copper and zinc. Mercury reacts with alloy particles to form two products, i.e. the silver mercury phase and tin mercury phase. After this reaction, the unreacted particles are embedded in the matrix of reaction products with mercury.
- Lathe cut is made by cutting fillings of alloy from a pre-homogenized ingot which was heat treated at 420°C for many hours. The fillings are then reheated at 100°C for 1 hour for aging of the alloy.
- Spherical (spheroidal) alloy is formed when molten alloy is sprayed into a column filled with inert gas, this molten metal solidifies as fine droplets of alloy.
- Presence of zinc can result in delayed expansion after 3 to 5 days of restoration, if during manipulation, zinc containing amalgam comes in contact with moisture or saliva. This occurs due to formation of zinc oxide and hydrogen gas when zinc react with water. This expansion can result in extrusion of restoration beyond preparation margins and pulpal pain.
- According to ADA specification no. 1, amalgam should have minimum 1 hour compressive strength of 11,600 psi (80 MPa). Amalgam has higher compressive strength (7 times) than tensile or shear strength making it brittle material.
- Creep is the time dependent response of an already set material to stress. This response is in form of plastic deformation. By ADA specification no. 1, creep is limited to 3 percent in a set-amalgam.

- In amalgam, corrosion causes decrease in strength of a restoration, the advantageous fact of corrosion is that the byproducts that form, seal the preparation margin, resulting in self-sealing property of amalgam.
- In low copper amalgams, the most corrosion prone phase is gamma 2 (Sn7-8 Hg3) phase. In these alloys, corrosion products are tin oxides and tin chlorides. Here the corrosion proceeds from outer surface to interior of restoration making it porous and spongy.
- In high copper amalgams, corrosion products are similar to that of low copper alloys, in addition there is formation of copper chloride which corrode slower than low copper amalgams. High copper alloys corrode slower because they contain little or none of gamma 2 phase. Also the corrosion is not of penetrating type as in low copper alloys.
- Microleakage occurs when there is 2 to 20 micron wide gap between the amalgam and tooth structure.
- In the bonded amalgam technique, a dentin bonding system is used along with a viscous resin liner which physically mixes with the amalgam and forms a micromechanical union to increase amalgam's retention to tooth structure.
- For this monomer molecule having hydrophilic and hydrophobic ends of 4-methyloxy ethyl trimellitic anhydride (4-META) based systems are used.
- Handling of gallium alloys is difficult because they have tendency to stick to the instruments. This sticking problem can be reduced by adding a drop of absolute alcohol to the mix before trituration. Alcohol slowly evaporates and thus does not adversely affect the properties of the amalgam.
- Reverse curve is given in the teeth with broader contacts, to both widen the box yet remove less tooth structure. It is given to the proximal walls by curving them inwards towards the contact area. If excessive flare is given in these teeth, proximal walls will end past the axial angle of tooth through the cusps resulting in weakening of tooth structure and fracture of restoration.
- Eames preferred 1:1 ratio of alloy/mercury for best results. Generally, it is 5:8 or 5:7, if mercury content is more than required amount, resultant mix will be weaker, but if it is less, it might not sufficiently wet the alloy particles. Lathe cut amalgam alloys require more (45%) of mercury to wet than the spherical alloys (40%).
- Purpose of trituration is to remove oxide layers from the alloy particles so as to coat each alloy particle with mercury, resulting in a homogeneous mass for condensation.
- Signs of a good mix amalgam are shiny, homogeneous mass that adheres together. Undertrituration results in a crumbly mix that is very weak.
- Mulling is done so that all alloy particles are properly coated with mercury, in other words it is continuation of the trituration.
- Precarve burnishing is done after condensation so as to improve marginal adaptability of the restoration and remove excess mercury from overpacked amalgam.
- Postcarve burnishing is done after completion of carving with the help of small sized burnishers using light strokes. It helps in producing denser amalgam at margins, improves marginal seal and increases surface hardness.
- Finishing and polishing of the amalgam restorations should be done atleast 24 hours after the placement of the amalgam. Premature finishing and polishing interferes with the crystalline structure of the hardening amalgam. The result will be a weakened restoration. Polishing may not be essential for restorations with high-copper alloys because they have a tendency of self-polishing.
- Scrap amalgam during insertion and condensation should be carefully collected and stored under water, glycerin or spent X-ray fixer solution in tightly capped jar.
- Spent X-ray fixer is preferred for storage of amalgam scrap because it is source of both silver and sulfide ions which react with mercury present in scrap amalgam to form solid product and decrease the mercury vapor pressure.
- The accepted threshold limit for exposure to mercury vapor for a 40-hour work per week is 50 $\mu g/m^3$ (given by OSHA).

QUESTIONS

1. Define and classify amalgam. What is role of each constituent in amalgam alloy.
2. Write short notes on:
   a. Indications and contraindications of amalgam restoration
   b. Bonded amalgam.
   c. Gallium amalgam
   d. Reverse curve
   e. Mercury toxicity
   f. Failure of amalgam restorations.
   g. Steps of amalgam restoration.
3. Explain in detail the steps of tooth preparation for class II amalgam restoration.

4. What are different reasons for failure of amalgam restorations?

5. Enumerate the steps of tooth preparation. How would you obtain resistance and retention form in class II cavity for amalgam restoration.

6. Write in detail about the delayed expansion of silver amalgam.

7. Write short note on unicompositional alloys.

8. Write short note on amalgam alloy.

9. Describe causes and treatment of pain in a teeth after placing a restoration.

BIBLIOGRAPHY

1. Almquist TC, et al. Conservative amalgam restorations. J Prosthet Dent. 1973;29:524.

2. American Dental Association. Amalgam waste. ADA's best management practices. ADA News. 2004;35:1.

3. Bauer JG. A study of procedures for burnishing amalgam restorations. J Prosthet Dent. 1987;57:669.

4. Ben-Amar A, et al. Long-term sealing properties of Amalgam bond under amalgam restorations. Am J Dent. 1994;7:141-3.

5. Ben-Amar A, et al. The sealing of the tooth/amalgam interface by corrosion products. J Oral Rehabil. 1995;22:101-4.

6. Berry FA, et al. Microleakage of amalgam restorations using dentin bonding system primers. Am J Dent. 1996;9:174.

7. Berry TG, et al. Amalgam at the new millennium. J Am Dent Assoc. 1998;129:1547-56.

8. Bona AD, Summitt JB. The effect of amalgam bonding on resistance form of class II amalgam restorations. Quint Int. 1998;29:95.

9. Bouschor CF, Martin JR. A review of concepts of silver amalgam retention. JPD. 1976;36:532-7.

10. Bryant RW. The strength of fifteen amalgam alloys. Austr Dent J. 1979;24:244-52.

11. Calamia JR, Styner DL, Rattet AH. Effect of amalgam bond on cervical sensitivity. Am J Dent. 1996;8:283.

12. Corbin SB, Kohn WG. The benefits and risks of dental amalgam: current findings reviewed. J Am Dent Assoc. 1994;125:381-8.

13. Cowan R. Amalgam repair—a clinical technique. JPD. 1983;49:49.

14. Della Bona A, Summitt JB. The effect of amalgam bonding on resistance form of class II amalgam restorations. Quintessence Int. 1998;29:95.

15. Drummond JL, et al. Surface roughness of polished amalgams. Oper Dent. 1992;17:129.

16. Duncalf WV, Wilson NHF. Adaptation and condensation of amalgam restoration in class II preparation of conventional and conservative design. Quint Int.1992;23:499.

17. Dunne SM, et al. Current materials and techniques for direct restorations in posterior teeth: silver amalgam: part 1. Int Dent J. 1997;47:123-36.

18. Ehrlich J, Yaffe A. A modified cavity preparation for restorating interproximal caries. Compendium. 1987;8:62.

19. Elderton RJ. Cavosurface angles, amalgam margin angles and occlusal cavity preparations. BDJ. 1984;156:319.

20. Elderton RJ. The prevalence of failure of restorations: a literature review. J Dent. 1976;4:207.

21. Fusayama T. Cavity preparation and amalgam restoration in enamel. JPD. 1971;25:657-61.

22. Gilmore HW. Restorative materials and tooth preparation design. Dent Clin North Am. 1971;15:99.

23. Görücü J, et al. Effects of preparation designs and adhesive systems on retention of class II amalgam restorations. J Prosthet Dent. 1997;78:250.

24. Gottlieb EW, et al. Microleakage of conventional and high-copper amalgam restorations. J Prosthet Dent. 1985;53:355.

25. Grieve AR. Finishing cavity margins. BDJ. 1968;125:12-7.

26. Gwinnett AJ, et al. Adhesive restorations with amalgam: guidelines for the clinician. Quintessence Int. 1994;25:687.

27. Hasselrot L. Tunnel restorations. Swed Dent J. 1993;17:173.

28. Hilton TJ. Sealers, liners and bases. J Esthet Restor Dent. 2003;15:141.

29. Liberman R, et al. Long-term sealing properties of amalgam restorations: an in vitro study. Dent Mater. 1989;5:168-70.

30. Lindemuth JS, et al. Effect of restoration size on fracture resistance of bonded amalgam restorations. Oper Dent. 2000; 25:177.

31. Lovadino JR, et al. Influence of burnishing on amalgam adaptation to cavity walls. J Prosthet Dent. 1987;58:284.

32. Mahler DB, Adey JD. Factors influencing the creep of dental amalgam. J Dent Res. 1991;70:1394-1400.

33. Mahler DB, Engle JH. Clinical evaluation of amalgam bonding in class I and II restorations. J Am Dent Assoc. 2000;131:43.

34. Mahler DB, et al. Marginal fracture of amalgam restorations. J Dent Res. 1973;52:823-7.

35. Mahler DB. The amalgam-tooth interface. Oper Dent. 1996;21:230.

36. Mahler DB. The high-copper dental amalgam alloys. J Dent Res. 1997;76:537-421.

37. Mandel ID. Amalgam hazards: an assessment of research. J Am Dent Assoc. 1991;122:62-5.

38. Markley MR. Restorations of silver amalgam. J Am Dent Assoc. 1951;43:133.

39. May KN, et al. Burnished amalgam restorations: a two-year evaluation. J Prosthet Dent. 1983;49:193.

40. Molin C. Amalgam-fact and fiction. Scand J Dent Res. 1992;100:66-73.

41. Osborne JW, Summitt JB. Direct-placement gallium restorative alloy. A 3-year clinical evaluation. Quintessence Int. 1999;30:49-53.

42. Osborne JW, Summitt JB. Extension for prevention: is it relevant today? Am J Dent. 1998;11:189.

43. Plasmans P, et al. Long-term survival of extensive amalgam restorations. J Dent Res. 1998;77:453-60.

44. Suchatlampong C, et al. Early compressive strength and phase-formation of dental amalgam. Dent Mater. 1995;14:143-51.

45. Sweeney JT. Amalgam manipulation: manual vs. mechanical aids: II. comparison of clinical applications. J Am Dent Assoc. 1940;27:1940.

46. Symons AL, et al. Adaptation of eight modern dental amalgams to walls of Class I cavity preparations. J Oral Rehabil. 1987;14:55.

47. Venugopalan R, et al. The effect of water contamination on dimensional change and corrosion properties of a gallium alloy. Dent Mater. 1998;14:173-8.

48. Vrijhoef MM, Letzel H. Creep versus marginal fracture of amalgam restorations. J Oral Rehabil. 1986;13:299-303.

49. Williams PT, Hedge GL. Creep-fatigue as a possible cause of dental amalgam margin failure. J Dent Res. 1985;64:470-5.

50. Winkler MM, et al. Comparison of retentiveness of amalgam bonding agent types. Oper Dent. 1997;22:200-8.

Pin Retained Restorations

Chapter Outline

INTRODUCTION

Most of the teeth can be restored using amalgam or composites. But when the preparation size is very big due to caries or other reason and the remaining tooth structure is very less, it becomes difficult to achieve optimal resistance and retention form. In such cases, dentin lock and slots are prepared in the dentin. But when these retentive features are insufficient to provide desired retention, pin supported restorations are used. In these cases, pins support the restorative materials and resist their dislodgement in severely damaged teeth.

Definition (Fig. 21.1)

A pin retained restoration is defined as any restoration which requires the placement of pin/pins in the dentin in order to provide sufficient retention and resistance form to the restoration.

Advantages of pin amalgam restorations

- *Conservation of tooth material*: Pin amalgam restoration is more conservative than tooth preparation for cast restoration
- *Resistance and retention form*: Use of pin increases the resistance and retention of the restoration
- *Number of appointments*: One appointment is required for pin retained restoration whereas for cast restoration, at least two appointments are required
- *Cost factor*: Pin amalgam restoration is relatively inexpensive as compared to cast restoration.

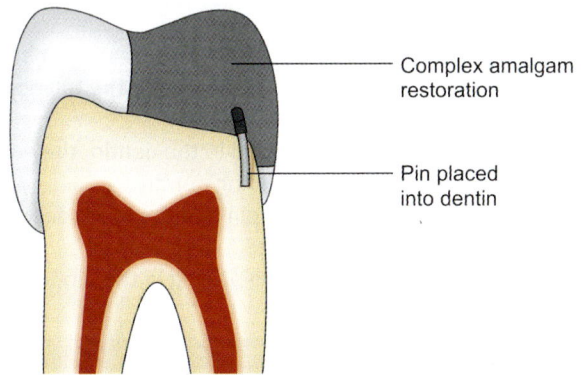

Complex amalgam restoration

Pin placed into dentin

Figure 21.1: Pin retained amalgam restoration

Disadvantages of pin amalgam restorations
➡ *Dentin fracture*: Use of pins in teeth where less dentin is present, may result in stresses in dentin in form of craze lines or cracks
➡ *Strength of amalgam*: Compressive strength is not increased by use of pins, but there is decrease in tensile and transverse strength of amalgam
➡ *Perforations*: Using bur or pin in wrong direction can cause pulpal exposure or perforation of external tooth surface
➡ *Microleakage*: If pin ends appear on or near to the surface of the restoration, it may result in microleakage around the pins
➡ *Tooth anatomy*: Sometimes, it is difficult to achieve optimal contours and occlusal contacts with these restorations.

INDICATIONS FOR PIN AMALGAM RESTORATIONS

- *Badly broken teeth*: In teeth where a large portion of tooth has been damaged, large restorations may be fractured or may be lost due to masticatory stresses. Use of pins helps in providing additional retention and resistance.
- *Badly broken nonvital tooth requiring endodontic treatment*: If endodontic treatment is indicated, pins are placed before initiating the treatment as they facilitate in securing of the rubber dam clamp.
- *Extended preparations*: In teeth requiring large interproximal restoration, restoration of cusp or extention of preparation beyond the line angles, use of pin provides additional strength especially when the margins of the restoration are not surrounded by enough tooth structure.
- *Foundation for full coverage restoration*: By using pins, amalgam core can be placed in less time and cost.

- *Extensive class V restorations*: Use of pins in extensive class V restoration to strengthen the restoration.
- *Time period and cost factors*: When patient cannot afford time for second appointment or expensive cast gold restoration, pin-retained amalgam restoration can be the restoration of choice.

CONTRAINDICATIONS OF PIN AMALGAM RESTORATIONS

- When patient has occlusal problems
- When esthetics is concerned
- When direct restoration is not possible because of functional or anatomical considerations.

RETENTIVE PINS

In 1958, Dr Miles Markley introduced stainless steel pins to provide retention and resistance form. Pins are available in different shapes, sizes and materials such as stainless steel, platinum-palladium, platinum iridium, plastic, aluminum and acrylic.

Types of pins
Pins can be classified as:
➡ Direct pins/nonparallel pins
◆ Cemented pins
◆ Friction locked pins
◆ Self-threading pins
➡ Indirect pins/parallel pins

- Direct pins are generally made of stainless steel and inserted into dentin after this restoration is placed directly over them. Pins can also be made from other materials like silver, titanium, stainless steel with gold plating, etc. These pins are also called as the non-parallel pins because they can be inserted directly into the tooth structure and need not be parallel.
- Indirect pins are made smaller in size when compared to their pinholes and they constitute an integral part of a cast restoration. These pins are also known as the parallel pins because the these pins are placed parallel to each other and also to the path of insertion of the restoration. Two types of pins are used in the parallel pin technique:
  - *Cast gold pins*: These pins have a smooth surface. For making restoration using parallel pins, place nylon bristles or plastic pins in the pinholes, over this build rest of the restoration in the conventional form with a blue inlay wax. Invest whole assembly and cast it with pins forming an integral part of the cast restoration.

– *Wrought precious metal pins*: Surface of these pins has been roughened by means of threaded or knurled patterns. Commonly used pins are alloys of gold, platinum, palladium or platinum-indium. In this pins are placed in the pinholes and included in the wax pattern. These pins are 20 to 30 percent more retentive than smooth cast pins.

Direct Pins

Cemented Pins (Fig. 21.2)

Cemented pins were introduced by Dr Merklay in 1958 for obtaining greater retention in large amalgam restorations. For these pins, the prepared pinholes should be 0.025 to 0.05 mm larger than the diameter of the pin. This difference in diameter provides space for cementing media. Pins are available in various diameters ranging from 0.018" to 0.030" with the corresponding pinholes of 0.020 to 0.032 inches.

The pin is checked for contour and length by placing in the tooth. If pin does not interfere with insertion into the pinhole and has the correct length, then it is cemented with glass ionomer or zinc phosphate cement. The depth of hole in dentin should be 3 to 4 mm.

Indications
→ In cases where least stresses or crazing is desired, e.g. endodontically treated teeth
→ When bulk of dentin to hold the pin is less
→ When dentin has lost its elasticity because of dehydration or sclerosis
→ When pin has to be placed near dentinoenamel junction.

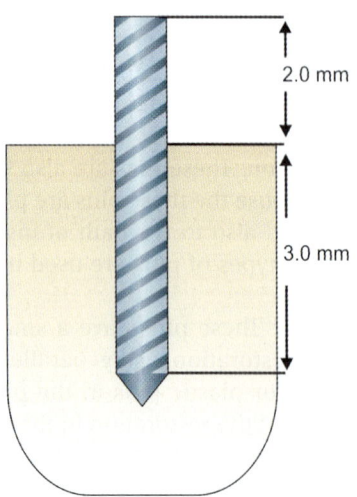

Figure 21.2: Cemented pin

Advantages
→ Cemented pins are 0.001 to 0.002 inches smaller than their pinholes. Thus they can be seated to the full depth of the hole
→ Since they are passively retained in the dentin, they produce no stress on the surrounding dentin
→ Cement present between the pin and the tooth decreases the chances of microleakage
→ They can be cut or bent before placing in the pinholes.

Disadvantages
→ Provide less retention
→ It is difficult to locate the pinhole after cement has been placed in it for cementation
→ A poorly cemented pin can be dislodged while inserting filling material
→ Requires more time for the mixing and hardening of the cement.

Techniques
→ Dry the prepared pin channels with endodontic paper points
→ Place the cement mix into the pin channel with a root canal file or/an explorer or a lentulospiral running at slow speed of 1000 rpm
→ Hold the pin in the forceps and coat with the cement
→ Insert the pin into the hole
→ Hold the pin in its position till it sets
→ Remove excess cement with an explorer.

Friction Locked Pins (Fig. 21.3)

Friction locked pins were introduced by Goldstein in 1966. These pins are 0.001" larger than their pinholes, hence utilize the elasticity of dentin for retention. They are 2 to 3 times more retentive than the cemented pins.

Indications
→ Vital teeth
→ Periodontally sound teeth
→ When direct access is possible so that the tapping force can be applied parallel to the long axis of the pin
→ When sufficient amount of dentin is available to surround the pin.

Advantages
→ Cementing media not required
→ Pins attain stability from the moment they are inserted
→ Better retention than the cemented pins.

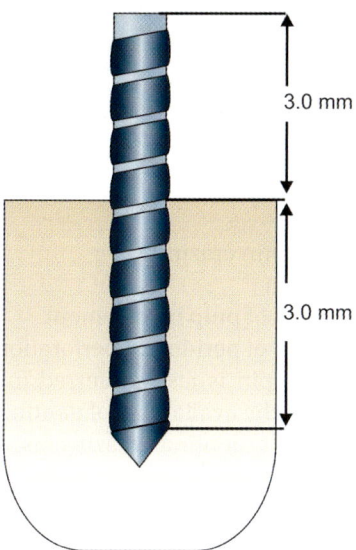

Figure 21.3: Friction locked pin

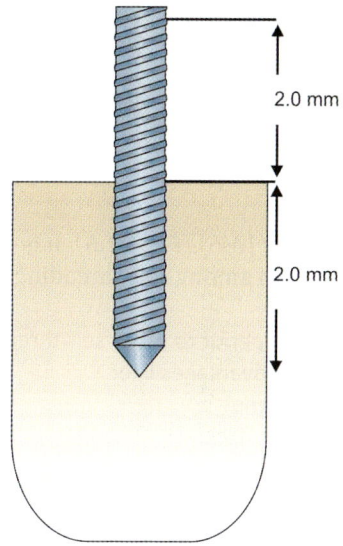

Figure 21.4: Self-threading pin

Disadvantages

- The length of the pin cannot be adjusted outside after insertion. Removed from dentin for cutting to the desired length once inserted
- Bending or contouring of the pin after it has been inserted into the pinhole results in further stresses
- Sometimes the pins do not reach full depth of the channel because of gouging
- Microleakage occurs if the overlying restoration leaks
- Stresses in dentin may result in form of cracks or craze lines.

Techniques of pin placement

- Cut the pin to the desired length before insertion since pin cannot be inserted for try-in and adjustment
- Insert the pin into a pin setter and carry to the pinhole. Apply force with mallet parallel to the long axis of the pin until pin reaches the desired length
- Remove excess length with a small round bur
- Bend the pin at a desirable angle with contouring pliers, if desired.

Self-threading Pin (Fig. 21.4)

They were introduces by Going in 1966. Self-threading pins are 0.0015" to 0.004" larger than their pinholes. The pins are retained due to the mechanical grasp of the threads into the dentin. The elastic property of the dentin allows insertion of a threaded pin into a hole of a smaller diameter. These are available in stainless steel or titanium but can be gold plated to increase their passivity.

Currently, threaded pins are most popular amongst the three pin systems because of their ease and rapidity of insertion and maximum retention offered. They are 3 to 6 times more retentive than the cemented pins. However, the amount of stresses induced in dentin in the form of cracks and craze lines are also more with the threaded pins.

Indications

- In vital teeth
- When maximum retention is desired
- When sufficient amount of dentin is available to surround the pins.

Advantages

- Ease of insertion
- Superior retention
- Require less depth for placement
- Require no cementing medium.

Disadvantages

- The pulpal stress is maximum when the pin is inserted perpendicular to the pulp
- Generate great stresses in dentin in form of craze or crack lines
- Pins may fail to seat completely
- If pin is forced into the pinhole it may strip the sides of the dentin resulting in a loose fit
- Microleakage is higher than the cemented pins if the overlying restoration leaks
- Pins may need to be bent, cut or contoured after placement which generate extra stress on the tooth or may loosen the pin.

Type of pin	Diameter of pinhole	Pin depth in dentin	Pin depth in amalgam
Cemented pin	0.025–0.05 mm larger than diameter of pin	3–4 mm	2 mm
Friction locked pin	0.025 mm smaller than diameter of pin	3 mm	2 mm
Self-threading pin	0.038–0.1 mm (0.015–0.004 inches) smaller than diameter of pin	2 mm	2 mm

Thread mate system (TMS) (**Fig. 21.5**): It is considered as the most widely used among self-threading pins.

TMS is considered superior to other self-threading pins because of its several advantages like:
→ Multipurpose designs
→ Wide variety of pin sizes
→ Good retention
→ Color-coding system for easy identification and use
→ Gold plating for good surface finish and also for reducing corrosion.

Types of pin sizes		
Type of pin		*Inches/mm*
→ Minuta	–	0.015/0.38
→ Minikin	–	0.019/0.48
→ Minim	–	0.024/0.61
→ Regular	–	0.031/0.78

- *Minuta*: Minuta is smallest of size among these self-threaded pins. It is too small to provide retention in the tooth. So, it is rarely used nowadays.
- *Minikin*: Minikin pin is considered as the pin of choice in grossly decayed posterior teeth. This pin causes:
  – Less risk of dentin crazing
  – Better retention
  – Lesser chances of pulp involvement
  – Lesser chances of peridontal perforation.
- *Minim pin*: This pin is also preferred in some cases, depending upon the availability of dentin:
  – It provides less dentinal crazing as compared to regular pins
  – It is used in cases where pinholes for minikin was over-prepared or threads strip during pin placement.
- *Regular*: Regular is largest diameter pin among thread mate system pins. It is rarely used because of its following disadvantages:
  – Great amount of stress and crazing around pins.
  – More chances of perforation in pulp chamber.

Pin Design

All of above-mentioned pins are available in the following designs
- Standard
- Self-shearing
- Two-in-one
- Link series
- Link plus series.

Standard Pin (Fig. 21.6)

The standard pin is a full length pin, i.e. 7 mm long which can be cut to the required length after placement. Pin provides a flat head for engagement with the hand wrench or the handpiece chuck. The self-shearing pin design is available in different lengths according to the diameters.

Self-shearing Pin (Fig. 21.7)

Self-shearing pin is designed such that on reaching the bottom of the pinhole, the head separates automatically at the shear line, leaving a portion of it to project from the dentin. Shearing occurs when there is resistance to turning because pin insertion is torque limited.

Two-in-one Design (Fig. 21.8)

In this, two pins join each other at a joint. This joint marks the shear line for the peripheral pin. Length of two-in-one

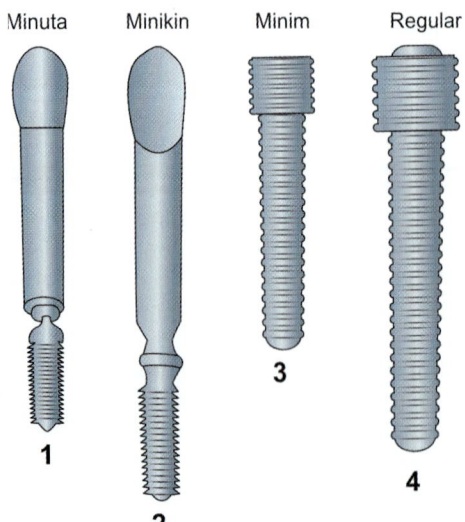

Figure 21.5: Different types of thread mate system pins

pin is approximately 8-9 mm with two pins of equal lengths. One pin is peripheral pin and the second pin is wrench attachment pin. It has a flat head to engage the hand wrench or the handpiece chuck. When the peripheral pin fixes to floor of pinhole, it shears off at the connecting joint leaving behind the wrench attachment pin along with its attachment. This pin can be reused for another pin channels.

Link Series (Fig. 21.9)

The disposable latch head design has a plastic sheath/head designed to fit in a slow speed contra-angle handpiece. The pin appears to lie freely in the plastic sheath. This helps in self-alignment as the pin penetrates into the pinhole. When the pin reaches the bottom of the pinhole, there is resistance to penetration which causes the separation of head from the pin at the shear line. The plastic sheath is then discarded. The plastic sheaths are color coded for easier identification of different sizes of pins.

Link Plus Series (Figs 21.10 and 21.11)

Link plus series pin design has following modifications from link series:
- Incorporation of sharper threads
- Tapered tip which readily fits in pinhole
- Shoulder stop.

With these modifications, it has been seen that there is great reduction in stresses in dentin while pin insertion.

Pin Insertion

Manual Insertion
- Attach the pin to hand wrench
- Insert it slowly into position
- Use tactile sense to determine whether pin has reached the bottom of pinhole.

Mechanical Insertion
- Engage the pin in the handpiece chuck. Pin may also have an attached latch head the pin for insertion into the handpiece
- Move handpiece at slow speed and insert the pin with light pressure
- When pin reaches bottom, there is increase in resistance and the pin shears off at the shear line or disengages from the handpiece.

The ideal pin length extending out of dentin should be 2.0 mm while providing space for 1 mm of restorative material around the pin and 2.0 mm occlusal to the pin.

PRINCIPLES AND TECHNIQUES OF PIN PLACEMENT

Pin Size

In general, increase in diameter of pin offers more retention but large sized pins can result in more stresses in dentin (**Figs 21.12A and B**).

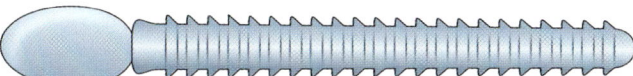

Figure 21.6: Standard pin

Figure 21.10: Link plus series

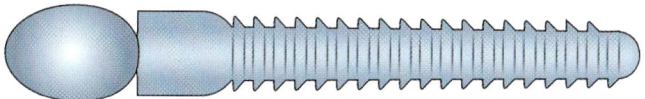

Figure 21.7: Self-shearing pin

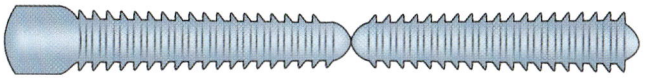

Figure 21.8: Two-in-one

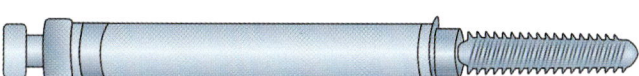

Figure 21.9: Link series

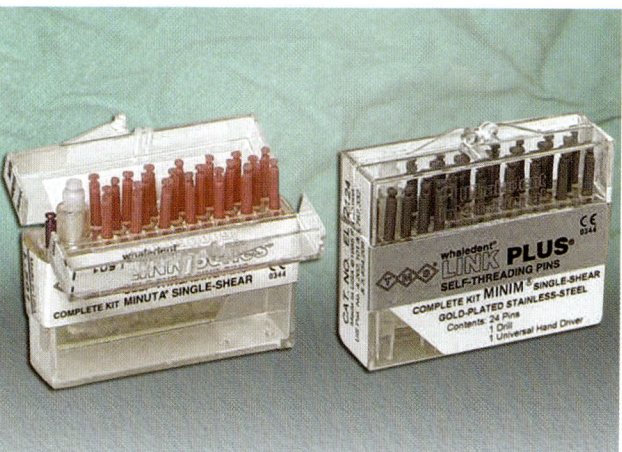

Figure 21.11: Self threading series

Pins are available in four color coded sizes		
Name	*Pin diameter*	*Color code*
→ Minuta	0.38 mm	Pink
→ Minikin	0.48 mm	Red
→ Minim	0.61 mm	Silver
→ Regular	0.78 mm	Gold

Selection of pin size depends upon following factors
→ Amount of dentin present
→ Amount of retention required.
For most of the posterior restorations, minikin or minim size of pins are used because they provide maximum retention without causing crazing in dentin.

Number of Pins

As far as possible, simple rule should be followed for use of number of pins, i.e. one pin per missing cusp and one pin for each missing axial line angle. unnecessary use of pins should be avoided as they can cause following (**Fig. 21.13**).
- Generate stress in the tooth resulting in fracture of tooth
- Voids in restoration
- Decrease the amount of available interpin dentin
- Decrease the strength of amalgam restoration.

Factor affecting choice for number of pins used
→ Amount of missing tooth structure
→ Amount of retention required
→ Amount of dentin present
→ Size and type of pin.

Interpin Distance (Fig. 21.14)

When more than two pins are to be used, interpin distance should be such that it prevents concentration of stresses in dentin and allows space for insertion of restorative material between pins. Interpin distance depends upon size and type of pins. For cemented pins it is 2 mm, for friction lock it is 4 mm and for threaded pins it is 5 mm.

Length of Pin into Dentin and Amalgam (Fig. 21.15)

In general, pin extension of 2 mm into dentin and amalgam provide maximum required retention. Pin extension more than 2 mm is avoided so as to preserve the strength of dentin and the restoration. Care should be taken when pins are placed in cuspal coverage areas, they should extend minimally into the restorative material. To prevent overextension of pins, depth limiting drills, or pin bender to reduce length of pin should be used.

Location of Pin Placement (Figs 21.16 and 21.17)

Following factors should be considered while selecting location of pins
- Knowledge of normal pulp anatomy to avoid pulpal exposure or external tooth perforations

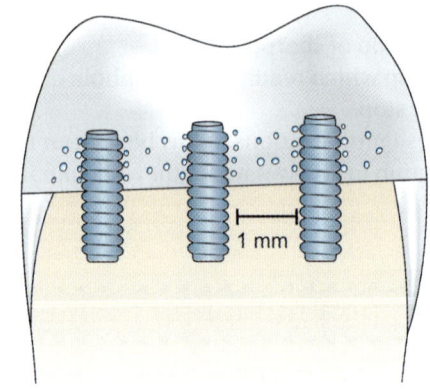

Figure 21.13: Unnecessary use of pins can cause stresses and voids in restoration

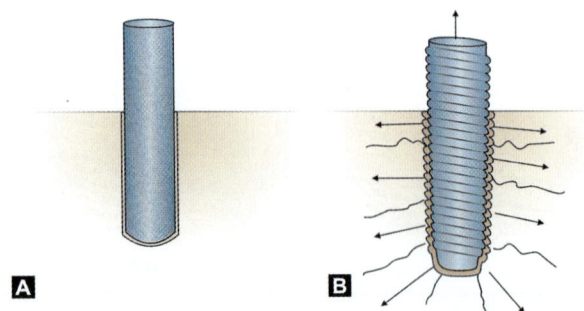

Figures 21.12A and B: If pin size is greater than pin channel it can cause stresses in the dentin (A) Pin diameter less than pin channel; (B) Showing stresses in dentin when pin diameter is more than pin channel

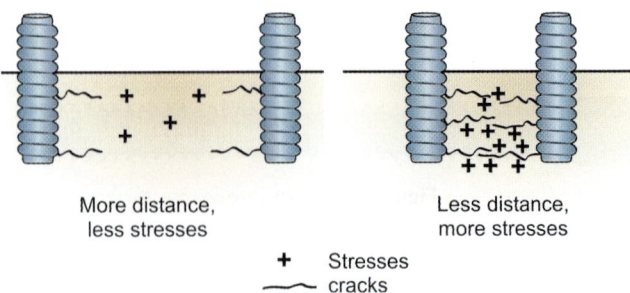

Figure 21.14: Lesser is the interpin distance, more are the stresses generated

- Avoid placing the pins directly under occlusal loads as this may weaken the amalgam
- Pinhole should be at least 0.5 mm inside the dentin to reduce the chances for crazing of the tooth structure
- Pinholes should be located on a flat surface, which should be perpendicular to the direction of the pinhole or on less angular surface
- When more than two pinholes are planned, they should be placed at different levels to prevent the stresses in same transverse plane of the tooth
- If two or more pins are to be placed, interpin distance should be such that it results in lower levels of stresses in dentin and restorative material around pins can be manipulated
- There should be at least 1 mm of sound dentin around circumference of the pin (**Figs 21.18A and B**).
- There should be at least 1 mm of dentin between pulp and the pin to avoid pulpal damage

- Intermittent radiographic monitoring should be done constantly, while preparing and placing the pins.

Preparation of Pinhole

- Pinholes are prepared using twist drills (**Figs 21.19A and B**). Commonly used drill for pinhole preparation is Kodex drill (**Fig. 21.20**). The drill is made of a high-speed steel that is swaged into aluminium shank. Drill performs cutting when rotated clockwise at slow speed. Suggested speed for drilling is 300 to 500 rpm to 1000 rpm
- Omni-depth gauge is used to measure accurate depth of the pinhole
- Mark the point where pin is supposed to be placed. Penetrate a small round bur (No. ¼) at low speed up

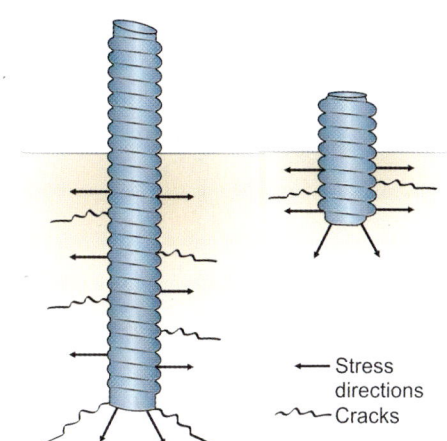

Figure 21.15: More is the pin in the restoration or dentin, more are the stresses

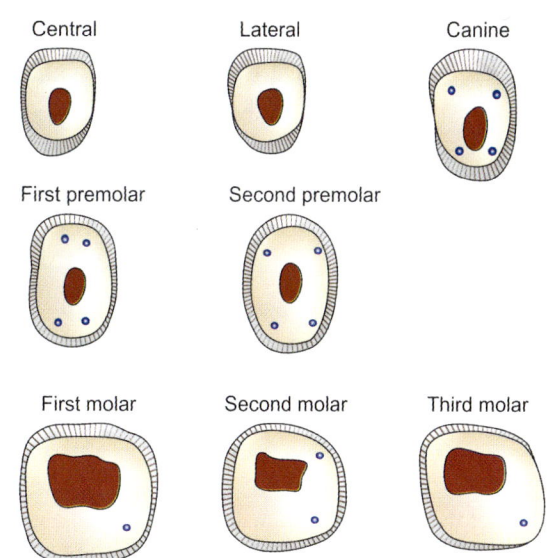

Figure 21.17: Ideal site for pin placement in mandibular teeth

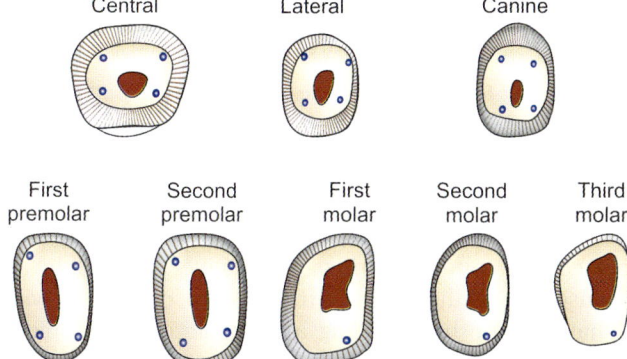

Figure 21.16: Ideal site for pin placement in maxillary teeth

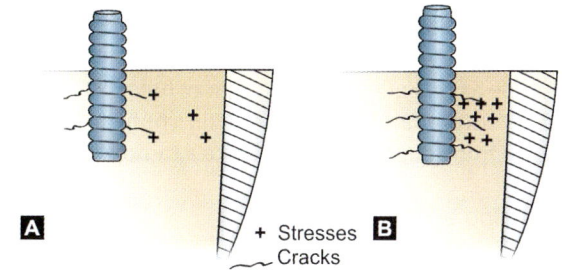

Figures 21.18A and B: (A) There should be at least 1 mm of sound dentin around pin circumference; (B) Lesser dentin present around pin results in more stresses

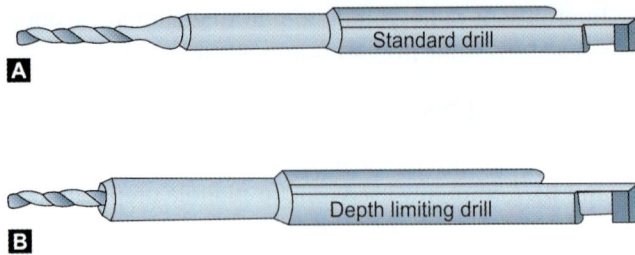

Figures 21.19A and B: Twist drills: (A) Standard drill; (B) Depth limiting drill

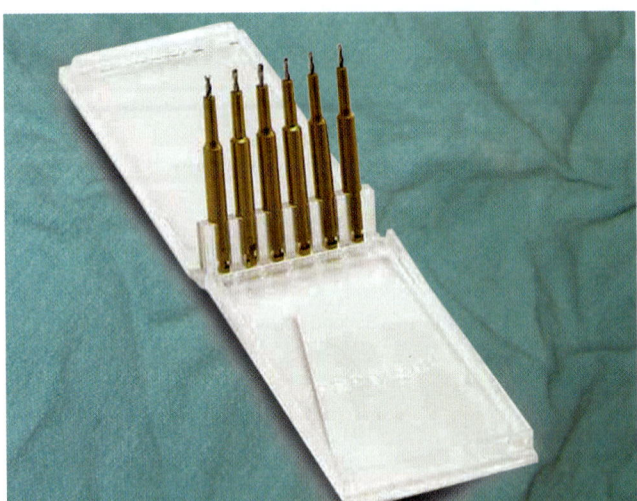

Figure 21.20: Kodex drill

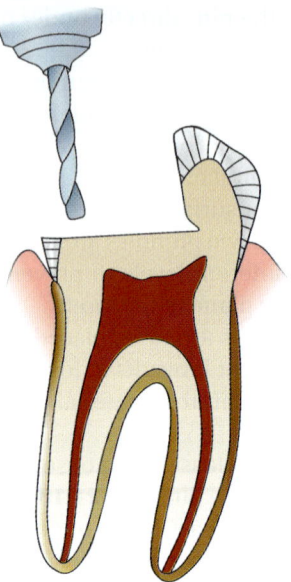

Figure 21.21: Direct the drill towards the desired location of pin placement

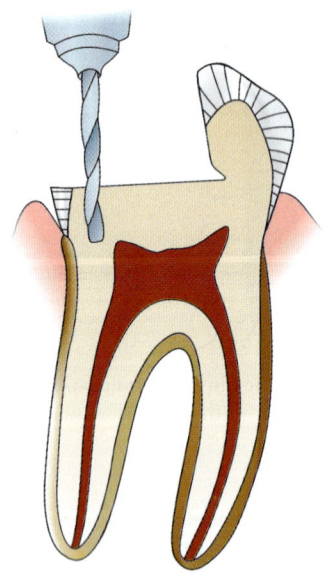

Figure 21.22: Preparation of pinhole

to half of its diameter. This will make pilot hole or lead hole which allows accurate positioning of the twist drill

- Direct the drill towards the desired location of pin placement (**Fig. 21.21**). Drill should be kept continuously moving only in one axis and one direction from the time of insertion till removal to avoid fracture of the drill in the pinhole and over cutting
- While cutting dentin, apply slight pressure (**Fig. 21.22**). During drilling, avoid slanting of the handpiece, or allowing the drill to rotate more at the bottom of the pinhole as this may results in a large hole
- After pin preparation is complete, confirm the depth using Omni-depth gauge and take a radiograph.

Pin Bending and Trimming

Ideally bending and trimming of pin if required should be done before their placement but it is not possible in friction locked and threaded pins. If possible, at least 1.5 mm of the pin should be exposed. At least 1.0 mm of

the space for restorative material around the periphery of the pin and at least 2.0 mm of space occlusal to the pin should be available (**Fig. 21.23**). Often bending is required to facilitate condensation of restorative material in an occlusogingival direction. To trim the pin, cut it short with a sharp fissure bur running in a high-speed handpiece keeping bur perpendicular to the pin. Stabilize the pin with a hemostat while lateral pressure is applied.

Placement of Pin Amalgam Restorations

Carry out the tooth preparation by excavating carious dentin and remove the weakend tooth structure. Prepare facial and lingual walls parallel, pulpal and gingival walls perpendicular to axial wall. Make dovetails, grooves boxes wherever required. Reduce the weakend cusp 1.5 to 2 mm having the shoulder finish. After final preparation, apply base or liner for pulp protection and to prevent postoperative discomfort. Then prepare pinholes for pins to provide resistance and retention. Place pins in the pinholes and prepare coves in the axial wall of the preparation to provide adequate space for amalgam condensation around pins (**Fig. 21.24**).

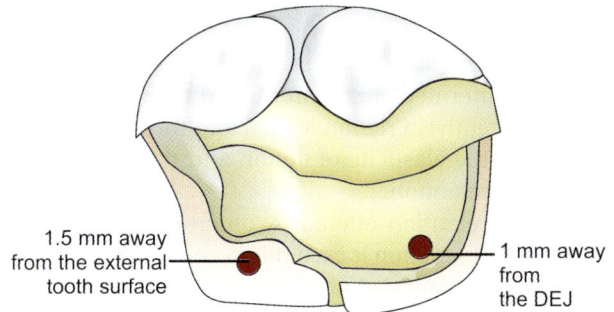

Figure 21.24: Tooth preparation for pin placement

Matrix Placement

In most of the cases, tofflemire retainer and band are used. When tofflemire matrix cannot be used, impression compound-supported copper band matrix or automatrix, which is a retainerless matrix system, can also be used.

Placement of Alloy

Spherical or admixed high copper alloy is preferred for restoration of these teeth because high early compressive strength and excellent clinical performance. Spherical alloys have higher early strength and can be condensed quicker with less pressure so as to have good adaptation of restoration around amalgam when compared with admixed alloys. But admixed alloys are preferred for proximal contacts because of their condensability and long working time which allows sufficient time for condensation, matrix removal and carving of the restoration. First pack and condense the amalgam restoration around pins and then all step areas and proximal box area. Each increment of amalgam is properly condensed to produce a flat surface. Amalgam must be properly condensed around the pins.

Carving of Amalgam

Remove excess of amalgam from the occlusal surface. Use discoid and hollenback carver to develop the anatomy of tooth. Marginal ridge must be at the same height as the adjacent marginal ridge.

Finishing and Polishing Procedure

The objective of polishing is refinement of the margins, development of the contour and smoothening of the surface. Polishing must be done after 24 hours of restoration placement. Round steel finishing bur or small wheel diamond is used to contour the occlusal restoration. Silica or aluminium oxide is applied by prophylactic cup to polish the surface.

FACTORS AFFECTING RETENTION OF PINS IN TOOTH STRUCTURE

Several factors are known to control the retention of pins in tooth structure. These include

Pin Diameter

Within limits, retention is directly proportional to diameter of pin. For example, retention doubles when the diameter of the pin increases from 0.0155 to 0.0190. However, overzealous increase in diameter may decrease amount of dentin and thus weaken the tool.

Pin Number

Within limits, increasing the number of pins increases the retention in dentin.

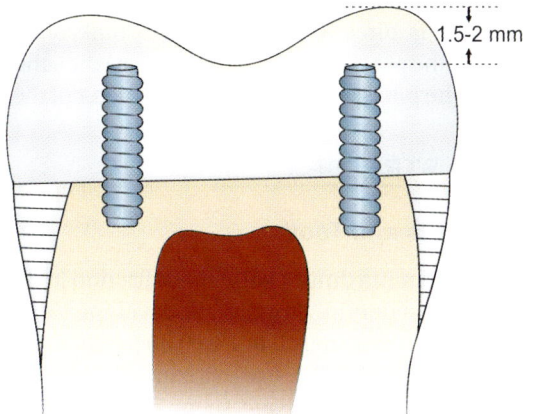

Figure 21.23: At least 1.5-2 mm space for restoration material should be present occlusal to pin

Pin Type

Cemented pins are the least retentive. Friction locked pins show intermediate retention and threaded pins are the most retentive. Friction locked and threaded pins are retained by the elasticity of dentin and this accounts for their higher retention.

Order of retention offered by different pin systems is threaded pins> friction locked pins > cemented pins.

Within the cemented pin type, serrated pins are more retentive than smooth surface pins.

Pin Depth in Dentin

Within limits, increasing the depth of pin in dentin increases the retention.

Cementing Agents

Zinc phosphate cement is more retentive than polycarboxylate and zinc-oxide eugenol cements. Glass ionomer cement is also more retentive. However, varnish reduces the retentive ability of the cemented pins.

Association Between Pin Channel and Pin Circumference

Poor quality in the manufacture of pins can result in problems like mismatch between the pin and drill diameters, variations in the inside diameter and thread shapes of the pins, etc.

Type of Dentin

Young resilient primary dentin offers more retention than secondary dentin.

FACTORS AFFECTING RETENTION OF PINS IN RESTORATIVE MATERIAL

The following factors affect the retention of pins in restoration material:

Pin Length

Within limits, increasing the length of the pin in restorative material increases retention.

Pin Number

Within limits, increasing the number of pins increases retention of the restoration. Excessive increase in the number of pins makes condensation of restorative material difficult and decreases the overall strength.

Pin Diameter

Within limits, retention increases with the increase in diameter of the pin.

Pin Orientation

It also affects retention, for example, pins placed in non-parallel increase retention.

Pin Shape

Retention cleats and square or pear shaped heads on the pins improve retention of pin.

Interpin Distance

Placing pins close to each other (minimum interpin distance 2 mm) increases retention. At distances lesser than 2 mm pin retention is reduced because of the less amount of material present in between the pins and increase in residual stresses in dentin.

Pin Restoration Interphases

An ideal interphases between the pin and material is one which is not interrupted. For example, when gold plated stainless steel pins are to be used with silver amalgam, gold should be pure for mercury to react with it. When silver plated stainless steel pins are used with amalgam, voids are seen at interphase because mercury (of amalgam) reacts with silver plating and dissolving it.

Surface Characteristics

Number of serrations present on the pin surface affect its retention.

Bulk of Material Surrounding the Pin

Pin retention is directly proportional to bulk of material surrounding the pin. Retention is almost lost when the material around the pin is less than half the diameter of the pin.

PINS AND STRESSES

Pins, Stresses and Tooth

Stresses are seen maximum with use of friction locked and threaded pins in dentin. Stresses are developed since pins are inserted into channels 0.001 to 0.004 smaller than the diameter of the pins. If the stresses exceed dentin's plastic limit, craze lines or cracks are seen. These fracture lines can cause pulpal involvement.

Threaded pins show only apical stresses whereas friction locked pins act as wedges which generate lateral stresses, cracked tooth syndrome, gross fractures, loose restorations, etc.

Cemented pins are shown to induce the least stresses, threaded pins induce intermediate stresses and friction locked pins induce the maximum stresses.

Stress tolerance of different types of dentin in a decreasing order is—secondary dentin > sclerosed dentin > tertiary dentin > calcific barrier. Cemented pins are therefore, the only preferred pins in endodontically treated teeth with nonvital dentin.

Pins, Stresses and Restorative Material

Pins did not strengthen or reinforce a restoration but aid in retention of restoration. Neither compressive strength nor transverse/tensile strength of amalgam is improved because of stress concentrations around the pins and cleavage planes set up in the restoration by the arrangement of pins. Pins are likely to reduce the strength of amalgam because of absence of any chemical union between the pin and restorative material at the interface.

FAILURE OF PIN RETAINED RESTORATIONS

The pin retained restoration may fail due to one of the following reasons.

Within the Restoration (Fig. 21.25)

Restoration may fracture, may be because of improper condensation or improper trituration.

Within Pin

Pin fracture may occur because of improper technique during pin placement (**Fig. 21.26**).

Broken pins can occur in following conditions
➡ During bending or if turned more than required in the pinhole
➡ Excessive force is applied while its placement
➡ Pin is rotated despite being fully seated in the pinhole.

Removal of broken pins and drills is difficult. It is best to choose another site about 1.5 mm away from the previous site and leave the broken pin as if it is not interfering in occlusion or condensation of amalgam.

At Pin Restoration Interface

Restoration may pull away from the restoration because of corrosion products at interface (**Fig. 21.27**).

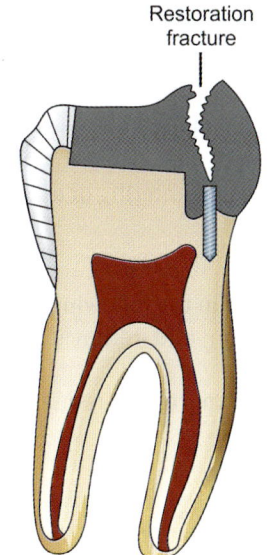

Figure 21.25: Restoration fracture

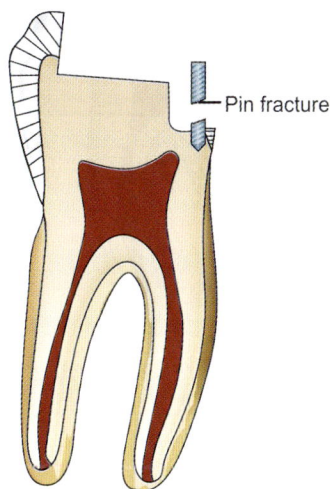

Figure 21.26: Pin fracture

At Pin Tooth Interface

Pin may separate along with restoration because of improper pin tooth joint (**Fig. 21.28**).

Within Tooth

Dentinal fracture (**Fig. 21.29**) can occur because of concentration of internal stresses because of improper selection of pin according to dentin type.

Broken Drills (Fig. 21.30)

Drill can break in the following conditions:
- Drill is stopped before being removed from the pinhole
- Stressed are applied laterally during drilling
- Dull drills are used
- Drill is stopped while entering or exiting from the tooth.

Loose Pins

Loose pins can occur in the following conditions:
- Repeated insertion and removal of drill during pin preparation
- Pin drill is rotated more than required
- Pinhole is too large

- Manufacturer's discrepancy, i.e. poor quality control between pin drill and pin size
- Pin failed to be driven in the pinhole resulting in stripped out or chipping of dentin or enamel.

To stabilize the pin, following can be done:
- Cement the existing pin in place
- Drill another hole of the same diameter 1.5 mm away from the present hole and insert the same pin.

Pulpal Penetration and Periodontal Perforation

Pin placement can also result in pulp and periodontal perforation (**Fig. 21.31**) and this is indicated with sudden

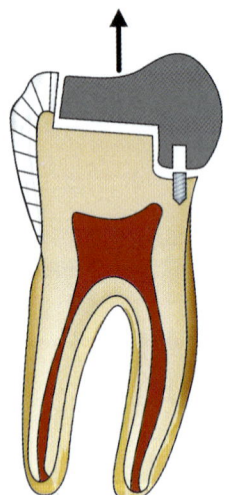

Figure 21.27: Restoration pulled away from the pin

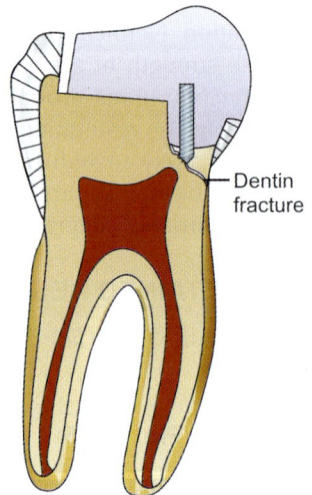

Figure 21.29: Dentin fracture

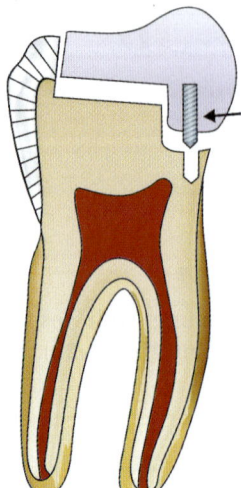

Figure 21.28: Separation of pin along with restoration

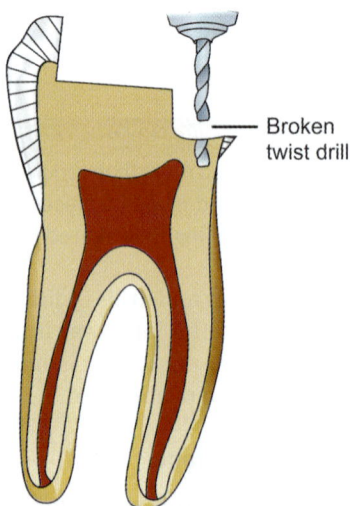

Figure 21.30: Broken twist drill

Pin placement for Maxillary teeth

Tooth	Site for placing pin	Areas to be avoided
Central and lateral incisor	Middle of labial gingival floor Incisal with minimum 2 mm of depth	Middle of lingual gingival floor. Proximolingual floor, with insufficient depth
Canine	Close to labial and lingual proximal part of tooth Incisal, close to incisal angle	Gingival pin close to groove or concavity
First and second premolars	Close to proximobuccal and lingual corner of the tooth	Middle of gingival floor buccally and lingually Mesiogingival floor
First and second molars	Gingival floor close to distolingual part of tooth	Gingival floor mesial to buccal part of tooth Any part of gingival floor occlusal to furcation
Third molar	Because of variable anatomy, pin is placed after radio-graphic evaluation	

Pin placement for Mandibular teeth

Tooth	Site for placing pin	Areas to be avoided
Central and lateral incisor	Because of less thickness of depth, pins are avoided except in teeth where pulp chamber is very much reduced	
Canine	Same as maxillary canine	Same as maxillary canine
First and second premolars	Close to labial and lingual proximal part of the tooth	Middle of gingival floor buccally and lingually
First and second molar	Distolingual portion of gingival floor Distobuccal and mesiolingual part of gingival floor	Mesiobuccal corner of gingival floor
Third molar	Because of variable anatomy, pin is placed after radio-graphic evaluation	

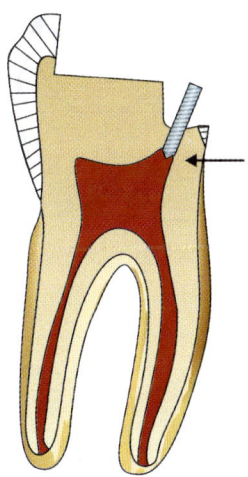

Figure 21.31: Pulp penetration while pin placement (arrow)

bleeding while operating the drill. Bleeding is more abundant if there is periodontal perforation (**Fig. 21.32**).

Penetration or perforation can be verified by radiograph. If pulpal penetration occurs and the tooth is asymptomatic and if very little and fresh bleeding is there, treat it by direct pulp capping and prepare a fresh hole. If tooth has extensive restorations or caries, root canal treatment should be done in case of pulpal exposure.

If periodontal perforation occurs occlusal to the gingival attachment, pin can be cut off and merged with tooth surface then prepare a cast restoration. Another method of management is to remove the pin, enlarge pinhole and restore it with amalgam. If perforation occurs apically, expose the area surgically, remove the bone, enlarge the pinhole and restore it with amalgam or with gold foil if possible.

Heat Generation

Generation of heat can be reduced by using 2.0 depth limiting drill and the smallest possible pin.

Microleakage

Microleakage around cemented pins occurs around whole circumference whereas it is semilunar in shape around threaded pins and friction locked pins. The dead space created by incomplete seating of pins may harbor bacteria and induce pulpal reaction.

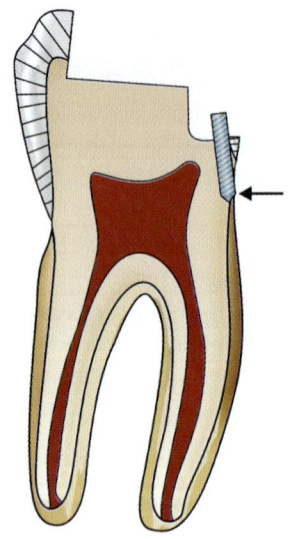

Figure 21.32: Perforation of periodontium (arrow)

PIN AMALGAM FOUNDATION

It is defined as a silver amalgam restorations using pin retention that is to be reduced to provide a core for subsequent cast restoration.

It is indicated for a tooth that is severely broken down and lacks the resistance and retention forms needed for an indirect restoration.

The principles of outline form dictate more conservative preparations for a pin amalgam foundation than for a pin amalgam restoration. The margins need not be extended to self-cleansing areas. However, for a pin amalgam foundation, cavosurface angles can range from 45 to 135° as they are not subjected to direct occlusal forces.

They rely mainly in secondary preparation retention features (pins, slots, coves and proximal retention locks) (**Fig. 21.33**). Minikin size of the pins should be used for the purpose of foundation.

ALTERNATIVES TO PINS FOR ADDITIONAL RETENTION IN AMALGAM RESTORATION

- Amalgapin
- Horizontal pin
- Slot
- Circumferential slot
- Lock.
- *Amalgapin*: Concept of amalgapin was given by Shavell in 1980 to allow amalgam to act as retentive pins. Amalgapins are vertical posts of amalgam anchored in dentin (**Fig. 21.34**). The pits prepared in dentin are shallow and little wider than pinholes and are called

'dentin chambers'. The post formed by amalgam in the dentin chamber is called 'amalgapin'. Dentin chamber is prepared by using inverted cone bur on gingival floor 0.5 mm in dentin with 1 to 2 mm depth and 0.5 to 1 mm width. Amalgapins increase the retention and resistance of complete restoration. They also increase the bulk of amalgam.

- *Horizontal pin*: It was decribed by Burgess. Horizontal pin should be placed 0.5 to 1.00 mm from DEJ. It should not be placed too close to the surface of amalgam restoration.
- *Slot (**Fig. 21.35**)*: Slot is a groove which is placed in the transverse plane. It is placed in dentin. It has 1.0 to 1.5 mm of depth which can be given in occlusal or gingival wall or both. It has four walls and is given all along the width of the occlusal or gingival walls.
- *Circumferential slot*: It is prepared with No. 331/2 inverted cone bur. It increases retention and resistance of the restoration.

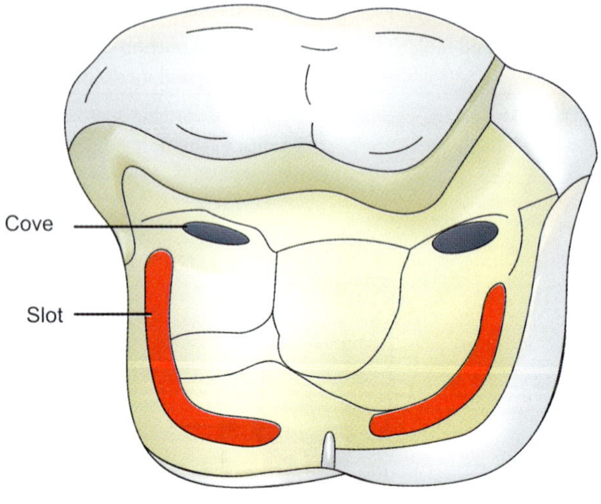

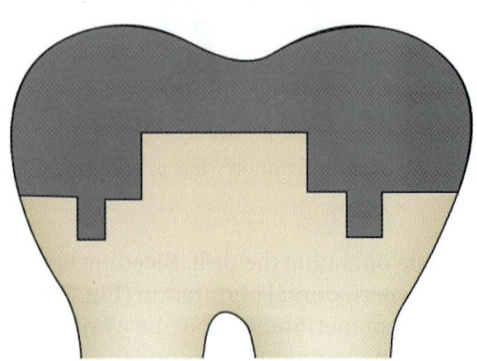

Figure 21.33: Slot and coves placed as secondary retentive features

Figure 21.34: Amalgapin

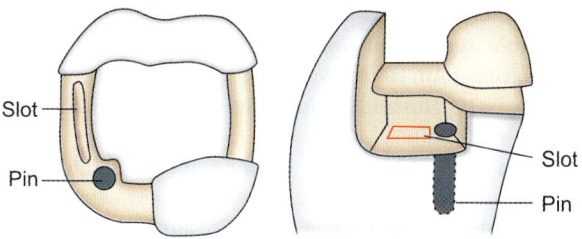

Figure 21.35: Slot and pin for providing secondary retention

- *Lock*: Lock is a groove whose length is in longitudinal plane. It is 0.2 to 0.3 mm wide and 0.5 mm deep into the dentin. It is usually prepared for class II amalgam restoration for increasing resistance and retention form.

 ## Key Points

- A pin retained restoration is defined as any restoration which requires the placement of pin/pins in the dentin in order to provide sufficient retention and resistance form to the restoration.
- Pin amalgam restoration is more conservative than tooth preparation for cast restoration. Pins increase the resistance and retention of the restoration.
- Pin retained restorations are indicated in badly broken teeth, teeth requiring large interproximal restoration, and in extensive class V restoration to strengthen the restoration.
- Pins are contraindicated in patients with occlusal problem, when esthetics is concerned and when direct restoration is not possible because of functional or anatomical considerations.
- Direct pins are generally made of stainless steel and inserted into dentin after this restoration is placed directly over them. Types of direct pins are cemented pins, self-threading pins and friction locked pins.
- Indirect pins are made smaller in size when compared to their pinholes and they constitute an integral part of a cast restoration. These pins are also known as the parallel pins because these pins are placed parallel to each other and also to the path of insertion of the restoration.
- Cemented pins were introduced by Dr Merklay in 1958. For these pins, the prepared pinholes should be 0.025 to 0.05 mm larger than the diameter of the pin. This difference in diameter provides space for cementing media. These are indicated in cases where least stresses or crazing is desired, e.g. endodontically treated teeth.

- Friction locked pins were introduced by Goldstein in 1966. These pins are .001" larger than their pinholes, hence utilize the elasticity of dentin for retention. They are 2 to 3 times more retentive than the cemented pins. These are indicated in vital teeth, and when sufficient amount of dentin is available to surround the pin.
- Self-threading pins were introduces by Going in 1966. These are 0.0015 to 0.004" larger than their pinholes. The pins are retained due to the mechanical grasp of the threads into the dentin. The elastic property of the dentin allows insertion of a threaded pin into a hole of a smaller diameter. They are 3 to 6 times more retentive than the cemented pins. They are indicated in vital teeth, when maximum retention is desired and when sufficient amount of dentin is present.
- Thread mate system is considered superior to other self-threading pins because of its multipurpose designs, better retention and color-coding system for easy identification and use.
- Minikin pin is considered as the pin of choice in grossly decayed posterior teeth because of the risk of dentin crazing, good retention and lesser chances of pulpal and periodontal perforation.
- Minim pin provides less dentinal crazing as compared to regular pins. It is used in cases where pinholes for minikin was over-prepared.
- Regular is the largest diameter pin. It is rarely used because of more stress and crazing around pins.
- Increase in diameter of pin offers more retention but large sized pins can result in more stresses in dentin.
- One pin per missing cusp and one pin for each missing axial line angle should be used.
- When more than two pins are to be used, interpin distance should be such that it prevents concentration of stresses in dentin and allows space for insertion of restorative material between pins. For cemented pins, it is 2 mm, for friction lock, it is 4 mm and for threaded pins, it is 5 mm.
- Pin extension of 2 mm into dentin and amalgam provide maximum required retention. To prevent overextension of pins, depth limiting drills, or pin bender to reduce length of pin should be used.
- Within limits, retention is directly proportional to diameter of pin. For example, retention doubles when the diameter of the pin increases from 0.0155 to 0.0190". However, overzealous increase in diameter may decrease amount of dentin and thus weaken the tool.
- Young resilient primary dentin offers more retention to the pins than secondary dentin.

- Placing pins close to each other (minimum interpin distance 2 mm) increases retention. At distances lesser than 2 mm pin retention is reduced because of the less amount of material present in between the pins and increase in residual stresses in dentin.
- Stresses are seen maximum with use of friction locked and threaded pins in dentin. Stresses are developed since pins are inserted into channels 0.001 to 0.004 smaller than the diameter of the pins. If the stresses exceed dentin's plastic limit, craze lines or cracks are seen. These fracture lines can cause pulpal involvement.
- Cemented pins are shown to induce the least stresses, threaded pins induce intermediate stresses and friction locked pins induce the maximum stresses.
- Stress tolerance of different types of dentin in a decreasing order is: secondary dentin > sclerosed dentin > tertiary dentin > calcific barrier. Cemented pins are therefore, the only preferred pins in endodontically treated teeth with nonvital dentin.
- Pin amalgam foundation is defined as a silver amalgam restorations using pin retention that is to be reduced to provide a core for subsequent cast restoration. It is indicated for a tooth that is severely broken down and lacks the resistance and retention forms needed for an indirect restoration.
- Concept of amalgapins was given by Shavell in 1980 to allow amalgam to act as retentive pins. Amalgapins are vertical posts of amalgam anchored in dentin.

QUESTIONS

1. What are indications and contraindications of pin retained restorations? Explain different pin types.
2. Short notes on
   a. TMS pins
   b. Pin design
   c. Principles of pin placement.
3. Explain in detail the factors affecting retention pins in tooth structure and restorative material.
4. What are different causes of failure of pin retained restorations?

BIBLIOGRAPHY

1. Abraham G, Baum L. Intentional implantation of pins into the dental pulp. J South Cal Dent Assoc. 1972;40:914-20.
2. Bailey JH. Retention design for amalgam restorations: pins versus slots. J Prosthet Dent. 1991;65:71-4.
3. Barkmeier WW, Cooley RL. Self-shearing retentive pins: a laboratory evaluation of pin channel penetration before shearing. J Am Dent Assoc. 1979;99:476-9.
4. Burgess JO. Horizontal pins. A Study of tooth reinforcement. JPD. 1985;53:317.
5. Butchart DGM, Grieve AR, Kamel JH. Retention of composite restorations. A comparison between a threaded pin and a dentin bonding agent. Br Dent J. 1988;165:217.
6. Butchart DGM, Llyord CH. The retention of self threading pin embedded in various restorative materials. Dent Mater. 1986;2:125.
7. Butchart DGM. A new self-threading dentin pin. Br Dent J. 1983;155:83.
8. Caputo AA, Standlee JP. Pins and posts—why, when and how. Dent Clin North Am. 1976;20:299-311.
9. Cecconi BT, Asgar K. Pins in amalgam: a study of reinforcement. JPD. 1971;26:159.
10. Chan CC, Chan KC. The retentive strength of slots with different width and depth versus pins. JPD. 1987;58:552.
11. Chan CC, Chan KC. The retentive strength of slots with different width and depth versus pins. J Prosthet Dent. 1987;58:552-7.
12. Chan KC. A proposed retentive pin. JPD. 1978;40:166.
13. Christensen GJ. Achieving optimum retention for restoration. J Am Dent Assoc. 2004;135:1143-5.
14. Collard EW, Caputo AA, Standlee JP. Rationale for pin retained amalgam restorations. Dent Clin North Am. 1970;14:43.
15. Cookey RL, Barkmeier WW. Temperature rise in the pulp chamber caused by twist drills. JPD. 1980;44:426.
16. Covey DA, Moon PC. Shear bond strength of amalgam to dentin. Am J Dent. 1991;4:19.
17. Currens WE, Korostoff E, Von Fraunhofer JA. Penetration of shearing and nonshearing pins into dentin. JPD. 1980;44:430.
18. Dawson PE. Pin retained amalgam. Dent Clin North Am. 1970;14:63.
19. Dilts WE, Coury TL. A conservative approach to the placement of retentive pins. Dent Clin North Am. 1976;20:397.
20. Dilts WE, Coury TL. Conservative approach to the placement of retentive pins. Dent Clin North Am. 1976;20:397-402.
21. Dilts WE, et al. Retention of self-threading pins. J Can Dent Assoc. 1981;47:119-20.
22. Duperon DF, Kasloff Z. Effects of three types of pins on compressive strength of dental amalgam. J Canad Dent Assoc. 1971;11:422.
23. Eames WB, Solly MJ. Five threaded pins compared for insertion and retention. Oper Dent. 1980;5:66-71.
24. Evans JR, Wetz Jh. The pin-amalgam restoration, Part 1-A Review. JPD. 1977;37:37.
25. Fischer GM, et al. Amalgam retention using pins, boxes and Amalgambond. Am J Dent. 1993;6:173-5.

26. Going RE. Pin-retained amalgam. J Am Dent Assoc. 1966;73:619-24.

27. Goldstein PM. Retention pins are friction locked without use of cement. JADA. 1966;73:1106.

28. Gourley JV. Favorable locations for pins in molars. Oper Dent. 1980;5:2-6.

29. Moffa JP, et al. Pins—a comparison of their retentive properties. J Am Dent Assoc. 1969;78:529-35.

30. Mondelli J, Vieira DF. The strength of Class II amalgam restorations with and without pins. J Prosthet Dent. 1972;28:179-88.

31. Outhwaite WC, et al. Pin vs. slot retention in extensive amalgam restorations. J Prosthet Dent. 1979;41:396-400.

32. Robbins JW, et al. Retention and resistance features for complex amalgam restorations. J Am Dent Assoc. 1989;118:437-42.

33. Van Nieuwenhuysen JP, Vreven J. Maillefer and TMS pins compared for retention and penetration. Oper Dent. 1985;10:150.

34. Wacker DR, Baum L. Retentive pins: their use and misuse. Dent Clin North Am. 1985;29:327-40.

35. Webb LE, Staka WF, Phillips CL. Tooth crazing associated with threaded pins: A three dimensional model. JPD. 1989;61:624.

36. Wilson PR, Bione HM. Ultrasonic removal of dentin pins. J Dent. 1993;21:285.

22

CHAPTER

Direct Filling Gold

Chapter Outline

INTRODUCTION

Gold is one of the oldest dental material, having been used for restoration of teeth. Earlier Phoenicians used gold wire to splint the teeth, and afterwards, the Etruscans and then the Romans initiated making fixed bridges from gold strip. The use of gold in restorations remains considerable today, however, with an increasingly wide range of alternative materials available in dentistry, there is choice for a replacement of older and discolored fillings.

In spite of these restorative materials, direct filling gold restoration still forms one of the best of the available restorative material, especially if:
- It is used only where indicated
- Proper manipulation is done
- Clinician has skill of using it.

If foil is not used correctly, it is one of the least successful restoration. Direct gold is pure 24 karat gold that can be compacted directly into the tooth preparations. Direct filling gold restorations are used to restore class I, II, III, V and class VI preparations. If done properly, direct gold restoration lasts for a lifetime, because of outstanding biocompatibility of gold in oral environment and its excellent marginal integrity.

PROPERTIES OF DIRECT FILLING GOLD

- Cohesiveness, this property depends on purity of gold. The best gold for restorations is about 999 parts in 1000 parts of pure gold.
- Softness during manipulation.
- Malleability (Gold be reduced by beating to 1/250,000 of an inch in thickness).

- Ductility (One grain of pure gold may be drawn into a wire nearly five hundred feet long).
- Hardness in bulk form—Brinell hardness number (BHN) is 25, which rises to 75 during condensation.
- Tensile strength is 19,000 psi which rises to 32,000 psi.
- Coefficient of thermal expansion is $14.4 \times 10^{-6}/°C$. This is almost similar to that of tooth.
- Gold has high thermal conductivity.
- Density of pure gold is 19.3 g/cm^3, while that of compacted gold is 16.5 gm per cubic centimeter.

Advantages of direct filling gold
⇢ Gold foil restorations can last for a long-time if correctly done
⇢ The resilience of dentin and the adaptability of gold allow an almost perfect seal between the tooth structure and gold
⇢ Malleability of gold makes it possible to add gold in very small amounts that are building up the filling
⇢ Malleability also provides permanent self sealing margins
⇢ Being a noble metal, gold does not tarnish and corrode
⇢ Coefficient of thermal expansion near to the dentin, so shows no shrinkage or expansion when placed in preparation
⇢ No cementing medium is required for restoration
⇢ Gold can withstand compressive forces even in thin layers, hence deeper tooth preparation is not required
⇢ If properly polished, the gold surface is plaque repulsive
⇢ It does not cause tooth discoloration because of good adaptation to the preparation margins and walls
⇢ The direct gold restoration is insoluble in oral fluids
⇢ The polish and smoothness lasts longer when compared with other restorative materials
⇢ Direct filling gold restorations are compatible with pulp and the periodontium. Direct gold restoration can be completed in one appointment.

Disadvantages of direct filling gold
⇢ These restorations are technique sensitive, and to achieve excellence, great skill, patience and time is required
⇢ Improper placement of gold foil can damage the pulp or periodontal tissues
⇢ The welding technique, with or without a mallet, can do pulpal trauma
⇢ Because of the high thermal conductivity of gold, larger restoration can increase sensitivity
⇢ A larger restoration is very difficult to finish and polish
⇢ Gold foil is more expensive than any other restoration material. The cost is high because of the high cost of gold and the work involved.

⇢ Multiple restorations are hectic because it is time-consuming.
⇢ It cannot be placed where esthetics is required.
⇢ Gold is indicated only when the lesion is small in size and present in nonstress bearing areas.
⇢ If gold and amalgam fillings are right next to each other, "galvanic shock" can occur. It happens when interactions between the metals and saliva result in electric current. This can result in discomfort to patient.

INDICATIONS FOR THE USE OF DIRECT FILLING GOLD

The extent of the decay is perhaps the principal guiding factor in determining indication of use of direct filling gold restoration. Foil is best adapted to teeth in which the lesion has just started, and to most of the eroded areas present on the labial and buccal surfaces of teeth.

According to Stibbs, the smaller the lesion, greater the indication, and greater the need for conservative permanent restorations, the greater the indication for foil.

For Restoration of Tooth Preparations

Direct filling gold restorations are indicated for incipient or early lesions, small in size and present in nonstress bearing areas. These may include:

- Small Class I preparations of all teeth
- Class II preparations with minimal proximal caries of premolars and on mesial surface of molars
- Class III preparations of all teeth specially when esthetics is not important.
- Class V preparations of all teeth
- Class VI preparations of teeth where high occlusal stress is not present.

Erosion

Direct filling gold restoration are done for small erosions on all the surfaces of premolars, canines and incisors where esthetics concern is limited.

To Repair Margins

It is used to repair endodontic openings in gold crowns or for gold crown margins, onlays and inlays.

For Hypoplastic Defect

Direct filling gold is used for hypoplastic or other defects on the facial or lingual areas

CONTRAINDICATIONS FOR THE USE OF DIRECT FILLING GOLD

Direct gold fillings are contraindicated in the following conditions:

Young Patients

It is not desirable to do direct filling gold restoration in young patient because:
- It is time consuming
- Periodontal membranes and alveolar processes do not offer the resistance to the hand pressure and mallet blows, necessary to insure a well-condensed mass of gold.

Limited Accessibility

It makes the manipulation of gold difficult so defies its use.

Size of the Lesion

If large amount of tooth is destroyed, it is not indicated to use direct filling gold.

Poor Periodontal Condition

In patients suffering from pyorrhea to the degree that they have lost considerable of the alveolar process and supporting tissues gold is not indicated.

Temperament of Patient

Some nervous patients are unable to tolerate the continuous blow of the mallet, direct filling gold restoration should not be used in them.

Handicapped Patient

Since these restorations are time consuming, they should not be used in such patients.

Esthetics

If esthetics is of prime importance, direct filling gold is not indicated.

Heavy Occlusal Stresses

Since gold cannot withstand heavy ooclusal forces, it should be avoided in stress bearing areas.

Prognosis of the Tooth

It should not be used when expected functional period of the tooth is not more than two years.

TYPES OF GOLD

Types of gold
➡ Gold foil
◆ Sheets
◆ Gold foil cylinder
◆ Gold pellets
◆ Platinized gold foil
◆ Corrugated foil
◆ Laminated foil.
➡ Crystalline gold or electrolytic precipitated
◆ Mat gold
◆ Mat foil
◆ Electraloy.
➡ Powdered gold.

Gold Foil

Gold foil or fibrous gold is one of the oldest form. Gold leaf used in ornamentation, is about 0.1 μm thick. Dental foil (the usual No 4) is six times thicker, in other words 0.6 μm. Gold is available in several types:
- Sheets
- Gold foil cylinder
- Gold pellets
- Platinized gold foil
- Corrugated gold foil
- Laminated gold foil.

Preparation of Different Forms of Gold Foil

Sheets: The gold foil is made by beating pure gold into thin sheets of size 10 × 10 cm (4 × 4 inch). The thickness of gold foil is 1.5 micron. The foils are supplied in books which are separated by thin paper pages. Each book has approximately twelve gold foils.

The book of gold, either 1/8 or 1/10 of an ounce is ruled off and sizes are cut with the help of scissors. The book is divided into such sizes that represent 1/2, 1/4, 1/8, 1/16, 1/32, 1/64 and 1/128 of a sheet of gold that weighs 4 grains (**Fig. 22.1**). No. 3 gold foil weighs 3 gm, No. 2 gold foil weighs 2 gm, No. 4 gold foil weighs 4 gm, and so on. Since size of 4 × 4 inch foil is too large for its use in preparation. Before insertion into the tooth preparation, it is cut, rolled into ropes, cylinders or pellet.

Gold foil cylinder: To make cylinder, one end of the ribbon is held with an instrument and rolled again and again until the other end is reached. Gold cylinders commonly used are of 1/4 and 1/8 of a sheet of gold. Cylinders of noncohesive gold are used in the noncohesive state and never annealed for cohesive use.

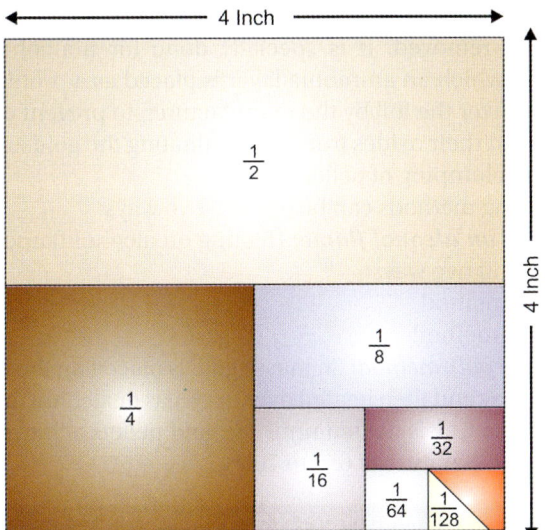

Figure 22.1: Sections of gold foil sheet

Gold pellets: They can be mechanical or handmade. To make gold pellets, a piece of foil is placed in the palm of the hand and each end is folded towards the center, this incompletely formed pellet is now transferred between the thumb and index finger and pellet is formed. Pellets are usually made cohesive before use. The rolled pellets can be stored in a gold foil box along with a cotton dipped in 18 percent ammonia (to prevent the formation of oxide layer on the pellets).

Platinized gold foil: This type of foil is made up by sandwiching a sheet of platinum between two sheets of gold foil and then hammered until a final platinized gold is formed. The platinum content in foil is 15 percent. Purpose of adding platinum to gold is to increase the hardness of the restoration. This allows its use in areas of high occlusal stress like cusp tips and incisal edge of anterior teeth.

Corrugated gold foil: Corrugated gold foil is made by putting thin sheets of paper in between gold foil sheets, and igniting them. Paper in between the gold foil gets burnt and charred leading to corrugated appearance of gold foil. Gold foil remains unharmed.

Laminated gold foil: Laminated gold foil is manufactured by combination of 2 to 3 gold foils together. It is more resistant to applied forces. It is based on the concept that a gold foil is usually formed from ingot with pattern of crystals running in specific direction. When two or more gold foils with crystals running in different direction are combined together, the resultant product is laminated gold foils.

Crystalline Gold or Electrolytic Precipitate

Types of Crystalline Gold

Crystalline, sponge, or mat gold: This is electrolytically precipitated type of gold. In other words, Mat is a microcrystalline form, produced by electrodeposition. To prepare mat gold, pure gold is sintered in an oven, which helps to hold the crystalline gold together. Then gold is heated slightly below the melting point so that partial fusion occurs. The resultant material is a spongy structure of loosely aligned crystals, the crystals being dendritic or fern like in shape about 0.1 mm long. These crystals adapt very nicely to the preparation walls. Mat gold can be used plain or sandwiched in gold foil to make it easier to handle. This is available in the form of strips which are cut by dental surgeon into desired size. This form of gold is mainly used for building up of the internal restoration because it can be easily compacted and adapted to internal walls of the preparation. It is not recommended on the external surface of the restoration.

Mat foil: Mat foil is formed, by placing the mat gold in between No. 3 or 4 gold foil and the resultant product is sintered by heating just below the melting point of gold. Then, it is cut into strips of different sizes. Advantage of using gold sheets is that gold sheets hold the crystalline gold together when it is placed and condensed into the prepared tooth. But since it is difficult to condense, it is not used nowadays. In restoring with mat gold foil, there is no need of veneering the restoration with gold foil.

Electraloy: It is the newest form of direct filling gold. It is produced by electrolytic precipitation method. In this, hardness and strength of gold is increased by adding minute quantities such as calcium (0.1%) without lessening desirable manipulative characteristics. Then this crystalline structure is sandwiched between two gold foils to improve handling properties. Electraloy on condensation produces the hardest direct filling gold surface.

Powdered Gold or Gold-dent or Granular Gold

These irregularly shaped, precondensed pellets or clusters of particles are prepared by combination of comminution, chemical precipitation and atomization from the molten state. The average particle size is of 15 microns. The atomized particles with organic matrix are wrapped in No. 2 or No. 3 foil. Each pellet consists of approximately 10 times more gold than a gold foil pellet. With some of the preparations, a volatile liquid is provided to act as a carrying medium to convey the pellet to the preparation. Before condensation, matrix is burned away so that only pure gold is left. Powdered gold does not require very sharp line angles and point angles in preparation because they are difficult to handle.

FORMS OF GOLD

Pure gold can be supplied in two forms
1. Cohesive
2. Noncohesive.

Cohesive Form

Gold can be easily welded together at room temperature if surface is clean. Ideally the manufacture should supply gold foil free from surface contaminants to place it in preparation. But it is difficult to maintain cohesive form of gold as some gases such as carbonic acid, phosphoric acid and hydrogen sulfide gets accumulated during storage.

But some manufacturers, supply the gold foil with protective gas film like ammonia. This film has two advantages:
1. Can be easily removed by degassing
2. Minimizes the absorption of other gases.

But before placing in preparation, one should always take care to degass the gold so as to make it free from any surface contaminants.

Noncohesive Form

This is that form of gold which loses its cohesive property. This is because of absorption of contaminants like sulphur, phosphorus and iron on the surface which can not be removed by heating. Noncohesive forms have lesser strength and hardness as compared to cohesive forms.

STORAGE OF GOLD

The gold is packed into the preparation under pressure so that during welding, minimal porosity occurs. Welding occurs by cohesion of pure clean surfaces of gold due to metallic bonding. For successful welding, the gold must be in a cohesive state. Gold foil comes in both cohesive and noncohesive state. These gases must be removed from the surface of gold by a process called degassing or annealing before gold is compressed into preparation.

Degassing or Annealing

In degassing, there is removal of the volatile protective coating present on pure gold surface. So we can say that degassing is a better term instead of annealing because in annealing, along with the removal of surface contamination, internal stress relief or recrystallization also occurs

but in degassing procedure only surface contamination is to be removed. It is specially done for noncohesive gold, in which an ammonia layer is placed as a protective coating over the foil by the manufacturer, to prevent other gases and their oxides from contaminating the gold and to prevent clumping of pellets.

Degassing methods can be done in two ways:

Heating on alcohol flame: Heating on alcohol flame can be done in two ways:
1. Bulk method
2. Piece method.

   1. *In bulk method:* En masse gold is placed on the mica tray and then heated over open gas or alcohol flame. The tray is heated until the gold pellets achieve the temperature of 650 to 700ºC.

The advantages of bulk method are
→ Takes less time
→ Convenient.

The disadvantages of bulk method are
→ Sticking of gold pieces
→ Unused gold may be left and it can be wasted due to contamination
→ Risk of overheating.

   2. *In piece method:* The gold foil is held with an instrument and heated over clean blue flame of absolute or 90 percent ethyl alcohol. Temperature of the flame is about 1300°F. The heating is done until the gold becomes a dull red.

Advantages of piece method
→ Less wastage
→ Desired size of piece can be selected.

Disadvantage of piece method
→ Time consuming

Electric annealer: In electric annealer, the gold is heated for 10 minutes at 850°F and then it is cooled for placing in the prepared tooth.

One must take care to prevent overheating or the underheating as both of these can hamper qualities of gold.

Consequences of overheating
→ Contamination from tray can occur
→ Metal may melt
→ Particles may adhere to each other instead of the surfaces
→ It becomes brittle
→ Difficult to select the annealed goldpiece that will fit into the cavity.

PRINCIPLES OF TOOTH PREPARATIONS FOR DIRECT FILLING GOLD RESTORATIONS

There are a few fundamental prerequisites to be considered to produce a lifetime gold restoration:
- Proper tooth preparation
- Dry operative field
- Proper manipulation of the material
- Protection of supporting and surrounding tissues.

Complying with these requisites is facilitated by:
- Rubberdam supplemented by a suitable retractor
- Set of good cutting instruments, hand and rotary
- Good tooth preparation that satisfies the requirements laid down by GV Black
- Tooth preparation according to type of gold used. Since gold is available in different forms for use viz; foil in pellet, sheet, or laminated form, mat, powdered gold. Each requires a specific technique if optimum results are to be achieved
- Instruments for preparing and compacting or condensing the gold
- Instruments for proper finishing of the restoration.

Preparation design for gold has following requisites:
- Controlled outline form to meet the patient's needs in terms of esthetics
- Mechanical retention
- Accessibility for proper instrumentation
- Pulp protection.

Operating field: The operative field can be best isolated by rubberdam. Most commonly used mechanical retractor is the Ferrier No. 212, since it is less traumatic to the tissues.

Class I Tooth Preparation

The outline form for class I tooth preparation involves removal of all carious fissures and extending them to the point of immunity. It is similar to amalgam except that, because of presence of sharp corners it looks more angular (**Fig. 22.2**).

The external walls of the preparation must be parallel with respect to each other. In case of extensive occlusal preparations, proximal walls (Mesial and distal walls) can be slightly diverging.

If additional retention is required in the dentin, undercuts are placed in the facial and lingual walls by small

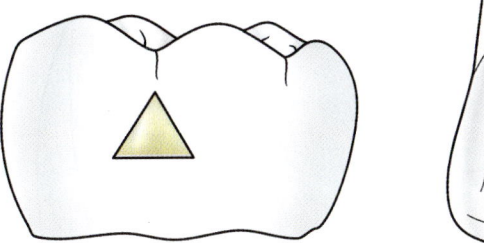

Figure 22.2: Tooth preparation for direct filling gold should have sharp corners and angular in looks

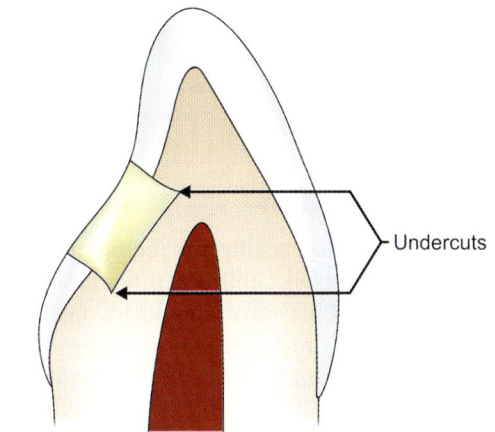

Figure 22.3: Undercuts in dentin are prepared for additional retention

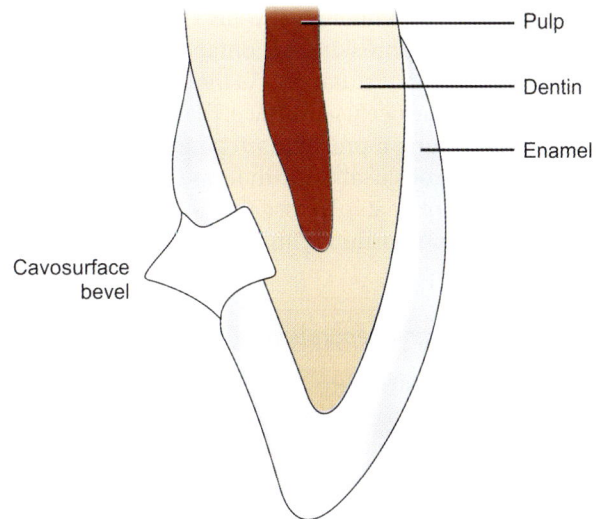

Figure 22.4: Bevels should be placed at carosurface margins

inverted cone bur (**Fig. 22.3**). Small bevels may be placed at the cavosurface margins for easy finishing (**Fig. 22.4**). This allows 40 to 45° metal margins which can be burnished against the tooth surface (**Figs 22.5A and B**).

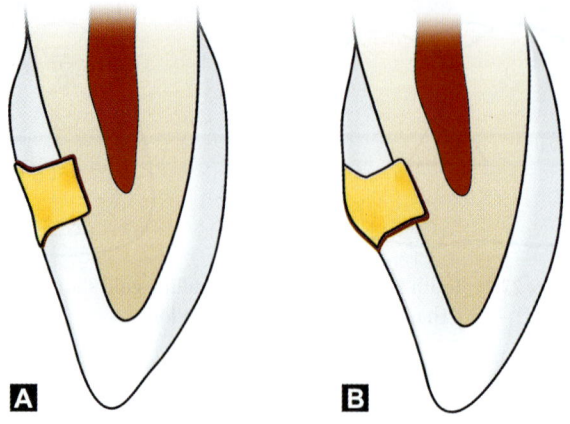

Figures 22.5A and B: (A) Proper bevelling and lingual concavity of class I restoration; (B) Improper overextended lingual contour

Class II Tooth Preparation

Class II preparations especially for incipient caries are ideal situations for gold foil. Outline of preparation is made using no.330 bur. Outline form should involve adjacent deep pits and fissures. The deep pits and fissures which are separated by at least 1 mm thick healthy dentin are filled as separate preparations. The proximal box for direct filling gold is made as done in amalgam except that it is more conservative in nature. The most susceptible areas for the secondary caries are the lingo-gingival and buccogingival angles. Buccal and lingual walls should be extended to contact area but breaking of contact is not required as in case of amalgam restoration. As the lingual and buccal walls approach the occlusal surface, they converge toward each other, forming a proximal preparation that is much narrower at the occlusal third than at the gingival third. This forms a narrow step across the occlusal surface that blends in fine proportion with the proximal part of the preparation.

Advantages of this Preparation

• Saving of tooth structure
• Protection of pulp horns
• Preservation of tooth strength.

The gingival margin should be just cervical to the contact areas. Retention grooves may be placed in dentin of the proximal and gingival walls. Retention is provided by sharp line angles and point angles.

Class III Tooth Preparation

For making class III preparation, at least 0.25 mm tooth separation is made.

For class III preparation, various designs like Ferrier design, Loma Linda design, Ingraham design, Lund and Baum design and Woodbury design have been suggested. Out of these, most commonly used design for tooth preparation is Ferrier design because of its advantages in conserving the tooth structure, providing accessibility for restoration and esthetics.

1. *Ferrier design:* Teeth are separated using rubber dam preferably six anterior teeth are included to avoid interference by the rubberdam. This is indicated for small carious lesions present on distal surfaces of anterior teeth, which are less visible.

In this the carious lesion is approached from the labial surface with a small round bur (no. ½). After this, a small inverted cone bur is used and a cut is made from the center labially and then lingually to outline and roughly form the gingival wall (**Figs 22.6A and B**). This also creates the linguogingival cavosurface angle in the form of a shoulder. The preparation is made triangular in shape. The incisal margin is kept cervical to the contact area to provide access for instrumentation. It meets the facial and lingual margins in a smooth curve. The 6½-2½-9 hoe is used both as a chisel and as a hoe to plane the preparation walls and establish the remainder of the outline form (**Figs 22.7A and B**). The resistance, retention and convenience form is made using the same instrument, by removal of the carious dentin and finishing of the enamel wall. Angle former is used to accentuate point angles and axiogingival line angle (**Figs 22.8A and B**).

The axial wall is made flat in all the directions and is about 0.5 mm deep into dentin. The axial wall provides resistance form. Linguoincisal curve provide convenience for condensation of gold. All enamel margins are slightly beveled to remove only overhanging

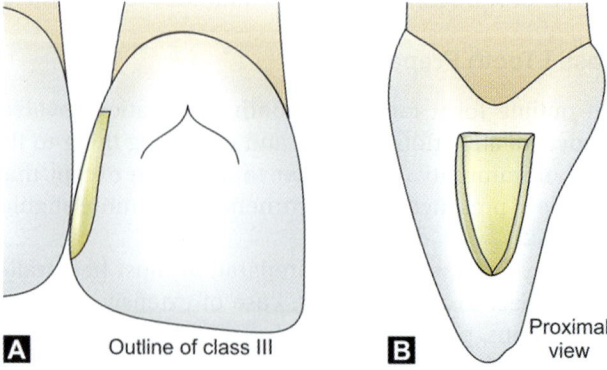

Figures 22.6A and B: (A) Outline of class III preparation; (B) Proximal view of class III tooth preparation

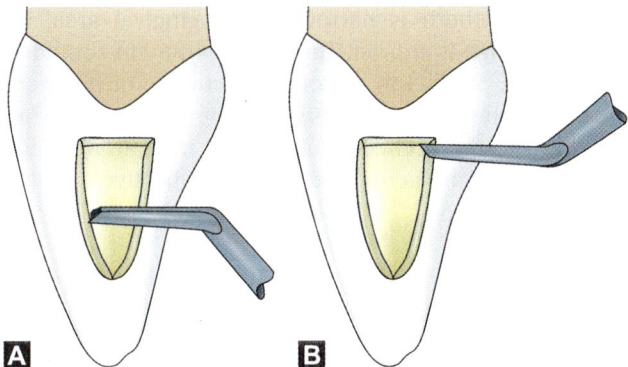

Figures 22.7A and B: Hoe is used to plane the preparation walls

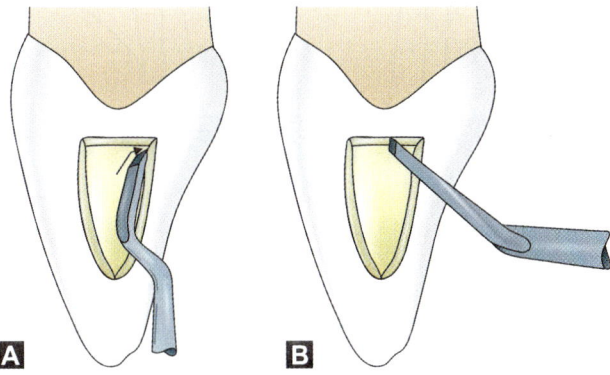

Figures 22.8A and B: Angle former is used to accentuate: (A) Point angles and to form; (B) Acute axiogingival line angle

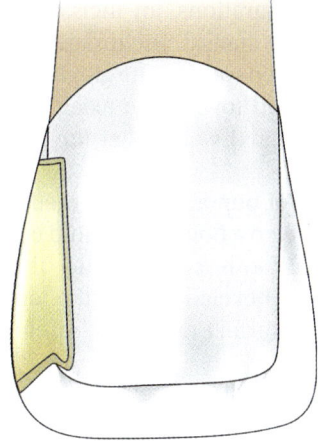

Figure 22.9: Completed class III tooth preparation

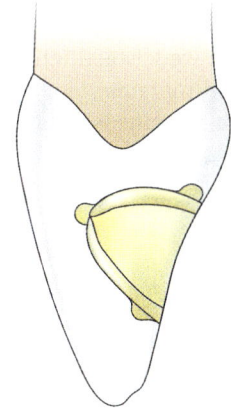

Figure 22.10: Class III tooth preparation showing retention points

unsupported enamel rods. The inward sloping dentin of the gingival wall, the incisal undercut in the dentin, sharp line angles and point angles provide retention.

Salient features of this preparation (Fig. 22.9)

- The labial outline form is straight line
- Labiogingival angle is placed under the free gingiva
- On the incisal third it presents a curve
- The lingual outline form closely follows the labial and meets the gingival in a square and sharp angle, forming "gingival shoulder"
- The gingival outline form is cut straight across at right angles to the long axis of the tooth
- Gingival cavosurface angle meets the labial in a definite angle.

2. *Loma linda design:* This design is used in cases where:
   - Lingual marginal ridge is involved
   - Facial surface has to be preserved
   - Esthetics is most important.

   In this method, access is made through lingual approach. Cavosurface angle is not beveled. For retention small grooves are made in three opposite directions (**Fig. 22.10**).

3. *Ingraham design:* This preparation is indicated when:
   - There is incipient proximal lesion
   - Esthetic is most important
   - Patient has low caries susceptibility
   - Oral hygiene is good.

   The shape of the preparation is parallelogram which is confined to the contact area. In this, lesion is approached from the lingual side with a inverted cone bur. To make the point angles, angle formers are used.

Class IV Tooth Preparation

Indications of using direct filling gold in class IV preparations:
- Bite is favorable
- Sufficient thickness of the incisal edge to permit a step.

In class IV preparations, an incisal or lingual step is substituted for the incisal anchorage that is used in a simple proximal preparation. The gingival wall is the same, but may be inclined toward the axial wall more acutely. The labial and lingual walls meet the axial wall at right angles.

With the help of bur, a step is formed by cutting away the lingual enamel to a point that would occupy the incisal two thirds of the tooth mesiodistally. The labial enamel wall of the step is beveled toward the labial cavosurface angle. All the cavosurface angles are carefully beveled.

Class V Tooth Preparation

The outline form of the class V preparation for direct gold is trapezoidal in shape (**Fig. 22.11**). The preparation is extended well out to the mesial and distal angles of the tooth, somewhat beyond the lesion. The outline form is obtained by the use of a small inverted cone bur (**Figs 22.12A to D**). Preparation is finished with a 6 ½-2 ½-9 hoe (**Fig. 22.13**) and wedelstaedt chisel is used to refine the occlusal wall and margins (**Fig. 22.14**). If beveling of gingival cavosurface margins is indicated, it is done with the help of chisel (**Fig. 22.15**).

Since the tooth is narrow in the gingival area, the gingival outline is shorter. The occlusal margin should be straight and parallel to the occlusal surface of the teeth. The mesial and distal margins should be straight and when they meet at the occlusal and gingival margin, the angle formed should be acute and obtuse respectively. In the

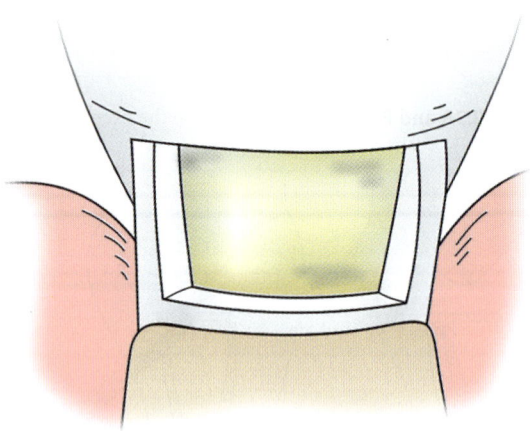

Figure 22.11: Outline form of class V tooth preparation

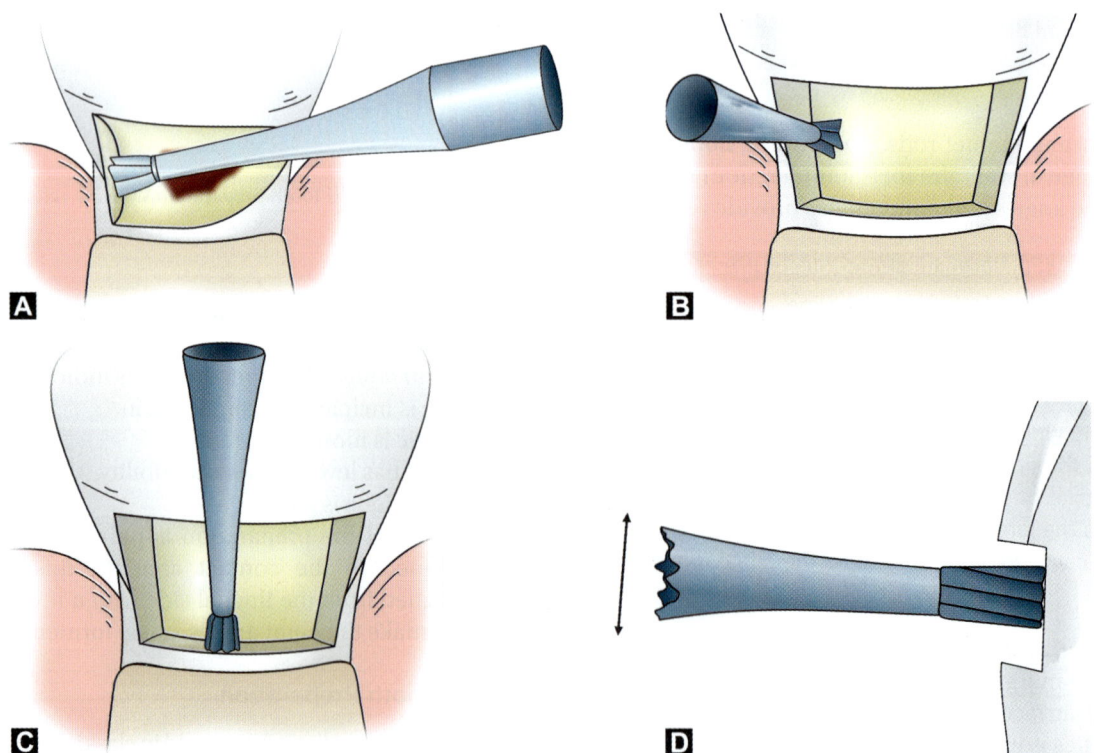

Figures 22.12A to D: (A) Penetration of inverted cone bur for class V tooth preparation; (B) Forming incisal wall; (C) Forming gingival wall; (D) Establishing initial axial wall depth, using end of the bur

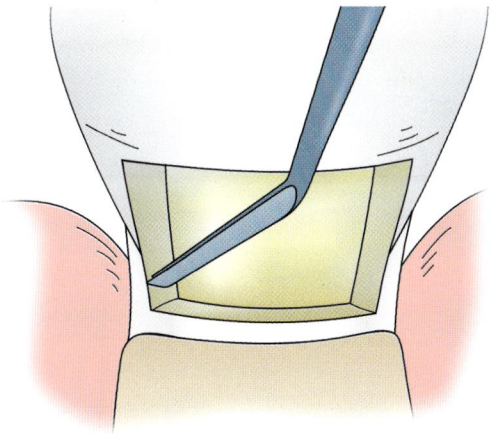

Figure 22.13: Hoe is used to plane the preparation walls

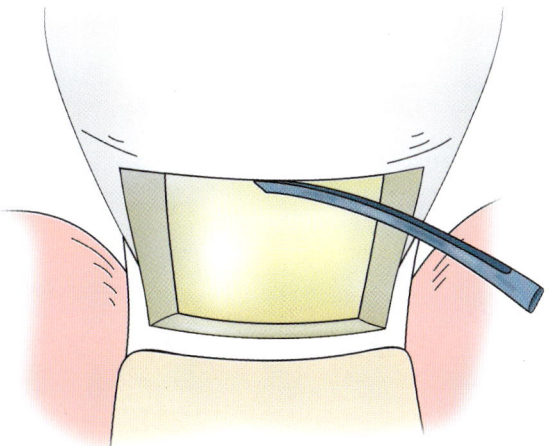

Figure 22.14: Wedelstaedt chisel is used to refine occlusal wall

outline form, the angles should be sharp and well defined. Retention is provided by convergence of the occlusal and gingival walls, acute axiogingival line angle (**Fig. 22.16**).

Variations in Class V Preparation (Figs 22.17A to D)

When caries in upper incisors are near the gingivalline, the curvature of the gum tissue would make a straight gingival wall unpleasant. In these cases, curve the gingival and incisal wall to follow the gum line (**Figs 22.17A and B**).

The incisal outline may be modified to follow the contour of the soft tissue mesiodistally when caries extends occlusally.

Sometimes fine chalky lines runup the mesial and distal angles of the labial surfaces of the tooth into the embrasures much farther than in the normal preparation. In these cases, curvature of the occlusal or incisal wall is made to include these lines without cutting too much of the tooth structure in the middle third area (**Figs 22.17C and D**).

STEPS OF DIRECT FILLING GOLD RESTORATION

Steps of direct filling gold restoration
⟹ Building of restoration
⟹ Paving of restoration
⟹ Compaction of restoration
⟹ Finishing of restoration:
◆ Burnishing
◆ Contouring
◆ Polishing
◆ Final burnishing.

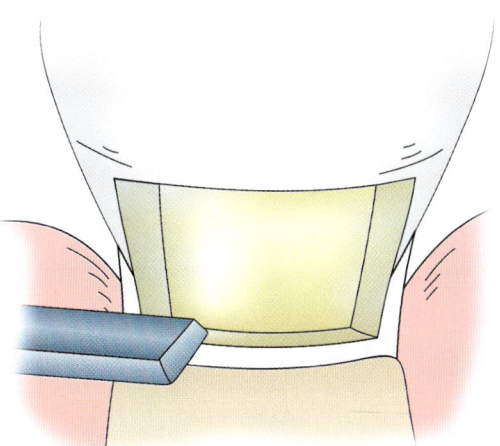

Figure 22.15: Preparation of gingival cavosurface margins using chisel

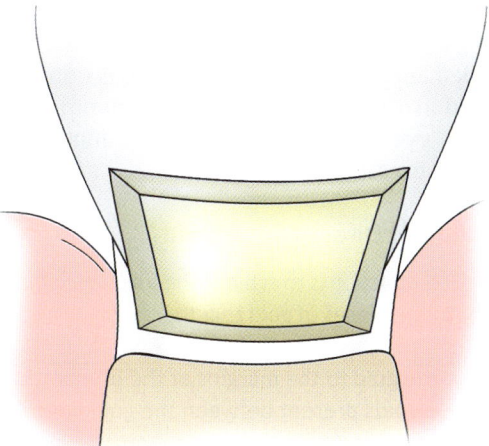

Figure 22.16: Completed class V tooth preparation

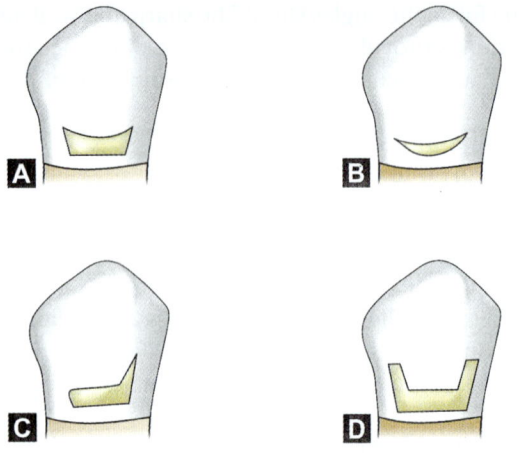

Figures 22.17A to D: Modifications of class V preparation for direct filling gold (A) Curved incisal outline to display less of gold; (B) Cresent shaped preparation with curved incisal and gingival outlines to have aesthetic look; (C) Normal trapezoidal shape of preparation with unilateral extension; (D) Normal trapezoidal shaped preparation with bilateral extensions

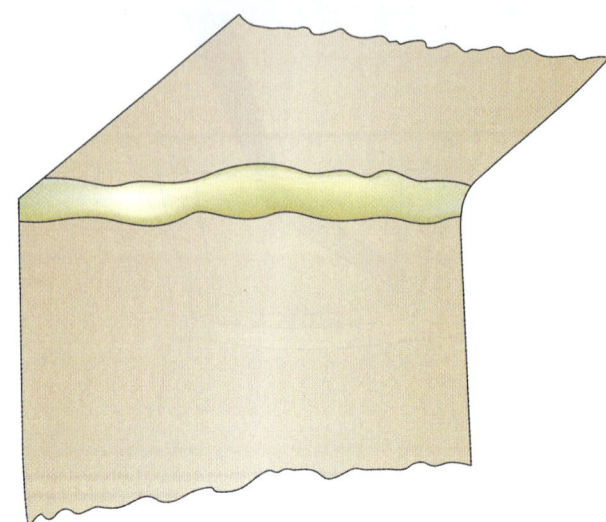

Figure 22.18: Tie formation

Building of Restoration

Gold is placed in the preparation in the form of three step build up. These are:

1. *Tie formation:* In this, two opposite starting points are filled with gold so as to form a tie which acts as a foundation for gold restoration (**Fig. 22.18**).
2. *Wall Banking:* In this, each wall is build from its floor or axial wall to the cavosurface margin (**Fig. 22.19**). It should be performed in other walls also simultaneously.
3. *Formation of shoulder:* This is made by joining two opposite walls with the help of direct filling gold (**Fig. 22.20**).

Paving of Restoration

A controlled amount of excess is built up is done to allow for restoration of normal contour and a smooth surface. In other words, every part of the cavosurface angle should be covered with excess gold.

Compaction of Direct Filling Gold

The aim of compaction is to achieve the following objectives:
- To cohere the pieces of gold together to make a cohesive mass
- To adapt the gold to the margins of the preparation
- To remove voids present between the gold pieces
- To increase the strength the restoration
- To increase the hardness by cold working.

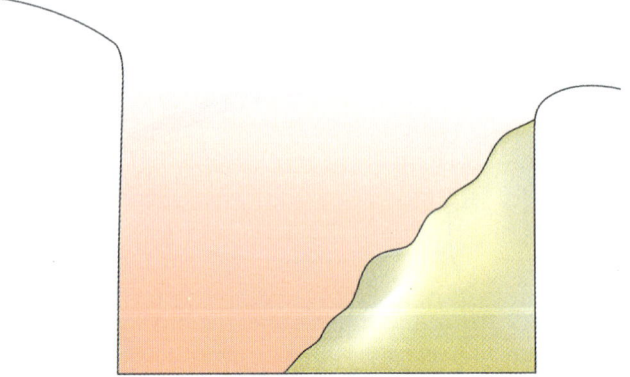

Figure 22.19: Wall banking

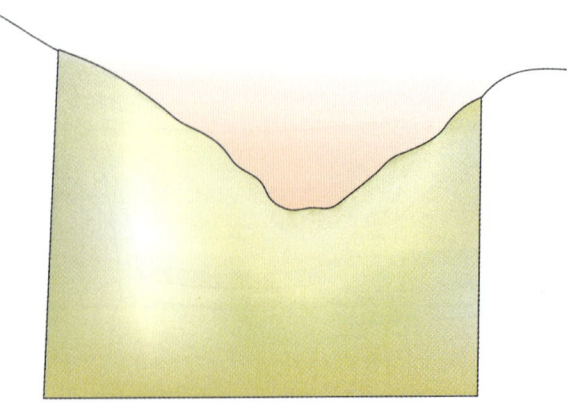

Figure 22.20: Formation of shoulder

Compaction of Gold Depends upon Following Factors

Compacting instrument: Compaction of gold can be done either by hand pressure, hand mallet, pneumatic mallet, automatic mallet, or electromallet. In hand condensation, gold is packed into the prepared tooth in the right direction with the help of condenser. The end of the condenser shank is blunt to receive blows from the mallet and it is about 15 cm in length.

In *hand mallet method*, gold is condensed by tapping mallet.

In *automatic mallet*, programed force is applied which is controlled by a spring present inside the mallet. When the desired force is attained the spring is released.

In *pneumatic condenser* compaction strokes are controlled by a rheostat attached to an electric motor. The condensation pressure is controlled by a button present on the back of handpiece. Condenser consists of working tip and a shank of about 2.5 cm and it fits in the malleting handpiece.

Electromallet compaction of gold is most efficient way of condensing gold. Here the vibrating condenser head is used to compact the gold.

While compaction of the gold, most important factors are the direction, amount, and pattern of application of the compacting force.

Direction: Compacting force should be such that it takes the advantage of property of gold to flow under pressure, in the direction of the force. The handle of the condenser should be at about 45° to preparation wall (**Fig. 22.21**).

Amount of force: Different types of condenser nibs are available like round (0.4 to 0.55 mm in diameter), rectangular (1 × 1.3 mm) or parallelogram shaped (0.5 × 1 mm). Common to all working ends are the pyramidal serrations so as to avoid slipping of the gold while compaction. Shank of the condenser can be straight, curved, monoangled or offset.

Under the constant malleting force if the nib area is small, greater pressure is applied per square cm, because area of a circle is directly proportional to the square of the diameter. If the diameter of the nib is doubled, the compaction force per square cm is decreased by four times.

Pattern of using force: It is important to step the condenser in a controlled pattern (**Fig. 22.22**). It has been seen that overlapping, one-half the diameter of the working end produces the finest restoration. This results in uniform compaction and a dense mass, optimal flow of metal, and sealing of preparation walls.

A goldpiece is placed in the initiating point which is generally in the corner of the preparation (**Fig. 22.23**). Malleting is

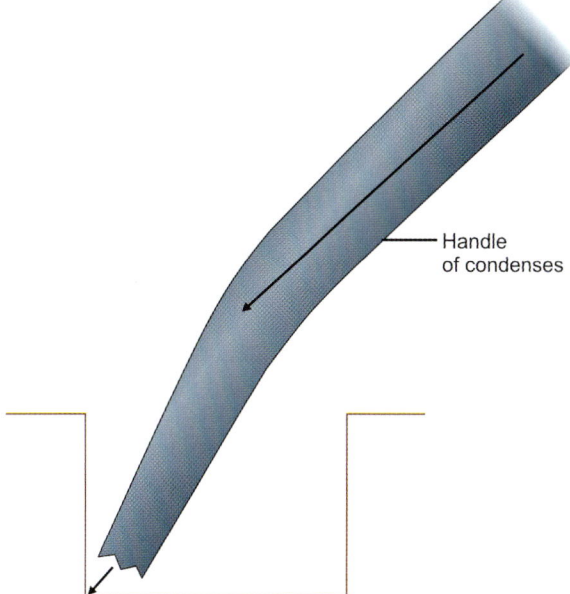

Figure 22.21: Handle of condenser should always be 45° to preparation wall

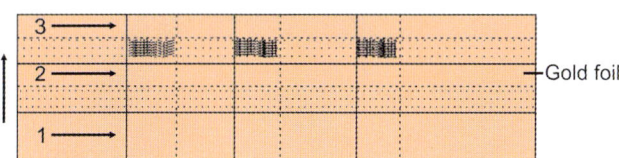

Figure 22.22: Stepping of one half of diameter of working end results in uniform compaction of gold

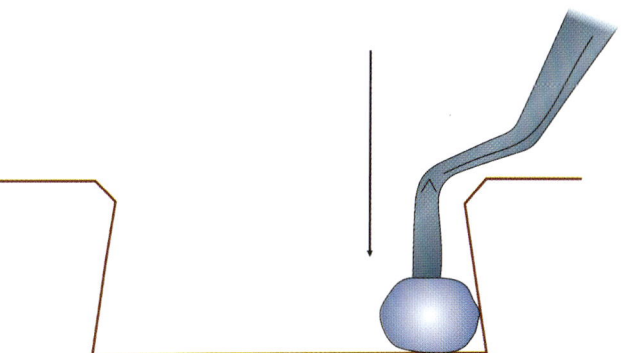

Figure 22.23: First goldpiece is placed in the corner of the prepared tooth

started using the condenser in the center of the mass. Force of condensation should be 45° to preparation walls and floor for maximum adaptation of gold to the preparation (**Fig.**

22.24). To the already condensed gold, force of condensation should be 90 degrees, this prevents the displacement of already condensed goldpieces (**Fig. 22.25**). Condensation is done with rocking motion of the instrument from the plane, perpendicular to the plane of the wall (**Fig. 22.26**). During condensation, as the condenser is moved towards periphery, each succeeding step of the condenser should overlap the half of the previous step. This is called as "stepping" (**Fig. 22.27**). Stepping helps in maximum adaptation of the gold to the preparation walls and reduction in number of voids. In spite of careful compaction, some void spaces may occur in the compacted gold and along the preparation walls. This is called bridging. Bridging should be minimum for a successful restoration.

Each type of gold requires different technique for manipulation. For example, if mat or powdered gold 'is compacted in the same manner as foil, there are chances of getting incomplete sealing of preparation walls, and incomplete compaction of the gold. For mat gold,

condensers with a slightly larger face and finer serrations give better results. For powdered or granular pellets, heavy pressure is required for malleting and they need to be opened up in the preparation before compaction begins, to minimize voids in the mass.

Finishing of Restoration

Burnishing (Fig. 22.28)

The first step in finishing of the gold restoration is burnishing. A specially designed Spratley burnisher is moved with pressure over the restoration to close the voids.

Contouring

- Since there is excess of restoration built up to allow normal contour, this excess restoration is removed with very sharp knives, files and abrasive stones (**Fig. 22.29**).
- Marginal excess can be removed using gold foil carver (**Fig. 22.30**).

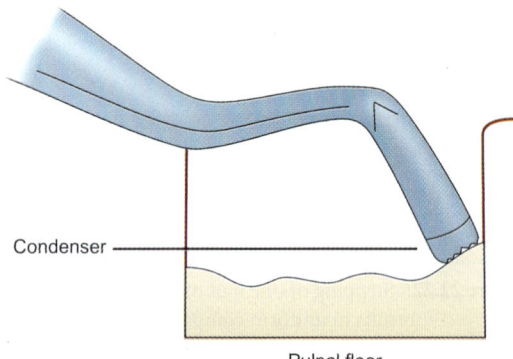

Figure 22.24: Condensing gold holding condenser at 45° angle to the preparation walls

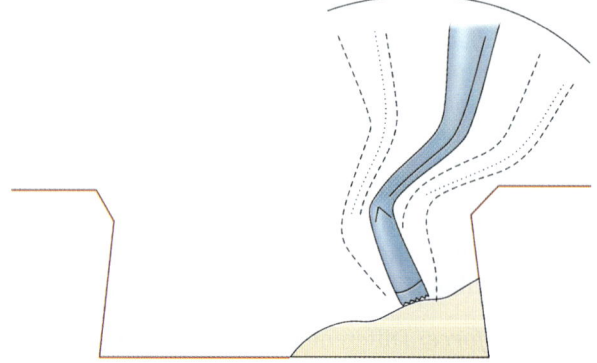

Figure 22.26: Rocking motion of the instrument for compaction of gold

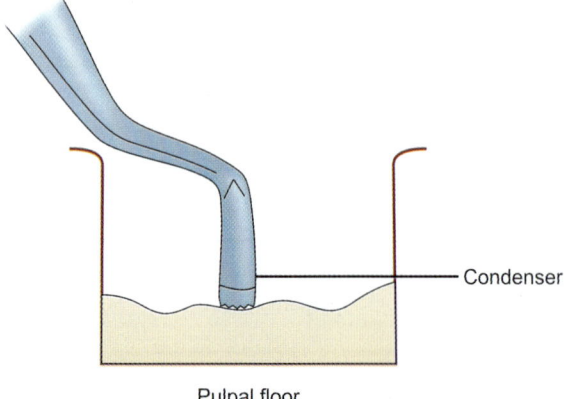

Figure 22.25: Force of condensation at 90° angle to the previously condensed gold

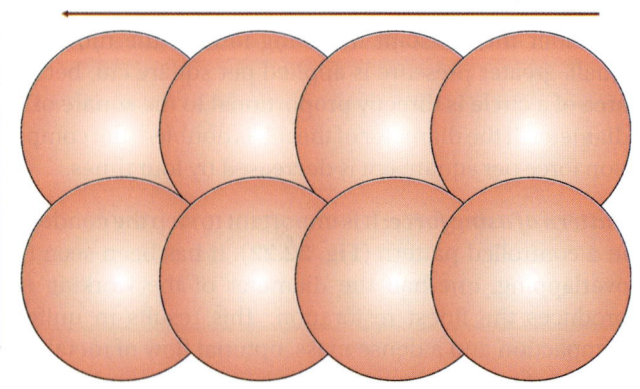

Figure 22.27: Stepping during gold condensation

- Smoothening of the restoration is done by disks with light pressure. Care must be taken while disking to not cut into the surface of the tooth. Careless finishing can also injure the adjoining soft tissues.

Polishing

- The fine garnet disks and cuttle disks are moved from the metal to the tooth for final finishing. To prevent the temperature elevation in the restoration, one must use lubricants and air coolants.
- For polishing, silica, pumice or metallic oxide compounds can be used. For final polish, a satin finish is preferable to a high gloss.

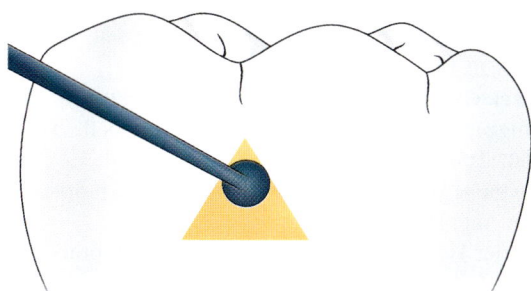

Figure 22.28: Burnisher is moved on the gold restoration to close the voids

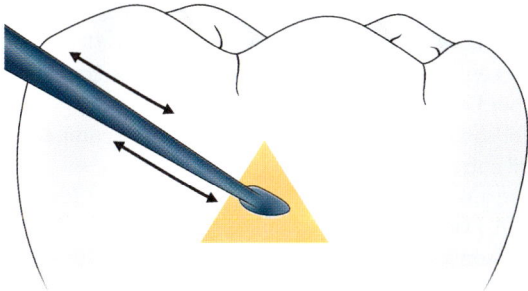

Figure 22.29: Contouring of gold restoration using gold file

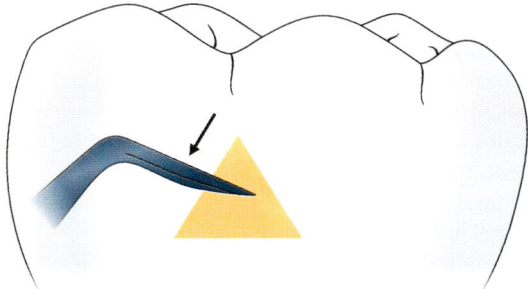

Figure 22.30: Marginal excess is removed using carver

Final Burnishing

Final burnishing is done to make the surface of the restoration shiny smooth free of voids.

Advantages of finishing and polishing
➡ Polished restorations do not tarnish or corrode in oral fluids
➡ They promote the health of the gingival tissue which is in contact with the restoration
➡ Polished restoration minimizes reflection of the light rays and creates a more esthetic and harmonious end result.

FUTURE OF GOLD IN DENTISTRY

The historical development work on use of gold in operative dentistry has provided a wide range of gold-based dental alloys. If requirements like function, esthetics, biocompatibility, longevity, and ease of manufacture are considered, the optimum material for dental restorations is high gold alloy. However, attention is also increasing on the alternative materials because of its technique sensitivity, high cost and less esthetics.

 Key Points

- According to Stibbs, the smaller the lesion the greater the indication and greater the need for conservative permanent restorations, the greater the indication for foil.
- Direct filling gold restoration is not indicated in young patient, poor accessibility, large size of lesion, and if esthetics is not required.
- Gold foil or fibrous gold is one of the oldest form.
- The gold foil is made by beating pure gold into thin sheets of size 10 × 10 cm (4 × 4 inch). The thickness of gold foil is 1.5 micron. The foils are supplied in books which are separated by thin paper pages. Each book has approximately twelve gold foils.
- Platinized gold foil is made up by sandwiching a sheet of platinum between two sheets of gold foil and then hammered until a final platinized gold is formed. Purpose of adding platinum to gold is to increase the hardness of the restoration.
- To prepare mat gold, pure gold is sintered in an oven, which helps to hold the crystalline gold together. Then gold is heated slightly below the melting point so that partial fusion occurs. The resultant material is a spongy structure of loosely aligned crystals, the crystals being dendritic or fern like in shape about 0.1 mm long.
- Electraloy is produced by electrolytic precipitation method. In this hardness and strength of gold is in-

creased by adding calcium (0.1%). Then this crystalline structure is sandwiched between two gold foils to improve handling properties.

- Noncohesive form of gold is that form which loses its cohesive property. This is because of absorption of contaminants like sulphur, phosphorus and iron on the surface which can not be removed by heating. Noncohesive forms have lesser strength and hardness as compared to cohesive forms.

- In degassing of gold, there is removal of the volatile protective coating present on pure gold surface. Degassing is a better term instead of annealing because in annealing, along with the removal of surface contamination, internal stress relief or recrystallization also occurs but in degassing procedure only surface contamination is to be removed.

- For class III preparation, various designs like Ferrier design, Loma Linda design, Ingraham design, Lund and Baum design and Woodbury design have been suggested. Out of these, most commonly used design for tooth preparation is Ferrier design because of its advantages in conserving the tooth structure, providing accessibility for restoration and esthetics.

- While compaction of the gold, most important factors are the direction, amount, and pattern of application of the compacting force. Compacting force should be such that it takes the advantage of property of gold to flow under pressure, in the direction of the force. The handle of the condenser should be at about 45° to preparation wall.

- Pattern of compacting force should be such that each succeeding step of the condenser should overlap the half of the previous step. This is called as "stepping".

- Stepping helps in maximum adaptation of the gold to the preparation walls and reduction in number of voids.

- Each type of gold requires different technique for manipulation. For example, if mat or powdered gold is compacted in the same manner as foil, there are chances of getting incomplete sealing of preparation walls, and incomplete compaction of the gold. For mat gold, condensers with a slightly larger face and finer serrations give better results. For powdered or granular pellets, heavy pressure is required for malleting and they need to be opened up in the preparation before compaction begins, to minimize voids in the mass.

QUESTIONS

1. What are the properties and indications of direct filling gold (DFG)?

2. Short notes on:
   a. Gold foil
   b. Degassing/Annealing of gold
   c. Steps of direct filling gold restoration.

3. Write various stages and steps of tooth preparation according to modern concept. Describe in brief class V tooth preparation for gold foil.

BIBLIOGRAPHY

1. Alperstein KS, Yearwood L, Boston D, E-Z Gold. The new Goldent. Oper Dent. 1996;21:36.
2. Baum L. Gold foil (filling gold) in dental practice. DCNA. 1965.p.109.
3. Baum L. Gold foil (filling golds) in dental practice. Dent Clin North Am. 1965.p.199.
4. Baum L. Gold foil. Oper Dent. 1984;9:42.
5. Birkett GH. Is there a future for gold foil. Oper Dent. 1985;20:41.
6. Black GV. The nature of blows and the relation of size of plugger points force as used in filling teeth. Dent Rev. 1907;21:499.
7. Dwinelle WH. Crystalline gold, its varieties, properties, and use. Am J Dent. 1855;5:249.
8. Ferrier WI. The use of gold foil in general practice. J Am Dent Assoc. 1941;28:691.
9. Ferrier WI. The use of gold foil in general practice. JADA. 1941; 28:691.
10. Ferrier WI. Treatment of proximal cavities in anterior teeth with gold foil. J Am Dent Assoc. 1934;21:571.
11. Germain HAST Jr, Rusz JE Jr. Restoring Class 6 abrasion/erosion lesions with direct gold. Oper Dent. 1996;21:49.
12. Harken BJ. Gold foil. A potential practice builder in the 80s. Oper Dent. 1985;10:28.
13. Hodson JT, Stibbs GD. Structural density of compacted gold foil and mat gold. J Dent Res. 1962;41:339.
14. Hodson JT. Structure and properties of gold foil and mat gold. J Dent Res. 1963;42:575.
15. Hodson JT. Structure and properties of gold foil and mat gold. JDR. 1963;42:575.
16. Lund MR, Baum L. Powered gold as a restorative material. J Prosthet Dent. 1963;13:1151.
17. Smith GE, et al. A study of the degree of adaptation possible in retention holes, convenience points and point angles in Class III cavity preparations. J Am Acad Gold Foil Oper. 1972;15:13.
18. Smith GE. Condenser selection for pure gold compaction. J Am Acad Gold Foil Oper. 1972;15:53.
19. Stibbs GD. Direct golds in dental restorative therapy. Oper Dent. 1980;5:107.
20. Thomas JJ, et al. Effects of gold foil condensation on human dental pulp. J Am Dent Assoc. 1969;78:788.
21. Trueman WH. An essay upon the relative advantage of crystallized gold and gold foil as a material for filling teeth. Dent Cosmos. 1868;10:128.

Cast Metal Restorations

Chapter Outline

INTRODUCTION

Various defects of teeth can be restored using different restorative materials like amalgam, composite resins, direct filling gold and cast metal restorative materials. Each material has its own indications, contraindications, advantages and disadvantages. When sufficient tooth structure is not present for the support of restoration, then cast metal restorations are indicated. Cast metal restorations were introduced in dentistry about 100 years ago and soon they became a subject of great interest to both dentists and patients. Most advantageous properties of gold alloy is its malleability, and when properly manipulated, it has wear similar to that of tooth structure. Cast gold restorations became most popular from the year 1930s to the 1970s because of their acceptable functions and restorative longevity. Most of the cast metal restorations are made from alloys formed by combination of gold with other metals such as silver, copper, zinc, platinum and palladium. Casting procedures have been used for replacement of teeth by means of fixed and removable partial denture prosthesis, and full mouth restorations.

In operative dentistry, cast metal restorations are mainly used in three forms:

1. Inlay
2. Onlay
3. Partial crown.

After 1970s, restorative materials providing esthetics came into light, i.e. and after that there was increase in awareness of tooth colored restorations in comparison to cast gold restorations.

History of casting of objects in gold by the wax elimination process dates back to four or five thousand years ago by Chinese. Italian artisan Benvenuto Cellini described the use of this technique to make statues and artistic pieces. Dr Taggart developed the technique of casting gold inlays by the invested wax pattern method, and introduced this to the profession in 1907.

There are two techniques of fabrication of cast metal restorations (**Fig. 23.1**)

1. Direct technique.
2. Indirect technique.

In direct technique, the wax pattern is directly prepared from the tooth preparation in mouth, invested and cast. In indirect technique, the wax pattern is fabricated from the model prepared from the impression taken.

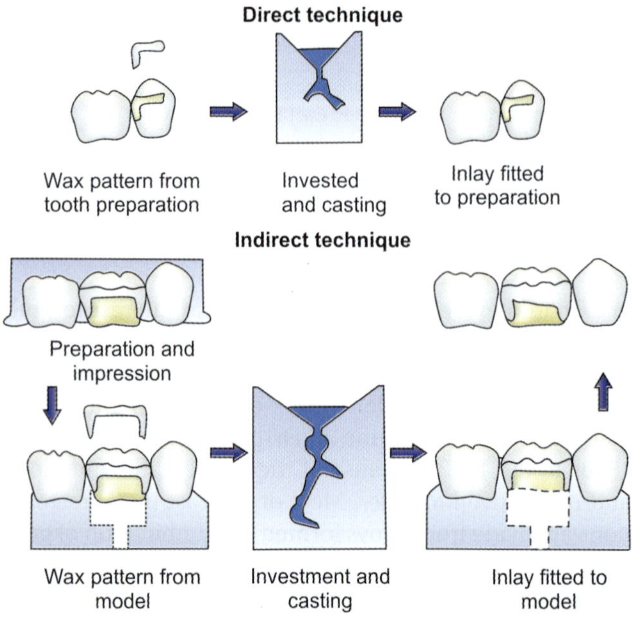

- **Inlay:** An inlay is an indirect intracoronal restoration which is fabricated extraorally and cemented in the prepared tooth. Inlay is designed to restore occlusal and proximal surfaces of posterior teeth without involving the cusps.
- **Onlay:** An onlay is a combination of intracoronal and extracoronal cast restoration which covers one or more cusps.
- **Class II inlay:** Class II inlay essentially involves proximal surface or surfaces of a posterior tooth, usually involve occlusal surface and may involve facial and/or lingual surface(s) and covers none or may cover all but one cusp of a tooth (**Fig. 23.2**).
- **Class II onlay:** Class II onlay involves the proximal surface or surfaces, and may involve facial and/or lingual surfaces of a posterior tooth and covers all the cusps (**Fig. 23.3**).
- **Partial crown:** In partial crown, a part of the crown remains uncovered and rest of the crown is covered like three quarter crown and seven-eighth crown.
- **Crown:** A crown completely covers the coronal portion of the tooth (**Figs 23.4 and 23.5**).

Alloys Used for Dental Use

Noble metals are metals that are resistant to corrosion and oxidation in moist air.

Base metals are metals that oxidize or corrode relatively easily.

Recent alloys are titanium and titanium alloys.

Desirable Properties of Dental Casting Alloys

- ***Biocompatibility***: The alloy material should be biocompatible, i.e it should be able to tolerate oral conditions and should not react with the oral fluids to release harmful products into the mouth.

Direct technique

Wax pattern from tooth preparation   Invested and casting   Inlay fitted to preparation

Indirect technique

Preparation and impression

Wax pattern from model   Investment and casting   Inlay fitted to model

Figure 23.1: Direct and indirect technique of cast metal restoration

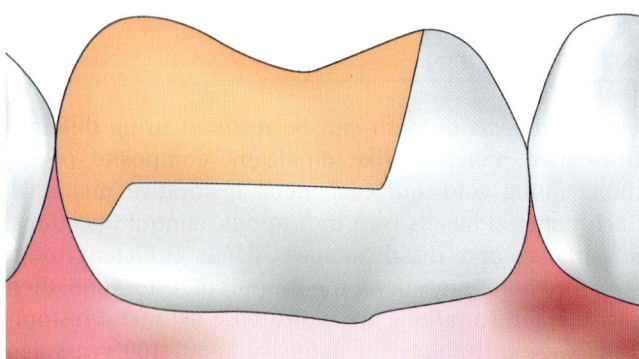

Figure 23.2: Class II inlay

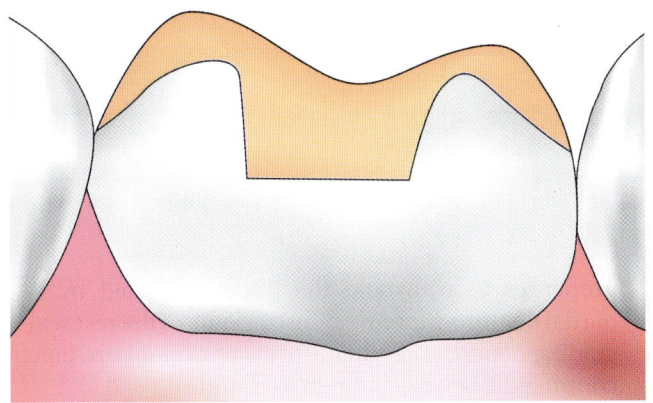

Figure 23.3: Class II onlay

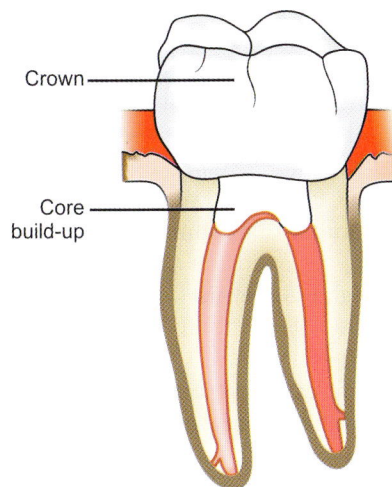

Figure 23.4: Crown given on root canal treated tooth

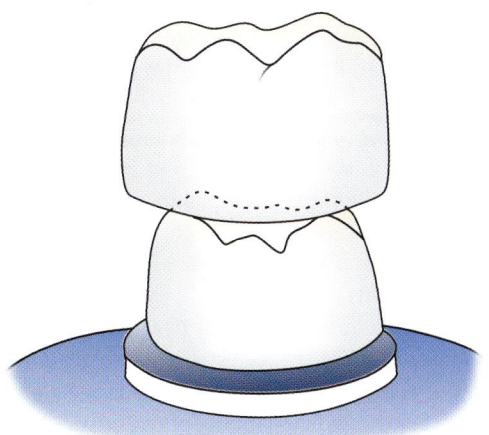

Figure 23.5: Crown placed on prepared tooth

- *Corrosion resistance:* The alloy material should either be inert so as to not to react in oral environment (like noble metal alloys) or should produce a passive film on its surface to inhibit any reaction (like chromium and titanium).
- *Melting temperature*: The casting alloys should be easy to melt and cast and should have a lower melting range.
- *Wear and sag resistance*: The alloys should have a high wear resistance as well as high sag resistance (especially for metal—ceramic alloys)
- *Strength*: The casting alloys should have high strength
- *Finishing and polishing*: The casting alloys should be easy to finish and polish.
- *Thermal requirements*: This is especially required for metal ceramic restorations in which the metals or alloys should have coefficient of thermal expansion closely matching that of porcelain.

Classification and Composition of Dental Casting Alloys (Tables 23.1 and 23.2)

According to noble metal content:

According to function: In 1927, the Bureau of Standard divided gold casting alloys into type I to IV:
- *Type I*: (soft)
  - Soft, weak and ductile
  - Used in low stress areas
  - Simple inlays in class I, III or V cavities
  - Highly burnishable
  - Used rarely nowadays.
- *Type II*: (medium)
  - Harder and stronger than type I
  - Ductility same as type I though yield strength high
  - Used in moderate stress areas
  - Thick three quarter crowns, pontics and full crowns
  - Less burnishable.
- *Type III*: (hard)
  - Used in high stress areas
  - Less burnishable than type I and II.
  - Can be age hardened
  - High stress inlays, full crowns, pontics, short span FPD's.

Table 23.1: Classification by American dental association (1984)

Alloy type	Noble metal content
High noble metal	Contains ≥ 40 wt% gold and ≥ 60 wt% of noble metal elements
Noble metal	Contains ≥ 25 wt% of noble metal elements
Predominantly base metal	Contains ≤ 25 wt% of noble metal elements

Table 23.2: Composition of various types of gold alloys

	Au(%)	Ag(%)	Cu(%)	Pd(%)	Zn and Ga(%)
Type I	83	10	6	0.5	Traces
Type II	77	14	7	1	Traces
Type III	75	11	9	3.5	Traces
Type IV	56	25	14	4	Traces

- Type IV: (extra hard)
  - Used in very high stress areas
  - Lowest gold content
  - Least ductile
  - Responsive to age hardening
  - High stress inlays, bars and clasps, long span FPD's.

Gold being very expensive, it is being replaced with base metal alloys and titanium. Base metal alloys were introduced in 1930 and include both cobalt—chromium and nickel chromium formulations. The advantages of base metal alloys are its reduced weights and improved mechanical properties.

Titanium alloys: Nowadays, titanium and titanium alloys are also used for cast metal restorations. This is because of its being passive in nature, highly biocompatible, having low density, modulus, coefficient of thermal expansion and relatively high strength.

But extensive use of titanium is limited by its certain disadvantages like high melting point, porosity in casting, difficulty in finishing, polishing and welding and also use of costly equipment.

Since this chapter deals mainly with cast gold restorations, detailed description of base metal alloys and titanium alloys is beyond the scope of this book.

INDICATIONS OF METAL INLAY AND ONLAY

- In extensive proximal surface caries in posterior teeth involving buccal and lingual line angles
- To maintain and restore proper interproximal contact and contour and for occlusal plane correction
- In patients with good oral hygiene and low caries index
- Postendodontic restorations are preferably restored by onlay to strengthen the remaining tooth structure and to distribute occlusal forces
- In teeth with extensive restoration, sometimes fracture line is present in enamel and dentin. Inlay/onlay can brace the tooth and prevent fragmentation of the tooth
- When there are other teeth present which are already restored with cast metal restorations
- Abutment teeth of removable partial denture are indicated for onlay because they provide superior physical properties to withstand the forces imparted by the partial denture. Moreover, the contours of the rest seats, guiding planes, and other aspects of contour are better controlled when the indirect technique is used
- In posterior teeth with heavy occlusal forces and attrition.

CONTRAINDICATIONS OF METAL INLAY AND ONLAY

- Where esthetics is prime consideration because metal inlay and onlay display metal color
- Patient having high caries index
- When patient cannot come for second visit
- In young patients, usually direct restorations are preferred since indirect restoration require longer and more number of appointments. Also the chances of iatrogenic pulp exposure are more in these patients because of high pulp horns
- Where expected life of a tooth is short, i.e. periodontally involved teeth
- In cases where extensive caries are present on facial, lingual and multiple surfaces. In such cases, full crown is indicated
- For patient of low economic status, inlay and onlay are not given because of higher costs
- In patients having restorations with different metals since dissimilar metals cause galvanic currents when they come in contact with each other
- When there are extensive occlusal wear facets involving the remaining marginal ridge of the tooth.

Advantages of cast metal restorations
➡ Since they are fabricated by indirect technique, there is better reproduction of contacts and contours
➡ Cast metal restorations are much more wear resistant than direct composite restorations, especially when restoring the occlusal surface
➡ More biocompatible with better tissue response
➡ Strengthens remaining tooth structure. In grossly carious lesion the remaining tooth structure is weakened and can be strengthened by capping of the cusp.
➡ Less chairside time is required

- Since cast metal restorations are build in bulk and not in increments, there are less chances of voids and internal stresses
- Extraoral polishing is easy.

Disadvantages of cast metal restorations
- It requires patient's subsequent appointment, with need for temporary restoration
- More expensive than direct restorations
- They are more technique sensitive
- Repair is difficult with these restorations
- Bonding of these restoration to tooth is weak at tooth cement casting junction. It can lead to microleakage with time
- Cast metal restorations are not acceptable esthetically.

PRINCIPLES OF TOOTH PREPARATION FOR CAST METAL INLAY

Preparation of inlay requires some fundamental steps. Each step has equal importance and although some steps are easier to accomplish, each step should be given the same careful attention for successful results.

Steps of inlay preparation (Figs 23.6 to 23.8)
- Tooth preparation
- Impression taking
- Die making
- Wax pattern
- Investing of the pattern and creating the mold
- Gold casting.

Among these the single step which can contribute to a large number of failures and which requires special efforts from the clinician is the tooth preparation. An optimally prepared tooth should meet the standard criteria of outline form, resistance and retention form, and other requirements given by GV Black. Ultimately, this accurate, smooth, optimally tapered preparation with distinct margins and internal line angles makes it possible to carry out each of the other step with accuracy.

The purpose of proper diagnosis and treatment plan is lost if care is not taken during tooth preparation. The preparation to receive a gold inlay should not only be designed to gain perfection of margins and restore occlusion, but should be made to enhance the strength of the tooth as well.

Cast metal restorations involve making of a wax pattern which should be removed from cast or die without any distortion. Hence, some fundamental basic designs are incorporated during preparation of class II inlay. These are

Basic designs of cast metal restoration
- Path of draw
- Inlay taper
- Circumferential tie
♦ Bevels
♦ Flares

Path of Draw

Preparation should have single insertion path opposite to the occlusal load and parallel to the long axis of tooth (**Figs 23.9A and B**). This helps in retention of the restoration (**Fig. 23.10**).

Inlay Taper

To have unhindered removal and placement of the wax pattern and seating of the final casting, intracoronal and extracoronal tooth preparation should have some taper. Ideally, a intracoronal tooth preparation should have slight diverging walls from gingival to occlusal surface. This is the concept of taper (**Fig. 23.11**).

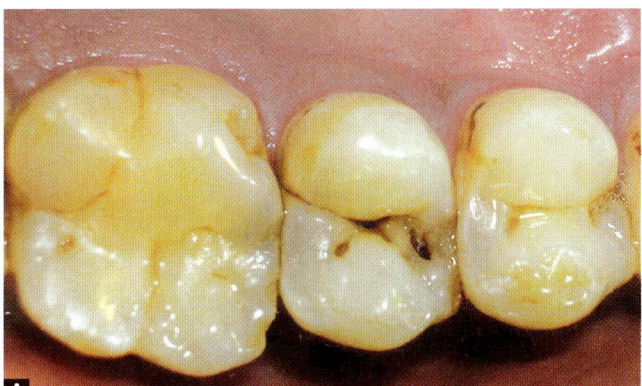
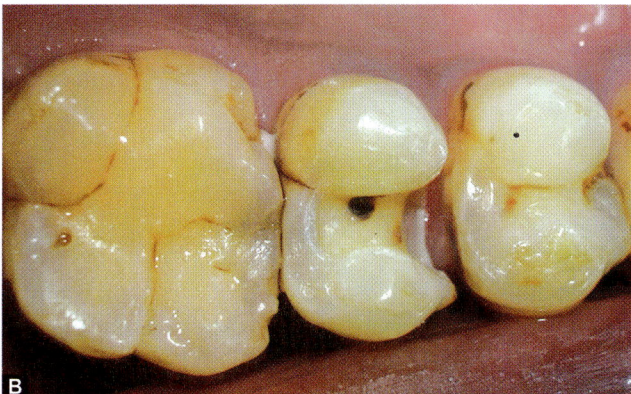

Figures 23.6A and B

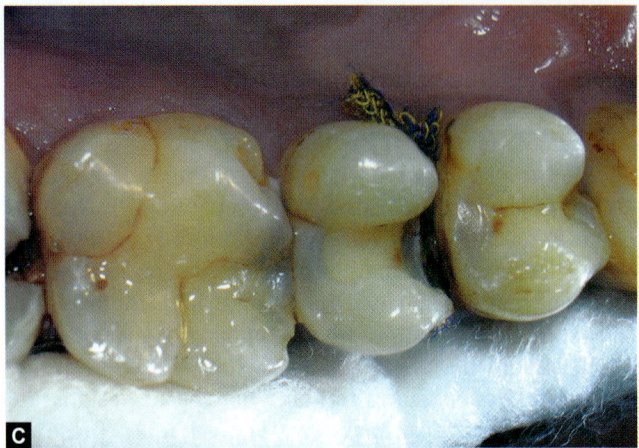

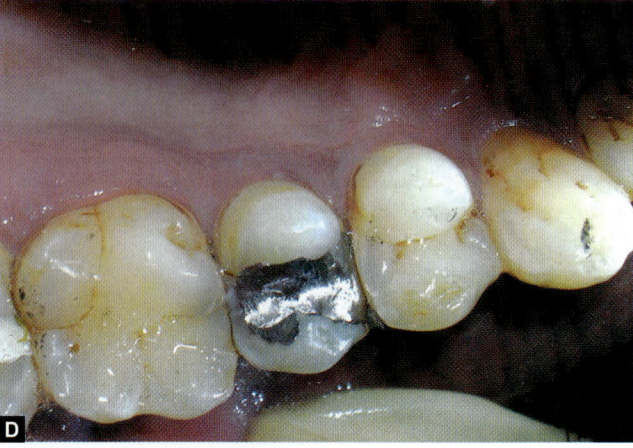

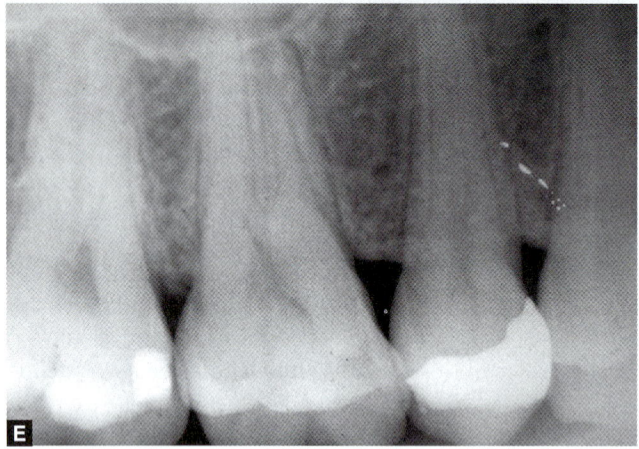

Figures 23.6C to E

Figures 23.6A to E: (A) Class II caries in 25; (B) Tooth preparation for cast metal inlay; (C) Completed tooth preparation;
(D) Inlay in place; (E) Radiograph showing inlay on 25

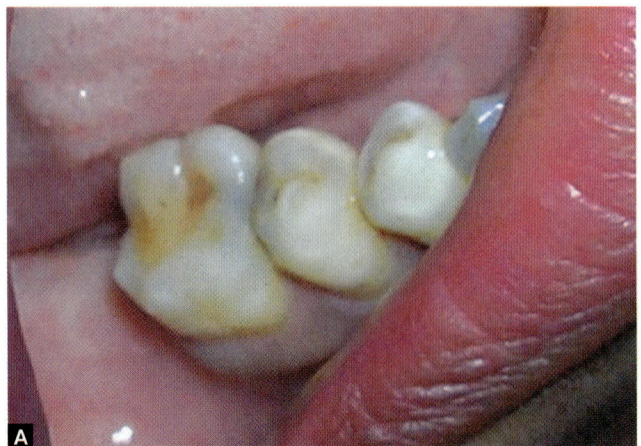

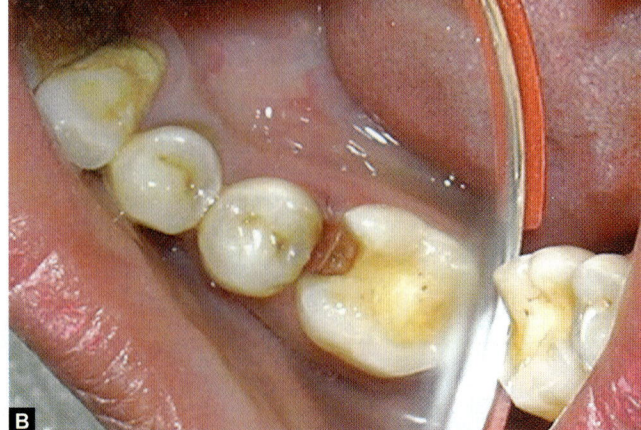

Figures 23.7A and B

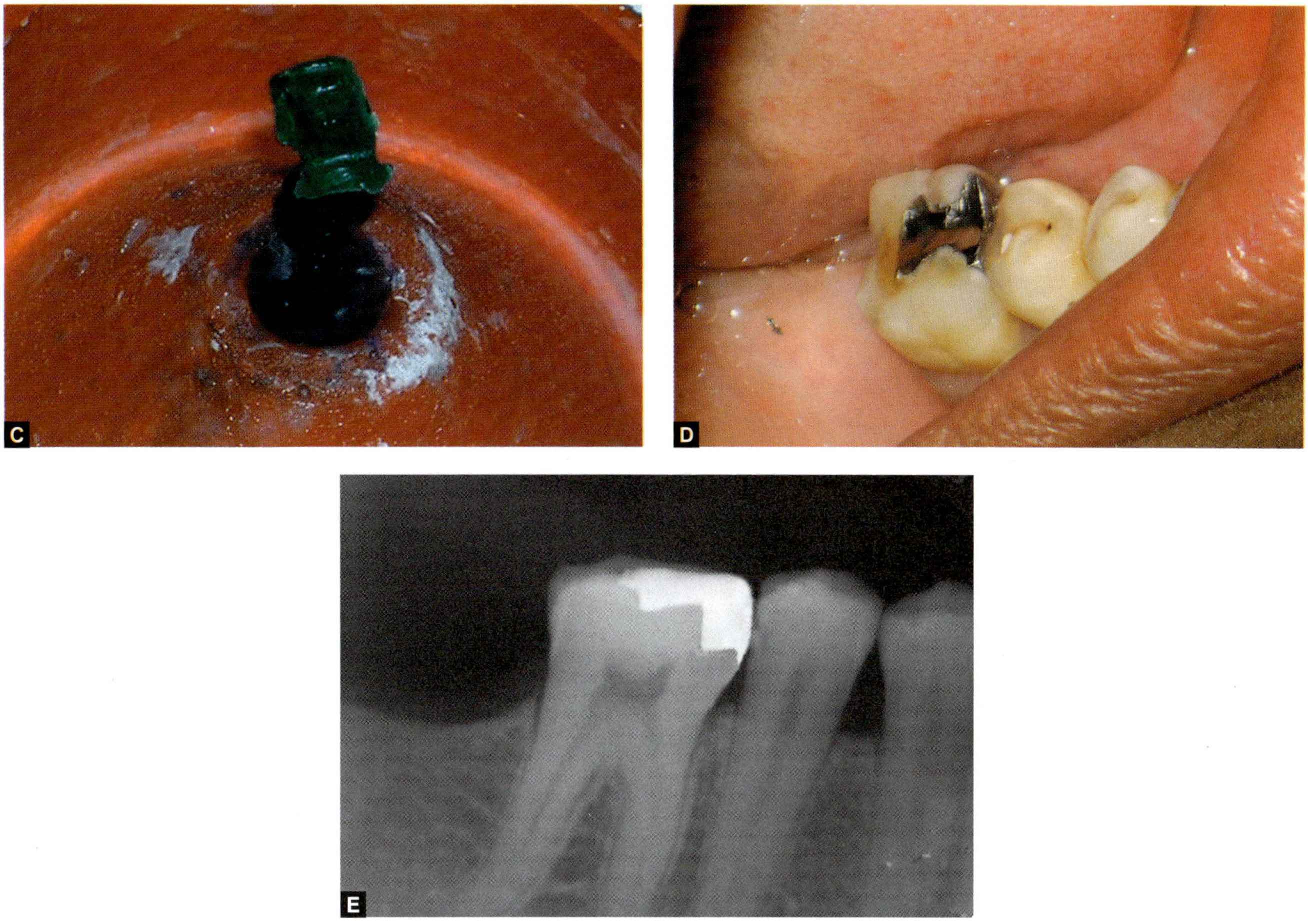

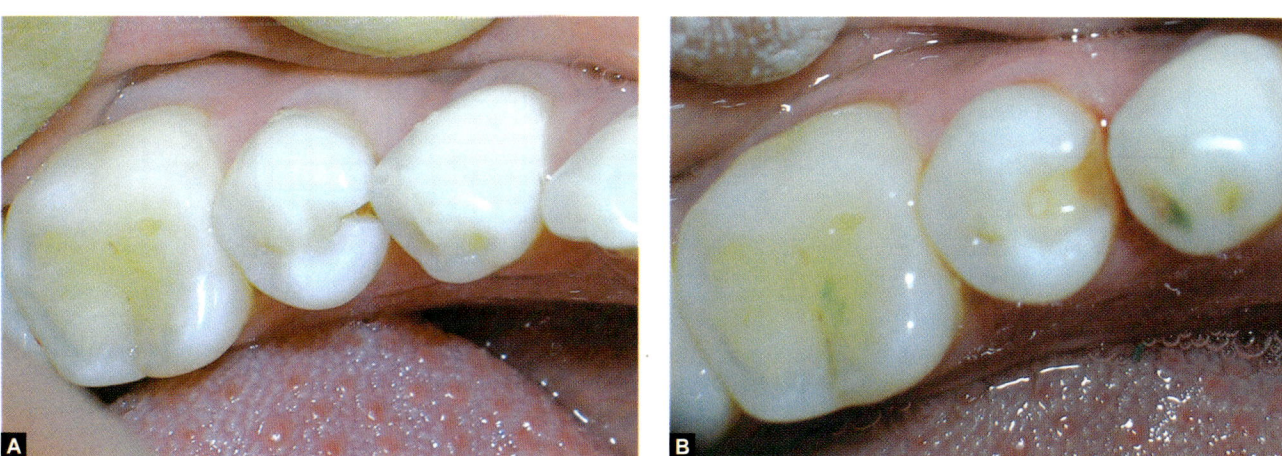

Figures 23.7C to E

Figures 23.7A to E: (A) Caries on mesial surface of 36; (B) Tooth preparation completed; (C) Wax pattern;
(D) Inlay placed on first molar; (E) Radiograph showing inlay in place on 36

Figures 23.8A and B

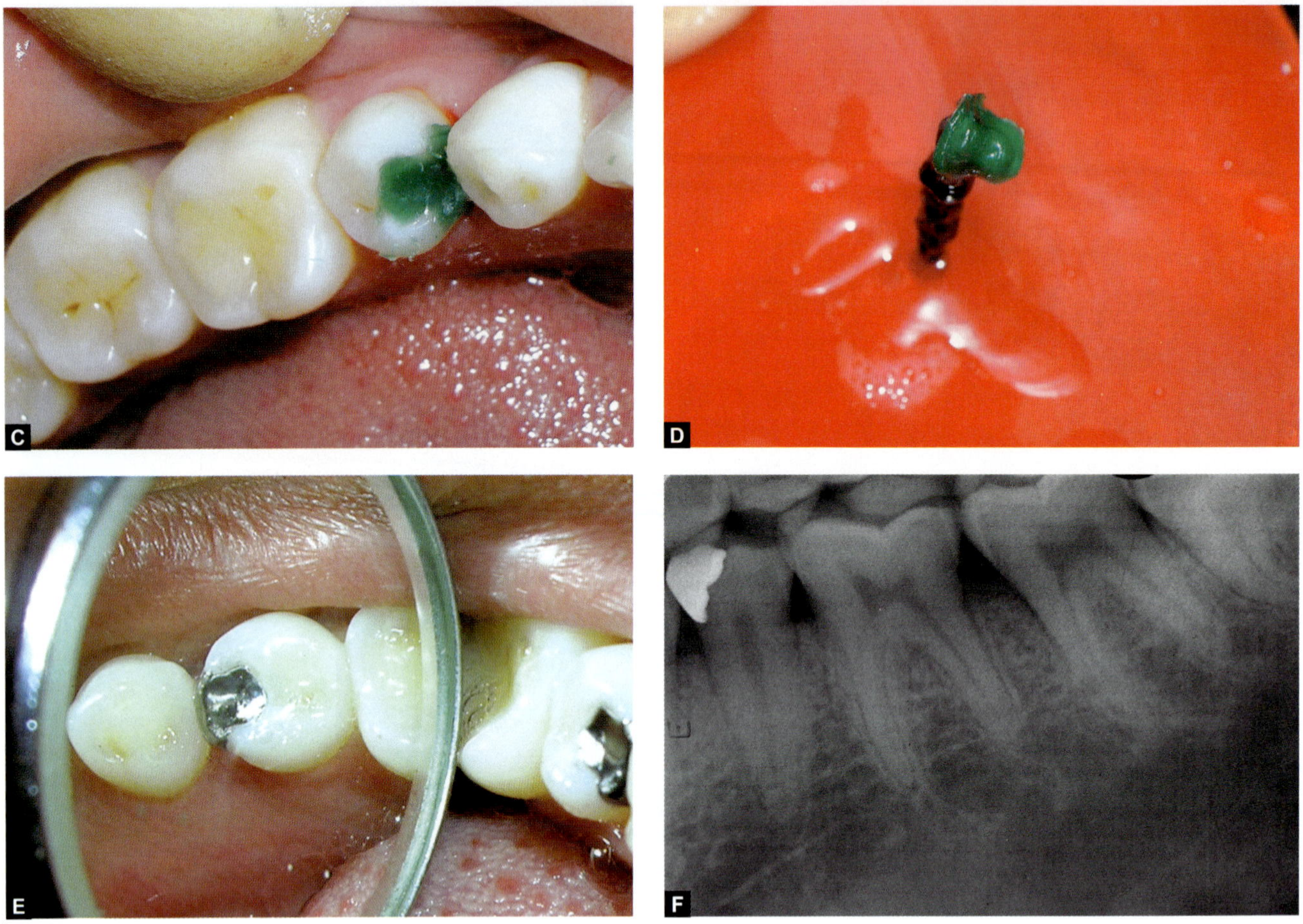

Figures 23.8C to F

Figures 23.8A to F: (A) Class II caries on 35; (B) Tooth preparation for inlay; (C) Wax pattern fabrication; (D) Spruing; (E) Metal inlay placed on 35; (F) Radiograph showing inlay placed on 35

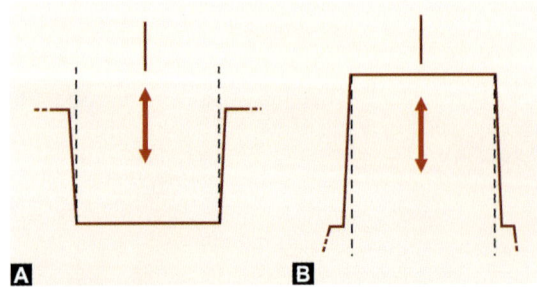

Figures 23.9A and B: Inlay preparation should have single path of insertion parallel to long axis of tooth

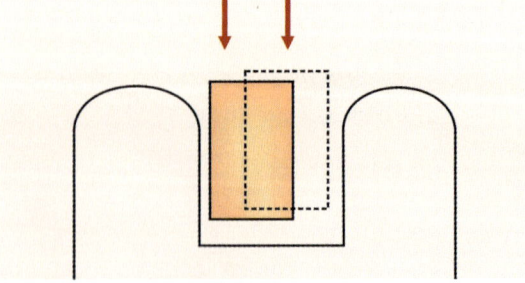

Figure 23.10: With multiple paths of insertion, there is no retention for inlay even if walls are parallel to each other

If possible, throughout the tooth preparation, the cutting instrument should be kept parallel to the long axis of the tooth and thus the preparation develops a line of withdrawal. This line of withdrawal also describes the path of insertion and removal of the casting and is the axis of taper. The optimal taper lie in the range of 2° to 5° per wall. If longitudinal walls of preparation are short, a maximum of 2° taper is given, and if longitudinal height of preparation is more, then taper should also be increased, but never exceed 10° (**Fig. 23.12**). Also the preparation should never

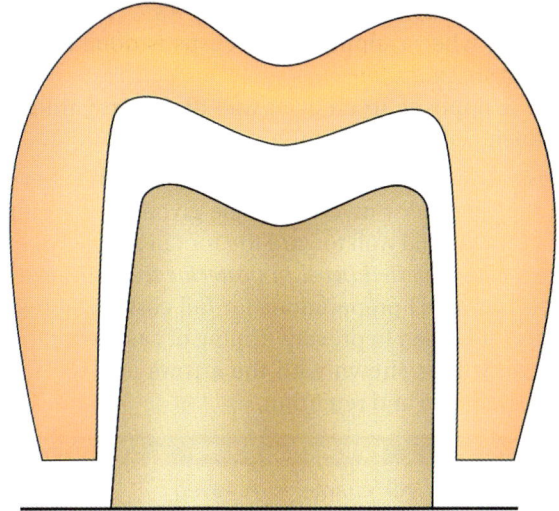

Figure 23.11: A 2°–5° of taper provides optimal retention for inlay

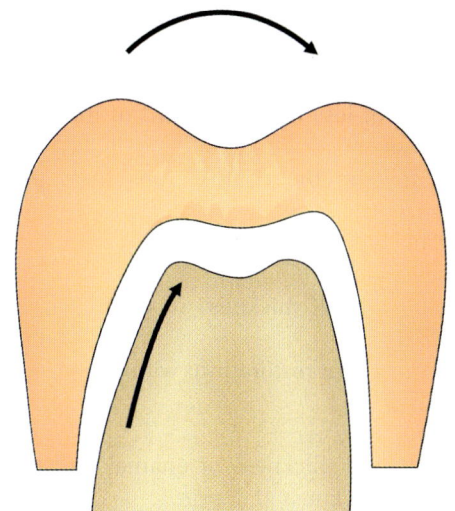

Figure 23.12: Giving more than required taper in preparation walls results in reduced retention of inlay

have one side with more taper than the other since it can result in more than one path of insertion (**Fig. 23.13**). For shallow preparations, the axis of taper is usually parallel to the long axis of the tooth and for class V preparations, the axis of taper is perpendicular to the long axis of the tooth. The angle formed by the convergence of the tapered preparation walls to a point of their intersection is bisected by line of withdrawal.

Circumferential Tie

Circumferential tie refers to the design of cavosurface margin of an inlay tooth preparation. This junction between tooth, cement and inlay is the weakest part of the cast metal restoration. For the success of restoration, the margins of restoration should be designed so as to achieve its maximum adaptation to tooth structure. Cavosurface margins of an inlay preparation can be of two types:
1. Bevels
2. Flares.

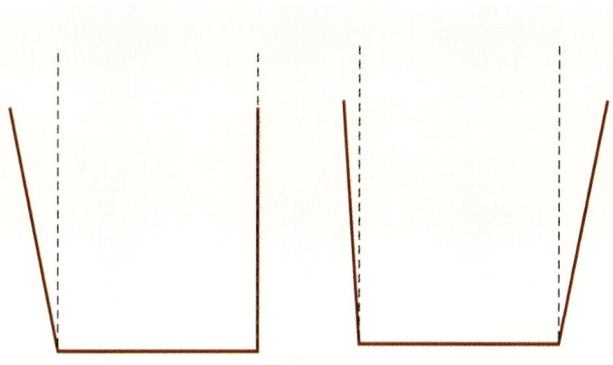

Figure 23.13: Uneven taper of preparation walls result in failure of inlay

Bevels

Bevel is defined as plane of cavity wall or floor directed away from cavity preparation.

An accurate wax pattern and casting may not have precise adaptation to the margins of tooth preparation if bevel is not given. Objective of bevel is to form a metal wedge of 30° to 35°, thus enhancing the chance to achieve closure at the interface of cast gold and tooth by burnishing (**Fig. 23.14**). By beveling, a strong enamel margin with an angle of 140° to 150° can be produced.

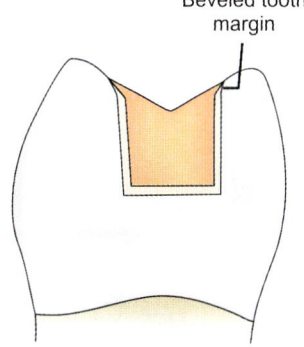

Beveled tooth margin

Figure 23.14: Bevel helps in better adaptation of restoration to the tooth surface

Types of bevel (Fig. 23.15): According to surface and area involved, bevels can be:

- Ultrashort or partial bevel
  - Beveling of less than two-third of the total enamel thickness.
  - Used to trim the enamel rods from preparation margins.
  - Used in type I casting alloys.
- Short bevel
  - Beveling of full thickness of enamel wall but not dentin.
  - Used mostly for restorations with type I and II casting alloys.
- Long bevel
  - Includes full thickness of enamel and half or less than half thickness of dentin.
  - Preserves the internal 'boxed up' resistance and retention features of the preparations.
  - Used in types I, II and III of cast gold alloys.
- Full bevel
  - Includes full enamel and dentinal wall.
  - It deprives the preparation of its internal resistance
  - Full bevel should be avoided except in cases where it is a must.
- Hollow ground (concave) bevel
  - Hollow ground is concave in shape and not a bevel in true sense.
  - It is rarely used.

- Counter bevel
  - Used when capping of the cusps is done to protect and support them.
  - It is opposite to an axial wall of the preparation on the facial or lingual surface of the tooth.
- *Reverse or inverted bevel in anterior teeth*: It is beveling in the reverse or inverted shape given on the gingival seat in the axial wall toward the root in anterior teeth.
- *Reverse or inverted bevel in posterior teeth*: In posterior teeth (in MOD preparations for full cast metal restorations), it is used to prevent tipping of cast restoration in the directions shown with the arrows and to increase the resistance and retention.

Functions of bevels
➡ By beveling, weak enamel is removed
➡ Beveling produce obtuse angled tooth margins. Resultant cavosurface angle of 135° to 140° forms the strongest and the bulkiest configuration
➡ Acute angled metal margins (35°-45°) allow the metal margins to be burnished against tooth surface (**Fig. 23.16**)
➡ Beveling increases retention, resistance, aesthetics and color matching for composite resin restoration
➡ It improves junctional relationship between the restorative material and tooth (**Fig. 23.17**)
➡ Bevels are the flexible extensions, i.e. they allow inclusion of faults, wear facets, etc. without overextending the preparation margins

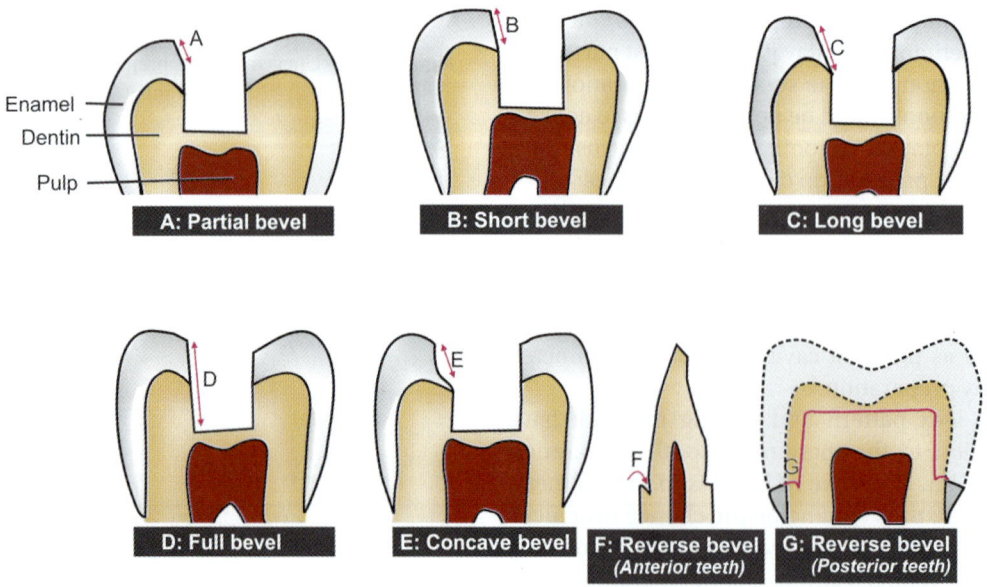

Figure 23.15: Different types of bevels

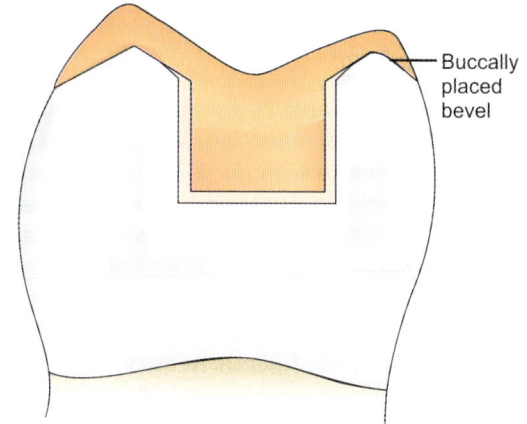

Figure 23.16: Bevels allow better finishing and burnishing of metal margins against tooth

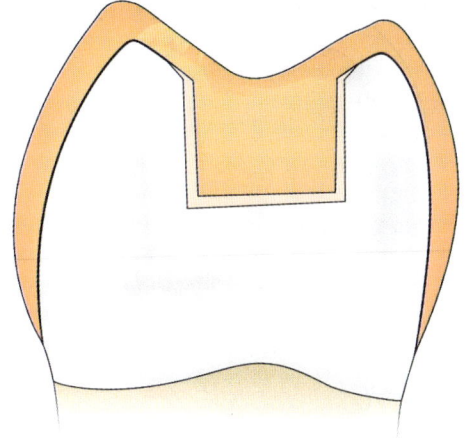

Figure 23.18: Lap sliding fit of restoration because of bevel

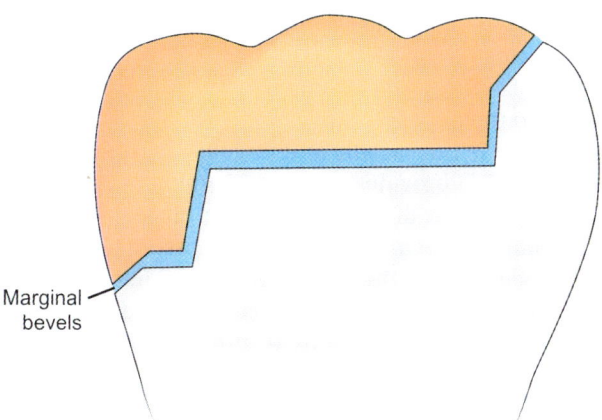

Figure 23.17: Marginal bevels reduce the space between tooth structure and the restoration, thus help in better retention

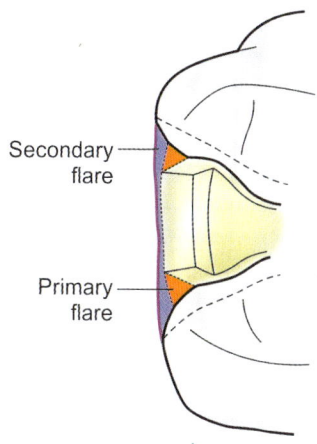

Figure 23.19: Primary flare and secondary flare

- Gingival margins become finishable and cleanasable because of gingival bevels
- Counter bevel increases the resistance form to remaining tooth structure
- Because of beveling, the gingival margin has a lap sliding fit which provides better fit at this region (**Fig. 23.18**).

Flares

Flares are concave or flat peripheral portions of the facial or lingual proximal walls. They are of two types:

Primary flare

- It is basic part of circumferential tie
- It is like a long bevel and is directed 45° to the inner dentinal wall proper (**Figs 23.19 and 23.20**)

- Primary flare is indicated when normal contacts are present
- When there is minimal extension of caries in buccolingual direction.

Secondry flare:

- It is a flat plane superimposed peripherally to the primary flare (**Fig. 23.19**).
- It may have different angulations, involvement and extent depending upon requirement
- Secondary flare is not given in the areas where esthetics is more important.

Indications of secondary flares:

- When broad contact area is present
- To include the faults present on facial and lingual walls beyond primary flare (**Fig. 23.21**).

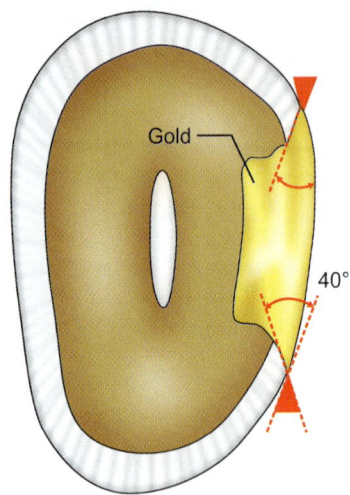

Figure 23.20: In class II metal inlay, proximal box should have flares so as to have metal of 40°

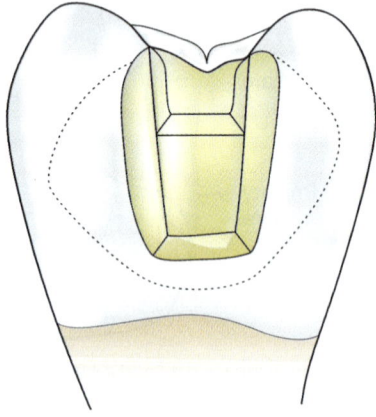

Figure 23.21: Secondary flare is extended beyond primary flare to involve all faults and defects

- When caries is widely extended in buccolingual direction
- To include the undercuts present at cervical aspect of facial and lingual walls.

Advantages of secondary flare:
- Secondary flare ensures cavosurface margins to extend into embrasures (self-cleansing area)
- Permits easy burnishing and finishing of the restoration
- Produce more obtuse angled and stronger cavosurface margin.

STEPS OF TOOTH PREPARATION FOR INLAY

The following steps are involved in the tooth preparation for class II inlay

Initial Tooth Preparation

Occlusal Outline Form

Anesthetize the tooth and apply a rubber dam to give better visibility, tissue retraction, and ease of operation. Penetrate the tooth with no. 271 bur held parallel to long axis of the tooth to initial depth of 1.5mm. The entry point should be closest to the involved marginal ridge (for example, mesial) (**Fig. 23.22**).

First establish the occlusal outline. Keeping the bur parallel, extend the tooth preparation while maintaining the initial pulpal depth of 1.5 mm. At the same time as the occlusal outline is being established, a flat pulpal floor of proper depth and the occlusal walls of a uniform taper are being prepared with the same bur (**Fig. 23.23**). Care is used to avoid overcutting (**Fig. 23.24**). Whilec maintaining the established pulpal depth and with the bur held parallel to the long axis of the tooth, extend the preparation towards the contact area of the tooth, ending short by 0.8 mm of cutting through the marginal ridge. Now extend the bur to the opposite side of marginal ridge (distal side) and move the bur facially and lingually to make occlusal dovetail which provides retention to the restoration (**Fig. 23.25**). Conserve the marginal ridge on the sound side of the tooth and if any faulty shallow fissure is present, it should be managed during preparation either by enameloplasty or including it using cavosurface bevel.

The width of the isthmus of the preparation on the occlusal surface should be maintained to a minimal extension for conservation of tooth structure.

Outline form should be carried onto smooth areas of the buccal and lingual slopes of the cusps of the tooth. This

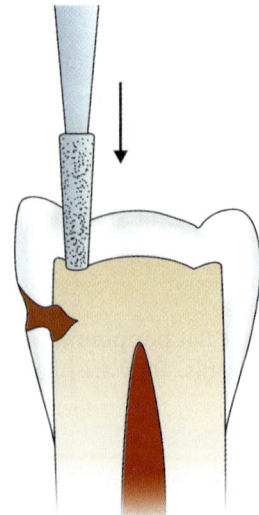

Figure 23.22: Penetrate the bur closest to the involved marginal ridge

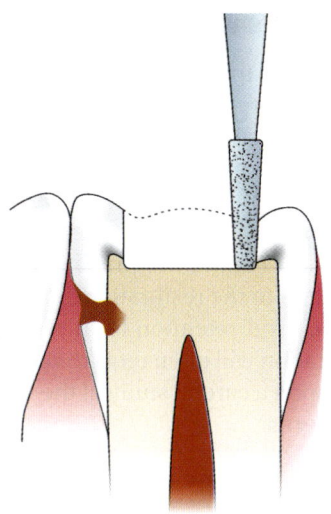

Figure 23.23: Keeping the same depth (1.5 mm), establish the occlusal outline

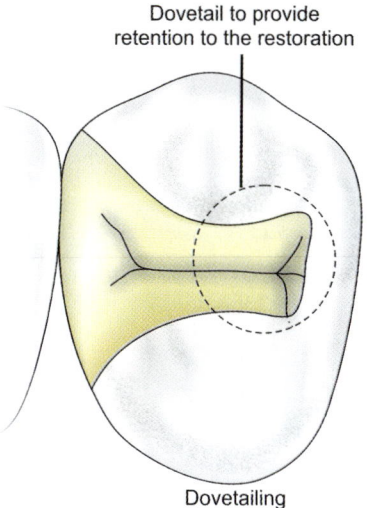

Figure 23.25: Extension of preparation and dovetail

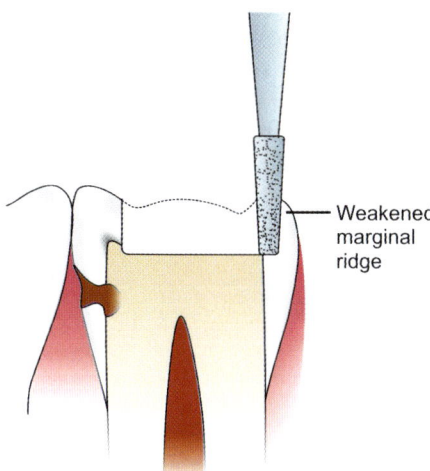

Figure 23.24: Overcutting can result in weakening of marginal ridge

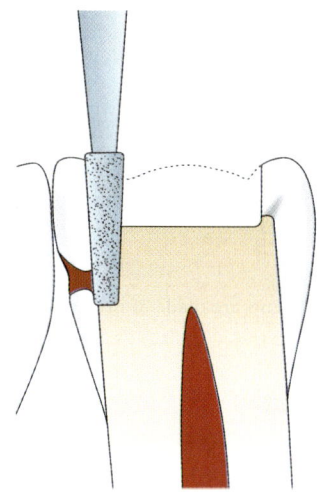

Figure 23.26: The proximal ditch is given after occlusal preparation

extension will place the margins of the casting in areas where they may be easily finished.

Proximal Box Preparation

Using the same bur, isolate the mesial enamel by proximal ditch cut. Width of this cut should be 0.8 mm with 0.5 mm in dentin and 0.3 mm in enamel. Extend this ditch facially and lingually to the sound tooth structure and proceed gingivally (**Fig. 23.26**).

Gingival extension should remove any caries present on the gingival floor and it should provide atleast 0.5 mm

clearance from the adjacent tooth (**Fig. 23.27**). To break the contact from the adjacent tooth, make two cuts with no. 271 bur; one on facial limit and other at lingual limit of the proximal box (**Fig. 23.28**). Extend these cuts gingivally till the bur is through the proximal surface. Keep a small slice of enamel at the contact area to prevent accidental damage to the adjacent tooth. If there is any doubt that accidental damage to the adjacent tooth can occur, use a metal matrix band interdentally. This will offer some protection to the adjacent tooth.

The remaining thin slice of unsupported enamel wall can be removed using hand instruments (**Fig. 23.29**). In

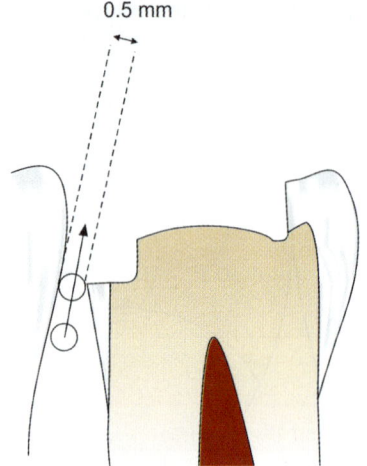

0.5 mm

Figure 23.27: The gingival floor should provide atleast 0.5 mm clearance from the adjacent tooth

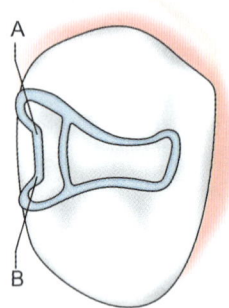

A

B

Figure 23.28: Two cuts are made to isolate the proximal enamel

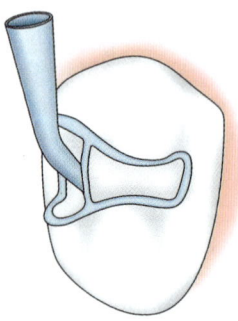

Figure 23.29: Isolated enamel wall is broken of by using a spoon excavator

that way the flat gingival floor of proper depth is formed at the same time as the proximal and axial walls are being formed. The gingival wall is usually established at approximately right angle to the long axis of the tooth. Gingival bevel is generally placed about one millimeter.

Resistance and Retention Form

- A nicely designed inlay preparation should have proximal box form for retention and flat pulpal and gingival walls for resistance to form.
- The extrathickness of gold provided by the box form and the occlusal step of the preparation helps in increasing its resistance and retention.
- The occlusal dovetail of the preparation also provides added retention to the restoration.
- The resistance and retention form of the occlusal step of the preparation will often require variations in design depending upon a careful study of the size and position of the pulp horns.

Final Tooth Preparation

During final preparation, clean the prepared tooth with air/water spray or with cotton pellet and inspect it for detection and removal of debris and examine for correction of all cavosurface angles and margins. Remove remaining caries and/or old restorative material. In large preparations with soft caries, the removal of carious dentin is done with spoon excavator or slow speed round bur (**Fig. 23.30**). In this, two step pulpal floor is made, i.e. only portion of tooth which is affected by caries is removed, leaving the remaining preparation floor untouched.

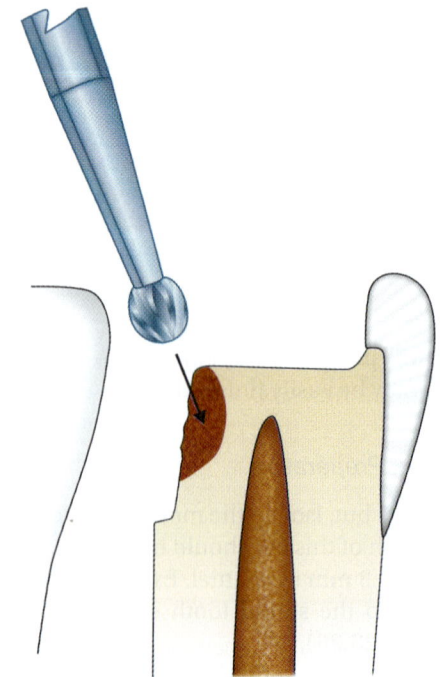

Figure 23.30: Removal of remaining caries using a large round bur

Use pulp protective materials whenever indicated (**Fig. 23.31**).

Placement of Grooves, Bevels and Flares

Retention grooves if needed are placed in the facioaxial and linguoaxial line angles using number 169 L carbide bur (**Figs 23.32 and 23.33**).

Gingival Bevel

It is advantageous to place a gingival bevel of approximately 45° in inlay preparations (**Fig. 23.34**). It should be made smooth and uniformly placed with the help of double ended gingival marginal trimmers. The gingival bevel should include one-half the width of the gingival wall. A properly placed gingival bevel eliminates the possibility of leaving weak or unsupported enamel on gingival wall. It provides a stronger obtuse angle of tooth structure which aids in finishing of the casting and a design which lends itself to a more efficient sealing of the margins of the restoration. Failure to bevel the gingival margin can result in formation of weak margins because of presence of undermined rods (**Fig. 23.35**). Gingival bevels more than 45° results in over extension of the gingival and proximal margins which causes difficulty in impression making, fabricating the wax pattern and finishing of the restoration.

Occlusal Bevels

It is suggested that the occlusal bevel should be about 0° beginning at the occlusal one-third of the adjacent occlusal walls (**Fig. 23.36**). The purpose of the bevel is to remove any irregularities in the preparation or unsupported enamel

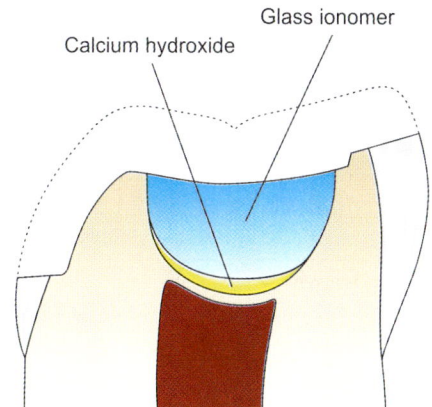

Figure 23.31: Pulp protection in deep preparation is provided by placing calcium hydroxide as liner and glass ionomer as base

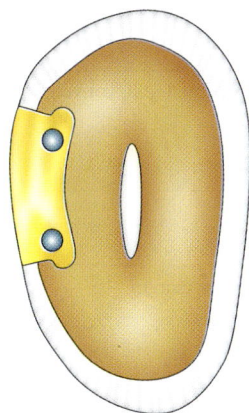

Figure 23.33: Placement of facioaxial and linguoaxial retentive grooves

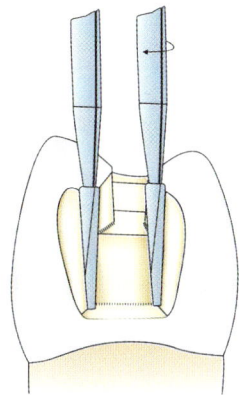

Figure 23.32: Retention grooves are placed in linguo and facioaxial line angles

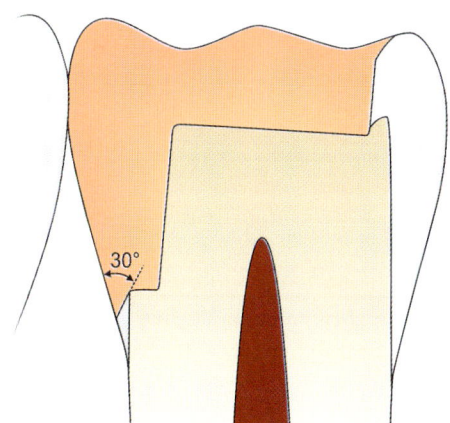

Figure 23.34: Bevel in gingival margin of proximal box

Difference between cavity preparation for silver amalgam and cast restorations

Silver amalgam	Cast restoration
• Intercuspal width is one-fourth of intercuspal distance • Outline form is narrow	• Intercuspal width is one-third of intercuspal distance • Outline form is wide
• Depth is more in this preparation	• Less depth
• Preparation walls converge occlusally	• Preparation walls are parallel
• Buccal and lingual proximal walls converge occlusally	• Buccal and lingual walls are parallel
• Butt joint at cavosurface margin Butt joint	• Cavosurface bevel is given Cavosurface bevel
• Rounded line and point angles • Bevelled axiopulpal line angle	• Well defined line and point angles • Rounded axiopulpal line angle
• No reverse bevel is given	• Reverse bevel is given Reverse bevel
• No grooves are given, only locks are given	• Grooves are given in facioaxial and linguoaxial line angles Grooves

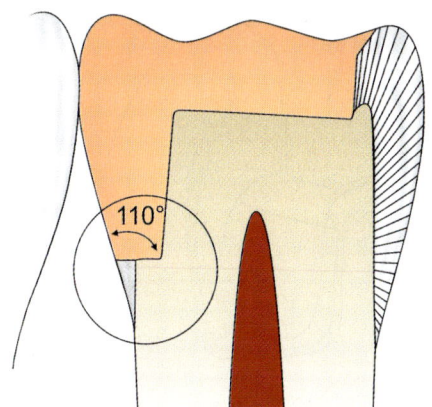

Figure 23.35: If no bevel is given, unsupported enamel rods can cause restoration failure

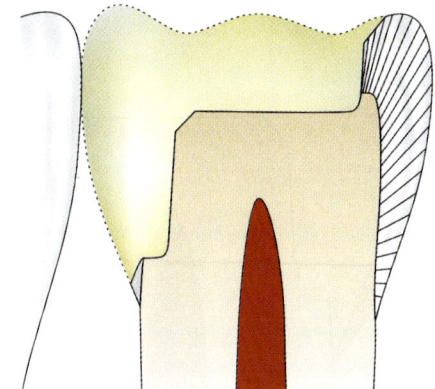

Figure 23.37: Bevel helps in removing unsupported enamel rods at cavosurface margins

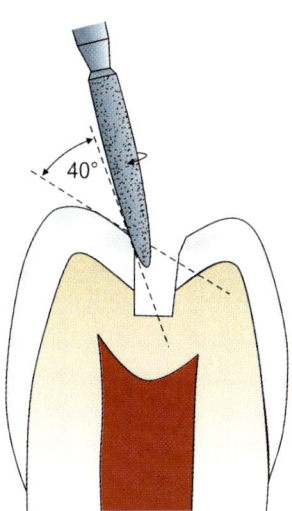

Figure 23.36: Occlusal bevel

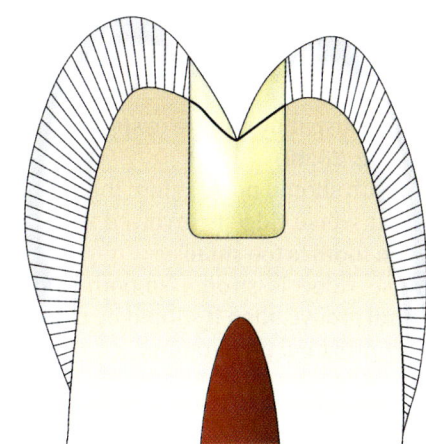

Figure 23.38: When cusps are steep, no occlusal bevel is placed especially in case of narrow preparation because here while occlusal preparation enamel rods of inner one-third of inclined plane get bevelled automatically

rods at the cavosurface margin (**Fig. 23.37**). This gives the cavosurface margin a smooth, flowing outline. When the cusps are steep, little or no bevel is placed (**Fig. 23.38**), but when shallow cusps are present, a more distinct bevel is placed.

When it is required to cover a cusp with cast metal, prepare a hollow ground bevel using a #7404 twelve fluted, round ended bur. This allows bulk of the restoration at the cavosurface margin. Finally finishing of walls and margins is done by removing all unsupported enamel.

The final stage of inlay preparation is to clean the preparation thoroughly with water and air spray. Then dry it with moist air (**Fig. 23.39**).

The surrounding margins of a preparation designed to accept a cast metal restoration should form an obtuse angle with the surface of the tooth. This gives the advantage of being able to finish an acute angle of tough malleable gold alloy against an obtuse angle of tooth structure.

MODIFICATIONS IN CLASS II TOOTH PREPARATION FOR INLAY

In Mandibular First Premolar

As we know, anatomy of the mandibular first premolar is different which requires special attention during tooth preparation. For example:

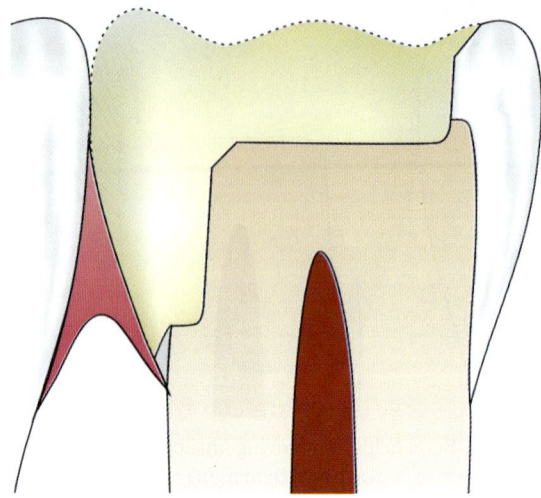

Figure 23.39: Completed inlay tooth preparation

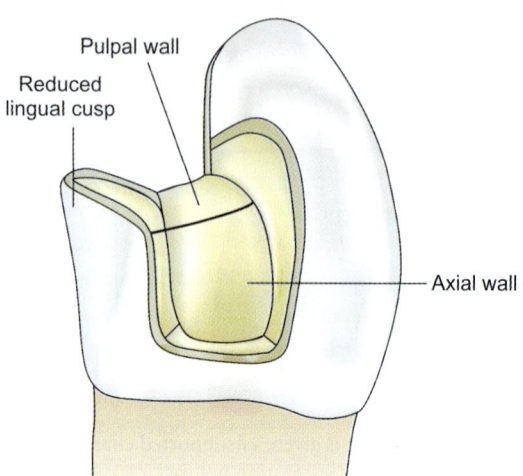

Figure 23.40: Reduction of lingual cusp of mandibular premolar without involving the pulp

- Small lingual cusp may require cusp capping whenever indicated (**Fig. 23.40**)
- Occlusal depth should not be more than 2 mm
- Occlusal transverse ridge is involved when it is defective or when tooth is too small
- If transverse ridge is strong, smooth and without a faulty central groove, then it should be conserved while preparing a proximal preparation.

Esthetic Reasons

In teeth which are esthetically important, for example, maxillary premolars and first molars, the class II preparation involving mesioproximal side indicates less mesiofacial flare for the minimal or no metal exposure.

In Maxillary Molars with Unaffected and Strong Oblique Ridge

In maxillary molars, oblique ridge provides strength to the tooth. If the oblique ridge is sound and unaffected by caries, then it is always preferred to preserve it while doing tooth preparation. This helps in maintaining the strength of the tooth. In this way, if tooth preparation is to be done on both mesial and distal sides, two separate preparations are made instead of one MOD (**Fig. 23.41**).

Mesiocclusal preparation is same as described above. But some points are kept in mind while doing preparation on the distal side, especially when the palatal

developmental groove is carious or prone to caries. To obtain adequate retention and resistance form, following can be done:

- Wall of the preparation should be almost parallel or have maximum of 2° occlusal divergence.
- Involve distopalatal cusp in the casting, if indicated.
- Palatal groove extension should not be very close to the distal proximal side, as this will result in weakening of the distopalatal cusp.
- Prepare mesioaxial and distoaxial grooves in the palatal groove extension and palatal and facial retention grooves in the mesial or distal box. Cusp capping prevents fracture of the underlying tooth structure since occlusal margins of the preparation are placed away from strong occlusal forces.

Class II Preparation with Gingival Extensions to Include the Root Surface Lesion

Gingival extension should be achieved by lengthening the gingival bevel in cases of root surface lesions (**Figs 23.42A and B**).

Capping of Cusp

Cusp capping is indicated when occlusal caries is extensive involving most of the cusp, resulting in weakened cusps and/undermined enamel. When removal of carious structure results in loss of the occlusal surface more than

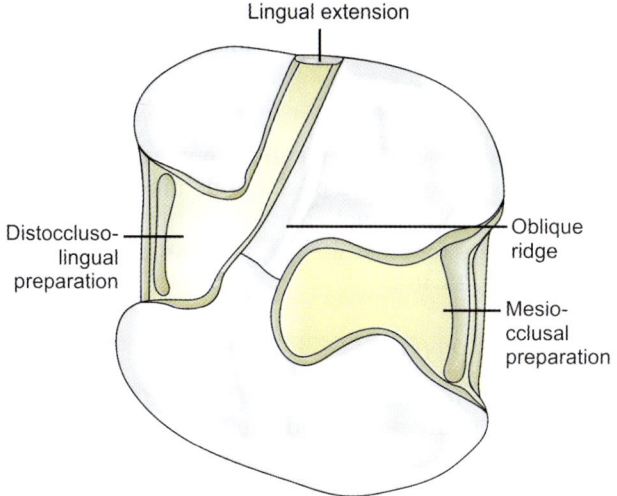

Figure 23.41: If oblique ridge is unaffected by caries, two separate preparations can be made on both sides of ridge instead of one MOD

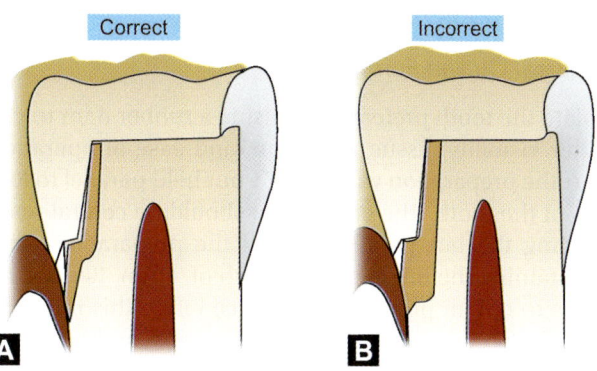

Figure 23.42: In cases of root surface lesion, gingival extension should be achieved by lengthening the gingival bevel

half the distance from primary groove to the cusp tip, the capping of the cusps is desirable and capping is mandatory if two-thirds or more of this distance, is involved.

Steps

- Cusp reduction should be started after making a groove (**Fig. 23.43**). Groove helps in accurate and uniform cutting. Different cusps require reduction according to the situation of a particular cusp, in other words all cusps do not require equal reduction
- While reducing the adjacent cusp, lingual or buccal developmental groove should be involved in cutting
- For increasing retention and resistance, grooves are made at the proximal walls of the box.
- Prepare a reverse bevel or counter bevel on the facial or lingual side of the reduced facial or lingual cusp respectively (**Fig. 23.44**). This bevel is not given in the areas where aesthetics is a prime concern like facial margins on maxillary premolars and the first molar.

TOOTH PREPARATION FOR CAST METAL ONLAY (FIGS 23.45A TO C)

Onlays are indicated where reinforcement of the cusps is indicated like in cases where all the cusps of a posterior teeth are damaged or have become weak either due to caries or previous faulty resteration or after endodoutic therapy.

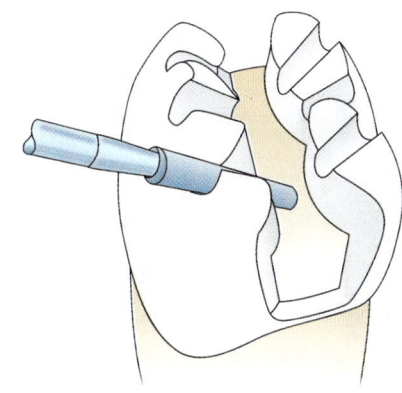

Figure 23.43: Cusp capping should be done after making grooves so as to have accurate and uniform cutting

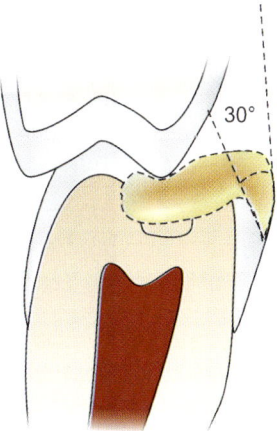

Figure 23.44: Make reverse bevel on lingual side of the reduced facial cusp or facial side of lingual cusp

Steps of Tooth Preparation for Onlay

Occlusal Outline Form

Isolate the tooth preferably by using a rubber dam to give better visibility, tissue retraction, and ease of operation. Start the preparation with no. 271 bur held parallel to long axis of the tooth. The entry point should be central fossa. Keeping the bur parallel, extend the preparation while maintaining the initial pulpal depth of 2 mm. Reduce the cusps to obtain proper convenience form. This improves both the access and the visibility for subsequent steps in tooth preparation. Care is taken to circumvent the cusps and extend the preparation adequately. Occlusal divergence depends on the occlusocervical depth of the preparation and is related to retention form of the prepared tooth. Usually the occlusal walls should have a uniform taper with 3° to 5° occlusal divergence.

Proximal Box Preparation

Using the same bur, extend the preparation on mesial and distal side to expose proximal dentinoenamel junction. Isolate the proximal enamel by proximal ditch cut. Proximal boxes for onlay are prepared in same way as that for inlay (**Fig. 23.46**).

Cusp Reduction (Fig. 23.47)

Cusp reduction is done using no. 271 carbide bur. Cusp reduction should be started after making grooves of 1.5 mm (for nonfunctional cusp) and 2 mm (functional

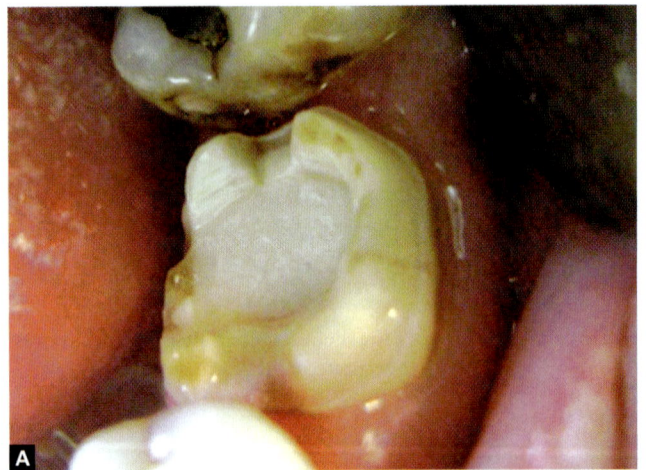
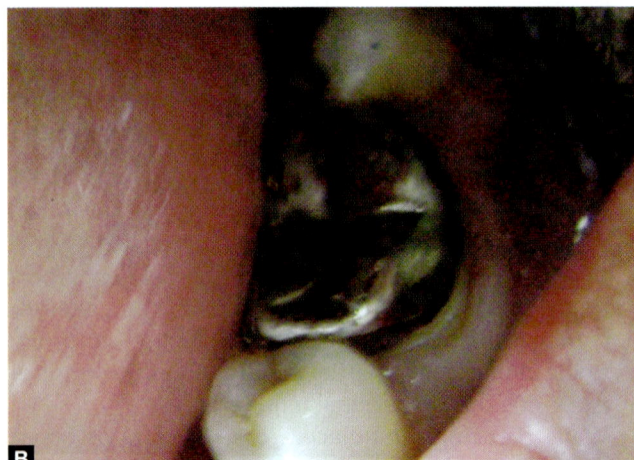
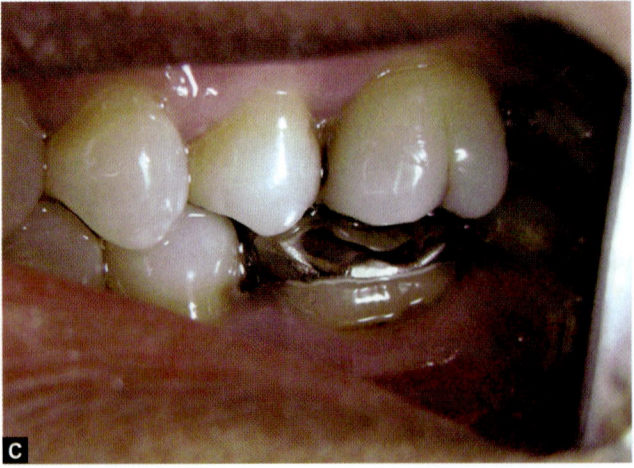

Figures 23.45A to C: (A) Tooth preparation for onlay; (B) Onlay in place; (C) Onlay in occlusion

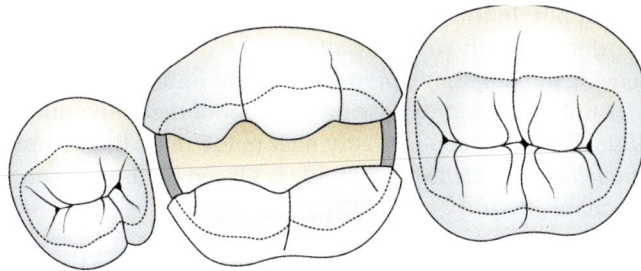

Figure 23.46: Proximal box for onlay are extended beyond contact area

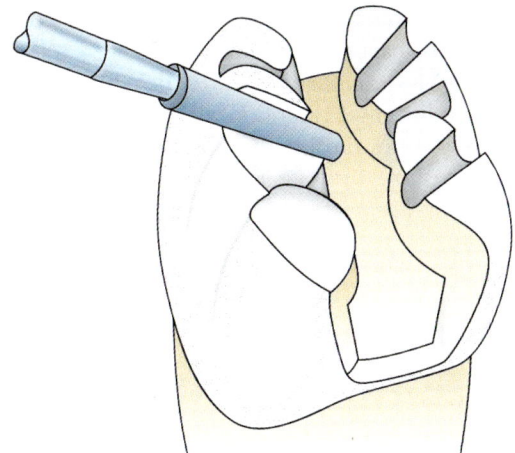

Figure 23.47: Cusps are reduced according to occlusal anatomy of the tooth

are given bevel by holding the bur at 30° angle with the tooth surface. Counter bevels should be wide enough so that cavosurface margins extend at least 1 mm beyond the occlusal contacts with opposing teeth (**Fig. 23.49**). The exceptions for the giving bevel are facial cusp of maxillary premolars and first molar because esthetics is a prime concern in these areas.

Retraction cord is correctly applied in the gingiva before giving bevels and flares to the preparation. Prepare gingival bevels and flares of the proximal enamel wall in the same way as in inlay preparation.

A nicely designed onlay preparation should have proximal box forms for retention and flat pulpal and gingival

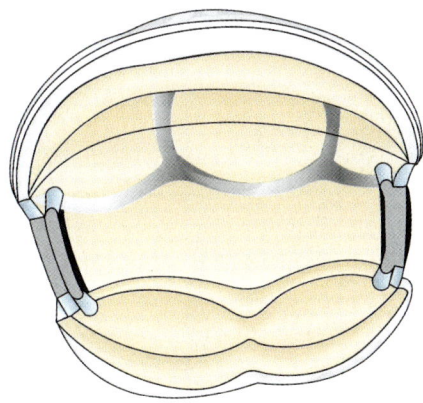

Figure 23.48: Onlay preparation with retention grooves in facioaxial and linguoaxial line angles

cusp) depth on the cuspal crest. Groove helps in accurate and uniform cutting. While reducing the adjacent cusp, involve lingual or buccal developmental groove in cutting.

Retention and Resistance Form

For increasing retention and resistance, grooves are made at the proximal walls of the box. Grooves are made in the facioaxial and linguoaxial line angles in the dentin so as to have added retention. Direction of placement of the grooves should be parallel with the path of withdrawal of wax pattern (**Fig. 23.48**). Prepare a reverse bevel or counter bevel on the facial or lingual side of the reduced facial or lingual cusp respectively. For this, usually a flame shaped, diamond point is used. Facial and lingual surfaces

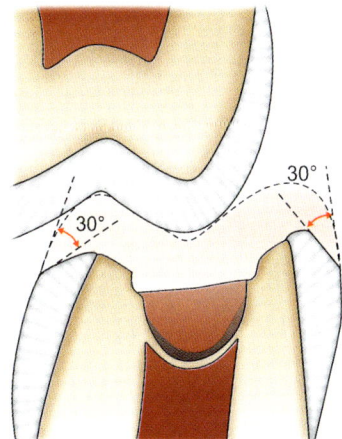

Figure 23.49: Cavorsurface margin of counter bevel should be clear of occlusal contact

walls for resistance to dislodging forces (**Figs 23.50 and 23.51**).

Final Preparation

Clean the preparation with air/water spray or with cotton pellet and inspect it for detection and removal of debris and examine for correction of all cavosurface angles and margins. Remove remaining caries and/or old restorative material.

In the large preparations with soft caries, the removal of carious dentin is done with spoon excavator or slow speed round bur. In this, two-step pulpal floor is made, i.e. only portion of tooth which is affected by caries is removed, leaving the remaining preparation floor untouched.

Apply a protective base on the floor of the preparation. If the caries is deep and very near to the pulp, then 1 mm thick layer of calcium hydroxide is placed before applying a suitable base.

ADDITIONAL RETENTION AND RESISTANCE FORM FEATURES FOR CAST RESTORATION

In addition to primary retention forms like parallelism of walls, circumferential tie, masticatory forces directed to seat the restoration and dovetail, etc. following auxillary means of retention can be used to provide additional retention to the cast restorations.

- *Grooves (Figs 23.52A and B)*: Grooves are placed to provide additional retention and resistance to lateral displacement of mesial, distal, facial or lingual part of the restoration.

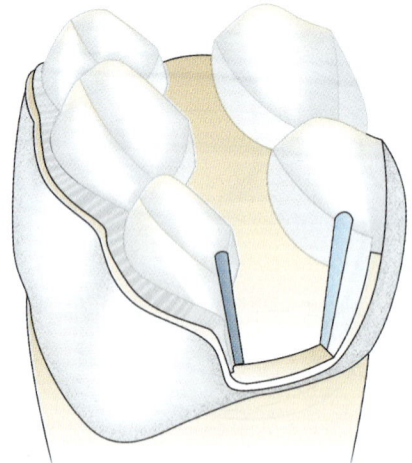

Figure 23.50: Completed onlay preparation showing rounded occlusal line angle, precise internal angles, properly tapered walls with smooth finish lines

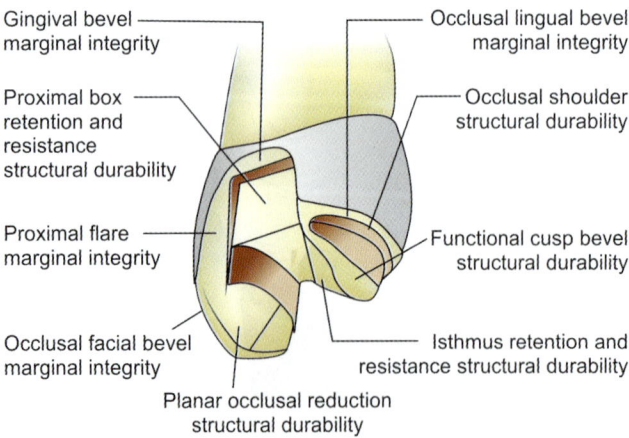

Gingival bevel marginal integrity

Occlusal lingual bevel marginal integrity

Proximal box retention and resistance structural durability

Occlusal shoulder structural durability

Proximal flare marginal integrity

Functional cusp bevel structural durability

Occlusal facial bevel marginal integrity

Isthmus retention and resistance structural durability

Planar occlusal reduction structural durability

Figure 23.51: Completed onlay preparation with all features

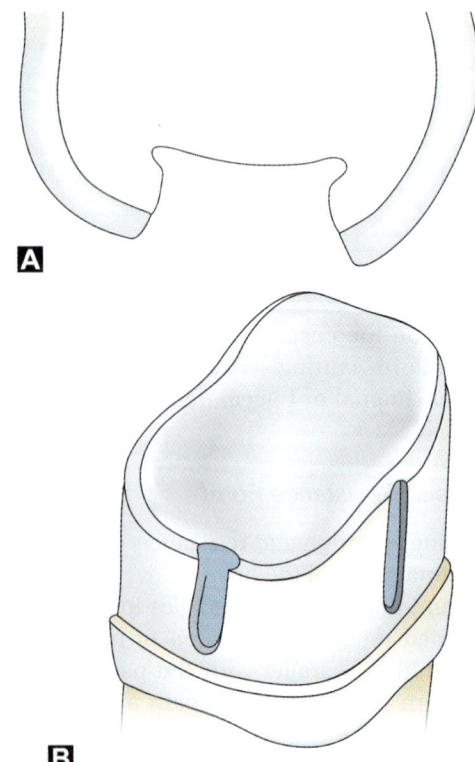

A

B

Figures 23.52A and B: Grooves placed in cast restoration

Internal grooves are given when preparation is shallow and small. They are contraindicated when preparation is deep with the danger of pulp involvement.

External grooves are indicated in extracoronal preparations which lack retention because of short preparation with severe taper or excessive width. They are placed at the periphery of preparation so as to prevent displacement of restoration.

- *Reverse bevel (Fig. 23.53)*: It is indicated for class I, II and III restorations. It is used when sufficient dimensions of gingival floor are present so as to accommodate it. It is placed at gingival floor forming an inclined plane directed gingivally and axially.
- *Internal box (Fig. 23.54)*: It is prepared in dentin which forms vertical walls with definite line and point angles.

It is indicated when sufficient dentin bulk is present. It increases the retention 8 to 10 times and thus placed at the periphery of preparation close to marginal ridge. It should be at least 2 mm in dimension. Internal box is contraindicated in class IV and V preparations.
- *External box (Fig. 23.55)*: It is a box like preparation opening to the axial surface of the tooth. It may have three, four or five walls with a floor. The peripheral portion of these walls can be flared or beveled.
- *Pins*: Various pins can be used to increase the retention of cast restorations. These can be cemented, threaded, parallel, cast and wrought.
- *Slot (Fig. 23.56)*: Slot is an internal cavity prepared with in the floor of preparation. It is indicated in tooth preparation with shallow depth, and when dovetail cannot

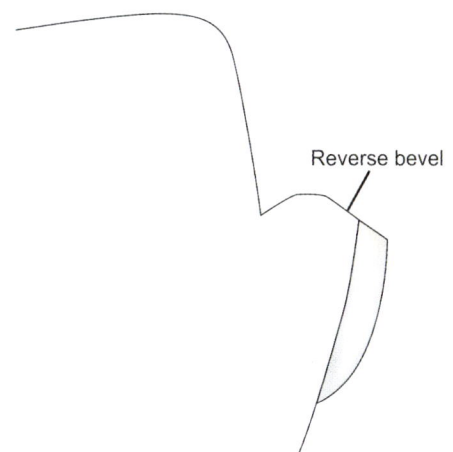

Figure 23.53: Reverse bevel

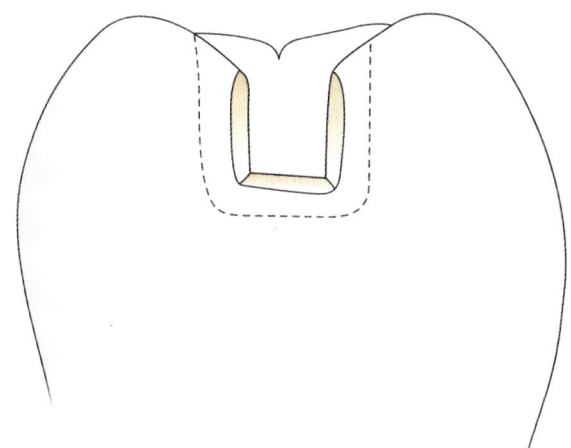

Figure 23.55: External box

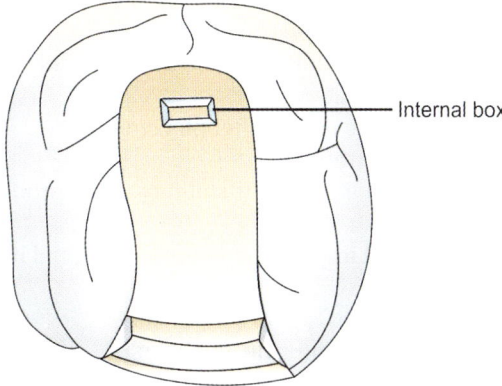

Figure 23.54: Internal box

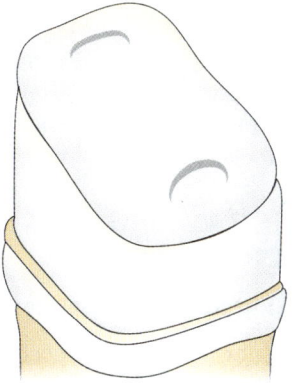

Figure 23.56: Slot

Designs of margins of cast restoratiaons (**Fig. 23.57**)

Design of margin	Advantages	Disadvantages	Indications
• Full shoulder	• Good edge strength due to more bulk	• Excessive tooth cutting	• Facial margin of metal (**Fig. 23.57A**) ceramic and ceramic crowns
• Shoulder with bevel	• Good edge strength due to more bulk of material along with the advantages of bevel	• Involves excessive tooth cutting	• Facial margin of metal ceramic crown with supragingival margins (**Fig. 23.57B**)
• Chamfer	• Easy to control extension and clear cut margins with sufficient bulk • Better finishing and polishing of margins	• More chances of unsupported enamel rods	• Cast metal restorations margins of metal ceramic (**Fig. 23.57C**)
• Bevel	• Less cutting of enamel • Removal of unsupported enamel rods • Better finishing of metal margins	• Apical margins have to be extended into gingival sulcus	• Margins of types I, II and III gold casting alloy restorations
• Chisel edge	• Conservative enamel cutting	• Indefinite and difficult to control location of the margins	• For malposed and titled teeth • Rarely used
• Feather edge	• Least cutting of enamel is required	• Poor strength due to inadequate bulk • Difficult to control and finish the margins	• Must be avoided

be prepared because of restricted occlusal anatomy. They have depth of 2 to 3 mm and are prepared using round and tapered fissure bur.

- Skirt is a specific extension which involves a part of axial wall of the tooth preparation. It is indicated when restoration has short/missing facial or lingual wall and when defect is more extensive. Skirt is also indicated in cases where contact and contour of the tooth is to be changed.
- *Collar*: It is the surface extension which involves facial or lingual surfaces of one or more cusps. It helps in increasing retention and resistance in case of grossly decayed teeth, in short teeth and in the teeth where pins are contraindicated, collar is prepared 1.5-2 mm deep.
- *Cusp capping*: Cusp capping also helps in increasing resistance and retention form, provided sufficient height of cusp is present to offer locking mechanism.
- *Reciprocal retention*: In case of cemented preparations, if restoration is not locked from the opposite end of locked side, movements of the free end create stresses in the locked end. To reduce this, reciprocal retention is provided by placing retention mode at every end of the preparation in the form of grooves, dovetail or internal box.

TECHNIQUE FOR MAKING CAST METAL RESTORATION

Impression Taking for Cast Metal Restoration

For achieving better results, the occlusal contacts in maximum intercuspal position and in all lateral and protrusive movements should be evaluated before and

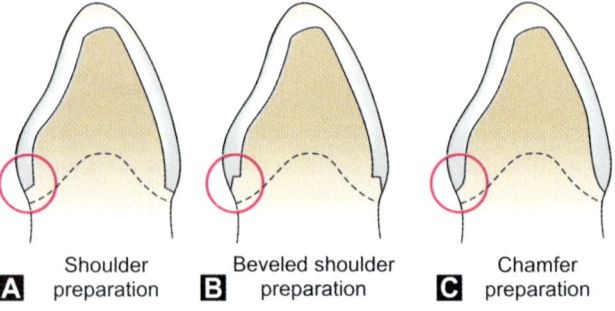

| A Shoulder preparation | B Beveled shoulder preparation | C Chamfer preparation |

Figures 23.57A to C: Different designs of preparations for cast restorations at gingival margin

after tooth preparation. After the tooth preparation, the impression of the prepared and adjacent teeth is taken using an elastomeric impression material (**Fig. 23.58**).

Before taking impression, gingival retraction cord should be applied first for better recording of gingival margins of the preparation (**Fig. 23.59**).

Requirements of a material to be used for final impression are that it should:

- Be able to become elastic after placement
- Have adequate strength
- Have dimensional accuracy, stability and reproduction of details.

Commonly used impression materials for final impression are:

- Polysulfide
- Silicone (polyvinyl siloxane impression)
- Polyether impression materials
- Agar.

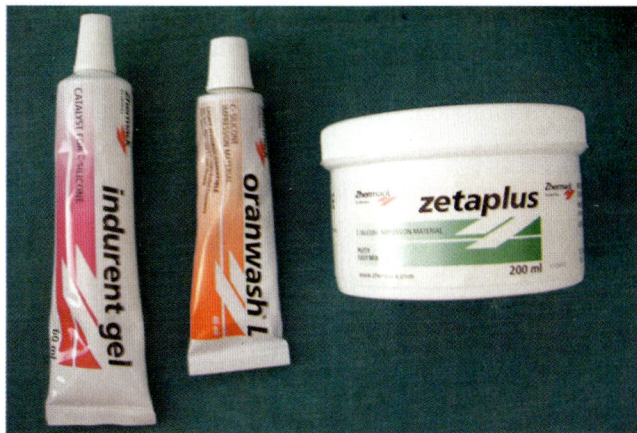

Figure 23.58: Rubber base impression material

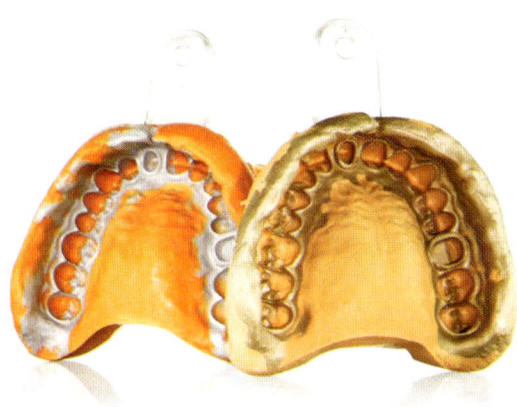

Figure 23.59: A proper impression should incorporate all the details of the preparation

Alginate hydrocolloid are mostly used for the impression of opposing arch and rubber impression material are used for the impression of prepared arch.

Record of Interocclusal Relationship

For single tooth inlay procedure, simple hinge type articulators are sufficient. But for restoring multiple teeth with cast metal restorations, the semi-adjustable articulators are used. Final adjustments in centric occlusion and various mandibular movements are made in the mouth before cementation to assure complete functionally harmonius restoration.

Temporary (Interim) Restoration

Interim restoration is given to the prepared tooth for the time period between tooth preparation and cementing the restoration so as to protect and stabilize it and to provide comfort to the patient.

An interim restoration should have the following features:
- Nonirritating
- Esthetically satisfactory
- Easy to clean and maintain
- Protect and maintain the health of periodontium
- Adequate strength and retention to withstand the masticatory forces.

Normally, the interim restorations are made up of acrylic resin. They can be prepared by direct and indirect methods.

Direct Technique

- Take preoperative impression of the patient
- Prepare the tooth
- Pour the tooth colored selfcure acrylic resin in the preoperative alginate impression in the prepared tooth area
- Seat the impression onto the prepared tooth and remove it after resin is cured
- Do final finishing and polishing of temporary restoration.

Advantage: Takes less time.

Disadvantage: Pulp and periodontal tissue may get trauma from heat produced by direct polymerization of the acrylic and its monomer.

Indirect Technique

- Take preoperative alginate impression (called impression no. 1). Preserve this impression in humid conditions by covering with wet cotton.
- Take an impression of the prepared tooth with alginate (called impression no. 2).
- Pour the impression no. 2 with fast setting plaster. Remove any defect if present in the cast and apply cold-mold seal separating media over the prepared tooth and about 5 mm around it.
- Mix tooth colored acrylic resin and pour it over impression no. 1 only in the prepared tooth area
- Now carefully seat the cast prepared by impression no. 2 in the impression no. 1 so as to give shape to the resin for making temporary restoration.
- Remove excessive resin from the embrasure areas.
- Wait for resin to cure completely and remove the cast after it is cured.
- Take out resin crown from impression no. 1 and do the final finishing and polishing.

Advantages
- Better marginal accuracy.
- Since polymerization takes place outside the mouth,

pulp and periodontal tissues are not traumatized by heat of polymerization and monomer.

- Resin cannot be locked on preparation surface of tooth in small undercuts and in the cervical areas.
- Less chairside time.

Working Cast

Working cast is an accurate replica of the prepared and adjacent unprepared teeth over which cast metal restoration can be fabricated.

For making working cast, commonly Type IV or V stones are used since they have superior properties. For making a working cast with removable dies, twice pouring of cast is required from an elastic impression. The first cast prepares the removable die and the second cast establishes the intraarch relationship called 'master cast'. These casts are known as split casts.

Working Die

Die Materials

Die is the positive replica of a prepared tooth. Dies should replicate the tooth preparation in the most minute details along with all accessible unprepared area of the tooth. Though various die materials are available with different properties, the ideal die material should:

- Be compatible with the impression materials
- Have a smooth nonabradable surface
- Produce accurate details of impression
- Have adequate strength
- Be easy and quick to fabricate
- Have contrasting color to that of inlay wax.

Commonly used materials for making die are:

- Dental stones
- Electroformed dies
- Epoxy resins
- Divestment.

Dental Stones

The material used to fabricate the die and working casts are usually gypsum products. Most commonly used are type IV dental stone (high strength) and type V dental stone (high strength and high expansion). Higher setting expansion of type V stone compensates for larger solidification shrinkage of base metal alloys.

Electroformed Dies

Electrodeposition of copper or silver on the impression gives a high strength, adequate hardness and good abrasion resistance to the cast.

Electroforming   *(Electroplasting/Electrodeposition)*: This is a process by which a thin coating of metal is deposited on the impression after which a gypsum cast is poured into the impression. The cast obtained will have hard metallic surface.

Metals used for electroforming are:

- Copper
- Silver.

Indications

- Individual tooth impression
- Full (upper/lower) arch impression.

Epoxy resins: They are supplied in two—paste and liquid systems which are mixed before insertion into the impression. They are mixed just before using the material.

On mixing, they form a viscous paste and poured into impression. The abrasive resistance, strength, and reproduction of details are much better than that of gypsum products.

Divestment: Divestment is a combination of die material and investing material. Divestment is mixed with a colloidal silica liquid, then a die is prepared from the mix and a wax pattern is made on it. After this, the wax pattern with die is invested in divestment. This is highly accurate technique for extracoronal cast gold restorations.

Wax Pattern Fabrication

There are two methods for wax pattern fabrication

- ***Direct wax pattern method:*** In this, wax pattern is prepared in the oral cavity.
- ***Indirect wax pattern method:*** In this wax pattern is prepared outside the oral cavity.

Direct Wax Pattern Method

Direct wax pattern produces better fitting than indirect method. This method is possible only in inlays and onlays and not in crowns and bridges, etc.

Direct wax pattern using matrix band

- Isolate the tooth using cotton rolls
- Apply matrix band and retainer. Coat the internal surface of band using separating media like vaseline
- For making direct wax pattern, type I inlay wax is used
- Soften the inlay wax by heating and moving it over a alcohol flame
- Compress the softened inlay wax into the prepared tooth for few minutes with finger pressure. This technique is called 'compression technique'
- Since cooling of wax to the mouth temperature results in shrinkage, it can be compensated by holding the wax

in the preparation under finger pressure until it reaches mouth temperature

- Remove excess of wax and do the carving. With a hot egg burnisher, contour the occlusal portion of the wax pattern
- Now remove the matrix band and retainer carefully without disturbing the wax pattern
- Ask the patient to bite in centric occlusion for a few seconds after placing a thin layer of cotton soaked in warm water
- Examine the occlusal surface for high points and remove them. Do the occlusal carving
- Pass a floss through the contact area while holding the pattern in place
- Smoothen the proximal surface of the pattern with fine soft silk
- Evaluate and correct all the margins of the pattern. Burnish and remove any excess wax over the axial margins with a warm hollenback waxing instrument
- Finally, examine the pattern. There should be a slight excess of wax over the gingival margin. Add positive contact by applying soft wax
- Once the satisfactory wax pattern is formed, attach the sprue former and reservoir to the thickest point of the wax pattern
- Remove the wax pattern from the preparation and examine it for marginal integrity.

Direct wax pattern without use of matrix band

Here, the technique is same except that matrix band is not used during fabrication of wax pattern. In this, after the carving of occlusal portion is done, use dental floss to remove extra wax from the proximal portion and to produce proper contact and contour.

Advantages
- Less chances of discrepancies
- Less laboratory time.

Disadvantages
- Requires more chair sidetime
- Requires more skill
- Finishing and polishing done on prepared tooth.

Indirect Wax Pattern Method

Indications
- Large preparations like onlays, full coverage crowns and MOD restoration
- Insufficient access and visibility
- When minute details like skirts and collars are present.

Steps for Fabricating
- Use Type II inlay wax for indirect wax pattern
- Lubricate the die using any lubricating fluid. The lubricator should produce a very thin separator film
- Adapt the inlay wax to the die by flowing or by the compression technique
- Do the carving using a warm instrument
- Attach a sprue former to the wax pattern to the thickest portion as in direct method.

Advantages
- Less chair side time
- Finishing and polishing can be done on die.

Disadvantages
- More laboratory work
- Errors in cast can result in inadequate casting.

Spruing (Fig. 23.60)

Principles of Optimal Sprue Design

- Sprue former provides a channel so that molten metal flows into mold space after the wax pattern has been eliminated.
- ***A sprue former can be made up of***
  - Wax
  - Plastic
  - Metal

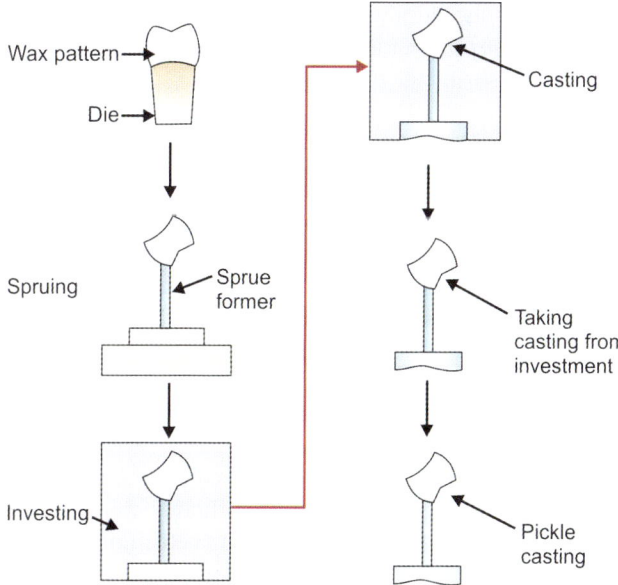

Figure 23.60: Steps of casting process

- **Functions of sprue former:** A sprue former:
  - Forms a channel through which molten metal can enter during casting.
  - Provides a reservoir of molten metal to compensate for metal shrinkage during solidification.
  - Forms a channel for elimination of wax.
- **Sprue diameter:** Sprue diameter usually depends upon the size of wax pattern. It should be either equal or greater than the thickest part of wax pattern.
- **Attachment of sprue former:** Sprue former should be attached to the thickest portions of wax pattern. This helps in minimizing the turbulence of molten alloy. It also reduces residual stresses in wax while attachment of sprue former. It also ensures that molten metal has filled thinner section of the mold.
- **Sprue length:** Length of sprue former should be long enough so that the end of wax pattern is 1/8th to 1/4th of an inch away from the open end of casting ring. This permits the investment to withstand the impact of molten alloy and it also allows gases to escape.
- **Direction of sprue:** The sprue former should not be attached to thin or delicate parts of wax pattern as molten alloy may fracture investment in that area and may cause failure of casting. It should always be attached at an angle of 45° to the bulkiest portion of the wax pattern.

  The sprue former attachment to wax pattern should be flared for high density gold alloys but constricted for base metal alloys (low density alloys).
- Reservoir should always be added to sprue former for constant supply of molten metal. This helps in reducing localized shrinkage porosity.

Washing of Wax Pattern

Washing of wax pattern: Before investment, the wax pattern should be washed and covered with detergent. Soap and 3 percent hydrogen peroxide is applied with a brush to remove cavity debris and blood which could result in rough casting. It is then rinsed with water. After washing, a layer of detergent is applied to reduce surface tension and aid in flow of the investment material over the wax pattern eliminating small bubbles that may remain. These agents are also called wetting agents. Soap is not a good wetting agent as it reacts with calcium sulphate of the binder forming a precipitate. Synthetic detergents are common like lissapol, teepol, cetavelon cetrimide, etc. The pattern must be left to dry for 10 minutes before investing takes place.

Investing (Fig. 23.61)

Once the wax pattern is cleaned, it is surrounded by an investment that hardens and forms the mold in which casting is made.

Principles of investing

- Type of ring
  - For hygroscopic expansion technique - rubber ring
  - For thermal expansion-metal ring
- Selection of ring liner
  A ring liner
  - Allows mold expansion
  - Decreases loss of heat
  - Permits separation of ring after casting
  Ring liners used nowadays are:
  - Asbestos
  - Non asbestos
    i. Cellulose (paper)
    ii. Ceramic
    iii. Combination of above.
  The casting ring liner is kept 3 mm short of the both ends of the ring. The minimum liner thickness is 1 mm.
- *Attaching the ring and crucible former:* The next step is to attach the ring to the crucible former such that the wax pattern can be invested.

Casting crucibles are of three types:
1. *Clay:* For noble and highly noble alloys.
2. *Carbon:* For high noble alloys for crown and bridge; and for higher fusing, gold based metal ceramic alloys.

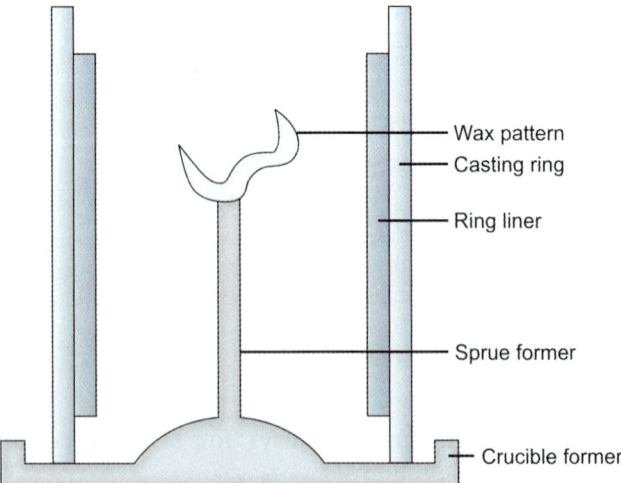

Figure 23.61: Arrangement in casting ring ready for investing

3. *Quartz (Zirconia-alumina)*: For high fusing alloys of any type, especially for alloys having higher melting range and sensitive to carbon contamination.

For example, High palladium alloys for crown and bridge, Palladium silver alloys for metal ceramic copings and nickel/cobalt based alloys.

Two main methods of investing the wax pattern are:
1. Hand investing
2. Vacuum investing.
- *Hand investing*
  - The investment powder is incorporated to the liquid in the mixing bowl in the proper powder-liquid ratio. (Usually 50 g of calcium sulfate-bonded investment powder or 60 g of phosphate-bonded investment powder is sufficient to fill an inlay ring). Here, the mixing for the investment material is done by hand followed by mechanically mixing under vacuum (as in case of phosphate bonded investments)
  - The mixing is done in accordance with the manufacturer's instructions
  - The pattern is painted with a layer of investment and the remainder is vibrated slowly into the ring
  - The ring is tilted once the investment reaches the level of pattern, minimizing entrapment of air
  - After that, the investment is allowed to set
  - If hygroscopic expansion technique is used, the ring is placed in 37°C water bath for one hour.
- *Vacuum investing*: For prevention of air entrapment during investing, vacuum investing is done.

It is further of two types:
1. *Mechanical vacuum investing*: In this type, the mixing of investment and its filing into the ring is done mechanically under vacuum
2. *Manual vacuum investing*: Here the investment is spatulated by hand under vacuum and then the ring is filled. The manual investing is more appropriate as greater control during addition of investment.

Disadvantages of hand investing
- Increased porosity in the investment
- Less reproduction of detail than vacuum investing
- Less tensile strength
- Less smoother cast than that obtained by vacuum investing.

Casting Procedure

Casting is a process by which a pattern for a restoration is converted to replicate in a dental alloy. Casting procedure includes burnout for wax elimination, expansion of investment to compensate for setting shrinkage and placement of gold alloy into the mold.

The casting procedure was not popular in dentistry until 1907, when WH Taggart introduced this technique and casting machine.

Burnout of Wax Pattern/Wax Elimination and Heating

Burnout is done approximately one hour after investing. If delayed, it is kept in 100 percent humidor. Ring should never be dried. For proper elimination, the mold is set in the furnace with the sprue hole placed downwards. This allows:
- The wax to be eliminated as liquid
- Oxygen can circulate more into the cavity to react with wax and form gases rather than fine carbon.

The heating should be gradual as 400°C in 20 min and maintained for 30 min. For next 30 min, the temperature is increased to 700°C and maintained for 30 min. (1 hr 20 min.) The casting procedure should be completed without permitting the mold to cool.

Temperature requirements for various investments
- For gypsum bonded investment:
  - In hygroscopic low heat technique – temperature required – 468°C for 60 to 90 mins. Casting done immediately after investment
  - In high heat thermal expansion technique-slow heating to 650°C in 60 mins, held for 15 to 20 mins.
    Gypsum investments disintegrate at 700°C to release sulphur gas which causes black and brittle castings.
- For phosphate bonded investments
  - Heated to 315°C for 30 mins and then to 750 to 900°C. Casting done within 1 min of its removal.

Methods of alloy melting: Various devices are used for melting of alloys. These can either be by torch or by electrical means.
- ***Torch melting:*** It uses
  - *Gas/air*: The gas used is mainly propane and has the lowest temperature of all sources. Used for small inlays and type I and II alloys
  - *Natural gas/oxygen*: Has high temperature and can be used for PFM alloys
  - *Air/acetylene*
  - *Acetylene/oxygen*: It has the highest temperature and is used for base metal alloys.
  - *Zones of flame*: Four zones are there
    i. *Mixing zone*:
       a. Dark in color
       b. Air and gas are mixed here before combustion
       c. No heat is present
    ii. *Combustion zone*:
       a. Surrounds the inner zone
       b. Green in color

c. Here, the gas and air is partially burned. This zone is definitely oxidizing in nature

d. Should always be kept away from the molten alloy during fusion.

iii. *Reducing zone*:

a. Dimly blue and located just beyond the tip of the green combustion zone is the reducing zone

b. Hottest part of the flame and it should be kept constantly on the alloy during melting.

iv. Oxidizing zone:

a. Zone in which final combustion between gas and surrounding air occurs

b. Not used for fusion of alloys

c. This portion of the flame should not be used to melt the alloy.

- *Electric melting*: It uses
  i. Resistance heating system
  ii. Induction heating system
  iii. Electric arc heating system

Casting machines: Different types of casting machines are used for casting of dental alloys.

Basically two types of casting machines are:
1. Centrifugal casting machine
2. Air pressure casting machine

Centrifugal casting machine: It is very popular and cheap in cost, giving good results for small castings. Here, the centrifugal force is used to accelerate the flow of molten metal into the mold space. Sequence of steps to be followed in gold alloy casting is as follows:

- Heat the ring in which wax pattern has been invested to 1200°F and keep it at this temperature for 15 minutes in the furnace
- Move the arm of the casting machine by 2 to 3 turns in clockwise direction and lock it so that the arm does not rotate back
- Heat the gold alloy in the crucible of the casting machine until it becomes bright orange in color and has a shiny appearance
- Place the casting ring in the cradle of the casting machine. The end of the ring with the sprue should be towards the crucible. Move up the crucible as close as possible to the casting ring
- When the gold alloy is fully melt, release the lock of the casting arm so as to force the molten gold into the mold by centrifugal force
- Remove the ring from the casting machine and keep it in the water keeping sprue end upward and above the water level, and dry, till the ring is cooled.
- Recover the casting and clean it with a bristle toothbrush and water to remove investment from the casting.

Advantages of centrifugal casting machine:
- Simplicity of design and operation
- Opportunity to cast both small and large castings on same machine.

Air pressure casting machine:
In this, compressed air or gases like carbon dioxide or nitrogen is used to force the molten alloy into the mold. This type of machine is preferred for small castings.

Other casting machines are:
- Electrical resistance heated casting machine
- Induction casting machine
- Direct current arc melting machine
- Titanium casting.

Cleaning of Casting

After completion of casting, the casting ring is removed from the casting machine and quenched.

Quenching involves rapid cooling at room temperature water bath or ice water bath. It does not allow sufficient time for atomic movements to form an ordered structure. This disordered structure is retained at room temperature, making it soft and ductile. This helps in final adjustments easier.

Advantages of Quenching

- Easy removal of casting from casting ring due to cracking of investment material.
- Keeps the gold alloy in annealed state for easy burnishing and polishing.

Pickling: The surface of casting usually appears dark due to presence of oxides and other contaminants. This type of film can be removed by method known as 'pickling'. Pickling is process in which discolored casting is heated with an acid in test tube or beaker.

Solution preferred for pickling are
- Fifty percent hydrochloric acid solution (best suited for gypsum bonded investment).
- Fifty percent sulfuric acid.

Precautions to be taken during pickling
- Casting should not be heated and then dropped into the pickling solution as margins of casting may be distorted during heating
- Casting should not be held with steel instruments as this may contaminate the pickling solution and casting
- Acid solution should not be boiled rather it should be heated
- Use fresh solution every time.

Trying in the Casting

- Before the 'trying in' procedure, remove the temporary restoration and cement completely and carefully
- Place a four layered gauze piece as a throat screen during trying in and removal of small indirect restoration till the cementation of the casting
- Place the casting on the tooth using light pressure. If it does not seat properly, do not force it in the preparation. Overcontoured proximal surfaces may also prevent seating of the casting
- Check the occlusion by asking patient to bite on bite paper. High points in restoration results in perforation of articulating paper. Improper occluding contacts make the tooth unstable and tend to deflect it (**Figs 23.62A and B**)
- Evaluate the embrasures and judge the points where proximal recontouring is required. Contacts can be present too occlusally, broad faciolingually or occlusocervically (**Figs 23.63A to D**)

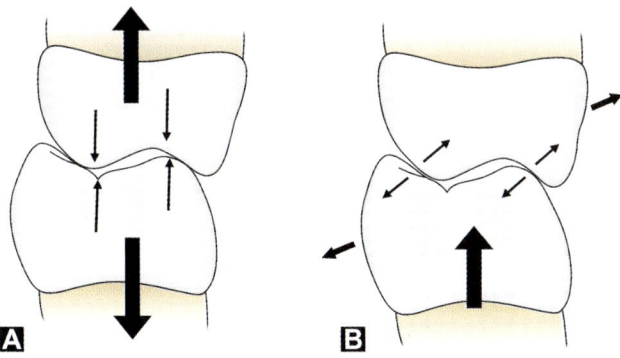

Figures 23.62A and B: (A) Proper occlusion tends to stabilize the cast; (B) Improper occlusion tends to deflect the tooth

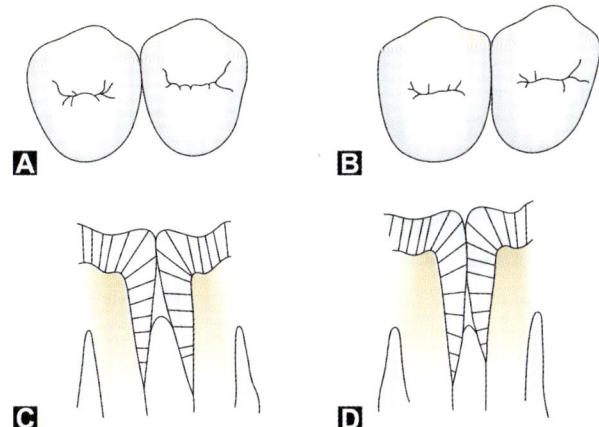

Figures 23.63A to D: (A) Proper contact; (B) Contact too broad faciolingually; (C) Contact too occlusally; (D) Contact too broad occlusocervically

- Pass the dental floss through the contact to find out the tightness of the contact and its locations.
- Adjust the contact area so that casting seats passively. Fine carborundum particles, impregnated rubber disks or wheels can be used for adjusting the proximal contact and contours.

What should be done if casting is short of proximal contact with adjacent tooth?
➡ To treat this problem, a solder of 650 or higher is added to the casting. The difference between soldius temperature of inlay and liquiduos temperature of solder should be 100°F.

Steps of soldering
➡ Treat the proximal surface of casting with abrasive wheel to remove traces of any polishing agents, as they may act as antiflux.
➡ Cut a strip of solder, it should extend 1 mm beyond contact area.
➡ Apply borax type flux on the contact area of the casting and on both the surfaces of the piece of solder.
➡ Place the solder at proper place on the contact area requiring build-up and direct the pinpoint flame of bunsen burner to the solder with the help of blow pipe so that the solder melts and flows.
➡ Apply melt solder on to the casting.
➡ Trim and polish the contact

Cementation of the Casting (Figs 23.64 to 23.66)

- Clean the casting thoroughly before cementation
- Isolate the prepared tooth, clean it and apply a thin layer of varnish in the preparation
- Apply warm air to the gingival sulcus of the prepared tooth to dry it
- Apply a thin layer of luting cement on the surfaces of the casting which will be in contact with the tooth surface and on the tooth preparation surface
- Seat the casting with the help of hand pressure using a suitable instrument
- Ask the patient to bite on a small cotton pellet which is placed on the occlusal surface of the casting
- Clean the area with dry cotton for removing the remnants of set cement
- Recheck the occlusion for harmony of centric occlusion
- Finally, check the gingival sulcus for any remnants of cement to avoid irritation to the supporting tissues.

To prevent postcementation pain:
- Do not desiccate the tooth
- Use the proper powder-to-liquid ratio of luting cement
- Do not remove the smear layer

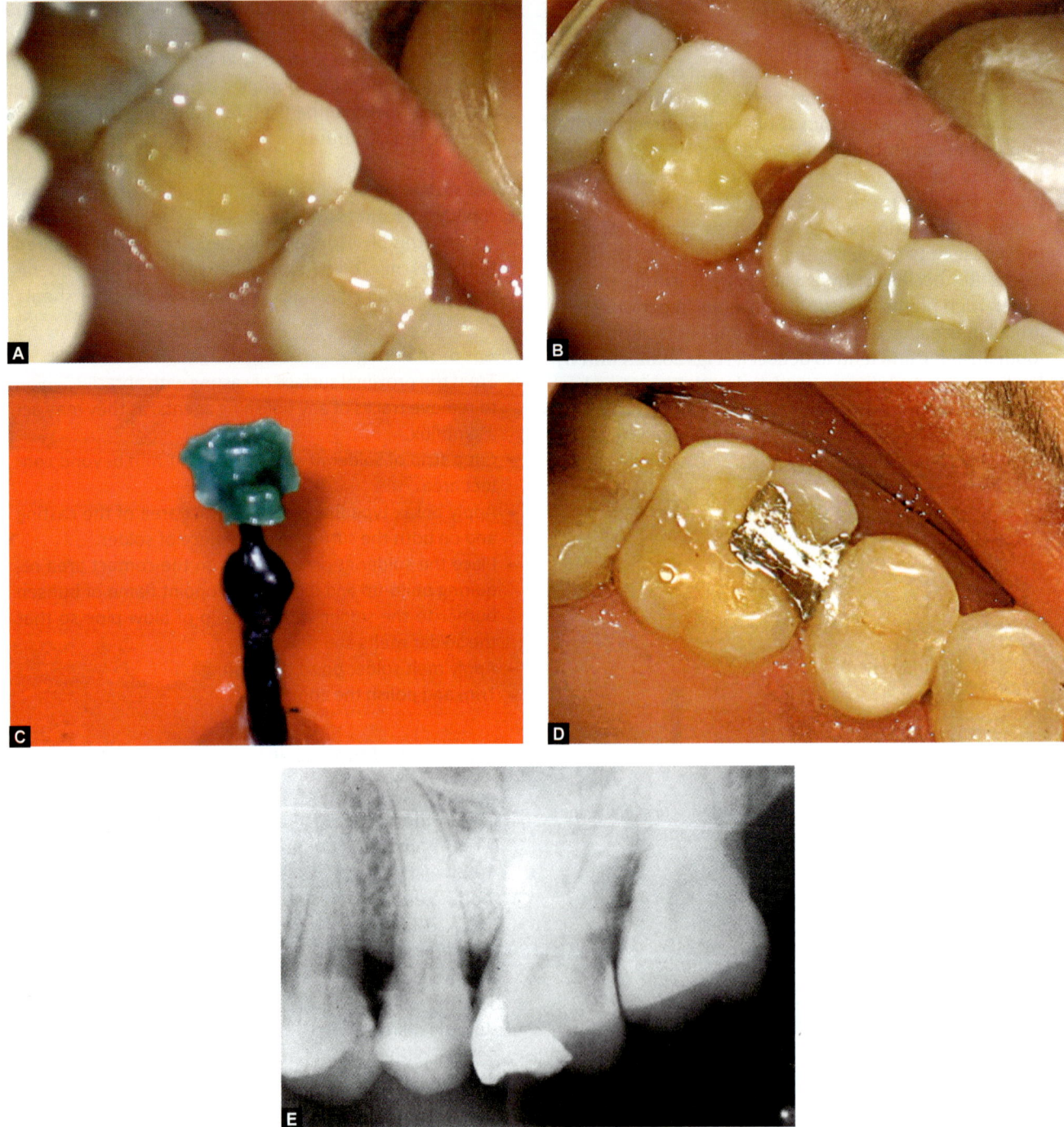

Figures 23.64A to E: (A) Class II caries in 26; (B) Tooth preparation for cast metal inlay; (C) Wax pattern and spruing; (D) Metal inlay in place; (E) Radiograph showing cast metal inlay on 26

- Use a base material on deep areas of the preparation
- Apply a resin dentin-desensitizer
- Avoid overfilling the casting with cement

- Seat the casting gently
- Protect the cement from moisture contamination
- Clean up excess cement only after it has fully set; this

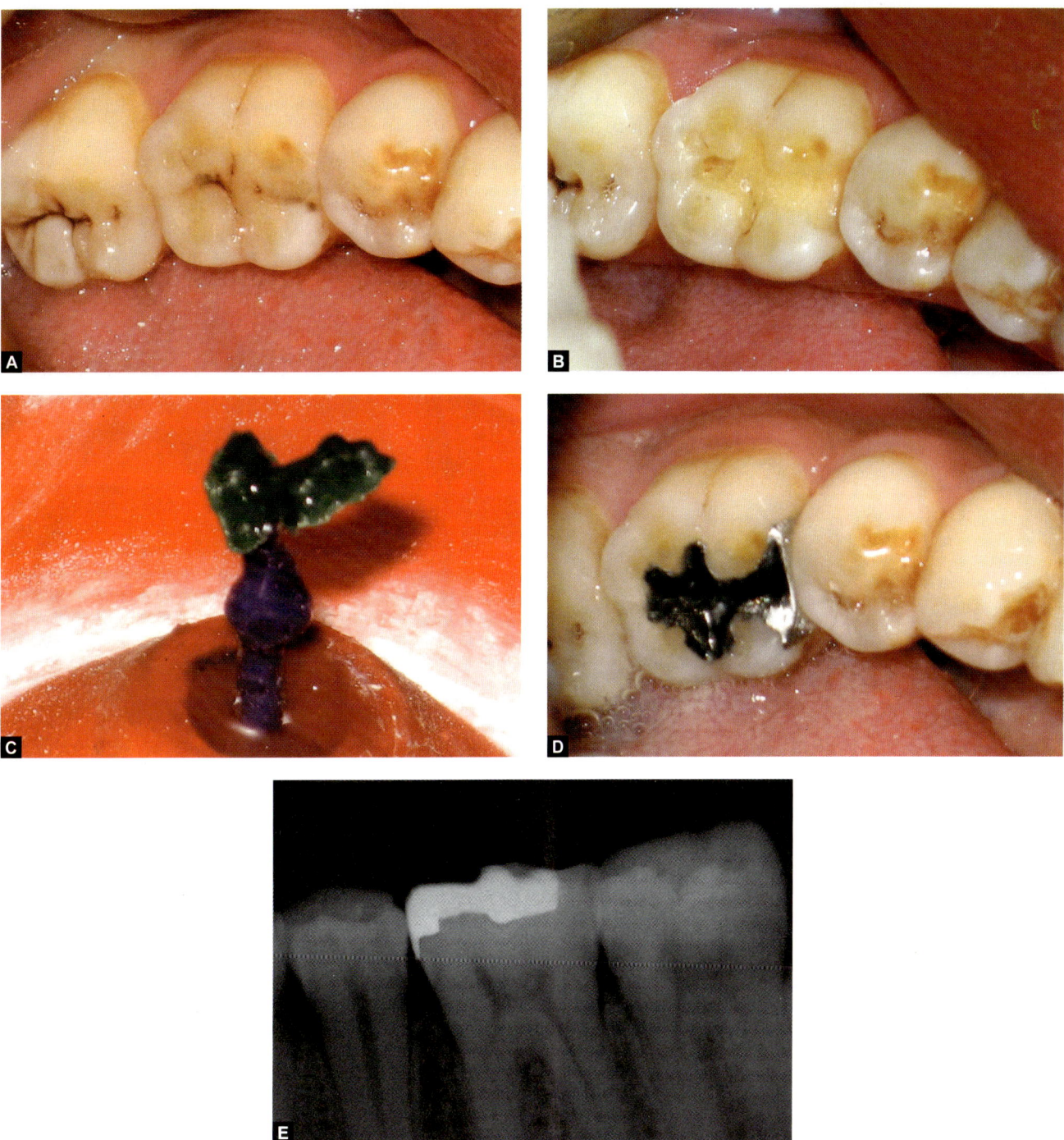

Figures 23.65A to E: (A) Class II caries in 36; (B) Tooth preparation of 36 for cast metal inlay; (C) Wax pattern and spruing; (D) Metal inlay cemented on 36; (E) Radiograph showing cast metal inlay in place

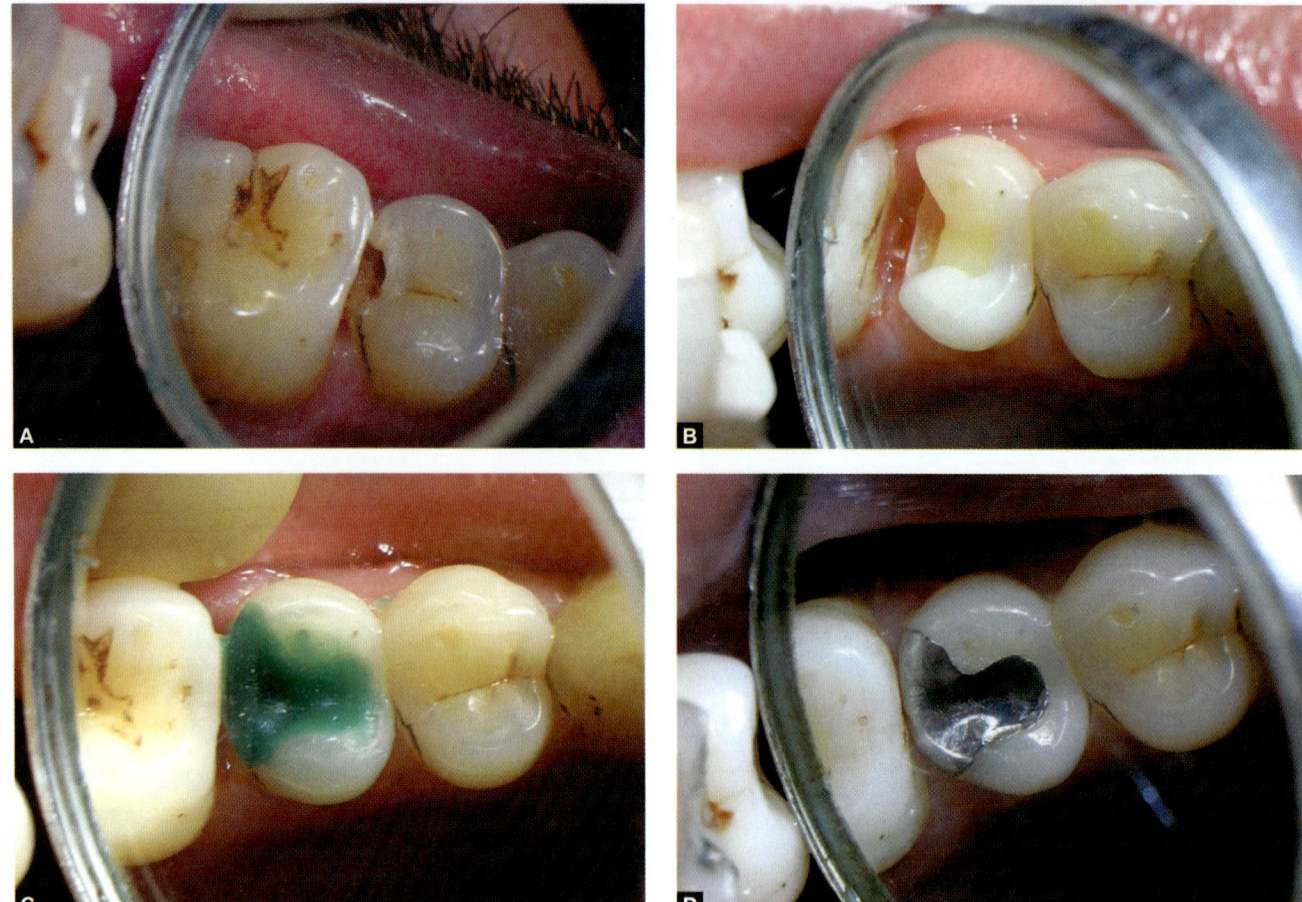

Figures 23.66A to D: (A) Class II caries of 15; (B) Tooth preparation of 15 for cast inlay; (C) Wax pattern fabrication; (D) Metal inlay in place

prevents the cement from being pulled out from underneath margins.

CASTING DEFECTS

The various steps in making of casting should be followed systematically, otherwise chances of casting defects are increased.

Casting defects are of many types and may be classified as:

Surface Roughness and Irregularities

Surface roughness is generalized roughness of the surface of the casting while surface irregularities are isolated imperfections such as nodules, ridges, fins and spines.

Causes

- Inadequate water/powder ratio
- Too rapid heating of investment
- Prolonged heating of investment
- Underheating causes incomplete elimination of wax
- Air bubbles on the pattern during investment
- Direction of sprue former
- Placement of several patterns in a ring together
- High temperature of molten alloy
- High casting pressure
- Presence of foreign bodies.

Prevention

- Powder and water ratio should be adequate
- Heating should be done gradually as too rapid heating would cause flaking of the investment material
- Gypsum bonded investment should not be heated above 700°C as it would cause disintegration of the investment material
- Ring should be heated for adequate period of time for complete elimination of wax

- Air bubbles can be avoided by vibrating the mixture before and after mixing. Vacuum investing technique should be used to avoid air bubbles
- The direction of sprue former should be adjusted to 45°
- Several pattern should not be placed close together in a single ring as expansion of wax can cause breakdown of intervening investment material
- High temperature of molten alloy cause surface roughness
- Casting pressure should be according to manufacture's recommendation given for various types of casting machines
- Foreign bodies should be avoided during investment of material.

Distortion

Distortion of casting usually occurs due to distortion of inlay wax pattern. The coefficient of thermal expansion of inlay wax is high. Distortion of wax pattern increases if it is improperly handled. Time lag between making of pattern and investing is also crucial during casting.

Causes

- Distortion of wax pattern
- Mishandling of pattern
- Due to unequal movement of walls of wax pattern while the investment is setting.

Prevention

- Proper manipulation of wax pattern
- Wax pattern should be immediately invested after fabrication.

Incomplete Casting and Rounded Margins (Fig. 23.67)

Causes

- Inadequate heating of the alloy
- Inadequate casting pressure
- Improper length and diameter of sprue
- Improper burnout of wax pattern
- Insufficient molten alloy.

Prevention

- Alloy should be heated above fusion temperature, i.e. 570°C
- Casting pressure should be adequate to force the molten alloy
- Proper length and diameter of sprue former

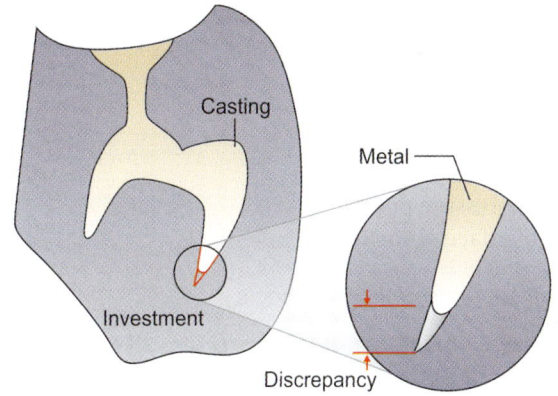

Figure 23.67: Incomplete casting

- Proper burnout of wax pattern should be done so that no carbon residues is left in the mold
- Adequate amount of molten alloy should be available for casting.

Discoloration

The casting usually appears dark after removing from the investment due to presence of oxides. This can be removed by a process known as 'Pickling'.

Causes

- **Prolonged heating:** Heating the investment above 700°C usually cause breakdown of the investment as well as formation of sulfur compounds, which causes blackening of the cast
- Sulfur content of torch flame also affects the casting
- Underheating of the investment also leaves the wax residues in the casting, affects the color of the casting
- Contamination with copper during the process of pickling causes discoloration.

Prevention

- Avoid prolonged heating of the investment
- Change the source of flame
- Proper heating should be done
- Tips of tongs must be covered with rubber to avoid contamination with copper during pickling.

Porosity

Porosity is considered as a major defect in the casting which can occur on the internal as well as on the external surface of the casting. It usually weakens the casting. Various types of porosities can be:

- Solidification shrinkage porosity
  - Localized shrinkage porosity
  - Microporosity.
- Gaseous defects
  - Gas inclusion porosity
  - Pinhole porosity.
- Backpressure porosity
- Subsurface porosity.

Solidification Shrinkage Defects

Localized shrinkage porosity (Figs 23.68A and B): This type of porosity occurs due to shrinkage of molten alloy when alloy solidifies from molten state. This can be avoided by providing adequate molten alloy to compensate casting shrinkage.

Causes

- If direction of sprue former is at 90°, then it will cause 'hot spot' in the casting, i.e. alloy will remain in molten state at that spot whilst solidifies everywhere else
- Diameter of sprue is too narrow
- Length of sprue former is long, i.e. molten alloy prematurely solidifies in the sprue before reaching to mold
- Absence of reservoir.

Prevention

- Direction of sprue former should be at 45°
- Avoid using excessively long and narrow sprue former.
- Use reservoir.

Microporosity

It is usually seen in fine grain molten metal alloy castings. This usually happens due to solidification shrinkage of molten alloy.

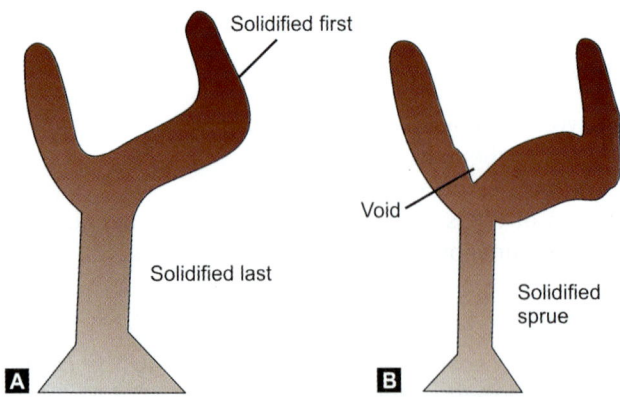

Figures 23.68A and B: Localized shrinkage porosity: (A) Proper sequence of hardening; (B) Improper sequence of hardening resulting in suckback porosity

Causes

- Too low casting temperature
- Rapid solidification of molten alloy.

Prevention

- Increase the casting temperature
- Increase the melting temperature of alloy.

Gaseous Defects

Two types of defects are seen
1. *Gas inclusion porosity*: Gas inclusion porosity is spherical voids larger in size than pinhole porosity.
2. *Pinhole porosity*: Spherical voids, smaller in size than gas inclusion porosity.

Causes

These are usually caused by entrapment of gas in alloy various causes are:
- Not using the reducing zone of flame
- Poor adjustment of torch flame.

Prevention

- Use reducing zone of the flame
- Position of torch flame should be correctly adjusted.

Backpressure Porosity

It usually occurs on the inner surface of the casting due to entrapment of gases.

Causes

- Use of dense investment material
- Low casting temperature
- Low casting pressure
- Improper wax burnout.

Prevention

Use of porous investment material:
- Adequate casting temperature
- Adequate casting pressure
- Proper wax burnout.

Subsurface Porosity

Causes: Simultaneous nucleation of solid grains and gas bubbles when the metal freezes at mold walls.

Prevention: Can be prevented by controlling the flow at which molten alloy enters the mold space.

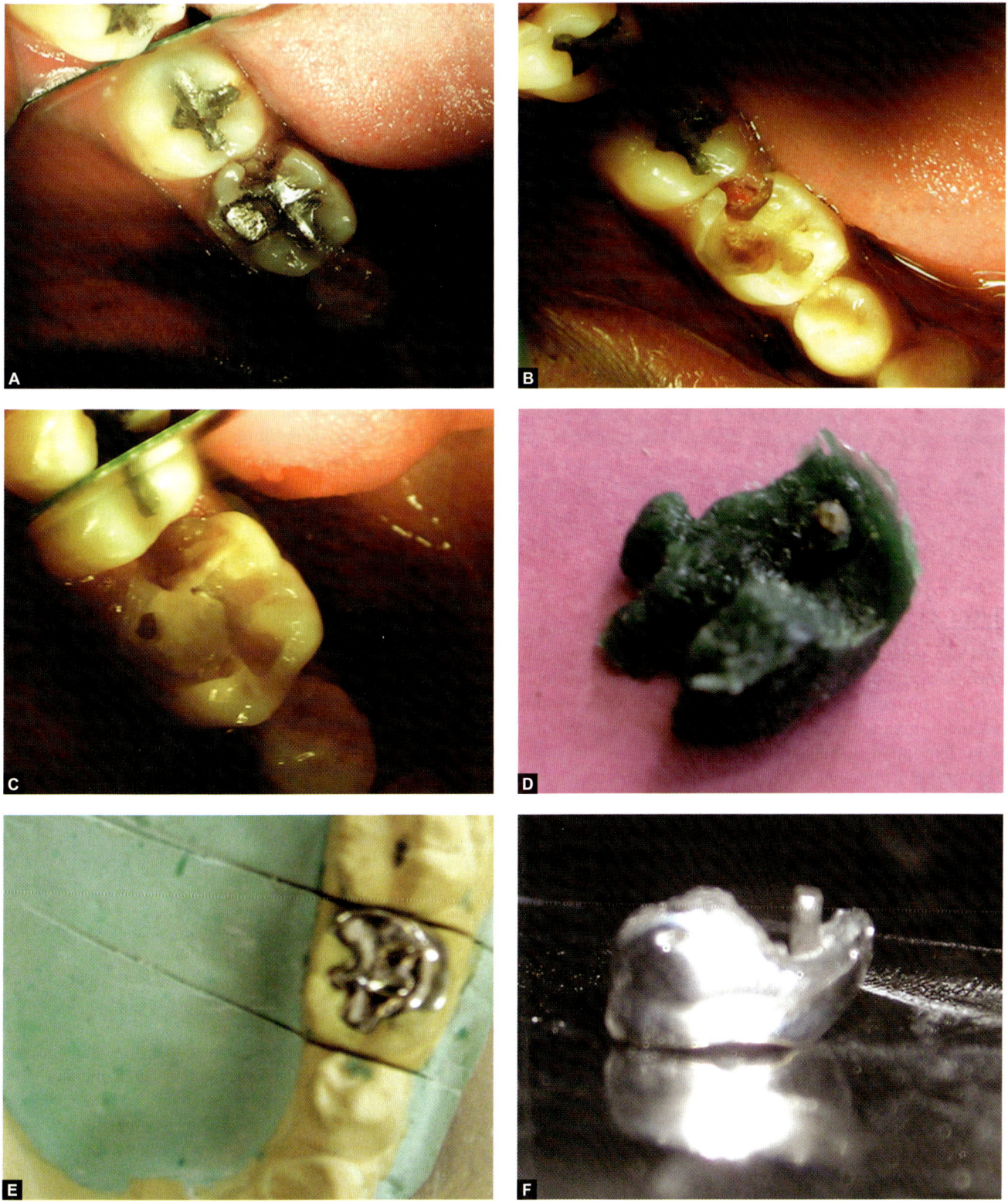

Figures 23.69A to F

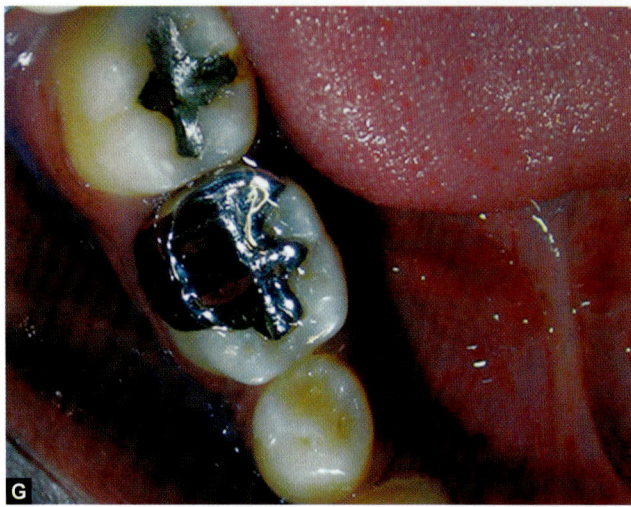

Figure 23.69G

Figures 23.69A to G: (A) Defective amalgam restoration of 36; (B) Restoration removed; (C) Tooth preparation and application of base; (D) Wax pattern with wrought pin; (E and F) Completed casting with wrought pin; (G) Cast metal inlay cemented on 36

PIN RETAINED CAST RESTORATIONS (FIGS 23.69A TO G)

Pins are generally used for providing additional retention. Cast pin channels are wider and have slightly divergent walls in comparison to the pin holes prepared for pin retained amalgam restorations. The cast pin channels are prepared with the help of tapering fissure bur having a diameter of 1 mm with the depth of about 2 to 3 mm.

Indications for Pin Retained Cast Restorations

Pin retained cast restorations are indicated in following cases
- When occlusogingival height is very short
- In cases of excessively tapered tooth preparation
- Cuspal fractures where large occlusal inlays and onlays are to be prepared
- When the proximal box is very long. The pin channel is prepared at the other end of occlusal lock
- In full crown preparation when one wall is very short and another wall is very long. In these cases, pin channel is prepared towards the shorter wall
- For shallow and wide preparations, when it is not possible to place surface extensions for retention
- In very thin and fragile teeth where extensive tooth preparation can be detrimental
- In absence of gingival floor, resistance and retention can be achieved by use of pins.

 Key Points

- An inlay is an indirect intracoronal restoration which is fabricated extraorally and cemented in the prepared tooth. Inlay may cover none, or all but one cusp of a tooth.
- An onlay is a combination of intracoronal and extracoronal cast restoration which covers one or more cusps.
- Class II inlay essentially involves proximal surface or surfaces of a posterior tooth, usually may involve occlusal surface and also may involve facial and/or lingual surface(s) and covers none or may cover all but one cusp of a tooth.
- Preparation should have single insertion path opposite to the occlusal load and parallel to the long axis of tooth. This helps in retention of the restoration.
- Concept of taper: A tooth preparation should have slight diverging walls from gingival to occlusal surface. The optimal taper should lie in the range of 2° to 5° per wall. But if longitudinal walls of preparation are short, a maximum of 2° taper is given, and if longitudinal height of preparation is more, then taper should also be increased, although it should never exceed 10°.
- Circumferential tie refers to the design of cavosurface margin of an inlay tooth preparation. This junction between tooth cement inlay is the weakest part of the cast metal restoration.
- Bevel is defined as the inclination that one surface makes with another when not at right angles. Objective of bevel is to form a metal wedge of 30o to 35°, thus enhancing the chance to achieve closure at the interface of cast gold and tooth.
- Flares are concave or flat peripheral portions of the facial or lingual proximal walls.
- Primary flare is basic part of circumferential tie. It is like a long bevel and is always directed 45° to the inner dentinal wall proper.
- Secondry flare is a flat plane superimposed peripherally to the primary flare. It may have different angulations, involvement and extent depending upon requirement. It is not given in the areas where esthetics is more important.
- The Gingival bevel should be placed 45° to inlay preparation. It should include one-half the width of the gingival wall. It eliminates the possibility of leaving weak or unsupported enamel on gingival wall and provides a stronger obtuse angle of tooth structure which aids in finishing of the casting and sealing of the margins of the restoration.
- Occlusal bevel should be 40° at the occlusal one-third of the adjacent occlusal wall to remove any irregularities

in the preparation or unsupported enamel rods at the cavosurface margin.

- Casting procedure includes the burnout for wax elimination, expansion of the investment to compensate for casting shrinkage and placement of the gold alloy into the mold.
- Surface roughness is generalized roughness on the surface of the casting while surface irregularities are isolated imperfections such as nodules, ridges, fins and spines.
- Distortion of casting usually occurs due to distortion of inlay wax pattern. The coefficient of thermal expansion of inlay wax is high. Distortion of wax pattern increases if it is improperly handled.
- The casting usually appears dark after removing from the investment due to presence of oxides. This can be usually be removed by process known as 'Pickling'.
- Porosity is considered as a major defect in the casting which can occur on the internal as well as on the external surface of the casting.

QUESTIONS

1. What are indications and contraindications of cast metal restorations?
2. Write short notes on:
   a. Difference in tooth preparation for class II amalgam and cast gold restoration
   b. Bevels
   c. Primary and secondary flares.
   d. Casting defects
   e. Additional retention and resistance form features for cast restoration.
3. What are different casting defects? What are their causes and how can we prevent them?
4. Write short note on compensation of casting shrinkage.
5. Write short note on:
   a. Porosity in casting
   b. Sprue
   c. Casting defects
   d. Die material
   e. Cavosurface bevel.
6. What are indication and contraindication for gold inlay? Discuss the difference in class II tooth preparation for gold inlay and silver amalgam preparation.
7. What are methods of preparing inlay wax pattern? Compare and contrast each method in detail.
8. Describe in brief indications, contraindications and advantages or disadvantages of gold inlay.

BIBLIOGRAPHY

1. Allan FC, Asgar K. Reaction of cobalt-chromium casting alloy with investment. JDR. 1966;45:1516.
2. Barreto MT, JonGoldberg A, Nitkin DA, Mumford G. Effect of investment on casting high fusing alloys. JPD. 1980;44: 504.
3. Blockhurst PJ, McLaverty VG, Kasloff Z. A castability standard for alloys used in restorative dentistry. Oper Dent. 1983;8:130.
4. Carson J, et al. A thermographic study of heat distribution during ultra-speed cavity preparation. J Dent Res. 1979;58(7):1681-4.
5. Fisher DW, et al. Indirect temporary restorations. J Am Dent Assoc. 1971;82:160-3.
6. Fisher DW, et al. Photoelastic analysis of inlay and onlay preparations. J Prosthet Dent. 1975;33:47-53.
7. Hasegawa J. Dental casting materials. Trans Acad Dent Mater. 1989;2:190-201.
8. Hood JA. Biomechanics of the intact, prepared and restored tooth: some clinical implications. Int Dent J. 1991;41:25-32.
9. Mori T. Study of gypsum-bonded casting investment. Part I and Part II. 1993;38:220-306.
10. Moulding MB, Loney RW. The effect of cooling techniques on intrapulpal temperature during direct fabrication of provisional restorations. Int J Prosthodont. 1991;4:332-6.
11. Myers RE. Time required to cast gold by centrifugal force. JADA. 1941;28:2001.
12. Palmer DW, Roydhouse RH, Skinner EW. Asbestos liner and casting accuracy. Dent Prog. 1961;1:156.
13. Pomes CE, Slack GI. Surface roughness of dental castings. JADA. 1950;41:545.
14. Rawson RD, Gregory GG, Lund MR. Photographic study of gold flow. JDR. 1972;51:1331.
15. Rosenstiel E. To bevel or not to bevel? BDJ. 1975;138:389.
16. Santos JF, Ballester RY. Delayed hygroscopic expansion of phosphate bonded investments. Dent Mater. 1987;3:165.
17. Smyd ES. Factors which influence casting accuracy: a universal casting technique. JADA. 1948;36:160.
18. Stevens L. The effect of time between mixing and heating on the expansion of phosphate-bonded investment. ADJ. 1986;31:207.
19. Sturdevant JR, et al. The 8-year clinical performance of 15 low-gold casting alloys. Dent Mater. 1987;3:347-52.
20. Taylor NO, Paffenbarger GC, Sweeny WT. Inlay casting golds. Physical properties and specification. JADA. 1932;19:36.
21. Tucker RV. Variation in inlay cavity design. JADA. 1972;84:616.
22. Vorhees FH. History and progress of the cast gold inlays. JADA. 1930;20:2111.
23. Wataha JC. Biocompatibility of dental casting alloys: a review. J Prosthet Dent. 2000;83:223-34.

Glass Ionomer Cement

Chapter Outline

INTRODUCTION

In dentistry, adhesion of restorative materials to tooth structure is an important objective. It is always required that a restoration should resemble the tooth in all respects. It should have identical properties and should bond to the surrounding enamel and dentin. The glass ionomer cements are one of the products developed to meet all these criteria.

Glass Ionomer Cement was introduced to dentistry 35 years ago (in 1972) by Wilson and Kent. Glass ionomers were first marketed in Europe in 1975 and became available in the United States in 1977. The first commercial glass ionomer was made by the De Trey Company and distributed by the Amalgamated Dental Co in England and by Caulk in the United States, known as ASPA (Aluminosilicate Polyacrylate). It consisted of an ion leachable aluminosilicate glass and an aqueous solution of a copolymer of acrylic acid.

The invention of the glass ionomer cement resulted from previous fundamental studies on silicate cements and studies where the phosphoric acid in dental silicate cements was replaced by organic chelating acids. It was supported by work on the zinc polycarboxylate cement in which Smith showed that dental cements exhibiting the property of adhesion could be prepared from polyacrylic acid. Glass ionomer cement for that reason has been described as a hybrid of dental silicate cements and zinc polycarboxylates (**Fig. 24.1**). Because of wide chemical diversity, the range of Glass ionomer cements is very wide. Extensive use of this cement to replace dentin, has given it different names: Dentin substitute, man-made dentin and artificial dentin.

History of Glass ionomer cements

- 1966: AD Wilson—examined cements prepared by mixing dental silicate glass powder with aqueous solutions of various organic acids (including polyacrylic acid)
- 1968, 1969: AD Wilson + Kent and Lewis—found that hydrolytically stable cements could be produced by employing novel glass formulations
- 1968: Kent—found that setting of these cements was controlled by Al_2O_3/SiO_2 ratio in the glass
- 1973, 1979: Kent et al—found a glass that was high in fluoride that gave a usable cement ASPA 1 (aluminosilicate polyacrylates)
- 1972 (reported in 1976): Wilson and Crisp—discovered that tartaric acid modified the cement forming reaction,

thus improving manipulation, extending working time and greatly sharpening setting rate. This refinement of ASPA I was termed ASPA II and constituted the first practical GIC

- 1975, 1977: Crisp and Wilson—developed copolymer of acrylic and itaconic acid that did not gel at high (50 percent) concentration in aqueous solution ASPA IV
- 1977: McLean and Wilson—ideal for restoration of class V erosion lesions
- 1977: Wilson et al—ASPA IVa—fine grained version for luting
- 1985: McLean et al—the original 1977 idea of using composite resin/ionomer laminate was revived in a modified form. GIC and enamel was etched – double etch technique composite resin was attached micromechanically to enamel and GIC bonded indirectly to dentin
- 1984: Hunt and Knight—tunnel preparation for Class II
- 1980: Sced and Wilson and 1983: Simmons—incorporated metallic oxides and metal alloy fillers, to improve strength of GIC
- 1985: McLean and Gasser—fused silver particles onto ionomer glass, giving cement radio-opacity, burnishability, smoother surface and increased wear resistance
- 1986: McLean—developed cermet cements for clinical use
- Late 1980s: Resin-modified glass ionomer cements.

CLASSIFICATION OF GLASS IONOMER CEMENTS

Traditional classification (based on application):
- Type I—Luting cements
- Type II—Restorative cements
    - Type II.1—Restorative esthetic
    - Type II.2—Restorative reinforced
- Type III—Liner or Base.

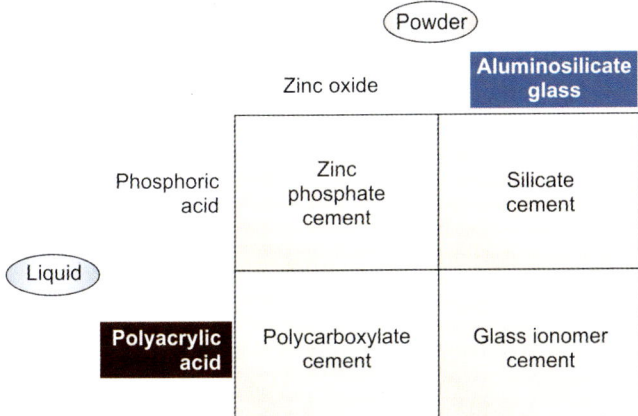

Figure 24.1: GIC, hybrid of silicate and zinc polycarboxylate cements

History of glass ionomer cements

Year	Name of scientists	Description
1972	Wilson and Kent	Development of GIC in London
1977	-	Introduced in USA as ASPA
		(Aluminosilicate Polyacrylate)
1980	Simmons	Miracle mix
1984	Hunt knight	Tunnel preparation
1985	McLean	Sandwich technique
1987	McLean and Gasser	Cermet
1994	McLean	Atraumatic Restorative
		technique (ART)

Newer classification:
- Type I—Luting cements
- Type II—Restorative esthetic or reinforced cements
- Type III—Liner or base:

Classification of GICs according to their use:
- Type I—For luting cements
- Type II—For restorations
- Type III—Liners and bases
- Type IV—Fissure sealants
- Type V—Orthodontic cements
- Type VI—Core build up.

GENERATION OF GLASS IONOMERS (FIG. 24.2)

First Generation of Glass Ionomer Cement

ASPA I

Discovery of the glass ionomer cement resulted as a hybrid of silicate cements and zinc polycarboxylates. But these initial cement pastes were impracticable, with slow setting and hydrolytic instability. There was less reactivity of the glass powder towards the polymer. Wilson and Kent in 1972 produced first glass that was high in fluoride, content called as ASPA. However, ASPA I showed slow setting, susceptibility to moisture and low translucency.

ASPA II

Wilson and Crisp in 1972 added D-tartaric acid to extend the working time and promote a snap set by helping ion extraction from the glass particles. The use of tartaric acid allowed the use of lower fluoride containing glasses, which were less opaque. This modification of ASPA I was called as ASPA II.

ASPA III

In ASPA II cement, polyacrylic acid was used as liquid which had a tendency to gel with time because of increase in intermolecular hydrogen bonds. In ASPA III cement, methyl alcohol was added to polyacrylic acid solutions because methyl alcohol inhibited the ordering of structures in solution and thereby gelation.

ASPA IV

Since copolymers of acrylic acids are less regular than polyacrylic acid, they are less liable to form intermolecular hydrogen bonds. To improve stability of cement, in ASPA IV cements, copolymer of acrylic and itaconic acid was added, which showed more stability.

Second Generation of Glass Ionomer Cement

Water Mixed GICs/Water Hardening Glass Ionomer Cements

Polyacid in solution form has shown an increase in viscosity of the liquid, making the manipulation of cement difficult. To solve this problem, use of polyacrylic acid in solid form for mixing with glass ionomer powder was made. Here the liquid component is either water or an aqueous solution of tartaric acid. These cements are called "water mixed" or "water hardened." Advantages of these cements are:
- More shelf life since there is no possibility of occurrence of gelation and hence less viscosity
- Improvement in the strength because polyacid concentration can be increased by this method.

Reinforced Glass Ionomer Cements

Strength of the glass ionomer cement can be improved by modifying the chemical composition of the original glass powder. It can be done by following:
- ***Disperse-phase glasses***: Here to improve the strength, glass was modified by phase separation. In this, glass was prepared with large amount dispersed phases of strengthening, crystallites like carborundum (Al_2O_3) and tielite (Al_2TiO_5).
- ***Fiber reinforced glasses***: To improve the flexural strength of the cement, alumina fibers, glass fiber, silica fiber and carbon fiber were added. But these materials showed difficulty to mix, and low resistance to abrasion.
- ***Metal reinforced glass ionomer cement***: In this metal powder or fibers were added to GIC to increase the flexural strength. Simmons gave the concept of "Miracle mix" by mixing amalgam alloy powder to glass ionomer cement. These cements show poor esthetics and resistance to burnishing and poor resistance to abrasion.

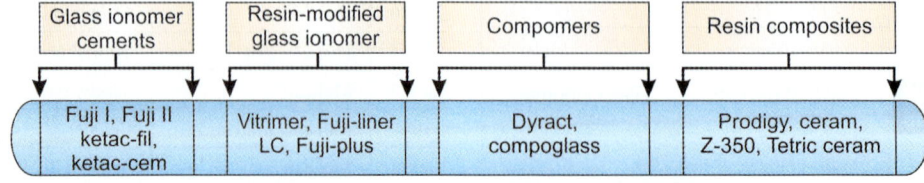

Figure 24.2: Glass ionomers and composite resins are different entities. RMGI is basically a glass ionomer with small amount of resin, where as compomers are polyacid modified composite resin

- **Cermet cements**: McLean and Gasser developed cermet cements by sintering the metal and glass powders together. It showed strong bonding of the metal to the glass. These cements have shown improved resistance to abrasion and higher flexural strength.

Resin-modified Glass Ionomer Cement (Fig. 24.3)

To solve the problem of moisture sensitivity and lack of control on working time, resin modification of glass ionomer cement was done. These materials are defined as hybrid materials which set by both acid–base reaction as well as a second curing process, which is initiated by light or chemical.

These are made by addition of small quantity of a resin like hydroxyethyl methacrylate (HEMA) or Bis–GMA in the liquid. In these cements, basic acid-base reaction is the same and only 4 to 6 percent of the cement is resin polymerized, this provides strength and protection to the continuing acid-base reaction from water sensitivity.

Highly Viscous Conventional Glass Ionomer Cement/High Viscosity Autocure Glass Ionomers

These highly viscous glass ionomers are mainly useful for atraumatic restorative treatment technique. These glass ionomers were developed to act as a substitute to amalgam for posterior restorations. In these cements, polyacrylic acid is made to finer grain size so that higher powder-liquid ratios can be used. For example, Ketac Molar and Fuji IX (**Fig. 24.4**).

Advantages of Highly Viscous Glass Ionomers

- Fast setting
- Low early moisture sensitivity
- Low solubility in oral fluids
- Finishing can be done in five minutes after placement.

Easily Mixable Glass Ionomer Cements

For simpler and easier manipulation of GICs, modifications have been made for dispensing glass ionomer cement.

- *Capsules (Figs 24.5A and B)*: These capsules contain premeasured powder and liquid to assure correct ratio for the mix. These capsules have angled nozzle which acts as a syringe for accurate placement of the cement into a preparation.
- *Paste dispensing system (Fig. 24.6)*: This is one of the recent development in dispensing system for the glass ionomer cement. It uses a cartridge and a material dispenser. In this system, an ultra fine glass powder is used to provide the cement in a paste consistency. Advantages of this system are optimum ratio, simple placement, and easy mixing.

Glass Ionomer Stabilization and Protection Material

This is recently developed glass ionomer cement which help in arresting the active carious lesions and to protect the teeth from caries in high risk patients. This is because of high fluoride release from this type of GIC. Fuji VII comes under this type of cement (**Fig. 24.7**).

GC Fuji VIII (Fig. 24.8)

GC Fuji VIII is radioopaque, reinforced glass ionomer cement used for restoration of anterior teeth. It has more translucency, thus more esthetic in nature. It is used for restoration of class III and V lesions.

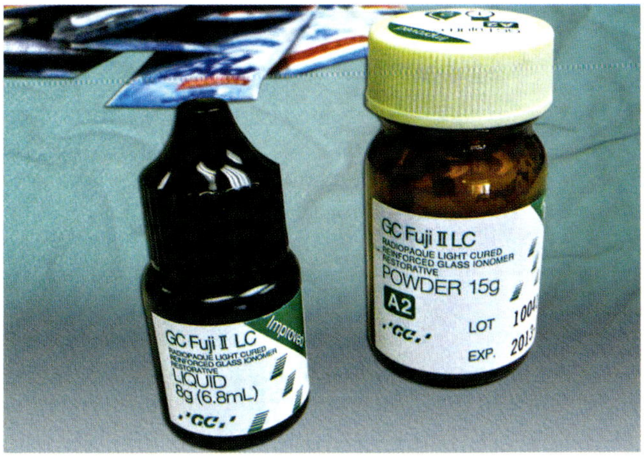

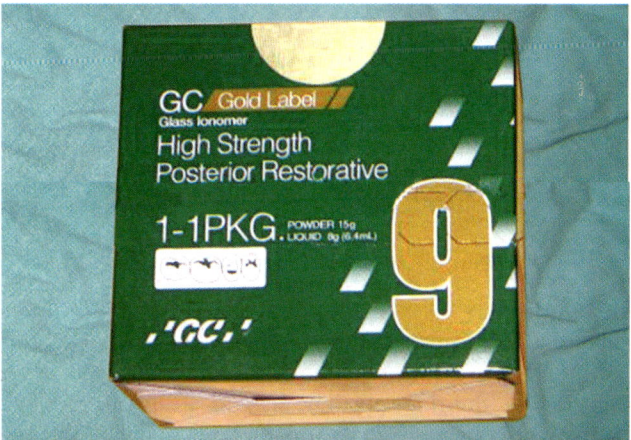

Figure 24.3: Resin modified glass ionomer cement

Figure 24.4: In highly viscous glass ionomers polyacrylic acid is made to finer grain size so as to have higher powder-liquid ratio

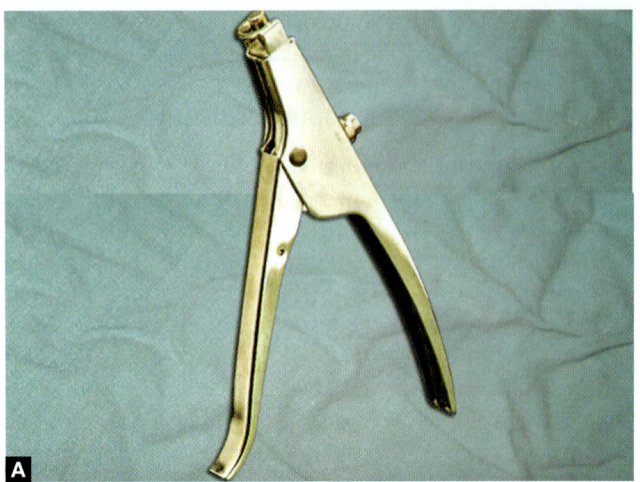

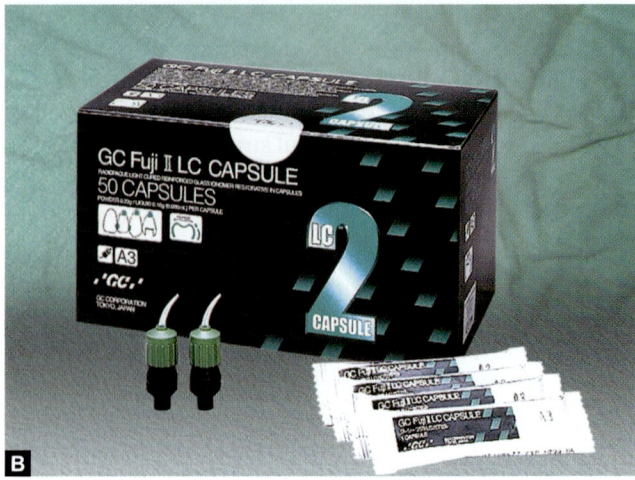

Figures 24.5A and B: Capsule dispenser and glass ionomer capsules

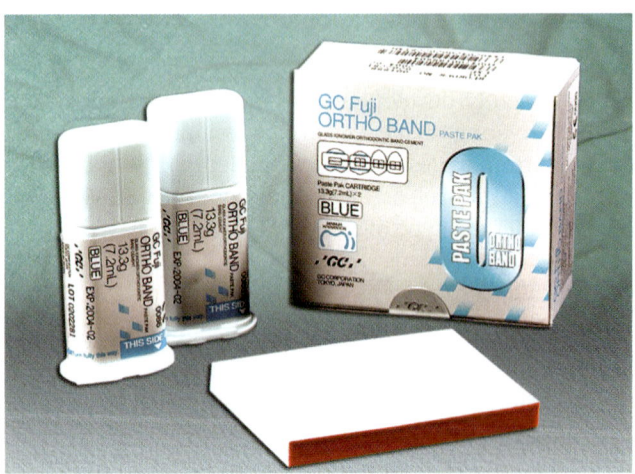

Figure 24.6: Glass ionomer in paste-paste system

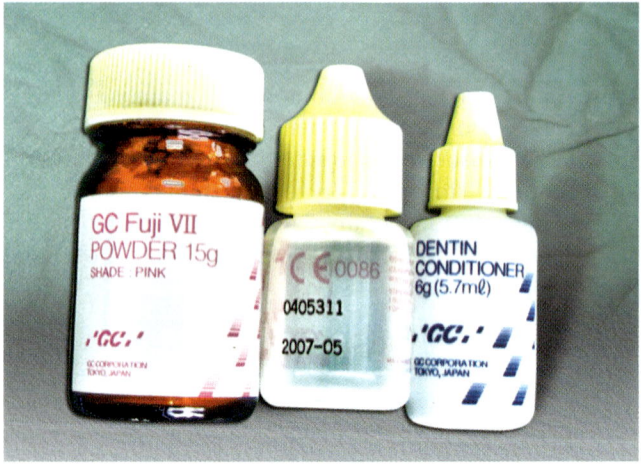

Figure 24.7: Type VII GIC is used in high caries risk patients because of its high fluoride release capacity

COMPOSITION OF GLASS IONOMER CEMENT

Glass ionomer cement usually comes in a mixture of a powder and a liquid.

GIC Powder

The powder is an acid-soluble calcium fluoroalumino-silicate glass similar to that of silicate but with a higher alumina-silicate ratio that increases its reactivity with liquid. The fluoride portion acts as a "ceramic flux". Lanthanum, strontium, barium or zinc oxide additives provide radiopacity. These powders are combined and fused (at temperatures 1100 to 1500°C) with a fluoride flux that serves to reduce their fusion temperature. The molten glass is then poured onto a steel tray. To fragment it, the mass is plunged into water and the resulting fragments are crushed, milled, and powdered. The particles are then sieved to separate them according to size. Particle size varies according to manufacturer, however sizes usually range from 20 microns for luting to 50 microns for restorative products. For cementation purposes, a glass particle size of 13 to 19 microns is optimal. The powder contains fluoride in a 10 to 23 percent concentration resulting from the calcium fluoride, sodium fluoride and aluminum fluoride. The fluoride flux also contributes to the final fluoride concentration.

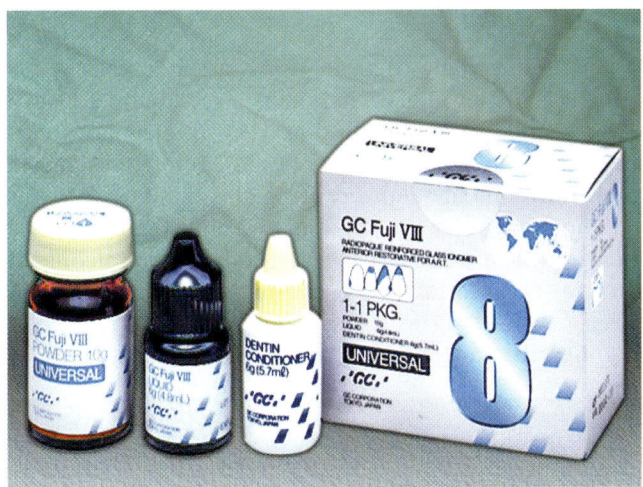

Figure 24.8: Radioopaque, reinforced anterior glass ionomer cement

cement to harden and loose its moisture sensitivity faster. This occurs because polymaleic acid has more carboxyl (COOH) groups which lead to more rapid polycarboxylate crosslinking. This also allows more conventional, less reactive glasses to be used which results in a more esthetic final set cement.

Tartaric acid is also present in the liquid. It improves handling characteristics and increases the working time, but it shortens the setting time. The viscosity of tartaric acid-containing cement does not generally change over shelf-life of the cement (**Figs 24.9 and 24.10**). However, a viscosity change can occur if the cement is out of date.

Water Settable Glass Ionomer

As a means of extending the working time of the GIC, freeze-dried polyacid powder and glass powder are placed

The percentages of the raw materials in powder are	
➡ Silica	41.9 percent
➡ Alumina	28.6 percent
➡ Aluminum fluoride	1.6 percent
➡ Calcium fluoride	15.7 percent
➡ Sodium fluoride	9.3 percent
➡ Aluminum phosphate	3.8 percent

GIC Liquid

The liquid is an aqueous solution of polymer and copolymer of acrylic acid.

Originally, the liquids for GIC were aqueous solutions of polyacrylic acid in a concentration of about 40 percent to 50 percent. The liquid was quite viscous and had tendency to gel over time.

Composition of liquid	
➡ Polyacrylic acid (Itaconic acid, maleic acid)	40–55 percent
➡ Tartaric acid	6–15 percent
➡ Water	30 percent

To decrease the viscosity of liquid, itaconic, and tri-carboxylic acids were added to the liquid. These acids tend to:
➡ Decrease the viscosity
➡ Promote reactivity between the glass and the liquid
➡ Prevent gelation of the liquid which can result from hydrogen bonding between two polyacrylic acid chains.

Polymaleic acid is often present in the liquid. It is a stronger acid than polyacrylic acid and causes the

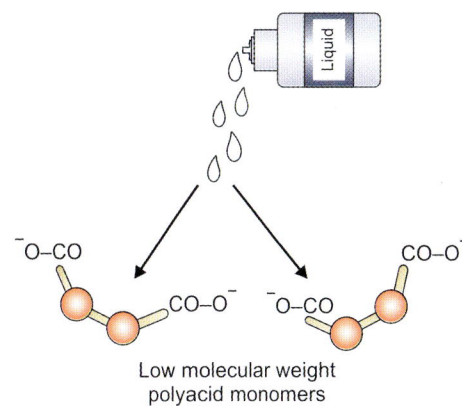

Figure 24.9: Only two carboxyl group are present in tartaric acid to react with powder

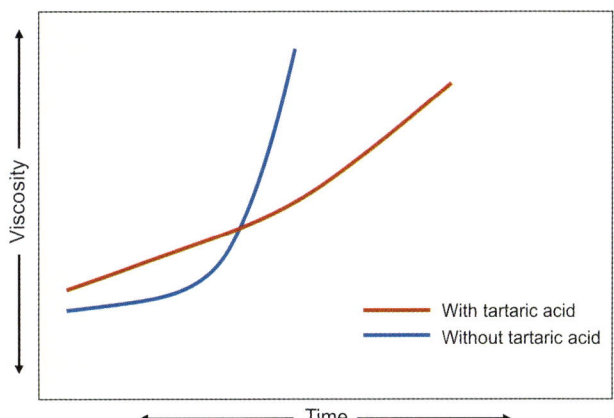

Figure 24.10: Effect of tartaric acid on viscosity of GIC liquid

in the same bottle as the powder. The liquid consists of water or water with tartaric acid. When the powders are mixed with water, the acid powder dissolves to reconstitute the liquid acid and this process is followed by the acid-base reaction. This type of cement is referred to occasionally as water settable glass ionomer or anhydrous glass ionomer.

Metal Reinforced Glass Ionomer Cement

In order to reinforce the physical properties of glass-ionomer, metal particles in powder or fiber form are added to glass powder. This cement is of two types.

Miracle Mix (Silver Alloy Admix Glass Ionomer Cement) (Fig. 24.11)

It was introduced by Simmons in 1983. In this, silver alloy powder is blended with glass ionomer powder in ratio of 1:6 and mixed with glass ionomer liquid. This increases the compressive strength, tensile strength and abrasion resistance to some extent.

Advantages
⇒ Better abrasion resistance
⇒ Better compressive strength
⇒ More tensile strength

Disadvantages
⇒ Difficult to achieve homogeneous mix of silver alloy and glass
⇒ Poor esthetics
⇒ Poor burnishing
⇒ Sensitivity to moisture contamination during setting.

Cermet Cement

It is introduced by McLean and Gasser in 1987. This cement is fusion of glass ionomer to metal powders like silver or gold through sintering. Here the cement ionomers are manufactured by sintering compressed pellets made from fine metal powder and glass ionomer powder at temperature of 800°C. The sintered metal and glass fit is then ground into fine form which results in ceramicometal particles of fused metal and ground glass. Most accepted metal for sintering with glass ionomer is silver or gold. Titanium dioxide (5%) is added to improve the color.

Advantages
⇒ Better abrasion resistance
⇒ Higher flexure strength.

Disadvantage
⇒ Poor esthetics.

Resin-modified Glass Ionomer

It was first introduced as Vitrebond (3m) in powder—liquid system to incorporate the best properties of both glass ionomer cement and composite resin (**Fig. 24.12**). In this system, powder is fluorosilicate glass with photoinitiator or chemical initiator. The liquid contains 15 to 25 percent resin component in the form of HEMA, a polyacrylic acid copolymer along with photoinitiator and water.

Advantages of Resin-modified Glass Ionomer Cements (Fig. 24.13)

RMGIs show combined advantages of both composites and glass ionomers.

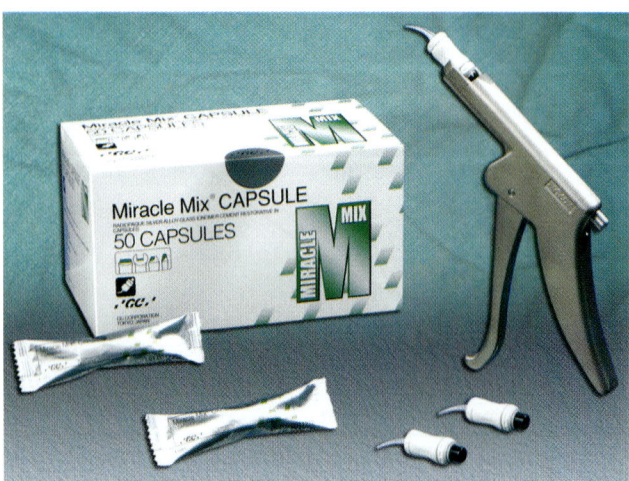

Figure 24.11: Miracle mix (silver alloy admix glass ionomer cement)

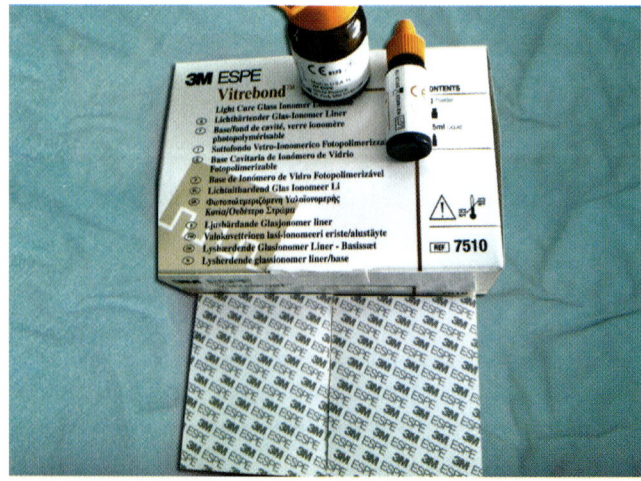

Figure 24.12: Resin modified glass ionomer cement

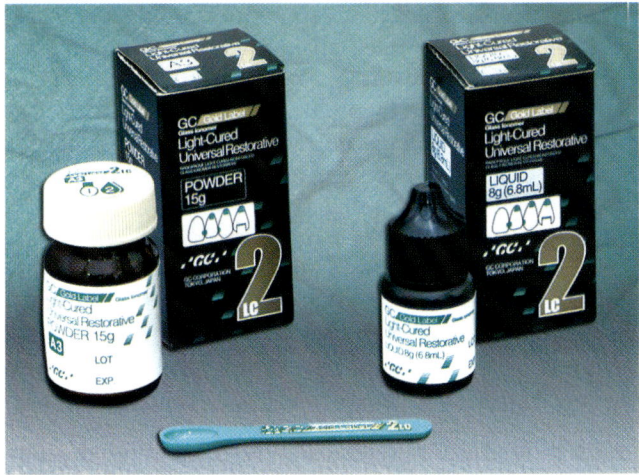

Figure 24.13: Resin modified (light cure) glass ionomer cement

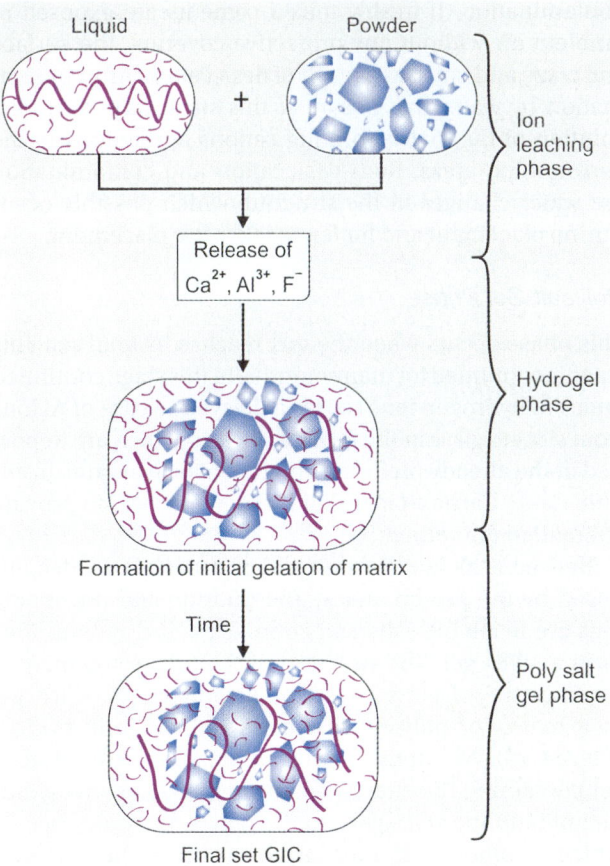

Figure 24.14: Setting reaction of glass ionomer cement

Advantages

- Extended working time
- Control on setting
- Good adaptation
- Chemical adhesion to enamel and dentin
- Fluoride release
- Improved esthetics.
- Low interfacial shrinkage stress
- Superior strength characteristics.

Disadvantages of resin-modified composites

- Shrinkage on setting
- Limited depth of cure especially with more opaque lining cements
- Intrinsic color change.

SETTING REACTION

Setting Reaction of Autocure Glass Ionomer Cement

Basically in autocure glass ionomer cement, setting reaction is an acid-base reaction between the acidic polyelectrolyte and the aluminosilicate glass. It occurs in three different but overlapping stages (**Fig. 24.14**).

Three stages of GIC setting rection

- Ion-leaching phase
- Hydrogel phase
- Polysalt gel phase.

Ion-leaching Phase

This phase occurs when powder and liquid are mixed. When the powder and aqueous acidic solution are mixed,

the polyacid attacks the glass particles (called leaching) to release cations like Ca^{2+} and Al^{3+}. These ions react with the fluoride ions to form CaF_2 and AlF^{3-}. Soon because of continued increase in acidity, CaF2 dissociates and reacts with acrylic copolymer to form a stable matrix. At this stage, the mix appears glossy in nature and it can adhere to the tooth structure.

At the end of this stage, gloss of the mix decreases and it becomes less adhesive to tooth structure.

Hydrogel Phase

In this phase, calcium ions are released rapidly. These liberated ions react with the acid and cross-link with the polyacrylic acid, i.e. calcium bridges to form a calcium polycarboxylate gel in which the non-reacted glass is embedded. The initial setting of the cement is because of this reaction. At this stage, the cement appears rigid and opaque. Water plays a critical role in the setting of GIC. It serves as the reaction medium initially and then slowly hydrates the crosslinked agents thereby yielding stable gel structure which is stronger and less susceptible to moisture contamination. If freshly mixed cements are exposed to ambient air without any protective covering, the surface will craze and crack as a result of desiccation. Any contamination by water that occurs at this stage can cause dissolution of the matrix forming cations and anions to the surrounding areas. Both desiccation and contamination are water changes in the structure which possibly occur during placement and for few weeks after placement.

Polysalt Gel Phase

This phase occurs when the mix reaches its final set. This stage is continued for many months. In this stage continued attack of hydrogen ions causes a delayed release of Al ions from silicate glass in the form of AlF ions which are deposited in the already preformed matrix to form a water-insoluble Ca-Al-Carboxylate gel. It is the Al ions which provide strength to the cement.

Between 20 and 30 percent of the glass is decomposed by the proton attack. The fluoride and phosphate ions are insoluble salts and complexes. The sodium ions form a silica gel. The structure of the fully set cement is a composite of glass particles surrounded by silica gel in a matrix of polyanions crosslinked by ionic bridges (**Fig. 24.15**). Within the matrix, are small particles of silica gel containing fluorite crystallites. Finally, a slow hydration of both the silica gel and the polycarboxylates occurs which results in a further improvement in the cement's physical properties. This reaction may continue for several months. Two clinically important results of this reaction are that the physical properties of the glass ionomer cements take a relatively long time to fully develop because of the cement's long setting reaction and that the cement is sensitive to moisture contamination and to desiccation because the glass particles are covered with a Hydrogel.

Calcium ions react with polycarboxylate chains initially and rapidly than the trivalent aluminum ions which are involved in secondary stage of reaction.

Calcium polycarboxylates are formed rapidly because:
- Calcium ions are released in greater quantity by the action of the hydrogen ions because attack on the glass particles occurs preferentially at the calcium rich sites.
- The calcium ions have a bivalent, rather than trivalent, charge which allows them to migrate faster into the aqueous cement phase.
- The calcium cations do not form stable complexes with the fluoride ions as do the aluminum cations. This means that the calcium is more readily available to crosslink the polyanion chains.

Setting Reaction of Resin-modified Glass Ionomers

Basically, in these cements two types of setting reactions occur:
- Acid-base neutralization reaction
- Free radical methacrylate cure

Because of these two reactions, following can be accounted:

1. Formation of two different matrices – an ionomer salt Hydrogel and a poly HEMA matrix. This whole system can inhibit the acid-base reaction.
2. Also there occurs multiple crosslinking chain formation which can occur by acid base reaction, light cure mechanism and resin autocure mechanism.

When powder and liquid are mixed and light is activated, a photoinitiated setting reaction starts. Now the methacrylate group of polymer grafts into polyacrylic acid chain and methacrylate groups of HEMA. This crosslinking of HEMA and of methacrylate group of polymer causes hardening of the cement (**Fig. 24.16**). But acid-base reaction continues for some days.

Setting Time

The GIC sets within 6 to 8 minutes from the start of mixing. Setting time is less for type I materials than type

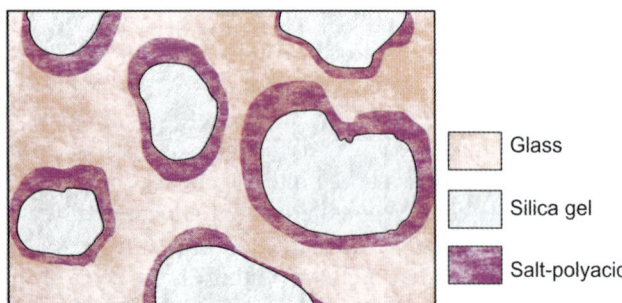

Figure 24.15: Diagrammatic representation of finally set GIC

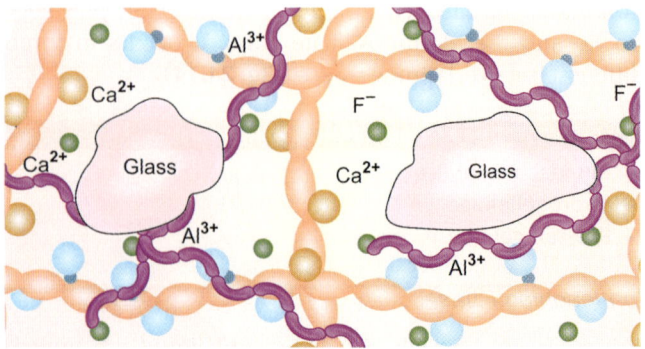

Figure 24.16: Setting reaction of resin modified glass ionomers

II materials. The setting can be slowed when the cement is mixed on a cool glass slab.

- Setting time for type I GIC—5 to 7 minutes
- Setting time for type II GIC—10 minutes .

Film Thickness

The film thickness of GICs is similar to or less than that of zinc phosphate cement and is suitable for cementation.

INDICATIONS OF GLASS IONOMER CEMENT

- Restoration of permanent teeth
  - Class V, Class III, small class I tooth preparations
  - Abrasion/Erosion
  - Root caries.
- Restoration of deciduous teeth
  - Class I to Class VI tooth preparations
  - Rampant and nursing bottle caries
- Luting or cementing
  - Metal restorations (Inlay, onlay, crowns)
  - Nonmetal restorations (composite inlays and onlays)
  - Veneers
  - Pins and posts
  - Orthodontic bonds and brackets.
- Preventive restorations
  - Tunnel preparation
  - Pit and fissure sealants
- Protective liner under composite and amalgam
- Bonding agent
- Dentin substitute
- Core build up
- Splinting
- Glazing
- Endodontics
  - Repair of external root resorption
  - Repair of perforation.
- Other restorative technique
  - Sandwich technique
  - Atraumatic restorative treatment
  - Bonded restorations.

CONTRAINDICATIONS OF GLASS IONOMER CEMENTS

- In stress bearing areas like class I, class II and class IV preparations
- In cuspal replacement cases
- In patients with xerostomia
- In mouth breathers because restoration may become opaque, brittle and fracture over a time
- In areas requiring esthetics like veneering of anterior teeth.

Advantages of GIC

- Inherent adhesion to tooth structure because of chemical bonding to enamel and dentin through ion exchange
- Biocompatible because large sized polyacrylic acid molecules prevent the acid from producing pulpal response
- Little shrinkage and good marginal seal
- Anticariogenic because of fluoride release. This fluoride can also be recharged from topical fluoride applications
- Good color matching and translucency makes it esthetic
- Minimal tooth preparation required hence easy to use on children
- Less soluble than other cements
- Less technique sensitive than composite resins.

Disadvantages of GIC

- Brittle and low fracture resistance
- Low wear resistance
- Water sensitivity during setting phase affects physical properties and esthetics
- Some newer products release less fluoride than conventional GIC
- Opaque which makes glass ionomer cement less esthetic than composites
- Not inherently radiopaque
- Require moisture control during manipulation and placement.

PROPERTIES OF GLASS IONOMER CEMENT

Physical Properties

Glass ionomer cements have high compressive strength, but low fracture toughness, flexure strength, high modulus of elasticity and wear resistance, thus we can mark them as hard but brittle material. Because of this nature, glass ionomer cements should not be used in high stress bearing areas. Modified GICs like cermet cements have more strength but their fracture resistance remains low. The resin modified glass ionomers have more flexural and tensile strength and lower modulus of elasticity when compared to conventional glass ionomer cements. This makes them more resistant to fracture but their wear resistance is still not improved much.

Biocompatibility

Glass ionomer cements are considered as biocompatible dental materials because of following reasons:

- Polyacrylic acid present in the liquid is a weak acid
- Dissociated hydrogen ions present in GIC are further bound to the polymer chains electrostatically.
- The long polymer chains tangle on one another, this prevents their penetration into the dentin tubules.

The postoperative sensitivity after GIC placement is usually seen with "water-mixed" forms of the GICs. This is because of low viscosity and low initial pH of these cements.

Type I glass ionomer cement show more sensitivity than type II cements because of following factors:

→ Seating of the restoration results in pressure which further increases sensitivity.
→ Use of a low powder-to-liquid ratio mix.
→ Luting GICs are placed over a large surface area of cut dentin.
→ Microleakage because of early moisture contamination can result in sensitivity.

Water Sensitivity

Conventional glass ionomer cement is very sensitive to moisture contamination during the initial stage of setting reaction and to desiccation when the cement begins to harden (**Fig. 24.17**). Moisture contamination has shown to affect the properties of cement markedly.

If moisture contamination occurs in first 24 hours of setting, calcium and aluminum ions leach out of the cement, thus they are prevented from forming polycarboxylates. This results in formation of chalky and eroded rough surface of restoration with low surface hardness. Similarly if early desiccation occurs during initial setting of the cement, it retards the setting reaction since water plays an important role in setting reaction. If desiccation occurs in later stages, it prevents increase in strength of the cement because hydration of the silica based hydrogel and the polycarboxylates cannot occur. It can also result in crazing, decreased esthetics and early deterioration of the cement.

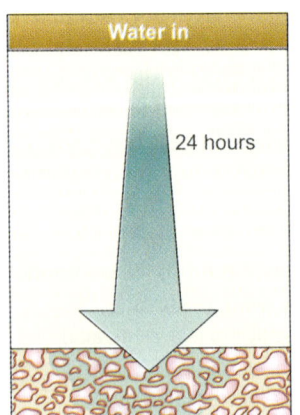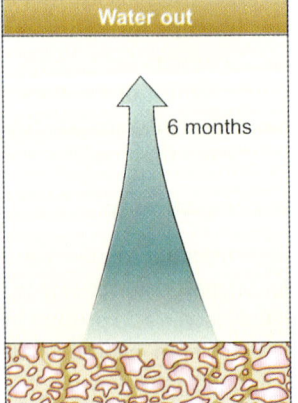

Figure 24.17: GIC shows sensitivity to water uptake and loss during initial setting stage. This may affect its physical properties

Therefore, one should always apply a low viscosity bonding resin, varnish or vaseline as a protective agent as soon as possible following cement placement to prevent both moisture contamination and desiccation across the surface of the GIC.

Adhesion

Glass ionomer cements are known chemical adhesives to tooth structure. The exact mechanism by which glass ionomer cements bond to tooth structure is not known, though it is said that chelation between the carboxyl groups of the cement and calcium of the tooth structure is responsible for their bonding. According to Wilson, adhesion of the glass ionomer cement is due to displacement of calcium and phosphate ions of the tooth structure because of the action of the carboxylate ions of cement. This results in formation of an intermediate aluminum and calcium phosphate layer which forms bond at the tooth/cement interface (**Figs 24.18 and 24.19**). Many studies have also shown that in adhesion of glass ionomer cement, both ionic and hydrogen bonding play role. Since enamel has higher percentage of inorganic content, bonding of GIC to enamel is stronger than to dentin. Though glass ionomer cement can bond directly to enamel and dentin even in the presence of a smear layer, but it has been shown that removal of smear layer results in better bonding. It is always preferred to condition the tooth surface before bonding for improving bonding of GIC. Conditioning causes removal of the smear layer without removing smear layer plugs from the dentin tubule orifices, or calcium ions.

Conditioning of tooth causes improved bonding because of following reasons:

→ It removes the smear layer, thus GIC can wet the dentin surface better
→ There is direct bond between the tooth and the cement, not with the smear layer
→ Conditioning also helps in ion exchange and increases surface energy which further increases the bonding.

Commonly used conditioner for glass ionomer cement is polyacrylic acid (10 to 25%) applied for 10 to 15 seconds. After using conditioner, use of dilute solution of ferric chloride on tooth has shown to improve the bonding by deposition of Fe^{3+} ions which further increase the ionic interaction between the cement and dentin. It chemically bonds to dentin/enamel, precious metals and porcelain restorations.

Fluoride Release

It has been shown in many studies that GICs contain fluoride in 10 to 23 percent concentration. This fluoride lies

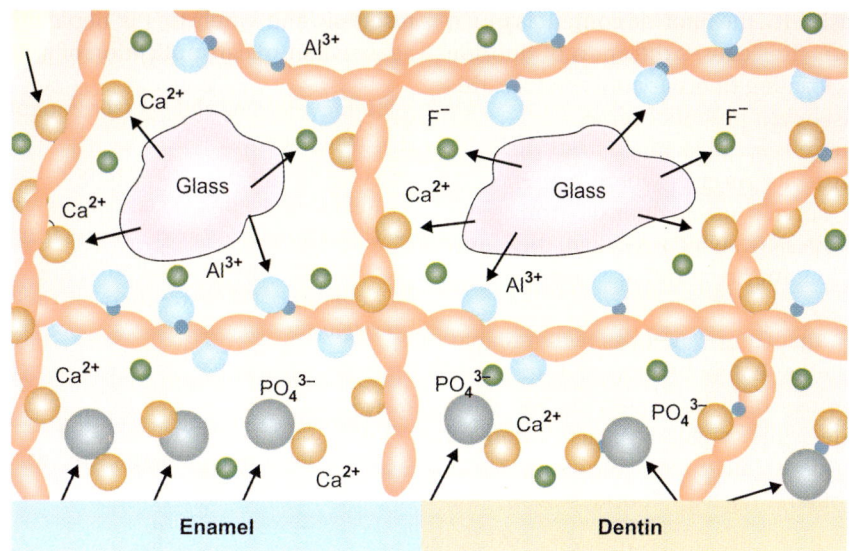

Figure 24.18: Chemical adhesion of GIC to tooth structure

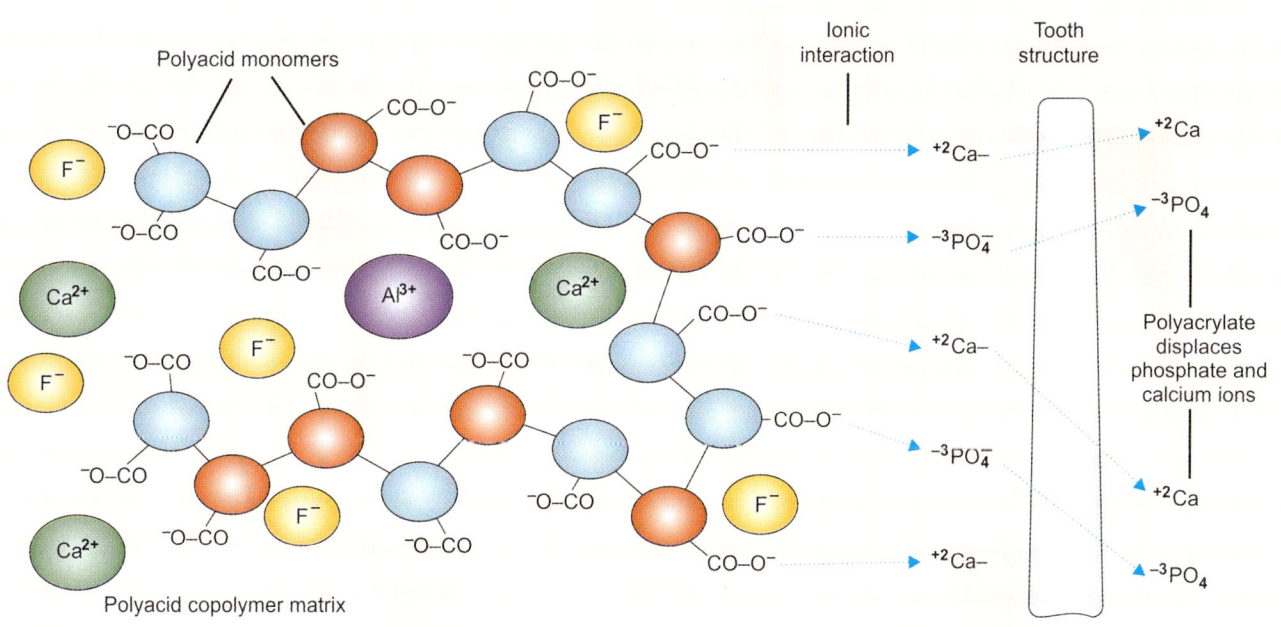

Figure 24.19: Diagrammatic representation of adhesion between GIC and tooth structure

free in the matrix and it is released from the glass powder at the time of mixing. When the powder and liquid of GIC are mixed, the setting reaction is initiated, in which the fluoride ions are released from the powder along with calcium, aluminum and sodium ions to build up the cement matrix as ions, salt compounds, etc. which later on deliver the fluoride from the set cement. The pattern of fluoride release by GIC is that it tends to peak in first 24 hours after the mixing. After this rate of release of fluoride decreases over many weeks and finally it stabilizes at a constant level in 3 to 4 months. In fresh GIC, the fluoride content is much more than that of tooth. This causes diffusion of fluoride from GIC to the tooth forming fluoroapatite crystals. This helps the tooth to resist development of caries.

In GIC, the fluoride release takes place from the interior of the restoration to its surface, where it then goes into solution. At the surface level, fluoride from glass ionomers diffuse into the saliva which gets lost, thus anti-cariogenicity of glass ionomer restoration at the margins decreases with time.

Studies have shown that GICs can act as rechargeable, fluoride releasing systems. It has been seen that application of topical fluorides help in recharging the glass ionomers with fluorides. This capacity of glass ionomers to recharge with fluoride is called reservoir effect. These recharged glass ionomers release fluorides from the reservoir and when this is depleted, it can be recharged again with topical application of fluorides (**Fig. 24.20**).

Fluoride releasing ability of glass ionomers also depends on following factors:
- Hand mixed glass ionomers release less fluoride than mechanically mixed glass ionomers
- On addition of resin monomers to its composition, fluoride release decreases significantly
- Covering of GIC restoration with a sealant reduces fluoride release.

Esthetics

In glass ionomer cements, the translucency gets better over the first 24 hours. These cements have shown good

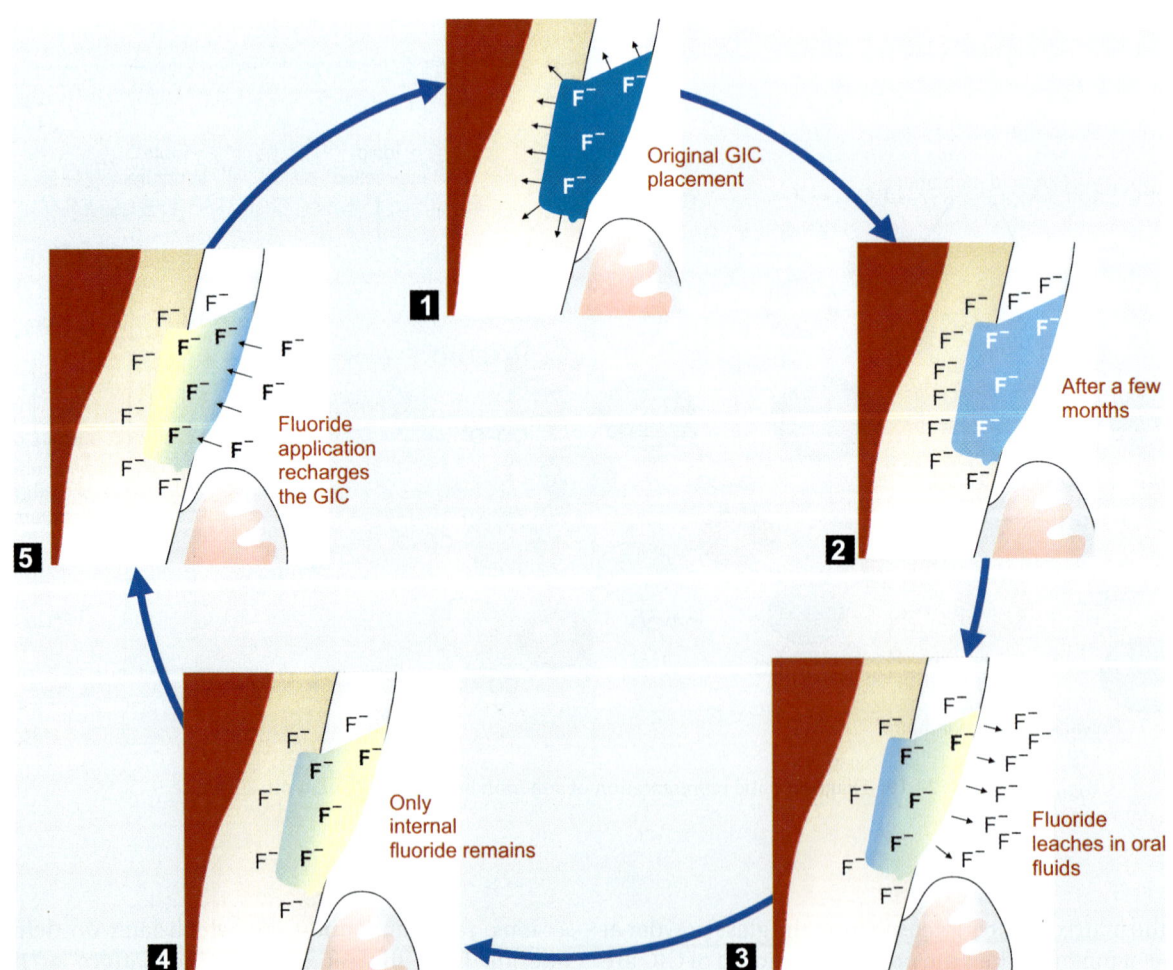

Figure 24.20: Diagram showing reservoir effect of glass ionomers: (1) Fluoride ions leach out from GIC into tooth; (2) Balance of fluoride between tooth and restoration; (3) Fluoride enters in saliva; (4) Both tooth and restoration are short of fluoride; (5) Topical application of fluoride replenish the cement

color stability. Initially the glass ionomer cements were very opaque because of presence of high fluoride content.

Increase in translucency of glass ionomers was developed by:
- Reduction in fluoride content
- Use of more translucent glasses
- Use of tartaric acid, polymaleic acid, etc. for improving the properties of cement
- Addition of resin in the RMGIs.

Though glass ionomer cements are reasonably tooth-colored and available in different shades (formed by addition of pigments like metal oxides, ferric oxide), they are still considered inferior to composites.

Margin Adaptation and Leakage

Coefficient of thermal expansion of glass ionomer cement is 0.8 that of tooth structure. In other words, it is almost similar to that of tooth, this is responsible for good marginal adaptation of glass ionomer restorations.

Radiopacity

Conventional glass ionomer cements are radiolucent, but metal modified and RMGIs are radiopaque because of presence of silver and heavy metal salts respectively.

USES OF GLASS IONOMER CEMENTS

As Pit and Fissure Sealants

Use of glass ionomer cements as fissure sealants is recommended because of anticariogenicity and adhesive properties. GIC is mixed to a more fluid consistency to allow it to flow into the depths of the pits and fissures of the posterior teeth. Seppa et al showed the advantages of glass ionomer as compared to composite resin sealants because of chances of contamination in erupting teeth (for composite resins) and their maintenance in the bottom of the fissure.

As Liners and Bases (Figs 24.21 and 24.22)

Glass ionomer cements (GICs) has number of advantages to be used like a liner. It is adhesive in nature and releases fluoride which not only prevent decay but also minimizes the appearance of secondary caries. It can be used beneath both composite resin and amalgam.

As Luting Agents (Fig. 24.23)

Glass ionomer luting cement is suited for permanent cementation of crowns, bridges, veneers and orthodontic

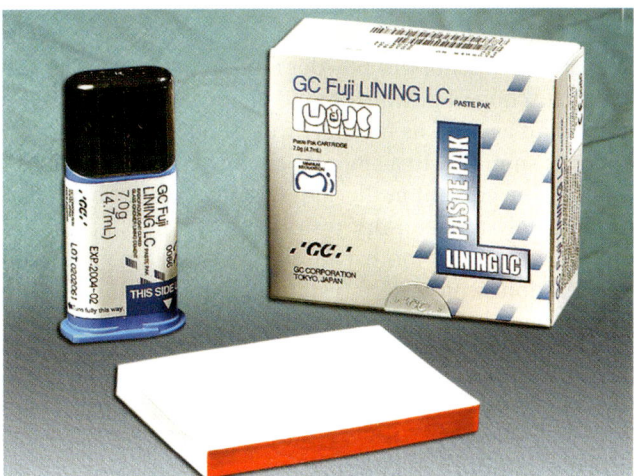

Figure 24.21: Glass ionomer cement used as liner and base in paste form

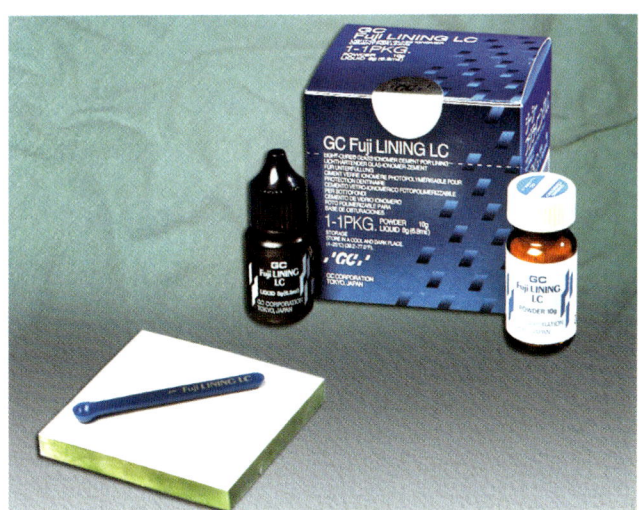

Figure 24.22: Glass ionomer cement used as liner/base in powder liquid form

bands. It chemically bonds to dentin/enamel, precious metals and porcelain restorations. It mechanically bonds to composite restorative materials. It reduces the incidence of microleakage when used to cement composite inlays or onlays. It is easy to mix with good flow properties.

Reasons for using glass ionomer as luting agent
- Chemical adhesion to tooth structure
- Anticariogenicity due to continuous fluoride release
- Fine film thickness
- Low solubility
- Sufficient tensile strength and abrasion resistance
- Biocompatibility to both pulp and gingival tissue.

Manipulation

Dispense two scoops of powder and three drops of liquid. The first scoop of powder should be incorporated into the liquid and as soon as it is fully wet, add the second scoop and mix smoothly to a smooth, creamy state (**Figs 24.24A and B**). The cement in this glossy state should be applied immediately to clean dry restoration which is seated on the dried prepared tooth. One should avoid the vital tooth dehydration which can result in hypersensitivity. The excess cement is trimmed away at its rubbery stage, just prior to the final set.

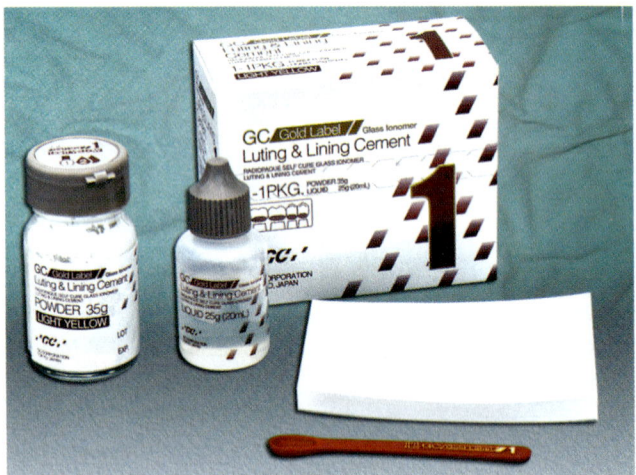

Figure 24.23: Glass ionomer cement used for luting inlays, onlays, crowns, veneers

As Orthodontic Brackets Adhesives (Figs 24.25 and 24.26)

Glass ionomer cements are commonly used because they bond directly to tooth tissue by the interaction of polyacrylate ions and hydroxyapatite crystals, thereby avoiding acid etching. Also they have anticariogenic affect due to their fluoride releasing action. However, their use in orthodontic bracket bonding has been limited due to inferior mechanical properties, in particular bond strength.

For Restorations of Class III and Class V Lesions (Fig. 24.27)

Lesions which are not under occlusal load can be successfully restored with a glass ionomer alone.

Fissure Sealing

If manipulated well, GIC has shown long-term success for fissure sealing. The recent high viscosity glass ionomer is preferred because of high strength and also it can be placed under finger pressure to adapt the cement into the depths of the fissure.

Restoration of Root Caries

Glass ionomer cement is the material of choice for restoration of root caries because of its adhesion to dentin, anticariogenicity, nearly esthetic and ease of use.

High Caries Risk Patients

High viscosity glass ionomers are used in caries management of patients with high-risk for caries because of their

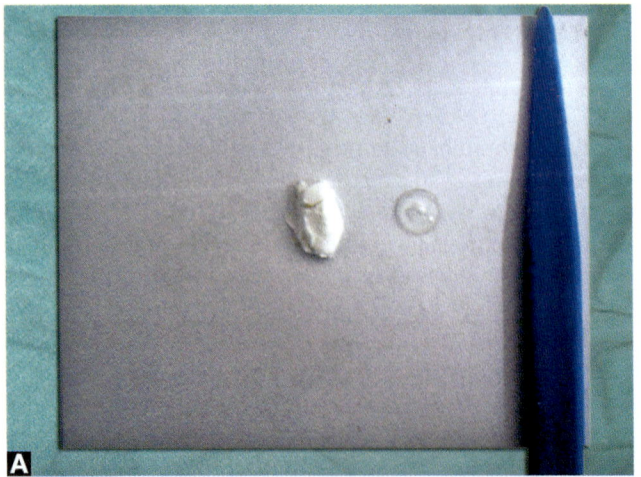

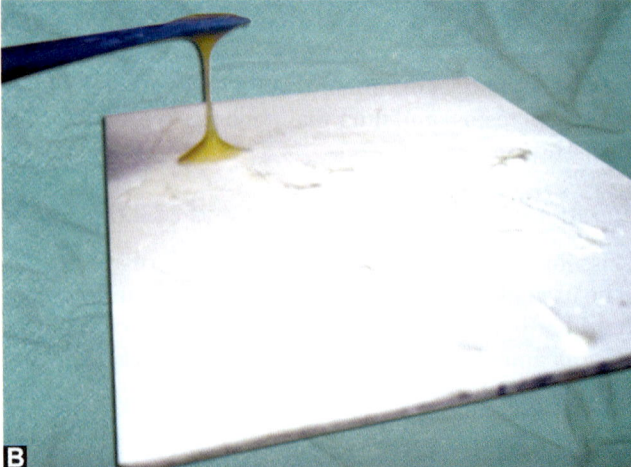

Figures 24.24A and B: Manipulation of GIC for luting consistency: (A) Dispensing of powder and liquid; (B) Smooth creamy mix for luting purpose

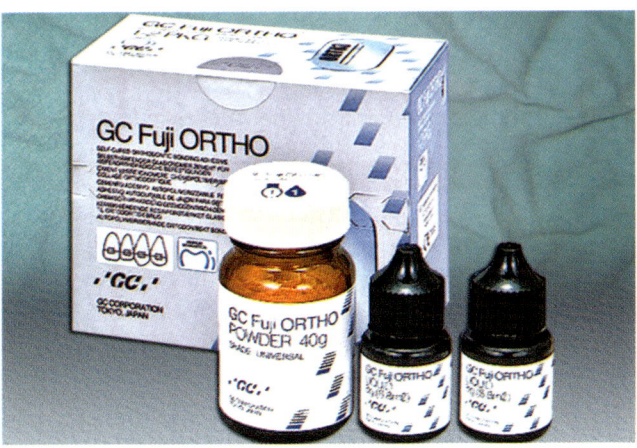

Figure 24.25: Glass ionomer cement used for joining orthodontic brackets in powder liquid form

For Core Build Up (Fig. 24.28)

Glass ionomers cements can be used for building cores. In general, silver containing GICs are preferred. It is believed that silver within the material enhances its physical and mechanical properties. However, many studies have shown GICs are inadequately strong to support major core buildups. Hence the recommendation that a tooth should have atleast two structurally intact walls if a GIC core is to be considered.

Atraumatic Restorative Treatment (ART)

Atraumatic restorative treatment (ART) was introduced in South Africa by Jo Frencken in 1996. This technique was first evaluated in Tanzania in 1980, and since then it has become very popular. It allows restorative treatments in

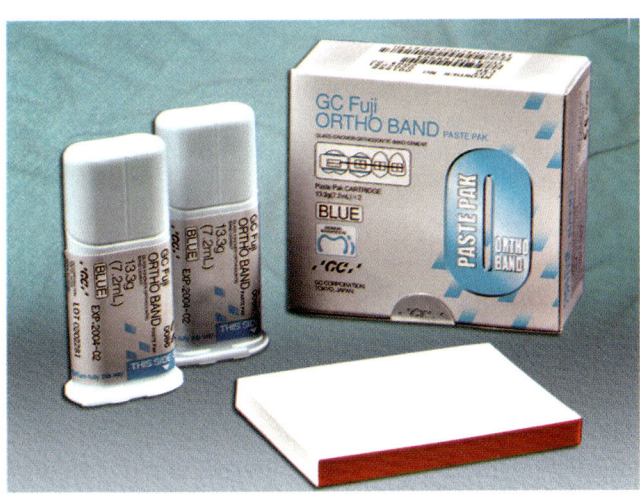

Figure 24.26: Glass ionomer cement for orthodontic use in paste form

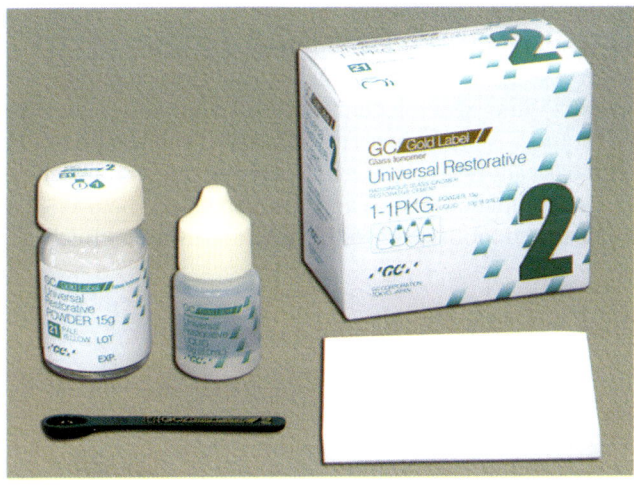

Figure 24.27: Glass ionomer cement for restoration of conservative tooth preparations

adhesion, adequate abrasion resistance, and fluoride releasing properties.

Emergency Temporary Restorations

Fractured cusps or restorations can be temporarily stabilized using glass ionomers because of their property of adhesion which gives retention even if mechanical support is absent. GIC is used in covering the exposed dentin to provide patient comfort with minimal chair time.

For Intermediate Restorations

Because of their adhesive nature and satisfactory esthetics, GICs are also used as interim restorations.

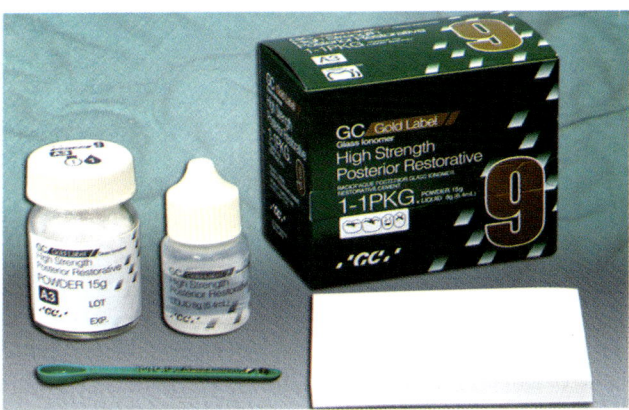

Figure 24.28: High strength glass ionomer used as core build up material

places with no electricity and without the aid of sophisticated dental equipment. ART restores tooth decay without using the drill or injecting a local anesthetic. It involves the removal of carious lesions by hand instruments such as spoon excavators, sometimes together with a caries softening gel. After the caries is removed, the tooth is restored with high viscosity glass ionomer cement.

Indications of ART technique
→ Areas without electricity and sophisticated dental aids
→ Children from poor families
→ In homes for mentally and physically disabled, and the elderly patients
→ Small to moderate pit and fissure caries.

Steps for ART Technique (Figs 24.29A to D)

In this technique, the patient is placed in a supine position, and the operator is comfortably seated. The carious lesion is excavated without anesthesia.
- Tooth is isolated using cotton rolls
- Access is made by breaking off undermined enamel
- After removal of soft demineralized dentin by excavation, tooth is restored using a modified GIC. This modified GIC is basically reinforced GIC so as to give increased strength under functional loads and is radiopaque in nature.
- Restored tooth is contoured and occlusion is checked

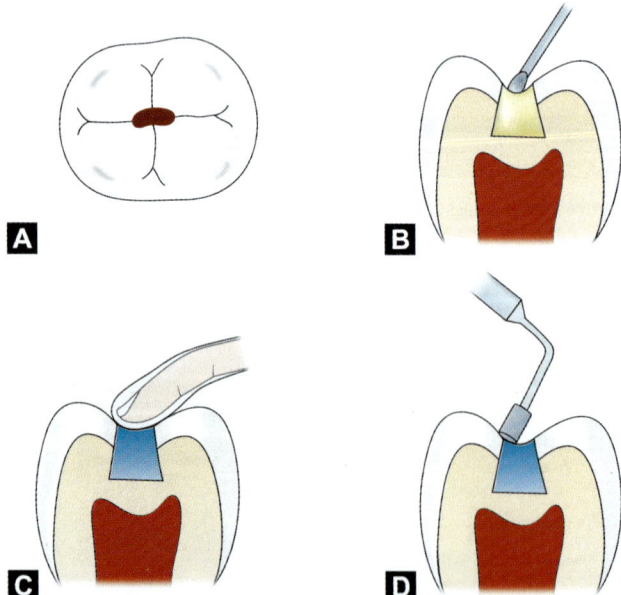

Figures 24.29A to D: Steps of ART technique: (A) Tooth with carious lesion; (B) Caries are excavated using spoon excavator; (C) GIC is placed in the prepared tooth; (D) Adjust the restoration while it is still in the workable state

- Since no rotary instruments can be used, all adjustments should be completed while the restorative material is in a workable state.
- Restoration is covered using petroleum jelly.

Advantages of ART technique
→ Mechanics needed for ART, does not require complicated mechanical instrument
→ Employs use of already present hand instruments
→ Minimal discomfort to patient
→ Causes less pain
→ No need of injecting local anesthetic
→ Low-cost of the treatment
→ Safe and cost-effective treatment
→ Minimum intervention procedure
→ Advantages of glass ionomer cements in form of adhesion, biocompatibility and anticariogenicity
→ Use of operators with minimal training.

Disadvantages of ART technique
→ Poor access and visibility especially in posterior region
→ Hand fatigue during instrumentation.
→ ART technique is now called as PRR technique introduced by simonsen and Stallard in 1978.

Sandwich Technique

The term "sandwich technique" refers to a laminated restoration using glass ionomer to replace dentin and composite resin to replace enamel. This technique was developed by McLean et al in 1985. Because of this technique, we get the advantages of both the materials that is caries resistance, chemical adhesion to dentin, fluoride release, reduced microleakage and remineralization of glass ionomer with the enamel bonding, surface finish, durability, and esthetic superiority of composite resin. Also composite resin bonds micromechanically to set glass ionomers and chemically to the HEMA in resin-modified glass ionomers.

Synonyms of sandwich technique
→ Replacement dentin technique
→ Bilayered technique
→ Laminate restoration technique.

The bond strength between conventional GIC and composite is limited by the low cohesive strength of glass ionomers due to the lack of chemical bonding. This is because of difference in the setting reactions between composite resin and conventional GIC.

Resin modified glass ionomer cement (RMGIC) have shown improved mechanical and physical properties over conventional GICs. Also they have shown a true adhesive bond to resin composites when compared to conventional GIC.

Indications of sandwich technique
➡ Large Class III, IV, V and class I and II lesions
➡ For laminate veneers.

Steps of Sandwich Technique

- Isolate the tooth to be prepared
- Prepare the tooth. Keep the cavosurface margins involving dentin as butt joint. Bevel the enamel margins to increase the composite resin bonding
- Provide pulp protection using calcium hydroxide base, if indicated. Usually it is avoided since it reduces the area for adhesion of glass ionomer cement
- Condition the prepared tooth using polyacrylic acid for optimal adhesion of GIC
- Place freshly mixed fast setting GIC in the prepared tooth
- It is only necessary to etch a GIC with acid if the restoration has been in place for sometime and has fully matured. If the GIC is freshly placed and is immature, bonding can be achieved simply by washing the GIC surface because water causes washout of GIC matrix from around the filler particles which gives microscopically rough surface to which the composite will attach
- Now coat the surface of prepared tooth either with an unfilled resin or a dentin bonding agent for optimal adhesion and cure it for 20 seconds (**Fig. 24.30**)
- Place composite and cure in usual manner
- Do finishing and polishing of the restoration and finally recure it for 20 seconds.

To have optimal results from sandwich technique, the following should be done:

- Use high strength glass ionomer available
- Before placing glass ionomer, condition the tooth preparation to have better adhesion

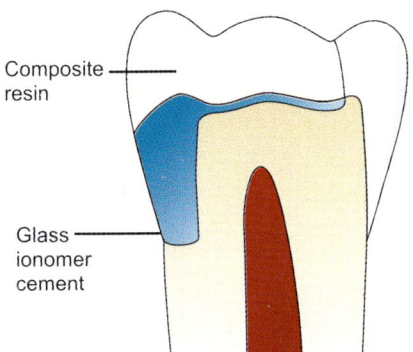

Figure 24.30: Sandwich technique: Glass ionomer is placed in prepared tooth, over which composite resin is placed as laminate

- Avoid placing subbase like calcium hydroxide as it reduces surface area of adhesion
- Before placing composite over glass ionomer, let the glass ionomer set fully
- Place composite restorative in sufficient bulk to provide the flexibility and resistance form to the restoration
- Before placing composite, remove the glass ionomer from margins to expose the enamel as composite-enamel bond is strongest
- The glass ionomer cement should be radio-opaque in nature
- The contact area should be built with composite resins, not glass ionomers.

Advantages of sandwich technique
➡ The open sandwich technique used for deep class II forms where the cervical margin lacks enamel, has shown improved resistance to microleakage and caries in comparison to resin bonding at dentin margins.
➡ Better strength esthetics and finish of composite resins.
➡ Fluoride release from GIC.
➡ Reduced bulk of composite resins pose less polymerization shrinkage.
➡ Minimizes the number of increments of composite resin to be placed, so saves time.
➡ Use of GIC eliminates acid etching of dentin and thus reduces postoperative sensitivity caused by incomplete sealing of etched dentin.
➡ Good pulpal response because of biocompatibility of GIC.

Disadvantages
➡ Technique sensitive
➡ Time consuming.

CLINICAL STEPS FOR PLACEMENT OF GLASS IONOMER CEMENT

Steps for placement of GIC
➡ Isolation
➡ Instrumentation and tooth preparation
➡ Mixing of GIC
➡ Restoration
➡ Finishing and polishing
➡ Surface protection.

Isolation

Saliva control is important for successful glass ionomer restorations. If moisture contaminates the cement during manipulation and setting, the gel will weaken and wash out prematurely. Commonly used methods for isolation are rubber dam, retraction cords, cotton rolls and saliva ejectors.

Instrumentation

Following instruments are normally used during restoration with GICs:
- Rubber dam
- Mouth mirror
- Explorer
- Cotton pliers
- Matrix material
- No. 330, ¼, ½ 1,2 burs
- Curved chisel
- Monoangle hoe
- Gingival marginal trimmer (small)
- Wooden wedge.

Tooth Preparation

Tooth preparation for glass ionomer cement is done in two ways:
1. Mechanical preparation
2. Chemical preparation (conditioning).

Mechanical Preparation

Glass ionomer can be used for class III, class V, small class I and II tooth preparations.

Class III Tooth Preparation

Glass ionomer is the material of choice to restore the class III lesion when caries extends onto the root surface.

Indications for class III glass ionomer restorations:
→ In patients with high caries index
→ When caries extend onto the root surface
→ In areas with low occlusal stress
→ When labial enamel is intact.

- *Outline form*: Using a small inverted cone bur, make an access through the lingual marginal ridge (**Figs 24.31A and B**). Extend the bur towards incisal or gingival area depending on caries. This helps in maintaining esthetics and exposing less material to dehydration. Do not try to break the contact, this helps in preserving the facial enamel. Prepare butt-joint cavosuface margins since glass ionomer is a brittle material, it cannot be placed over the bevels.
- *Retention and resistance form*: Since retention in glass ionomer is chemical in nature, so placing undercuts and dovetail is not mandatory. For retention, deepen

the outline to provide atleast 1 mm bulk for the cement.

Small grooves incisially or cervically may provide additional retention form when required.
- *Convenience form*: Lingual wall is sometimes broken for access in maxillary teeth. Teeth may be mechanically separated for convenience form.
- *Pulpal protection*: Any area where less than 0.5 mm of remaining dentin is present, fast setting calcium hydroxide liner is placed for pulp protection.

Varnish is not used, since there is no need to prevent chemical invasion.

Class V Tooth Preparation

Indications for use of glass ionomers in class V restorations (**Fig. 24.32**) are:
→ Patients with high caries incidence
→ When esthetics is not of primary concern
→ In root surface lesions.

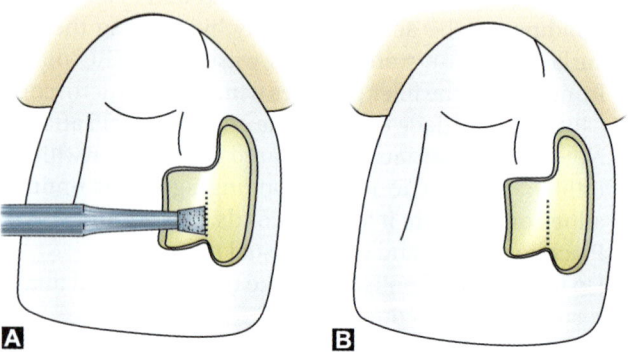

A   **B**

Figures 24.31A and B: Class III tooth preparation for GIC: (A) Access is made through the lingual marginal ridge; (B) Completed tooth preparation

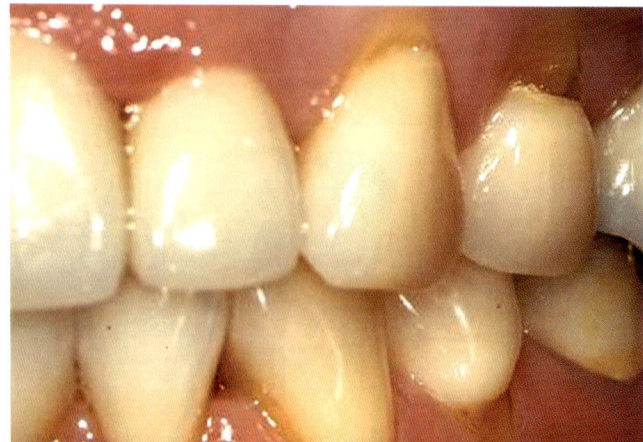

Figure 24.32: Abrasion of 24 can be restored with glass ionomer

The class V lesion can be present only in enamel or both in enamel and cementum (**Figs 24.33A and B**). Steps for tooth preparation of class V lesions are:

- *Outline form*: External outline form is limited to the extension of the lesion. Prepare the tooth using high speed round bur along with air water coolant. Take care to manage sulcular fluid do not make further preparation in cases of cervical abrasion or erosion where most part is in cementum.
- *Retention and resistance form*: Retention is primarily achieved by chemical bonding, so nothing special is required for added retention. Prepare rounded grooves into occlusal and cervical dentin wall if required in wider tooth (**Figs 24.34A and B**).
- *Convenience form*: Lip and cheek retractors and tongue guards are generally used for convenience of operation though use of rubber dam is preferred.
- *Pulp protection:* Same as for class III.

Class I Tooth Preparation

Glass ionomer are only used for small pit and fissure lesions which do not have high occlusal stresses.

Indications for Use of Glass Ionomers as Pit and Fissure Sealants.
- Deep pits and fissures (**Fig. 24.35**)
- Recently erupted teeth in patients with high caries index.

Outline form: Use a small round bur to enter in the fissure and remove carious dentin. After this, use fine tapered fissure bur to widen the fissures (**Fig. 24.36**). This fissure widening helps in better flow and increased retention of glass ionomer cement (**Fig. 24.37**).

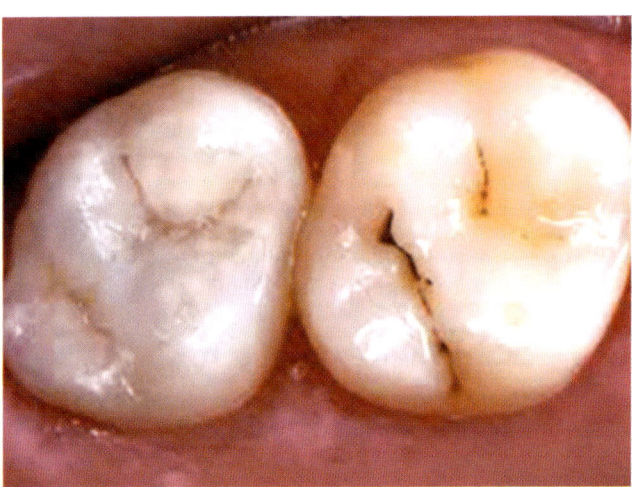

Figure 24.35: Deep pits are indicated for glass ionomers

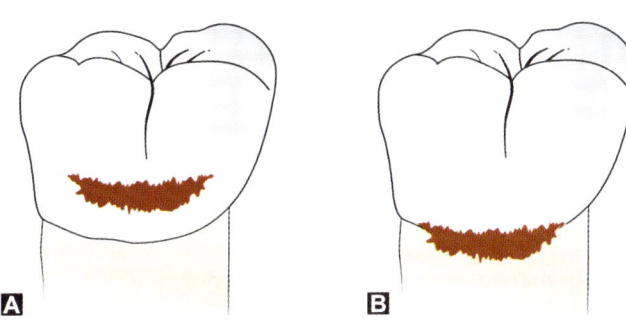

Figures 24.33A and B: The cervical lesion can be present only in:
(A) Enamel; (B) Both in enamel and cementum

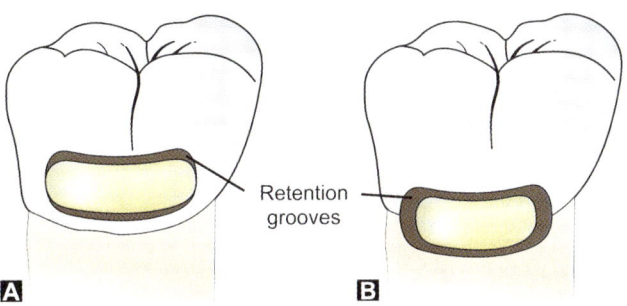

Retention grooves

Figures 24.34A and B: For retention, grooves can be made only:
(A) On occlusal and gingival walls; (B) On all the four walls

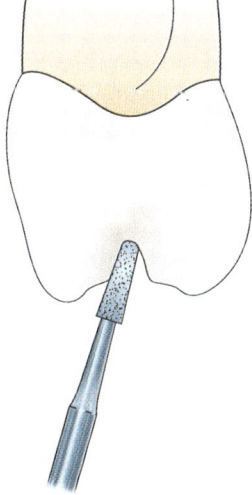

Figure 24.36: Widen the deep fissure using tapered fissure bur

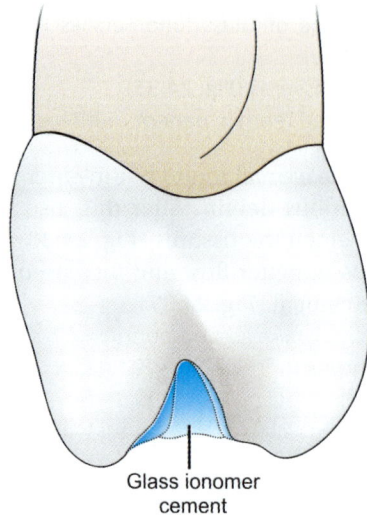

Glass ionomer
cement

Figure 24.37: Place GIC in widened fissure

Retention form: Since glass ionomer cement bonds chemically to tooth structure, so no special retention aid is required.

Convenience form: Widen the fissures properly for better flow of the glass ionomer.

Use of rubber dam is always preferred for convenience form.

Class II Tooth Preparation

Since glass ionomer cements lack fracture toughness and they are porus in nature, their use is limited in class II restorations.

Internal Preparation on Occlusal Fossa

In this, occlusal fossa is penetrated using small round burs leaving atleast 2 mm width of marginal ridge intact. Commonly used material for such preparations is silver cermet ionomer.

Tunnel Restoration

A tunnel preparation is made for removal of proximal caries by making an access through occlusal surface while leaving the marginal ridge intact. Though the concept of tunnel preparation is very simple, yet the preparation is not that simple because it is too conservative to prepare, fill and finish.

This technique was first used in primary molars by Jinks in 1963. Hunt and Knight later on used this technique for restoration of small proximal carious lesions.

Indications
➤ Indicated when life expectancy of tooth is not more than 5 years like in deciduous teeth or mobile teeth in geriatric patients
➤ Incipient proximal lesions of posterior teeth (**Fig. 24.38**)
➤ Low caries index of patient.

Contraindication
➤ When proximal decay undermines the marginal ridge.

Advantages of tunnel preparation
➤ Conservative tooth preparation
➤ Preservation of marginal ridge
➤ Less damage to adjacent tooth structure
➤ If carious structure is more extensive, than originally thought, tunnel preparation can be easily converted to traditional class II design
➤ Results in more esthetic restoration
➤ Less microleakage
➤ Less chances of proximal overhang
➤ Since caries usually start below contact point, contact area is preserved
➤ Cost-effective.

Disadvantages
➤ Difficult to fill and finish
➤ Difficult to practice
➤ Needs precise control during preparation
➤ More chances of developing secondary caries
➤ Reduces strength of marginal ridge
➤ More chances of injury to pulp or periodontium
➤ Limited access and visibility
➤ Anatomical landmarks are not clear
➤ Poor marginal adaptability of restoration
➤ Risk of incomplete removal of caries.

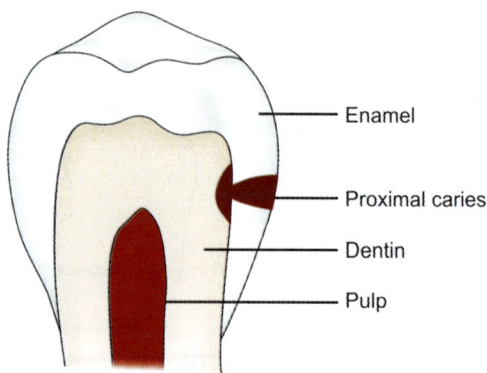

Enamel

Proximal caries

Dentin

Pulp

Figure 24.38: Tunnel preparation is indicated in small proximal lesions

Armamentarium: Before initiating the restoration, one should be ready with isolation materials (retraction cord, rubber dam material), mylar strip, instruments like explorers, condensers, plastic instruments, carvers, etc.

Technique

- Before initiating the treatment, one should evaluate the tooth properly to determine location and extent of caries (**Fig. 24.39**). Bitewing radiograph is taken to know that the access area does not involve any pulp horn.
- Isolate and dry the tooth to be restored with tunnel preparation.
- Place a wedge below the carious proximal portion
- Penetrate the occlusal surface of tooth with a round bur. Entry of bur should be 2 mm inside the marginal ridge (**Fig. 24.40**). Angle of bur should be 45° to the carious lesion (**Fig. 24.41**).

- After enamel has been penetrated, spoon excavator is used to remove the caries. Use periodontal probe to measure the depth of lesion. Widen the preparation using tapered fissure bur.
- Now remove the caries by cutting into proximal lesion and remove the wedge to see the extent of preparation
- Once the complete caries removal is confirmed, place a matrix band and wedge on the proximal surface so as to avoid overhanging restoration and injury to gingiva (**Fig. 24.42**).
- Use restorative material and condense it from occlusal surface, avoiding any void (**Fig. 24.43**).
- Remove wedge and matrix and do final finishing and polishing of the restoration (**Fig. 24.44**).

Precautions while making tunnel preparation: Since tunnel preparation is almost a blind procedure, following precautions should be taken while preparing it so as to have an optimal restoration:

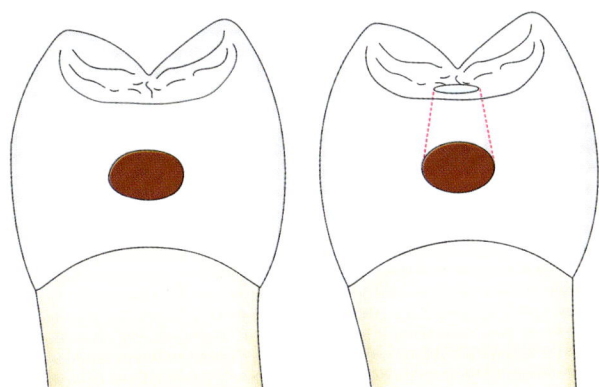

Figure 24.39: Before initiating the preparation, one should know extent of dental caries

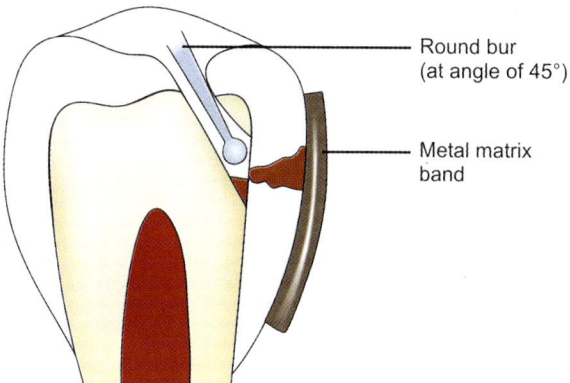

Figure 24.41: Entry of bur should be at 45° to the lesion

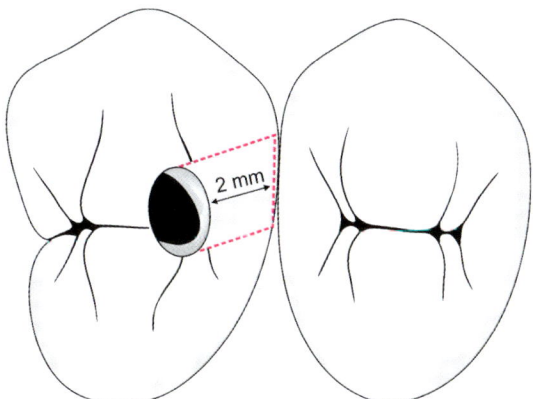

Figure 24.40: Entry of bur should be 2 mm inside the marginal ridge

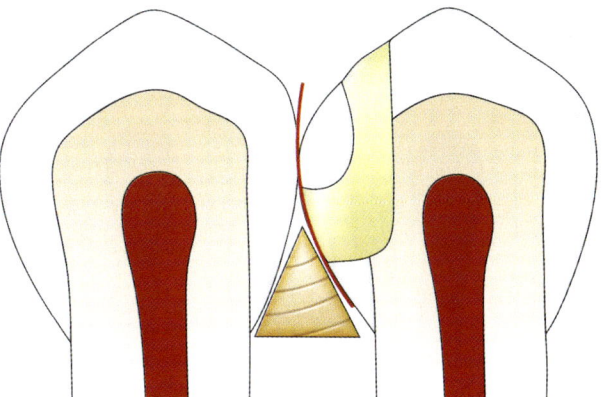

Figure 24.42: Completed tunnel preparation

- Always predetermine the angulation of the bur before initiating the procedure. This can be done by sticking three pieces of 2.0 cm long straight wire, each at slightly different angles, on the buccal surface of the tooth to be restored. The wires are fixed such that one end of the wire should cross the center of the caries and other end should extend beyond the occlusal surface, i.e. the point from where the tunnel preparation is to be started. Once the wires are temporarily fixed on the tooth surface, take a radiograph with 1 mm square wire gauge mounted on X-ray film. By this, correct angulation and distance between the center of the lesion and the occlusal pit of the affected side can be determined.
- On reaching dentinoenamel junction, one should take radiograph of tooth along with the bur present in the tunnel preparation. This helps in determining correct angulation of the bur.

- Maintain a constant angulation of the bur so that the prepared tunnel is in a straight line to assist caries removal, and condensation of the restorative material.
- After completion of the preparation, take a radiograph to confirm the complete removal of the carious lesion and soft dentin.

Chemical Preparation for GIC (Fig. 24.45)

For better adhesion of GIC to tooth structure, many conditioning agents have been used. These are 50 percent citric acid, 10 percent EDTA, 20 percent polyacrylic acid, 3 percent hydrogen peroxide and 25 percent tannic acid. Polyacrylic acid is the most commonly used conditioner.

In Resin-modified glass ionomers, an added step of priming the tooth surface is done in which primer is applied in a thin coat and light cured for 20 to 40 seconds.

Mixing of Cement

Mixing should be done using the powder: liquid ratio as recommended by the manufacturer. The powder to liquid ratio is important and varies from manufacturer to manufacturer. A reduction in powder to liquid ratio can result in poor physical properties.

Mixing should be done
➡ At room temperature 21 to 25°C
➡ With humidity of 40 to 60 percent
➡ For 45 to 60 seconds
➡ On a cool (not below the dew point) and dry glass slab or paper pad
➡ With the help of a flat and firm plastic spatula.

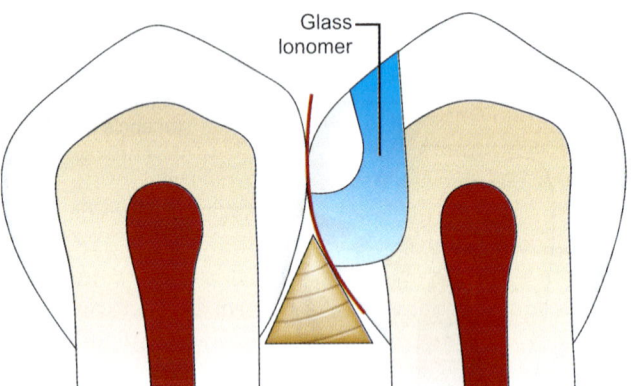

Figure 24.43: Placement of GIC in the prepared tunnel

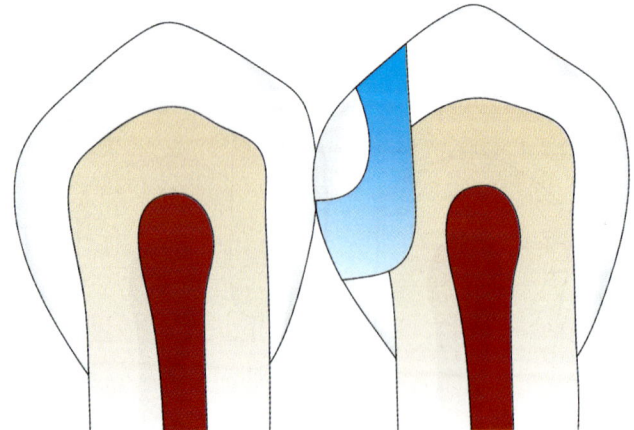

Figure 24.44: Completed tunnel restoration using glass ionomer cement

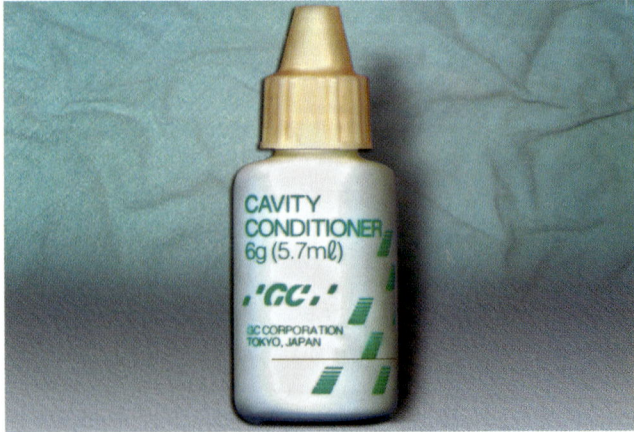

Figure 24.45: Conditioner used for chemical preparation for glass ionomer

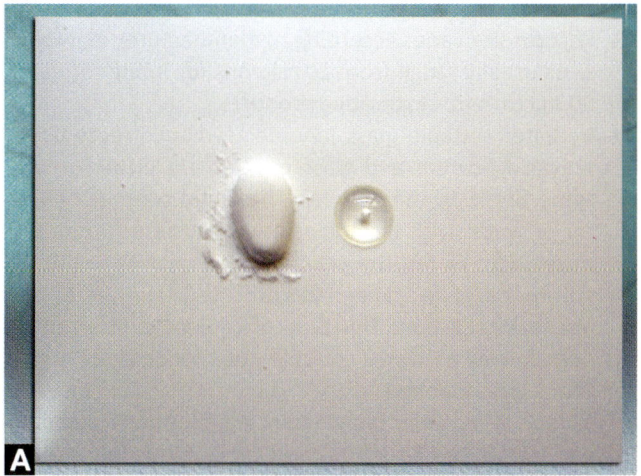
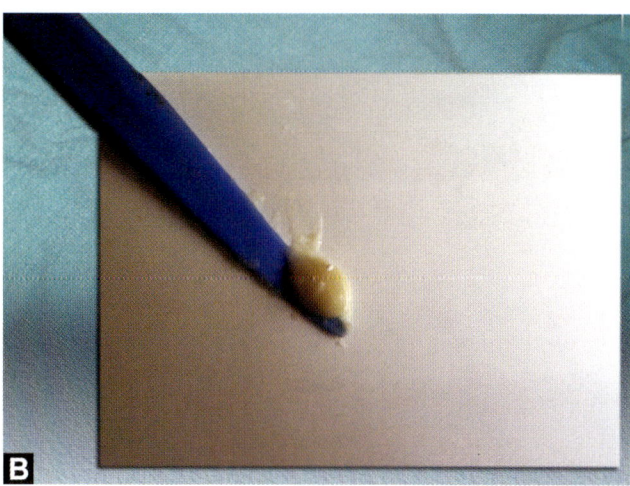

Figures 24.46A and B: Mixing of GIC: (A) Dispensing of powder and liquid of GIC for mixing; (B) Freshly mixed GIC ready to be used for restoration

Glass slab is better than paper pad for mixing as it can be cooled to prolong the working time if required. It should be noted that an excessively chilled slab can cause a reduction in the cement compressive strength and modulus of elasticity.

It is not necessary to mix the cement over a large area on the glass slab because the setting reaction is only mildly exothermic.

For mixing, divide the dispensed cement powder into two equal portions. Mix the first portion into the liquid in 20 seconds and then add the remaining powder and mix for another 20 seconds. Mixing should be completed within 40 to 60 seconds (**Figs 24.46A and B**). Working time for glass ionomer cement is 60 to 90 second. Loss of gloss on the surface of the mixed cement shows end of working time and start of setting reaction. The cement should be used before it loses its glossiness. If the glossiness is lost, the cement would not wet the tooth surface well and bond strength will be reduced.

Restoration

After mixing, glass ionomer cement is carried with the help of cement carrier for placement into the prepared tooth. For optimal restoration and to reduce the number of voids, use of matrix is always advisable. After placing the cement, the gross excess is removed immediately and final contouring is done. In case of chemically cure glass ionomer, matrix is held till the initial hardening of cement starts but in case of light cure glass ionomers, photoactivation can be done for accelerated setting.

Finishing and Polishing

As we know, surface of glass ionomers is sensitive to both moisture contamination and dessication. During initial phase of cement setting, it is always preferred to delay finishing and polishing of glass ionomer cements. It is delayed for atleast 24 hours after the cement placement because by then, the surface of restoration attains ionic equilibrium in the environment. But in case of resin modified glass ionomer cements, finishing is started after their placement.

After placing the restoration, gross finishing is done following the matrix removal. Before starting the finishing procedure, the surface of restoration is coated with protective agent. A sharp knife is used to remove the extra cement. For this, rotary or hand cutting instruments can also be used though it is believed that hand cutting instruments can tear or pull the restoration margins leading to marginal break-down. Final finishing of restoration is done with the help of superfine diamond points, soflex disk and abrasive strips in moist condition. After final finishing and polishing is done, surface of restoration is protected using petroleum jelly, varnish or bonding agent.

Surface Protection

Since glass ionomers show sensitivity to both moisture contamination and surface desiccation, the newly placed restoration should always be protected immediately after matrix removal so as to prevent water exchange. It can be done with the help of resin bonding agent, cocoa butter, petroleum jelly or varnish (**Fig. 24.47**). Among these, resin

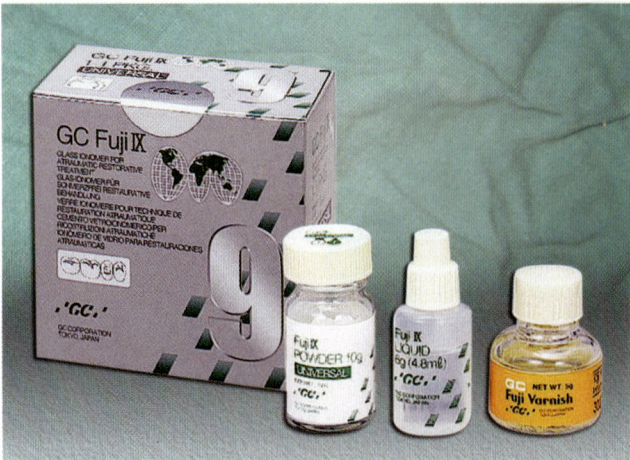

Figure 24.47: Varnish

bonding agents provide the best surface protection as they fill the microporosities of the surface and stay for longer time in comparison to other agents.

Commercial brands of glass ionomer cement	
Fuji II LC	World's first resin modified glass ionomer restorative material
Fuji bond LC	Resin reinforced glass ionomer
Fuji plus capsule	World's first resin modified glass ionomer luting cement in capsules
Fuji CEM	World's first paste-paste glass ionomer. This fast system uses a specially designed dispenser and prepackaged cartridges of cement
Fuji IX GP fast	World's first packable condensable glass ionomer for posterior restorations
Fuji VII	World's first command setting glass ionomer without a resin component.

Key Points

- Glass ionomer cement was introduced to the dentistry in 1972 by Wilson and Kent.
- The first commercial glass ionomer was made by the De Trey Company and distributed by the Amalgamated Dental Co in England and by Caulk in the United States, known as Alumino silicate polyacrylate (ASPA).
- The powder is an acid-soluble calcium fluoroaluminosilicate glass similar to that of silicate but with a higher aluminasilicate ratio that increases its reactivity with liquid. The fluoride portion acts as a "ceramic flux".

- Particle size varies according to manufacturer, however sizes usually range from 20 microns for luting forms to 50 microns for restorative products.
- in water settable glass ionomer cement, freeze-dried polyacid powder and glass powder are placed in the same bottle as the powder. The liquid consists of water or water with tartaric acid. When the powders are mixed with water, the acid powder dissolves to reconstitute the liquid acid and this process is followed by the acid-base reaction. This type of cement is referred to occasionally as water settable glass ionomer or anhydrous glass ionomer.
- Miracle Mix (Silver alloy admix glass ionomer cement) was introduced by Simmons in 1983. In this, silver alloy powder is blended with glass ionomer powder in ratio of 1:6 and mixed with glass ionomer liquid. This increases the compressive strength, tensile strength and abrasion resistance to some extent.
- Cermet Cement was introduced by Mclean and Gasser in 1987. Here the cement ionomers are manufactured by sintering the compressed pellets made from fine metal powder and glass ionomer powder at temperature of 800° c. The sintered metal and glass fit is then ground into fine form which results in ceramicometal particles of fused metal and ground glass.
- In RMGI, the powder is fluorosilicate glass with initiator. The liquid contains 15 to 25 percent resin component in the form of HEMA, a polyacrylic acid copolymer along with photoinitiator and water.
- According to Wilson, adhesion of the glass ionomer cement is due to displacement of calcium and phosphate ions of the tooth structure because of the action of the carboxylate ions of cement. This results in formation of an intermediate aluminum and calcium phosphate layer which forms bond at the tooth/cement interface.
- In the initial stages, GIC releases fluoride which lies free in the matrix and is released from the glass powder at the time of mixing. When the powder and liquid of GIC are mixed, the setting reaction is initiated, in which the fluoride ions are released from the powder along with calcium, aluminum and sodium ions to build up the cement matrix, this later on delivers the fluoride from the set cement.
- The fluoride release by GIC tends to peak in first 24 hours after the mixing, after this rate of release of fluoride decreases over many weeks and finally it stabilizes at a constant level in 3 to 4 months.
- GICs can act as rechargeable, fluoride releasing systems. Application of topical fluoride helps in recharging

the glass ionomers with fluorides. This capacity of glass ionomers to recharge with fluoride is called reservoir effect. These recharged glass ionomers release fluorides from the reservoir and when this is depleted, it can be recharged again with topical application of fluorides.

- Initially the glass ionomer cements were very opaque because of presence of high fluoride content. But by reducing fluoride content, use of more translucent glasses, and addition of resins in RMGI have helped in increasing the translucency of glass ionomers.
- Atraumatic restorative treatment (ART) was introduced in South Africa by Jo Frencken in 1996. It allows restorative treatments in places with no electricity and without the aid of sophisticated dental equipment.
- Atraumatic restorative treatment (ART) restores tooth decay without using the drill or injecting a local anaesthetic. It involves the removal of carious lesions by hand instruments such as spoon excavators, sometimes together with a caries softening gel. After the caries is removed, the tooth is restored with high viscous glass ionomer cement.
- The term "sandwich technique" refers to a laminated restoration using glass ionomer to replace dentin and composite resin to replace enamel. This technique was developed by McLean et al in 1985.
- A tunnel preparation is made for removal of proximal caries by making an access through occlusal surface while leaving the marginal ridge intact. This technique was first used in primary molars by Jinks in 1963.
- For better adhesion of GIC to tooth structure, many conditioning agents have been used. These are 50 percent citric acid, 10 percent EDTA, 20 percent polyacrylic acid, 3 percent hydrogen peroxide and 25 percent tannic acid. Polyacrylic acid is the most commonly used conditioner.
- For mixing glass ionomer cement, glass slab is better than paper pad for mixing as it can be cooled to prolong the working time if required.
- It is not necessary to mix the glass ionomer cement over a large area on the glass slab because the setting reaction is only mildly exothermic.
- Since glass ionomers show sensitivity to both moisture contamination and surface desiccation, the newly placed restoration should always be protected (using bonding agent, cocoa butter, petroleum jelly or varnish) immediately so as to prevent water exchange.

QUESTIONS

1. Classify GICs. What are their advantages and disadvantages?
2. What is composition of glass ionomer cement? Write in detail setting reaction of GIC.
3. Short notes on:
   a. Fluoride release property of GIC
   b. ART technique
   c. Sandwich technique
   d. Adhesion of GIC
   e. Tunnel restoration.
4. Classify various cements used in dentistry. Describe in detail about the composition, setting reaction, advantages, disadvantages, properties and uses of glass ionomer cement.

BIBLIOGRAPHY

1. Cho E, Kopel H, White SN. Moisture susceptibility of resin-modified glass-ionomer materials. Quint Int. 1995;26:351.
2. Davidson CL. Glass ionomer bases under posterior composites. J Esthet Dent. 1994;6:223.
3. El-Kalia IH, Garcia Godoy F. Mechanical properties of compomer restorative material. Oper Dent. 1999;24:2.
4. Forsten L. Fluoride release of glass ionomers. J Esth Dent. 1994;6:216.
5. Frencken JE, Pilot T, Songpaisan Y, et al. Atraumatic restorative treatment (ART): rationale, technique and development. J Public Health Dent. 1996;56:135.
6. Frencken JE, Songpaisan Y, Phantumvanit P, et al. An atraumatic restorative treatment (ART) technique: evolution after one years. Int Dent J. 1994;44:460.
7. Garcia GF, Marshall TO, Mount GJ. Microleakage of glass ionomer tunnel restorations. Am J Dent. 1998;1:53.
8. Guggenberger R, et al. New trends in glass-ionomer chemistry, Biomaterials. 1998;19:479-83.
9. Hunt PR. A modified class II cavity preparation for glass ionomer restorative materials Quintessence. 1984;10:1011.
10. Kent BE, Lewis BG, Wilson AD. The properties of a glass ionomer cement. BDJ. 1973;135:322-6.
11. Kerby RE, Knobloch L, Thakur A. Strength properties of visible light cured resin modified glass ionomer cements. Oper Dent. 1997;22:79.
12. Maki L, Ge L, Kimura M. Clinical evaluation of a light cured glass ionomer cements for filling. JDR. 1994;73:135.
13. McCabe JF. Resin-modified glass-ionomers, Biomaterials. 1998;19:521-7.
14. McCabe JF. Resin modified glass ionomer. Biomaterials: 1998;19:521.
15. Mclean JW, Gasser O. Glass cermet cements. Quint Int. 1985;16:333.
16. McLean JW. Evolution of glass ionomer cements: a personal view. J Esthet Dent. 1994;6:195.
17. Mclean JW. The clinical use of Glass Ionomer Cements. DCNA. July 1992.
18. Meyer JM, et al. Compomers: between glass-ionomer cements and composites, Biomaterials. 1998;19:529-9.
19. Mitra SB, et al. Setting reaction of Vitrebond light cure glass ionomer liner/base. Trans Acad Dent Mater. 1992;5:1-22.

20. Mount GJ. Clinical placement of modern glass ionomer cements. Quint Int. 1993;24(2):99.

21. Mount GJ. Glass ionomer cements. Past present and future. Oper Dent. 1994;19:82.

22. Mount GJ. Restoration with glass-ionomer cement: requirements for clinical success. Oper Dent. 1981;6:59-65.

23. Mount GJ. Restoration with glass ionomer cements. Requirement for clinical success. Oper Dent. 1985;6:59.

24. Mount GJ. Some physical and biological properties of glass ionomer cement. Int Dent J. 1995;45:135.

25. Myor IA. Glass ionomer cement restorations and secondary caries–a preliminary report. Quint Int. 1996;27:171.

26. Nicholson JW, Croll TP. Glass ionomer cements in restorative dentistry. Quint Int. 1997;28:705.

27. Silvey RG, Myers GE. Clinical study of dental cements: VII. a study of bridge retainers luted with three different dental cements. J Dent Res. 1978;57:703-7.

28. Simmons JJ. The miracle mixture: glass ionomel and alloy powder. Tex Dent J. 1983;100:10-2.

29. Smith DC. Development of glass-ionomer cement systems. Biomaterials. 1998;19:467-78.

Dental Ceramics

Chapter Outline

INTRODUCTION

Ceramics are popular due to the demand for esthetics and durability of the restorations. Dental ceramics mainly consist of glasses, porcelains or highly crystalline structures. The physical and mechanical properties of ceramics are much closer to enamel than those of acrylic resins and metals. Ceramics also have coefficient of thermal expansion very close to that of tooth, excellant wear resistance and durability, all these qualities make ceramics as choice of restorations in areas demanding esthetics and durability. Though ceramics are strong, resilient and temperature resistant, but these are also brittle and thus may fracture when flexed, or when quickly heated and cooled.

Commonly used ceramic materials are feldspathic porcelain, castable ceramic (Dicor) and new machinable glass ceramic (Dicor MGC) used with CEREC systems. While seating on the prepared tooth, the cementing surface of the ceramic restoration is etched with aids to remove all the glossy matrix.

Hydrofluoric acid is commonly used acid for feldspathic porcelain whereas ammonium bifluoride is used to etch Dicor and Dicor MGC.

The treatment with acid also causes increase in surface area for micromechanical bonding of cement between ceramics and tooth surface.

DEFINITIONS

Ceramic

An inorganic compound with nonmetallic properties typically composed of metallic or semimetallic and nonmetallic elements.

Dental Ceramic

An inorganic compound with nonmetallic properties typically composed of oxygen and one or more metallic (or semimetallic) elements, e.g. aluminum, calcium, magnesium and zirconium, etc. that is formulated to produce the ceramic based prosthesis.

Feldspathic Porcelain

A ceramic consists of a glass matrix phase and one or more crystalline phases.

Glass Ceramic

A ceramic composed of a glass matrix phase and at least one crystal phase which is formed by controlled crystallization of the glass.

Glaze Ceramic

A special ceramic powder when mixed with a liquid applied to a ceramic surface and heated to an appropriate temperature for a sufficient time, forms a smooth glossy layer on ceramic surface.

Metal Ceramic Restoration

Restoration made with a metal substrate to which porcelain is bonded for esthetic enhancement with an intermediate metal oxide layer.

Aluminous Porcelain

A ceramic consisting of a glass matrix phase and at least 35 vol% alumina.

Body Porcelain

A veneering ceramic used for ceramic or metal-ceramic restoration.

Castable Ceramic

A glass or other ceramic especially used for casting into a refractory mold to produce a core coping or framework for a ceramic restoration.

CAD-CAM Ceramic

This type of ceramic is used for making whole or part of an all-ceramic restoration by use of a computer-aided design (CAD) and computer-aided manufacturing (CAM) process.

History of dental ceramics		
1728	Pierre Fauchard	Suggested the use of porcelain in dentistry
1789	Duchateau and DeChemant	Introduced porcelain tooth material for bridge work and denture
1808	Fonzi	Terrometallic porcelain (held in place by platinum foil)
1837	Ash	Improved version of porcelain tooth material
1900-05	–	Introduction of first electric porcelain furnace
1903	Dr Charles land	Introduction of first ceramic crown using platinum foil matrix and high fusing porcelain
1962	Weinstein and Weinstein	Introduction of porcelain fused to metal restorations
1963	Vita	Commercial production of porcelain
1965	Mclean and Hughes	Improved the fracture resistance by introducing aluminous porcelain
1984	Adair and Grossman	Introduction of castable glass ceramic (Dicor)

Classification of dental ceramics
→ According to use:
◆ Metal ceramics
◆ Ceramic denture teeth

- Anterior bridge porcelain
- Jacket crown, veneer, inlay porcelain.
- According to fusion temperature:
  - High fusing ceramics—1300°C (2372°F)
  - Medium fusing ceramics—1101°C to 1300°C (2013°F-2372°F)
  - Low fusing ceramics—850°C to 1100°C (1562°F-2012°F)
  - Ultra low fusing ceramics—< 850°C (1562°F).
- According to composition:
  - Pure alumina
  - Pure zirconia
  - Silica glass
  - Leucite based glass ceramic
  - Lithia based glass ceramic.
- According to processing method:
  - Sintering
  - Partial sintering and glass infiltration
  - CAD-CAM
  - Copy milling.

COMPOSITION

Dental porcelains are basically glassy materials. Molten glass solidifies with liquid structure rather than crystalline structure during cooling. The structure formed is known as vitreous and process is known as vitrification. The principal anion which is responsible for forming bonds with multivalent cations such as silicon and boron is O^{2-} ion. These ions are considered as glass formers. Other oxides such as potassium, sodium, calcium or aluminum oxides are added in glass to obtain additional desirable properties (**Fig. 25.1**).

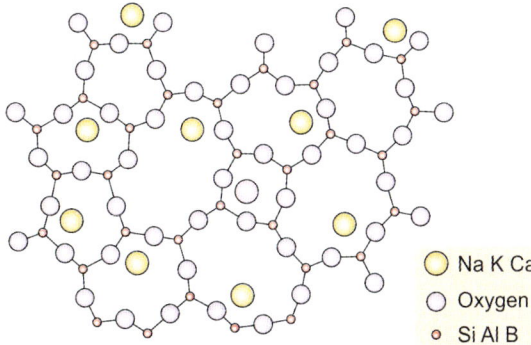

Figure 25.1: Matrix of porcelain

- ○ Na K Ca
- ○ Oxygen
- ○ Si Al B

High Fusing Porcelains

The basic ingredients of these types of porcelains are:
- Feldspar
- Kaolin (clay)
- Quartz.

Feldspar

- Primary constituent
- Present in concentration of 75 to 80 percent
- Sodium or potassium form is mainly used but in dental, potassium feldspar is preferred
- Potassium feldspar is selected because of increased resistance to pyroplastic flow and increased viscosity
- Undergo incongruent melting at 1150°C to 1530°C to form a liquid and crystalline material, i.e potassium alumino silicate known as leucite.

Kaolin

- Present in concentration of 4 to 5 percent
- Main function of Kaolin is to act as binder
- Lowers the translucency of porcelain.

Quartz

- Present in concentration of 13-14 percent
- Main function is to act as strengthener
- Also increases the translucency of porcelain.

Medium and Low Fusing Ceramics

The medium and low fusing ceramics are formed by process known as fritting and product obtained is termed as frit.

The basic ingredients for medium and low fusing ceramics are same as those of high fusing but in addition, certain glass modifiers are also added.

Glass Modifiers

- Most commonly used are potassium, sodium and calcium oxides
- Act as fluxes and reduces the softening temperature of glass
- Also lowers the viscosity of glass.

Intermediate Oxides

- Most commonly used is aluminum oxide (Al_2O_3)
- Lowers the softening temperature along with viscosity of glass.

Boric Oxide (B_2O_3)

- Acts as glass former and glass modifier
- Lowers the melting point and viscosity of glass
- Matrix of B_2O_3 is formed by 3-dimensional arrangement of BO_3 triangles.

Opacifying Agents

Most commonly used agents are:
- Zirconium oxide
- Titanium oxide
- Cerium oxide.

Coloring Agents

Various coloring agents used to obtain proper hue and chroma. Their main objective is to obtain various shades needed to simulate natural teeth.

Metallic pigments	Color
➡ Ferric oxide	Gray
➡ Titanium oxide	Yellowish brown
➡ Manganese oxide	Lavender
➡ Cobalt oxide	Blue
➡ Nickel oxide	Brown
➡ Chromium-alumina	Pink
➡ Copper oxide	Green

Stains or Color Modifiers

- Used to create markings like enamel check lines, decalcification spots, etc.
- Used for creating gingival effects and in highlighting body color of porcelain.

METHODS OF STRENGTHENING PORCELAIN

Chemical Strengthening (Fig. 25.2)

This is one of the effective methods of introducing residual compressive stresses into the surface of a ceramic. Chemical strengthening is usually carried out by replacing small sized cations in the surface layer with large sized cations while matrix remains the same. This is also known as low temperature ionic crowding. Sodium ions present in the matrix are replaced by large size potassium ions by placing porcelain crown in bath of potassium nitrate. The potassium ion is 35 percent larger in size than sodium ion, so, creates residual compressive stresses. This is available under commercial name GC Tuf-coat (GC).

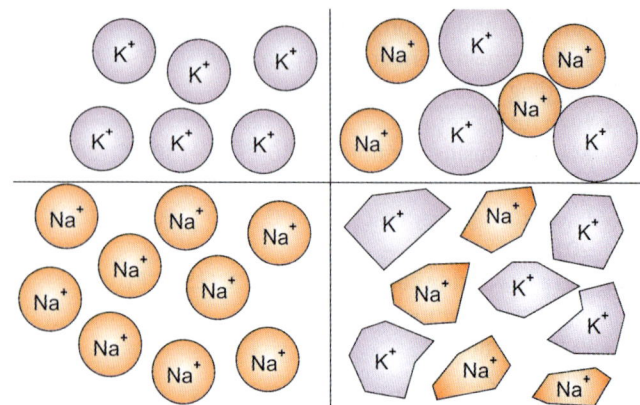

Figure 25.2: Chemical strengthening of porcelain where sodium ions are replaced by larger sized potassium ions

Dispersion Strengthening

Dispersion strengthening is process in which strengthening is done with dispersed phase of different material with a capability of blocking a crack from propagating the material.

Dispersion strengthening of ceramic can be obtained by increasing the crystal content of alumina, leucite and zirconia.

For example, if alumina is added to glass, the glass is toughened and strengthened as crack cannot pass through tough crystalline particle such as alumina easily, while it can pass through glass easily.

Thermal Tempering

It is most common method for strengthening glass. This process creates residual compressive stresses in the glass by heating and when it is in molten state, it is immediately quenched. This quenching (rapid cooling) produces a rigid glass surrounding a soft molten metal.

For dental use, ceramics are quenched (rapid cooled) in silicone oils or other special liquids.

Reduce the Number of Firing Cycles

The main function of firing cycle is to sinter the powder particles together and produce a relatively smooth surface. Several chemical reactions occur at the time of firing cycles. If number of firing cycles is increased, the leucite content of porcelain also increases which further increases the coefficient of thermal expansion of porcelain. The expansion mismatch between porcelain and metal creates stresses on cooling which can cause crack formation in the porcelain. Thus reduction in number of firing cycles can help in reducing crack formation.

Creating Residual Compressive Stresses

This is also one of the important methods for developing residual compressive stresses in the ceramic. In metal ceramic crowns, metal should have high coefficient of thermal expansion than porcelain so that on cooling, metal contracts slightly more than that of porcelain, creates stresses and provides strength for porcelain.

This rule also applies to all ceramic systems in which inner layer (core) has high coefficient of thermal expansion than outer layers, creating stresses and strengthening the porcelain.

Transformation Toughening

In this process, small and tough particles are uniformly dispersed in the matrix so that cracks cannot pass through these crystals.

Ceramics can be toughened by variety of crystalline particles such as:
- Alumina
- Leucite
- Lithium di-silicate.

In case of zirconia based ceramics, zirconia crystals undergo change from tetragonal crystal to monoclinic phase upon stressing and cause transformation toughening.

Advantages of ceramics
⇢ Highly esthetic
⇢ No display of metal
⇢ Strong once bonded to tooth
⇢ Does not stain
⇢ Low thermal conductivity
⇢ Suitable for large tooth preparations
⇢ Long lasting
⇢ Low coefficient of thermal expansion
⇢ Biocompatible.

Disadvantages of ceramics
⇢ More costly than amalgam or composite
⇢ Accurate occlusion can be difficult to achieve
⇢ Takes two appointments
⇢ Intraoral finishing and polishing is a time-consuming procedure
⇢ Fragile and brittle
⇢ Abrasive to the opposing enamel
⇢ Very technique sensitive

⇢ Finishing of the margins is difficult in the less accessible interproximal areas
⇢ Need special and expensive laboratory equipment.

METAL CERAMIC RESTORATIONS (FIG. 25.3)

All ceramic restorations though look very natural but are very brittle and subject to fracture. All metal restorations are very strong but they cannot be used in areas where esthetics is the main concern. In metal ceramic restoration, advantages of esthetics of porcelain and strength of metal are combined.

For proper bonding between metal and porcelain, alloys and porcelain used should have following properties:
- Porcelain and alloys should be able to form a strong bond since the most common cause for the failure of metal ceramic restoration is debonding of porcelain from the metal.
- Both porcelain and alloy should have almost similar coefficient of thermal expansion so that porcelain does not crack or separate from alloy on cooling (**Fig. 25.4**).
- Porcelain should fuse at a much lower temperature than the melting temperature of the metal. The alloy should not deform at porcelain fusing temperature.
- Alloy should have a high modulus of elasticity so that it can share greater proportion of stress than the adjacent porcelain.

Porcelain-metal Bond (see Fig. 25.3)

There are generally two types of bonding present between metal and ceramic:
1. Micromechanical bonding
2. Chemical bonding.

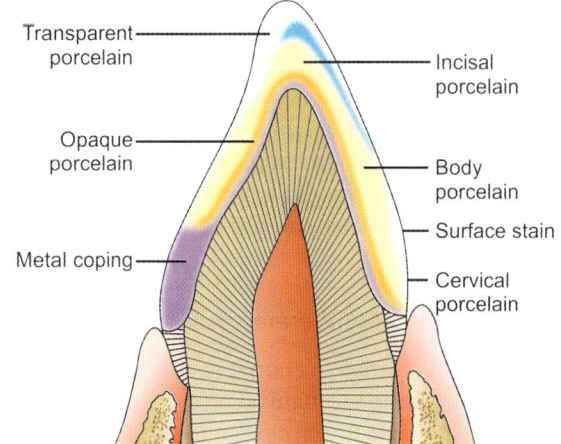

Figure 25.3: Diagrammatic representation of metal ceramic restoration

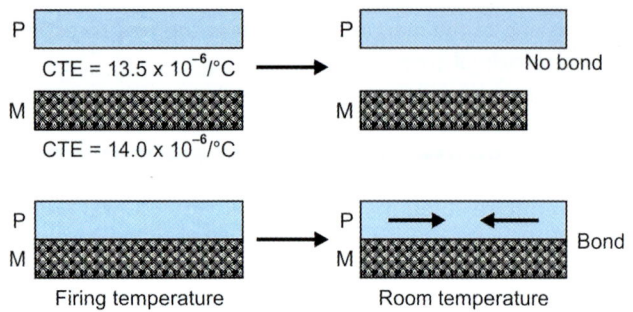

Figure 25.4: For optimal bonding of metal and ceramic, they should have equal coefficient of thermal expansion

Micromechanical Bonding

The fused ceramic flows over the metal covering and adapts to minute irregularities present on metal surface and form micromechanical bonds. The irregularities present on metal surface should be regular without any sharp line angles so as to avoid stress concentration which can result in fracture of porcelain. This ability of the fused porcelain to intimately adapt to the metal surface is called "wetting". Irregularities on the coping surface can be produced by sand blasting.

Chemical Bonding

Chemical bonding occurs between the ceramic and the surface oxide layer present on the base metals such as iron, indium and tin of gold alloys. Fused porcelain diffuses into the metallic oxide layer and vice versa.

In metal ceramic bonding:

- The metal should not interact with ceramic as it will visibly discolor it and affect the esthetics
- Metal-porcelain bond must be durable and stable at interface to withstand masticatory stresses.

In a metal ceramic restoration, on the facial side the thickness of the metal is about 0.3 to 0.4 mm thick which is covered with opaque porcelain of about 0.3 to 0.4 mm thickness. The body porcelain is about 1 mm thick on the labial side and the transparent porcelain is about 0.3 to 0.5 mm thick at incisal third. At the middle-third of the crown it is about 0.2 to 0.3 mm thick and at the cervical third it is about 0.1 mm thick.

Composition of Metal Ceramic Alloys and Ceramics

The alloys used for metal ceramic restorations should not only have acceptable mechanical properties but also coefficient of thermal expansion similar to the porcelain. Most of the nickel-chromium alloys for metal ceramic restorations contain 62 to 76 percent nickel and 13 to 28 percent

chromium along with cobalt, beryllium, molybdenum and ruthum.

The cobalt chromium alloy contains by weight 52 to 68 percent cobalt, 24 to 33 percent chromium and 2 to 7 percent molybdenum.

Failures of Metal Ceramic Restorations

- Most of the metal ceramic restorations fail because of bond fracture at the metal oxide interface (**Fig. 25.5**). Other reasons for failure of metal ceramic restorations are:
  - Fusion of porcelain grains inside the coping
  - Thin margins of metal buckle due to contraction of porcelain
  - Elastic deformation of nonrigid metal structure
  - Casting contamination by low fusing alloy components from the metallic die
  - Forceful fitting may result in elastic deformation of the metal and breakdown in porcelain bond.

CONDENSATION OF PORCELAIN

Complete the condensation of wet porcelain powder and remove excess water or liquid with clean tissue or blotting paper. This helps in maximum incorporation of porcelain powder and proper condensation of porcelain powder particles.

Condensation of porcelain helps in
➡ Lowering the firing shrinkage
➡ Reducing the porosity in fired porcelain

Wet porcelain powder condensation can be done by following methods:

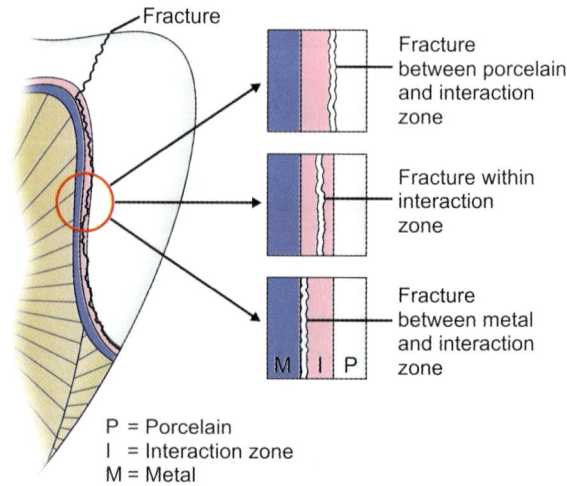

P = Porcelain
I = Interaction zone
M = Metal

Figure 25.5: Interfacial zone fracture

- *Vibration method*: Mild vibrations help in packing the wet powder densely. This is most useful method in removing excess water from the mix.
- *Spatulation method*: In this method, a small spatula is used to smoothen the wet powder and the wet particles condense together by which the excess water comes to the surface from where it can be removed.
- *Brush technique*: In this method, dry porcelain powder is added to the surface with the help of a brush which absorbs the extra water, making the condensation of wet particles.

FIRING OF PORCELAIN

Porcelain powder in shape of the restoration is placed in 'fire clay tray' and fired in a furnace. In the initial stage, preheating is done. In preheating, the porcelain is kept for 10 minutes in the outer low temperature chamber of the furnace and the door of the furnace is kept open so that water vapor and gases produced due to organic combustion can escape. Presence of water vapor and/or gases in furnace at a high temperature, can damage the casting. At approximately 870°C, (650°C for low fusing porcelain) combustion of organic matter is completed. The tray is pushed in the center of the furnace and firing cycle is initiated after closing the door of the furnace. Degree of condensation of porcelain and density of the final restoration is also affected by the size of the powder particles of the porcelain. Since porcelain is a poor thermal conductor, therefore, too rapid heating may over fuse the outer layers but inner layers remain partially fused.

Stages of Firing

Porcelain undergoes different stages during firing known as bisque stages.

Low Bisque Stage

In low bisque stage, porcelain becomes rigid and porous and readily absorbs water. Particles lack strength, though porcelain exhibits very little shrinkage during this stage.

Medium Bisque Stage

Though there is complete cohesion of powder particles, but the surface is still porous and lack translucency and high glaze. There is definite shrinkage in this stage.

High Bisque Stage

Here the porcelain mass exhibits smooth surface and the shrinkage is complete. Slight porosity may be seen in this stage. Now the porcelain is very strong.

During firing in the first phase, the water is lost, i.e. drying takes place. After drying stage, the temperature and time is controlled till final fusing, glazing and shading stages. As the temperature is raised, the porcelain particles fuse together by sintering. By densification, volume is reduced.

COOLING

After firing is done, porcelain is cooled. It is always preferable to do cooling slowly since rapid cooling may result in crazing or cracking of the surface. Slow cooling is done by placing the restoration under a glass cover to protect it from cold wind and dirt contamination.

GRINDING FOR FINAL ADJUSTMENTS

Grinding of surface of the polished porcelain required for intraoral minor adjustments results in decrease in the strength, increase in the discoloration and plaque accumulation. If grinding is unavoidable, it is done using very fine diamond round bur in an air rotor along with water coolant. Once the grinding is done, the ground rough surface should be polished using very fine finishing disks, porcelain laminate, polishing laminate, or polishing kit.

GLAZING

Glazes, shades and stains are added to provide natural appearance.

Glaze layer is kept atleast 50 micron thick. Glazing helps in

- Reduction of surface flaws.
- Sealing of surface porosities.
- Increase in porcelain strength as it prevents crack propagation.

Types of Glazing

- *Self-glazing*: In this technique, the completed restoration is heated to the glazing temperature. This results in formation of a glossy film by a viscous flow on the porcelain surface.
- *Add-on glazing*: In add-on glazing, the uncolored glasses with fusion temperature lesser than porcelain restoration are used which form an external glossy layer.

Self-glazing is preferred over add on glaze because add on glaze produces unnatural glossy appearance. Moreover it is difficult to apply and has less durability.

ALL CERAMIC SYSTEM

To overcome the disadvantages of porcelain fused to metal, all ceramic materials have been introduced with new technique and technology. Due to new advancement in technology, all ceramic system have high strength and precision fit close to that of ceramometal in addition to esthetics.

Classification of all ceramic systems

- → Traditional powder slurry ceramic
  - ◆ Alumina reinforced ceramic (Hi-ceram)
  - ◆ Leucite reinforced ceramic (Optec-HSP).
- → Infiltrated ceramic
  - ◆ In ceram
  - ◆ In ceram spinel.
- → Castable ceramic
  - ◆ Dicor.
- → Pressable ceramic
  - ◆ IPS empress 1 and 2.
- → Machinable ceramic
  - ◆ Cerec vitablocks mark I and II
  - ◆ Dicor MGC
  - ◆ Celay.

Traditional Powder Slurry Ceramic

These are supplied in powders which are mixed with water to form 'slurry'. This slurry formed can be built up in different layers on a die to form the restoration. This type of ceramic can be classified in two types:

Alumina Reinforced Ceramic

This type of ceramic is based on dispersion strengthening—one of the method used for strengthening of ceramic. Alumina crystals are dispersed uniformly in glass matrix to increase strength, toughness and elasticity of the material. In case of aluminous ceramic, the concentration of alumina crystals and glass powder are mixed and prefritted at 1200°C. Then this crystal glass mixture is grounded and incorporated into glass matrix, for example, Hi-ceram.

Leucite Reinforced Ceramic

In this type, leucite crystals (potassium alumino silicate) are dispersed in glassy matrix. Leucite is added in feldspathic porcelain to match the thermal contraction of ceramic to the metal but it also acts as reinforcing filler because of very high tensile strength. The leucite and glassy components are fused together and baked at 1020°C to form the ceramic. These ceramics have high strength and good translucency. In addition, surface stains or pigments can also be added to enhance esthetics, for example, Optec-HSP.

Infiltrated Ceramic (Fig. 25.6)

To overcome the disadvantages of aluminous porcelain, a new system is introduced known as infilterable ceramic in which alumina/spinel is used as the core material.

In Ceram

Composition: This type of ceramic is available in two components:
1. Powder: Aluminum oxide
2. Low viscosity glass.

In this, aluminum oxide is fabricated on a porous substrate in which low viscosity glass is heated at high temperature, to be infiltrated in this matrix.

Procedure

- Alumina powder is mixed with water to form slurry known as 'Slip' which is painted on die. This procedure leaves a layer of solid alumina on the surface
- Sintering is done at 1120°C for 10 hours to form porous core
- Glass is selected and applied on the porous core and firing is done at 1100°C for 3 to 5 hours
- The molten glass infiltrates by capillary action into core
- This results in high strength composite structure, i.e. In ceram.

In Ceram Spinel

In this spinel (aluminum and magnesium oxide) is used as the core material. It has better translucency than In ceram (High opacity due to higher concentration of alumina crystals).

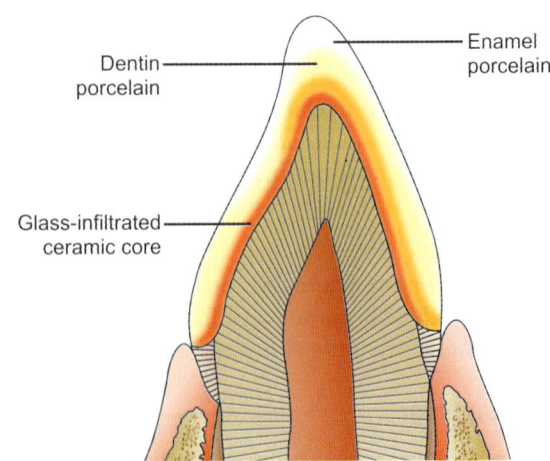

Dentin porcelain

Enamel porcelain

Glass-infiltrated ceramic core

Figure 25.6: In-ceram crown

This type of ceramic can be used for crowns—both anterior and posterior crowns.

Castable Ceramic (Fig. 25.7)

Castable ceramic was first introduced in 1984. In this, a glass ceramic is a material which is modified into the desired shape and size as a glass and heat treatment is given to induce crystallization. The process of crystallization is known as ceramming.

Composition

After ceramming, the material contains:
- 55 percent—Tetrasilicic fluoride crystals
- 45 percent—Glass ceramic.

In 1984, castable ceramic was marketed under the trade name DICOR.

Advantages of dicor
⇒ Satisfactory marginal fit
⇒ High strength
⇒ Higher surface hardness
⇒ Wear resistance similar to enamel
⇒ Dicor inlays are stronger than procelain inlays made on refractory dies.

Pressable Ceramic

This type of ceramic is available as core ingot which is heated at high temperature and pressed into a mold. The pressing process is done for duration of 45 mintues at high temperature to get ceramic substructure which further can be shaded with stains or by glazing.

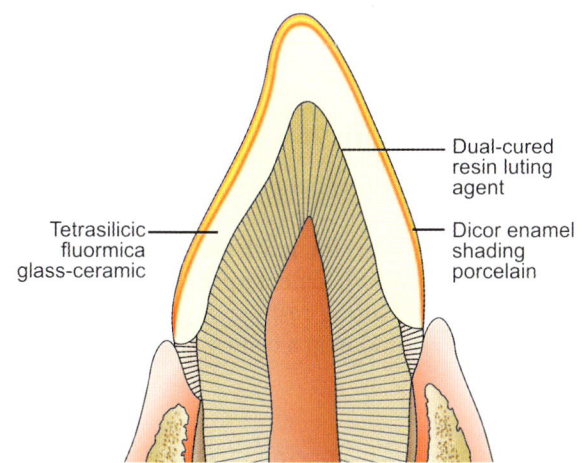

Figure 25.7: Dicor glass-ceramic crown

(labels on figure:)
Tetrasilicic fluormica glass-ceramic
Dual-cured resin luting agent
Dicor enamel shading porcelain

Two Types of Pressable Ceramics are Available

1. *IPS Empress 1:* Contains 35 vol. percent of leucite crystals
2. *IPS Empress 2:* Contains 70 vol. percent of lithia disilicate crystals.

Advantages of pressable ceramics
⇒ Lack of metal
⇒ High flexural strength
⇒ Excellent fit
⇒ Excellent esthetics.

Disadvantage
Prone to fracture in posterior areas.

Machinable Ceramic

These ceramics are supplied in the form of ceramic blocks under various shades. Later on, these blocks are fabricated into inlays, onlays and crown with the help of CAD-CAM or copymilling.

Computer Generated Ceramic Restorations

Recent advances in technology have resulted into many computerized devices which can fabricate ceramic inlays and onlays, crown and bridge copings out of very high-quality ceramic blocks. Indirect computer generated ceramic restorations can be made chair side in CEREC® SYSTEM–CAD (Computer aided design), CAM (Computer aided manufacturing). The CEREC® system was the first commercially available CAD/CAM system developed for the rapid chairside design and fabrication of ceramic restorations. Machined ceramics are unique to dentistry in that they do not require the addition of glasses to achieve proper morphology. Instead, the morphology can be milled or carved out of the same, single block of pure, uniform and inclusion-free ceramic. Using a special camera, an accurate picture of the tooth is taken which is transferred and displayed on a color computer screen, where CAD technology is used to design the restoration. Then CAM takes over and automatically creates the restoration in a matter of minutes.

Advantages
⇒ Total time required for an inlay or onlay from tooth preparation to cementation is about one hour
⇒ A single appointment restoration
⇒ Conventional impression, multiple sittings and temporary restorations are not required
⇒ Quality of the ceramic restorative material is very good. Blocks of very good quality machinable ceramics are used for milling. They come in various natural tooth shades

➡ No laboratory expenses in inlays and onlays
➡ A natural looking filling with excellent esthetics
➡ Results in a restoration that is antiabrasive, bio- compatible and resistant to plaque.

Disadvantages

➡ High cost of the equipment
➡ Special training is required
➡ More conservative tooth preparation is required
➡ Computer prepares rough occlusal anatomy without consideration of opposing occlusal anatomy
➡ Requires final occlusal adjustments.

Examples

- *Vitablocks mark I and II:* These have similar properties to feldspathic porcelain and are developed by Cerec- CAD System. VitaBlocs Mark II has high strength than VITABLOCS Mark I. These materials can be used for inlays, onlays and crowns.
- *Dicor MGC:* The CAD-CAM Ceramic Dicor MGC has high concentration of tetrasilicicfluormica crystals (i.e. 70%) than castable dicor ceramic (i.e. 55%). It has properties similar to that of dicor ceramic except for less translucency.
- *Procera allceram:* This type of crown contains sintered and highly packed aluminum oxide (99.9%) as core material which is combined as all ceram veneering porcelain. This is one of the hardest ceramics used in dentistry for anterior and posterior crowns, inlays and onlays.

CERAMIC INLAYS AND ONLAYS

Ceramic inlay is the most conservative ceramic restoration and enables most of the remaining enamel to be preserved. A ceramic inlay fits within the contours of the tooth and is cemented to the remaining tooth structure. An onlay fits within the contours of the tooth and covers part or all of the occlusal surface needed to be restored.

For patients demanding esthetic restorations, ceramic inlays and onlays provide a durable alternative to posterior composite resins. Bonding to porcelain is accomplished by etching the tooth with hydrofluoric acid and the use of a silane coupling agent.

Indications

- When esthetics is main concern
- Patient having good oral hygiene status
- Suitable for large preparations
- When accessibility and isolation of tooth are easy to achieve

- When there are no excessive undercuts in the tooth preparation
- When preparation margins are on enamel and sound tooth structure making it feasible for bonding.

Contraindications

- In patients with poor oral hygiene
- Patient with multiple active caries
- Because of their brittle nature, they are contraindicated in patients with excessive occlusal loading, such as bruxers
- When esthetic is not main requirement
- In cases with minimal tooth loss
- When moisture control is difficult to achieve
- In cases with excessive attrition of teeth
- Inadequate enamel for bonding
- When marked undercuts are present in the tooth preparation.

Advantages

➡ Excellent esthetic
➡ Low thermal conductivity
➡ Long lasting
➡ Chemically inert
➡ Low coefficient of thermal expansion
➡ Biocompatible nature.

Disadvantages

➡ More expensive than amalgam or composite
➡ Requires special and expensive laboratory equipment
➡ Takes two appointments
➡ Intraoral finishing and polishing is a time consuming procedure
➡ Fragile and brittle, so, intraoral occlusal adjustment is not possible before it is bonded to place
➡ Abrasive to the opposing enamel
➡ Highly technique sensitive.

Tooth Preparation (Fig. 25.8)

Isolate the tooth using rubber dam for visibility and moisture control.

Before applying the dam, mark and assess the occlusal contact relationship with articulating film. To avoid chipping or wear of the luting resin, avoid placement of the margins of the restoration at a centric contact.

Outline Form

Outline form is usually governed by the existing restoration and caries. It is grossly similar to that for conventional metal inlays and onlays except that bevels and flares are

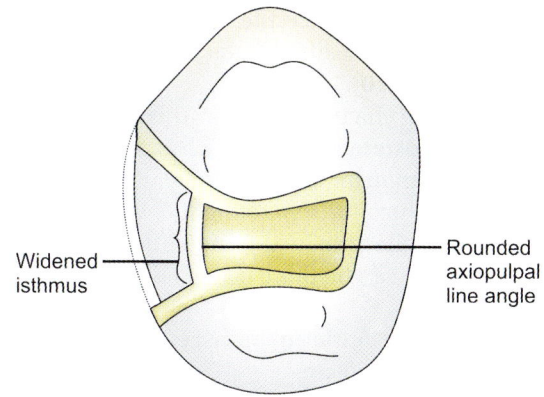

Figure 25.8: Maxillary premolar with ceramic inlay preparation showing rounded angle and widened isthmus

not given here. In Initial tooth preparation the carbide burs are used. Bur should be held tapering to make straight facial and lingual walls that diverge occlusally to allow the insertion and removal of restoration. During final tooth preparations, coarse diamond preparation points are used. Always remove the undermined or weakened enamel. Do the central groove reduction (approximately 1.5-2 mm) following the anatomy of the unprepared tooth. This provides additional bulk for the ceramic so as to have strength. The outline form should avoid occlusal contacts.

There should be at least 1.5 mm of clearance in all excursions to prevent ceramic fracture. Preparation walls should exhibit 6 to 8 degree of occlusal divergence per wall. Increased degree of taper in ceramics is given because ceramic restoration are adhesively bonded to tooth structure, restoration should passively seat in the tooth preparation.

Extend the proximal box to have a minimum of 0.6 mm of clearance for impression making. Isthmus width should be minimum of 1.5 mm to prevent fracture. Margins of the preparation should be kept supragingival. The width of the gingival floor of the box should be approximately 1.0 mm.

All internal angles should be rounded and preparation walls should be smooth and even. All cavosurface margins should be made butt angled. Bevels are contraindicated because bulk is needed to prevent fracture. A distinct heavy chamfer is recommended for ceramic onlay margins.

Remove any caries not included in the outline form using an excavator or a round bur in the low-speed handpiece.

Provide pulp protection by placing resin modified glass ionomer cement base in excavated tissue in the gingival wall.

Refine the margins with finishing burs and hand instruments, do trimming of any excess glass ionomer base because smooth, distinct margins are needed to a precisely fitting ceramic restoration.

PORCELAIN LAMINATE VENEERS

Porcelain veneer was introduced about 25 years back. The esthetic results of ceramic veneers are excellent in comparison to resin veneers.

Indications

Porcelain laminate veneers can be used in following conditions:
- Extrinsic permanent staining, not masked by bleaching techniques.
- Intrinsic staining caused by:
  – Physiological aging
  – Erosion and abrasion
  – Trauma
  – Amelogenesis imperfecta
  – Fluorosis
  – Enamel hypoplasia
  – Tetracycline staining.
- Nonvital tooth
- To correct malformed tooth like peg shaped lateral incisors
- To repair fractured incisal edges
- For treatment of diastema.

Contraindications

- Patient with high caries risk
- Teeth with poor periodontal condition
- Tooth with gingival recession
- In cases where the preparation has to be extended up to cervical tooth structure
- In malaligned teeth (rotated and overlapped teeth)
- In deep bite cases (because of unfavorable occlusal forces)
- In severely discolored teeth (crown is better option in these teeth)
- In tooth with interproximal caries
- Poorly motivated patient.

Advantages
→ Conservative tooth preparation (only about 0.5 mm of facial reduction is needed)
→ Since tooth preparation is confined to the enamel layer. Local anesthesia is not usually required
→ Excellent esthetics and color match
→ Chemically inert, so resistance to fluid absorption

- Biocompatible in nature
- Good abrasion resistance.

Disadvantages

- Fragile and brittle in nature
- Difficult to repair or modify after cementation
- Expensive than amalgam or composite
- Need special and expensive laboratory equipment
- Intraoral finishing and polishing is a time consuming procedure
- Highly technique sensitive
- Needs precise tooth preparation.

Tooth Preparation

- For achieving optimal esthetics, maximum reduction should be carried out with minimum penetration into the dentin because gingival third and proximal line angles are often overcontoured with these restorations.
- Make depth cuts with a round bur to have uniform cutting (**Figs 25.9A and B**).
- Generally a minimum of 0.5 mm depth is required, though amount of reduction depends upon the extent of discoloration.
- The tooth preparation should follow the anatomic contours of the tooth.
- The margin should follow the gingival crest. This results in veneering of whole discolored enamel without unnecessary involvement of the gingival sulcus.

- Wherever possible, place the margins of the preparation labial to the proximal contact area to preserve it in enamel (**Fig. 25.10**).
- Place the "long chamfer" margin. This design results in an obtuse cavosurface angle, which exposes the enamel rods at the margin for better etching.
- Provide clearance for separating the working cast and for accessing the proximal margins for finishing and polishing. This can be done using a diamond finishing strip.
- If possible, avoid cutting of incisal edge as this provides support to the porcelain.
- If it is required to increase the incisal edge length, extend the preparation to the lingual without any undercuts because an undercut will prevent placement of the veneer.
- Finally confirm that all prepared surfaces are rounded so as to prevent areas of stress concentration in the porcelain (**Fig. 25.11**).

FULL CERAMIC CROWNS

Indications

- In areas with a high esthetic requirement where a more conservative restoration would be inadequate.
- In teeth with proximal and/or facial caries that cannot be restored with composite resin.
- In teeth with sufficient coronal structure to support the restoration especially in the incisal area.

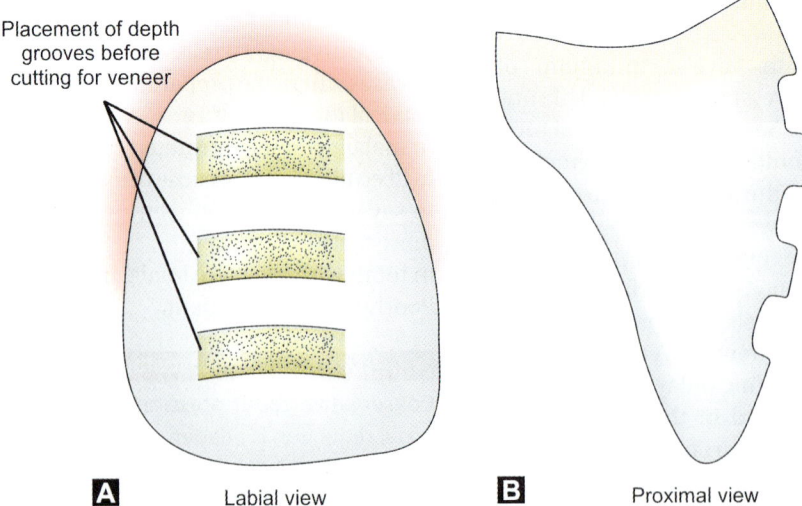

Placement of depth grooves before cutting for veneer

A   Labial view   **B**   Proximal view

Figures 25.9A and B: Depth grooves prepared in central incisor prior to cutting for veneer: (A) Labial view; (B) Proximal view

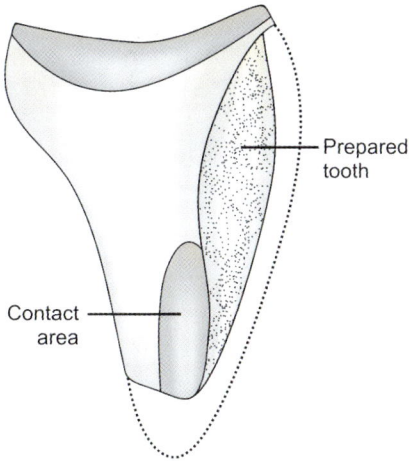

Figure 25.10: Proximally, the veneer should terminate 0.2 mm labial to contact area so as to preserve maximum enamel

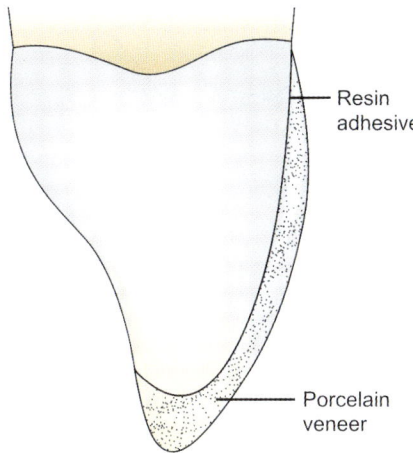

Figure 25.11: Ceramic veneer bonded to tooth surface

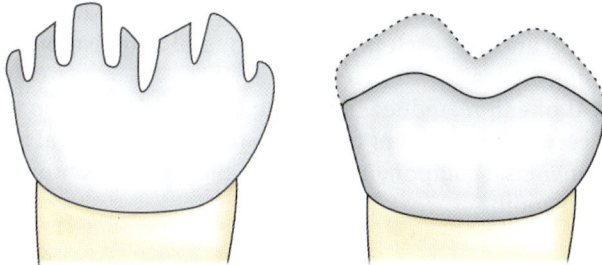

Figure 25.12: Occlusal reduction

➡ Lack of reinforcement by a metal substructure permits slightly more conservative reduction of the facial surface than with the metal-ceramic crown.

<table>
<tr><td>Disadvantages</td></tr>
</table>

➡ Reduced strength of the restoration because of the absence of a reinforcing metal substructure
➡ Requires more tooth cutting because of the need for a shoulder type margin circumferentially
➡ Difficult to achieve well fitting margins in some cases
➡ Cannot be modified once prepared.
➡ Proper preparation design is essential to ensure mechanical success
➡ Needs butt joint cavosurface angle to minimize the risk of fracture
➡ The preparation should provide support for the porcelain along its entire incisal edge. Therefore, it cannot be given in severely damaged tooth
➡ These restorations are not effective as retainers for a fixed partial denture.

Tooth Preparation

Occlusal Reduction (Fig. 25.12)

• Ideally there should be 1.5 to 2 mm of clearance incisally/occlusally for porcelain in all excursive movements of the mandible. This results in an esthetically pleasing restoration with adequate strength.
• Place depth grooves in the occlusal surface of approximately 1.3 mm deep (to allow for additional loss of tooth structure during finishing).
• The grooves should be directed perpendicular to the long axis of the opposing tooth to provide adequate support for the porcelain crown.

Facial Reduction

• Place depth grooves and reduce the facial surface. The depth of these grooves should be approximately 0.8 mm to allow finishing.

Contraindications

• When a more conservative restoration can be used.
• In posterior teeth with increased occlusal load and reduced esthetic requirement where metal ceramics crowns are preferred.
• If occlusal loading is unfavorable.
• If sufficient enamel is not present to provide adequate support.

<table>
<tr><td>Advantages</td></tr>
</table>

➡ Excellent esthetics
➡ Translucency similar to that of natural tooth structure
➡ Biocompatibility

- One depth groove is placed in the middle of the facial wall and one each in the mesiobuccal and distobuccal line angles.
- At one time, reduce half of the facial surface. Keep the cervical component parallel to path of withdrawal and an incisal component parallel to the original contour of the tooth.

Lingual Reduction (Fig. 25.13)

- Place depth grooves and reduce the lingual surface. The depth of these grooves should be approximately 0.8 mm to allow finishing.
- Use the football shaped diamond for lingual reduction.
- Do the lingual reduction until a clearance of 1 mm in all mandibular excursive movements is achieved.
- Do the shoulder preparation, from the center of the lingual wall towards the proximal, until the lingual shoulder meets the facial shoulder.

Chamfer Preparation (Fig. 25.14)

- For subgingival margins, do the chamfer preparation after placing the retraction cord
- Avoid making a sloping shoulder which may result in unfavorable loading of the porcelain and thus tensile failure
- Take care that no unsupported enamel remains to avoid fracture
- The completed chamfer should be 1 mm wide, smooth, continuous and free of any rough edges.

Finishing

- Finish and smoothen the prepared surfaces (**Fig. 25.15**)
- There should not be sharp line angles, which can cause fracture because of wedging action
- Do margin refinement if needed.

FABRICATION OF CERAMIC RESTORATIONS

Techniques used for fabrication of ceramic restorations are:
- Firing on platinum foil
- Using refractory techniques
- Lost wax technique
- Machined restoration using CAD-CAM technology.

Firing on Platinum Foil

Ceramic inlays and onlays are commonly fabricated by firing dental porcelains on refractory dies. Firing is the oldest method amongst different fabrication techniques. This is no longer preferred nowadays. In this technique,

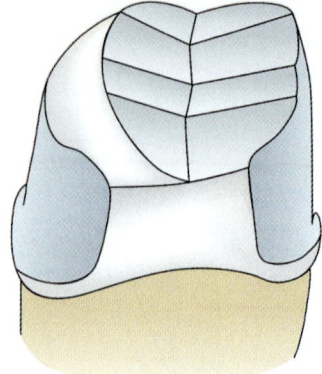

Figure 25.13: Buccal and lingual axial reduction

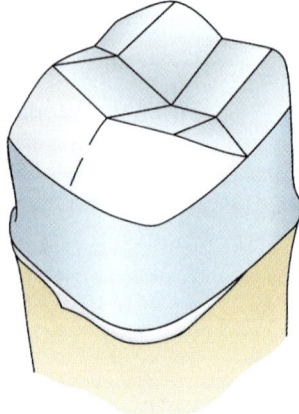

Figure 25.14: Chamfer preparation and axial finishing

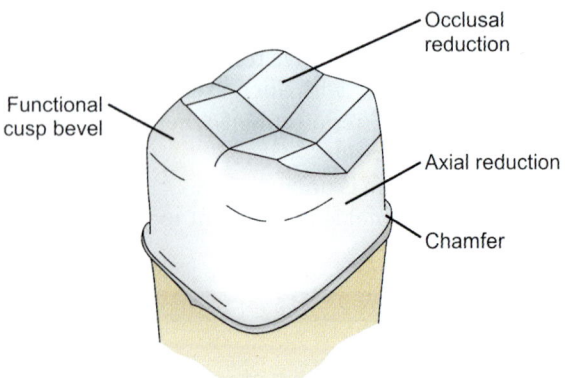

Figure 25.15: Finished tooth preparation for crown

platinum foil is adapted over the die. Feldspathic porcelain is applied over the layer of platinum foil. Then along with foil, porcelain layer is removed from the die and fired in oven. Before cementation, remove the platinum foil.

Advantages
- Ease of fabrication
- Easy accessibility in proximal areas of preparation.

Disadvantages
- More chances of inaccuracies
- Technique sensitive.

Fabrication Using Refractory Die

This is most commonly used method for fabricating inlays, onlays and veneers.

Steps

- Complete the tooth preparation as per requirement.
- Take the final impression, wash and remove excess water removed from the impression surface using cotton pellets.
- Pour the impression using Type IV stone and prepare 'Master' working cast.
- Die is duplicated very accurately in refractory investment material which can withstand porcelain firing temperature.
- Mix the porcelain powder with distilled water or binder provided by manufacturer, pour it in the desired form on the refractory die.
- Recover the restoration from refractory die and fitted on master die.
- Do final adjustments, finishing and polishing.

Lost Wax Technique

- Complete the tooth preparation, take the impression, pour 'master' die and cast using die stone.
- Make a wax pattern and invest it in phosphate bonded investment.
- Burn out the wax using a wax eliminating furnace.
- Heat the transparent casting glass at 1100°C till the casting glass is turned into white, opaque, semicrystalline material. A special casting machine is used to melt the glass ingot.
- The molten glass is slowly cast into the mold using centrifugal casting machine. After cooling, clean the restoration of all the investment.
- Seat the restoration on master die and working cast for adjustment of contour, final adjustment and finishing.

- Once the fitting is confirmed, final adjustment and finishing procedures are done, shading porcelains are applied and fired for better color matching and final finishing and glazing.

Machined Restorations Using CAD-CAM

- After completion of the tooth preparation, a scanning device collects the information on the shape and size of the preparation. This step is called as "optical impression". A video image of the prepared tooth is displayed to ensure proper positioning of the scanning device.
- The system projects an image of the tooth preparation and surrounding structures on a monitor.
- Once the restoration has been designed, the computer directs a micromilling device (CAM portion of the system) to mill the restoration out of a ceramic block. These blocks of "machinable ceramics" specially used for CAM devices are fabricated under ideal conditions. The blocks are among the strongest ceramics available for use with physical properties almost similar to enamel.
- The restoration is removed from the milling device, ready for try in and cementation.

Cementation

- Isolate the prepared tooth to prevent contamination from saliva and gingival fluid.
- Condition the tooth surface for 15 seconds using phosphoric acid.
- Apply dentin bonding agent and cure it.
- For ceramic inlays/onlays, use hydrofluoric acid to etch the fitting surface of the preparation for one minute. Rinse and dry it.
- Etched ceramic is treated with silanating agents. These agents chemically bond to silica in composite and porcelain.
- Apply luting resin to the fitting surface and seat the restoration. Remove the extra cement and cure it for one minute.
- After cementation, examine all the margins. Use fine diamond instruments to finish margins of restoration. Polishing of ceramic restoration is completed with diamond polishing paste with bristle brush.

 Key Points

- Dental ceramic is an inorganic compound with nonmetallic properties typically composed of oxygen and one or more metallic (or semimetallic) elements, e.g. aluminum, calcium, magnesium and zirconium, etc. that is formulated to produce the ceramic based prosthesis.

- Dental porcelains are basically glassy materials. Molten glass solidifies with liquid structure rather than crystalline structure during cooling. The structure formed is known as vitreous and process is known as vitrification.
- Chemical strengthening is usually carried out by replacing small sized cations (Sodium) in the surface layer with large sized cations (Potassium) while matrix remains the same. This is also known as low temperature ionic crowding. The potassium ion is 35 percent larger in size than sodium ion, so, creates residual compressive stresses.
- Dispersion strengthening is process in which strengthening is done with dispersed phase of different material with a capability of blocking a crack from propagating the material. It is obtained by increasing the crystal content of alumina, leucite and zirconia.
- Thermal tempering creates residual compressive stresses in the glass by heating and when it is in molten state, it is immediately quenched. This quenching produces a rigid glass surrounding a soft molten metal.
- In transformation toughening, small and tough particles are uniformly dispersed in the matrix so that cracks cannot pass through these crystals.
- In porcelain fused to metal systems, for optimal bonding, porcelain and alloy should have almost similar coefficient of thermal expansion so that porcelain does not crack or separate from alloy on cooling.
- Most of the nickel-chromium alloys for metal ceramic restorations contain 62 to 76 percent nickel and 13 to 28 percent chromium along with cobalt, beryllium, molybdenum and ruthenium.
- The cobalt chromium alloy contain by weight 52 to 68 percent cobalt, 24 to 33 percent chromium and 2 to 7 percent molybdenum.
- Porcelain undergoes different stages during firing known as bisque stages.
- In low bisque stage, porcelain becomes rigid and porous and readily absorbs water. Particles lack strength, though porcelain exhibits very little shrinkage during this stage.
- In high bisque stage the porcelain mass exhibits smooth surface and the shrinkage is complete. Slight porosity may be seen in this stage.
- In self-glazing, the completed restoration is heated to the glazing temperature. This results in formation of a glossy film by a viscous flow on the porcelain surface.
- In add on glazing, the uncolored glasses with fusion temperature lesser than porcelain restoration are used which form an external glossy layer.
- In alumina reinforced ceramic, dispersion strengthening method is used for strengthening of ceramic. Here alumina crystals are dispersed uniformly in glass matrix to increase strength, toughness and elasticity of the material.
- In leucite reinforced ceramic, leucite crystals (potassium alumino silicate) are dispersed in glassy matrix to match the thermal contraction of ceramic to the metal and increase the tensile strength.
- Castable ceramic is a material which is modified into the desired shape and size as a glass and heat treatment is given to induce crystallization. The process of crystallization is known as ceramming.
- The pressable ceramic is available as core ingot which is heated at high temperature and pressed into a mold. The pressing process is done for duration of 45 mintues at high temperature to get ceramic substructure which in further can be shaded with stains or by glazing.
- Machinable ceramic are supplied in the form of ceramic blocks in various shades. Later on, these blocks are fabricated into inlays, onlays and crown with the help of CAD-CAM or copy milling.
- Indirect computer generated ceramic restorations can be made chairside in CEREC® SYSTEM–CAD (Computer aided design), CAM (Computer aided manufacturing). Here using a special camera, an accurate picture of the tooth is taken which is transferred and displayed on a color computer screen, where CAD technology is used to design the restoration. Then CAM takes over and automatically creates the restoration in a matter of minutes.
- In tooth preparation for ceramic restorations, there should be at least 1.5 mm of clearance in all excursions to prevent ceramic fracture. Preparation walls should exhibit 6 to 8 degree of occlusal divergence per wall so that restoration seats passively in the tooth preparation.

QUESTIONS

1. What are methods of strengthening dental ceramics?
2. Short notes on:
   a. Metal ceramic restorations
   b. Veneers
   c. CAD-CAM
   d. Porcelain laminate veneers
   e. All ceramic system
   f. Ceramic inlays and onlays.

BIBLIOGRAPHY

1. Al-Hiyasat AS, et al. Three-body wear associated with three ceramics and enamel. J Prosthet Dent. 1999;82:476-81.
2. Anderson M, Oden A. A new all ceramic crown. A densely sintered, high purity alumina copying with porcelain. Acta Odont Scant. 1993;51:9.

3. Anderson M, Razzoog ME, Oden A, et al. Procera. A new way to achieve an all ceramic crown. Quint Int. 1998;29:285.

4. Anusavice KJ, Zhang NZ. Chemical durability of Dicor and Lithia based glass ceramics. Dent Mater. 1997;13:13.

5. Anusavice KJ. Recent developments in restorative dental ceramics. JADA. 1993;124:72.

6. Banks RG. Conservative posterior ceramic restorations: a literature review. J Prosthet Dent. 1990;63:619-26.

7. Barnes DM, Blank LW, Gingell JC, Latta MA. Clinical evaluation of castable ceramic veneers. J Esthet Dent. 1992;4: 21.

8. Burgoyne AR, et al. *In vitro* two-body wear of inlay-onlay composite resin restoratives. J Prosthet Dent. 1991;65:206-14.

9. Burke FJT, Qualtrough AJE. Aesthetic inlays. Composite or ceramic? BDJ. 1994;176:53.

10. Calamia JR, Simonsen RJ. Effects of coupling agents on bond strength of etched porcelain. JDR (Spl. Issue): 1984;63:179.

11. Cattell MJ, et al. The transverse strength, reliability and microstructural features of four dental ceramics—part I. J Dent. 1997;25:399-407.

12. Christensen GJ. Ceramic v/s porcelain fused-to-metal crowns: give your patients a choice. JADA. 1994;125:311.

13. Christensen GJ. Veneering of teeth. State of the art. DCNA. 1985;29:373.

14. Christensen GJ. Why all-ceramic crowns? JADA. 1997;128: 1453.

15. David SB, LoPresti JT. Tooth-colored posterior restorations using cerec method (CAD/CAM) generated ceramic inlays. Compend. Contin Educ Dent. 1994;15:802.

16. Eidenbenz S, Lehner Ch R, Scharer P. Copy milling ceramic inlays from resin analogs: A practicable approach with the CELAY system. Int J Prosth. 1994;7:134.

17. El-Mowafy O, Brochu JF. Longevity and clinical performance of IPS-Empress ceramic restorations—a literature review. J Can Dent Assoc. 2002;8:233-7.

18. Estafan D, et al. Scanning electron microscope evaluation of CEREC II and CEREC III inlays. Gen Dent. 2003;51:450-4.

19. Ferrari M, et al. Influence of tissue characteristics at margins on leakage of Class II indirect porcelain restorations. Am J Dent. 1999;12:134-42.

20. Fradeani M, et al. Longitudinal study of pressed glass-ceramic inlays for four and a half years. J Prosthet Dent. 1997;78:346-53.

21. Hager B, Oden A, Andersson B, et al. Procera allceram laminates: A clinical report. J Prosth Dent. 2001;85:231.

22. Hayashi M, et al. Eight-year clinical evaluation of fired ceramic inlays. Oper Dent. 2000;25:473-81.

23. Haywood VB, Heymann HO, Kusy RP, et al. Polishing porcelain veneers: An SEM and specular reflectance analysis. Dent Mater. 1988;4:116.

24. Ibsen RL, Yu XY. Establishing cuspid, guided occlusion with bonded porcelain. Esthet Dent.1989;80.

25. Jensen ME, Redford DA, Williams BT, et al. Posterior etched porcelain restorations: An *in vitro* study. Compend Contin Educ Dent. 1987;8:615.

26. Krejci I, et al. Wear of ceramic inlays, their enamel antagonists, and luting cements. J Prosthet Dent. 1993;69:425-30.

27. Krejci I, Krejci D, Lutz F. Clinical evaluation of a new pressed glass ceramic inlay material over 1.5 years. Quint Int. 1992;23:181.

28. Leinfelder KF, Isenberg BP, Essig ME. A new method for generating ceramic restorations: A CAD/CAM system. JADA. 1989;118:703.

29. MacCulloch WT. Advances in dental ceramics Br Dent J. 1968;124:361-5.

30. Mount GJ. Glass ionomer cements: clinical considerations. In Clinical dentistry. New York, 1984, Harper & Row.

31. Nicholson JW, Wasson EA. The setting of glass-polyalkenoate ("glass-ionomer") cements. Trans Acad Dent Mater. 1992;5:1-14.

32. Sturdevant JR, et al. Margin gap size of ceramic inlays using second-generation CAD/CAM equipment. J Esthet Dent. 1999;11:206-14.

33. Van Dijken JW, et al. Fired ceramic inlays: a 6-year follow up. J Dent. 1998;26:219-25.

Tooth Hypersensitivity

Chapter Outline

INTRODUCTION

The term tooth hypersensitivity, dentinal sensitivity or hypersensitivity is often used intermittently to describe clinical condition of an exaggerated response to an exogenous stimulus.

The exogenous stimuli may include thermal, tactile or osmotic changes. While extreme stimuli can make all the teeth hurt, the term hypersensitivity means painful response to stimuli not normally associated with pain. The response to a stimulus varies from person to person due to difference in pain tolerance, environment factors and psychology of patient. Tooth hypersensitivity can fit the criteria of several pain terms described by Merskey (1979), for the International Association for the Study of Pain (IASP). Pain is described "as an unpleasant sensory and emotional experience associated with actual or potential tissue damage."

DEFINITION

Dentin hypersensitivity is defined as "sharp, short pain arising from exposed dentin in response to stimuli typically thermal, chemical, tactile or osmotic and which cannot be ascribed to any other form of dental defect or pathology (Holland et al, 1997).

Historic review

- Leeuwenhoek (1678) described "tooth canals in dentin"
- JD White (1855) proposed that dentinal pain was caused by movement of fluid in dentinal tubules
- Lukomsky (1941) advocated sodium fluoride as a desensitizing obtundent
- Brannstrom (1962) described hydrodynamic theory of dentinal pain
- Kleinberg (1986) summarized different approaches that are used to treat hypersensitivity.

Tooth hypersensitivity is not associated with actual tissue damage in the acute sense but can involve potential tissue damage with constant erosion of the enamel or cementum along with the concomitant pulpal response.

NEUROPHYSIOLOGY OF TEETH

The dental pulp is richly innervated. According to conduction velocities, the nerve units can be classified into A group—having the conduction velocity more than 2 m/s and C group—with conduction velocity less than 2 m/s.

The sharp, better localized pain is mediated by A delta fibers, whereas C fiber activation seems to be connected with the dull radiating pain sensation. Myelinated A fiber seems to be responsible for dentin sensitivity.

MECHANISM OF DENTIN SENSITIVITY

Theories of Dentin Sensitivity

Neural Theory

The neural theory attributes to activation of nerve ending lying within the dentinal tubules. These nerve signals are then conducted along the parent primary afferent nerve fibers in the pulp, into the dental nerve branches and then into the brain (**Fig. 26.1**). Neural theory considered that entire length of tubule contains free nerve endings.

Theories of dentin sensitivity
⇒ Neural theory
⇒ Odontoblastic transduction theory
⇒ Hydrodynamic theory.

Odontoblastic Transduction Theory

The theory assumed that odontoblasts extend to the periphery. The stimuli initially excite the process or body of the odontoblast. The membrane of odontoblasts may come into close apposition with that of nerve endings in the pulp or in the dentinal tubule and the odontoblast transmits the excitation of these associated nerve endings. However, in the most recent study; Thomas (1984) indicated that the odontoblastic process is restricted to the inner third of the dentinal tubules. Accordingly it seems that the outer part of the dentinal tubules does not contain any cellular elements but is only filled with dentinal fluid.

Hydrodynamic Theory

This theory proposes that a stimulus causes displacement of the fluid that exists in the dentinal tubules. The displacement occurs in either an outward or inward direction and this mechanical disturbance activates the nerve endings present in the dentin or pulp.

Brannstrom (1962) suggested that the displacement of the tubule contents is rapid enough to deform nerve fiber in pulp or predentin or damage odontoblast cell. Both of these effects appear capable of producing pain (**Fig. 26.2**).

Currently most investigators accept that dentin sensitivity is due to the hydrodynamic fluid shift, which occurs across exposed dentin with open tubules (**Fig. 26.3**). This rapid fluid movement in turn activates the mechanoreceptor nerves of A group in the pulp (**Fig. 26.4**).

Mathews et al (1994) noted that stimuli such as cold causes fluid flow away from the pulp, produces more rapid and greater pulp nerve responses than those such as heat, which causes an inward flow. This certainly would explain the rapid and severe response to cold stimuli compared to the slow dull response to heat.

The dehydration of dentin by air blasts or absorbent paper causes outward fluid movement and stimulates the mechanoreceptor of the odontoblast, causing pain. Prolonged air blast causes formation of protein plug into the dentinal tubules, reducing the fluid movement and thus decreasing pain (**Fig. 26.5**).

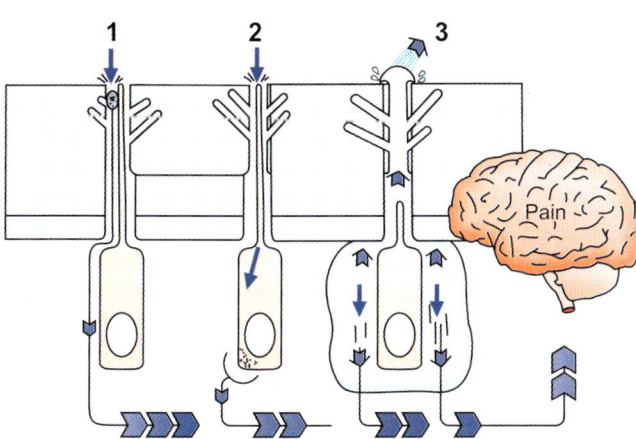

Figure 26.1: Theories of dentin hypersensitivity. (1) Neural theory: Stimulus applied to dentin causes direct excitation of the nerve fibers, (2) Odontoblastic transduction theory: Stimulus is transmitted along the odontoblast and passes to the sensory nerve endings through synapse, (3) Hydrodynamic theory: Stimulus causes displacement of fluid present in dentinal tubules which further excite nerve fibers

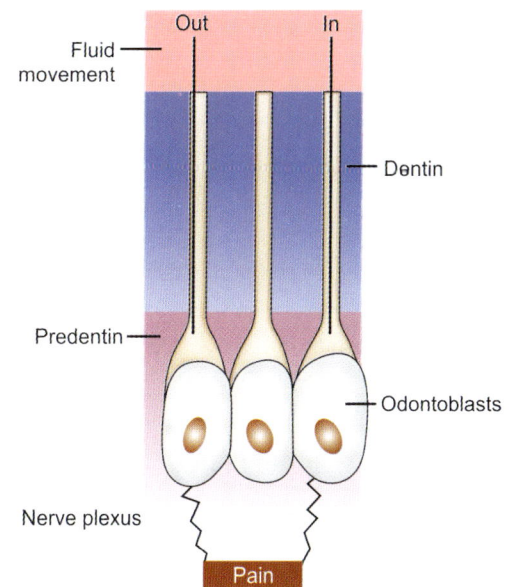

Figure 26.2: Hydrodynamic theory showing pain because of fluid movement

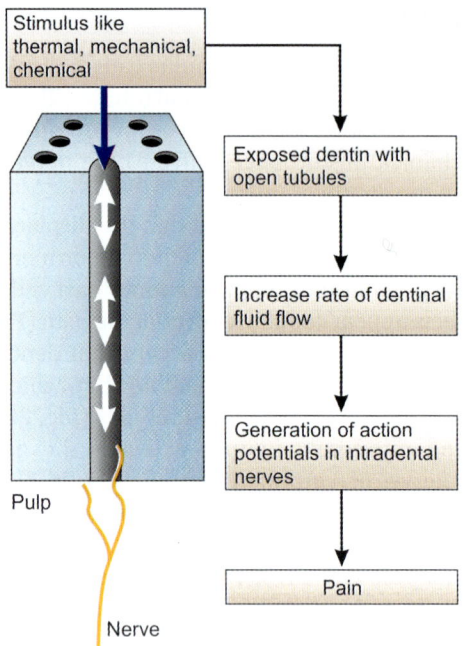

Figure 26.3: Hydrodynamic theory of dentin hypersensitivity

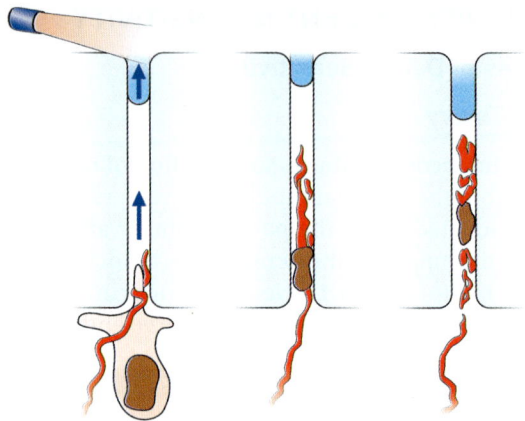

Figure 26.5: Effect of air blast on dentin, pain produced by different stimuli

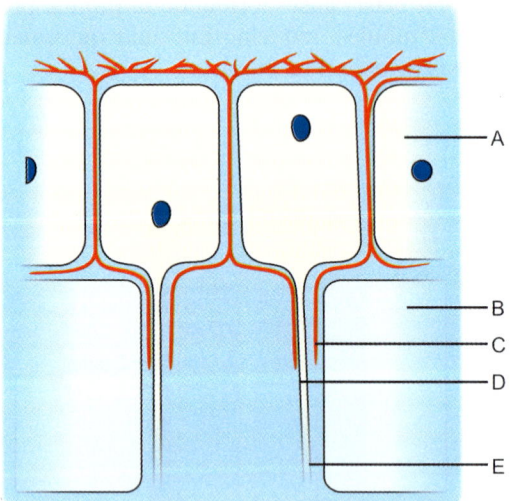

Figure 26.4: Hydrodynamic theory: A. Odontoblast; B. Dentin; C. A-δ nerve fiber; D. Odontoblastic process; E. Stimulation of A-δ nerve fiber from fluid movement

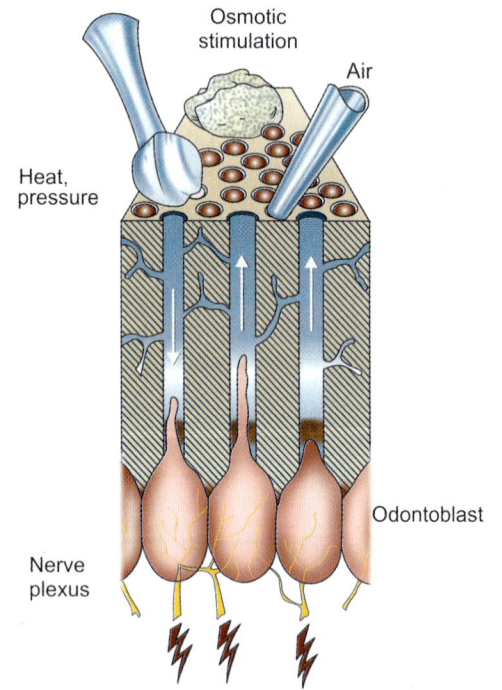

Figure 26.6: Different stimuli resulting in fluid movement and subsequent pain

INCIDENCE AND DISTRIBUTION OF DENTIN HYPERSENSITIVITY

The pain produced when sugar or salt solutions are placed in contact with exposed dentin can also be explained by dentinal fluid movement. Dentinal fluid is of relatively low osmolarity, which have tendency to flow towards solution of higher osmolarity, i.e. salt or sugar solution (**Fig. 26.6**).

The prevalence studies for dentin hypersensitivity are limited in number. The available prevalence data varies considerably and dentin hypersensitivity has been stated to range from 8 to 30 percent of adult population.

- Most sufferers range from 20-40 years of age and a peak occurrence is found at the end of the third decade.
- In general, a slightly higher incidence of dentin hypersensitivity is reported in females than in males.
- The reduced incidence of dentin hypersensitivity in older individuals reflects age changes in dentin and the dental pulp. Sclerosis of dentin, the laying down of secondary dentin and fibrosis of the pulp would interfere with the hydrodynamic transmission of stimuli through exposed dentin.

Intraoral Distribution

- Hypersensitivity is most commonly noted on buccal cervical zones of permanent teeth. Although all tooth type may be affected, canines and premolars in either jaw are the most frequently involved.
- Regarding the side of mouth, in right handed tooth brushers, the dentin hypersensitivity is greater on the left sided teeth compared with the equivalent contralateral teeth.

ETIOLOGY AND PREDISPOSING FACTORS (FIG. 26.7)

The primary underlying cause for dentin hypersensitivity is exposed dentinal tubules. Dentin may become exposed by two processes; either by loss of covering periodontal structures (gingival recession), or by loss of enamel.

The most common clinical cause for exposed dentinal tubules is gingival recession (**Fig. 26.8**). Various factors which can cause recession are inadequate attached gingiva, improper brushing technique, periodontal surgery, overzealous tooth cleansing habits, oral habits, etc.

Common reasons for gingival recession
➡ Inadequate attached gingiva
➡ Prominent roots
➡ Toothbrush abrasion
➡ Oral habits resulting in gingiva laceration, i.e. traumatic tooth picking, eating hard foods
➡ Excessive tooth cleaning
➡ Excessive flossing
➡ Gingival recession secondary to specific diseases, i.e. NUG, periodontitis, herpetic gingivostomatitis
➡ Crown preparation.

The recession may or may not be associated with bone loss. If bone loss occurs, more dentinal tubules get exposed. When gingival recession occurs, the outer protective layer of root dentin, i.e. cementum gets abraded or eroded away (**Fig. 26.9**).

This leaves the exposed underlying dentin, which consists of protoplasmic projections of odontoblasts within the pulp chamber (**Fig. 26.10**). These cells contain nerve endings and when disturbed, nerves depolarize and this is interpreted as pain (**Fig. 26.11**).

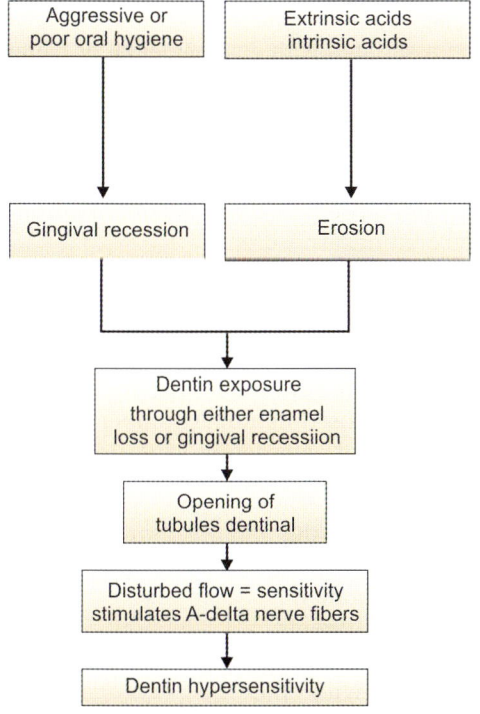

Figure 26.7: Etiology of dentin hypersensitivity

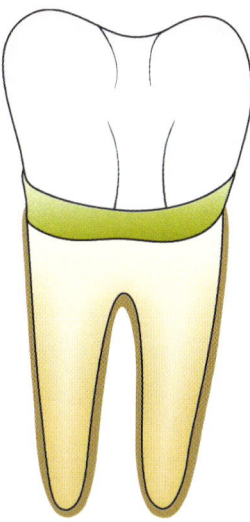

Figure 26.8: Recession of gingiva

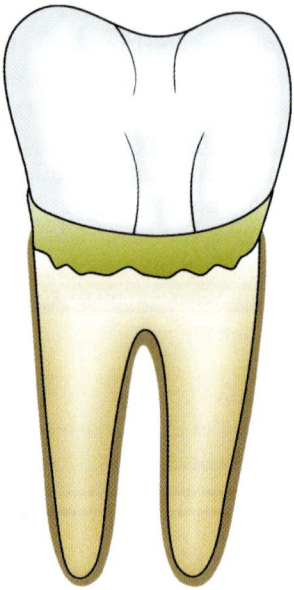

Figure 26.9: Erosion of cementum

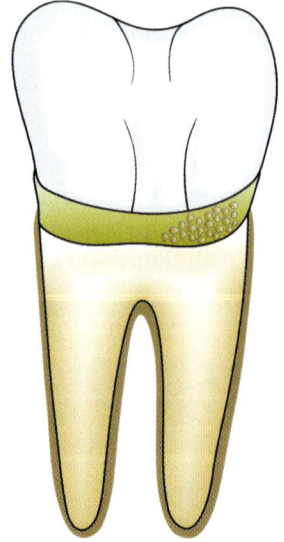

Figure 26.10: Exposure of dentinal tubules

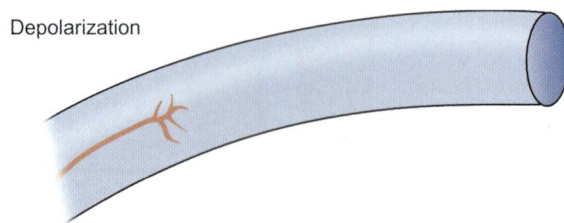

Figure 26.11: Depolarization of nerve ending causing pain

Once the dentinal tubules are exposed, there are oral processes which keep them exposed. These include poor plaque control, enamel wear, improper oral hygiene technique, cervical erosions, enamel wear and exposure to acids.

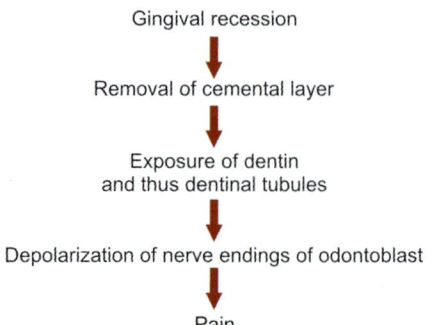

Gingival recession

↓

Removal of cemental layer

↓

Exposure of dentin
and thus dentinal tubules

↓

Depolarization of nerve endings of odontoblast

↓

Pain

Reasons for continued dentinal tubular exposure

→ Poor plaque control, i.e. acidic bacterial byproducts
→ Excess oral acids, i.e. soda, fruit juice, swimming pool chlorine, bulimia
→ Cervical decay
→ Toothbrush abrasion
→ Tartar control toothpaste. The other reason for exposure of dentinal tubules is due to loss of enamel.

Causes of loss of enamel

→ Attrition by exaggerated occlusal functions like bruxism
→ Abrasion from dietary components or improper brushing technique
→ Erosion associated with environmental or dietary components particularly acids.

Since dentinal tubules get sclerosed of their own and plug themselves up in the oral environment, treatment should focus on eliminating factors associated with continued dentinal exposure.

DIFFERENTIAL DIAGNOSIS (FIG. 26.12)

Dentin hypersensitivity is perhaps a symptom complex rather than a true disease and results from stimulus transmission across exposed dentin. A number of dental conditions are associated with dentin exposure and therefore, may produce the same symptoms.

Such conditions include:
- Chipped teeth
- Fractured restoration
- Restorative treatments
- Dental caries
- Cracked tooth syndrome
- Other enamel invaginations.

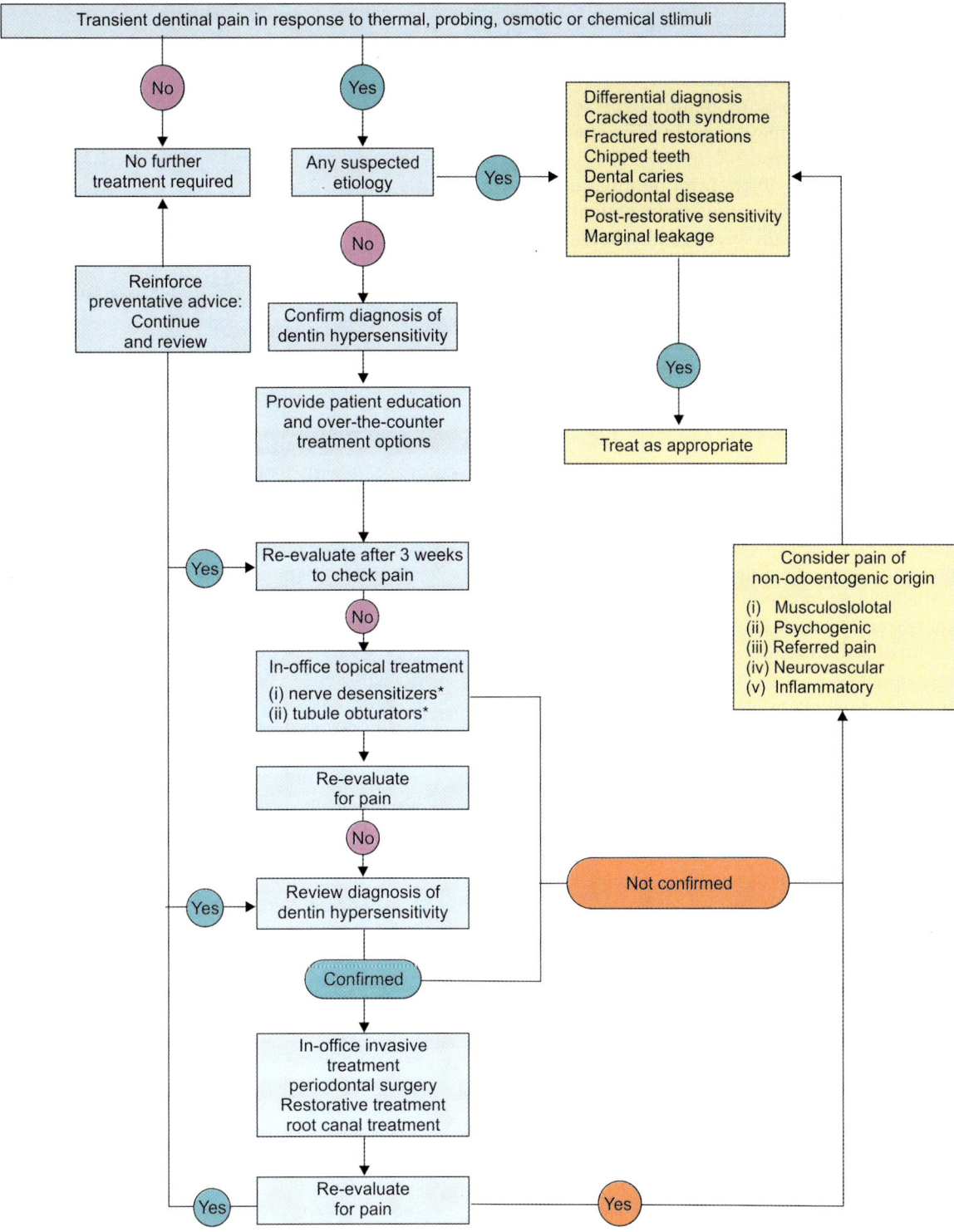

Figure 26.12: Treatment of dentin hypersensitivity

DIAGNOSIS

- A careful history together with a thorough clinical and radiographic examination is necessary before arriving at a definitive diagnosis of dentin hypersensitivity. However, the problem may be made difficult when two or more conditions coexist.
- Tooth hypersensitivity differs from dentinal or pulpal pain. In case of dentin hypersensitivity, patient's ability to locate the source of pain is very good, whereas in case of pulpal pain, it is very poor.
- The character of the pain does not outlast the stimulus; the pain is intensified by thermal changes, sweet and sour.
- Intensity of pain is usually mild to moderate.
- The pain can be duplicated by hot or cold application or by scratching the dentin. The pulpal pain is explosive, intermittent and throbbing and can be affected by hot or cold.

TREATMENT STRATEGIES

Hypersensitivity can resolve without the treatment or may require several weeks of desensitizing agents before improvement is seen. Treatment of dentin hypersensitivity is challenging for both patient and the clinician mainly for two main reasons:

1. It is difficult to measure or compare pain among different patients.
2. It is difficult for patient to change the habits that initially caused the problem.

Management of Tooth Hypersensitivity

It is well known that hypersensitivity often resolves without treatment. This is probably related to the fact that dentin permeability decreases spontaneously because of occurrence of natural processes in the oral cavity.

Natural process contributing to desensitization
➡ Formation of reparative dentin by the pulp
➡ Obturation of tubules by the formation of mineral deposits (Dental sclerosis)
➡ Calculus formation on the surface of the dentin.

Two principal treatment options (Fig. 26.13)
➡ Plug the dentinal tubules preventing the fluid flow
➡ Desensitize the nerve, ma ing it less responsive to stimulation. All the current modalities address these two options.

Treatment of dentin hypersensitivity can be divided into
➡ Home care with dentifrices
➡ Inoffice treatment procedure
➡ Patient education.

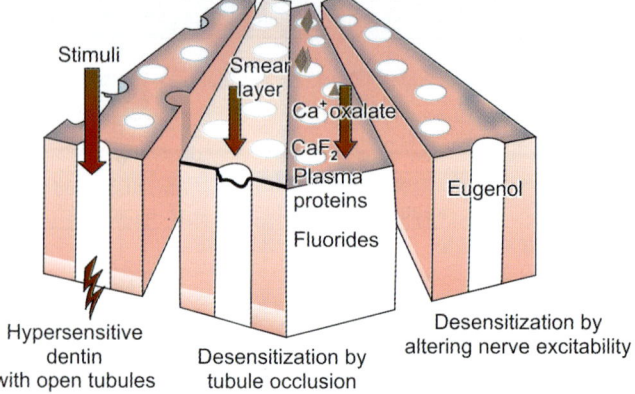

Figure 26.13: Different treatment modalities for dentin hypersensitivity

Management of dentin hypersensitivity
➡ Home care with dentifrices:
• Strontium chloride dentifrices
• Potassium nitrate dentifrices
• Fluoride dentifrices.
➡ In office treatment procedure:
• Varnishes
• Corticosteroids
• Treatments that partially obturate dentinal tubules.
i. Burnishing of dentin
ii. Silver nitrate
iii. Zinc chloride—potassium ferrocyanide
iv. Formalin
v. Calcium compounds.
a. Calcium hydroxide
b. Dibasic calcium phosphate.
vi. Fluoride compounds
a. Sodium fluoride
b. Sodium silicofluoride
c. Stannous fluoride.
vii. Iontophoresis
viii. Strontium chloride
ix. Potassium oxalate.
• Tubule sealant
i. Restorative resins
ii. Dentin bonding agents.
• Miscellaneous
i. Laser.
➡ Patient education:
• Dietary counseling
• Tooth brushing technique
• Plaque control.

Home Care with Dentifrices (Fig. 26.14)

Dentifrice has been defined as a substance used with a toothbrush to aid in cleaning the accessible surfaces of the

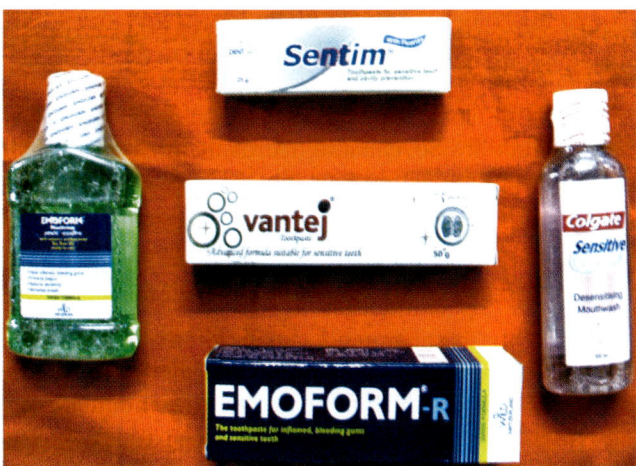

Figure 26.14: Commonly used home care products for dentin hypersensitivity

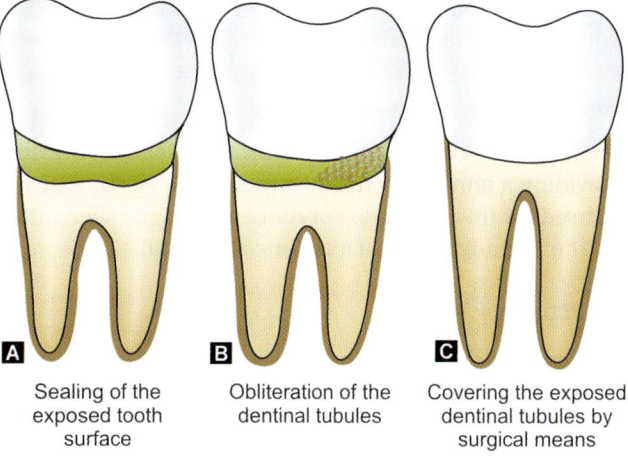

A	B	C
Sealing of the exposed tooth surface	Obliteration of the dentinal tubules	Covering the exposed dentinal tubules by surgical means

Figures 26.15A to C: In office treatment procedures for dentin hypersensitivity

teeth. Dentifrice components include abrasive, surfactant, humectant, thickener, flavor, sweetener, coloring agent and water.

After professional diagnosis, dentinal hypersensitivity can be treated simply and inexpensively by home use of desensitizing dentifrices. The habit of toothbrushing with a dentifrice for cosmetic reasons is well established in the population, thus compliance with this regimen can be easily made.

Strontium Chloride Dentifrices

Ten percent strontium chloride desensitizing dentifrices have been found to be effective in relieving the pain of tooth hypersensitivity.

Potassium Nitrate Dentifrices

Five percent potassium nitrate dentifrices have been found to alleviate pain related to tooth hypersensitivity.

Fluoride Dentifrices

Sodium monofluorophosphates dentifrices are the effective mode of treating tooth hypersensitivity.

In-office Treatment Procedure

Rationale of Therapy

According to hydrodynamic theory of hypersensitivity, a rapid movement of fluid in the dentinal tubules is capable of activating intradental sensory nerves. Therefore, treatment of hypersensitive teeth should be directed towards reducing the anatomical diameter of the tubules,

obliteration of the tubules or to surgically cover the exposed dentinal tubules so as to limit fluid movement (**Figs 26.15A to C**).

Criteria for selecting desensitizing agent
→ Provides immediate and lasting relief from pain
→ Easy to apply
→ Well tolerated by patients
→ Not injurious to the pulp
→ Does not stain the tooth
→ Relatively inexpensive.

Treatment Options to Reduce the Diameter of Dentinal Tubules can be

- Formation of a smear layer by burnishing the exposed root surface (smear layer consists of small amorphous particles of dentin, minerals and organic matrix—denatured collagen).
- Application of agents that form insoluble precipitates within the tubules.
- Impregnation of tubules with plastic resins.
- Application of dental bonding agents to seal off the tubules.
- Covering the exposed dentinal tubules by surgical means.

It must be recognized that single procedure may not be consistently effective in the treatment of hypersensitivity; therefore, the dentist must be familiar with alternative methods of treatment. Prior to treating sensitive root surfaces, hard/soft deposits should be removed from the teeth. Root planning on sensitive dentin may cause considerable discomfort, in this case, teeth should be anesthetized prior to treatment and teeth should be isolated and dried with warm air.

Varnishes

Open tubules can be covered with a thin film of varnish, providing a temporary relief; varnish such as copalite can be used for this purpose. For more sustained relief a fluoride containing varnish Duraflor can be applied.

Corticosteroids

Corticosteroids containing one percent prednisolone in combination with 25 percent parachorophenol, 25 percent methacresylacetate and 50 percent gum camphor was found to be effective in preventing postoperative thermal sensitivity.

The use of corticosteroids is based, on the assumption that hypersensitivity is linked to pulpal inflammation; hence, more information is needed regarding the relationship between these two conditions.

Partial Obliteration of Dentinal Tubules

Burnishing of dentin: Burnishing of dentin with a toothpick or orange wood stick results in the formation of a smear layer. This layer partially occludes the dentinal tubules which help in reducing the hypersensitivity.

Formation of insoluble precipitates to block tubules: Certain soluble salts react with ions in tooth structure to form crystals on the surface of the dentin. To be effective, crystallization should occur in 1-2 minutes and the crystals should be small enough to enter the tubules and must also be large enough to partially obturate the tubules.

- Calcium oxalate dihydrate crystals are formed when potassium oxalate is applied to dentin; these crystals are very effective in reducing permeability.
- Silver nitrate ($AgNO_3$) has ability to precipitate protein constituents of odontoblast processes, thereby partially blocking the tubules.
- Zinc chloride—potassium ferrocyanide: When applied forms precipitate, which is highly crystalline and covers the dentin surface.
- Formalin 40 percent is topically applied by means of cotton pellets or orangewood sticks on teeth. It had been proposed by Grossman in 1935 as the desensitizing agent of choice in treating anterior tooth because, unlike $AgNO_3$, it does not produce stain.
- Calcium compounds have been popular agent for many years for the treatment of hypersensitivity. The exact mechanism of action is unknown but evidence suggests that:

- It may block dentinal tubules
- May promote peritubular dentin formation
- On increasing the concentration of calcium ions around nerve fibers, may result in decreased nerve excitability. So, calcium hydroxide might be capable of suppressing nerve activity.
  - i. A paste of $Ca(OH)_2$ and sterile distilled water applied on exposed root surface and allowed to remain for 3-5 minutes, can give immediate relief in 75 percent of cases.
  - ii. Dibasic calcium phosphate when burnished with round toothpick forms mineral deposits near the surface of the tubules and found to be effective in 93 percent of patients.
- Recaldent (CPP-ACP)

CPP-ACP (complex of casein phosphopeptides and amorphous calcium phosphate). CPPs are group of peptides derived from casein. Casein is the part of protein which naturally occurs in milk, CPP is responsible for high availability of Ca^{2+} from milk. In normal state calcium phosphate forms a crystalline structure at neutral pH and thus becomes insoluble. But CPP keeps calcium and phosphorus in ionic form (amorphous state). In this state, calcium and phosphate ions can enter the tooth enamel and thus promote remineralization of tooth. Recently, a sugar free, water based crème containing RECALDENT™ (CPP-ACP) has been made available under the name GC tooth mousse (**Fig. 26.16**).

- *Fluoride compounds:* Lukomsky (1941) was the first to propose sodium fluoride as desensitizing agent, because dentinal fluid is saturated with respect to calcium and phosphate ions. Application of NaF leads

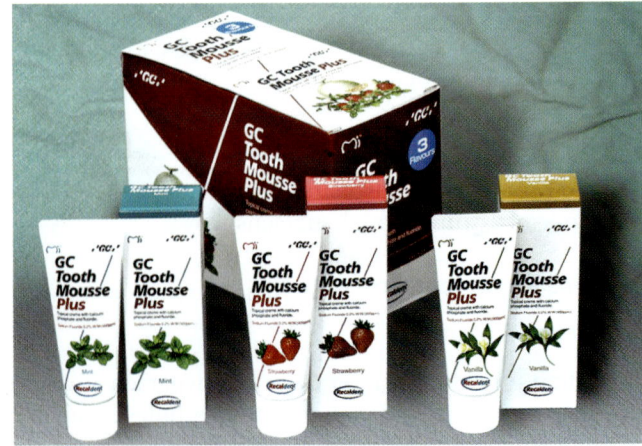

Figure 26.16: GC tooth mousse for tooth remineralization, thereby reducing hypersensitivity

to precipitation of calcium fluoride crystals, thus, reducing the functional radius of the dentinal tubules.

– *Acidulated sodium fluoride:* Concentration of fluoride in dentin treated with acidulated sodium fluoride is found to be significantly higher than dentin treated with sodium fluoride.

– *Sodium silicofluoride:* Silicic acid forms a gel with the calcium of the tooth and produces an insulating barrier. Thus application of 0.6 percent sodium silicofluoride is much more potent than 2 percent solution of sodium fluoride as desensitizing agent.

– *Stannous fluoride*: Ten percent solution of stannous fluoride forms dense layer of tin and fluoride containing globular particles blocking the dentinal tubules. 0.4 percent stannous fluoride is also an effective agent, however, requires prolonged use (up to 4 weeks) to achieve satisfactory results.

• *Fluoride iontophoresis:* Iontophoresis is a term applied to the use of an electrical potential to transfer ions into the body for therapeutic purposes. The objective of fluoride iontophoresis is to drive fluoride ions more deeply into the dentinal tubules that cannot be achieved with topical application of fluoride alone.

• *Strontium chloride:* Studies have shown that topical application of concentrated strontium chloride on an abraded dentin surface produces a deposit of strontium that penetrates dentin to a depth of approximately 10 to 20 μm and extend into the dentinal tubules.

• *Oxalates:* Oxalates are relatively inexpensive, easy to apply and well tolerated by patients. Potassium oxalate and ferric oxalate solution make available oxalate ions that can react with calcium ions in the dentin fluid to form insoluble calcium oxalate crystals that are deposited in the apertures of the dentinal tubules.

Dental Resins and Adhesives

The objective in employing resins and adhesives is to seal the dentinal tubules to prevent pain producing stimuli from reaching the pulp. Several investigators have demonstrated immediate and enduring relief of pain for periods of up to 18 months following treatment. Although not intended for treatment of generalized areas of root sensitivity, this can be an effective method of treatment when other forms of therapy have failed.

GLUMA is a dentin bonding system that includes glutaraldehyde primer and 35 percent HEMA (hydroxyethyl methacrylate). It provides an attachment to dentin that is immediate and strong. GLUMA has been found to be highly effective when other methods of treatment failed to provide relief (**Fig. 26.17**).

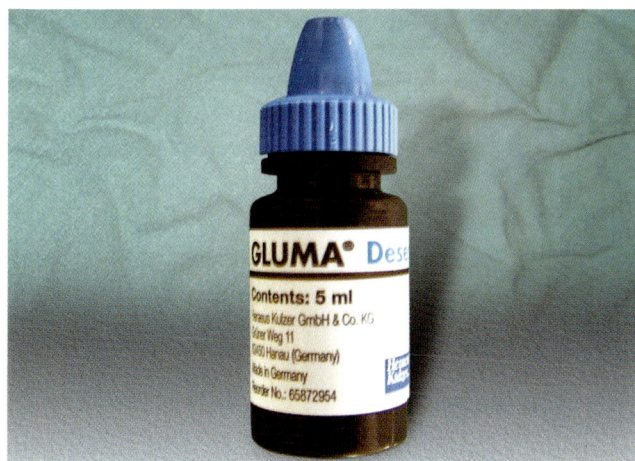

Figure 26.17: GLUMA desensitizing solution

Lasers

Treatment of Dentin Hypersensitivity by Lasers

Kimura Y et al (2000) reviewed treatment of dentin hypersensitivity by lasers. The lasers used for the treatment of dentin hypersensitivity are divided into two groups:

1. *Low output power (low level) lasers*: Helium-neon [He-Ne] and gallium/aluminum/arsenide (GaAIAs) [diode] lasers

2. *Middle output power lasers*: Nd:YAG and CO_2 lasers.

Laser effects are considered to be due to the effects of sealing of dentinal tubules, nerve analgesia or placebo effect. The sealing effect is considered to be durable, whereas nerve analgesia or placebo effects are not.

Patient Education

Dietary Counseling

Dietary acids are capable of causing erosive loss of tooth structure, thereby removing cementum and resulting in opening of the dentinal tubules. Consequently, dietary counseling should focus on the quantity and frequency of acid intake and intake occurring in relation to tooth brushing. Any treatment may fail if these factors are not controlled. A written diet history should be obtained on patients with dentinal hypersensitivity in order to advise those concerning eating habits.

Because of the presence of a smear layer on dentin, teeth are not usually sensitive immediately following scaling and root planning. However, removal of the smear layer may result from exposure to certain components of the diet. Studies have shown that citrus fruit juices, apple juice and yoghurt are capable of dissolving the smear layer.

Because loss of dentin is greatly increased when brushing is performed immediately after exposure of the tooth surface to dietary acids, patients should be cautioned against brushing their teeth soon after ingestion of citrus food.

Toothbrushing Technique

Because incorrect toothbrushing appears to be an etiologic factor in dentin hypersensitivity, instruction about proper brushing techniques can prevent further loss of dentin and the hypersensitivity.

Plaque Control

Saliva contains calcium and phosphate ions and is therefore able to contribute to the formation of mineral deposits within exposed dentinal tubules. The presence of plaque may interfere with this process, as plaque bacteria, by producing acid, are capable of dissolving any mineral precipitates that form, thus opening tubules.

Professional interest in the cause and treatment of dentinal hypersensitivity has been evident in the dental literature for approximately 150 years or more. Dentinal hypersensitivity satisfies all the criteria to be classified as a true pain syndrome. Myelinated A fibers mostly A-delta type seems to be responsible for the sensitivity of dentin. Of the various theories proposed, the hydrodynamic theory is the most accepted explanation for the mechanism of dentin hypersensitivity. Management of the condition requires determination of etiologic factors and predisposing influences. Desensitizing toothpastes containing potassium nitrate, strontium chloride and sodium monofluorophosphate have proven to be effective in the management of hypersensitivity. Partial obturation of open tubules the most widely practiced in office treatment of dentinal hypersensitivity.

 Key Points

- Pain is described "as an unpleasant sensory and emotional experience associated with actual or potential tissue damage."
- Dentin hypersensitivity is defined as "sharp, short pain arising from exposed dentin in response to stimuli typically thermal, chemical, tactile or osmotic and which cannot be ascribed to any other form of dental defect or pathology.

- The sharp, better localized pain is mediated by A delta fibers, whereas C fibers activation seems to be connected with the dull radiating pain sensation. Myelinated A fiber seems to be responsible for dentin sensitivity.
- The dehydration of dentin by air blasts or absorbent paper causes outward fluid movement and stimulates the mechanoreceptor of the odontoblast, causing pain. Prolonged air blast causes formation of protein plug into the dentinal tubules, reducing the fluid movement and thus decreasing pain.
- The most common reason for exposed dentinal tubules is gingival recession which can be due to inadequate attached gingiva, improper brushing technique, periodontal surgery, overzealous tooth cleansing habits, oral habits, etc.
- Tooth hypersensitivity differs from dentinal or pulpal pain. In case of dentin hypersensitivity, patient's ability to locate the source of pain is very good, whereas in case of pulpal pain, it is very poor.
- To treat dentin hypersensitivity different ways to reduce the diameter of dentinal tubules are formation of a smear layer by burnishing the exposed root surface, application of agents that form insoluble precipitates within the tubules, application of dental bonding agents and covering the exposed dentinal tubules by surgical means.
- The objective of fluoride iontophoresis is to drive fluoride ions more deeply into the dentinal tubules that cannot be achieved with topical application of fluoride alone.
- GLUMA is a dentin bonding system that includes glutaraldehyde primer and 35 percent HEMA (hydroxyethyl methacrylate). It provides an immediate and strong attachment to dentin.
- Laser causes desensitization because of sealing of dentinal tubules, nerve analgesia or placebo effect.

QUESTIONS

1. Write short notes on:
   a. Management of dentin hypersensitivity
   b. Theories of dentin hypersensitivity.

BIBLIOGRAPHY

1. Butler WT. Dentin matrix proteins. Eur J Oral Sci. 1998;106:204.
2. Trowbridge HO, Silver DR. A review of current approaches for in-office management of tooth hypersensitivity. Dent Clin North Am. 1990;107:65-9.

Management of Discolored Teeth

INTRODUCTION

In the pursuit of looking good, man has always tried to beautify his face. Since the alignment and appearance of teeth influence the personality, they have received considerable attention.

Tooth discoloration varies in etiology, appearance, localization, severity and adherence to tooth structure. It may be classified as intrinsic, extrinsic and combination of both. Intrinsic discoloration is caused by incorporation of chromatogenic material into dentin and enamel during odontogenesis or after tooth eruption. Exposure to high levels of fluoride, tetracycline administration, inherited developmental disorders and trauma to the developing tooth may result in pre-eruptive discoloration. After

eruption of the tooth, aging and pulp necrosis are the main causes of intrinsic discoloration.

Coffee, tea, red wine, carrots and tobacco give rise to extrinsic stains. Wear of the tooth structure, deposition of secondary dentin due to aging or as a consequence of pulp inflammation and dentin sclerosis affect the light-transmitting properties of teeth, resulting in a gradual darkening of the teeth.

Scaling and polishing of the teeth removes many extrinsic stains. For more stubborn extrinsic discoloration and intrinsic stain, a variety of tooth whitening options are available today. These include over-the-counter whitening systems, whitening tooth pastes and the latest option laser tooth whitening.

Currently available tooth whitening options are:
- Office bleaching procedures
- At home bleaching kits
- Composite veneers
- Porcelain veneers
- Whitening toothpastes.

Among these procedures, bleaching procedures are more conservative than restorative methods, simple to perform and less expensive. This chapter reviews discoloration and its correction. Following aspects of discoloration and bleaching procedures are discussed in this chapter:
- Etiology and types of discoloration
- Commonly used medicaments for bleaching
- External bleaching technique, i.e. bleaching in teeth with vital pulp
- Internal bleaching technique, i.e. usually performed in nonvital teeth
- Efficacy and performance of each procedure
- Possible complications and safety of various procedures.

Before discussing bleaching of the discolored teeth, we should be familiar with the color of natural healthy teeth. Teeth are polychromatic so color varies among the gingival, incisal and cervical areas according to the thickness, reflections of different colors and translucency of enamel and dentin (**Fig. 27.1**). Color of healthy teeth is primarily determined by the translucency and color of dentin and is modified by:
- Color of enamel covering the crown
- Translucency of enamel which varies with different degrees of calcification

- Thickness of enamel which is greater at the occlusal/incisal edge of the tooth and thinner at the cervical third. That is why teeth are more darker on cervical one third than at middle or incisal one-third.

Normal color of primary teeth is bluish white whereas color of permanent teeth is grayish yellow, grayish white or yellowish white.

CLASSIFICATION OF DISCOLORATION

Tooth discoloration varies with etiology, appearance, localization, severity and adherence to the tooth structure. It may be classified as extrinsic or intrinsic discoloration or combination. Feinman et al 1987, describes extrinsic discoloration as that occurring when an agent or stain damages the enamel surface of the teeth. Extrinsic staining can be easily removed by a normal prophylactic cleaning. Intrinsic staining is defined as endogenous staining that has been incorporated into the tooth matrix and thus can not be removed by prophylaxis. Combination of both is multifactorial in nature, e.g. nicotine staining.

Classification of discoloration
➡ Intrinsic discoloration
➡ Extrinsic discoloration
➡ Combination of both.

Etiology of tooth discoloration

Intrinsic Stains
- ➡ Preeruptive causes
  - ◆ Disease
    - i. Alkaptonuria
    - ii. Hematological disorders
    - iii. Disease of enamel and dentin
    - iv. Liver diseases.
  - ◆ Medications
    - i. Tetracycline stains and other antibiotic use
    - ii. Fluorosis stain.
- ➡ Posteruptive causes of discoloration
  - ◆ Pulpal changes
  - ◆ Trauma
  - ◆ Dentin hypercalcification
  - ◆ Dental caries
  - ◆ Restorative materials and operative procedures
  - ◆ Aging
  - ◆ Functional and parafunctional changes.

Extrinsic Stains
- ➡ Daily acquired stains
  - ◆ Plaque
  - ◆ Food and beverages
  - ◆ Tobacco use

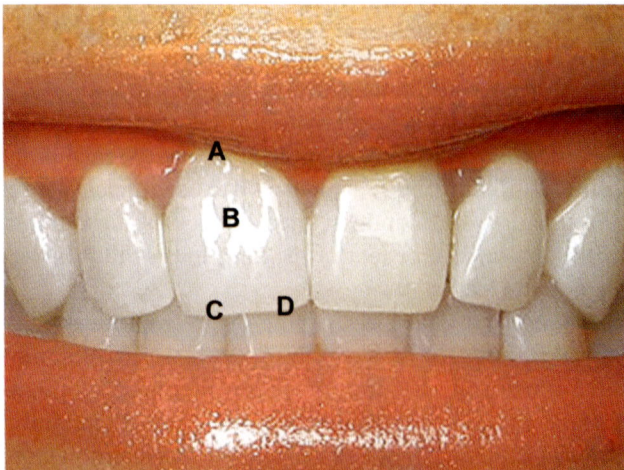

Figure 27.1: Normal anatomical landmarks of tooth: A. Cervical margin; B. Body of tooth; C. Incisal edge; D. Translucency of enamel

- Poor oral hygiene
- Swimmer's calculus
- Gingival hemorrhage.
- Chemicals
  - Chlorhexidine
  - Metallic stains.

ETIOLOGY OF TOOTH DISCOLORATION

Intrinsic Stains

Pre-eruptive Causes

These are incorporated into the deeper layers of enamel and dentin during odontogenesis and alter the development and appearance of the enamel and dentin.

Alkaptonuria: Dark brown pigmentation of primary teeth is commonly seen in alkaptonuria. It is an autosomal recessive disorder resulting in complete oxidation of tyrosine and phenylalanine causing increased level of homogentisic acid.

Hematological Disorders

- **Erythroblastosis fetalis**: It is a blood disorder of neonates due to Rh incompatibility. In this, stain does not involve teeth or portions of teeth developing after cessation of hemolysis shortly after birth. Stain is usually green, brown or bluish in color.
- **Congenital porphyria**: It is an inborn error of porphyrin metabolism, characterized by overproduction of uroporphyrin. Deciduous and permanent teeth may show a red or brownish discoloration. Under ultraviolet light, teeth show red fluorescence.
- **Sickle cell anemia**: It is inherited blood dyscrasia characterized by increased hemolysis of red blood cells. In sickle cell anemia infrequently the stains of the teeth are similar to those of erythroblastosis fetalis, but discoloration is more severe, involves both dentitions and does not resolve with time.

Disease of Enamel and Dentin

Developmental defects in enamel formation
Amelogenesis imperfecta
Fluorosis
Vitamin and mineral deficiency
Chromosomal anomalies
Inherited diseases
Tetracycline
Childhood illness
Malnutrition
Metabolic disorders.

Amelogenesis imperfecta (AI): It comprises of a group of conditions, that demonstrate developmental alteration in the structure of the enamel in the absence of a systemic disorder. Amelogenesis imperfecta (AI) has been classified mainly into hypoplastic, hypocalcified and hypomaturation type (**Fig. 27.2**).

Fluorosis: In fluorosis, staining is due to excessive fluoride uptake during development of enamel. Excess fluoride induces a metabolic change in ameloblast and the resultant enamel has a defective matrix and an irregular, hypomineralized structure (**Fig. 27.3**).

Staining manifests as:
- Gray or white opaque areas on teeth.
- Yellow to brown discoloration on a smooth enamel surface.
- Moderate and severe changes showing pitting and brownish discoloration of surface.

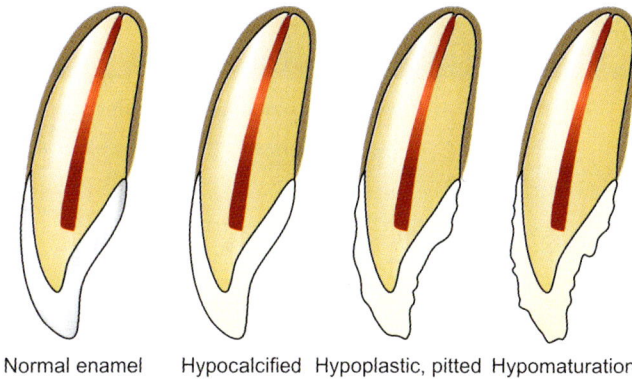

Normal enamel   Hypocalcified enamel   Hypoplastic, pitted enamel   Hypomaturation enamel

Figure 27.2: Amelogenesis imperfecta

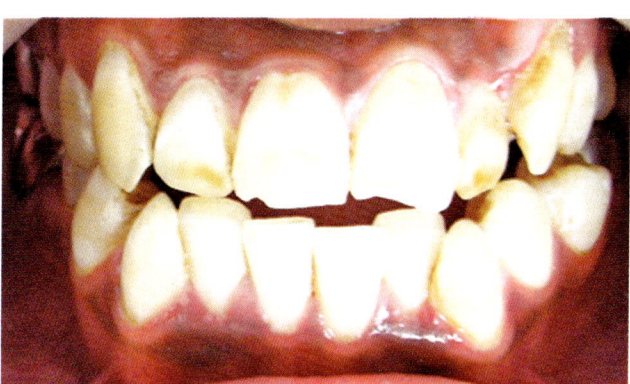

Figure 27.3: Fluorosis of teeth

- Severely corroded appearance with dark brown discoloration and loss of most of enamel (**Fig. 27.4**).
- Enamel hypoplasia and hypocalcification due to other causes (**Figs 27.5A to C**).
- Vitamin D deficiency results in characteristic white patch hypoplasia in teeth.
- Vitamin C deficiency together with vitamin A deficiency during formative periods of dentition resulting in pitting type appearance of teeth.

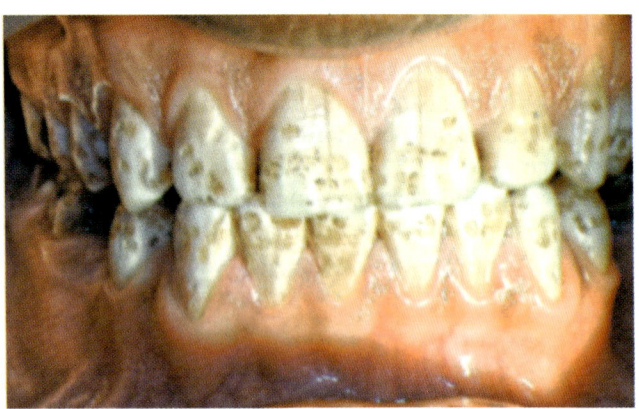

Figure 27.4: Brownish discoloration with pitting

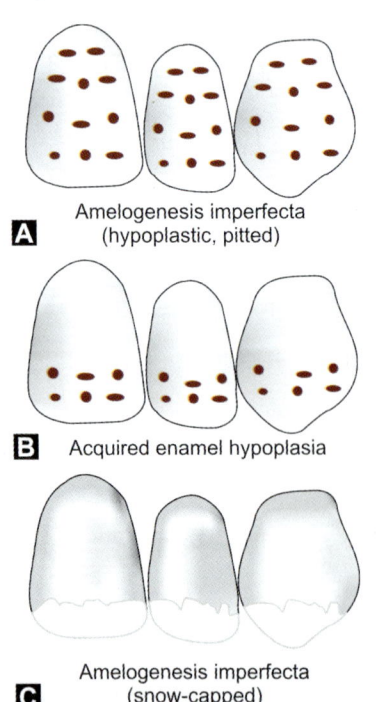

Figures 27.5A to C: (A) Amelogenesis imperfecta (hypoplastic, pitted); (B) Acquired enamel hypoplasia; (C) Amelogenesis imperfecta (snow-capped)

- Childhood illnesses during odontogenesis, such as exanthematous fevers, malnutrition, metabolic disorder, etc. also affect teeth.

Defects in Dentin Formation

- Dentinogenesis imperfecta
- Erythropoietic porphyria
- Tetracycline and minocycline (excessive intake)
- Hyperbilirubinemia.

Dentinogenesis imperfecta (DI) (Figs 27.6A to C): It is an autosomal dominant developmental disturbance of the dentin which occurs along or in conjunction with amelogenesis imperfecta. Color of teeth in DI varies from gray to brownish violet to yellowish brown with a characteristic usual translucent or opalescent hue.

Tetracycline and Minocycline: Unsightly discoloration of both dentitions results from excessive intake of tetracycline and minocycline during the development of teeth. Chelation of tetracycline molecule with calcium in hydroxyapatite crystals forms tetracycline orthophosphate which is responsible for discolored teeth (**Fig. 27.7**).

Classification of staining according to developmental stage, banding and color (Jordun and Boksman 1984).

- First degree (mild)—Yellow to gray, uniformly spread through the tooth. No banding.

Severity of pigmentation with tetracycline depends on three factors
➥ Time and duration of administrations
➥ Type of tetracycline administered
➥ Dosage.

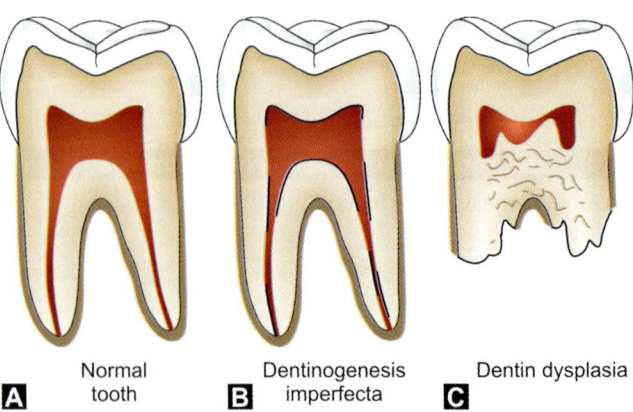

Figures 27.6A to C: (A) Normal tooth; (B) Dentinogenesis imperfectal; (C) Dentin dysplasia

- Second degree (moderate)—Yellow brown to dark grey, slight banding, if present.
- Third degree (severe staining)—Blue gray or black and is accompanied by significant banding across tooth.
- Fourth degree—Stains that are so dark that bleaching is ineffective, totally.

Posteruptive Causes

- **Pulpal changes**: Pulp necrosis usually results from bacterial, mechanical or chemical irritation to pulp. In this disintegration products enter dentinal tubules and cause discoloration (**Fig. 27.8**).
- **Trauma**: Accidental injury to tooth can cause pulpal and enamel degenerative changes that may alter color of teeth (**Fig. 27.9**). Pulpal hemorrhage leads to grayish discoloration and nonvital appearance. Injury causes hemorrhage which results in lysis of RBCs and liberation of iron sulfide which enter dentinal tubules and discolor surrounding tooth.
- **Dentin hypercalcification**: Dentin hypercalcification results when there are excessive irregular elements in the pulp chamber and canal walls. It causes decrease in translucency and yellowish or yellow brown discoloration of the teeth.

- **Dental caries**: In general, teeth present a discolored appearance around areas of bacterial stagnation and leaking restorations (**Fig. 27.10**).
- **Restorative materials and dental procedures**: Discoloration can also result from the use of endodontic sealers and restorative materials.
- **Aging**: Color changes in teeth with age result from surface and subsurface changes. Age related discoloration are because of:
  - *Enamel changes:* Both thinning and texture changes occur in enamel.
  - *Dentin deposition:* Secondary and tertiary dentin deposits, pulp stones cause changes in the color of teeth (**Fig. 27.11**).
- **Functional and parafunctional changes**: Tooth wear may give a darker appearance to the teeth because of loss of tooth surface and exposure of dentin which is yellower and is susceptible to color changes by absorption of oral fluids and deposition of reparative dentin.

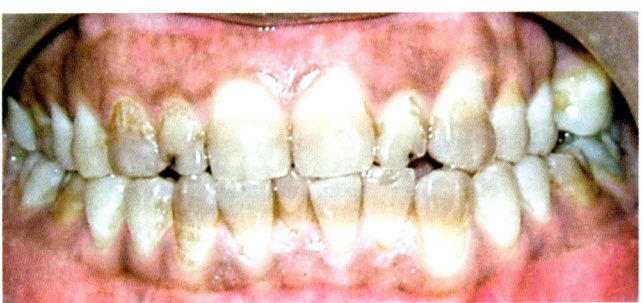

Figure 27.7: Tetracycline stains

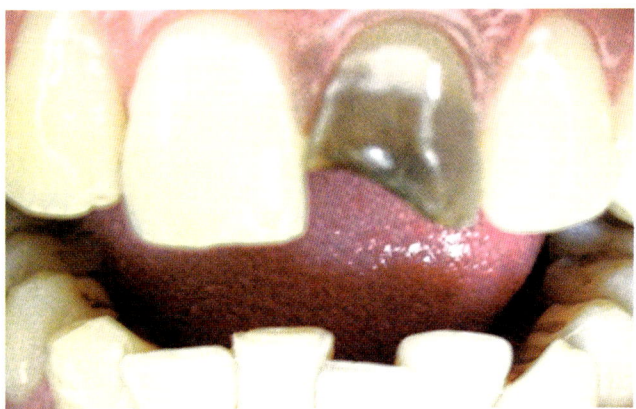

Figure 27.9: Discolored 21 with history of trauma and subsequent pulpal death

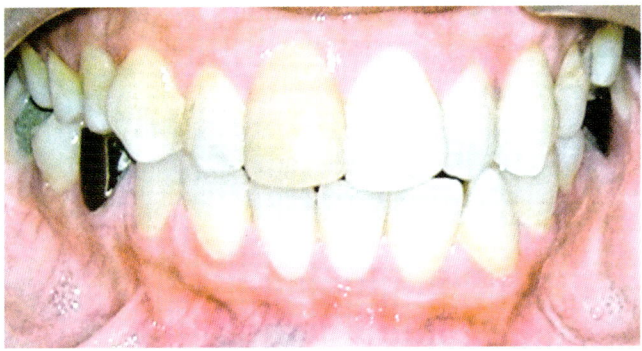

Figure 27.8: Discolored nonvital 11

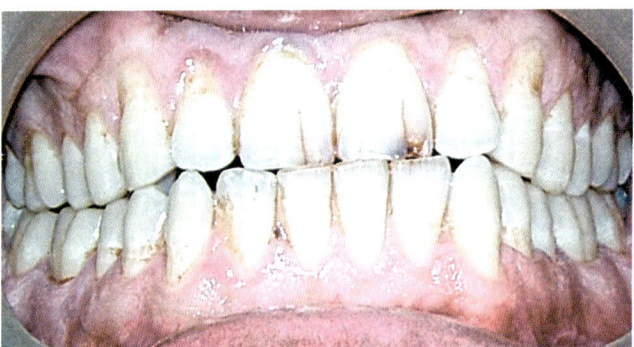

Figure 27.10: Discolored 11, 21 because of caries

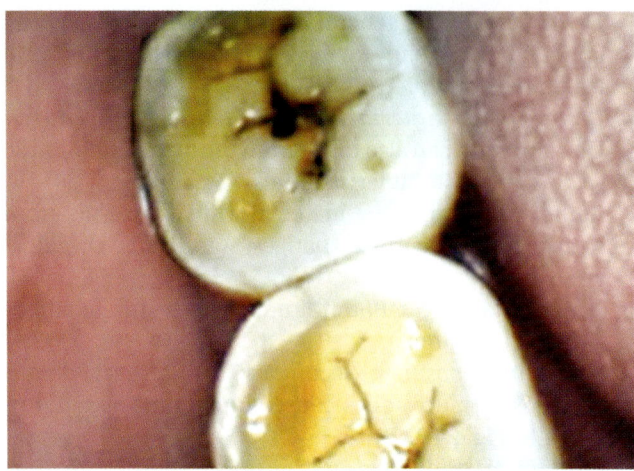

Figure 27.11: Yellowish discoloration of teeth because of secondary/tertiary dentin deposition

Extrinsic Stains

Daily Acquired Stains

- **Plaque**: Pellicle and plaque on tooth surface gives rise to yellowish appearance of teeth
- **Food and beverages**: Tea, coffee, red wine, curry and colas if taken in excess cause discoloration
- Tobacco use results in brown to black appearance of teeth.
- **Poor oral hygiene manifests as**:
  - Green stain
  - Brown stain
  - Orange stain.
- **Swimmer's calculus**: It is yellow to dark brown stain present on facial and lingual surfaces of anterior teeth. It occurs due to prolonged exposure to pool water.
- **Gingival hemorrhage**.

Chemicals

- **Chlorhexidine stain**: The stains produced by use of chlorhexidine are yellowish brown to brownish in nature.
- **Metallic stains**: These are caused by metals and metallic salts introduced into oral cavity in form of metal containing dust inhaled by industry workers or through orally administered drugs.

Etiology and color of tooth discoloration

Intrinsic discoloration	Color
Amelogenesis imperfecta	Brown, black
Dentinogenesis Imperfecta	Brown, blue
Porphyria	Brown, purple-brown blue green
Tetracyclin	Brown, gray, black
Fluorides	Light brown, dark brown
Pulp canal obliteration	Yellow
Pulp necrosis	Gray, black, gray-brown
Extrinsic discoloration	
Coffee, tea	Brown to black
Poor oral hygiene	Yellow to brown
Smoking, Tobacco chewing	Yellowish brown to black
Iatrogenic	
Tissue remnants in pulp chamber	Brown, gray, black
Dental materials	Brown, black, gray
Endodontic materials	Black, gray
Endodontic materials	Black, gray
Trauma during pulp extirpation	Gray, black

Stains caused by different metals

- Copper dust—Green stain
- Iron dust—Brown stain
- Mercury—Greenish black stain
- Nickel—Green stain
- Silver—Black stain.

Classification of extrinsic stains (Nathoo in 1997)

- N1 type dental stain (direct dental stain)—Here colored materials bind to the tooth surface to cause discoloration. Tooth has same color, as that of chromogen.
- N2 type dental stain (direct dental stain)—Here chromogen changes color after binding to the tooth.
- N3 type dental stain (Indirect dental stain)—In this type prechromogen (colorless) binds to the tooth and undergoes a chemical reaction to cause a stain.

BLEACHING

Bleaching is a procedure which involves lightening of the color of a tooth through the application of a chemical agent to oxidize the organic pigmentation in the tooth.

HISTORY OF TOOTH BLEACHING

Bleaching of discolored, pulpless teeth was first described in 1864 and a variety of medicaments such as chloride, sodium hypochlorite, sodium perborate and hydrogen peroxide has been used, alone or in combination, with or without heat activation.

The Walking Bleach technique was introduced in 1961. It involved placement of a mixture of sodium perborate and water into the pulp chamber. This technique was later modified and water replaced by 30 to 50 percent hydrogen peroxide. Now popular, night guard vital bleaching technique described the use of 10 percent carbamide peroxide in mouth guard to be worn overnight for lightening tooth color. Later in 1996, Reyto did the tooth whitening by lasers.

CONTRAINDICATIONS FOR BLEACHING

Poor Case Selection

- Patient having emotional or psychological problems are not right choice for bleaching.
- In case selection, if clinician has opinion that bleaching is not in patient's best interest, he should decline doing that.

Dentin Hypersensitivity

Hypersensitive teeth need extraprotection before going for bleaching.

Extensively Restored Teeth

These teeth are not good candidate for bleaching because:
- They do not have enough enamel to respond properly to bleaching.
- Teeth heavily restored with visible, tooth colored restorations are poor candidates as composite restorations do not lighten, infact they become more evident after bleaching.

Teeth with Hypoplastic Marks and Cracks

Application of bleaching agents increase the contrast between white opaque spots and normal tooth structure:
    In these cases, bleaching can be done in conjunction with:
- Microabrasion
- Selected ameloplasty
- Composite resin bonding.

Defective and Leaky Restoration

Defective and leaky restorations are not good candidates for bleaching.

Contraindications of bleaching
→ Poor patient and case selection
◆ Psychologically or emotionally compromised patient.
→ Dentin hypersensitivity
→ Extensively restored tooth
→ Teeth with hypoplastic marks and cracks
→ Defective and leaky restorations.
◆ Discoloration from metallic salts particularly mercury
◆ Defective obturation.

- *Discoloration from metallic salts particularly silver amalgam:* The dentinal tubules of the tooth become virtually saturated with alloys and no amount of bleaching with available products will significantly improve the shade.
- *Defective obturation:* If root canal is not well obturated, then refilling must be done before attempting bleaching.

MEDICAMENTS USED AS BLEACHING AGENTS (FIGS 27.12A AND B)

An ideal bleaching agent should
→ Be easy to apply on the teeth
→ Have a neutral pH
→ Lighten the teeth efficiently
→ Remain in contact with oral soft tissues for short periods
→ Be required in minimum quantity to achieve desired results
→ Not irritate or dehydrate the oral tissues
→ Not cause damage to the teeth
→ Be well-controlled by the dentist to customize the treatment to the patient's need.

Tooth bleaching today is based upon hydrogen peroxide as an active agent. Hydrogen peroxide may be applied directly or produced in a chemical reaction from sodium perborate or carbamide peroxide. Hydrogen peroxide acts as a strong oxidizing agent through the formation of free radicals, reactive oxygen molecules and hydrogen peroxide anions. These reactive molecules attack the long chained, dark colored chromophore molecules and split them into smaller, less colored and more diffusible molecules.

Carbamide peroxide also yields urea which is further decomposed to CO_2 and ammonia. It is the high pH of ammonia which facilitates the bleaching procedure.

This can be explained by the fact that in basic solution, lower activation energy is required for formation of free radicals from hydrogen peroxide and the reaction rate is higher, resulting in improved yield rate compared with an acidic environment.

The outcome of bleaching procedure depends mainly on the concentration of bleaching agents, the ability of the agents to reach the chromophore molecules and the

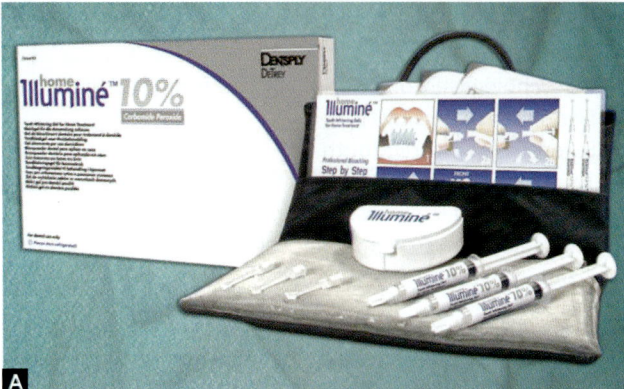

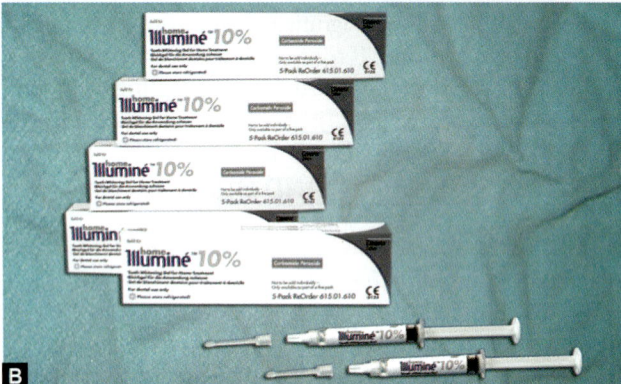

Figures 27.12A and B: Bleaching agent

duration and number of times the agent is in contact with chromophore molecules.

Constituents of Bleaching Material

- First generation bleaching materials were available in liquid form so could not remain long-time in bleaching tray, therefore they had to be replenished frequently.
- Second generation bleaching materials were viscous so they could stay in the bleaching tray for longer.
- Third generation bleaching materials have different colors and mode of activation.

CONSTITUENTS OF BLEACHING GELS

- Carbamide peroxide
- Hydrogen peroxide and sodium hydroxide (Li, 1998)
- Sodium perborate
- Thickening agent-carbopol or carboxy polymethylene
- Urea
- Surfactant and pigment dispersants
- Preservatives

- Vehicle-glycerine and dentifrice
- Flavors
- Fluoride and 3 percent potassium nitrate.

Carbamide Peroxide ($CH_6N_2O_3$)

It is a bifunctional derivative of carbonic acid. It is available as:
- Home bleaching
  - 5 percent carbamide peroxide
  - 10 percent carbamide peroxide
  - 15 percent carbamide peroxide
  - 20 percent carbamide peroxide.
- In office bleaching
  - 35 percent solution or gel of carbamide peroxide.

Hydrogen Peroxide (H_2O_2)

H_2O_2 breaks down to water and nascent oxygen. It also forms free radical perhydroxyl (HO_2) which is responsible for bleaching action.

Sodium Perborate

It comes as monohydrate, trihydrate or tetrahydrate. It contains 95 percent perborate, providing 10 percent available oxygen.

Thickening Agents

Carbopol (Carboxy polymethylene): Addition of cabopol in bleaching gels causes:
- Slow release of oxygen
- Increased viscosity of bleaching material, which further helps in longer retention of material in tray and need of less material
- Delayed effervescence–thicker products stay on the teeth for longer time to provide necessary time for the carbamide peroxide to diffuse into the tooth
- The slow diffusion into enamel may also allow tooth to be bleached more effectively.

Urea

It is added in bleaching solutions to:
- Stabilize the H_2O_2
- Elevate the pH of solution
- Anticariogenic effects.

Surfactants

Surfactant acts as surface wetting agent which allows the hydrogen peroxide to pass across gel tooth boundary.

Preservatives

Commonly used preservatives are phosphoric acid, citric acid or sodium stannate. They sequestrate metals such as Fe, Cu, Mg, accelerate breakdown of H_2O_2 and give gels better durability and stability.

Vehicle

- *Glycerine:* It is used to increase viscosity of preparation and ease of manipulation
- Dentifrice.

Flavors

They are added to improve patient acceptability.

Fluoride and 3 percent Potassium Nitrate

They are added to prevent sensitivity of teeth after bleaching.

FACTORS AFFECTING BLEACHING

Rate of color change is affected by:
- *Amount of time, the bleach is in contact with the teeth:* Increase in contact time, increases the bleaching effect
- *Cleanliness of tooth surface:* Cleaner the enamel surface, better is the effect of bleaching
- *Concentration of solution:* Increase in peroxide concentration, increases the effect of bleaching
- *Location and depth of discoloration.*
- *Temperature:* Increase in temperature increases the release of oxygen free radicals which increases bleaching effect
- *Rate of oxygen free radical release:* More is the oxygen free radical release, better is the effect of bleaching
- *Viscosity of solution:* Addition of agents like glycerine, glycol to increase the viscosity of bleaching solution decrease the efficacy of bleaching agent
- *Shelf life:* Carbamide peroxide has more shelf life (1–2yrs) than hydrogen peroxide (few weeks)
- *Sealed* preparation in nonvital teeth is important to maintain the concentration of bleaching agent
- *Frequency* with which bleaching solution is changed
- Degradation rate of bleaching agent that is rate of oxygen release
- *Age* of patient
- Original *shade and location* of discoloration.

MECHANISM OF BLEACHING (FIG. 27.13)

Mechanism of bleaching is mainly linked to degradation of high molecular weight complex organic molecules that reflect a specific wavelength of light that is responsible

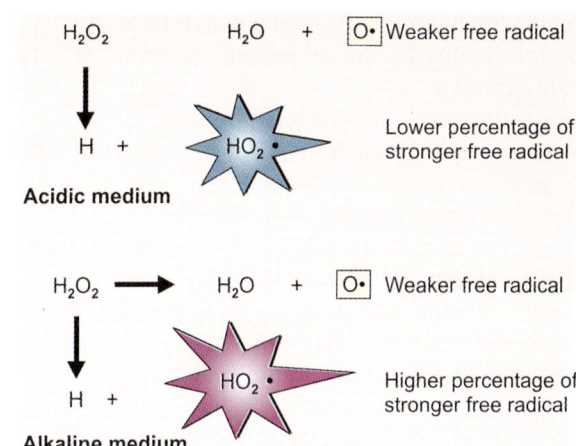

Figure 27.13: Diagram showing ionization of hydrogen peroxide in acidic and alkaline medium

for color of stain. The resulting degradation products are of lower molecular weight and composed of less complex molecules that reflect less light, resulting in a reduction or elimination of discoloration.

Bleaching technique

→ For vital teeth
 ◆ Home bleaching technique/Night guard vital bleaching.
 ◆ In-office bleaching
   i. Thermocatalytic
   ii. Nonthermocatalytic
   iii. Microbrasion.
 → For nonvital teeth
 ◆ Thermocatalytic in-office bleaching
 ◆ Walking bleach/Intracoronal bleaching
 ◆ Inside/outside bleaching
 ◆ Closed chamber bleaching/Extracoronal bleaching.
 → Laser assisted bleaching.

Home Bleaching Technique/Night Guard Bleaching

Indications for Use

- Mild generalized staining
- Age related discolorations
- Mild tetracycline staining
- Mild fluorosis
- Acquired superficial staining
- Stains from smoking tobacco
- Color changes related to pulpal trauma or necrosis.

Contraindications

- Teeth with insufficient enamel for bleaching
- Teeth with deep and surface cracks and fracture lines

- Teeth with inadequate or defective restorations
- Discolorations in the adolescent patients with large pulp chamber
- Severe fluorosis and pitting hypoplasia
- Noncompliant patients
- Pregnant or lactating patients
- Teeth with large anterior restorations
- Severe tetracycline staining
- Fractured or malaligned teeth
- Teeth exhibiting extreme sensitivity to heat, cold or sweets
- Teeth with opaque white spots
- Suspected or confirmed bulimia nervosa.

Advantages of Home Bleaching Technique

- Simple method for patients to use
- Simple for dentists to monitor
- Less chair time and cost effective
- Patient can bleach their teeth at their convenience.

Disadvantages of Home Bleaching Technique

- Patient compliance is mandatory
- Color change is dependent on amount of time the trays are worn
- Chances of abuse by using excessive amount of bleach for too many hours per day.

Factors that Guard the Prognosis for Home Bleaching

- History or presence of sensitive teeth
- Extremely dark gingival third of tooth visible during smiling
- Extensive white spots
- Translucent teeth
- Excessive gingival recession and exposed root surfaces.

Commonly used Solution for Night Guard Bleaching

- 10 percent carbamide peroxide with or without carbopol
- 15 percent carbamide peroxide
- Hydrogen peroxide (1 to 10%).

Steps of Tray Fabrication

- Take the impression and make a stone model
- Trim the model
- Place the stock out resin and cure it
- Apply separating media
- Choose the tray sheet material
- Nature of material used for fabrication of bleaching tray is flexible plastic. Most common tray material used is ethyl vinyl acetate

- Cast the plastic in vacuum tray forming machines
- Trim and polish the tray
- Checking the tray for correct fit, retention and over extension
- Demonstrate the amount of bleaching material to be placed.

Thickness of Tray (Fig. 27.14)

- Standard thickness of tray is 0.035 inch
- Thicker tray, i.e. 0.05 inch is indicated in patients with breaking habit
- Thinner tray, i.e. 0.02 inch thick is indicated in patients who gag.

Treatment Regimen

When and how long to keep the trays in the mouth, depends on patients lifestyle preference and schedule? Wearing the tray during day time allows replenishment of the gel after 1 to 2 hours for maximum concentration. Overnight use causes decrease in loss of material due to decreased salivary flow at night and decreased occlusal pressure. Patient is recalled 1 to 2 weeks after wearing the tray.

Maintenance After Tooth Bleaching

Additional re-bleaching can be done every 3 to 4 yrs if necessary with re-bleaching duration of 1 week.

Side Effects of Home Bleaching

- Gingival irritation—Painful gums after a few days of wearing trays.
- Soft tissue irritation—From excessive wearing of the trays or applying too much bleach to the trays.

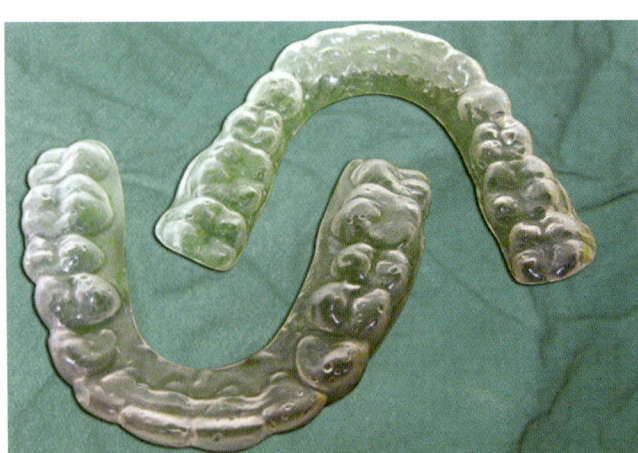

Figure 27.14: Bleaching trays

- Altered taste sensation—Metallic taste immediately after removing trays.
- Tooth sensitivity—Most common side effect.

In-office Bleaching

Thermocatalytic Vital Tooth Bleaching

Equipment needed for in-office bleaching are:
- Power bleach material
- Tissue protector
- Energizing/activating source
- Protective clothing and eye wear
- Mechanical timer.

Light Sources Used for In-office Bleach

Various available light sources are:
- Conventional bleaching light
- Tungsten halogen curing light
- Xenon plasma arc light
- Argon and CO_2 lasers
- Diode laser light.

Conventional Bleaching Light
- Uses heat and light to activate bleaching material
- More heat is generated during bleaching
- Causes tooth dehydration
- Uncomfortable for patient
- Slower in action.

Tungsten-Halogen Curing Light
- Uses light and heat to activate bleaching solution
- Application of light 40 to 60 seconds per application per tooth
- Time consuming.

Xenon Plasma Arc Light
- High intensity light, so more heat is liberated during bleaching
- Application requires 3 seconds per tooth

- Faster bleaching
- Action is thermal and stimulates the catalyst in chemicals
- Greater potential for thermal trauma to pulp and surrounding soft tissues.

Argon and CO_2 Laser
- True laser light stimulate the catalyst in chemical so there is no thermal effect
- Requires 10 seconds per application per tooth.

Diode Laser Light
- True laser light produced from a solid state source
- Ultra fast
- Requires 3 to 5 seconds to activate bleaching agent.
- No heat is generated during bleaching.

Indications of In-office Bleaching (Figs 27.15A to D)

- Superficial stains
- Moderate to mild stains.

Contraindications of In-office Bleaching

- Tetracycline stains
- Extensive restorations
- Severe discolorations
- Extensive caries
- Patient sensitive to bleaching agents.

Advantages of In-office Bleaching

- Patient preference
- Less time than overall time needed for home bleaching
- Patient motivation
- Protection of soft tissues.

Disadvantages of In-office Bleaching

- More chair time
- More expensive
- Unpredictable and deterioration of color is quicker

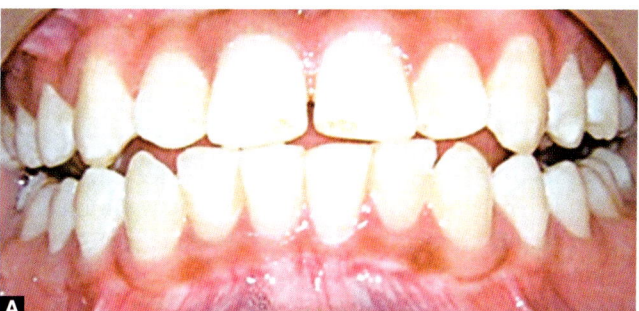
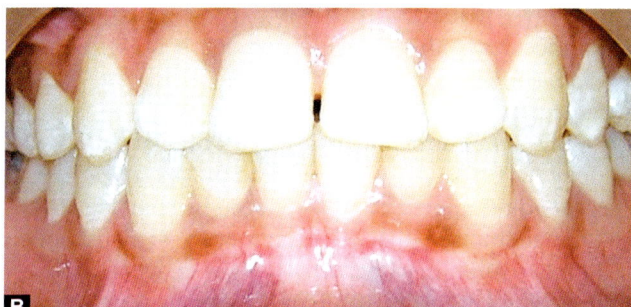

Figures 27.15A and B

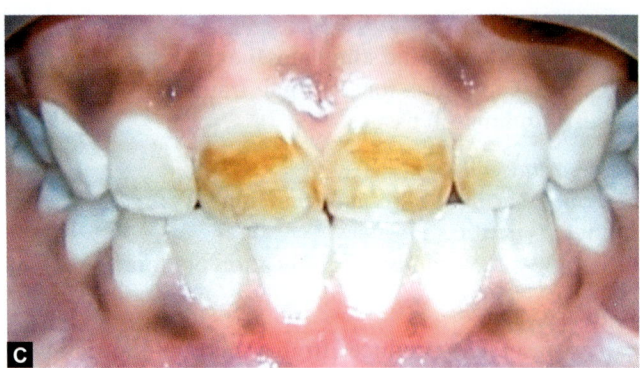

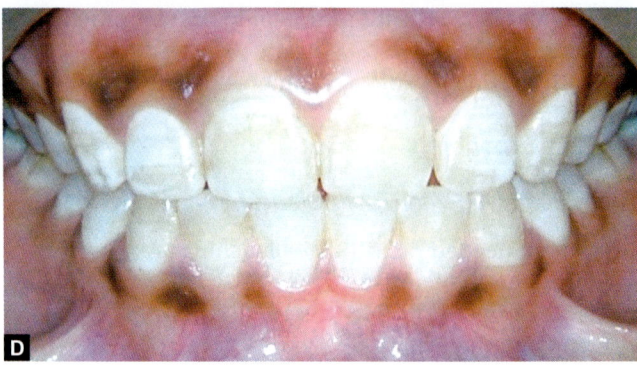

Figures 27.15C and D

Figures 27.15A to D: (A) Discolored teeth; (B) After bleaching; (C) Discolored teeth; (D) After bleaching

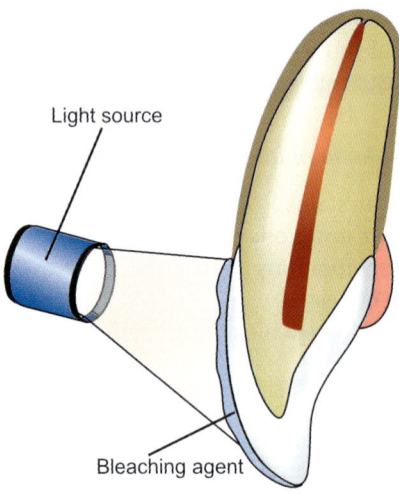

Figure 27.16: Power bleaching technique

- More frequent and longer appointment
- Dehydration of teeth
- Serious safety considerations
- Not much research to support its use
- Discomfort of rubber dam.

Procedure

- Pumice the teeth to clean off any debris present on the tooth surface
- Isolate the teeth with rubber dam
- Saturate the cotton or gauze piece with bleaching solution (30-35% H_2O_2) and place it on the teeth
- Depending upon light, expose the tooth/teeth (**Fig. 27.16**)
- Change solution in between after every 4 to 5 minutes
- Remove solution with the help of wet gauge
- Repeat the procedure until desired shade is produced

- Remove solution and irrigate teeth thoroughly with warm water
- Polish teeth and apply neutral sodium fluoride gel
- Instruct the patient to avoid coffee, tea, etc. for 2 weeks
- Second and third appointment is given after 3 to 6 weeks. This will allow pulp to settle.

Non-thermocatalytic Bleaching

In this technique, heat source is not used.

Commonly used solutions for bleaching	
Name	*Composition*
➡ Superoxol	5 parts H_2O_2:1 part ether
➡ McInnes solution	5 parts of HCl (36%)
	Etches the enamel
	1 part of 0.2 percent ether
	Cleans the tooth surface
	5 parts 30 percent H_2O_2
	Bleaches the enamel.

- ➡ Modified MC Innes solution
- ➡ In this sodium hydroxide is added. Because of its highly alkaline nature, it dissolves calcium of tooth at slower rate.
  - ◆ H_2O_2 (30%)
  - ◆ NaOH (20%)
- ➡ Mix in equal parts, i.e. (1:1) along with ether (0.2%)

Steps

- Isolate the teeth using rubber dam
- Apply bleaching agent on the teeth for five minutes
- Wash the teeth with warm water and reapply the bleaching agent until the desired color is achieved
- Wash the teeth and polish them.

Microabrasion

It is a procedure in which a microscopic layer of enamel is simultaneously eroded and abraded with a special compound (usually contains 18 percent of hydrochloric acid) leaving a perfectly intact enamel surface behind.

Indications

- Developmental intrinsic stains and discolorations limited to superficial enamel only
- Enamel discolorations as a result of hypominera-lization or hypermineralization
- Decalcification lesions from stasis of plaque and from orthodontic bands
- Areas of enamel fluorosis
- Multicolored superficial stains and some irregular surface texture.

Contraindications

- Age related staining
- Deep enamel hypoplastic lesions
- Areas of deep enamel and dentin stains
- Amelogenesis imperfecta and dentinogenesis imperfecta cases
- Tetracycline staining
- Carious lesions underlying regions of decalcification.

Advantages

- Minimum discomfort to patient
- Can be easily done in less time by operator
- Useful in removing superficial stains
- The surface of treated tooth is shiny and smooth in nature.

Disadvantages

- Not effective for deeper stains
- Removes enamel layer
- Yellow discoloration of teeth has been reported in some cases after treatment.

Protocol (Figs 27.17A and B)

- Clinically evaluate the teeth
- Clean teeth with rubber cup and prophylaxis paste
- Apply petroleum jelly to the tissues and isolate the area with rubber dam
- Apply microabrasion compound to areas in 60 seconds intervals with appropriate rinsing
- Repeat the procedure if necessary. Check the teeth when wet
- Rinse teeth for 30 seconds and dry
- Apply topical fluoride to the teeth for four minutes
- Re-evaluate the color of the teeth. More than one visit may be necessary sometimes.

Bleaching of Nonvital Teeth

Thermocatalytic Technique of Bleaching for Nonvital Teeth

- Isolate the tooth to be bleached using rubber dam
- Place bleaching agent (superoxol and sodium perborate separately or in combination) in the tooth chamber
- Heat the bleaching solution using bleaching stick/light curing unit
- Repeat the procedure till the desired tooth color is achieved
- Wash the tooth with water and seal the chamber using dry cotton and temporary restorations
- Recall the patient after 1 to 3 weeks

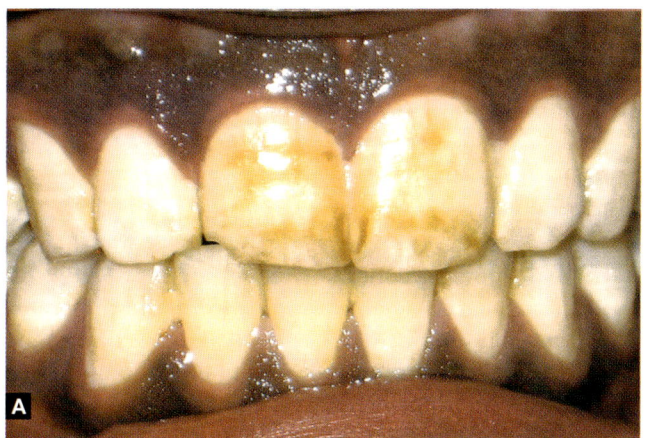
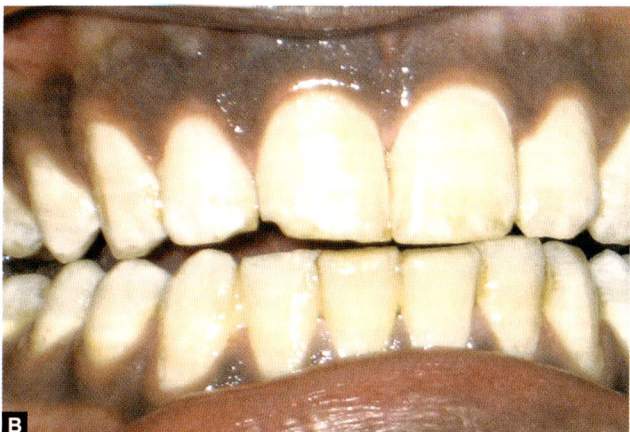

Figures 27.17A and B: (A) Discolored 11 and 21; (B) After microabrasion

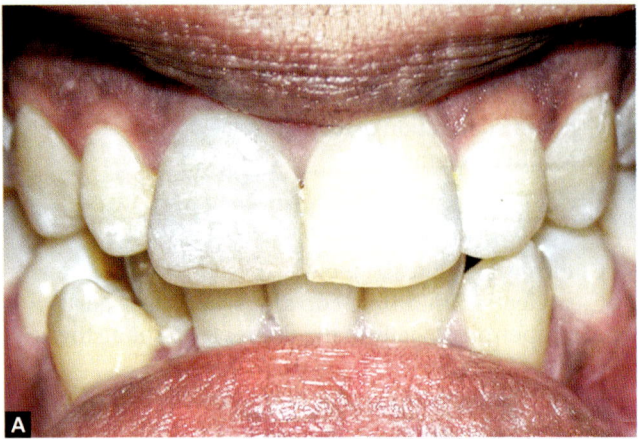 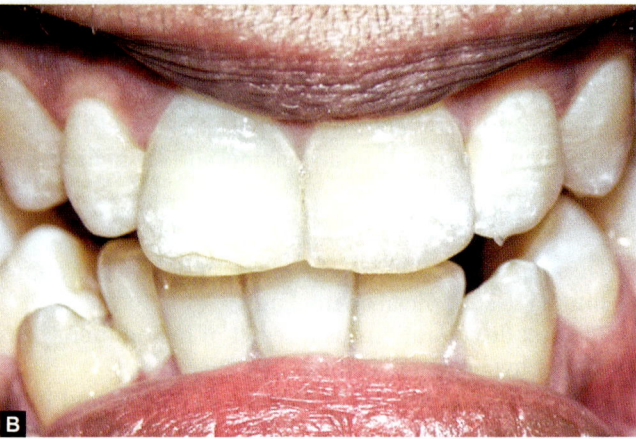

Figures 27.18A and B: (A) Discolored nonvital 11; (B) 11 after walking bleach

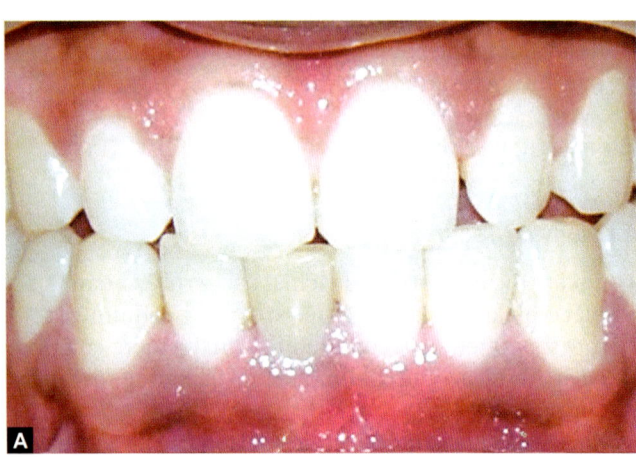 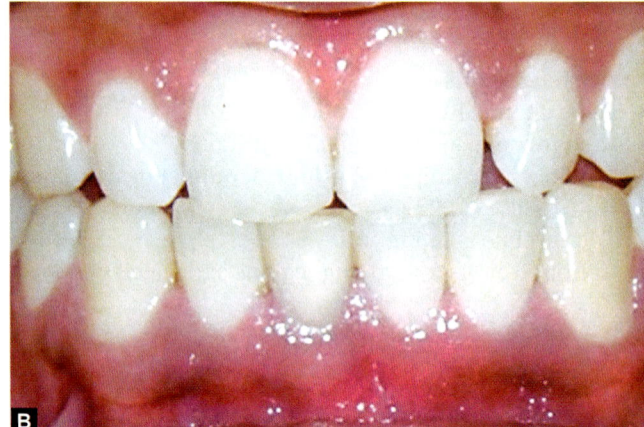

Figures 27.19A and B: (A) Discolored 41; (B) Management of 41 with walking bleach

- Do the permanent restoration of tooth using suitable composite resins afterwards.

Intracoronal Bleaching/Walking Bleach of Nonvital Teeth

It involves use of chemical agents within the coronal portion of an endodontically treated tooth to remove tooth discoloration.

Indications of Intracoronal Bleaching
- Discolorations of pulp chamber origin (**Figs 27.18 and 27.19**)
- Moderate to severe tetracycline staining
- Dentin discoloration
- Discolorations not agreeable to extracoronal bleaching.

Contraindications of Intracoronal Bleaching
- Superficial enamel discoloration
- Defective enamel formation

- Presence of caries
- Unpredictable prognosis of tooth.

Steps
- Take the radiographs to assess the quality of obtura-tion. If found unsatisfactory, retreatment should be done
- Evaluate the quality and shade of restoration if present. If restoration is defective, replace it
- Evaluate tooth color with shade guide
- Isolate the tooth with rubber dam
- Prepare the access cavity, remove the coronal gutta percha, expose the dentin and refine the cavity (**Fig. 27.20**)
- Place mechanical barriers of 2 mm thick, preferably of glass ionomer cement, zinc phosphate, IRM, poly-carboxylate cement on root canal filling material (**Fig. 27.21**). The coronal height of barrier should protect the dentinal tubules and conform to the external epithelial attachment

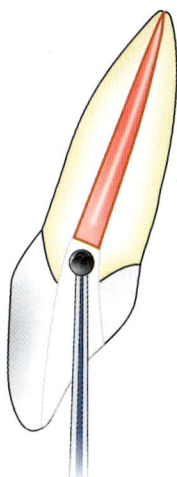

Figure 27.20: Removal of coronal gutta-percha using rotary instrument

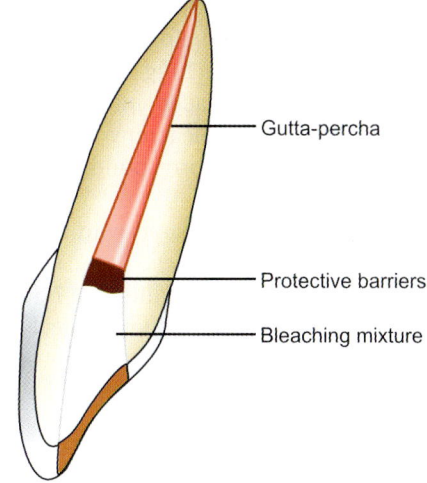

Figure 27.22: Placement of bleaching mixture into pulp chamber and sealing of cavity using temporary restoration

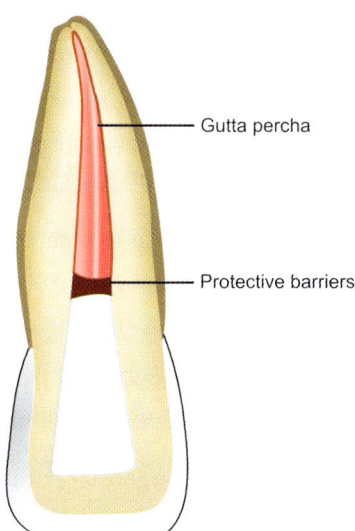

Figure 27.21: Placement of protective barrier over gutta-percha

- Now mix sodium perborate with an inert liquid (local anaesthetic, saline or water) and place this paste into pulp chamber (**Fig. 27.22**)
- After removing the excess bleaching paste, place a temporary restoration over it
- Recall the patient after 1 to 2 weeks, repeat the treatment until desired shade is achieved
- Restore access cavity with composite after 2 weeks.

Complications of Intracoronal Bleaching
- External root resorption
- Chemical burns if using 30 to 35 percent H_2O_2
- Decrease bond strength of composite.

Precautions to be Taken for Safer Nonvital Bleaching
- Isolate tooth effectively
- Protect oral mucosa
- Verify adequate endodontic obturation
- Use protective barriers
- Avoid acid etching
- Avoid strong oxidizers
- Avoid heat
- Recall periodically.

Synonyms

➡ Internal/External bleaching, modified walking bleach technique.

Inside/Outside Bleaching Technique

This technique involves intracoronal bleaching technique along with home bleaching technique. This is done to make the bleaching program more effective. This combination of bleaching treatment is helpful in treating difficult stains, for specific problems like single dark vital or nonvital tooth and to treat stains of different origin present on the same tooth.

Procedure
- Assess the obturation by taking radiographs.
- Isolate the tooth and prepare the access cavity by removing gutta-percha 2 to 3 mm below the cemento-enamel junction.
- Place the mechanical barrier, clean the access cavity and place a cotton pellet in the chamber to avoid food packing into it.
- Evaluate the shade of tooth.

- Check the fitting of bleaching tray and advise the patient to remove the cotton pellet before bleaching.
- Instructions for home bleaching are given. Bleaching syringe can be directly placed into chamber before seating the tray or extrableaching material can be placed into the tray space corresponding to tooth with open chamber (**Fig. 27.23**).
- After bleaching, tooth is irrigated with water, cleaned and again a cotton pellet is placed in the empty space.
- Reassessment of shade is done after 4 to 7 days.
- When the desired shade is achieved, seal the access cavity initially with temporary restoration and finally with composite restoration after at least two weeks.

Advantages
- More surface area for bleach to penetrate
- Treatment time in days rather than weeks
- Decreases the incidence of cervical resorption
- Uses lower concentration of carbamide peroxide.

Disadvantages
- Noncompliant patients
- Over–bleaching by overzealous application
- Chances for cervical resorption is reduced but still exists.

Closed Chamber Bleaching/Extracoronal Bleaching

In this technique, instead of removing the existing restoration, the bleaching paste is applied to the tooth via bleaching tray.

Indications of Closed Chamber Technique
- In case of totally calcified canals in a traumatized tooth

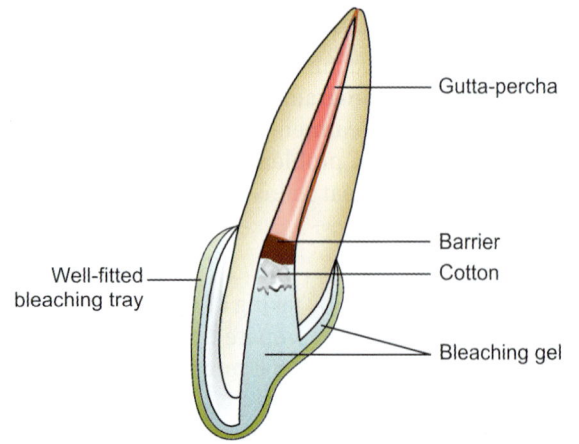

Figure 27.23: Inside/outside techniques in this tray is sealed over an open internal access opening, with a cotton pellet place in open access cavity

- As a maintenance bleaching treatment several years after initial intracoronal bleaching
- Treatment for adolescents with incomplete gingival maturation
- A single dark nonvital tooth where the surrounding teeth are sufficiently light or where other vital teeth are also to be bleached.

Laser Assisted Bleaching Technique

This technique achieves power bleaching process with the help of efficient energy source with minimum side effects. Laser whitening gel contains thermally absorbed crystals, fumed silica and 35 percent H_2O_2. In this, gel is applied and is activated by light source which further activates the crystals present in gel, allowing dissociation of oxygen and therefore better penetration into enamel matrix. Following laser have been approved by FDA for tooth bleaching:
- Argon laser
- CO_2 laser
- GaAlAs diode laser.

Argon Laser

- Emits wavelength of 480 nm in visible part of spectrum
- Activates the bleaching gel and makes the darker tooth surface lighter
- Less thermal effects on pulp as compared to other heat lamps.

CO_2 Laser

- Emits a wavelength of 10,600 nm
- Used to enhance the effect of whitening produced by argon laser
- Deeper penetration than argon laser thus more efficient tooth whitening
- More deleterious effects on pulp than argon laser.

GaAlAs Diode Laser (Gallium Aluminum–Arsenic)

Emits a wavelength of 980 nm.

Tetracyclin Discoloration

Minocyclin can discolor the teeth permanently due to its ability to form complexes with calcium of dentin.

Classification (Lordon and Boskman)

- *First degree*: Light yellow to light gray color without banding
- *Second degree*: Darker than yellow and gray color without banding

- *Third degree*: Severe staining of dark gray or blue color with banding.

Management of Tetracycline Discoloration

- Bleaching is seen successful for yellow stains than brownish-black stains
- 30 percent H_2O_2 along with thermostatically controlled heat source is applied for superficial stains
- For deeper stains, discolored teeth are treated endodontically and then bleached from with in
- Endodontically treated teeth can also be treated by veneers or crowns.

EFFECTS OF BLEACHING AGENTS ON TOOTH AND ITS SUPPORTING STRUCTURES

Tooth Hypersensitivity

Tooth sensitivity is common side effect of external tooth bleaching. Higher incidences of tooth sensitivity (67%-78%) are seen after in office bleaching with hydrogen peroxide in combination with heat. The mechanism responsible for external tooth bleaching though is not fully established, but it has been shown that peroxide penetrated enamel, dentin and pulp. This penetration was more in restored teeth than that of intact teeth.

Effects on Enamel

Studies have shown that 10 percent carbamide peroxide significantly decreased enamel hardness. But application of fluoride showed improved remineralization after bleaching.

Effects on Dentin

Bleaching has shown to cause uniform change in color through dentin.

Effects on Pulp

Penetration of bleaching agent into pulp through enamel and dentin occur resulting in tooth sensitivity. Studies have shown that 3 percent solution of H_2O_2 can cause:
- Transient reduction in pulpal blood flow
- Occlusion of pulpal blood vessels.

Effects on Cementum

Recent studies have shown that cementum is not affected by materials used for home bleaching. But cervical resorption and external root resorption in teeth has been seen in teeth treated by intracoronal bleaching using 30 to 35 percent H_2O_2.

Effects on Restorative Materials

Application of Bleaching on Composites has Shown Following Changes

- Increased surface hardness
- Surface roughening and etching
- Decrease in tensile strength
- Increased microleakage
- No significant color change of composite material itself other than the removal of extrinsic stains around existing restoration.

Effect of Bleaching Agents on Other Materials

- No effect on gold restorations
- Microstructural changes in amalgam
- Alteration in the matrix of glass ionomers
- IRM on exposure to H_2O_2 becomes cracked and swollen
- Provisional crowns made from methyl methacrylate discolor and turn orange.

Mucosal Irritation

A high concentration of hydrogen peroxide (30–35%) is caustic to mucous membrane and may cause burns and bleaching of the gingiva. So the bleaching tray must be designed to prevent gingival exposure by use of firmly fitted tray that may have contact only with teeth.

Genotoxicity and Carcinogenicity

Hydrogen peroxide shows genotoxic effect as free radicals released from hydrogen peroxide (hydroxy radicals, perhydroxyl ions and superoxide anions) are capable of attacking DNA.

Effects of bleaching agents on tooth and its supporting structures
➡ Tooth sensitivity
➡ Alteration of enamel surface
➡ Effects on dentin
➡ Effects of bleaching on pulp
➡ Effects on cementum
➡ Effects on restorative materials
➡ Mucosal irritation
➡ Genotoxicity and carcinogenicity
➡ Toxicity.

Toxicity

The acute effects of hydrogen peroxide ingestion are dependent on the amount and the concentration of hydrogen peroxide solution ingested. The effects are more severe, when higher concentrations are used.

Signs and symptoms usually seen are ulceration of the buccal mucosa, esophagus and stomach, nausea, vomiting, abdominal distention and sore throat. It is therefore important to keep syringes with bleaching agents out of reach of children to prevent any possible accident.

Bleaching is safe, economical, conservative and effective method of decoloring the stained teeth due to various reasons.

It should always be given a thought before going for more invasive procedure like veneering or full ceramic coverage, depending upon specific case.

Advantages of bleaching	Disadvantages of bleaching
• Noninvasive approach for tooth whitening • Immediate effect • In multitreatment approach, shade of veneer/crown selected can be much lighter than required.	• Tooth sensitivity • Expensive • Unpredictable • Long duration of treatment. • Root resorption in nonvital teeth

Key Points

- Color of healthy teeth is determined by the color of dentin and is modified by color, thickness and translucency of enamel.
- Normal color of primary teeth is bluish white whereas color of permanent teeth is grayish yellow, grayish white or yellowish white.
- Bleaching is a procedure which involves lightening of the color of a tooth through the application of a chemical agent to oxidize the organic pigmentation in the tooth.
- Tooth bleaching today is based upon hydrogen peroxide as an active agent. Hydrogen peroxide may be applied directly or produced in a chemical reaction from sodium perborate or carbamide peroxide.
- Hydrogen peroxide acts as a strong oxidizing agent through the formation of free radicals, reactive oxygen molecules and hydrogen peroxide anions. These reactive molecules attack the long chained, dark colored chromophore molecules and split them into smaller, less colored and more diffusible molecules.
- The outcome of bleaching procedure depends mainly on the concentration of bleaching agents, the ability of the agents to reach the chromophore molecules and the duration and number of times the agent is in contact with chromophore molecules.
- Commonly used solution for night guard bleaching are 10 percent carbamide peroxide with or without carbopol, 15 percent carbamide peroxide and hydrogen peroxide (1–10%).
- Microbrasion is a procedure in which a microscopic layer of enamel is simultaneously eroded and abraded with a special compound (usually contains 18% of hydrochloric acid) leaving a perfectly intact enamel surface behind.
- Laser bleaching gel contains thermally absorbed crystals, fumed silica and 35 percent H_2O_2. In this, gel is applied and is activated by light source which in further activates the crystals present in gel, allowing dissociation of oxygen and therefore better penetration into enamel matrix.
- Lasers used for tooth bleaching are argon laser, CO_2 laser and GaAlAs diode laser.

QUESTIONS

1. How will you bleach a nonvital 11 which has history of trauma five years back?
2. Write short notes on:
    a. Thermocatalytic technique of bleaching for nonvital teeth
    b. Walking bleach technique
    c. Mechanism of bleaching
    d. Side effects of bleaching
    e. Composition of McInnes solution.
3. Explain about in-office bleaching technique.
4. What are ideal properties of bleaching materials? Mention about various constituents of the bleaching material.
5. What are various factors affection bleaching process?

BIBLIOGRAPHY

1. Abou-Rass M. The elimination of tetracycline discoloration by intentional endodontics and internal bleaching. J Endod. 1982;8:101-6.
2. Arens D. The role of bleaching in esthetics. Dent Clin North Am. 1989;33:319-36.
3. Ari H, Ungor M. In vitro comparison of different types of sodium perborate used for intracoronal bleaching of discolored teeth. Int Endod J. 2002;35:433-6.
4. Attin T, Paque F, Ajam F, Lennon AM. Review of the current status of tooth whitening with the walking bleach technique. Int Endod J. 2003;36:313-29.

5. Croll TP. Enamel microabrasion for removal of superficial dysmineralization and decalcification defects. J Am Dent Assoc. 1990;120:411-5.

6. Davis MC, Walton RE, Rivera EM. Sealer distribution in coronal dentin. J Endod. 2002;28:464-6.

7. Dishman MV, Covey DA, Baughan LW. The e¡ects of peroxide bleaching on compos¬ite to enamel bond strength. Dent Mat. 1994;9:3--6.

8. Glockner K, Hulla H, Ebeleseder K, Stadler P. Five-year folllow-up of internal bleach¬ing. Braz Dent J. 1999;10:105-10.

9. Kaneko J, Inoue S, Kawakami S, Sano H. Bleaching effect of sodium percarbonate on discolored pulpless teeth in vitro. J Endod. 2000;26:25-8.

10. Kim ST, Abbot PV, McGinley P. The effects of Ledermix paste on discolouration of mature teeth. Int Endod J. 2000;33:227-32.

11. Rostein I. Tooth discoloration and bleaching. In: Ingle JI, Bakland LK, eds. Endodontics. 5th ed. Hamilton, Ontario, Canada: BC Decker Inc. 2002:845-60.

12. Rotstein I, Mor C, Friedman S. Prognosis of intracoronal bleaching with sodium perborate preparations in vitro: 1-year study. J Endod. 1993;19:10-2.

13. Seghi RR, Denry I. Effect of external bleaching on indentation and abrasion characteristics of human enamel in vitro. J Dent Res. 1992;7:1340-4.

14. Smith JJ, Cunningham CJ, Montgomery S. Cervical canal leakage after internal bleaching procedures. J Endod. 1992;18:476-81.

15. StewartGG.Bleachingdiscolouredpulplessteeth.J Am Dent Assoc. 1965;70:325-8.

16. Teixeira EC, Hara AT, Serra MC. Use of 37% carbamide peroxide in the walking bleach technique: a case report. Quintessence Int. 2004;35:97-102.

17. Titley KC, Torneck CD, Smith DC, Applebaum NB. Adhesion of a glass ionomer cement to bleached and unbleached bovine dentin. Endod Dent Traumatol. 1989;5:132-8.

18. van der Burgt TP, Eronat C, Plaesschaert AJM. Staining patterns in teeth discolored by endodontic sealers. J Endod. 1986;12:187-91.

19. Vogel RI. Intrinsic and extrinsic discoloration of the dentition. J Oral Med. 1975;30:99-104.

20. Watts A, Addy M. Tooth discoloration and staining: a review of the literature. Br Dent J. 2001;190:309-16.

21. Westlake A. Bleaching teeth by electricity. Am J Dent Sci. 1895;29:101.

Minimally Intervention Dentistry

Chapter Outline

- Early Diagnosis
- New Caries Classification Based on Site and Size of Lesion
- Assessment of Individual Caries Risk
  (High, Moderate, Low)
- Decreasing the Risk of Further Demineralization and Arresting
  Active Lesion
- Remineralization of Initial Lesions and Reduction in Cariogenic
  Bacteria

- Bioactive Glasses—NovaMin
- Recaldent (CPP-ACP)
- Minimal Intervention of Cavitated Lesions
  - Dental Materials Used for Minimally Invasive Treatment
  - Minimally Invasive Treatment Options for Cavitated Lesions
- Repair Instead of Replacement of the Restoration
- Disease Control

INTRODUCTION

The "extension for prevention" approach to dental disease management, with GV Black's tooth preparation designs has been the basis of 20th century dentistry.

GV Black published lots of papers on tooth preparation and restoration techniques between 1869 and 1915. Conventional design of the tooth preparation include a self-cleansing outline form, resistance form, retention form, convenience form, removal of caries and finish of the enamel walls, margins. Till the middle of the 19th century, the exact etiology of dental caries was not known. Tooth preparations were designed without specifications. Materials used at that time had little standardization which resulted in their poor performance. Black advised the placement of the cavosurfaces in "self-cleansable areas". This led to the term "extension for prevention," which could be summarized as "the removal of the enamel margin by cutting from a point of greater liability to a point of lesser liability to recurrence of caries". But this traditional restorative approach does not help in management of complex restorative challenges in older patients like erosion, abrasion, demineralization, rampant caries, sound and decayed retained roots, recurrent caries, etc. Black recommended the removal of the entire pits and fissures and the placement of an amalgam regardless of the size of the carious lesion. Rationale for removal of the pits and fissures was prevention of future caries.

The major advancement which is associated with bonding has greatest impact on MID. In 1955, Buonocore described etching of enamel surfaces to make it retentive for a restoration. In 1962, Bowen introduced Bis-GMA. These two developments led to the creation of tooth conservation or minimally invasive surgical dentistry.

> Minimum intervention dentistry is defined as a philosophy of professional care which deals with the first occurrence, earliest detection and earliest cure of the disease on microlevels, followed by minimally invasive treatment to repair irreversible damage caused by that disease (**Fig. 28.1**).

Based on minimal intervention theory, caries is an infectious microbial disease resulting in dissolution of calcified tissues of teeth. Caries starts with imbalance between remineralization and demineralization on the tooth surface and progresses into initial reversible lesion (noncavitated) and later as irreversible lesion (cavitated) along with loss of tooth structure, esthetics, masticatory function, phonetic and biological functions. The period of transition from a reversible lesion to a cavitated one depends on its location on the tooth.

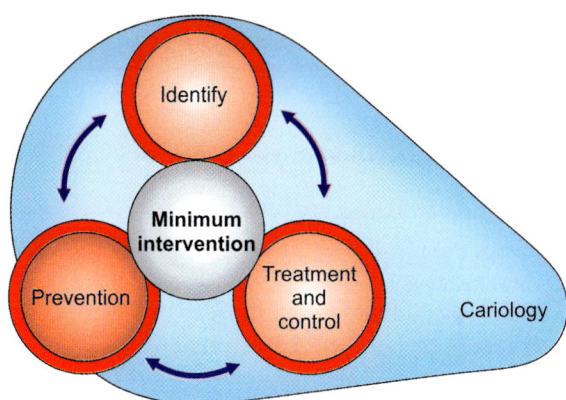

Figure 28.1: Concept of MID

Concepts of minimally intervention dentistry (given by Tyas et al)
→ Early caries diagnosis
→ Classification of caries depth and progression
→ Assessment of individual caries risk (high, moderate, low)
→ Reduction in cariogenic bacteria to eliminate the risk of further demineralization and cavitation and arresting of active lesions
→ Remineralization of early lesions
→ Minimal surgical intervention of caries lesions
→ Repair rather than the replacement of defective restorations
→ Assessing disease management outcomes at intervals.

EARLY DIAGNOSIS

The goal of minimally intervention dentistry is to halt the disease first and then to restore lost structure and function. To achieve this goal, an accurate diagnosis of the disease is mandatory. It is important to note that caries activity cannot be determined at one stage only, it has to be monitored over the time by taking radiographs and clinical checkups. Recent developments in technologies like electrical conductance methods, quantitative laser fluorescence, laser fluorescence, tuned aperture computed tomography and optical coherence tomography have helped in early diagnosis of the lesion. For complete diagnosis along with detection of the carious lesion one should also assess the caries activity which may be even more important.

NEW CARIES CLASSIFICATION BASED ON SITE AND SIZE OF LESION

Because of importance of site and size of carious lesions for treatment, Mount et al gave a new classification of dental

caries by combining both site and size of the lesion (**Fig. 28.2**). The basis of classification system given by Mount and Hume is that it is only essential to make entry into the lesions and remove infected areas which are infected and broken down to an extent where remineralization is not possible.

Firstly, lesions are classified according to their location:
- *Site 1:* Pits and fissures
- *Site 2:* Contact area between two teeth
- *Site 3:* Cervical area in contact with gingival tissues.

Secondly, the classification identifies carious lesions according to various sizes:
- *Size 0:* Carious lesion without cavitation, can be remineralized.
- *Size 1:* Small cavitation, just beyond healing through remineralization.
- *Size 2:* Moderate cavitation not extended to cusps.
- *Size 3:* Enlarged cavitation with at least one cusp which is undermined and which needs protection from occlusal load.
- *Size 4:* Extensive decay with atleast one lost cusp or incisal edge.

Difference between caries classification given by GV black and G mount	
GV Black classification	*MI classification of G Mount (1997)*
→ Provision of specifications for preconceived preparation designs for amalgam.	• Direct recommendation for appropriate treatment according to classification code
→ Preparation designs do not take extent of active caries into various tooth tisssues.	• Considers both site as well as size of the carious lesion.

Size / Site	Minimal 1	Moderate 2	Enlarged 3	Extensive 4
Pit/fissure 1	1.1	1.2	1.3	1.4
Contact area 2	2.1	2.2	2.3	2.4
Cervical 3	3.1	3.2	3.3	3.4

Figure 28.2: Mount and Hume classification combining both size and site of the carious lesion

This classification shows the differences in caries progression in different locations and sizes of decay and thus helps in guiding for the treatment of new carious lesions, especially for monitoring and intervention purposes.

Minimally invasive procedure mandates that "leave the groove intact unless there is caries on the surface, even if it is stained". If the groove is intact, it can be sealed at the end of the procedure. For treatment of proximal caries, conservative "slot" preparation can be made instead of design given by Black, which requires that the margins be brought into a cleansable area of the interproximal embrasure.

The teeth, requiring replacement of a cusp can be restored using indirect composite or porcelain restorations. These large, indirect esthetic restorations can be prepared with minimal destruction of additional sound tooth structure. These restorations can be fabricated using either indirect laboratory techniques or using computer aided design and computer-assisted manufacturing (CAD/CAM).

The philosophy of minimal surgical intervention also involves anterior esthetic procedures (e.g. diastema closure) rather than aggressively preparing the tooth for a porcelain laminate or full coverage porcelain crown.

ASSESSMENT OF INDIVIDUAL CARIES RISK (HIGH, MODERATE, LOW)

Assessment of individual caries risk is one of the important tool which helps the clinician to make a treatment plan for each individual. In caries risk assessment, one identifies the children/patients who are at higher risk for dental caries and thus require more dental care than the individuals with low or moderate caries risk.

While assessing the caries risk for an individual, clinician should identify some risk factors which have contributory effect on dental disease.

Following factors are commonly seen in patients with high risk caries
→ Status of oral hygiene
♦ Poor oral hygiene
♦ Nonfluoridated toothpaste
♦ Low frequency of tooth cleaning
♦ Orthodontic treatment
♦ Partial dentures
→ Dental history
♦ History of multiple restorations
♦ Frequent replacement of restorations
→ Medical factors
♦ Medications causing xerostomia
♦ Gastric reflux
♦ Sugar containing medication
♦ Sjögren's syndrome
→ Behavioral factors
♦ Bottle feeding at night
♦ Eating disorders
♦ Frequent intake of snacks
♦ More intake of sticky foods
→ Socioeconomic factors
♦ Low education status
♦ Poverty
♦ No fluoride supplement.

DECREASING THE RISK OF FURTHER DEMINERALIZATION AND ARRESTING ACTIVE LESION

According to minimal invasive dentistry, one should employ the use of chemicals and other medicaments which can reduce the rate of progress of tooth demineralization. These agents can also help in remineralization of affected dentin which is left behind after removal of infected dentin (**Figs 28.3A to C**). Application of fluorides has also shown to arrest the existing carious lesion.

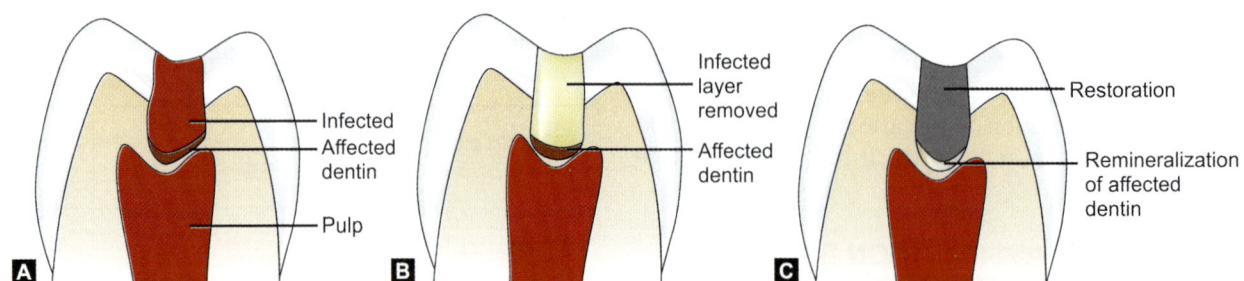

Figures 28.3A to C: Remineralization of affected dentin and arresting carious progression: (A) Tooth with deep caries in close proximity to pulp; (B) Removal of infected dentin and leaving behind affected dentin for remineralization; (C) Remineralization of affected dentin and protective restoration of tooth

REMINERALIZATION OF INITIAL LESIONS AND REDUCTION IN CARIOGENIC BACTERIA (FIGS 28.4 AND 28.5)

Dental caries pass through the series of demineralization and remineralization cycles depending on the microenvironment. When the pH is less than 5.5, demineralization occurs. Presence of fluoride enhances the uptake of calcium and phosphate ions and makes the tooth more resistant to demineralization. It has been shown in many studies that a noncavitated lesion can be made reversible. But once cavitation occurs, caries removal and restoration is indicated.

In the noncavitated lesion, one should always try to remineralize the tooth by

- Decreasing the frequency of intake of refined carbohydrates
- Following plaque control measures
- Ensuring optimum salivary flow
- Patient education
- Application of chlorhexidine as an antimicrobial which acts by reducing the number of cariogenic bacteria
- Application of topical fluorides.

Commonly used agent for remineralization of teeth is fluorides, though some new materials have also been introduced in dentistry in an attempt to remineralize the teeth. These are:

- Bioactive glasses—NovaMin
- Recaldent (CPP-ACP).

Bioactive Glasses—NovaMin (Fig. 28.6)

It was introduced in 1969 by Hench. It contains calcium sodium phosphosilicate. On coming in contact with water, NovaMin releases active calcium and phosphorus ions resulting in remineralization. Sodium present in NovaMin increases the pH of oral cavity, this further enhances remineralization since precipitation of crystals occur on teeth at pH $\geq$ 7. A minimum of 40 to 50 minutes of exposure time is required for remineralization to occur, so the person using NovaMin dentifrice should be refrained from rinsing, drinking or eating after toothbrushing.

Recaldent (CPP-ACP)

CPP-ACP is acronym for a complex of casein phosphopeptides and amorphous calcium phosphate. CPPs are

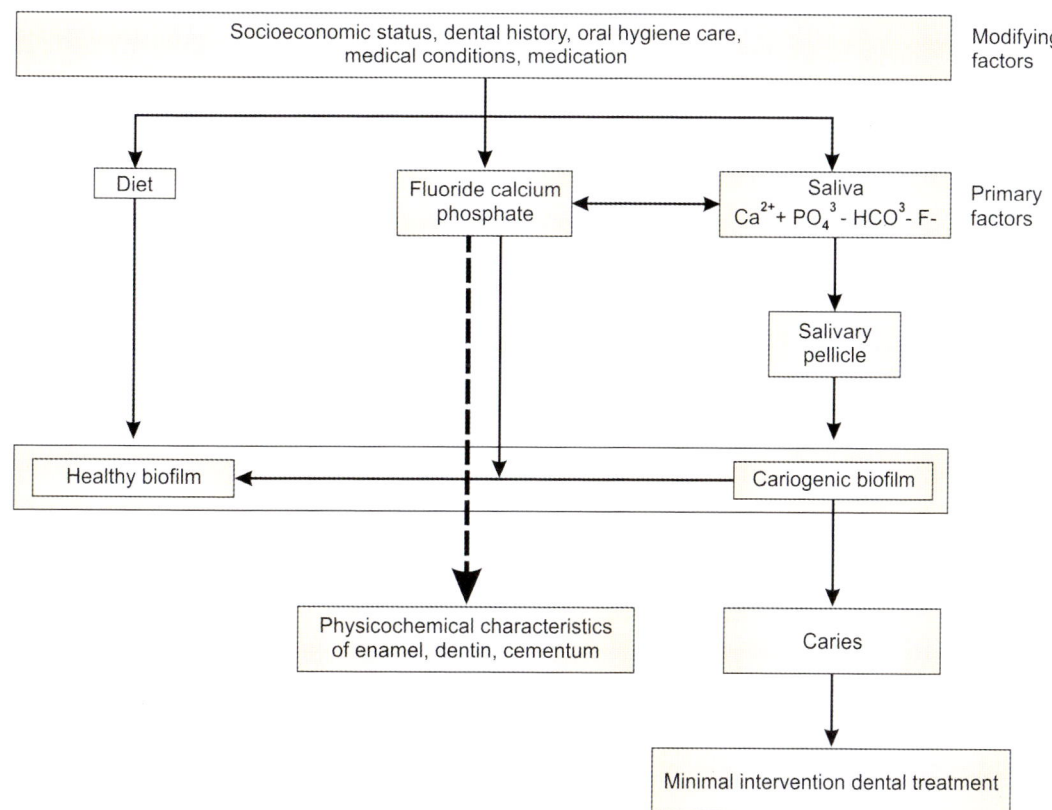

Figure 28.4: Factors affecting tooth demineralization, remineralization and treatment planning

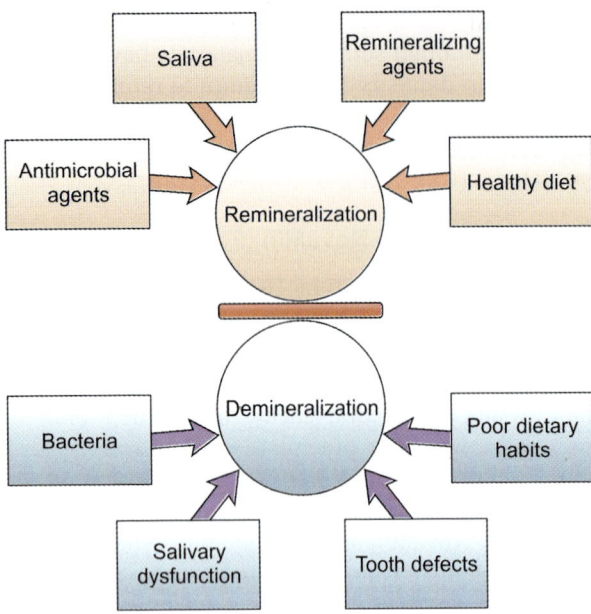

Figure 28.5: Factors affecting remineralization and demineralization of teeth

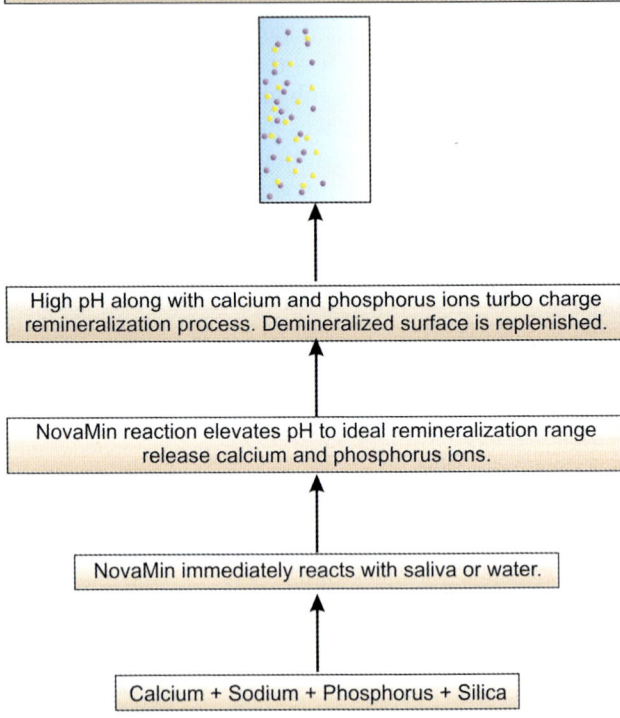

Figure 28.6: Mechanism of action of NovaMin

group of peptides derived from casein. Casein is the part of protein which naturally occurs in milk, CPP is responsible for high availability of Ca^{2+} from milk. In normal state calcium phosphate forms a crystalline structure at neutral pH and thus becomes insoluble. But CPP keeps calcium and phosphorus in ionic form (amorphous state). In this state, calcium and phosphate ions can enter the tooth enamel and thus promote remineralization of tooth.

CPP-ACP technology has been trademarked as; RECALDENT™. It is available as chewing gum. Recently, a sugar-free, water based creme containing RECALDENT™ (CPP-ACP) has been made available under the name GC tooth mousse (**Fig. 28.7**).

MINIMAL INTERVENTION OF CAVITATED LESIONS

One should try to preserve maximum of natural tooth structure whether preparing for the smallest or the largest carious lesion. The tooth preparation design and selection of dental material depend on occlusal load and wear factors. Nowadays, classification of tooth preparation designs given by Mount and Hume is followed rather than as given by GV Black. In earlier days, tooth preparations were made when caries were diagnosed at an advanced state rather than the incipient lesions which are commonly detected these days. Moreover earlier the choice of restorative materials was amalgam, which has been replaced nowadays by adhesive materials. Other factor is instrumentation, which was mainly slow rotary instrumentation and use of hand instruments. Now it is high-speed rotary, modifications in bur design and other techniques which cause minimal removal of tooth structure (**Figs 28.8 and 28.9**)

Dental Materials Used for Minimally Invasive Treatment

Introduction of adhesive materials have played a major role in minimally intervention dentistry because they do not require the incorporation of mechanical retention features. Various adhesive restorations are glass ionomer cements, resin-based composites, dentin bonding agents and combination of composites and GICs.

Glass Ionomer Cement (Fig. 28.10)

Glass ionomer cement has various advantages like chemical adhesion to tooth structure, esthetics and anticariogenicity. Added advantage of glass ionomer cement is that set cement is "rechargeable". This means it can take up fluoride from the environment, which is provided by exposure to fluoride treatments and tooth-paste. Disadvantages of glass ionomer cement include technique sensitivity. Recently resin modified glass ionomer cements have been introduced which are easier to place, light cured and have improved esthetic qualities (**Fig. 28.11**).

Composites Resins (Fig. 28.12)

These materials show effective bonding to enamel and dentin. In these, tooth preparations are designed to conserve maximum tooth structure because these materials adhere to tooth via micromechanical retention achieved by etching enamel and dentin and formation of a hybrid layer. Newer flowable resin based composites have low viscosity and are commonly used for smaller, preventive resin type preparations, along with class V preparations.

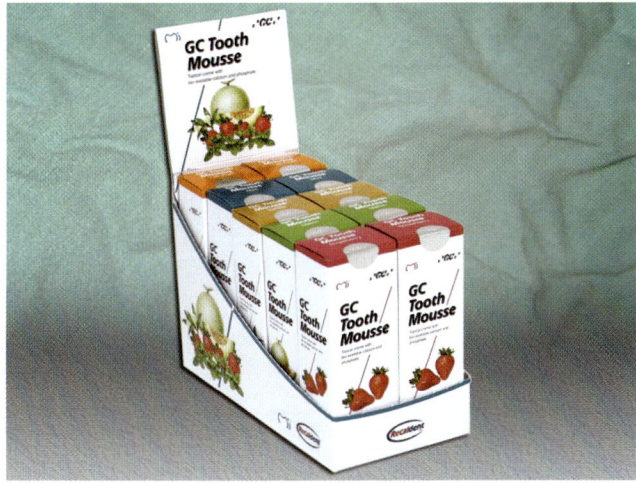

Figure 28.7: GC tooth mousse for remineralization of teeth

Minimally invasive treatment options for cavitated lesions

- Atraumatic restorative technique.
- Sandwich technique.
- Chemomechanical caries removal (CMCR).
- Pit and fissure sealants and preventive resin restorations.
- Tunnel, box and slot preparation.
- Tooth preparation using air abrasion.
- Tooth preparation using lasers.

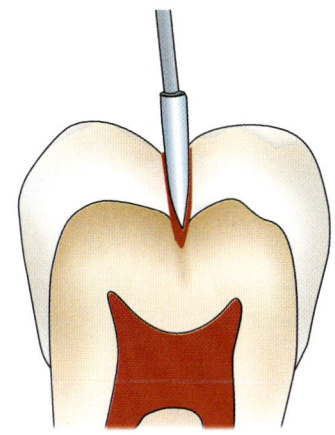

Figure 28.8: Conservative tooth preparation using tapered diamond abrasive

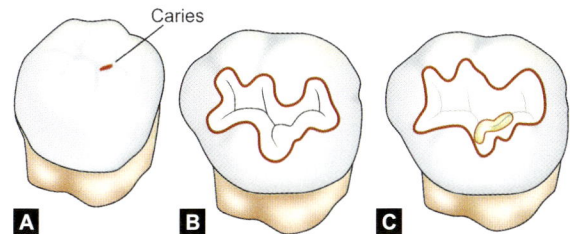

Figures 28.9A to C: (A) Caries; (B) Conventional tooth preparation; (C) Minimal intervention preparation

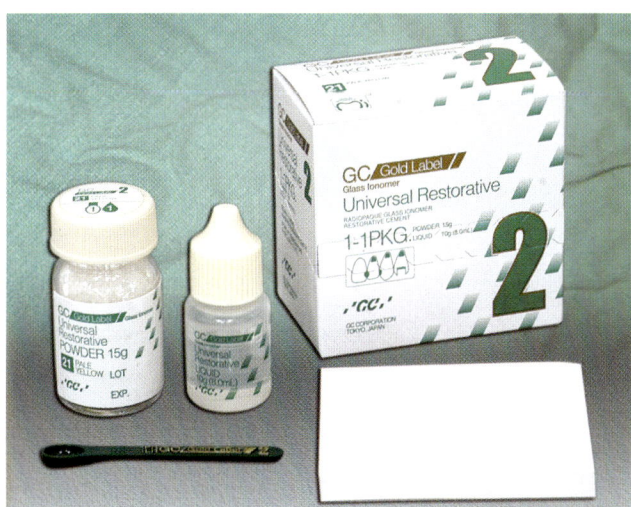

Figure 28.10: Conservative tooth preparation and restoration with glass ionomer cement

Minimally Invasive Treatment Options for Cavitated Lesions

Atraumatic Restorative Technique

Atraumatic restorative technique (ART) was pioneered in mid-1980s in Zimbabwe and Tanzania in the need for basic treatment of carious teeth in communities with limited resources. In this excavation of caries is done using hand instruments and then tooth is restored using glass ionomer cement, an adhesive material (**Figs 28.13A to C**).

Sandwich Technique

This technique was given by McLean in 1985. It takes the advantage of the physical properties of both GIC and composite resins. This technique is especially useful in situations when strength and pleasing esthetics are essential. In this, first the tooth is restored with GIC because of its chemical adhesion to dentin and fluoride release. Over it, composite resin is placed so as to have better occlusal wear and esthetics (**Figs 28.14 and 28.15**).

Composite resin bonds micromechanically to set glass ionomers and chemically to hydroxyethylmethacrylate in resin modified glass ionomers. If a composite restoration is to be done over a conventional glass ionomer, then both glass ionomer and enamel are etched before placing bonding agent and composite resin. But if composite is being placed over a resin modified glass ionomer, then it is not compulsory to etch the resin-modified glass ionomer, due to chemical HEMA bond.

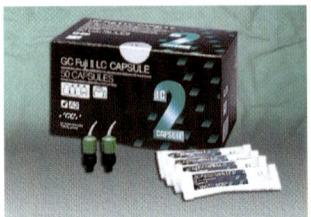
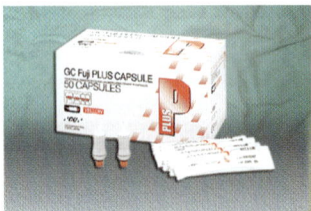
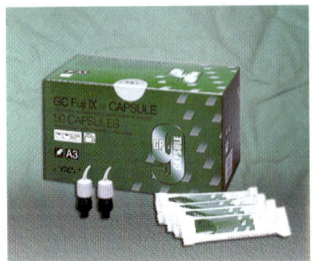
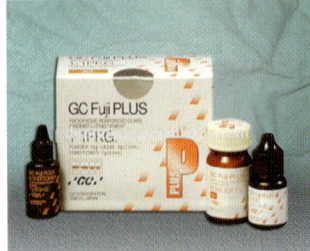

Figure 28.11: Light cure GICs are easier to place and have improved esthetic qualities

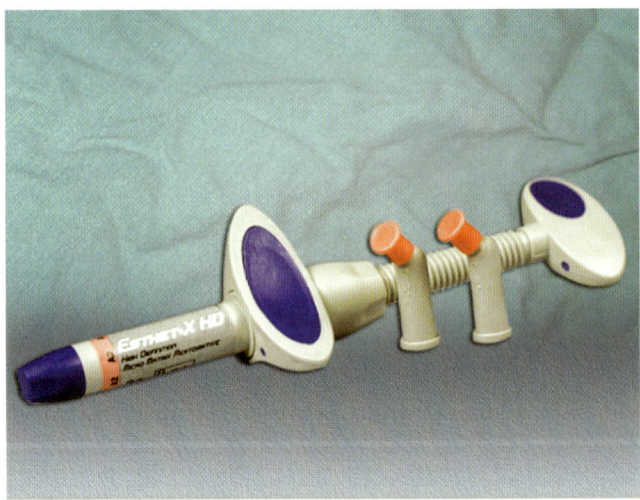

Figure 28.12: Composite resin

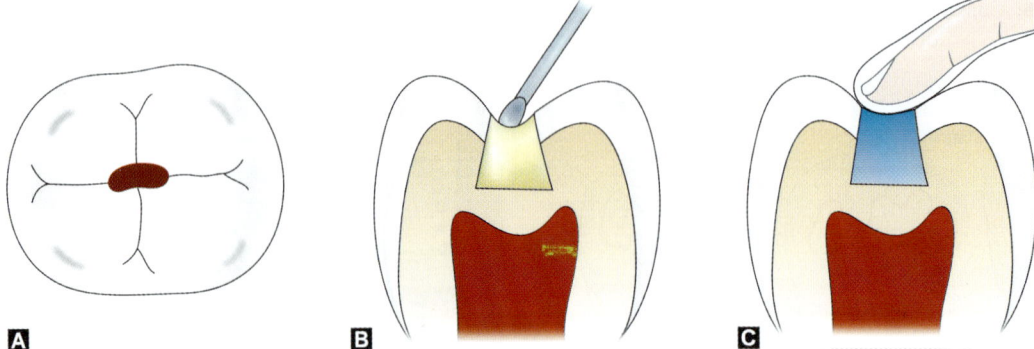

Figures 28.13A to C: The ART technique of tooth restoration (A) Carious lesion in posterior tooth; (B) Excavation of caries using hand instruments; (C) Restoration of tooth using glass ionomer cement

Chemomechanical Caries Removal

Chemomechanical caries removal (CMCR) involves the selective removal of carious dentin. Reagents commonly available in market are Caridex and Carisolv.

Caridex consists ot two solutions viz; Solution I containing sodium hypochlorite and Solution II containing glycine, aminobutyric acid, sodium chloride and sodium hydroxide.

The two solutions are mixed immediately before use. The solution is applied to the carious lesion by means of applicator. Application is done until the sound dentin appears. Carisolv is available in two syringes, one containing the sodium hypochlorite and other a pink viscous gel consisting of lysine, leucine and glutamic acid amino acids, together with carboxymethylcellulose to make it viscous and erythrocin to make it readily visible in use.

The contents of the two syringes are mixed together immediately before use. The gel is applied to the carious lesion with hand instruments and after 30 seconds, carious dentin can be gently removed.

Pit and Fissure Sealants and Preventive Resin Restorations

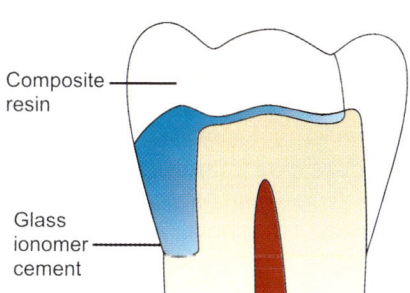

Figure 28.14: Sandwich technique

For occlusal surface, preparation in minimally intervention dentistry includes placement of pit and fissure sealants and preventive resin restorations. A fissure sealant is a material which is placed in pits and fissures of teeth so as to prevent or arrest the development of caries. Plaque accumulation and caries susceptibility is greatest during eruption of teeth and deep pits and fissures are vulnerable to caries attack. Thus, a fissure sealant should be placed as soon as possible after tooth eruption.

Materials used for pit and fissure sealants are composite resins, glass ionomer cement, compomers and fluorides releasing sealants.

Preventive resin restorations are placed in teeth with the rationale that placement of a resin sealant isolates the carious lesion from the surface biofilm. But use of preventive resin restorations should be limited to fissures where lesion is confined to enamel and that dentin lesions should not be restored using minimally invasive technique.

Tunnel, Box and Slot Preparation

For proximal lesions, modified preparation designs include tunnel, box or slot preparations.

Tunnel and slot preparations are conservative preparations in which slot preparation is indicated for lesions which are less than 2.5 mm from the marginal ridge whereas if the lesion is more than 2.5 mm from the marginal ridge, a tunnel preparation is indicated.

In the tunnel preparation, access to carious lesion is made from the occlusal surface, while preserving the marginal ridge. Entry point for these preparations should not be under occlusal load. For tooth preparation, small tapered bur with long shank is directed at the lesion and the preparation is completed using small round burs and hand instruments.

For tunnel preparation, we preserve the marginal ridge and the proximal surface enamel (**Fig. 28.16**). Whereas in box or slot preparations, there is removal of the marginal ridge, but the preparation does not include the occlusal

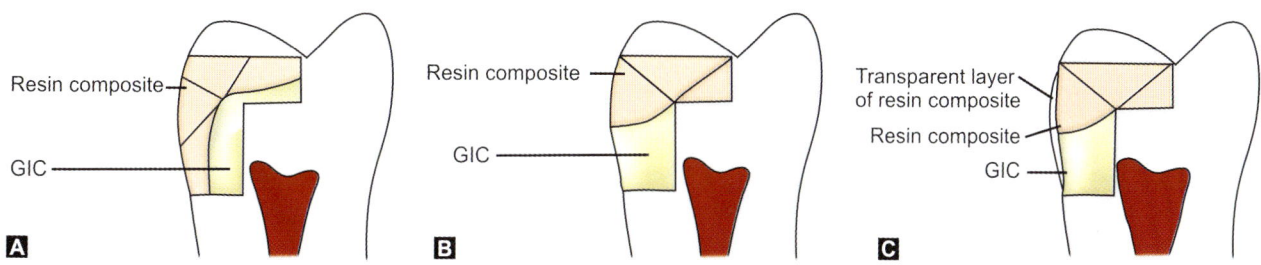

Figures 28.15A to C: (A) Closed sandwich technique; (B) Open sandwich technique; (C) Centripetal sandwich technique

pits and fissures if caries removal in these areas is not required (**Fig. 28.17**).

Tooth Preparations Using Air Abrasion

In this technique, kinetic energy is used to remove carious lesion. Here powerful fine stream of moving aluminum oxide particles is directed against the surface to be removed. The abrasive particles hit the tooth with high velocity and a small amount of tooth structure is removed. Commonly used particle sizes are either 27 or 50 micrometers in diameter. The speed of the abrasive particles when they hit the target depends upon air pressure, size of particles, powder flow, nozzle diameter, the angle of the tip and the distance of tip from the tooth. Usually the distance from the tooth ranges from 0.5 to 2 millimeters. As the distance increases, the cutting efficiency decreases. An added advantage is that tooth preparations achieved using air abrasion show rounded internal contours when compared with those prepared with a handpiece and straight burs. Air abrasion is not indicated in patients with dust allergy, asthma, chronic obstructive lung disease, open wounds, advanced periodontal disease, fresh extractions and recent placement of orthodontic appliances.

Tooth Preparation Using Lasers (Fig. 28.18)

Commonly used lasers for tooth preparation are erbium: yttrium-aluminum-garnet lasers and erbium, chromium: yttrium-scandium-gallium-garnet lasers. These lasers can remove soft caries as well as hard tissue. Lasers have shown to remove caries selectively while leaving the sound enamel and dentin. They can be used without application of local anesthetics. Other advantages include no vibration, little noise, no smell and tooth preparation almost similar to that prepared by using air abrasion technique.

REPAIR INSTEAD OF REPLACEMENT OF THE RESTORATION

Old restorations are replaced instead of being repaired when there is presence of secondary caries, fracture of restoration or failure of existing restoration. But it has been seen that repairing defective restorations rather than replacing them is a more conservative option for treatment if indicated. The decision to repair rather than replace a restoration should be based on the patient's risk of developing caries, the professional's judgment of advantages vs. risks and conservative principles of tooth preparation.

When treating an old restoration, one should consider the following options before performing their replacement
➡ Recontour and/or polish
➡ Seal margins
➡ Repair local defect
➡ Replace restoration.

Restoration is indicated for replacement when any of following occurs
➡ Secondary caries which cannot be removed during repair procedure
➡ Need for esthetics
➡ Presence of pulpal pathology.

DISEASE CONTROL

We know that dental caries is an infectious disease. Different efforts which must be made in order to decrease the incidence of caries include identification and monitoring of bacterias, diet analysis and modification, use of topical fluorides and antimicrobial agents. For caries control, caries vaccines and bacterial replacement therapy have also come up in the show.

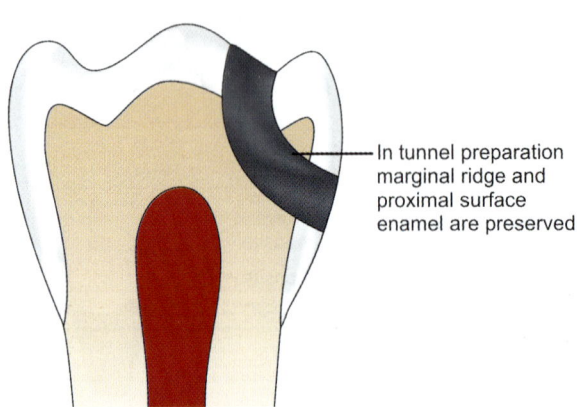

Figure 28.16: Tunnel preparation

In tunnel preparation marginal ridge and proximal surface enamel are preserved

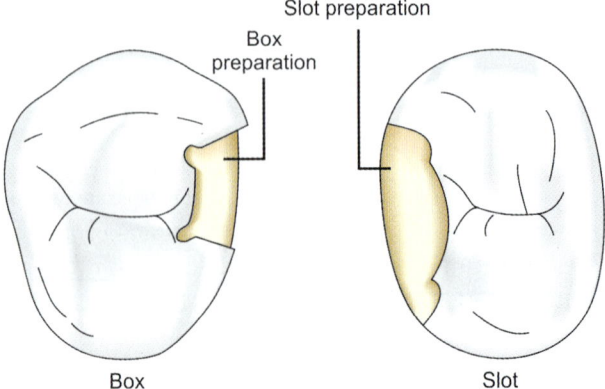

Slot preparation

Box preparation

Box

Slot

Figure 28.17: Box and slot preparation

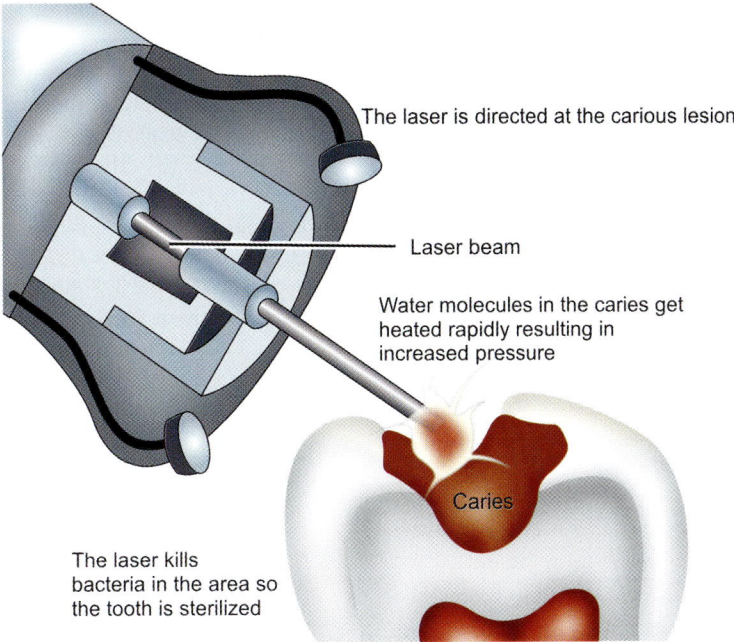

The laser is directed at the carious lesion

Laser beam

Water molecules in the caries get heated rapidly resulting in increased pressure

Caries

The laser kills bacteria in the area so the tooth is sterilized

Figure 28.18: Management of caries using LASER

Vital Pulp Therapy

In minimally intervention dentistry for deep carious lesions, vital pulp therapy is indicated which involves stepwise remineralization using biocompatible dental materials. Before initiating the treatment, clinician must determine the extent of decay and the feasibility of vital pulp therapy. Only the minimal marginal enamel is removed to gain entry into the carious lesion and remove the infected dentin.

CONCLUSION

Minimally intervention dentistry (MID) is the natural evolution of dentistry. As new materials and techniques are developed, dentistry is changed to make use of most conservative techniques. In general, the minimally intervention dentistry should fulfil following objectives of dental care which involve:

- Categorizing the patients for risk of developing dental caries depending upon existing oral health conditions.
- Applying aggressive caries preventive measures like implementation of fluoride therapy, antimicrobial therapy, diet modification and calcium supplementation to reduce the caries risk.
- Conservative use of intervention procedures.

 Key Points

- Black gave the term "extension for prevention," which means "the removal of the enamel margin by cutting from a point of greater liability to a point of lesser liability to recurrence of caries".
- The major advancement in adhesive dentistry has the greatest impact on MID. In 1955, Buonocore described etching of enamel, and in 1962, Bowen introduced Bis-GMA. These two developments showed the way to minimally invasive dentistry.
- Minimum intervention dentistry is defined as a philosophy of professional care which deals with the first occurrence, earliest detection and earliest cure of the disease on microlevels, followed by minimally invasive treatment to repair irreversible damage caused by that disease.
- Mount and Hume gave a new classification of dental caries by combining both site and size of the lesion. The basis of this classification is that it is only essential to make entry into the lesions and remove infected areas which are infected to an extent where remineralization is not possible.
- Minimally invasive procedure mandates that "leave the groove intact unless there is caries on the surface, even if it is stained".

- Agents used for remineralization of teeth are fluorides, bioactive glasses—NovaMin and Recaldent (CPP-ACP).
- Bioactive Glasses—NovaMin contains calcium sodium phosphosilicate. On coming in contact with water, NovaMin releases active calcium and phosphorus ions resulting in remineralization. Sodium increases the pH of oral cavity which further enhances remineralization.
- CPP-ACP is acronym for a complex of casein phosphopeptides and amorphous calcium phosphate. CPP keeps calcium and phosphorus in ionic form (amorphous state). In this state, calcium and phosphate ions can enter the tooth enamel and thus promote remineralization of tooth.
- Materials used for pit and fissure sealants are composite resins, glass ionomer cement, compomers and fluorides releasing sealants.
- Tunnel and slot preparations are conservative preparations in which slot preparation is indicated for lesions which are less than 2.5 mm from the marginal ridge whereas if the lesion is more than 2.5 mm from the marginal ridge, a tunnel preparation is indicated.
- Commonly used lasers for tooth preparation are erbium:yttrium-aluminum-garnet lasers and erbium, chromium:yttrium-scandium-gallium-garnet lasers These lasers can remove soft caries as well as hard tissue.

QUESTIONS

1. Write in detail about the concept of minimal intervention dentistry.
2. Write short notes on:
   a. Concepts of minimal intervention dentistry.
   b. Mount and Hume classification of caries.
   c. Minimal invasive options for carious lesions.
   d. Various tooth remineralization options.

BIBLIOGRAPHY

1. Ardu S, Perround R, Krejci I. Extended sealing of interproximal caries lesions. Quint Int. 2006;37:423.
2. Banerjee A, Watson TF. Air abrasion: its uses and abuses. Dent Update. 2002;29:340.
3. Beelay JA, Yip HK, Stevenson AG. Chemomechanical caries removal: a review of the techniques and latest developments. BDJ. 2000;188:427.
4. Christensen GJ. The advantages of minimally invasive dentistry. JADA. 2005;136:1563.
5. Ericson D. What is minimally invasive dentistry? Oral Health Prev. Dent. 2004;2:287.
6. Frencken JE, Pilot T, Songpaisan Y, et al. Atraumatic restorative treatment (ART): rationale, technique and development. J Public Health Dent. 1996;56:135.
7. Frencken JE, Songpaisan Y, Phantumvanit P, et al. An atraumatic restorative treatment (ART) technique: evolution after one year. Int Dent J. 1994;44:460.
8. Gungor K, Erten H, Akarslan ZZ, et al. Approximal carious lesion depth assessment with insight and ultra speed films. Oper Dent. 2005;30:58.
9. Hamilton JC, Gregory WA, Valentine JB. Diagnodent measurement and correlation with the depth and volume of minimally invasive cavity preparation. Oper Dent. 2006;31:291.
10. Kakaboura A, Masomas C, Staikou O, Vougiouklakis GA. Comparative clinical study on the carisoly™ caries removal method. Quint Int. 2003;34:269.
11. Latta MA, Naughton WT. Bonding and curing considerations for incipient and hidden caries. DCNA. 2005;49:889.
12. Mickenautsch S, Rudolph MJ, Oganbodede EO, et al. The impact of the ART approach on the treatment profile in a mobile dental system (MDS) in South Africa. Int Dent J. 1999;49:132.
13. Murdoch-Kinch CA, Mclean ME. Minimally Invasive Dentistry. JADA. 2003;134:87.
14. Smales RJ, Yip HK. The atraumatic restorative treatment (ART) approach for the management of dental caries. Quint Int. 2002;2:97.
15. Strand GV, Nordbu H, Leirskar J. Tunnel restoration placed in routine practice and observed for 24 to 54 months. Quint Int. 2002;2:103.
16. Whitehouse J. Minimally invasive dentistry: Clinical application. Dent Today. 2004;23:56.

29

CHAPTER

Cervical Lesions

Chapter Outline

INTRODUCTION

There are many lesions which affect the teeth apart from dental caries. Cervical lesions are those which occur because of loss of hard tooth tissue at the cemento-enamel junction. According to GV Black, these lesions may be included under class V lesions because they are found at the gingival third of the facial and lingual surfaces of anterior and posterior teeth, though they can affect mesial and distal surface also. In general, cervical lesions may occur either due to caries or other noncarious reasons which include abrasion, erosion and abfraction. Noncarious cervical lesions are etiologically and pathogenetically different from caries. Approximately 60 to 70 percent of cervical lesions fall under this category. These are usually seen as physiological changes, though may be associated with other factors like trauma, bad habits, dietary habits, etc.

CLASSIFICATION OF CERVICAL LESIONS

Classification of cervical lesion is based upon the etiology of the lesion:

- Carious cervical lesion (**Fig. 29.1**)
- Noncarious cervical lesion
  - Erosion lesions
  - Abrasion lesions
  - Abfraction lesions.

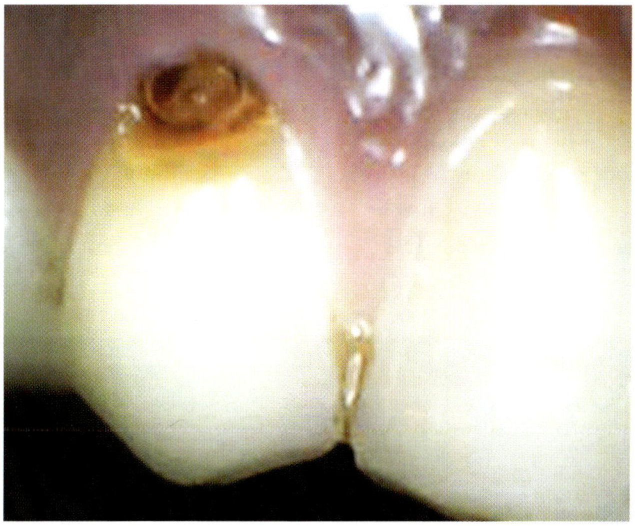

Figure 29.1: Cervical caries

CARIOUS CERVICAL LESIONS

Carious cervical lesions are smooth surface lesions which are commonly seen in patients undergoing radiation therapy for treatment of malignancy or in patients with poor oral hygiene. Root surface carious lesions are commonly seen on the root surfaces exposed to oral environment.

They usually occur at or apical to the cementoenamel junction (CEJ). Most common reason for their occurrence is gingival recession, though there may be other reasons also. Carious cervical lesion can occur independently or in areas of abrasion, erosion and abfraction. These lesions are usually seen in the region of plaque accumulation, i.e. near the gingiva or under proximal contacts.

Etiology of the carious lesion
➡ Periodontal disease
➡ Gingival recession
➡ Xerostomia
➡ Poor oral hygiene
➡ Malocclusion
➡ Abfraction lesions
➡ Tipped teeth which make areas of teeth inaccessible for cleaning
➡ Advanced age
➡ Medications that decrease the salivary flow
➡ Radiation therapy.

Clinical Features (Fig. 29.2)

- Commonly seen when there is periodontal attachment loss exposing the root surface.
- Usual site of occurrence is at or apical to the CEJ
- A cervical carious lesion can be shallow saucer shaped or deep notch shaped
- Cross section of lesion shows a 'V' shape with a wide area of origin towards enamel and the apex of 'V' facing towards pulp. Once the caries penetrate the

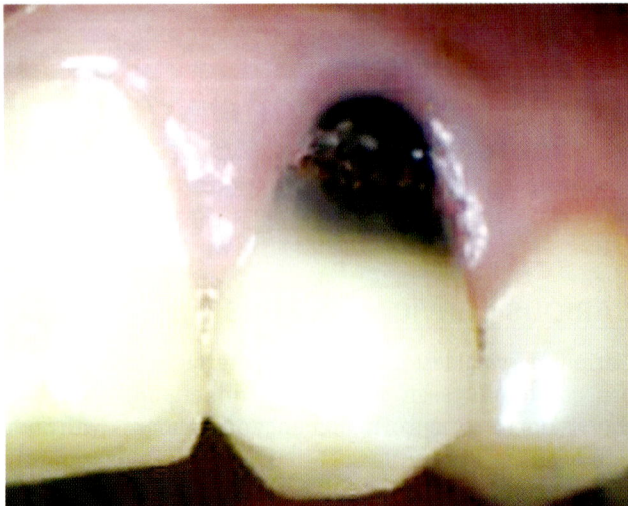

Figure 29.2: Cervical caries

dentinoenamel junction, they spread rapidly laterally and towards pulp
- More commonly seen in males than females.

Diagnosis

Diagnosis is best carried out with an explorer after cleaning the tooth surface. Radiographs can be used as adjuncts but they should be free from overlapping or burnout. (For details see chapter 5).

NONCARIOUS CERVICAL LESION

Noncarious cervical lesions are defined as any gradual loss of tooth structure characterized by the formation of smooth, polished surfaces, irrespective of their etiology. In these, loss of tooth structure occurs due to other lesions rather than caries. Noncarious cervical lesions can also be described as 'wasting disease of the teeth'. These lesions include abrasion, erosion and abfraction. These can occur pathologically, though they are seen in general associated with the aging process. These may show independently or simultaneously. These are usually seen in more than 50 percent of the population. Noncarious cervical lesions cannot be referred as inflammatory lesions or developmental abnormalities but considered as regressive alteration of the teeth. The clinical picture of these lesions can vary from shallow grooves to broad scooped out lesions, to large notched or wedge shaped defects. Improper diagnosis and thus treatment can cause continuous loss of tooth structure, dentin hypersensitivity, pulpal involvement or even the loss of tooth. The recent studies have shown improvements in the field of understanding etiology, diagnosis, treatment and prevention of these lesions.

Classification

Erosion

Definition: It is defined as a loss of tooth substance caused by a chemical process that does not involve known bacterial action. In general, erosion appears as sharply defined wedge shaped or irregular depression caused by chemicals in the cervical area usually on the facial tooth surface (**Figs 29.3 and 29.4**).

It is classified according to the source of the acid, i.e. either intrinsic or extrinsic.

Intrinsic sources of acids originate in the stomach and are associated with eating disorders, such as anorexia and bulimia nervosa, or with acid reflux and regurgitation.

Extrinsic sources are acids contained in dietary components, such as carbonated soft drinks and fruit and fruit juices.

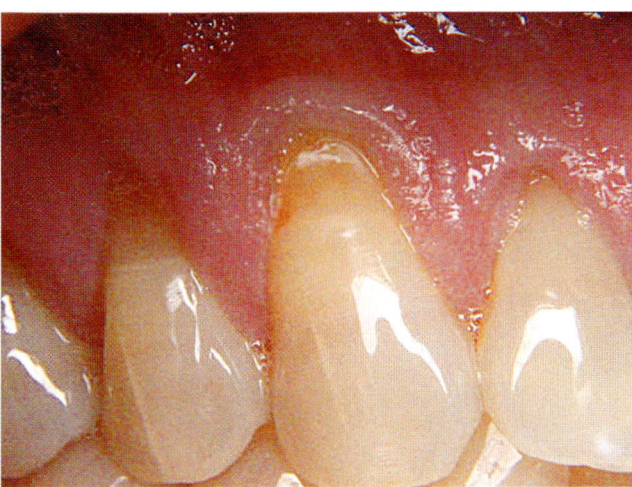

Figure 29.3: Erosion

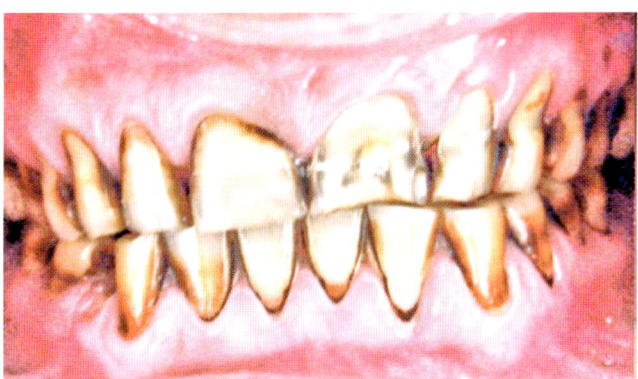

Figure 29.4: Erosion of teeth

Etiology of erosion
- *Intrinsic erosion:* It occurs due to involvement of endogenous acids, mainly due to regurgitation of gastric acid into the oral cavity. This may occur in certain conditions such as:
  - Eating disorder
    i. Anorexia nervosa
    ii. Bulimia nervosa
  - Vomiting
    i. Recurrent vomiting
    ii. Psychogenic vomiting syndrome
    iii. Drug induced vomiting
  - Pregnancy morning sickness
  - Gastrointestinal disorder
    i. Peptic ulcer
    ii. Gastroenteritis
    iii. Hiatus hernia
  - Chronic alcoholism

- *Extrinsic erosion:* Occurs due to acids from
  - Environmental origin
  - Dietary origin
  - Medicinal origin
  - Environmental erosion
    i. Professional wine tasters, battery, electroplating chemical manufacture
    ii. Swimmers
  - *Dietary origin*: High intake of
    i. Citrus fruit and juices
    ii. Carbonated beverages
    iii. Acidic fruit flavored candies
    iv. Pickled foods
  - Medicinal origin
    i. Aspirin
    ii. Vitamin C
    iii. Iron tonics
    iv. Acidic mouthwashes.

Abrasion (Fig. 29.5)

Abrasion is derived from Latin word abradere which means to scrap off. Abrasion is the loss of tooth substance through some abnormal mechanical process other than tooth contact.

Definition: It is defined as the loss of tooth substance induced by mechanical wear other than that of mastication (**Fig. 29.6**).

Etiology of abrasion: Various etiological factors are:
- Faulty oral hygiene practice
  - Horizontal brushing technique or improper brushing technique

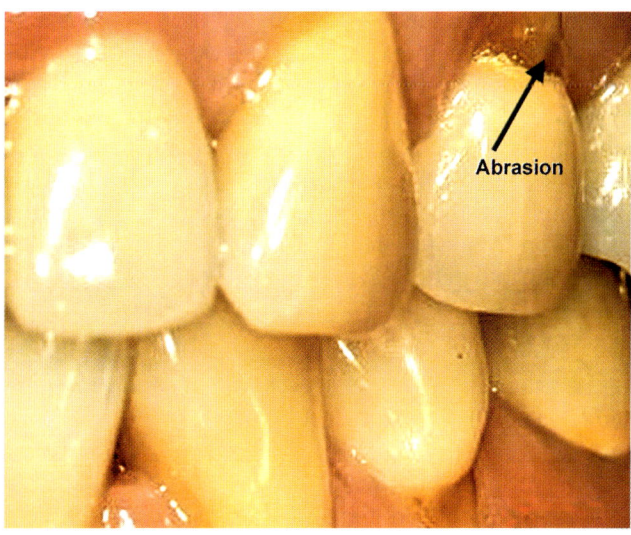

Figure 29.5: Abrasion of canine

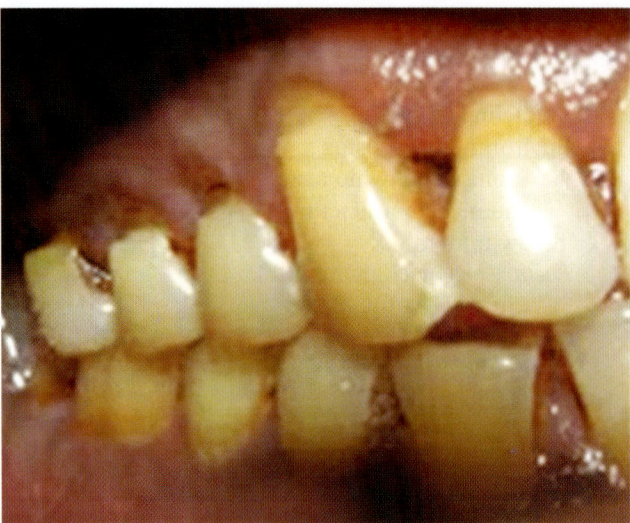

Figure 29.6: Abrasion of teeth

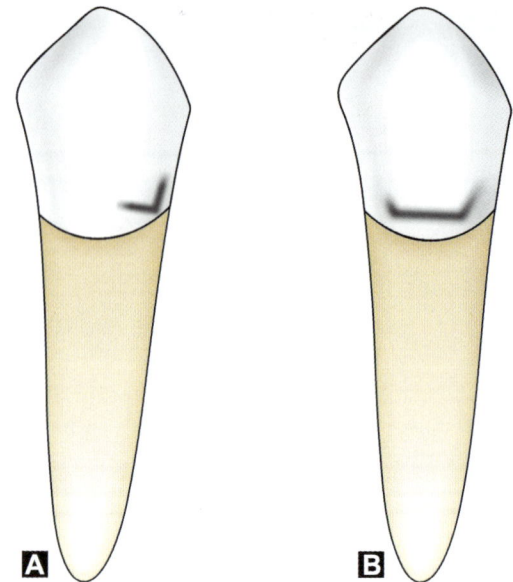

Figures 29.7A and B: Abfraction lesion is seen as wedge shaped lesion with sharp angles

- – Overzealous brushing
- – Use of toothbrush with hard bristles
- – Use of abrasive toothpaste/toothpowder
- – Excessive time, force and frequency of brushing
- – Excessive use of interproximal brushes
- Abnormal oral habits
- – Use of toothpicks
- – Finger nail biting

Abfraction Lesion

These are wedge type defects usually occur in cervical areas of tooth due to excessive occlusal stresses or parafunctional habits such as bruxism.

Abfractions are the microfractures which appear in the enamel on cervical area of tooth, and flexe under heavy loads. Abfraction lesion appears as a wedge shaped defect with sharp line angles (**Figs 29.7A and B**). In the early stages they may appear as minor irregular cracks or fracture lines or wedge shaped defects in the cervical region of the tooth. But in later stages, they appear as grooves extending into dentin (**Fig. 29.8**).

Etiology (Fig. 29.9)

In 1984, Lee and Eakle described lateral forces as the cause of the breakdown of the tooth structure. Grippo showed that the forces could be static, such as those produced by swallowing and clenching, or cyclic, those generated during chewing action. The abfractive lesions are caused by flexure and ultimate material fatigue of susceptible teeth at

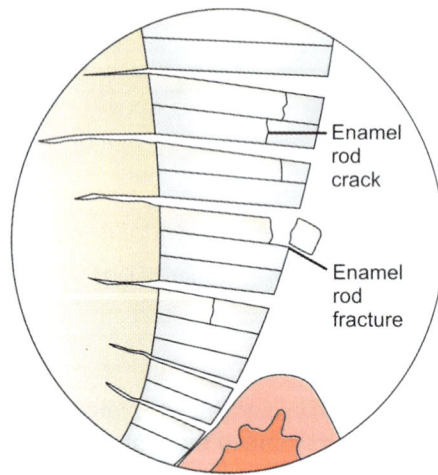

Figure 29.8: Abfraction lesions may appear as minor cracks in early stages but in latter stages they appear as grooves extending into dentin

locations away from the point of loading. The breakdown is dependent on the magnitude, duration, frequency and location of the forces.

If a tooth has an abfraction, the occlusal loading on the tooth can be tested in centric occlusion and in excursive movements with occlusal marking paper. The tooth with abfraction will show a heavy marking on one of the inclines of a cusp. This damaging lateral force produces stress lines in the tooth and results in tooth breakdown.

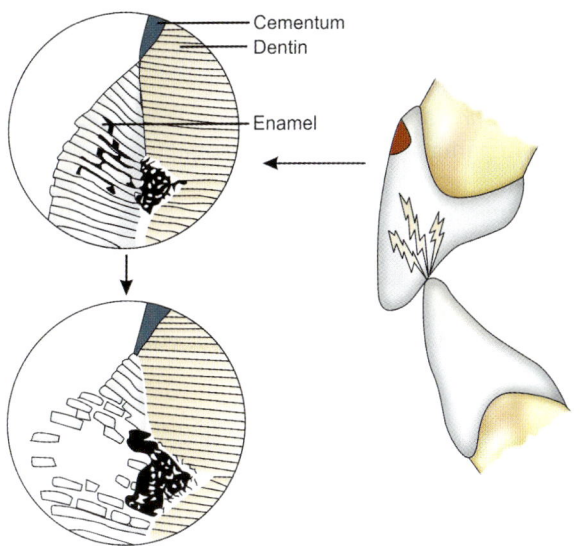

Figure 29.9: Abfraction occurs when tooth flexes under occlusal loading, resulting in microfracture of enamel and dentin

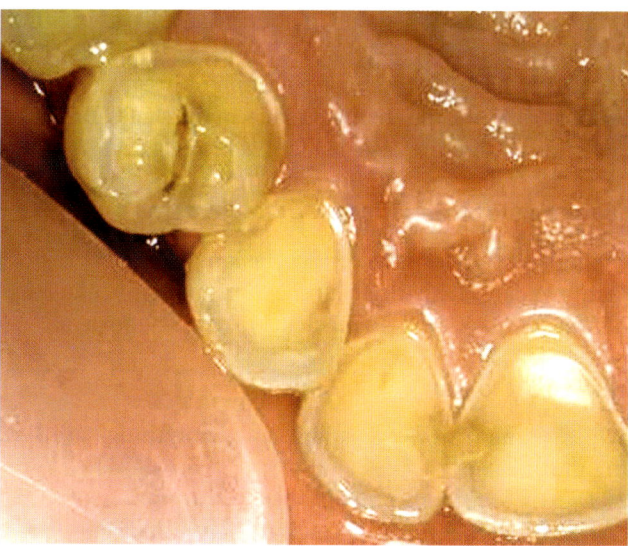

Figure 29.10: Erosion lesion shows broad, saucer shaped depression on the tooth surface

If during lateral excursions, there is cuspid rise, the loading forces of the excursive movement will be directed into the canines. Abfractions are commonly found in cases where malaligned canines cause initial lateral guidance forces to be exerted on the lingual incline of the buccal cusp of the maxillary premolar.

Clinical Features of Noncarious Cervical Lesions

Erosion (Fig. 29.10)

- Broad saucer shaped or irregular depressions in the cervical area usually on the facial tooth surface
- The surface appears smooth, hard and polished
- Commonly seen at gingival third of the labial surface of anterior teeth
- Erosive lesion is generally glazed and has no demarcation from adjacent surface
- The tooth is sensitive to chemical, physical and mechanical stimuli.

Abrasion (Figs 29.11 and 29.12)

- Abrasion results in saucer shaped or wedge shaped indentation with a smooth, shiny surface
- Commonly affected teeth are canines and premolars
- Usually occurs on the exposed root surfaces but may also occur elsewhere, such as on incisal surface in pipe smokers and tailors holding needle with anterior teeth

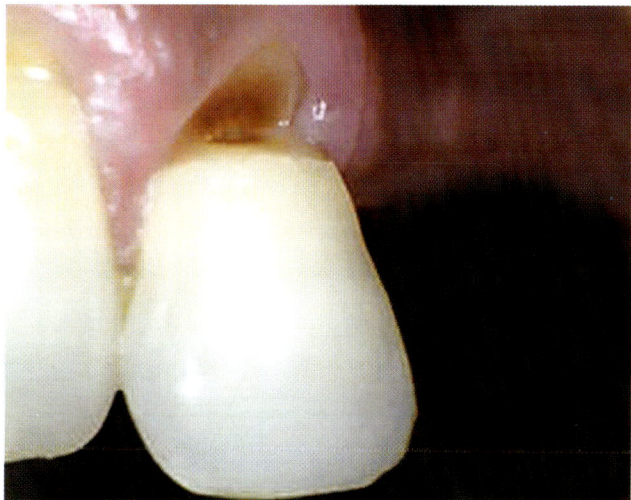

Figure 29.11: Abrasion lesion is wedge shaped indentation with sharply defined margins

- Most commonly seen toothbrush abrasions are unilateral in nature
- Lesion has sharply defined margins and internal angles.

Abfraction

- Usually a single tooth is involved in abfraction lesion.
- Seen as sharply defined wedge shaped depression.

- Most commonly seen on the buccal surface of mandibular teeth.
- In early stages, lesion appears as minor irregular crack or fracture line on the enamel surface. In late stages, it appears as notch extending into dentin (**Figs 29.13A and B**).

Diagnosis of Noncarious Cervical Lesions

Diagnosis of noncarious cervical lesions starts with history taking. A careful history taking and proper clinical examination are mandatory to reach at correct diagnosis.

History of the Patient

While taking history of patient, following things are kept in mind:
- *Dietary habits of patient:* Overconsumption of citrus fruits, aerated drinks, pickled food and vitamin C sources can cause erosive tooth loss.

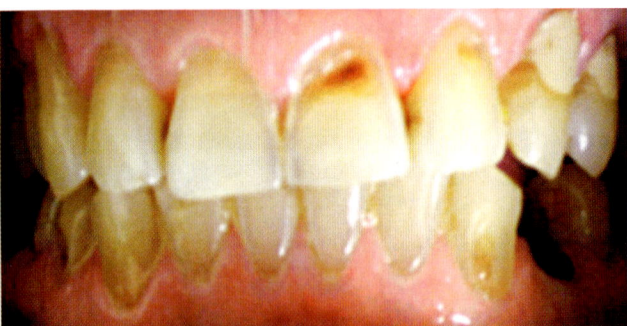

Figure 29.12: Abrasion of teeth

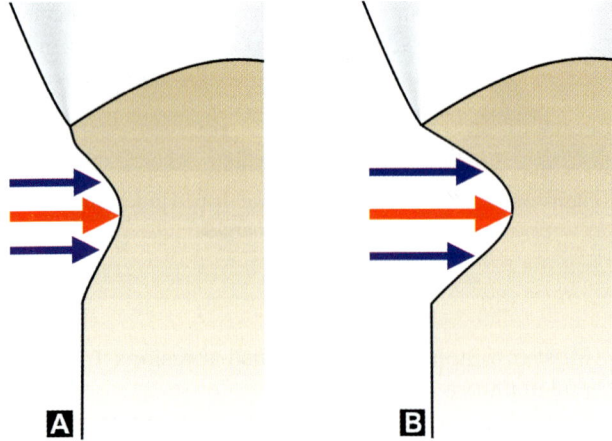

Figures 29.13A and B: In abfraction, concentration of stresses increase in center rather than at periphery. This results in notch shaped appearance of the lesion

- *Occupation of patient:* Erosion is most commonly seen in patients working in metal plating or battery manufacture industries.
- *General health of patient:* Erosion is most commonly seen in patients with gastrointestinal ulcers and hiatus hernia.
- *Brushing habits:* Dentist should ask about brushing technique, brush, type and nature of dentifrice as these factors are responsible for abrasion of teeth.
- *Abnormal habits:* Bruxism, clenching, grinding or any other habit which poses deleterious effect on occlusion should be asked about.

Examination

- The clinician should look for the clinical appearance of teeth for erosion, abrasion and/or abfraction which can be broad, shallow saucer shaped defect or notched 'V' shaped defect with sharp margins or wedge shaped defect.
- Look for any abnormal signs of traumatic occlusion like mobile teeth, tilted teeth, abnormal tooth wear, cross bite, deep bite, poorly occluding teeth, with malalignment and open contacts, etc. These occlusal problems can result in noncarious cervical tooth loss.

Radiographs

In patients with abnormal occlusal problems and subsequently cervical tooth loss, following can be seen on the radiographs:
- Root resorptions, hypercementosis
- Widening of periodontal ligament
- Vertical bone loss
- Thickening of lamina dura
- Calcification of pulp space.

Differential diagnosis of cervical lesions			
	Incipient caries	Arrested caries	Intrinsic stains or developmental enamel defects
Color	Chalky white	Brown or black	Shiny white
Surface texture (when dried)	Porous	Firm and smooth	Firm and smooth
Site (most common)	At the area of plaque accumulation	At the area of plaque accumulation	Anywhere

MANAGEMENT OF CERVICAL LESIONS

One of the important steps for the treatment of noncarious cervical lesion is careful concern of the etiology and progression of the lesion. To reach at accurate diagnosis careful history of the patient should be taken. Without determination of the etiological factors, successful results of treatment may not be obtained.

Management of noncarious cervical lesion is done in two phases

➟ Preventive management
➟ Restorative management.

Preventive Management

The primary objective of preventive management is removal of the etiological factors. After taking history regarding dietary habits, brushing habits, abnormal habits like bruxism, following preventive measures should be taken to prevent unusual tooth loss:

- Proper toothbrushing technique using soft bristle toothbrush
- Use of less abrasive dentifrice
- Correct occlusal disharmony to reduce occlusal stresses
- Restrict intake of acidic foods and acid producing diet
- Use of sodium bicarbonate mouthrinse in patients with gastric regurgitation
- Use of orthodontic appliances to prevent bruxism and clenching
- Correct ill fitting metal clasps or denture
- Correction of abnormal habits like holding pins or pipes, nail biting, etc.
- Topical fluoride application
- Psychiatric consultation in patients with anorexia nervosa.

Restorative Management

Restoration of noncarious cervical lesion is important for the following reasons:

- To maintain the structural integrity of the tooth
- To treat sensitivity of the tooth
- To maintain esthetics
- To protect pulp
- To maintain the health of the periodontium
- To prevent caries.

The first step for the treatment of cervical lesion is restoration of the defective part of tooth, but if there has been pulpal involvement or if cervical lesion is associated with severe gingival recession or periodontal defect, the tooth may require endodontic or periodontal therapy respectively or the combination of both so as to achieve better prognosis.

Though noncarious cervical lesion can be restored using either of the restorative material used for carious cervical lesion, i.e. composites, silver amalgam, glass ionomer or direct filling gold, choice of materials are composites or resin modified glass ionomer cements because they:

- Require minimum tooth preparation
- Achieve retention by forming a bond with tooth tissues
- Offer good esthetics.

However, where esthetics is not of much concern like in posterior teeth, the material of choice for restoration is silver amalgam or direct filling gold because of their superior physical properties and durability.

Although the type of tooth preparation for restoration of a cervical lesion is class V for all restorative materials, there are certain modifications in preparation design for different restorative materials.

Restoration of Cervical Lesions Using Composite Resins

Composite resins are most commonly used restorative material for restoration of cervical lesions. As we know composites are mainly of three types based on the size, amount and composition of the inorganic filler:

1. Conventional composites
2. Microfilled composites
3. Hybrid composites.

Of the above three types of composites, microfilled composites are the material of choice for restoration of cervical lesions. Microfilled composites are esthetically better, offer better finish and have low modulus of elasticity which allows them to flex during tooth flexure. These qualities make them suitable choice for restoring cervical lesions where cervical flexure can be significant.

Advantages of composites

➟ Conservation of tooth structure
➟ Esthetically acceptable
➟ Bonding with enamel and dentin, hence have good retention
➟ Can be finished immediately after curing.

Disadvantages of composites

➟ Microleakage problem usually on root surfaces
➟ Costlier than amalgam
➟ More technique sensitive
➟ High LCTE may result in marginal percolation around composite restorations.

> **Microleakage is a major problem while restoring a cervical lesion. This microleakage can lead to**
>
> → Postoperative sensitivity
> → Secondary caries
> → Pulpal damage
> → Staining
> → Accelerated deterioration of restorative material.

Basically three types of designs of tooth preparation for composites are made:

1. *Conventional class V tooth preparation:* Indicated for cervical lesion present exclusively or partially on the root surface of a tooth.
2. *Beveled conventional class V tooth preparation:* Indicated either for a large lesion or for the replacement of an existing, defective class V restoration which earlier was used as a conventional preparation.
3. *Modified class V tooth preparation:* Indicated for small to moderate cervical lesions.

Following steps are done during tooth preparation for composite restoration:

- Remove the defective, friable tooth structure.
- Create cavosurface angle of 90 degrees (for root surface) or greater (for crown portion of teeth).
- Roughen the prepared tooth surface. Sometimes, retention groove is placed in nonenamel area (**Figs 29.14 and 29.15**). It helps in increasing resistance to marginal leakage because groove placement assists in resisting the effects of polymerization shrinkage and tooth flexure.
- Clean the tooth surface with pumice prophylaxis.

- Select an appropriate shade matching the tooth.
- Isolate the tooth preferably using rubber dam.
- Etch the tooth surface using a suitable etchant.
- Apply bonding agent as per manufacturer instructions.
- Use composite resin (preferably microfilled and flowable composite) and cure it. (For detail refer chapter 17 page number 307)
- Do final finishing and polishing of the restoration.

Restoration of Cervical Lesion Using Glass Ionomer Cement (Figs 29.16A to D)

For past many years, Glass ionomer cements have been used to restore cervical lesion. Their advantageous property is their capacity to release fluoride when exposed to oral cavity. This anticariogenic quality makes glass ionomer restorations more resistant to secondary caries.

Both self-cured and light cured types of glass ionomers are available. But resin modified light cured glass ionomers are preferred because of their:

- Extended working time
- Improved physical properties
- Better esthetics.

Tooth preparation for glass ionomer cements involves following steps:

- Remove the defective, friable tooth structure
- Roughen the prepared tooth surface
- Clean the tooth surface using 10 percent polyacrylic acid for 10 to 15 seconds. This is done to remove the smear layer
- Isolate the tooth preferably using rubber dam

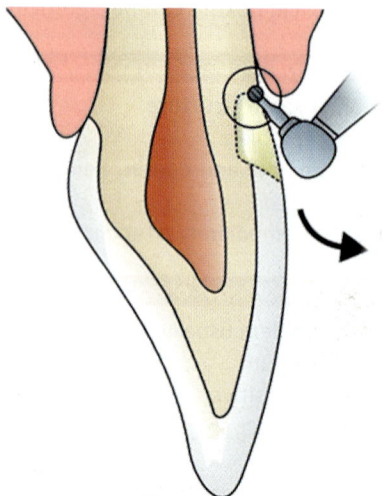

Figure 29.14: Preparation of retentive grooves for composite restoration

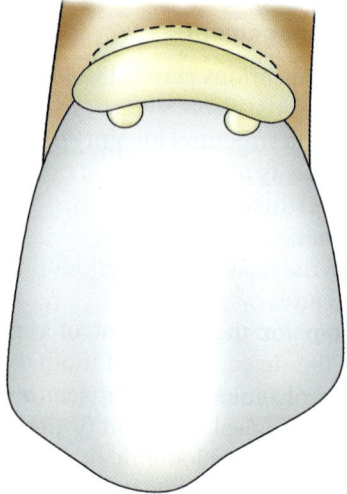

Figure 29.15: Completed class V preparation for composites

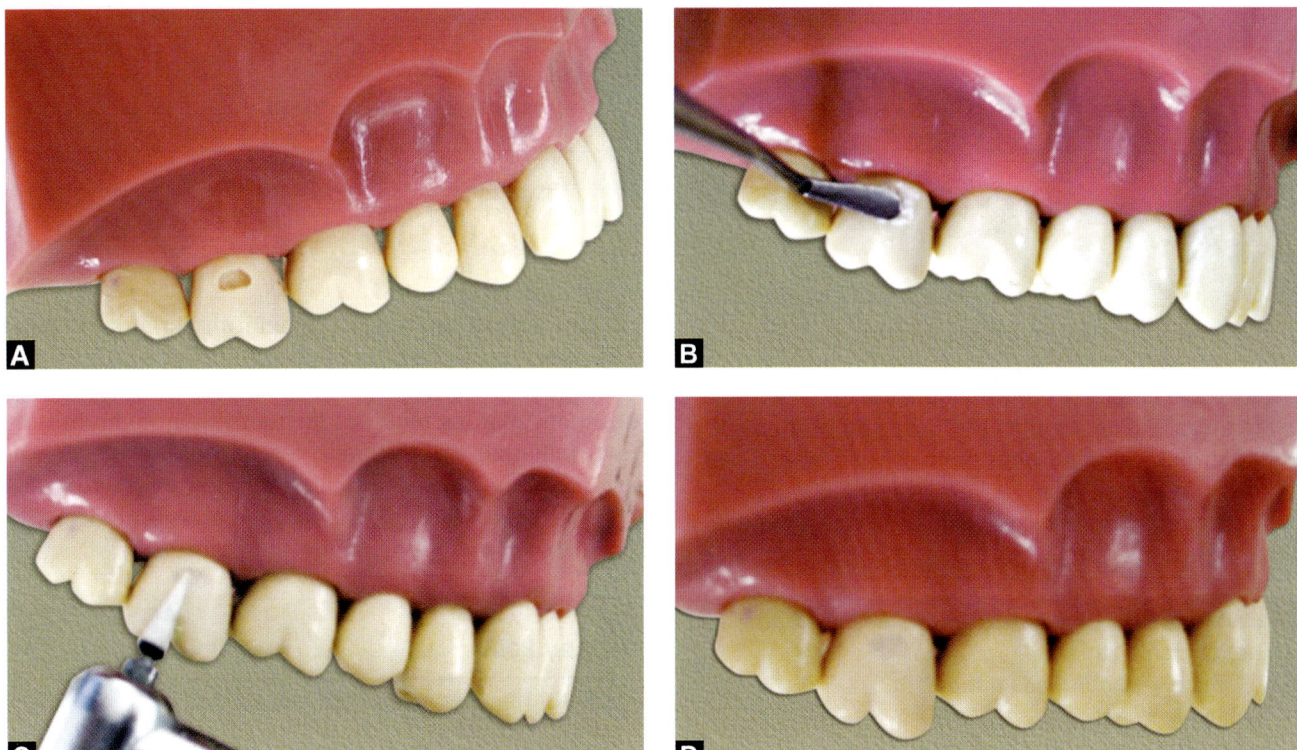

Figures 29.16A to D: Glass ionomer restoration in a cervical lesion: (A) Completed tooth preparation; (B) Placement of GIC; (C) Finishing of restoration; (D) Final restoration

- Take glass ionomer cement, mix and place it in the prepared tooth
- Do final finishing and polishing of the restoration.

Advantages of glass ionomer cement
→ Inherent adhesion to tooth structure
→ Biocompatible
→ Fluoride release and hence act as anticariogenic
→ Minimal tooth preparation required, hence easy to use on children.

Disadvantages of glass ionomer cement
→ Water sensitive during setting phase
→ White and crazed surface
→ Opaque
→ Not inherently radiopaque
→ Less esthetic than composite.

Restoration of Cervical Lesion Using Silver Amalgam (Fig. 29.17)

Amalgam is normally used for cervical lesions in the following conditions:

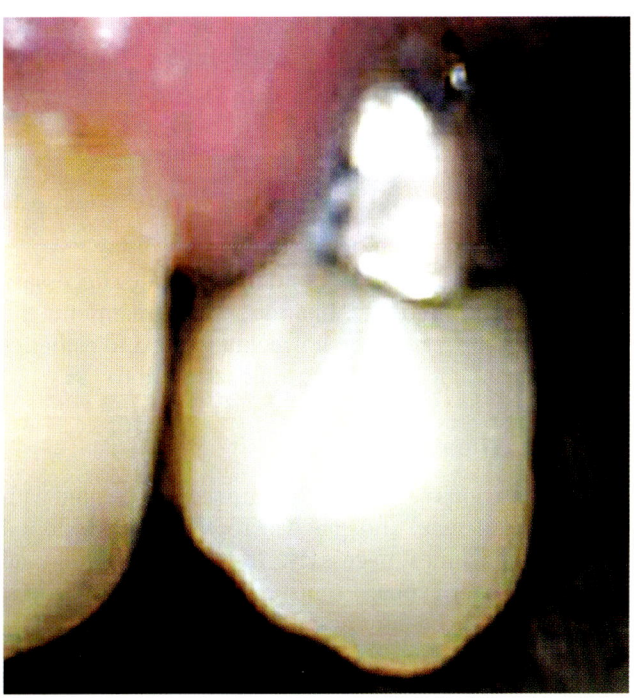

Figure 29.17: Silver amalgam restoration for cervical lesion of premolar

Comparison between Erasion, Abrasion and Abfraction

	Erosion	*Abrasion*	*Abfraction*
Site	Lingual or facial	Facial	Facial
Appearance	Shallow, saucer shaped	Wedge V-shaped	Wedge shaped
Margins	Smooth	Sharp	Sharp
Enamel surface	Smooth, glazed, polished	Smooth, minor cracked appearance	Rough, sharp angles

- For areas which do not require esthetics
- For areas where access and visibility are limited
- When it is difficult to control moisture
- For areas that are significantly deep gingivally
- Partial denture abutment teeth, because amalgam is more resistant to wear.

Tooth preparation is same as that for class V conventional composite restoration.

Advantages of amalgam

- Ease of manipulation
- Satisfactory marginal adaptation
- Technique insensitivity
- Self sealing
- Good wear resistance
- Low cost.

Disadvantages of amalgam

- Less esthetic
- Extensive preparation to hold an amalgam filling
- Amalgam fillings can corrode or tarnish over time, causing discoloration
- Does not bond to tooth
- Poor tensile strength making it a brittle material.

Endodontic Treatment

When cervical lesion involves pulp, it becomes necessary for endodontic therapy. After root canal treatment, the tooth should be restored to normal function and esthetics by post placement and full coverage restoration.

Periodontal Treatment

When noncarious cervical lesions are seen associated with periodontal defects and gingival recession, periodontal treatment becomes necessary. It involves periodontal surgery to cover exposed roots using free gingival grafts, coronally advanced flaps or guided tissue regeneration.

Since many people are retaining their teeth for longer time, the incidence of cervical lesions (both carious and noncarious) have been increased. Most of the noncarious cervical lesions are seen in general in geriatric population. When tooth loss becomes significant it causes loss of esthetics and function, thus dentist should know all the treatment options required for tooth wear. Many restorative materials are available for restoration of cervical lesions, among these microfilled and flowable composites are considered in esthetic areas, and glass ionomers and amalgam are preferred in nonesthetic areas.

 Key Points

- Noncarious cervical lesions form 60 to 70 percent of total cervical lesions.
- Root surface carious lesions are seen on the root surfaces exposed to oral environment, usually at or apical to the cementoenamel junction (CEJ).
- Noncarious cervical lesions can also be described as 'wasting disease of the teeth'. These lesions include abrasion, erosion and abfraction.
- Noncarious cervical lesions cannot be referred as inflammatory lesions or developmental abnormalities but considered as regressive alteration of the teeth.
- Erosion is defined as a loss of tooth substance caused by a chemical process that does not involve known bacterial action.
- Abrasion is defined as the loss of tooth substance induced by mechanical wear other than that of mastication.
- Abfraction lesion is a wedge type defect which usually occur in cervical areas of tooth due to excessive occlusal stresses or parafunctional habits such as bruxism. It appears as a wedge shaped defect with sharp line angles.
- The abfraction lesion is caused by flexure and ultimate material fatigue of susceptible tooth at location away from the point of loading. The breakdown is dependent on the magnitude, duration, frequency and location of the forces.
- In patients with abnormal occlusal problems and cervical tooth loss, radiographically root resorptions, hypercementosis, widening of periodontal ligament, vertical bone loss and thickening of lamina dura is seen.
- The primary objective of management of non carious cervical lesion is removal of the etiological factors like

improvement of dietary habits, brushing habits, correction of abnormal habits like bruxism.

- Microfilled composites are the material of choice for restoration of cervical lesions because they are esthetic in nature, offer better finish and have low modulus of elasticity which allows them to flex during tooth flexure.
- Glass ionomer cements are used to restore cervical lesion mainly because of their fluoride release quality (anticariogenicity) and chemical bonding to tooth structure.
- Amalgam is indicated for cervical lesions when esthetics is not important, moisture control is difficult and for partial denture abutment teeth, because amalgam is more resistant to wear.

QUESTIONS

1. Classify cervical lesions. Explain mechanism of abfraction in detail.
2. Write short notes on:
   a. Cervical lesions
   b. Differential diagnosis of noncarious cervical lesions.
   c. Management of cervical lesions.

BIBLIOGRAPHY

1. Ferrari M, Davidson CL. Sealing capacity of a resin modified glass ionomer and resin composite placed *in vivo* in class V restorations. Oper Dent. 1996;21:69.
2. Fuller JL, Johnson WW. Citric acid consumption and the human dentition. JADA. 1977;95:80.
3. Gallien GS, Kaplan I, Ownes BM. A review of non-carious dental cervical lesions. Compend. Cont Educ Dent. 1994;16:552.
4. Grimaldi JR, Hood J. Lateral deformation of the tooth crown under axial cuspal loading. JDR. 1973;52:584 (Abst. no.10).
5. Grippo JO, et al. Attrition, abrasion, corrosion, and abfraction revisited: a new perspective on tooth surface lesions. J Am Dent Assoc. 2004;135:1109-18.
6. Grippo JO. Abfractions: a new classification of hard tissue lesions of teeth. J Esthet Dent. 1991;3:14-9.
7. Harrison JL, Roeder LB. Dental erosion caused by color beverages. Gen Dent. 1991;39:23.
8. High AS. An unusual pattern of dental erosion – case report. BDJ. 1977;143:403.
9. Hong FL, Nu ZY, Xie XM. Clinical classification and therapeutic design of dental cervical abrasion. Gerodontics. 1988;4:101.
10. Hood JAA. Stress/displacement analysis of a class V restoration in a premolar. JDR. 1979;58:1210.
11. Imfeld T. Dental erosion–definition, classification and links. Eur J Oral Sci. 1996;104:191.
12. James PMC, Parfitt GJ. Local effects of certain medicaments on the teeth. BDJ. 1953;2:1252.
13. Jarvinen V. Location of dental erosion in a referred population. Caries Res. 1992;26:391.
14. Konig KG. Root lesions. Int Dent J. 1990;40:283.
15. Toffeneti F, Vamini L, Tammaro S. Gingival recession and non-carious cervical lesions: A soft and hard tissue challenge. J Esth Dent. 1998;10:208.
16. Vandewalle KS, Vigil G. Guidelines for the restoration of class V lesions. Gen Dent. 1997;45:254.
17. Welsh EL, Hembree H. Microleakage at the gingival wall with four class V anterior restorative materials. J Prosth Dent. 1985;54:370.
18. Winstanley RB. The treatment of attrition, abrasion and erosion. 1986;2:5.
19. Xhonga FA, Wolcott RB, Sogniaes RF. Dental erosion II. Clinical measurement of dental erosion progress. JADA. 1972;84:577.
20. Xhonga FA. Bruxism and its effects on the teeth. J Oral Rehab. 1977;4:65.

30

CHAPTER

Selection of Restorative Materials

INTRODUCTION

Restoration of carious teeth presents the dentist with the dilemma of selecting a suitable restorative material. Dentist must make this selection with great care because, in future years, those restorations needing replacement will result in the loss of increasing amount of tooth structure. This sets up a cycle where the increasing cavity size limits the choice of the materials that may be used effectively. There are numerous factors to consider when restoring a tooth, e.g. the extent of the lesion, the strength of the remaining tooth structure, the preference of the dentist in using the material, and the financial cost of the procedure tooth related factors. This chapter reviews the information regarding selection of intracoronal restorative materials.

FACTORS REGULATING THE SELECTION OF RESTORATIVE MATERIALS

Teeth need restorative intervention most commonly due to carious destruction. This must accomplished with restoration of proper form, function, aesthetics and occlusal stability. To achieve these objectives selection of suitable restorative material is very important and varies with individual case. This selection depends upon many factors, characteristics of the tooth itself, the patient, the dentist, and the material.

Material Related Factors

The ideal restorative material should have the following features:
- Should resist occlusal forces
- Should resist the wear
- Should be indestructible in oral fluids
- Should be adequately adapted to the cavity walls
- Co-efficient of thermal expansion should be comparable to tooth structure
- Should exhibit low thermal conductivity
- Should be biocompatible
- Should be accomplished with minimal tooth preparation
- Should strengthen the remaining tooth structure
- Should be antibacterial
- Should be aesthetically pleasing
- Should be compatible with the pulpal and periodontal health
- Should be easily manipulated
- Should be economical.

Till date no material exhibits all the properties, although developments have been made to closely resemble these parameters.

Direct Filling Gold

It is considered as one of the most permanent restorative material, as it closely meets the properties of ideal restorative material. It is completely indestructible in the oral fluids. It can be well adapted to the cavity walls. Density of gold foil is low but is increased during condensation. Its co-efficient of thermal expansion is almost similar to tooth structure (**Table 30.1**). It is highly polished and not susceptible to corrosion. Before its use patients oral hygiene and physical condition must be considered. It is not suitable for very young, old and patients with periodontally compromised teeth, as it needs high condensation pressure and long operating time. Its use has declined because of its poor esthetics and reluctance of the dentist to explain to the patients, the benefits of the material.

Advantages of direct filling gold

➜ The resilience of dentin and the adaptability of gold allow an almost perfect seal between the tooth structure and gold
➜ Malleability of gold provides permanent self sealing margins
➜ Being a noble metal, gold does not tarnish and corrode
➜ Coefficient of thermal expansion close to dentin
➜ No cementing medium is required for restoration
➜ It does not cause tooth discoloration because of good adaptation to the preparation margins and walls
➜ The direct gold restoration is insoluble in oral fluids

Disadvantages of direct filling gold

➜ Technique sensitive
➜ Because of the high thermal conductivity of gold, larger restoration can increase sensitivity
➜ Gold foil is more expensive than any other restoration material
➜ It cannot be placed where aesthetics is required.

Indications for the Use of Direct Filling Gold

• Small Class I, II, V and VI preparations of teeth where high occlusal stress is not present
• To repair gold crown margins, onlays and inlays
• For hypoplastic or other defects on the facial or lingual areas

Contraindications for the Use of Direct Filling Gold

• In young patient because periodontal membranes and alveolar processes do not offer the resistance to the hand pressure and mallet blows, necessary to insure a well-condensed mass of gold
• When there is limited accessibility
• When aesthetics is of prime importance
• In stress bearing areas.

Dental Amalgam

Amalgam has been used successfully for many years, although its use has declined in recent years because of increased aesthetic demand and concerns regarding mercury toxicity. Amalgam can be easily manipulated, less technique sensitive and at the same time isolation is not critical, especially in zinc free restorations. Bactericidal property of amalgam decrease biofilm formation and bacterial colonization. It has good wear resistance and can sustain high occlusal loads, even if all contacts are on restoration. It has low tensile strength and thus requires specific tooth preparation thereby sacrificing more tooth structure. It has high thermal conductivity requiring pulp protection in deep cavities. This may be the reason of initial postoperative sensitivity. Coefficient of thermal expansion of amalgam is almost double than tooth structure, which invites percolation due to temperature changes (**Fig. 30.1**). Cuspal deflection in amalgam is associated with condensation forces and slight expansion during setting.

Table 30.1: Linear coefficients of thermal expansion (LCTE)

Restorative dental materials/Tooth tissues	LCTE (ppm /°C)
Tooth tissues	
• Enamel	11.4
• Dentin	8.3
Restorative dental materials	
• Dental amalgam	25
• Glass ionomer	11.0
• Gold foil	14–15
• Ceramics	14
• Packable composites	28–35

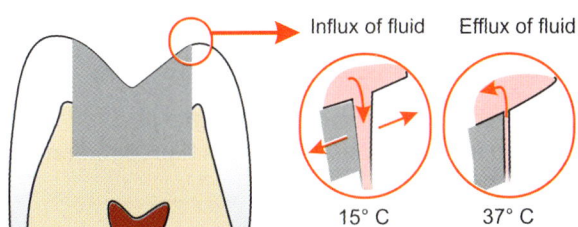

Figure 30.1: Percolation along the margins of an amalgam restoration due to its difference in linear coefficient of thermal expansion from tooth structure during intraoral temperature changes. Fluid influx occurs during cooling (contraction). Fluid efflux occurs during heating (expansion)

Mercuroscopic expansion occurs with internal phase changes and creep leading to extrusion at the margins. This is the cause of marginal fracture inviting failure in low copper alloys. On the other hand creep may have some beneficial effects as it may also decreases marginal gaps over time. Mode of failure in high copper alloys is the bulk fracture. Other reasons of failure are secondary caries. Amalgam undergoes corrosion in oral cavity, which helps in self sealing of the restorations, thus decreasing microleakage over time.

Advantages of silver amalgam
→ Ease of manipulation
→ Physical characteristics of amalgam are comparable to enamel and dentin
→ Less technique sensitive
→ Self sealing
→ Biocompatible
→ Good wear resistance
→ Low cost
→ Bonded amalgam restorations can also bond to tooth structure.

Disadvantages of silver amalgam
→ Less aesthetic
→ Extensive preparation to hold an amalgam filling
→ Amalgam fillings can corrode or tarnish overtime, causing discoloration
→ Does not bond to tooth
→ Amalgam is not strong enough to reinforce the weakened tooth structure
→ Poor tensile strength making it a brittle material.

Indications of Amalgam Restoration

- Class I, II, V and VI preparations where aesthetic is not required, and isolation is difficult
- Used as a foundation in cases of grossly decayed teeth while planning for cast restoration
- Used as a postendodontic restoration.

Contraindications of Amalgam Restoration

- When esthetics is the prime concern
- Small to moderate class I and class II preparations.

Glass Ionomer Cements

GIC was introduced by Wilson and Kent in 1972. They are tooth colored restorations containing fluoride and can be used in deciduous teeth, as liner and bases, for cementation, as pit and fissure sealant, and in patients with high caries risk. Wear resistance of GIC has low strength and is not suitable for stress bearing area. They are hydrophilic and provide good adhesion even in the presence of moisture, chemically retained in the cavity and are affected by water absorption and desiccation, so must be are protected by varnish or light cured resin after placement. The water trapped within their hydrogel matrix refracts light, making the GICs opaque. The glass-ionomer cement seals the open dentin tubules and prevents the hydrodynamic pressure that is the source of tooth sensitivity following composite placement. Unlike composite resins, GICs can be "recharged" with fluoride after the restoration is set. To improve handling characteristics, wear resistance, and esthetics water hydrophilic monomers were added to liquid and filler particles were added to powder. These materials are characterized as resin modified glass ionomers. These are dual cured as they undergoes acid base reactions during setting and are light cured after placement. Light curing improves the early strength of the restoration and affords greater protection of the maturing hydrogel matrix. Although they have improved translucency, their mechanical properties are inadequate to serve as posterior restorative materials.

Advantages of GIC
→ Adhesion to tooth structure because of chemical bonding
→ Biocompatible because large sized polyacrylic acid molecules prevent the acid from producing pulpal response
→ Anticariogenic because of fluoride release
→ Minimal tooth preparation required hence easy to use on children
→ Less technique sensitive than composite resins.

Disadvantages of GIC
→ Brittle and low fracture resistance
→ Low wear resistance
→ Water sensitivity during setting phase affects physical properties and esthetics
→ Opaque which makes glass ionomer cement less esthetic than composites
→ Not inherently radiopaque.

Indications of Glass Ionomer Cement

- Restoration of Class V, III, and small Class I tooth preparations
- Restoration of deciduous teeth
- For luting inlay, onlay, crowns, veneers, pins and posts
- As protective liner under composite and amalgam
- Core build up
- In other restorative technique like sandwich technique, atraumatic restorative treatment and bonded restorations.

Contraindications of Glass Ionomer Cements

- In stress bearing areas like class I, Class II and class IV preparations
- In cuspal replacement cases
- In patients with xerostomia
- In mouth breathers because restoration may become opaque, brittle and fracture over a time
- In areas requiring esthetics like veneering of anterior teeth.

Composites

Composites are used mostly to restore anterior teeth and small to moderate sized class I and class II lesions in posterior teeth where occlusal loading is not severe. These are most esthetic direct restorative materials with color and translucency being similar to tooth. Their adhesive property requires minimal tooth structure removal and strengthens the remaining tooth structure. Contemporary restorative composites have embraced nanotechnology, are available in various shade and opacities. Even with significant improvements, polymerization shrinkage and resulting stress are still a major clinical consideration for composite restorations. An important part of sensitivity in posterior teeth restored with direct composite restorations is the configuration factor, more is the C-factor more are the polymerization stresses. This leads to marginal degradation, microleakage, staining, enamel cracks, postoperative sensitivity and cuspal deflection. Cuspal deflection varies with the size of the cavity and occlusal loading, being more in MODs than MO or DO cavity. Composites favor increased biofilm formation. Indirect composites were developed to decrease the effects of polymerization shrinkage as these are cured outside the oral cavity using heat and pressure. Though many composite resins are described as fluoride releasing, once fully set, actual free fluoride release is minimal. Being hydrophobic these requires proper isolation and should not be placed in areas where moisture control is difficult. The use of a flowable base to relieve the internal stress generated during the curing process has been effective at eliminating post treatment sensitivity of posterior composite restorations. The most common flowable base used under composite resins is glass-ionomer cement.

Advantages of composites

- Maximum conservation of tooth structure possible
- Esthetically acceptable
- Composites have low thermal conductivity, thus no insulation base is required to protect underlying pulp
- It can be repaired rather than replaced
- Composite restoration show low microleakage than unfilled resins
- Composite restorations can bond directly to the tooth, making the tooth stronger than it would be with an amalgam filling
- Indirect composite fillings and inlays are heat-cured, increasing their strength.

Disadvantages of composites

- Because of polymerization shrinkage, gap formation on margins may occur, usually on root surfaces. This can result in secondary caries and staining
- More difficult, time consuming
- Expensive than amalgam
- More technique sensitive
- Low wear resistance.

Indications of Composite Restorations

- For restoration of mild to moderate class I and class II tooth preparations of all teeth
- Restoration of class III, IV and V preparations of all teeth specially when esthetics is important
- Esthetic improvement procedures like laminates, veneers, and diastema closures
- As a pit and fissure sealants
- For periodontal splinting of weakened teeth or mobile teeth
- For repair of fractured ceramic crowns
- For bonding orthodontic appliances.

Contraindications of Composites

- When isolation of operating field is difficult
- Where very high occlusal forces are present
- When clinician does not possess the necessary technical skill for the restoration
- When lesion extends up to the root surface
- Patients with high caries susceptibility
- When preparation extends subgingivally
- Patients with poor oral hygiene.

Cast Gold Inlays

Among all available materials for restoration of posterior teeth cast gold are more advantageous. These can resist wear and sustain high occlusal loads, thus suitable for high stress bearing area. They can be used to restore or alter occlusal contacts and can assure tight contact. These are indestructible in the oral cavity and are free from dimensional changes after placement. Their shortcomings are poor esthetic, high thermal conductivity, poor adaptation to the cavity walls, and need of cementing media. These require more time and second appointment though most of the work is accomplished in the laboratory. They are technique sensitive and may produce wedging or splitting forces on tooth.

Ceramics Inlays

Ceramics are used to fabricate tooth colored restorations. This is the very hard and strong material, but being brittle may fracture under heavy masticatory loads. Strength of ceramics depends greatly on quality of bond to underlying tooth structure, and thickness of the material thus necessitating greater tooth reduction. These are highly resistant to wear but can wear opposing tooth structure if surface is rough. Ceramics are highly biocompatible.

TOOTH RELATED FACTORS

Characteristics of the Carious Lesion

The choice of restorative material depends upon the tooth type, its location in the arch, forces acting on the tooth, the surface(s) to be restored, and lesion depth. If anterior tooth is involved than choice is made among esthetic materials, in case posterior tooth is involved than material with high strength is used.

Status of the Pulp

If there is no threat to the health of the pulp by carious lesion, caries is removed avoiding pulpal exposure and then restore the tooth with permanent restoration. Pulp capping is performed in the teeth with questionable pulpal condition. If pulp is irreversibly involved then endodontic treatment is done.

Status of the Periodontium

The operative procedure must be performed only after evaluating the health status of the periodontium. If periodontium is not healthy than direct filling gold is not the material of choice as it need high forces of condensation.

Size, Form and Structure of Teeth

When open proximal contacts are to be restored, re-establishment of the space or slight alteration in the usual size of the tooth is to be decided. Recontouring of interproximal surfaces is usually done with cast gold or metal ceramic restorations, as they have greater convenience and accuracy, as mostly these are made by indirect method. Amalgam often fails to close the contact and produce an ideal interproximal contour due to its physical properties, technique of placement and condensation.

PATIENT RELATED FACTORS

- Age of the patient
- Physical condition of the patient
- Hygienic condition of the mouth
- Strength and character of the bite
- Esthetic appearance
- Cooperation and will power of the patient
- Expense of the operation
- Bruxism/habits
- Systemic conditions that can change the amount of saliva and its chemistry.

Site Specific Selection

For Anterior Teeth

For restoration of anterior teeth preoperative occlusal assessment is very important along with esthetic considerations. Proximal restorations in anterior teeth are subjected to horizontal force that tends to displace the restoration in labio-proximo-linguo or linguo-proximo-labio direction and vertical force that tends to rotate the restoration proximally. The amount of these forces depends upon the location, extent and type of occluding contacts between anterior teeth during function. Metallic restorations are usually not indicated for anterior teeth, but the distal surface of canine due to its location exhibits the unique stress pattern and may require a metallic restoration. These cavities are more satisfactorily restored with amalgam than with any other material except gold foil. When using composites for other class III and class IV restorations, ideally it should not be loaded directly. For class III cavities demanding more esthetics microfilled composite can be used. In class IV cavities where esthetics is essential, but the restoration is also subjected to stress, the use of a microfilled composite as a veneer over a hybrid composite core is suggested.

For Posterior Teeth

The choice of material for posterior restoration depend on individual clinical situation including patient's age, caries risk, esthetic requirements, ability to isolate the area and functional demands from the restoration. A thorough evaluation of patients, occlusion, functional and parafunctional habits is critical. Cast metal is preferred in situations demanding alterations of occlusal contact or to build open contact. In patients with heavy occlusal forces or bruxism, metallic (amalgam, cast metal) restorations are suitable. Composite restorations in these situations undergo

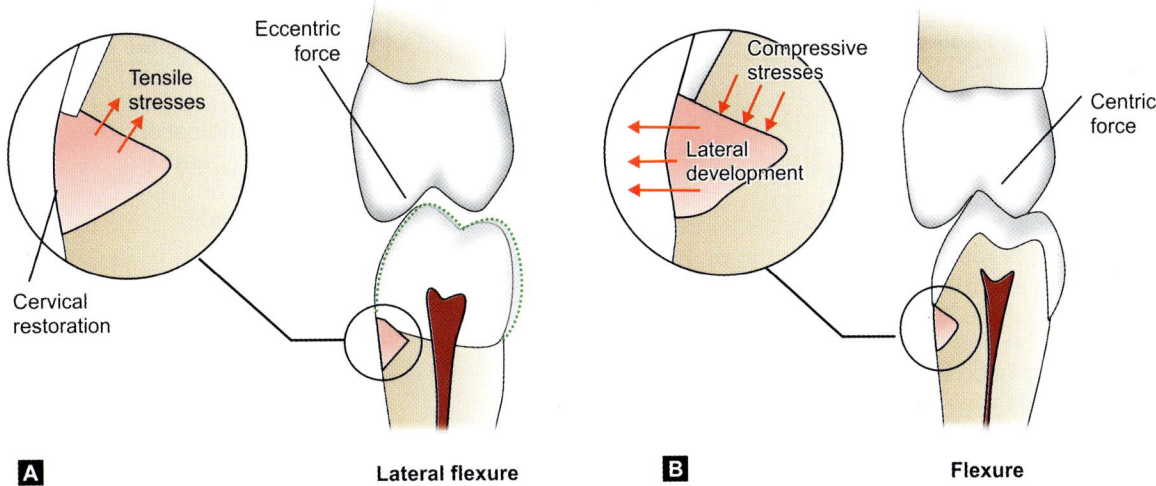

Figures 30.2A and B: (A) Eccentric forces produce tensile stresses at marginal interface with restoration, resulting in lateral flexure; (B) Tooth flexure causing cervical stresses

more wear. Whereas ceramic restoration can wear the opposing tooth structure or metallic restoration. Wear of composite depends on the size and location of the lesion. Use of composite is preferred for sealing of pit and fissures, preventive resin restorations, restoration of moderate sized class I and class II lesions. While doing composite, it should be kept in mind that occlusal contacts must be shared by healthy tooth structure and gingival extension is in the enamel rather than on cementum. Glass ionomers are useful for the high caries risk patient, as they release fluoride and are recharged with fluoride but their poor wear resistance and low fracture toughness limits their use for posterior restorations in permanent teeth. However, these can be used under composite restorations in cases of deep cavity or with subgingival margin. Resin modified GIC and compomers with better esthetics, improved mechanical properties and caries protecting are suitable for restoring deciduous teeth.

For Class V Cavities

When selecting a restorative material for class V cavities its complex morphology, isolation of the preparation site and that it may end in enamel, dentine or cementum must be considered. In addition, occlusal forces cause stress accumulation in the cervical area, resulting in tooth flexure that may lead, micro-leakage or loss of bonded class V restorations without retentive features (**Figs 30.2A and B**). In this region High-fluoride–releasing restorative materials are the logical choices for simple Class V restorations in

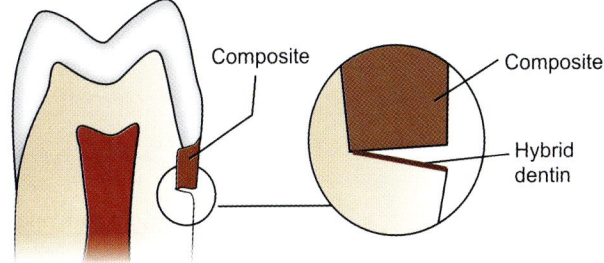

Figure 30.3: V-shaped gap formation on root surface

caries-active patients. If the restorations are in nonesthetic areas, resin-modified glass ionomer is the preferred restorative material. If the lesions are in esthetic areas, with all enamel margins composite is the material of choice. If composite is used when the lesion extends on root surface, polymerization shrinkage can cause a V-shaped gap because forces of polymerization are greater than initial bond strength of composite to root surface (**Fig. 30.3**). In these situations sandwich technique can be used, in which resin modified glass ionomer restorative material may be placed on the internal aspect of the tooth preparation, followed by a layer of resin-based composite on the surface of the restoration. Among composites microfilled composites are suitable for restoration of class V cavities, as these restorations can flex rather than debond, when tooth undergoes cervical flexure.

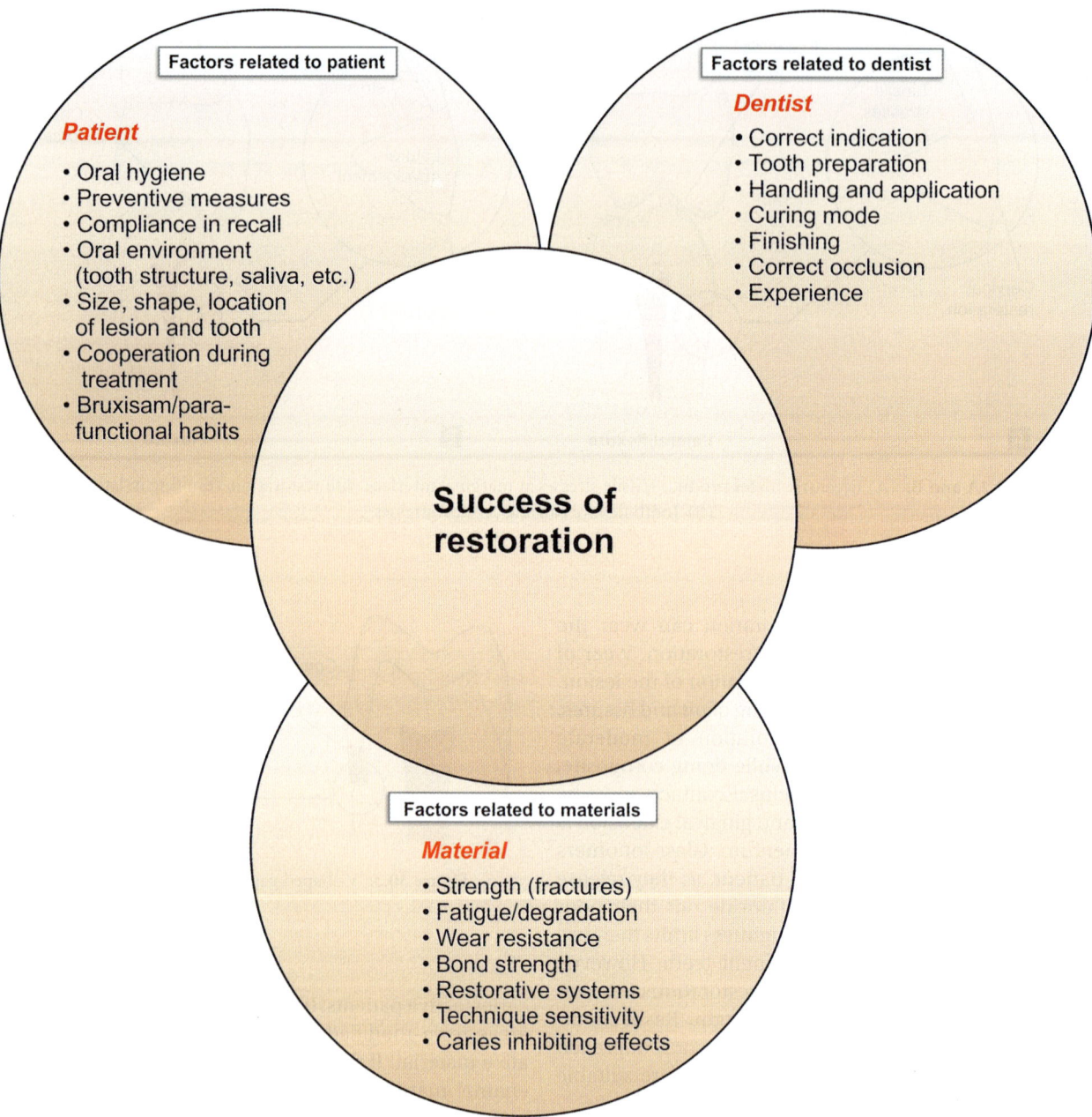

Figure 30.4: Factors affecting success of restoration

Factors Effecting Success of Restoration (Fig. 30.4)

The primary reason for the failure and replacement of restorations is secondary caries irrespective of the type of restorative material used. Other causes include, fracture, and wear, marginal defects and postoperative sensitivity. These factors can be reduced to minimal by the quality of the restoration done and the home care measures taken by the patient. The longevity of restorations depends on the selection of materials; clinical technique used patient care.

Summary of intracoronal restorative materials

Material	Indications	Contraindications	Advantages	Disadvantages
Direct filling gold	• Initial Class III cavities especially on distal surface of canines • Class V lesions for patients of all ages	• Teeth with poor peri-odontal health • High caries activity • Risk patients	• Marginal integrity • Longevity	• Time-consuming • Poor esthetics
Silver Amalgam	• Class I, II, V lesions • Class III lesions on distal surface of canines • Caries control restorations, as foundations	• Small defects • Very large intracoronal restorations	• Self sealing property • Good strength • Isolation is not critical • Easy manipulation	• Color is not acceptable • Marginal breakdown • Concerns about Hg toxicity • Need of specific cavity design removing more tooth structure
Glass ionomer cement	• Class I, II and V lesions in patients with high caries activity • Crown repairs	• Areas of high esthetic need • Areas of difficult moisture control • High stress bearing areas	• High fluoride release • Can be recharged with fluoride • No postoperative sensitivity • Less time consuming	• Opaque • Fluoride uptake
Resin modified glass ionomer Cement	• High caries activity • Repair of crowns • Pediatric patients	• Occlusal stress • Locations where color stability is necessary	• High fluoride release • Tri-cured • Sets in dark	• Somewhat difficult to use • Color changes with time.
Compomer	• Moderate to high caries activity • Repair of crowns • Pediatric patients	• Occlusal stress • Locations where color stability is necessary	• Moderate fluoride release • Easy to use	• Aesthetically better than GIC but color degrades over time
Resin composite	• Class I to Class VI lesions • Areas of high esthetic need • Patients sensitive to metal • Tooth splinting • Veneers • Laminates • Core build ups • Diastema closure	• If patient is allergic • Patients with heavy occlusal force, e.g. bruxers and clenchers • If isolation is not possible	• Esthetics • Preservation of tooth structure • May strengthen tooth • Insulating, can be repaired	• Wear resistance is low • No cariostatic activity • Polymerization shrinkage • Postoperative sensitivity • Marginal leakage • Secondary caries • Technique sensitive
Composite inlay	• Class II lesions where high esthetics is desired • Patients sensitive to metals	• Parafunctional habits • Poor oral hygiene • Technical difficulty of placement • Short teeth • Subgingival margins	• Good esthetics • Provide ability to refine margins • Achieve properly contoured contacts • Possess shock absorption capability • Gentle to opposing dentition • Easily repaired intraorally	• Wear easily • Less strength than ceramic
Cast gold inlays	• Large Restorations • For additional strength • Dental Rehabilitation • Diastema Closure • Occlusal plane correction. • Removable prosthodontic abutment .	• High caries activity • Young patients • Esthetics • Small Restorations	• Reproduces anatomy well • Longevity • Wear rate similar to enamel • Strength • Biocompatibility • Control of contours and contacts	• Number of appointments and higher chairside time • Cost • Poor esthetics • Technique sensitive • Considerations for temporary restorations • High thermal conductivity

Contd...

Contd...

Material	Indications	Contraindications	Advantages	Disadvantages
Ceramic inlays	• Class II and V locations where high esthetics is desired • Metal allergies • Large carious lesions	• Teeth that are grossly broken down • Patients with parafuntional habits • High caries activity • Gold/composite restoration in opposite arch • Subgingival margins	• Excellent esthetics • Ability to refine margins • Properly contoured contacts	• May create tooth sensitivity if bonding agents are not used properly • May fracture during service

Key Points

- Gold closely met the properties of an ideal restorative material.
- Amalgam has a low tensile strength, thereby requires a butt joint or 900 cavosurface angle.
- Mercuroscopic expansion in amalgam occurs because of internal phase change and creep.
- Glass ionomer cements can be recharged with fluorides after it sets.
- With composites polymerization shrinkage is the main concern.
- Choice of composite for restoring class V cavity is microfilled composite and for class III and class IV is a layer of microfilled over hybrid composite.
- Flowable base under composites act as a stress breaker.
- Cast gold can be used to restore occlusal contacts.
- Ceramics being brittle can fracture under heavy masticatory loads.
- Ceramics can wear opposing tooth structure if surface is rough.

QUESTIONS

1. Explain factors affecting selection of restorative materials?
2. Discuss the choice of material for restoration of class III and class IV cavities?
3. Write down the factors affecting success of a restoration?
4. For restoration of class II cavities, which material will you prefer, amalgam or composite?

BIBLIOGRAPHY

1. Anusavice KJ. Phillips' science of dental materials. 2006; 11th edition.
2. Attar N, Onen A. Fluoride release and uptake characteristics of aesthetic restorative materials. J Oral Rehabil. 2002;29:791-8.
3. Craig RG, Powers JM, Restorative dental materials; 2002;11th edition.
4. González-López S, Vilchez Díaz MA, de Haro-Gasquet F, Ceballos L, de Haro-Muñoz C. Cuspal flexure of teeth with composite restorations subjected to occlusal loading. J Adhes Dent. 2007;9(1):11-5
5. Herbert D Coy. The selection and purpose of dental restorative materials in operative dentistry. Dent Clin North Am 1957;65-80.
6. Karaoğlanoğlu S, Akgül N, Ozdabak HN, et al. Effectiveness of surface protection for glass-ionomer, resin-modified glass-ionomer and polyacid-modified composite resins. Dent Mater J. 2009;28:96-101.
7. Macghee William HO. A textbook of operative dentistry. 4th edition.
8. Manhart J, Garcia-Godoy F, Hickel R. Direct posterior restorations:clinical results and new developments. Dent Clin North Am 2002;46:303-39.
9. Marzouk MA, Simonton AL, Gross RD. Modern theory and practice 2003; 3rd edition.
10. Osborne JW. Creep as a mechanism for sealing amalgams. Oper Dent. 2006;31(2):161-4.
11. Sidhu SK. Clinical evaluations of resin-modified glass-ionomer restorations. Dent Mater. 2010;26:7-12.
12. Sturdevan CM, Heymann HO, Sturdevant JR. Art and science of operative dentistry. 2002; 4th edition
13. Willershausen B, Callaway A, Ernst CP, Stender E. The influence of oral bacteria on the surfaces of resin-based dental restorative materials: an in vitro study. Int Dent J. 1999;49(4):231-9.
14. Williams PT, Hedge GL. Creep-fatigue as a possible cause of dental amalgam margin failure. J Dent Res. 1985; 64(3):470-5.
15. Wilson AD, Kent BE. A new translucent cement for dentistry. The glass ionomer cement. Br Dent J. 1972;132:133-5.

Evidence-based Dentistry

Chapter Outline

- Steps Involved in Practicing Evidence-based Dentistry
  - Framing Clinical Questions
- Clinical Application of Evidence-Based Approach

INTRODUCTION

In today's world, dentistry is changing at a surprising rate. Each new day, we are inundated with information on new procedures, materials and techniques. Out of these, few procedures, techniques and materials have undergone controlled clinical research. Keeping up-to-date with latest advancement in dentistry and managing patients with complex needs, are bit challenging for practicing dentists.

Dentistry has evolved through three phases. The three phases are

1. *Age of expertise*: Knowledge gained through experience.
2. *Age of professionalism*: Knowledge gained through experience. It is maintained and disseminated.
3. *Age of evidence*: Currently, evidence based practice is required for development of clinical practice.

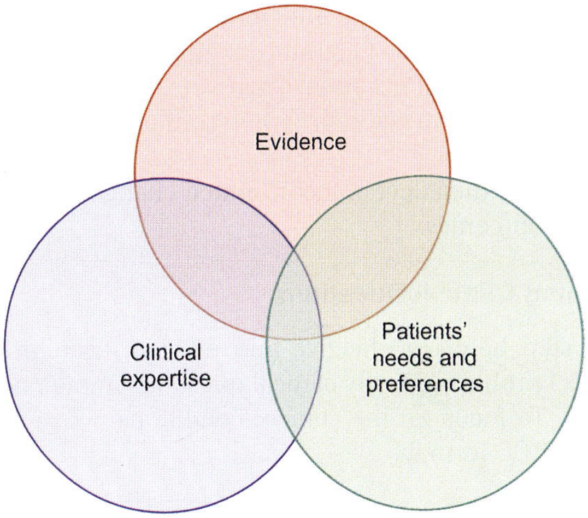

DEFINITION

David Sackett (founder person for evidence based practice) has defined it as an integrated individual clinical expertise with best available external clinical evidence from systematic research.

American dental association (ADA) has defined it as "An approach to oral health care that requires the judicious integration of systematic assessments of clinically relevant scientific evidence, relating to patient's oral and medical conditions and history, together with dentist's clinical expertise and the patient's treatment needs and preferences (**Fig. 31.1**).

Figure 31.1: Concept of evidence based dentistry

Why evidence based dentistry is required

- Helps in bridging the gap between clinical knowledge that is commonly practiced and dental knowledge that derives from research and clinical trials, etc.
- Helps the dentist in deciding the etiology of the disease and effective treatment for the disease
- Helps in reducing variations of patients care
- Helps in updating the knowledge of practitioner
- Helps in utilizing the best possible treatment available for patient.

Advantages of evidence-based approach

The advantages of evidence-based approach over other assessment methods are:
- ➡ Simple and objective in nature
- ➡ Based on scientifically proven data
- ➡ Patient oriented
- ➡ Includes clinical experience of various dentists in the world
- ➡ Always focuses on good judgments
- ➡ Practices transparent methodology
- ➡ More comprehensive
- ➡ Easy to apply.

STEPS INVOLVED IN PRACTICING EVIDENCE-BASED DENTISTRY (FLOW CHART 31.1)

- Identify clinical problem
- Frame/ask clinical questions related to the problem
- Search for evidence to find pertinent literature
- Critical appraisal of literature available
- Use relevant information; if needed to conduct research
- Utilize the relevant information results of research into clinical practice
- Evaluate the effect of incorporated changes on healthcare outcomes.

Framing Clinical Questions

This step helps in effective and efficient searching for clinical problem. Mostly clinical questions framed are too broad. To focus on the clinical conditions, we generally prefer PICO format.

Flow chart 31.1: Steps involved in practicing evidence based dentistry

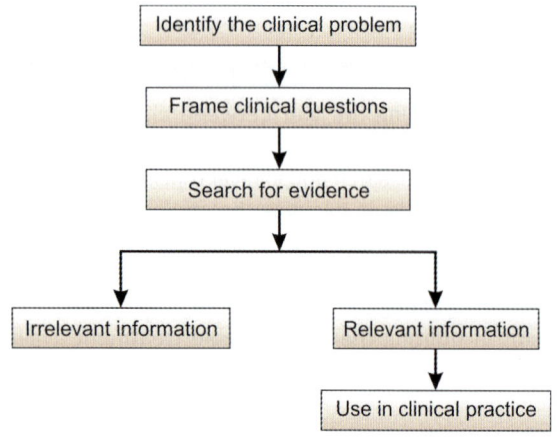

PICO format

- ➡ P – The patient or problem
- ➡ I – Intervention
- ➡ C – Comparison
- ➡ O – Outcome.

Purpose of using PICO in Framing Questions

- Helps in focusing the clinician to the most important single issue related to clinical problem.
- Helps in directing the patient to identify what actually the problem is? And what are the outcomes if specific type of treatment is given to the patient.
- Helps is simplifying the search related to clinical problem.
- How clinical questions are framed?
- By collecting clinical findings properly.
- Selection and interpretation of diagnostic tests.
- Select treatment which is more beneficial.
- Methods which prevent or reduce the risk of disease.
- Educate the patient about its after effects.

Search and Evaluate the Evidence (Fig. 31.2)

Search and evaluate the best evidence available. To achieve this, various studies and tools can be used:

Different methods for searching evidence
- Comparative studies
  - Prospective studies
    - i. Randomized controlled trials
    - ii. Nonrandomized controlled trials
    - iii. Cohort study
  - Retrospective studies
    - i. Case control study
- Descriptive studies
  - Cross-sectional study
  - Case report
  - Case series

Systematic review and metaanalysis using two or more randomized clinical trials is accepted as the best level of evidence. It is considered as the "Gold standard".

- ➡ **Systematic review** are generally outline of existing evidence on a specific topic. This review is more focused than narrative literature review and given by team of experts.
- ➡ **Meta-analysis:** This analysis is often used with systematic review. It combines the several individual studies into one analysis.

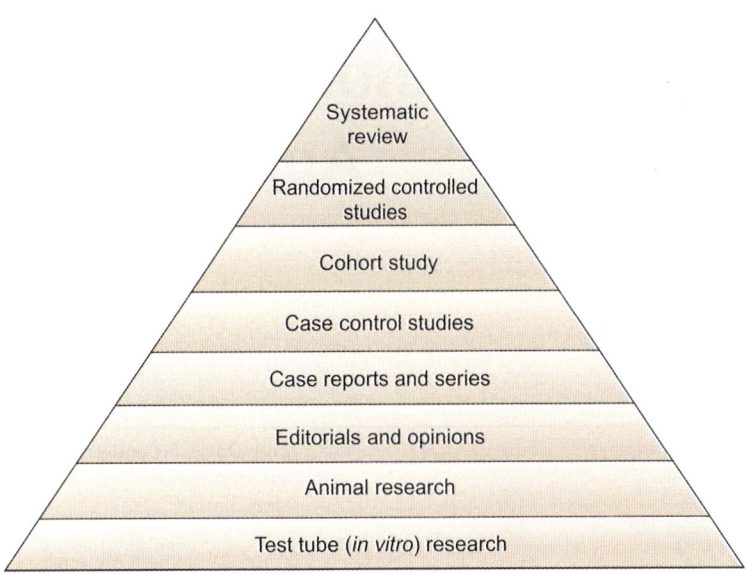

Figure 31 .2: To achieve best evidence available, different studies and tools are used

CLINICAL APPLICATION OF EVIDENCE-BASED APPROACH

The information gathered by critical evaluation of evidence is noted and assessed by its application to clinical practice and patient care. Certain points that should be taken into care while applying information on the patient are:

- *Diagnosis:* Diagnostic tests which are required should be easily available, accurate and affordable from patient point of view
- *Prognosis:* The information in the article should be clearly depicting outcome after treatment. The outcome/result is whether treatment is sufficient enough for patient to reassure or not
- *Therapy:* The knowledge gained from evidence should be used in improvement of therapy to the patient
- *Prevention:* Methods/techniques should be used to prevent the disease further
  Problems in implementation of evidence based dentistry (given by Richards and Lawrence 1998)
- Amount of evidence available
- Quality of evidence
- Dissemination of evidence
- Clinical practice based on authority rather than practice.

CONCLUSION

Evidence based dentistry helps in providing interpretation and application of various research findings.

In other words, they join the clinical research and the real practice dentistry. Also it provides the logic to treatment whenever there is some legal issue regarding procedure. To practice evidence based dentistry, the clinician must have up-to-date knowledge regarding new technologies and developments.

 Key Points

- Evidence based dentistry helps in bridging the gap between clinical knowledge that is commonly practiced and dental knowledge that is derived from research and clinical trials, etc.
- For framing clinical questions, PICO format is used. It means patient or problem, intervention, comparison and outcome.
- Systematic review is outline of existing evidence on a specific topic. This review is more focused than narrative literature review and given by team of experts.
- Meta-analysis is often used with systematic review. It combines the several individual studies into one analysis.

QUESTION

1. Short note on evidence based dentistry.

BIBLIOGRAPHY

1. Bero L, Grilli R, et al. Closing the gap between research and practice. BMJ. 1998;317:465-8.
2. Bickley S, Harrison J. How to find the evidence. J. orthod. 2003;30:72-8.
3. Greenhalgh T. How to read a paper. Getting your bearings (deciding what a paper is about) BMJ. 1997;315:243-6.

Nanodentistry and Its Applications

Chapter Outline

INTRODUCTION

Nano is derived from the Greek word for dwarf. The prefix "Nano" means ten to the minus ninth power 10^{-9}, or one billionth. It is usually combined with a noun to form words such as nanometer, nanotechnology or nanorobot. Nanotechnology is engineering of molecularly precise structures. These are the molecular machines of typically 0.1 micrometer (μm) or smaller than that.

The term 'nanotechnology' was coined by Prof Kerie E Drexler, a lecturer, researcher, and writer of nanotechnology. The aim of nanotechnology is to manipulate and control particles to create structures with unique properties and promises advances in medicine and dentistry.

DEFINITION

Nanotechnology is defined as "A field of science which aims to control individual atoms and molecules to create computer chips and other devices which are thousands of times smaller than those that the current technologies permit".

Basically, nanotechnology is about manipulating matter, atom by atom. For example, like robots assemble cars in factories from a set of predefined parts, nanorobots will assemble things from atomic and molecular building blocks. These nanorobots will have accurate control over matter. They will allow us to build crystals, molecule by molecule

as extremely fine-grained atomic structures, following a detailed blueprint. It seems to be very slow and tiresome process but billions of nanodevices working together on the same object will decrease the working time. In nanotechnology, the nanocomputers will be used to activate, control and deactivate nanomechanical devices. Nanocomputers will store and execute mission plans, receive and process external signals and stimuli, communicate with external control and monitoring devices, and have appropriate knowledge to ensure safe functioning of the nanomechanical devices. Programmable nanorobotic devices are proposed to perform precise interventions at the cellular and molecular level. Their use has been planned for pharmaceutical research and clinical diagnosis, and in dentistry.

Increasing interest in the future medical applications of nanotechnology is resulting in appearance of a new field called nanomedicine. This is the science and technology of diagnosing, treating, and preventing disease and traumatic injury, of relieving pain and preserving human health using nanoscale structured materials, biotechnology and genetic engineering, complex molecular machine systems and nanorobots. In the same way "nanodentistry" aims towards the maintenance of oral health by use of nanomaterials, biotechnology, tissue engineering, and nanorobotics. Nanorobots will be used to induce local anesthesia, treating sensitivity of teeth, for manipulation of tissues and to realign and straighten irregular set of teeth.

Nanotechnology is also applied in other areas of interest like:

- In pharmacological research
- In clinical diagnosis
- DNA sequences in cells, repairing brain damage
- Cryogenic storage of biological tissues
- Achieving near-instantaneous hemostasis
- Supplementing the immune system
- Resolving gross cellular insults.

ADVANTAGES OF NANOTECHNOLOGY

- The ability to exploit the atomic or molecular properties of materials
- Development of newer materials with better properties.

HOW ARE THE NANOPRODUCTS MADE?

There are two perceptions:
1. Building up particles by combining atomic elements.
2. Using equipment to create mechanical nanoscale objects.

MECHANISM OF ACTION

Dentifrobots

Nanorobots will be used in prevention of tooth decay. Subocclusal dwelling nanorobotic dentifrice delivered by mouthwash or toothpaste could patrol all supragingival and subgingival surfaces, metabolizing trapped organic matter into harmless and odorless vapors and performing continuous calculus debridement. Thus, properly planned dentifrobots can identify and destroy pathogenic bacteria present in the plaque allowing the harmless species of oral microflora to increase in a healthy ecosystem. With the use of this kind of daily care using dentifrobots can result in prevention of tooth decay and gingival disease.

Dentin Hypersensitivity

We know that dentin hypersensitivity is caused by pressure transmitted hydrodynamically to the pulp. These teeth have wide dentinal tubules. In treatment, nanorobots will selectively and specifically occlude the specific tubules giving quick and permanent cure.

Nanoanesthesia

To achieve nanoanesthesia, a colloidal suspension containing millions of active analgesic micrometer sized dental nanorobot particles are placed on the patient's gingiva. On coming in contact with the surface of the crown or mucosa, the nanorobots reach dentin by migrating into the gingival sulcus. On reaching the dentin, the nanorobots enter dentinal tubules and then towards pulp. This movement of nanorobots is guided by a combination of chemical gradients, temperature differentials and position of navigation, all controlled by onboard nanocomputer as directed by the dentist. It takes about two minutes for nanorobots to reach pulp. On reaching pulp, the dentist commands the analgesic dental nanorobots to shut down all sensitivity in selected tooth that requires treatment. This causes immediate anesthesia of that tooth. After completion of the procedure, the dentist commands the nanorobots via the same data links to restore all sensation.

Photosensitizers and Carriers

Quantum dots can be used as photosensitizers and carriers. They can bind to the antibody present on the surface of the target cell and when stimulated by UV light, they can give rise to reactive oxygen species and thus will be lethal to the target cell. Thus, can be used in treatment of cancer.

Major Tooth Repair

Nanodental techniques involve many tissue engineering procedures for major tooth repair. Major tooth repair involve several stages like using genetic engineering, tissue engineering and tissue regeneration and involving the growth of whole new teeth *in vitro* and their installation. Mainly manufacture and installation of a biologically autologous whole tooth that includes both mineral and cellular components leads to complete dentition replacement therapy.

Orthodontic Nanorobots

Orthodontic nanorobots can directly manipulate the periodontal tissue allowing fast and painless tooth straightening, rotation and vertical movement within minutes to hours.

Tooth Durability and Esthetics

Nanodentistry has introduced nanostructured composite material Sapphire which increases tooth durability and esthetics. Tooth durability and appearance may be improved by replacing upper enamel layers with pure sapphire and diamond which can be made more fracture resistant as nanostructured composites, possibly including embedded carbon nanotubes. Sapphire has 100 to 200 times the hardness and strength of ceramic. It is usually placed to replace the superficial enamel layers. Nanocomposites are produced by nonagglomerated discrete nanoparticles that are homogeneously distributed in resins. The nanofiller include an aluminosilicate powder with particle size of approximately 80 nm. They are superior to conventional composites in having superior hardness, modulus of elasticity, translucency, esthetics, high polish and 50 percent reduction in filling shrinkage.

Nanoimpression

An impression material will be manufactured by application of nanotechnology, and nanofillers will be integrated in the vinylpolysiloxanes producing a unique addition siloxane impression material. This material will provide better flow and hydrophilic properties hence fewer voids at margin and better model pouring.

Nanosolution

Nanosolutions will form unique and dispersible nanoparticles, which can be used in bonding agents. This will make the solution homogeneous and makes sure that the adhesive is perfectly mixed everytime.

Nanoencapsulation

South West Research Institute (SWRI) developed targeted release systems which will cover nanocapsules including novel vaccines, antibiotics and drug delivery with reduced side effects.

Other products developed by South West Research Institute:

- Protective clothing and masks, using antipathogenic nanoemulsions and nanoparticles
- Medical appendages for instantaneous healing, for example, biodegradable nanofibers delivery system for hemostatic and wound dressings with silk nanofibers.
- Bone targeting nanocarriers
- Calcium phosphate-based biomaterial will be developed which supports growth of cartilage and bone cells.

Bone Replacement Materials

Many hydroxyapatite nanoparticles have been developed, for example, VITOSSO (Orthovita, Inc, USA) HA +TCP to treat bone defects.

Nanoneedles

New suture needles have been developed having nanosized stainless steel crystals. These will help in making cell-surgery possible in the future.

SAFETY FACTOR OF NANOROBOTS

Two types of nanorobots are used mainly; nonpyrogenic nanorobots are composed of teflon, carbon powder and monocrystal sapphire, whereas pyrogenic nanorobots are composed of alumina, silica, copper and zinc.

If nanodevice surface pyrogenicity is unavoidable, the use of medical nanorobots is done to control the pyrogenic pathway. These nanorobots will release inhibitors or antagonists for the pyrogenic pathway in a targeted pattern to selectively absorb the endogenous pyrogens, then modify them and finally set them back into the body in a harmless inactivated form.

CHALLENGES FACED BY NANODENTISTRY

- Biocompatibility
- Simultaneous coordination of activities of large number of independent micron-scale robots
- Basic engineering problems run the range from precise positioning and assembly of molecular-scale parts to economical mass-production techniques
- Cost factor
- Social issues of public acceptance
- Ethics
- Human safety.

CHALLENGES FACED FOR RESEARCH IN NANOTECHNOLOGY

- Lack of engagement of private enterprises.
- Suboptimal funding.
- Problem of retention of trained manpower.
- Slow strategic decisions.

It sounds like science fiction but to treat even a mildest form of an oral disease, the dentists will ask the patients to rinse mouth with solution containing millions of microscopic particles called "nanoassemblers". These particles receiving signals from a computer controlled by the dentist, will reach the areas of patient's mouth and get rid of the disease and bacteria causing the disease.

Nanodentistry is the future of dentistry in which every procedure will be performed using equipment and devices based on nanotechnology. It will become possible to replace teeth in a single procedure with ultimate accuracy using a combination of nanomedicine and biotechnology.

Future of nanotechnology is forecast to change health care in a fundamental way:

- Fresh methods for diagnosis and prevention of the disease
- Therapeutic treatment according to patient's profile
- Drug delivery and gene therapy.

QUESTIONS

1. Short note:
   a. Nanodentistry with its future aspects.

BIBLIOGRAPHY

1. Absi EG, Addy M, Adams D. Dentine hypersensitivity. A study of the patency of dentinal tubules in sensitive and non-sensitive cervical dentine. J Clin Periodontol. 1987;14:280-4.

2. Addy M, West N. Etiology mechanisms and management of dentine hypersensitivity. Curr Opin Periodontol. 1994;2:71-7.

3. An application of Nanotechnology in advanced dental materials. JADA 2003;134:1382.

4. Arends J, Stokroos I, Jongebloed WG, Ruben J. The diameter of dentinal tubules in human coronal dentine after demineralization and air drying. A combined light microscopy and SEM study. Caries Res. 1995;29:118-21.

5. Ashley S. Nanobot construction crews. Sci Am. 2001;285:84-5.

6. Berger M. Nanotechnology in my tooth paste. Nanowork Spottlight; www.nanowork.com.

7. Beun S, Glorieux T, Devaux J, Vreven J, Leloup G. Characterization of nanofilled compared to universal and microfilled composites. Dent Mater. 2007;23(1):51-9.

8. Bogedal M, Gleiche M. Nanotechnology and its implications; www.nanoform.org.

9. Chen HF, Clarkson BH, Sunk, Mansfield JF. Self assembly of synthetic hydroxyapatite nanorods into enamel prism like structure. J Colloid Interface Sci. 2005;288(1);97-103.

10. Christopher Roman. Superior dental composites; www.nanoproducts.com.

11. Davis SS. Biomedical applications of nanotechnology—implications for drug targeting and gene therapy. Trends Biotechnol. 1997;15(6):217-24.

12. Dourda AO, Moule AJ, Young WG. A morphometric analysis of the cross-sectional area of dentine occupied by dentinal tubules in human third molar teeth. Int Endod J. 1994;27:184-9.

13. El-Shabouri MH. Positively charged nanoparticles for improving the oral bioavailability of cyclosporine. A Int J Pharm. 2002;249:101-8.

14. Farr C. Biotech in periodontics: Molecular engineering yields new therapies. Dent Today. 1997;16:92-7.

15. Fartash B, Tangerud T, Silness J, Arvidson K. Rehabilitation of mandibular edentulism by single crystal sapphire implants and overdentures: 3-12 year results in 86 patients. A dual center international study. Clin Oral Implants Res. 1996;7:220-9.

16. Freitas RA Jr. Exploratory design in medical nanotechnology: A mechanical artificial red cell .Artificial Cells Blood Substitute Immobile Biotechnology. 1998;26:30-2.

17. Freitas RA Jr. Nanodentistry. Journal of American Dental Association. 2000;131(11):1559-65.

18. Freitas RA jr. Nanotechnology, nanomedicine and nanosurgery. Int J Surg. 2005;3(4):243-6.

19. Frietas RA. Nanodentistry; JADA. 2000;131:1559-65.

20. Goracci G, Mori G. Micromorphological aspects of dentin. Minerva Stomatol. 1995;44:377-87.

21. Goverdhana S, Puntel M, Xiong W, Zirger JM, Barcia C, Curtin JF, et al. Regulatable gene expression systems for gene therapy applications: Progress and future challenges. Mol Ther. 2005;12(2):189-211.

22. Graham L. Identifying, diagnosing, and treating dentin hypersensitivity. Dent Today. 2005;24:72-3.

23. Guccione S, LiKC, Bednarski MD. Vascular-targeted nanoparticles for molecular imaging and therapy. Methods Enzymol. 2004;386:219-36.

24. Henkel. Nano active toothpaste; www.nannit-active.com.

25. Herzog A. Of genomics, cyborgs and nanotechnology: a look into the future of medicine. Conn Med. 2002;66:53-4.

26. Jain KK. Nanodiagnostics: application of nanotechnology in molecular diagnostics. Expert Rev Mol Diagn. 2003;3:153-61.

27. Jain KK. Nanotechnology in clinical laboratory diagnostics. Clin Chim Acta 2005;358:37-54.

28. Jhaveri HM, Balaji PR. Nanotechnology the future of dentistry; JIPS. 2005;5:15-7.

29. Lavenus S, Ricquier JC, Louarn G, Layrolle P. Cell interaction with nanopatterned surface of implants. Nanomedicine (Lond). 2010:5(6):937-47.

30. Le Gu´ehennec L, Soueidan A, Layrolle P, Amouriq Y. Surface treatments of titanium dental implants for rapid osseointegration, Dent Mater. 2007:23(7):844-54.

31. Li KC, Pandit SD, Guccione S, Guccione S, Bednarski MD. Molecular imaging applications in nanomedicine. Biomed Microdevices. 2004;6:113-6.

32. Lin H, Datar RH. Medical applications of nanotechnology. Natl Med J India. 2006;19:27-32.

33. Mitra SB, et al. An application of nanotechnology in advance dental materials, J Am Dent Assoc. 2003;134:1382-90.

34. Patil M, Mehta DS, Guvva S. Future impact of nanotechnology on medicine and dentistry. J Indian Soc Periodontol. 2008;12(2):34-40.

35. Pruzansky S.Letter to the editor. Effect of molecular genetics and genetic engineering on the practice of orthodontics. Am J Orthod. 1972;62:539-42.

36. Sahoo SK, Parveen S, Panda JJ. The present and future of nanotechnology in human health care. Nanomedicine: Nanotechnology, Biology, and Medicine. 2007;3:20-31.

37. Shellhart WC, Oesterle LJ. Uprighting molars without extrusion. J Am Dent Assoc. 1999;130:381-5.

38. Shi H, Tsai WB, Garrison MD, Ferrari S, Ratner BD. Template-imprinted nanostructured surfaces for protein recognition. Nature. 1999;398:593-7.

39. Sims MR. Brackets, epitopes and flash memory cards: a futuristic view of clinical orthodontics. Aust Orthod J. 1999;15:260-8.

40. Slavkin HC. Entering the era of molecular dentistry. J Am Dent Assoc. 1999 Mar;130:413-7.

41. Wells DJ. Gene therapy progress and prospects: electroporation and other physical methods. Gene Ther. 2004;11(18):1363-9.

42. West JL, Halas NJ. Applications of nanotechnology to biotechnology commentary. Curr Opin Biotechnol. 2000;11:215-7.

43. Whitesides GM, Love JC. The Art of Building Small. Scientific American. 2001;285(3):33-41.

44. Yunshin S, Park HN, Kim KH. Biologic evaluation of Chitosan Nanofiber Membrane for guided bone regeneration. Journal Periodontology. 2005;76:84-85.

Index

Page numbers followed by *f* refer to figure and *t* refer to table